PRINCIPLES AND PRACTICE OF CLINICAL ELECTROPHYSIOLOGY OF VISION

PRINCIPLES AND PRACTICE OF CLINICAL ELECTROPHYSIOLOGY OF VISION

Second Edition

Editors: John R. Heckenlively and Geoffrey B. Arden

Associate Editors: Steven Nusinowitz

Graham E. Holder

Michael Bach

THE MIT PRESS
CAMBRIDGE, MASSACHUSETTS
LONDON, ENGLAND

MIT Press books may be purchased at special quantity discounts for business or sales promotional use. For information, please email special_sales@mitpress.mit.edu or write to Special Sales Department, The MIT Press, 55 Hayward Street, Cambridge, MA 02142.

This book printed and bound in the United States of America.

Library of Congress Cataloging-in-Publication Data

Principles and practice of clinical electrophsyiology of vision
    / editors, John R. Heckenlively and Geoffrey B. Arden ;
    associate editors, Steven Nusinowitz, Graham E. Holder,
    and Michael Bach—2nd ed.
        p. ; cm.
    Includes bibliographical references and index.
    ISBN 0-262-08346-9
    1. Electroretinography. 2. Electrooculography. 3. Visual
evoked response. I. Heckenlively, John R. II. Arden,
Geoffrey B. (Geoffrey Bernard)
    [DNLM: 1. Electroretinography. 2. Electrooculography.
3. Electrophysiology. 4. Evoked Potentials, Visual. 5. Vision
Disorders—physiopathology. WW 143 P957 2006]
    RE79.E4P75   2006
    617.7′1547—dc22
                                        2006041876

10   9   8   7   6   5   4   3   2   1

CONTENTS

XV ANIMAL TESTING   897

FOREWORD

History of the ERG Through Early Human Recordings: A Preface
Ragnar Granit* (1900–1991)
Karolinska Institutet for Neurophysiology

It is of some interest to note that the electroretinogram (ERG) was discovered in two independent laboratories and that in both cases, it emerged from different but false assumptions. The Uppsala physiologist Professor Frithiof Holmgren was inspired by his famous teacher, DuBois-Reymond of Berlin, who discovered the electrical nature of the nerve impulse, then known as "the negative variation," as elicited by an electrical shock to a nerve.[1] With better recording instruments available in the early 20th century, the more precise term *action potential* came to be used, and Holmgren's question was "Could the negative variation also be obtained when a natural stimulus such as light was used?"

To this end, he placed recording electrodes on the front and at the back of a frog eye and was rewarded by observing a response to a light flash. At the time (1865), he thought that he had recorded an electrical mass discharge from the optic nerve, thus confirming DuBois-Reymond's discovery. I assume that Holmgren must have been worried by the fact that he also saw another electrical response at cessation of illumination, or why otherwise would he have started shifting his electrodes around the bulb to conclude in 1870 that the current distribution required the observed responses to have arisen in the retina itself? The date of understanding what he had recorded is thus 1870, the real birth date of the ERG.

Responsible for an independent discovery of the ERG were two young Scotsmen, Dewar and McKendrick.[1] The former later became the brilliant physicist Sir James Dewar, head of the Royal Institution in London, the latter ultimately professor of physiology at the University of Glasgow. The year was 1873, and in that year, photoconductivity in selenium had been first reported in Great Britain by Willoughby Smith.[1] The Edinburgh scientists, not knowing about Holmgren's findings, wondered whether some similar photoelectric effect initiated the activity in the retina.

To make a long story short, I quote the greater part of a letter from McKendrick to Holmgren:

Sir, I send along with this letter a number of papers of which I respectfully beg your acceptance. Among these you will find a Memoir by Mr. James Dewar and myself on the physiological action of Light, in which we give details regarding an experimental research we made as to the specific action of light on the retina. This research was begun, carried on and concluded, and the Memoir was actually printed, before we were aware of your most admirable work as published in the Uppsala Journal. You will observe that at the end of the Memoir we have added an Appendix in which we at once acknowledge your priority in the discovery. We have had your papers translated from Swedish, and it is satisfactory to know that our independent work corroborates yours in almost every particular.

. . . Meantime with every sentiment for you and in admiration of your work.[1]

Professor Granit won the Nobel Prize in Medicine in 1967 with corecipients George Wald and Haldan Keffer Hartline.

Dewar also succeeded in recording from the human eye, and so 1877 became the year of birth of the ERG of the human.

The slow galvanometers of that period prevented further development. Actually, the first author to describe the full phasic display of the ERG was Gotch[1] in 1903, who used the capillary electrometer and a frog eye, which, as we know now, is a more complex structure than that of mammals because it has to operate at a level of precision that the mammals can achieve only by recourse to cortical centers. But in that same year, Einthoven developed his string galvanometer, fast and sensitive enough for the recording of both ERGs and electrocardiograms (EKGs), the latter being Einthoven's main interest. It came to dominate instrumentation in electrophysiology for some 20 years, or until electronic amplification became available, and soon was applied everywhere. The first amplifiers for ERG were developed by the American physicist Chaffee and his team in 1923.[1] Again the frog eye was their preparation. From that time on, after sufficient amplification, any fast recording instrument could be used in neurophysiological experimentation, the most popular being at first the Matthews oscillograph, later the cathode ray.[1]

The pioneer Dewar was followed some 45 years later by Kahn and Lowenstein (1924)[1] and Hartline (1925).[2] The former pair realized that the Einthoven string galvanometer made recording of human ERGs possible. Their aim was clinical, but they concluded that the technique was too difficult for clinical purposes. Hartline, in the course of recording ERGs from different animals, also included the human. He had some good records but never returned to ERGs because he became permanently fascinated by the single-fiber preparation. I have followed his scientific development in the *Biographical Memoirs of Fellows of the Royal Society*.[2]

In the early 1930s, I was engaged in the Oxford laboratory of Sir Charles Sherrington in an analysis of the obviously complex EFG. For this end, I employed the more compact and sturdy Edelmann permanent magnetic string galvanometer, with which the risk of breaking strings was greatly reduced. It was used with a homemade amplifier base on a circuit I had received from Hartline, who, I believe, had it from K. S. Cole. E. D. Adrian had given me good advice on the choice of vacuum tubes. Two of my Oxford friends, Sybil Cooper and R. S. Creed,[1] collaborated to make an attempt at the human ERG, and we had records with b-waves on the order of 0.35 mV alike in the central and peripheral vision. At about the same time, some records were published by Sachs (1929) and Groppel, Haass, and Kohlrausch (1938).[1] In 1940 and 1941, Bernhard,[1] in the course of the electroencephalographic (EEG) work, also recorded ERGs from some subjects. Perhaps the advent of EEG contributed to making clinically-minded scientists less afraid of electrically based techniques. This development synchronized happily with the advent of more robust and easily handled commercial EEGs.

The long latency of the clinical application of around 1925 depended partly upon technical difficulties. It certainly had to await the advent of electronic amplification. But then, why did I not, for instance, try to mobilize ophthalmologists in Stockholm to come to my laboratory for the necessary instructions for clinical application? Actually, I was skeptical about the outcome. It seemed to me that there might well be significant information within the virtually monophasic human ERG, but it would be difficult to extract in comparison with what I had been able to do with the ERGs of cats and frogs 10 years earlier. But Karpe was insistent and of course received the necessary elementary advice from our laboratory. The work itself was carried out at the Ophthalmological Department of Karolinska Institutet. So by dint of hard work, Karpe became the first to prove that clinical ERG was both possible and worth doing. Thus, a new field of approach to ocular disease had been opened, and soon it was developed in many directions. We did not know at the time that during the war the able American psychologist Lorrin Riggs[1] had designed a contact lens electrode for the recording of ERG in man. Karpe designed one independently.

January 10, 1989

REFERENCES

1. Granit R: *Sensory Mechanisms of the Retina.* London, Oxford University Press, 1947.
2. Granit R, Ratliff F: *Haldan Ueffer Hartline*, 1903–1983: *Biographical Memoirs of Fellows of the Royal Society*, vol 31. London, The Royal Society, 1985, pp. 261–292.

PREFACE TO THE SECOND EDITION

We are very pleased to present a second edition of *The Principles and Practice of Clinical Electrophysiology of Vision*. It has been a considerable undertaking and has taken 5 years. We would like to take the opportunity to thank the authors who generously contributed their fine work and ideas. Most of the chapters have been rewritten, and many new topics have been added. As before, we have adopted the policy of having some differences of opinion between authors so that the reader will obtain the benefit of different points of view, and we have tried to cover a broad perspective, including historical introductions and a wealth of references for serious students. The first edition of this book sold out in 6 months, which would have been extremely gratifying to the editors and authors had the original printing been in a larger quantity! We now have a new publisher who has assured us that it is in the business for the long run and will keep up with demand. We are pleased with the publisher's track record in the field of neuroscience publication.

For the past 15 years, we have been asked repeatedly where any copy of the first edition could be obtained. The apparent demand for this material and the fact that there is indeed a great deal of new information in the field of clinical electrophysiology convinced us that we should try for a second edition despite the proliferation of online information. We have tried to include material that is likely to become more important in the next decade, in which period we hope that this edition will be helpful to workers in the field, both to orient themselves to what is new and to obtain a perspective of the subject and its remarkable development in the past century. In particular, we have added reports on multifocal techniques, the recent advances in analysis of abnormalities in disease, and the applications of these techniques to the study of genetic abnormalities in humans and animals.

The high quality of this reference book directly reflects the expertise and broad knowledge of its authors, to whom full credit must be given. Each of them took time from very full schedules to contribute their chapters, and we thank them most sincerely. We would also like to thank the many colleagues who contributed to this base of data and made this volume possible. In addition, the editorial staff at MIT Press (especially Ms. Barbara Murphy) was most supportive and deserve all our commendations. The role of ISCERG/ISCEV should be acknowledged in providing organizational support for the development of the field. The field of clinical electrophysiology has come a long way since Karpe did his initial human studies in the 1950's.

Geoffrey B. Arden
John R. Heckenlively

PREFACE TO THE FIRST EDITION

"Scribble, scribble, scribble," said the Duke of Gloucester to the author of *The Decline and Fall of the Roman Empire*. "Always another damn thick square book, eh, Mr. Gibbon?" When we first saw the height of the pillar of our page proofs, our feelings were mixed: pride at the industry of the contributors competed with wonder that Gibbon had recorded the thousand-year history of the entire civilized world in considerably fewer pages than seemed necessary to describe a specialized branch of applied clinical science is barely 50 years old (and, of course, Gibbon incorporated a much greater number of jokes in his volumes than do we).

The need for an authoritative text was borne on us by conversations with our colleagues when the possibility of the book was first raised some 4 years ago. There are several excellent works—some of them in English—that deal with various aspects of clinical electrophysiology and the eye. None of them completely meets the needs of the worker in the clinical laboratory, in the sense that detailed practical information on techniques and practical problems is needed in the same volume as the basic physiology and anatomy, the theoretical concepts, and the clinical findings. All these disciplines are encountered (if not mastered) by a practitioner in this field, and, in our experience, a *successful* practitioner must refer fairly frequently to such sources to understand and properly utilize the developments in the field. We have aimed at complete coverage for such persons, but of course we could not include articles on every topic. Many important aspects of cortical and lateral geniculate structure and function and the biophysics of excitable tissue have not been covered. We have regretfully not included many fascinating aspects of retinal biochemistry and cell biology. These we thought to be of lesser clinical relevance than the material on ancillary and clinical methods of examination.

The itch to be encyclopedic was not to be resisted, when several chapters, received early in the project, seemed to break ground either in the completeness of exposition or in the elegance with which difficult subjects were explained. We also were able to include as a contributor a founder of the field—Ragnar Granit—who recruited Goste Karpe to exploit the new electrophysiology for the purposes of clinical ophthalmology. This led to the burgeoning of the subject. Happily, this process continues, implying that any future book on this subject must be selective. Today, however, we have been able to present more than one contribution on the same topic, and thus not stifle discordant opinions, which are to be expected in so young a discipline. This is not to say we have not edited our contributors' results to minimize overlap, and we apologize to those of them who are smarting at out pruning. Our thanks are due to them all, and in reading their contributions we have ourselves learned a great deal about our own subject.

Our thanks also to our staff who assisted us, colleagues of the International Society for Clinical Electrophysiology of Vision who encouraged the project, and the people at

Mosby-Year Book who graciously allowed us to turn a book of 350 pages into one of more than 800!

Errors of omission are all our own, and especially, in the choice of authors: we have turned to a considerable extent to the younger contributors in the field, in the confident expectation that their increasing reputations will add luster to the book.

John R. Heckenlively
Geoffrey B. Arden

CONTRIBUTORS

ADACHI-USAMI, EMIKO   Department of Ophthalmology, Chiba University School of Medicine, Chiba, Japan

ALEXANDER, KENNETH R.   Laboratory of Clinical Psychophysics and Electrophysiology, Department of Ophthalmology and Visual Sciences, University of Illinois at Chicago, Chicago, IL

ANTAL, ANDREA   Department of Clinical Neurophysiology, Georg-August University of Göttingen, Göttingen, Germany

APKARIAN, P.   Department of Ophthalmology, University of Rotterdam, Rotterdam, The Netherlands

APTSIAURI, NATALIA   Department of Ophthalmology, University of Iowa, Iowa City, IA

ARDEN, GEOFFREY B.   Department of Optometry and Visual Science, City University, London, United Kingdom

BACH, MICHAEL   Electrophysiological Laboratory, Department of Ophthalmology, University of Freiburg, Freiburg, Germany

BARBER, COLIN   Queen's Medical Centre, Nottingham, United Kingdom

BERNINGER, THOMAS   Department of Ophthalmology, University Eye Hospital, Munich, Germany

BIRCH, DAVID G.   Retina Foundation of the Southwest, Dallas, TX, and UT Southwestern Medical Center, Dallas, TX

BIRCH, EILEEN E.   Retina Foundation of the Southwest, Dallas, TX, and UT Southwestern Medical Center, Dallas, TX

BODIS-WOLLNER, IVAN   Department of Ophthalmology, Mt. Sinai School of Medicine, New York, NY

BOUR, L. J.   Department of Neurology/Clinical Neurophysiology, Academic Medical Centre, University of Amsterdam, Amsterdam, The Netherlands

BRIGELL, MITCHELL   Pfizer Global Research and Development, Chicago, IL

BRODIE, SCOTT E.   Department of Ophthalmology, Mt. Sinai School of Medicine, New York, NY

BRUNKEN, WILLIAM J.   Department of Anatomy and Cellular Biology, Tufts University School of Medicine, Boston, MA

CARR, RONALD E.   Department of Ophthalmology, New York University Medical Center, New York, NY

CLARKE, MICHAEL P.   Department of Ophthalmology, Royal Victoria Infirmary, Newcastle upon Tyne, United Kingdom

CLAUDEPIERRE, THOMAS   Department of Anatomy and Cellular Biology, Tufts University School of Medicine, Boston, MA

CONWAY, BEVIL R.   Department of Neurobiology, Harvard Medical School, Boston, MA

COUPLAND, STUART   School of Psychology, University of Ottawa, Ottawa, Ontario, Canada

DE ROUCK, A. F.   Department of Ophthalmology, Ghent University Hospital, Ghent, Belgium

EDMUNDS, BETH   Dever's Eye Institute, Good Samaritan Hospital, Portland, OR

ESTÉVEZ, OSCAR   Department of Informatics, University of Amsterdam, Amsterdam, The Netherlands

FAHLE, MANFRED   Institute of Brain Research IV and the Unit for Human Neurobiology, Universität Bremen, Bremen, Germany

FAIN, GORDON L.   Departments of Physiological Science and Ophthalmology, University of California, Los Angeles, Los Angeles, CA

FALK, GERTRUDE   Biophysics Unit, Department of Physiology, University College London, London, United Kingdom

FISHMAN, GERALD A.   Department of Ophthalmology and Visual Sciences, University of Illinois at Chicago, Chicago, IL

FRANCIS, PETER J.   Department of Ophthalmology, Oregon Health and Science University, Portland, OR

FRISHMAN, LAURA J.   College of Optometry, University of Houston, Houston, TX

FRUMKES, THOMAS E.   Retired, Colorado

FULTON, ANNE B.   Department of Ophthalmology, Children's Hospital and Harvard Medical School, Boston, MA

GIRKEN, CHRISTOPHER A.   Department of Ophthalmology, University of Alabama at Birmingham, Birmingham, AL

GOURAS, PETER   Department of Ophthalmology, Columbia University, New York, NY

GRANIT, RAGNAR (deceased)   Nobel Laureate, Karolinska Institutet, Stockholm, Sweden

HAGEMAN, GREGORY S.   Department of Ophthalmology and Visual Services, University of Iowa, Iowa City, IA

HANSEN, RONALD. M.   Department of Ophthalmology, Children's Hospital and Harvard Medical School, Boston, MA

HARDING, GRAHAM F. A.   Neurosciences Research Institute, Aston University, Birmingham, United Kingdom

HAWLINA, MARKO   Department of Ophthalmology, University of Ljubljana, Ljubljana, Slovenia

HECKENLIVELY, JOHN R.   Department of Ophthalmology and Visual Sciences, Kellogg Eye Center, University of Michigan, Ann Arbor, MI

HÉON, ELISE   Department of Ophthalmology, University of Toronto, Toronto, Ontario, Canada

HOFFMANN, MICHAEL B.   Visual Processing Lab, Universitäts-Augenklinik, Magdeburg, Germany

HOGG, CHRIS   Electrophysiology Department, Moorfields Eye Hospital, London, United Kingdom

HOLDER, GRAHAM E. Department of Electrophysiology, Moorfields Eye Hospital, London, United Kingdom

HOOD, DONALD C. Department of Psychology, Columbia University, New York, NY

HUNTER, DALE D. Department of Neuroscience, Tufts University School of Medicine, Boston, MA

JOHNSON, LINCOLN V. Center for the Study of Macular Degeneration, Neuroscience Research Institute, University of California, Santa Barbara, Santa Barbara, CA

JOHNSON, MARY A. Department of Ophthalmology, University of Maryland, Baltimore, MD

KAWASAKI, KAZUO Professor Emeritus, University of Kanazawa, Japan

KEATING, DAVID Department of Cardiovascular and Medical Sciences, Faculty of Medicine, University of Glasgow, Glasgow, Scotland, United Kingdom

KHAN, NAHEED W. Kellogg Eye Center, University of Michigan, Ann Arbor, MI

KOENEKOOP, ROBERT K. Department of Ophthalmology, Montreal Children's Hospital Research Institute, Montreal, Quebec, Canada

KOLB, HELGA Moran Eye Center, University of Utah School of Medicine, Salt Lake City, UT

KONDO, MINEO Department of Ophthalmology, Nagoya University School of Medicine, Nagoya, Japan

LACHAPELLE, PIERRE Department of Ophthalmology, McGill University, Montreal, Quebec, Canada

LIVINGSTONE, MARGARET S. Department of Neurobiology, Harvard Medical School, Boston, MA

MACDONALD, IAN M. Department of Medical Genetics, University of Alberta, Edmonton, Alberta, Canada

MACKAY, CYNTHIA Eye Clinic, New York, NY

MANGLAPUS, MARY K. Department of Anatomy and Cellular Biology, Tufts University School of Medicine, Boston, MA

MARMOR, MICHAEL F. Department of Ophthalmology, Stanford University School of Medicine, Stanford, CA

MEIGEN, THOMAS Elektrophysiologisches Labor, Universitäts-Augenklinik, Würzburg, Würzburg, Germany

MITCHELL, KEITH W. Regional Medical Physics Department, University of Newcastle upon Tyne, Newcastle upon Tyne, United Kingdom

MIYAKE, YOZO Department of Ophthalmology, Nagoya University School of Medicine, Nagoya, Japan

MONTIANI-FERREIRA, FABIANO Department of Small Animal Clinical Sciences, Veterinary Medical Center, Michigan State University, East Lansing, MI

MUNIER, FRANCIS Unité de Génétique Moléculaire, Division Autonome de Génétique Médicale, Lausanne, Switzerland

NARFSTRÖM, KRISTINA Department of Veterinary Medicine and Surgery, College of Veterinary Medicine, University of Missouri-Columbia, Columbia, MO

NEWMAN, NANCY J. Departments of Ophthalmology, Neurology, and Neurological Surgery, Emory University School of Medicine, Atlanta, GA

NILSSON, SVEN ERIK G. Department of Ophthalmology, Linköping University, Linköping, Sweden

NUSINOWITZ, STEVEN Visual Physiology Laboratory and Department of Ophthalmology, Jules Stein Eye Institute, Los Angeles, CA

ODOM, J. VERNON West Virginia University Eye Institute, Robert C. Byrd Health Sciences Center of West Virginia, Morgantown, WV

OGUCHI, YOSHIHISA Department of Ophthalmology, Keio University School of Medicine, Tokyo, Japan

PARKS, STUART Eye Department, Gartnavel Hospital, Glasgow, United Kingdom

PEPPERBERG, DAVID R. Department of Ophthalmology and Visual Sciences, College of Medicine, University of Illinois at Chicago, Chicago, IL

PETERSEN-JONES, SIMON Department of Small Animal Clinical Sciences, Veterinary Medical Center, Michigan State University, East Lansing, MI

RIDDER, WILLIAM Basic and Visual Science Department, Southern California College of Optometry, Fullerton, CA

SEABRA, MIGUEL C. Department of Molecular Biology, Division of Biomedical Sciences, School of Medicine, Imperial College London, London, United Kingdom

SEAH, ALVIN B. H. Department of Ophthalmology, Emory University School of Medicine, Atlanta, GA

SEELIGER, MATHIAS W. University Eye Hospital, Tübingen, Germany

SHIRAO, YUTAKA Department of Ophthalmology, University of Kanazawa, Japan

SHIELLS, RICHARD Institute of Biological Science, University of Tsukuba, Tsukuba, Ibaraki, Japan

SIEVING, PAUL A. National Eye Institute, National Institutes of Health, Bethesda, MD

SMITH, W. CLAY Department of Ophthalmology, University of Florida College of Medicine, Gainesville, FL

STRAUSS, OLAF Department of Experimental Ophthalmology, Universitätsklinikum Hamburg-Eppendorf, Hamburg, Germany

TANABE, JHOJI Department of Ophthalmology, School of Medicine, Kanazawa University, Ishikawa, Japan

THOMPSON, DOROTHY Electrophysiology Department, Hospital for Sick Children, London, United Kingdom

TORMENE, ALMA PATRIZIA Dipartimento di Neuroscienze/Clinica Oculistica, University of Padova, Padova, Italy

TRICK, GARY L. Eye Care Services, Henry Ford Health System, Detroit, MI

TUNTIVANICH, NALINEE College of Veterinary Medicine, Michigan State University, East Lansing, MI

VAEGAN School of Optometry and Vision Science, University of New South Wales, Sydney, Sydney, New South Wales, Australia

VAN DER TWEEL, L. HENK (deceased) Laboratory of Medical Physics, University of Amsterdam, The Netherlands

WAKABAYASHI, KENJI Department of Ophthalmology, University of Kanazawa, Japan

WELEBER, RICHARD G. Casey Eye Institute, Oregon Health and Science University, Portland, OR

WILLOUGHBY, COLIN Unit of Ophthalmology, Department of Medicine, University of Liverpool, Liverpool, United Kingdom

WILSON, DAVID J. Department of Ophthalmology, Casey Eye Institute, Oregon Health and Science University Portland, OR

YAMAMOTO, SHUICHI Sakura Hospital, Toho University, Sakura, Japan

ZRENNER, EBERHART Department for Pathophysiology of Vision and Neuro-Ophthalmology, University Eye Hospital of Tübingen, Tübingen, Germany

I HISTORY AND BACKGROUND TO MODERN TESTING

1 History of the Electroretinogram

A. F. DE ROUCK

Early discoveries

In 1849, DuBois-Reymond[27] discovered in excised tench (fish) eyes a potential of about 6 mV when using an electrode placed behind the eye and a similar electrode placed on the surface of the cornea. He found that the cornea was positive with respect to the posterior pole of the eye. The existence of this standing potential was soon confirmed by other authors.

In 1865, Holmgren[39] discovered that an excised frog eye showed an electrical response to light, and in 1880 he found by removing the anterior segment of the eye and placing the corneal electrode directly on the retinal surface that the retina itself was the source of the response.[38,40]

About the same time, Dewar and McKendrick[26] independently reported the discovery of "action currents" with illumination of the eye; they concluded that there was a relationship between the amplitude of the electrical response and the logarithm of the stimulus intensity. Wavelengths that appeared brightest to the human eye evoked the largest amplitude response.

In 1877 Dewar[25] showed that electrical potentials could be recorded from an intact animal eye by applying the second (reference) electrode on the abraded skin. He also reported the first successful recording of a human electroretinogram (ERG). For this purpose, he used an elaborate instrumental setup.

A small trough of clay or paraffin was constructed around the margin of the orbit, so as to contain a quantity of salt solution, when the body was placed horizontally and the head properly secured. The terminal of a non-polarizable electrode was introduced into this solution and in order to complete the circuit, the other electrode was connected with a large gutta-percha trough containing salt solution, into which one of the hands was inserted.

The two electrodes were connected to a sensitive Thomson galvanometer. The resulting curves, however, were not published.

In 1880, Kuhne and Steiner,[47] working on isolated frog and fish retinas, claimed that the light-induced action currents originated in the receptor layer and not in the ganglion cell layer.

Early recording

The electrical measuring devices at the time, slow galvanometers, were unable to measure rapid changes in potential accurately. The responses were often practically invisible. Brücke and Garten[18] connected many eyes in series to construct a living battery to obtain more power. In an extensive series of investigations, they showed that the electrical responses of various vertebrate eyes were similar.

Gotch[32] described a capillary electrometer that allowed him to determine that there was a response in the frog eye at both the onset and cessation of the light stimulus. He was the first to call the latter wave the "off-effect" and to note the early negative portion of the response. He was able to produce accurate measurements of the latent period and to show that it decreases when the intensity of stimulation increases.

Einthoven and Jolly[28] obtained excellent detailed records of the frog eye by using a string galvanometer. They were the first to designate several portions of the ERG by letters (figure 1.1); an initial negative segment, the a-wave, is followed by a larger positive deflection, the b-wave, and later, by another slower positive potential, the c-wave. When the light stopped, the d-wave, or off-effect, appeared. The authors stated that the electrical potential is in fact an integrated mass response made up of a number of independent components.

Piper[55] realized that there are two main types of retinas; he found that eyes with large a-waves showed a good off-effect whereas those with small a-waves had poor off-effects. Piper's analysis of the ERG into three components, based partly on the work of Waller,[72] was also accepted by Kohlrausch.[46]

The first published human electroretinogram

Kahn and Löwenstein[43] published the first human ERG curve (figure 1.2) by employing a string galvanometer and leads from the cornea and a distal temporal point of an anesthetized eyeball. They attempted to use the ERG as part of the clinical examination of the human eye but concluded that the practical difficulties of their method made it unsuitable in the clinical setting.

About this same time, Hartline[36] used moist thread electrodes and saline-filled goggles to make contact with the eyes. Since this was uncomfortable for the patient, another method was developed. A simple cotton wick was applied to the cornea after local anesthesia, and the reference electrode was placed in the mouth. The string galvanometer revealed

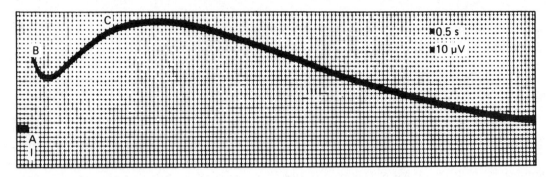

FIGURE 1.1   ERG recorded by Einthoven and Jolly (1908). The a-, b- and c-waves are designated. (From Einthoven W, Jolly W: *J Exp Physiol* 1908; 1:373–416.)

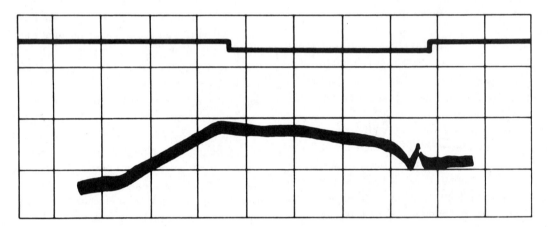

FIGURE 1.2   First human ERG (Kahn and Löwenstein). The curves are to be read from right to left (*squares*: 500 µV, 1.2 seconds).

(From Kahn R, Löwenstein A: *Graefes Arch Ophthalmol* 1924; 114:304–325.)

the same components as previously obtained in animal records. In 1929 Sachs[60] showed that the human ERG was dependent on the scotopic visual system of the retina.

In 1933, Cooper and associates[21] recorded the human ERG with a string galvanometer and a direct-coupled amplifier. They obtained good waves on single and multiple flash stimulation. Leads were taken from anesthetized conjunctiva and the mouth.

Gröppel et al.[35] used a nonpolarizable zinc electrode consisting of a short glass tube that contained an amalgamated zinc rod in a concentrated watery solution of zinc sulfate. The part near the eye was filled with Ringer's gelatin in which a small cotton wick was inserted. The reference electrode consisted of a glass funnel that was placed on the temple and a zinc electrode in Ringer's gelatin. The electrical potentials were magnified by a direct-coupled amplifier and photographically registered by a string galvanometer.

The development of the vacuum tube amplifier increased the precision with which an ERG could be obtained. The measuring instruments became fast enough to follow the rapid action potentials in nerves.

Electroretinogram components

Granit's (1933 to 1947) extensive investigations with improved techniques led to the analysis that is still in use.[34] By the use of chemical agents he was able to modify the ERG in ways that could be interpreted by postulating the existence of three processes (or potentials) that he called PI, PII, and PIII, named for the sequence of disappearance under ether anesthesia. The properties of these processes were summarized by Riggs (table 1.1).[58]

Granit's analysis indicated that the fast-developing corneal negative PIII forms the a-wave. The corneal positive PII (which is much larger) then develops, and the resultant of the PIII and PII produces the b-wave. As PII decreases, PI grows slowly and thus produces the c-wave.

Granit believed that PII originated in the neural pathway between the receptors and the ganglion cells and was correlated with optic nerve activity. A possibility suggested by Bartley[11] was that it arose in the bipolar cell layer. The short latency of PIII indicated that it developed very early in the chain of events constituting retinal activity, probably in the receptors themselves.

TABLE 1.1

A summary of the properties of electroretinograms and their relation to PI, PII, and PIII as described by Granit

Property	Process		
	PI	PII	PIII
Latency	Long	Medium	Short
Polarity	Positive	Positive	Negative
Electroretinogram wave accounted for	c-Wave	b-Wave	a- and d-Waves
Effect on nerve impulses	"Sensitizes" PII	Excitatory	Inhibitory
Result of light adaptation	Usually abolished	Greatly reduced	Not much change
Probable site of origin	?	Bipolar cells?	Rod and cone cells
Effect of asphyxia	Moderately susceptible	Very susceptible	Highly resistant
Effect of ether	Abolished first (reversible)	Abolished second (reversible)	Abolished last (irreversible)
Intensity of light to stimulate	High	Low	High
Effect of alcohol	?	Enhances	Diminishes
Effect of adrenalin	Enhances and prolongs	Diminishes and prolongs	?
Effect of KCl	None	Abolishes	Enhances, then inhibits

Adapted from Riggs LA: Electrical phenomenon in vision. In Hollaender A (ed): *Radiation Biology*, vol 3. New York, McGraw-Hill International Book Co, 1956, pp 581–619.

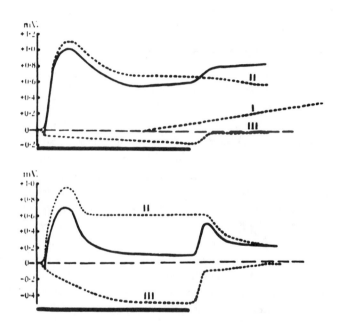

FIGURE 1.3   Analysis of the I-ERG (frog): upper, dark-adapted; lower, light-adapted; duration of stimulus, 2 seconds. (From Granit R, Riddell HA: *J Physiol* 1933; 77:207–240. Used by permission.)

The ERG off-response coincided with the end of PIII and the off-response in the optic nerve, and Granit suggested that PIII might represent a "central inhibitory state," release from which was associated with optic nerve discharge. He also showed that retinas dominated by cones respond to photic stimulation by generating a large a-wave (I retinas, "inhibitory" type, figure 1.3), whereas those dominated by rods generate large positive waves (E retinas, excitatory type, figure 1.4). The E-retina response in flickering light is characterized by a rather low fusion frequency, and the wavelets consist primarily of b-waves. The I retina responds with a series of a- and b-waves and has a much higher fusion frequency. However, rod (E) and cone (I) systems possess the same components, but their relative size may vary a great deal from species to species.

Noell[51–53] extensively studied the relationship of the cellular elements of the retina to ERG components and was the first to record both the slow and rapid changes associated with retinal illumination. He used three substances, sodium azide, iodoacetate, and sodium iodate, each of which had a specific effect upon the ERG and on the transretinal potential. Sodium azide increases both the transretinal potential and the c-wave, but not after the use of sodium iodate, which causes damage to this layer while leaving the remaining ERG components relatively unaffected. He concluded that the retinal pigment epithelium (RPE) develops the c-wave and the transretinal potential. The negative PIII could be differentiated into an early and late component with different time constants, with the faster arising from the receptors. The b-wave arose from a region lying between the inner portion of the receptors and the inner nuclear layer.

Microelectrodes

Intraretinal microelectrodes were first used to analyze the ERG by Tomita[68] and by Brindley.[14] The former discovered the subdivisions of Granit's PIII, while the latter documented the presence of the highly resistive R membrane formed by the tight junctions of the pigmented epithelium. These groups worked on amphibia, but Brown and Wiesel[15–17] and later Brown with a number of collaborators used Kuffler's closed-eye preparation to investigate the ERG of cats and primates.

Brown identified the "landmarks" encountered by a penetrating extracellular microelectrode and was thus able to judge the position of its tip relative to the RPE and the internal limiting membrane (ILM). He took advantage of the

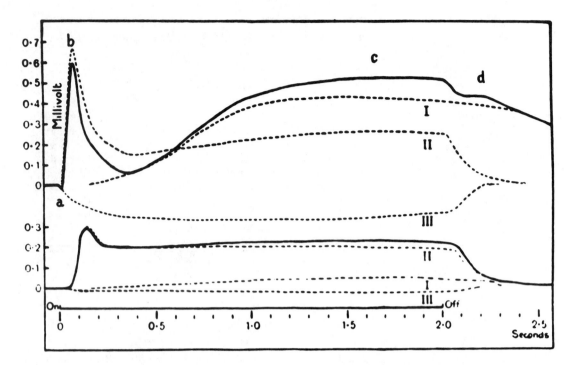

FIGURE 1.4 Analysis of the E-ERG (cat) at two intensities: upper, 14 mL; lower, 0.14 mL. The a-wave has been broadened slightly out of proportion to demonstrate its derivation more clearly. (From Granit R: *J Physiol* 1934; 81:1–28. Used by permission.)

dual blood supply of the retina and by blocking the central retinal artery was able to demonstrate that PIII was produced by the receptor layer. He utilized the anatomy of the foveola, which contains only photoreceptors, to further identify PIII and to distinguish between rod and cone receptor responses.

The generators of the b-wave sought by recording amplitude/depth characteristics of the responses. However, no clear distinction was made between voltage and current gradients, and the significance of the change in gradient was not understood; this was unfortunate since the published results clearly demonstrate that the b-wave is generated by a cell that extends from the outer to the inner limiting membranes, the significance of which was first detailed by Faber[29] who recognized the b-wave as a glial potential, which was confirmed the following year by Miller and Dowling,[48] who recorded intracellular Müller cell responses from mud puppy retinas and confirmed the localization by staining and identifying the cells.

Brown's group saw a number of other minor ERG components that were later described by others and, in particular, discovered the early receptor potential, a charge displacement in the outer limb due to the chemical changes in rhodopsin that occur in the first milliseconds after bleaching.

Following this work, intracellular recordings from individual retinal neurons[13,48,69,70] clarified the nature between extracellular and intracellular recordings and laid the foundation for the present spate of work on transduction, the mechanisms of the generation of photoreceptor potentials, and the interactions and synaptology of retinal neurons. The first of these, the discovery of the eponymously named S-potential by Svaetichin, remained for some years little understood; in fact, only since the recent developments of intravital staining and analysis of cultured cell recordings are we beginning to obtain quantitative estimates of retinal synaptic function.

Steinberg et al.,[65] in Brown's laboratory, investigated the slower responses from the RPE and demonstrated the mechanisms of production of the c-wave, fast oscillation, and the light peak. The microelectrode experiments also proved the site of origin of the c-wave and showed that it was caused by a reduction in potassium ion concentration in the subretinal space, which causes apical polarization of the RPE.

Clinical electroretinography

The development of clinical electroretinography was the consequence of a better understanding of the major components of the ERG, progress in the recording devices, and the introduction of the haptic (scleral) contact lens electrode by Riggs[33,57,62]; this consisted of a silver disk cemented into a hole in the contact lens. A fine flexible wire supported by beeswax was employed as a lead from the electrode. When the lens was inserted into the eyes, the silver made contact with the isotonic sodium chloride solution between it and the cornea.

The contact lens minimized the influence of irrelevant eye movements and reflex blinks. Even untrained patients could wear it because it allowed long experimental sessions without

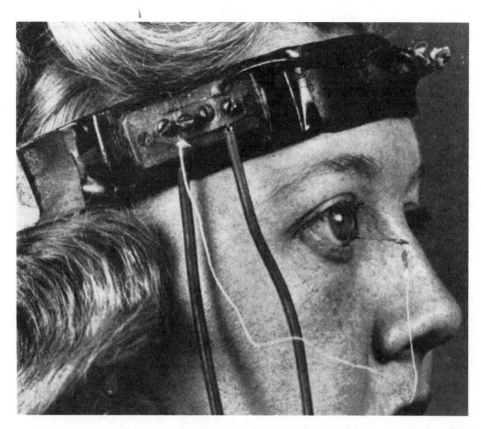

FIGURE 1.5   Contact lens electrode (Riggs).

discomfort for the subject. Another advantage was that the potentials were larger than those recorded with previous types of electrodes.

Karpe and Tansley[45] used a direct-coupled amplifier that was connected to an oscillograph with a camera. Later they used a condenser-coupled amplifier with a time constant of approximately 1.5 seconds. The records were made on moving photographic film.

Karpe[44] introduced ERG as a routine method in the ophthalmology clinic and used a similar electrode consisting of a silver rod screwed into a bottleneck in a plastic contact lens. The tube was filled with isotonic sodium chloride solution, and the reference electrode was a chlorided silver plate applied to the patient's forehead. Since then many models have been proposed, including those of Burian and Allen,[19] Jacobson,[41] Henkes and Van Balen,[37] and Sundmark.[66] In recent years, however, other types of corneal or scleral electrodes have been introduced that are generally more comfortable for the patient; these include soft contact lenses by Galloway[31] and Sole et al.,[64] a gold foil electrode by Arden et al.,[5] and a DTL microfiber electrode by Dawson, Trick, and Litzkow.[23]

Karpe[44] emphasized the importance of the ERG as an objective record of the function of the retina, one that is not dependent on the function of the optic nerve or the optic pathways and is minimally modified by clouding of the optic media (figure 1.5). He stressed the need for standardized procedures and established a normal range of response amplitudes as a function of age. With his technique the light-adapted ERG was sometimes too small to measure. It was merely possible to state whether the a-wave was present or absent. The dark-adapted ERG was much larger and dominated by the b-wave. Changes in amplitude were found to be clinically useful. Although this technique was important in the detection of some retinal diseases such as metallosis, tapetoretinal degenerations, vascular disturbances, and congenital functional anomalies, the early restriction of the human ERG to scotopic visual processes was a serious handicap for both clinical and experimental work.[59] This deficiency was remedied by Johnson and Bartlett[42] and Alpern and Faris,[4] who introduced intense short stimulus flashes that yielded photopic responses with durations well below those that gave maximal scotopic ones.

Another method of distinguishing cone from rod responses was pioneered by Motokawa and Mita,[49] who discovered a smaller positive deflection preceding the b-wave of the ERG in a moderately light-adapted human eye. They called it an x-wave but gave no interpretation of it.

Adrian[3] rediscovered the phenomenon independently (figure 1.6) and established that the scotopic b-wave was absent in red light and in a state of light adaptation, that it could be isolated in blue light, and that it was augmented

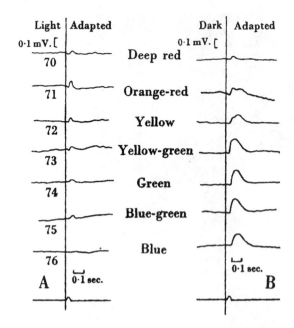

Light	Adapted	Dark	Adapted

0·1 mV. [⎡

70 — Deep red

71 — Orange-red

72 — Yellow

73 — Yellow-green

74 — Green

75 — Blue-green

76 — Blue

A 0·1 sec.   B 0·1 sec.

FIGURE 1.6 Human ERG responses to various wavelengths of light in the light-adapted (A) and dark-adapted state (B). (From Adrian ED: *J Physiol (Lond)* 1945; 104:84–104. Used by permission.)

considerably by dark adaptation. On the other hand, the x-wave (called "photopic response"), characterized by a shorter implicit time, was absent in blue light, could be isolated by red light, and did not increase during the later part of dark adaptation.[10] Adrian[2] showed that it is best developed in animals with a rich cone population (monkey, pigeon) and not in animals with few or no cones (cat, rabbit, guinea pig). Armington[7] demonstrated that the x-wave was augmented during the first minute of dark adaptation. Its spectral sensitivity did not correspond to the subjective scotopic or photopic curves, but had a maximum of 630 nm. Armington and Thiede[9] showed that either the x-wave or the b-wave may be selectively reduced in amplitude if the eye was adapted to light for which one component or the other possessed greater sensitivity.

Later studies[30] have shown that cone responses to red light were absent or severely reduced in protanopia and congenital achromatopsia and that cone responses to green light could be obtained as well.[33,56] The spectral sensitivity curve, determined by the method of flicker ERG, showed sensitivity losses at appropriate wavelengths for protanopes and deuteranopes.[22,24,54,59] Blue cone responses could only be isolated with more complex techniques.[61,71]

In 1954, Cobb and Morton[20] described rhythmic wavelets, now known as oscillatory potentials, on the ascending limb of the b-wave that appeared when bright flashes were used. Yonemura et al.[73] proved their clinical importance. They were absent in disturbances of the superficial retinal layers and often selectively reduced in circulatory disturbances and diabetic retinopathy.

In the last five decades, clinical developments have included an analysis of the timings of ERG components in disease[12]; an analysis of sensitivity from the voltage/log light intensity function[6,50]; and the use of computer averaging techniques to obtain small responses and to reduce the effect of noise, which allowed for the development of the visual evoked cortical potential and the pattern ERG and ultimately culminated in the recording of the "scotopic threshold response."[63] In addition, technical developments have led to the possibility of recording focal responses, pattern responses, and the slow c-wave in clinical situations; these topics are treated in separate sections of this book.

REFERENCES

1. Adrian ED: *Basis of Sensation.* Christophers, London, 1928.
2. Adrian ED: Rod and cone components in the electric response of the eye. *J Physiol (Lond)* 1946; 105:24–37.
3. Adrian ED: The electrical response of the human eye. *J Physiol (Lond)* 1945; 104:84–104.
4. Alpern M, Faris JS: Luminance—duration relationship in the electric response of the human retina. *J Opt Soc Am* 1956; 46:845–850.
5. Arden GB, Carter RM, Hogg C, Siegel IM, Margolis S: A gold foil electrode: Extending the horizons for clinical electroretinography. *Invest Ophthalmol* 1979; 18:421–426.
6. Arden GB, Carter RM, Hogg CR, Powell DJ, Ernst WJ, Clover GM, Lyness AL, Quinlan MP: A modified ERG technique and the results obtained in X-linked retinitis pigmentosa. *Br J Ophthalmol* 1983; 67:419–430.
7. Armington JC: A component of the human electroretinogram associated with red color vision. *J Opt Soc Am* 1952; 42:393–401.
8. Armington JC, Johnson EP, Riggs LA: The scotopic a-wave in the electrical response of the human eye. *J Physiol* 1952; 18:289–298.
9. Armington JC, Thiede FC: Selective adaptation of components of the human electoretinogram. *J Opt Soc Am* 1954; 44:779–786.
10. Auerbach E, Burian H: Studies on the photopicscotopic relationship in the human electroretinogram. *Am J Ophthalmol* 1955; 40:42–60.
11. Bartley SH: Some observations on the organization of the retinal response. *Am J Physiol* 1937; 120:184–189.
12. Berson EL, Gouras P, Hoff M: Temporal aspects of the electroretinogram. *Arch Ophthalmol* 1969; 81:207–214.
13. Bortoff A: Localisation of slow potentials in the Necturus retina. *Vision Res* 1964; 4:626–627.
14. Brindley GS: The passive electrical properties of the frog's retina, choroid and sclera for radial fields and currents. *J Physiol* 1956; 134:339–351.
15. Brown KT, Wiesel TN: Analysis of the intraretinal electroretinogram in the intact cat eye. *J Physiol* 1961; 158:229–256.
16. Brown KT, Wiesel TN: Intraretinal recording with micropipette electrodes in the intact cat eye. *J Physiol* 1959; 149:537–562.
17. Brown KT, Wiesel TN: Localisation of the origins electoretinogram components by intraretinal recording in the intact cat eye. *J Physiol* 1961; 158:257–280.

18. Brücke E, Garten S: Zur vergleichender Physiologie der Netzhautströme. *Pflugers Arch Ges Physiol* 1907; 120:290–310.

19. Burian HM, Allen L: A speculum contact lens electrode for electoretinography. *Electroencephalogr Clin Neurophysiol* 1954; 6:509–511.

20. Cobb WA, Morton HB: A new component of the human ERG. *J Physiol* 1953; 123:36–37.

21. Cooper S, Creed RS, Granit R: Note on the retinal action potential of the human eye. *J Physiol* 1933; 79:185–190.

22. Copenhaver RM, Gunkel RD: The spectral sensitivity of color-defective subjects determined by electroretinography. *Arch Ophthalmol* 1959; 62:55–68.

23. Dawson WW, Trick GL, Litzkow CA: Improved electrode for electroretinography. *Invest Ophthalmol* 1979; 18:988–991.

24. Denden A: Flimmerpotential zur Bestimmung der photopischen Spektralsensitivität bei normale Trichromasien und bei angeborenen Dichromatopsien. *Graefes Arch Ophthalmol* 1962; 165:1–19.

25. Dewar J: The physiological action of light. *Nature* 1877; 15:433–435.

26. Dewar J, McKendrick JG: On the physiological action of light. *Trans R Soc Edinb* 1873; 27:141–166.

27. DuBois-Reymond E: *Untersuchungen über die tierische Elektrizität*, vol 2. In Reumer G (ed): Berlin, 1849, p 256.

28. Einthoven W, Jolly W: The form and magnitude of the electrical response of the eye to stimulation at various intensities. *Q J Exp Physiol* 1908; 1:373–416.

29. Faber DS: *Analysis of the slow transretinal potentials in response to light* (Ph.D. thesis). University of New York at Buffalo, 1969.

30. Francois J, Verriest G, De Rouck A: Pathology of the x-wave of the human electroretinogram: I. Red-blindness and other congenital functional abnormalities. *Br J Ophthalmol* 1956; 40:430–443.

31. Galloway NR: *Ophthalmic Electrodiagnosis*. London, WB Saunders Co, 1975.

32. Gotch F: The time relations of the photo-electric changes in the eye ball of the frog. *J Physiol (Lond)* 1903; 29:388–410.

33. Gouras P: Electroretinography: Some basic principles. *Invest Ophthalmol* 1970; 9:557–569.

34. Granit R: *Sensory Mechanisms of the Retina With an Appendix on Electroretinography.* London, Oxford University Press, 1947.

35. Gröppel F, Haas F, Kohlrausch A: Aktionsströme und Gesichtsempfindungen des menschlichen Auges. *Z Sinnesphysiol* 1938; 67:207–226.

36. Hartline HK: The electrical response to illumination of the eye in intact animals, including the human subject and in decerebrate preparations. *Am J Physiol* 1925; 73:600–612.

37. Henkes HE, Van Balen ATM: Techniques of recording of the hitherto unrecordable ERG in the human eye. Presented at the ERG Symposium at Luhacovice, Belgium. *Acta Fac Med Univ Brunensis* 1959; 4:21–28.

38. Holmgren F: En method att objektivera effekten av zjusintryck pâ retina. *Ups Lakareforenings Forh* 1865; 1:177–191.

39. Holmgren F: Om retinastromme. *Ups Lakareforenings Forh* 1870; 6:419–455.

40. Holmgren F: Ueber die Retinaströme. *Untersuch Physiol Inst Univ Heidelberg* 1880; 3:278–326.

41. Jacobson J: A new contact lens electrode for clinical electroretinography. *AMA Arch Ophthalmol* 1958; 60:137.

42. Johnson EP, Bartlett NR: Effect of stimulus duration on electrical responses of the human retina. *J Ophthalmol Soc Am* 1956; 46:167–170.

43. Kahn R, Löwenstein A: Das Elektroretinogramm. *Graefes Arch Ophthalmol* 1924; 114:304–325.

44. Karpe G: Basis of clinical electroretinography. *Acta Ophthalmol* 1945; 24(suppl):1–118.

45. Karpe G, Tansley K: Relationship between the change in the electroretinogram and the subjective dark adaptation curve. *J Physiol* 1948; 107:272–279.

46. Kohlrausch A: Elektrische Erscheinungen am Auge, in Bethe A (ed): *Handbuch der normalen und pathologischen Physiologie*, vol 12. Berlin, Springer Publishing Co, 1931, pp 1393–1496.

47. Kuhne W, Steiner J: Ueber das electromotorische Verhalten der Netzhaut. *Untersuch Physiol Inst Univ Heidelberg* 1880; 3: 327–377.

48. Miller RF, Dowling JE: Intracellular responses of the Müller (glial) cells of mudpuppy retina: Their relation to b-wave of the electroretinogram. *J Neurophysiol* 1970; 33:323–341.

49. Motokawa K, Mita T: Ueber eine einfache Untersuchungsmethode und Eigenschaften der Aktionsströme der Netzhaut des Menschen. *Tohoku J Exp Med* 1942; 42:114–133.

50. Naka KI, Rushton WAH: S-potentials from colour units in the retina of fish (Cyprinidae). *J Physiol* 1966; 185:536–555.

51. Noell WK: Azide-sensitive potential difference across the eye bulb. *Am J Physiol* 1952; 170:217–238.

52. Noell WK: Electrophysiologic study of the retina during metabolic impairment. *Am J Ophthalmol* 1952; 35:126–132.

53. Noell WK: *Studies on the Electrophysiology and the Metabolism of the Retina.* Randolph Field, Tex, United States Air Force School of Aviation Medicine, Project No 21-129-0004, Report No 1, October 1953.

54. Padmos P, Van Norren D: Cone spectral sensitivity and chromatic adaptation as revealed by human flicker electroretinography. *Vision Res* 1971; 11:27–42.

55. Piper H: Ueber die Netzhautströme. *Arch Anat Physiol Leipzig* 1911; 85–132.

56. Rendahl I: Components of the human electroretinogram in normal eyes in deuteranopia and in deuteranomaly. *Acta Physiol* 1958; 44:189–202.

57. Riggs LA: Continuous and reproducible records of the electrical activity of the human retina. *Proc Soc Exp Biol Med* 1941; 48:204–207.

58. Riggs LA: Electrical phenomenon in vision. In Hollaender A (ed): *Radiation Biology*, vol 3. New York, McGraw-Hill International Book Co, 1956, pp 581–619.

59. Riggs LA, Berry RN, Wayner M: A comparison of electrical and psychophysical determinations of the spectral sensitivity of the human eye. *J Opt Soc Am* 1949; 39:427–436.

60. Sachs E: Die Aktionsströme des menschlichen Auges, ihre Beziehung zu Reiz und Empfindung. *Klin Wochenschr* 1929; 8:136–137.

61. Sawusch M, Pokorny J, Smith VC: Clinical electroretinography for short wavelength sensitive cones. *Invest Ophthalmol Vis Sci* 1987; 28:966–974.

62. Schubert G, Bornschein H: Beitrag zur Analyse des menschlichen Elektroretinogramms. *Ophthalmologica* 1952; 123:396–413.

63. Sieving PA, Frishman LJ, Steinberg RH: Scotopic threshold response of proximal retina in cat. *J Neurophysiol* 1986; 56:1049–1061.

64. Sole P, Lumbroso P, Alfieri R, Trapeau F: Présentation d'une nouvelle lentille porte-électrode permettant l enrégistrement couplé ERG-PEV. *Bull Soc Ophthalmol Fr* 1979; 79:217–219.

65. Steinberg RH, Schmidt R, Brown KT: Intracellular responses to light from cat pigment epithelium: Origin of the electroretinogram c-wave. *Nature* 1970; 227:728.

66. Sundmark E: The contact glass in human electroretinography. *Acta Ophthalmol Suppl (Copenh)* 1959; 52:1.

67. Therman PO: The neurophysiology of the retina in the light of chemical methods of modifying its excitability. *Acta Soc Sci Fenn* 1938; 11:1–73.

68. Tomita T: Studies on the intraretinal action potential; Part I. Relationship between the localisation of micropipette in the retina and the shape of the intraretinal action potential. *Jpn J Physiol* 1950; 1:110–117.

69. Tomita T: The electroretinogram as analysed by microelectrode studies. In Fuortes MGF (ed): *Handbook of Sensory Physiology*, vol 7, ed 2. Heidelberg, Springer-Verlag, 1972.

70. Tomita T, Kaneko A, Murakami M, et al: Spectral response curves of single cones in the carp. *Vision Res* 1967; 7:519–531.

71. Van Norren D, Padmos P: Human and macaque blue cones studies with electroretinography. *Vision Res* 1973; 13:1241–1254.

72. Waller AD: On the double nature of the photo-electrical response of the frog's retina. *Q J Exp Physiol* 1909; 2:169–185.

73. Yonemura D, Tsuzuki K, Aoki T: Clinical importance of the oscillatory potential in the human eye. *Acta Ophthalmol Suppl (Copenh)* 1962; 70:115–123.

2 History of Electro-Oculography

GEOFFREY B. ARDEN

THE POTENTIAL voltage difference that occurs between the cornea and fundus was known to DuBois-Reymond.[9] The main site of the voltage is across the retinal pigmented epithelium (RPE), and this was demonstrated by Dewar and Mc'Kendrick,[8] Kuhne and Steiner,[21] and de Haas[7]—all in the 19th century. Although illumination was known to affect the potential,[14,21] the capillary electrometers used in early work were not sufficiently sensitive or stable to analyze the changes in detail. With the advent of electronic amplification, condenser coupling prevented recording the changes caused by light. It was not until the 1940s that Noell[38] was able to employ stable dc recording systems and follow the slow changes; he related the c-wave of the electroretinogram (ERG) to the later and still slower responses and related the effects of poisons such as iodate and azide to the morphological sites of action.

The eye movement potential was studied in humans by numerous authors, some of whom[6,12,19,20,29,46] noted that the magnitude of the dipole was altered in illumination. The first complete description of the light-dark sequence was due to Kris,[19] but an analysis of the nature of the response and the recognition of its clinical utility is usually attributed to Arden.[1-4]

Since that time, research has moved along various lines; in animal work, the nature of the ionic channels and pumps in the apical and basal surfaces of the RPE has been greatly extended and related to water movement across the RPE. The most notable contributions are by Steinberg, Miller, Oakley, and other collaborators,* and the nature of the membrane changes that cause the c-wave, the "fast oscillation," and the light rise has been worked out in some detail.

The pharmacology of the dc potential and its relation to neurotransmitters have recently been reinvestigated by several authors.[11,24,42,47] The exact mechanisms of control still prove elusive, but this research has emphasized that interpretations from clinical work, especially the sensitivity to circulatory embarrassment,[5] are largely correct.

The eye movement potential in humans has also been frequently studied. It has been shown that cones contribute to the "light rise."[10] There have been attempts to describe the sequence of changes in terms of mathematical concepts, but this has not yet led to simplifications or to a reconciliation with cellular mechanisms. This is perhaps not surprising given that at least three separate mechanisms for current production have been identified in animal experiments, each with their own locations, while at each location, several different ionic mechanisms may be involved in current production.

Experimental clinical work has been more successful. Recently, the relationship of ERG and electro-oculographic (EOG) changes in inflammatory disease has recently been analyzed,[18] although the major clinical use of the EOG is that a reduced EOG and normal ERG are a diagnostic feature of Best's disease and some other forms of juvenile macular degeneration, as has been widely reported.[49] It is useful as an ancillary test in retinal degenerations and in cases of unexplained loss of vision. The influence of other agents on the EOG (mannitol and acetazolamide, a carbonic anhydrase inhibitor) has been studied by the Japanese school and clinical tests developed as a result.[27,28,50] Most recently, extension of this work has suggested that while acetazolamide acts directly on the membrane mechanisms, mannitol activates a "second messenger" system.[22]

Finally, continuing efforts have been made to reduce the population variability of the EOG as a clinical test. Some of these involve more lengthy periods of recording, but even if this results in greater precision, it is clinically difficult to justify. The original method envisaged a 12-minute period of dark adaptation followed by light adaptation for 10 minutes. The dark adaptation has been whittled down to "a period of reduced illumination sufficient to stabilize the voltage changes." In the author's experience, this sometimes takes as long as 60 minutes. Alternatively, more lengthy periods of dark adaptation have been suggested. Such modifications have their protagonists. As yet unconfirmed on a large scale, a recent report[43] shows that part of the problem is due to errors in eye movement control. All eye movement techniques assume that the ocular excursions are precise, there is a linear relation between voltage and the degree of eye motion, and that the changes in recorded voltage are due only to changes in the apparent ocular dipole which generates the current. If the real ocular excursion is measured, and appropriate corrections made, variability decreases.

---

*13, 15–17, 23, 25, 26, 30–37, 39–41, 44, 45, and 48.

REFERENCES

1. Arden GB, Barrada A: An analysis of the electro-oculograms of a series of normal subjects. *Br J Ophthalmol* 1962; 46:468–482.

2. Arden GB, Barrada A, Kelsey JH: A new clinical test of retinal function based upon the standing potential of the eye. *Br J Ophthalmol* 1962; 46:449–467.

3. Arden GB, Kelsey JH: Changes produced by light in the standing potential of the human eye. *J Physiol* 1962; 161:189–204.

4. Arden GB, Kelsey JH: Some observations on the relationship between the standing potential of the human eye and the bleaching and regeneration of visual purple. *J Physiol* 1962; 161:205–226.

5. Arden GB, Kolb K: Electrophysiological investigations in retinal metabolic disease: Their range and application. *Exp Eye Res* 1964; 3:334–347.

6. Aserinsky E: Effect of illumination and sleep on the amplitude of the electro-oculogram. *Arch Ophthalmol* 1955; 53:542–546.

7. de Haas HK: *Lichtprikkels en Retinastroomen in hun quantitatief Verband* (dissertation). University of Leiden, The Netherlands, 1903. Quoted by Kohlsrausch, A: Elektrische Erscheinungen am Auge. In *Handbuch der normalen und pathologischen Physiologie*, vol 12. Berlin, Springer-Verlag, 1931, pp 1394–1426.

8. Dewar J, Mc'Kendrick JG: On the physiological action of light. *Trans Royal Soc Ed* 1876; 27:141–166.

9. DuBois-Reymond RE: *Untersuchungen uber thierische Electricität*, vol 2. Berlin, G Reimer, 1849, p 256.

10. Elenius V, Aantaa E: Light induced increase in amplitude of electrooculogram evoked with blue and red lights in totally colour-blind and normal humans. *Arch Opthalmol* 1973; 90:60–63.

11. Frambach DA, Valentine JL, Weiter JJ: Modulation of rabbit retinal pigment epithelium electrogenic transport by alpha-1 adrenergic stimulation. *Invest Ophthalmol Vis Sci* 1988; 29:814–817.

12. François J, Verriest G, De Rouck A: Modification of the amplitude of the human electrooculogram by light and dark adaptation. *Br J Ophthalmol* 1955; 39:398–408.

13. Griff ER, Steinberg RH: Origin of the light peak: In vitro study of *Gekko gekko*. *J Physiol* 1982; 331:637–652.

14. Himstedt F, Nagel WA: Festschr D. Univ. Freiburg z 50 jahr. Reg.-Jubil. Sr. Kgl. Hocheit dl.1 Grossherzogs Friedrich von Baden. 1902, pp 262–263. Quoted by Kohlrausch A: Elektrische Erscheinungen am Auge, in *Handbuch der normalen und pathologischen Physiologie*, Vol 12. Berlin, Springer-Verlag, 1931, pp 1394–1426.

15. Hughes BA, Adorante JS, Miller SS, Lin H: Apical electrogenic $NaHCO_3$ cotransport: A mechanism for HCO_3 absorption across the retinal pigment epithelium. *J Gen Physiol* 1989; 94:124–150.

16. Hughes BA, Miller SS, Farber DB: Adenylate cyclase stimulation alters transport in frog retinal pigment epithelium. *Am J Physiol* 1987; 253:385–395.

17. Hughes BA, Miller SS, Joseph DP, Edelman JL: Cyclic AMP stimulates the Na-K pump of the bullfrog retinal pigment epithelium. *Am J Physiol* 1988; 254:84–98.

18. Ikeda H, Franchi A, Turner G, Shilling J, Graham E: Electroretinography and electro-oculography to localise abnormalities in early stage inflammatory disease. *Doc Ophthalmol* 1989; 73:387–394.

19. Kris C: Corneo-fundal potential variations during light and dark adaptation. *Nature* 1958; 182:1027.

20. Kolder H: Spontane und experimentelle Anderungen des Bestandpotentials des menschlichen Auges. *Pflugers Arch Gesamte Physiol* 1959; 268:258–272.

21. Kuhne W, Steiner J: Ueber electrische Vorgange im Sehorgane. *Untersuch Physiol Inst Univ Heidelberg* 1881; 4:64–160.

22. Leon JA, Arden GB, Bird AC: The standing potential in Bests's macular dystrophy: Baseline and drug-induced responses. *Invest Opthalmol Vis Sci* 1990; 31(suppl):497.

23. Lin H, Miller SS: $[K^+]_o$-induced changes in apical membrane voltage (Va) modulate pH_i in frog retinal pigment epithelium. *Invest Ophthalmol Vis Sci* 1989; (suppl):30.

24. Linsenmeier RA: Effects of light and darkness on oxygen distribution and consumption in the cat retina. *J Gen Physiol* 1986; 88:521–542.

25. Linsenmeier RA, Steinberg RH: Origin and sensitivity of the light peak of the intact cat eye. *J Physiol* 1982; 331:653–673.

26. Hughes BA, Miller SS, Machen TE: Effects of cyclic AMP on fluid absorption and ion transport across frog retinal epithelium. Measurements in the open-circuit state. *J Physiol* 1984; 83:875–899.

27. Madachi-Yamamoto S, Yonemura D, Kawasaki K: Diamox response of ocular standing potential as a clinical test for retinal pigment epithelial activity. *Acta Soc Ophthalmol Jpn* 1984; 88:1267–1272.

28. Madachi-Yamamoto S, Yonemura D, Kawasaki K: Hyperosmolarity response of ocular standing potential as a clinical test for retinal pigment epithelial activity. *Doc Ophthalmol* 1984; 57:153–162.

29. Miles WR: Modification of the human eye potential by dark and light adaptation. *Science* 1940; 91:456.

30. Miller SS, Edelman JL: Active ion transport pathways in the bovine retinal pigment epithelium. *J Physiol* 1990; 424:283–300.

31. Miller SS, Farber D: Cyclic AMP modulation of ion transport across frog retinal pigment epithelium. Measurements in the short-circuited state. *J Gen Physiol* 1984; 83:853–874.

32. Miller SS, Lin H: $[K^+]_o$-induced changes in apical membrane voltage (Va) modulate pH_i in frog retinal pigment epithelium. *Invest Ophthalmol Vis Sci* 1989; 30(suppl):168.

33. Miller SS, Steinberg RH: Potassium transport across the frog retinal pigment epithelium. *J Membr Biol* 1982; 67:199–209.

34. Miller SS, Steinberg RH: Active transport of ions across frog retinal pigment epithelium. *Exp Eye Res* 1977; 25:235–248.

35. Miller SS, Steinberg RH: Passive ionic properties of frog retinal pigment epithelium. *J Membr Biol* 1977; 36:337–372.

36. Miller SS, Steinberg RH: Potassium modulation of taurine transport across the frog retinal pigment epithelium. *J Gen Physiol* 1979; 74:237–259.

37. Miller SS, Steinberg RH, Oakley B II: The electrogenic sodium pump of the frog retinal pigment epithelium. *J Membr Biol* 1978; 44:259–279.

38. Noell WK: *Studies on the Electrophysiology and Metabolism of the Retina*. Randolph Field, Tex, US Air University School of Aviation Medicine Project Report No. 1, 1953.

39. Oakley B II: Potassium and the photoreceptor dependent pigment epithelial hyperpolarization. *J Gen Physiol* 1977; 70:405–424.

40. Oakley B II, Steinberg RH, Miller SS, Nilsson SE: The in vitro frog pigment epithelial cell hyperpolarization in response to light. *Invest Ophthalmol Vis Sci* 1977; 16:771–774.

41. Ostwald T, Steinberg RH: Localization of frog retinal pigment epithelium (Na-K)-ATPase. *Exp Eye Res* 1980; 31:351–360.

42. Pautler EL, Tengerdy C: Transport of acidic amino acids by the bovine pigment epithelium. *Exp Eye Res* 1986; 43:207–214.

43. Reimslag FCC, Verduyn-lunel HFE, Spekreijse H: The electrooculogram: A refinement of the method. *Doc Ophthalmol* 1989; 73:369–376.

44. Steinberg RH, Linsenmeier RA, Griff ER: Retinal pigment epithelial cell contributions to the electroretinogram and electrooculogram, in Osborne NN, Chader GJ (eds): *Progress in Retinal Research*, vol 4. New York, Pergamon Press, 1985, pp 33–66.

45. Steinberg RH, Miller SS, Stern WH: Initial observations on the isolated retinal pigment epithelium–choroid of the cat. *Invest Ophthalmol Vis Sci* 1978; 17:675–678.

46. Ten Doesschate G, Ten Doesschate J: The influence of the state of adaptation on the resting potential of the human eye. *Ophthalmologica* 1956; 132:308–320.

47. Textorius O, Nilsson SEG, Andersson B-E: Effects of intravitreal perfusion with dopamine in different concentrations on the DC electroretinogram and the standing potential of the albino rabbit eye. *Doc Ophthalmol* 1989; 73:149–162.

48. Tsuboi S: Measurement of the volume flow and hydraulic conductivity across the isolated dog retinal pigment epithelium. *Invest Ophthalmol Vis Sci* 1987; 28:1776–1782.

49. Weleber RG: Fast and slow oscillations of the electrooculogram in Best's macular dystrophy and retinitis pigmentosa. *Arch Ophthalmol* 1989; 107:530–537.

50. Yonemura D, Kawasaki K, Madachi-Yamamoto S: Hyperosmolarity response of ocular standing potential as a clinical response for retinal pigment epithelium activity. Chorioretinal dystrophies. *Doc Ophthalmol* 1984; 57:163–173.

3 History of Visual Evoked Cortical Testing

GRAHAM F. A. HARDING

HUMAN VISUAL evoked responses (VERs) have been known almost since the origin of human electroencephalography (EEG). In 1934 Adrian and Matthews[1] demonstrated that regularly repeated flashes of light elicited electrical responses from surface electrodes placed over the occipital cortex. By utilizing a sectored disk in front of a car headlight they demonstrated that photic following took place at the same rate as the frequency of the periodically repeated flashes of light. The rates of stimulation that they used varied between 8 and 12 per second, and their classic paper contains clear illustrations of the responses from Adrian's brain. These results were the origin of what is now known as the "steady-state evoked potential."

Early reports of responses to single flashes of light began with Monnier[39] who recorded both the electroretinogram (ERG) and cortical response from the scalp and stated that the most consistent component of the cortical response was a slow surface-positive monophasic potential occurring between 90 and 120 ms. He suggested that earlier components of the cortical response were much more difficult to record but consisted of a diphasic potential, initially positive, with a latency of approximately 40 ms. Cobb[8] following the development of Dawson's superimposition technique, produced averaged responses to 50 flashes of light of high intensity involving the full visual field. The initial components of the evoked potential appeared at times to vary between 35 and 60 ms in different individuals, but in a later study[10] the evoked potential was identified as a small positive deflection with a peak latency around 26 ms followed by a negative one at 45 ms and a larger positive wave around 79 ms. In a further study in 1952 Monnier[38] recorded cortical responses by using bipolar derivations around the occiput. The earliest visual evoked potential (VEP) component consisted of a small occipito-positive deflection with a peak latency of 35 ms. The highest amplitude and most consistent component occurred between 95 and 115 ms, being a positive potential, presumably P2 (see figure 3.1). Monnier introduced the concept of retinocortical time by simultaneously recording the ERG and determining retinal time by the latency of the b-wave. The latency to the peak of the first component of the cortical response was termed *cortical time*, and the retinocortical time was derived from subtracting the retinal time from the cortical time. In 1956 Calvet et al.[4] demonstrated an initial positive component around this 35-ms peak latency. Monnier in a later paper[37] also reported a positive deflection around 37.5 ms. There is little doubt that these concepts of retinocortical time were a gross oversimplification. There are great difficulties in identifying initial responses as distinct from gross responses by large groups of neurons.

Cobb and Dawson[9] studied the occipital potentials evoked by bright flashes of light in 11 adult subjects. They averaged between 55 and 220 flashes and demonstrated that the earliest component of the VEP had a latency of 20 to 25 ms with an average amplitude of between 1 and 1.5 μV. The following negative deflection at 45 ms was slightly larger, and this component they found to be enhanced when the subject paid attention to the stimulus. It was Ciganek[7] who produced the first morphological description of the human VEP to light flashes and the results obtained on 75 subjects; his classic illustration began the principle of labeling the components, and in addition the components were divided between early or primary components (waves 0 to III) and late components (waves IV to VII). The first component was positive at 28.6 ms, the second wave negative at 53 ms, the third wave positive at 73 ms, the fourth wave negative at 94 ms, the fifth wave positive at 114 ms, with a later positive wave around 134 ms. Ciganek also described an after-discharge that was sometimes obtained and appeared to be related to the alpha rhythm of the EEG.[6] This concept of labeling was quickly taken up by Gastaut and Regis,[20] but unfortunately the labeling systems were different. They described a typical response that was similar in form to that of Ciganek; in addition, they compared the normal VEP reported by a number of previous investigators.[3,13,43,49,51] They pointed out that although there was great variation in the presence and shape of many of the components the major positive P2 component was almost invariably present between 100- and 150-ms latency. The components they themselves identified consisted of wave 1, positive at 25 ms; wave 2, negative at 40 ms; wave 3, positive at 60 ms; and wave 4, negative at 80 ms. They found there was a good deal of variation between individuals in both latency and amplitude of these components. Wave 5 was by far the most constant and significant wave of the VEP, the

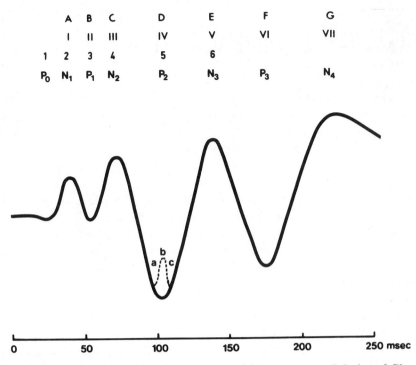

A	B	C		D	E	F		G
I	II	III		IV	V	VI		VII
1	2	3	4		5	6		
P_0	N_1	P_1	N_2		P_2	N_3	P_3	N_4

FIGURE 3.1 The figure illustrates the "stylized" VEP to flash stimulation in normal adults. The major positive component, often referred to as P2, can be seen at approximately at 105 ms. In this illustration positive is indicated downward and negative upward. Various systems of nomenclature have been used to identify the components of the VEP. The top row of alphabetic nomenclature is that of Dustman and Beck (1969), the second row of Roman numerals is that of Ciganek (1961), the third row is that of Gastaut and Regis (1967), and the lowest row is that of Harding (1974). It is this latter nomenclature that is now quite commonly used in describing the flash VEP. It should be noticed that the P2 component (wave 5 of Gastaut and Regis) can sometimes become a triphasic component showing peaks at both A and C.

amplitude appeared to vary between 30 and 50 µV, and it was usually monophasic, peaking at around 130 ms. On some occasions they found that this wave was biphasic, with an early peak at 120 ms, and a later positive peak around 180 ms.

Only 20% of the subjects tested demonstrated a complete VEP from wave 1 to wave 4, usually waves 1, 2, or 3 were missing for many of the subjects. For each individual there was little variability in terms of latency from one recording session to the next; indeed, for wave 5 the variation in latency was only ±2.5 ms. Between individuals, however, this wave varied by ±30 ms. They also showed that the separate components of wave 5 could be affected by opening and closing the eyes and by dark adaptation and suggested that the photopic system, that is the fovea, was associated with the early positive peak of wave 5 and the later positive peak associated with the scotopic system.

Over the ensuing years the complexity of labeling systems grew, and it is still not entirely resolved. However, most systems now identify the component as negative or positive and use either a mean latency for the wave as a subscript or alternatively a sequential numbering system. An example of labeling of a flash VEP is given in figure 3.1.

The early component of the VEP that were frequently mentioned by the pioneer workers have over subsequent years been the subject of much controversy. Some authors, for example, Allison et al.,[2] proposed that many of the early components reflect the ERG in view of its high amplitude and its complete domination of the anterior portions of the scalp.[42] However, other authors do not accept this hypothesis[52]; indeed, some authors such as Van Hasselt[50] suggest that even early components around 10-ms latency were arising from the optic nerve. Vaughan and Gross[53] suggested that the early wavelets in the VEP reflected geniculocalcarine input to the striate visual cortex. Corletto et al.,[14] undertaking depth recordings of the VEP before an ablation of the occipital poles in humans, noted persistence of initial components having peak latencies earlier than 45 ms. Spire and Hosobuchi,[47] using depth recordings, located a flash evoked potential of 22-ms peak latency in an area just anterior to the lateral geniculate body.

In a series of studies Harding and coworkers[24–26,42] identified the components of what they termed the visual evoked subcortical potential (VESP), which consists of a positive around 21 ms, a negative at 28 ms, and a positive at 35-ms latency. They demonstrated that the VESP could be elicited by both flash and pattern-reversal stimulation. In patients who had suffered direct optic nerve trauma in whom the ERG was still present, the VESP was absent when that eye was stimulated. This indicated, therefore, that the components were independent of the ERG. Equally, by a combination of binocular and monocular stimulation it could be demonstrated that these potentials were in fact arising postchiasmally. By using luminance-matched red-green color checkerboards it was possible to elicit clear responses that were maximal in response to checkerboards in which each element subtended 2 degrees. When black and white checkerboards were used, the responses were maximal in response to 12 minutes of visual angle checkerboard and showed clear tuning. These findings would be entirely consistent with the potential arising in the parvocellular layers of the lateral geniculate body.

The first study of the flash VEP across the life span was carried out by Dustman and Beck.[15] They found that in the first 6 years of life there was a steady increase in the amplitude of the response followed by a reduction until around the age of 15 years, after which the amplitude of the response was not significantly altered until the 60s or 70s. In older subjects there is an increase in the amplitude of early components and a decrease in the amplitude of later components.

Neonatal flash VEPs were first recorded in full-term infants by Ellingson.[18] However, in 1960[17] he published a comprehensive survey of the VEPs of both full-term and preterm babies and showed that in full-term infants the VEP was of relatively simple morphology consisting of an initial brief positive wave around 180 ms followed by a negative wave of fairly rounded form. However, the preterm infants prior to 35 weeks' gestational age showed only a broad negative deflection that had a longer peak latency than those seen in full-term infants. The initial positive wave appeared to develop in babies around 35 weeks' postmenstrual age (PMA), although the earliest it was seen was around 32 weeks. Flash VEPs have been recorded from human infants of 24 weeks' PMA.[5,48]

The inherent variability between subjects of the flash VEP and its crudity in representing a response to a gross change in luminance led to the development of pattern stimulation. Early pattern stimulation utilized the flashing of a patterned visual field. This technique has since become known as the flashed-on pattern, and it was by utilizing this technique that the early studies of the response to the commonly used black and white checkerboards or gratings were first investigated.[44] Such responses are of course a mixture of both luminance and contour as well as contrast and show a much closer correlation between the amplitude of the evoked potential and visual acuity.[31] Jeffreys[34] attempted to identify the pattern component of the resulting evoked potential by subtracting the luminance response from the flashed-on pattern response. It has also been shown that such patterns are of great use in studying abnormal evoked potentials such as those found in epilepsy.[33]

The type of reversing checkerboard pattern now commonly used owes its origin to the work of Spekreijse[45] and Cobb et al.[11] By utilizing these techniques it became possible to identify both the average response to a reversing checkerboard pattern as well as the response to the onset and offset of patterns. The reversal response is of relatively simple outline and consists of a negative peak around 75 ms, a positive component at 100 ms, and a later negative peak at 145 ms. These components are usually known by their polarity and their latency, the positive component therefore becoming the P100 component. All studies have shown that these responses have little variability within a subject and remarkably small variability between normal healthy subjects. This lack of variability has encouraged the use of this technique for studies of stimulus variables and subjective parameters in normal individuals and, in addition, in the clinical development of evoked potential testing. Indeed it was the paper of Halliday et al.[22] that provided the spur for many of the evoked potential laboratories that have since developed.

The response to pattern onset-offset is more complex, and certainly there are separate responses to both the onset and offset of patterns.[19] To obtain these separate responses the onset and offset of the stimulus have to be more than 100 ms apart, and under these circumstances it can be seen that the offset response is very similar to the pattern-reversal response. The onset response consists of three components: a positive response around 75 ms (C1), a negative response at 100 ms (C2), and a positive response around 150 ms (C3).[35,46] These components are only present when the lower half of the field is stimulated. The C2 component appears to be markedly affected by the contour or sharpness of the pattern and is most sensitive to defocusing. The C1 component appears to be related to the contrast present in the pattern.

During the years since their first description all the VEPs have been shown to be dependent to a greater or lesser degree on the integrity of the visual pathway and the normal functioning of the visual cortex. Lesions affecting the optic nerves may affect all forms of evoked potentials, although certainly demyelinating diseases are shown to affect the pattern-reversal response and the pattern onset-offset response far more than the flash response.[28] Gross lesions such as those seen in optic nerve trauma affect all the potentials, and it is under these circumstances and those of major eye injuries that the flash evoked potential comes into its own as an electrodiagnostic tool.[29] With abnormalities affecting the visual cortex the various types of evoked potentials may be differentially affected. Certainly, if the lesion involves the primary visual cortex, there is little doubt that the pattern-reversal P100 response and the C1 component of the pattern-onset response are clearly affected. Surprisingly for extrastriate abnormalities, particularly those affecting the association areas, the flash response is often that most affected.[28]

Needless to say, many of the early clinical studies involved the flash technique. Ebe et al.[16] carried out a study utilizing both the ERG and the VEP in a variety of patients including those with retinal disorders, optic atrophy, as well as cataracts. They showed that patients with macular losses had little change in either the ERG or the VEP whereas patients with retinitis pigmentosa showed reductions in both. In patients with optic atrophy the evoked potential was undetectable, and the ERG was normal although the patients were not blind. Vaughan and Katzman[54] confirmed that a normal ERG with an absence of the VER was indicative of optic nerve disease. Gerin et al.[21] showed that in patients with optic nerve lesions the latency of the first peak of the evoked potential was delayed; this was confirmed by Richey et al.[41]

Early attempts to relate the asymmetry of the VEP to hemianopic defects, ús by us at least two electrodes, one over each cerebral hemisphere, began with Cohn.[12] He suggested that there is a prominent amplitude asymmetry in the evoked response, and this was confirmed by Vaughan and Katzman.[54] Many studies followed, including those of Kooi et al.,[36] Jacobson et al.,[32] Harding et al.,[27] and Oosterhuis et al.[40] Such findings of course correlate with subjective sensation in that the patient is complaining of a hemianopic defect. There is little doubt that in other areas the relationship between flash response and sensation is much less clear. The development of pattern reversal and, even more, pattern onset-offset have allowed the precise interrelationship between evoked potentials and sensation to be developed. Particularly with pattern onset-offset there is a freedom that allows nongeometric patterns to be investigated, and therefore patterns that carry inherent meaning can also be studied, although it must be admitted that such studies are relatively rare.

REFERENCES

1. Adrian ED, Mathews BHC: The Berger rhythm: potential changes from the occipital lobes in man. *Brain* 1934; 57:365–385.
2. Allison T, Matsumya Y, Goff GD, et al: The scalp topography of human visual evoked potentials. *Electroencephalogr Clin Neurophysiol* 1977; 42:185–197.
3. Brazier MAB: Long persisting electrical traces in the brain of man and their possible relationship to higher nervous activity. *Electroencephalogr Clin Neurophysiol Suppl* 1960; 13:374–378.
4. Calvet J, Cathala HP, Hirsch J, Scherrer J: La rèsponse corticale visuelle de l'homme ètudiee par une methode d'integration. *CR Soc Biol (Paris)* 1956.
5. Chin KC, Taylor MJ, Menzies R, & Whyte H: Development of visual evoked potential in neonates. A study using light emitting diode goggles. *Arch Dis Child* 1985; 60:116–118.
6. Ciganek ML: A comparative study of visual and auditory EEG responses in man. *Electroencephalogr Clin Neurophysiol* 1965; 18:625–629.
7. Ciganek ML: The EEG response (evoked potential) to light stimulus in man. *Electroencephalogr Clin Neurophysiol* 1961; 13:165–172.
8. Cobb WA: On the form and latecny of the human cortical response to illumination of the retina. *Electroencephalogr Clin Neurophysiol* 1950; 2:104.
9. Cobb WA, Dawson GD: The latency and form in man of the occipital potentials evoked by bright flashes. *J Physiol* 1960; 152:108–121.
10. Cobb WA, Morton HB: The human retinogram in response to high intensity flashes. *Electroencephalogr Clin Neurophysiol* 1952; 4:547–556.
11. Cobb WA, Morton HB, Ettinger G: Cerebral potentials evoked by pattern reversal and vein suppression in visual rivalry. *Nature* 1967; 216:1123–1125.
12. Cohn R: Evoked visual cortical responses in homonymous hemianopic defects in men. *Electroencephalogr Clin Neurophysiol* 1963; 15:922.
13. Contamin F, Cathala HP: Rèsponses electrocorticales de l'homme normal èveille à des eclairs lumineux. Resultats obtenus à partir d'enregistrements sur le cuir chevelu à l'aide d'un dispositif d'integration. *Electroencephalogr Clin Neurophysiol* 1961; 13:674–694.
14. Corletto F, Gentilomo A, Rodadini A, Rossi GF, Zattoni J: Visual evoked potentials as recorded from the scalp and from the visual cortex before and after surgical removal of the occipital pole in man. *Electroencephalogr Clin Neurophysiol* 1967; 22:378–380.
15. Dustman RE, Beck EC: The effects of maturation and ageing on the waveform of visually evoked potentials. *Electroencephalogr Clin Neurophysiol* 1969; 26:2–11.
16. Ebe M, Mikami T, Ito H: Clinical evolution of electrical responses of retina and visual cortex in photic stimulation in ophthalmic diseases. *Tohoku J Exp Med* 1964; 84:92–103.
17. Ellingson RJ: Cortical electrical responses to visual stimulation in the human infant. *Electroencephalogr Clin Neurophysiol* 1960; 12:663–677.
18. Ellingson RJ: Electroencephalograms of normal full-term infants immediately after birth with observations on arousal and visual evoked responses. *Electroencephalogr Clin Neurophysiol* 1958; 10:31–50.
19. Estévez O, Spekreijse H: Relationship between pattern appearance-disappearance and pattern reversal. *Exp Brain Res* 1974; 19:233–238.
20. Gastaut H, Regis H: Visual evoked potentials recorded transcranially in man. In Proctor LD, Adey WR (eds): *The Analysis of Central Nervous System and Cardio-vascular System Data Using Computer Methods*. Washington, DC, NASA, 1965, pp 7–34.
21. Gerin P, Ravault MP, David C, et al: Occipital average response and lesions of optic nerve. *C R Soc Biol (Paris)* 1966; 160:1445–1453.
22. Halliday AM, McDonald WI, Mushin J: Delayed visual evoked response in optic neuritis. *Lancet* 1972; 1:982–985.
23. Harding GFA: The visual evoked response, in Roper-Hall MJ, et al (eds): *Advances in Ophthalmology*. Basel, S Karger AG, 1974, pp 2–28.
24. Harding GFA, Dhanesha U: The visual evoked subcortical potential to pattern reversal stimulation. *Clinical Vision Sciences* 1986; 1:179–184.
25. Harding GFA, Rubinstein MP: The scalp topography of the human visual evoked subcortical potential. *Investigative Ophthalmology and Visual Science* 1980; 19:318–321.

26. Harding GFA, Rubinstein MP: Early components of the visual evoked potential in man. Are they of subcortical origin? In Spekreijse H, Apkarian PA (eds): *Documenta Ophthalmologica Series*. No 27. The Hague, Junk Publishers, 1981, pp 49–65.

27. Harding GFA, Thomon CRS, Panayiotopoulos C: Evoked response diagnosis in visual field defects. *Proc Electrophysiol Technol Assoc* 1969; 16:159–163.

28. Harding GFA, Wright CE: Visual evoked potentials in acute optic neuritis. In Hess RF, Plant GT (eds): *Optic Neuritis*. Cambridge, England, Cambridge University Press, 1986, pp 230–254.

29. Harding GFA: Neurophysiology of vision and its clinical application, in Edwards K, Llewellyn R (eds): *Optometry*. London, Butterworth Publishers, 1988; pp 44–60.

30. Reference deleted by author.

31. Harter MR, White CT: Effects of contour sharpness and check size on visually evoked cortical potentials. *Vision Res* 1968; 8:701–711.

32. Jacobson HH, Hirose T, Susuki TA: Simultaneous ERG and VER in lesions of the optic pathway. *Invest Ophthalmol* 1968; 7:279–292.

33. Jeavons PM, Harding GFA: Photosensitive epilepsy. *Clinics in Developmental Medicine*. No 56. London, William Heinemann Books, 1975.

34. Jeffreys B: Separable components of human evoked responses to spatially patterned visual fields. *Electroencephalogr Clin Neurophysiol* 1968; 24:596.

35. Jeffreys DA, Axford JG: Source localisations of pattern specific components of human visual evoked potentials I & II. *Exp Brain Res* 1972; 16:1–40.

36. Kooi KA, Guvener AM, Bagchi BK: Visual evoked responses in lesions of the higher visual pathways. *Neurology* 1965; 15:841–854.

37. Monnier M: Le centre visuel cortical et l'organisation des perception visuelles. In *Problèmes Actuels d'Ophthalmologie*, vol 1. Basel, S Karger AG, 1951, pp 277–301.

38. Monnier M: Retinal, cortical and motor responses to photic stimulation in man. Retino-cortical time and opto-motor time. *J Neurophysiol* 1952; 15:469–486.

39. Monnier M: Retinal time, retino-cortical time, alpha blocking time and motor reaction time. *Electroencephalogr Clin Neurophysiol* 1949; 1:516–517.

40. Oosterhuis HJGH, Ponsen L, Jonkman EJ, Magnus O: The average visual response in patients with cerebrovas-cular disease. *Electroencephalogr Clin Neurophysiol* 1969; 27:23–34.

41. Richey ET, Kooi KA, Tourtelotte WW: Visually evoked responses in multiple sclerosis. *J Neurol Neurosurg* 1971; 34:275–280.

42. Rubinstein MP, Harding GFA: The visually evoked subcortical potential: Is it related to the electroretinogram? *Investigative Ophthalmology and Visual Science* 1981; 2:335–344.

43. Schwartz M, Shagass C: Recovery functions of human somato-sensory and visually evoked potential. *Ann N Y Acad Sci* 1964; 112:510–525.

44. Spehlmann R: The averaged electrical response to diffuse and to patterned light in the human. *Electroencephalogr Clin Neurophysiol* 1965; 19:560–569.

45. Spekreijse H: *Analysis of EEG Responses in Man*. The Hague, Junk, 1966.

46. Spekreijse H, Estévez O: The pattern appearance-disappearance response. *Trace* 1972; 6:13–19.

47. Spire JP, Hosobuchi Y: Depth electrode recording of the VER from the geniculate region in man. *Electroencephalogr Clin Neurophysiol* 1980; 47:8.

48. Taylor MJ, Menzies R, MacMillan LJ, Whyte HE: VEPs in normal full-term and premature neonates: Longitudinal versus cross-sectional data. *Electroencephalogr Clin Neurophysiol* 1987; 68:20–27.

49. Van Balen A, Henkes HE: Recording of the occipital lobe response in man after light stimulation. *Br J Ophthalmol* 1960; 44:449–460.

50. Van Hasselt PA: A short latency visual evoked potential recorded from the human mastoid process and auricle. *Electroencephalogr Clin Neurophysiol* 1972; 33:517–519.

51. Van Hoff MW: Open eye and closed eye occipito-cortico response to photic stimulation of the retina. *Acta Physiol Pharmacol Neerl* 1960; 9:443–451.

52. Vaughan HG: The perceptual and physiologic significance of visual evoked responses recorded from the scalp in man. In Burian HM, Jacobsen JH (eds): *Clinical Electroretinography*. Oxford, England, Pergammon Press, Inc, 1966, pp 203–223.

53. Vaughan HG, Gross CG: Cortical responses to light in unanes-thetized monkeys and their alteration by visual system lesions. *Exp Brain Res* 1969; 8:19–36.

54. Vaughan HG, Katzman R: Evoked response in visual disorders. *Ann NY Acad Sci* 1964; 112:305–319.

II ANATOMY OF THE RETINA, PRINCIPLES OF CELL BIOLOGY IN THE VISUAL PATHWAYS: FUNCTIONAL, PHYSIOLOGICAL, BIOCHEMICAL, MOLECULAR, BIOLOGICAL

4 The Photoreceptor–Retinal Pigmented Epithelium Interface

GREGORY S. HAGEMAN AND LINCOLN V. JOHNSON

THIS CHAPTER DEALS with the interface between the photosensitive outer segments of photoreceptor cells and the retinal pigmented epithelium (RPE). At this interface, photoreceptor cells and cells of the RPE, both highly polarized, abut one another. The photoreceptor cells are responsible for converting light into electrical signals through the process of transduction, a subject beyond the scope of this chapter; however, there are a number of excellent reviews that provide detailed descriptions of the process.[59,110,116] Photoreceptor cell outer segments, which contain the photosensitive visual pigments, are continually renewed through the addition of new membrane basally and intermittent (daily) shedding of old membrane from their apical tips. Shed outer segment membrane is ingested by the simple, cuboidal RPE cells, which are located directly adjacent to the photoreceptors and separate them from the choroidal vasculature. Interspersed between these two retinal layers is the interphotoreceptor matrix, a unique extracellular matrix that fills the "subretinal" space (figures 4.1 and 4.3). The matrix is composed of molecules that appear to play a role in mediating biochemical and physical interactions among the retina, RPE, and choroidal vasculature. Thus, the photoreceptor–RPE interface is an area of crucial importance to proper retinal function.

Embryological origins of the retina, retinal pigmented epithelium, and interphotoreceptor matrix

This section focuses primarily on human retinal development; references to other species are included where appropriate. A number of excellent reviews contain additional detail.[14,24,39,65,66,79,92,106,124,127,147] It should be noted that developmental stages of the human embryo have been defined on the basis of a variety of parameters including gestational time, crown–rump length, or heel length, and discrepancies in the time course of development are common in the literature. These discrepancies are complicated further by the fact that (1) the retina differentiates along a central-to-peripheral gradient, with an approximate 6-week lag,[71] (2) regional variations exist (e.g., the fovea), and (3) in some cases it is difficult to determine from which region of the developing retina published data have been derived.

DEVELOPMENT OF THE RETINA The optic primordium and optic sulcus are evident within the neural fold of the diencephalon at about 22 days of gestation. The retina develops subsequently as an evagination from this region at approximately 25 days (2.6 mm) of gestation. This out-pocketing enlarges to form the primary optic vesicle, which remains attached to the diencephalon by the optic stalk. At this stage, the cavity of the optic vesicle (future subretinal space) remains in communication with the ventricle of the brain through the optic stalk. The neural epithelium of the optic vesicle is a columnar epithelium containing an abundance of mitotically active cells.

During the fourth week of gestation (4.5 mm), the optic vesicle invaginates upon itself, and this results in the formation of the optic cup, a structure consisting of two neuroectodermally derived epithelial cell layers with their ventricular surfaces directly apposed. The cavity of the optic vesicle is all but obliterated during this time and remains only as a potential space, termed the *subretinal* or *interphotoreceptor space*. Although the molecular events that lead to invagination are not fully understood, recent evidence suggests that calcium[63] and extracellular matrix components[146] may be involved.

Although both layers of the retina differentiate from a continuous neural epithelium, their subsequent differentiation at both the cellular and molecular levels is quite diverse. The outermost layer of this neuroepithelium remains a single cellular layer and becomes the RPE. The innermost layer, the presumptive neural retina, thickens rapidly and becomes stratified; by 4 weeks (4 to 4.5 mm) of gestation, the neural retina is approximately 0.1 mm thick and consists of eight to nine distinct rows of cells. Both epithelial layers extend peripherally to form the ciliary body epithelium and posterior aspect of the iris. During the invagination process, the choroidal fissure, through which blood vessels pass into the interior of the eye, is formed along the ventral portion of the optic stalk.

During cellular differentiation of the neural retina, undifferentiated neuroblasts, which make up the entire thickness of the retina from the ventricular to the vitreal surfaces, typically lose their attachment to the vitreal surface and migrate to the ventricular surface where mitosis occurs. Following cell division, daughter cells migrate toward the vitreal

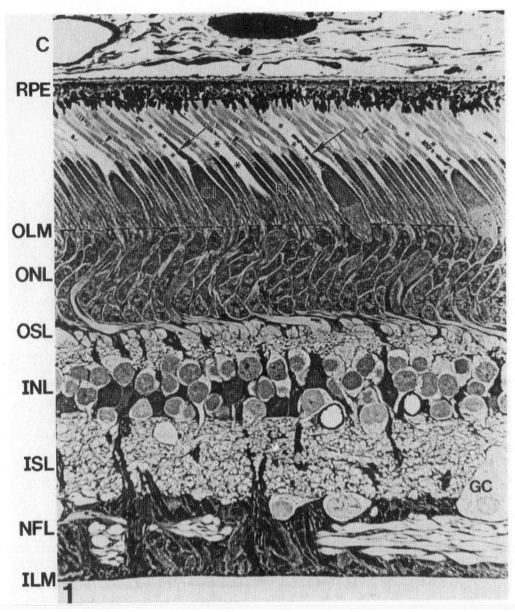

FIGURE 4.1 Light micrograph of a section of central retina from a monkey eye depicts the relationship between the choroid (C), retinal pigmented epithelium (RPE), interphotoreceptor matrix (asterisks), and neural retina. The neural retina is composed of a defined number of cell types arranged in a precise lamellar configuration. The apical surface of the neural retina contains highly polarized photoreceptor cells that abut the apical surface of the retinal pigmented epithelium. Interspersed between the apicies of these two retinal layers is the interphotoreceptor matrix (asterisks), a unique extracellular matrix that fills the subretinal space. Two types of photoreceptor cells can be identified morphologically. Cone photoreceptor inner segments (CI) are large in diameter, and the outer segments (arrows) are broader basally and tapered toward their apical tips. In contrast, rod photoreceptor inner (RI) and outer (arrowheads) segments retain a relatively uniform diameter that is smaller than that of cone photoreceptors (OLM = outer limiting membrane; ONL = outer nuclear layer (contains photoreceptor cell nuclei); OSL = outer synaptic layer; INL = inner nuclear layer [contains nuclei from Müller, amacrine, bipolar, and horizontal cells]; ISL = inner synaptic layer; GC = ganglion cell; NFL = nerve fiber layer; ILM = inner limiting membrane).

surface and ultimately reestablish connections with it. This process is repeated at each round of cell division, eventually resulting in the differentiation of a stratified neural epithelium. The glial or Müller cells can be distinguished at 4 weeks of gestation. By 5 weeks of gestation (5 to 7 mm) the nerve fiber layer is visible in the central retina (although this layer is lacking in the macula, even at birth[39]), as are ganglion cells.[114] The layer of Chievitz, a transient fiber layer that separates the retinoblast layer into two nucleated layers, also forms during the fifth week of gestation.[92,127]

By 7 to 8 weeks (20 to 23 mm) the inner neuroblast layer separates into two layers of nuclei that consist of potential ganglion cells (inner layer) and amacrine and Müller cells (outer layer). The ganglion cells give rise to nerve fibers that course toward the future optic nerve and form the nerve fiber layer. The inner limiting membrane also is clearly evident by this stage. During the ninth and tenth weeks of gestation (40 to 50 mm), photoreceptor, horizontal, and bipolar cells begin to differentiate within the outer neuroblast layer.[50,66,143] Horizontal and bipolar cells migrate into the layer of Chievitz and become separated from photoreceptor cells by the outer plexiform layer.[66] Amacrine and Müller cell bodies intermingle with those of horizontal and bipolar cells, and the transient layer of Chievitz is thereby obliterated; however, it persists in the macular region until birth. At this same time extensive junctional complexes, including gap junctions, macula adherens, zonula adherens, and zonula occludens, can be observed between cells of the neural retina and pigmented epithelium.[50,66] Between 12 and 15 weeks of gestation, cellular proliferation in the outer neuroblast layer ceases[127] except in the macular region.[104] The development of the macular region slows and begins to lag behind the development of the extramacular regions at this time. By 7 months of gestation, all layers except the macular region, which is not completely developed until 16 weeks postpartum, have assumed adult arrangement and proportion.

Development of photoreceptor cells

Photoreceptor cells are probably specified within the outer layers of the neural retina as early as 10 gestational weeks (40 to 50 mm),[149] but they are difficult to identify. By 12 weeks (83 mm) of gestation, however, cone photoreceptors are easily identified by their relatively large, slightly oval configuration, lightly stained or electron lucent cytoplasm, large juxtanuclear accumulation of smooth endoplasmic reticulum, and a single cilium.[66] Rod photoreceptors, which have distinct, dense nuclei, can be identified conclusively by 15 weeks (120 mm) of gestation.[66] At 18 weeks (156 mm) of gestation, a single layer of large, pale-staining cone photoreceptor cell bodies is visible in the outermost portion of the neural retina. The smaller rod photoreceptors comprise the remainder of the outer nuclear layer. Some synapses are established by cone photoreceptor pedicles by 12 weeks of gestation; however, synapses are not observed in association with rod photoreceptor cells until approximately 18 weeks of gestation. By 24 weeks, both types of photoreceptor cells are well polarized and have distinct inner segments that extend approximately 2 μm beyond the outer limiting membrane.[71] Rudimentary cone outer segments, which begin to develop at 16 weeks, are numerous and filled with whorls of tubular structures at this stage.[71] The majority of cone but not rod photoreceptor cell outer segments have stacks of disc membranes by 24 weeks of gestation. In contrast, rod photoreceptor cells contain a mixture of uniform and randomly oriented discs even at 28 weeks[71] and do not resemble adult outer segments until approximately 36 weeks.[149]

DEVELOPMENT OF THE FOVEA Although it has been recognized for some years that development of the human fovea lags behind that of the central retina, recent studies have provided detailed information regarding its development.[59,155] The fovea can be identified at approximately 22 weeks of gestation by the existence of a photoreceptor layer that contains only cones and by the presence of an unusually thick layer of ganglion cells. Following birth, the fovea continues to develop, a process that is characterized by deepening of the foveal depression, narrowing of the rod-free zone (foveola), and maturation and elongation of foveolar cone photoreceptor cells, including the differentiation of outer segments and development of basal axosomal processes that constitute Henle's fiber layer. The fovea is not fully differentiated until the third or fourth postnatal year (figure 4.2).

DEVELOPMENT OF THE RETINAL PIGMENTED EPITHELIUM At 5 to 6 weeks (15 to 20 mm) of gestation the presumptive retinal pigmented epithelium exists as a pseudostratified layer of columnar epithelial cells that have a dense cytoplasm, oval nuclei, and the first detectable pigment granules.[66] Mitoses are numerous and are located primarily in the farthest ventricular portion of this epithelium. By 7 weeks (20 mm) of gestation, basal and lateral infoldings of RPE cell plasma membrane and apical microvilli can be observed.[100] In addition, distinct "terminal bars" consisting of zonula occludens and zonula adherens, are evident.[100] By 8 weeks (27 to 31 mm) of gestation the RPE is established as a simple cuboidal epithelium. A close apposition between RPE and neural retinal cells is attained following invagination of the optic vesicle. Intercellular junctions, including both gap junctions and zonula adherens junctions, are present between these two cell layers at this time.[50]

DEVELOPMENT OF THE INTERPHOTORECEPTOR SPACE The interphotoreceptor space is the extracellular matrix-filled

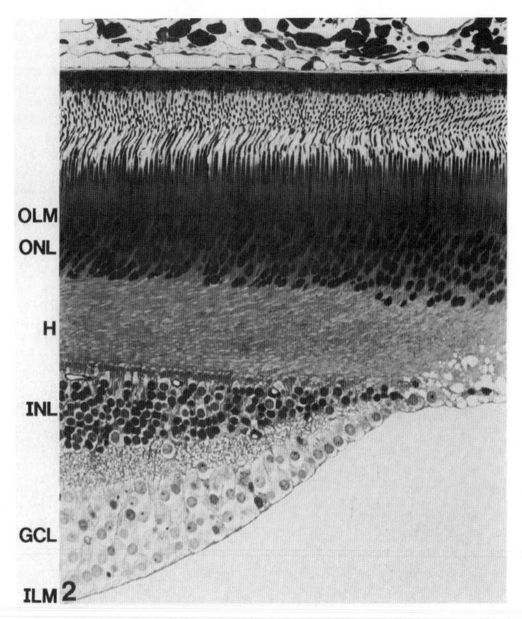

OLM
ONL
H
INL
GCL
ILM 2

FIGURE 4.2 Light micrograph of a section of a fovea of a monkey retina. In contrast to other regions of the neural retina, inner and outer segments of foveal cones are of a narrower diameter and appear more rodlike (compared with cones in figure 4.1). In the central fovea, only cone photoreceptor cell bodies are present within the outer nuclear layer (ONL). Henle's layer (H) consists of cone photoreceptor cell axons (OLM = outer limiting membrane; INL = inner nuclear layer; GCL = ganglion cell layer; ILM = inner limiting membrane).

remnant of the central cavity of the embryonic optic vesicle. It is within this interphotoreceptor space that important interactions between RPE cells and photoreceptor cells of the neural retina take place. Little information exists in humans pertaining to the development of the interphotoreceptor space or its contents, collectively referred to as the interphotoreceptor matrix. A.T. Johnson and coworkers,[71] however, have demonstrated that interstitial retinol-binding protein, a major component of the adult interphotoreceptor matrix, is first detectable in human retinas at approximately 20 weeks of gestation, a time that corresponds to photore-

ceptor cell outer segment differentiation. Between 15 and 18 weeks of gestation, intercellular junctions that form between RPE and neural retinal cells earlier in development gradually disappear, and an obvious interphotoreceptor space filled with a detectable flocculent material is visible at the tips of photoreceptor cell inner segments. By 24 weeks, the interphotoreceptor space widens, and distinct domains of flocculent interphotoreceptor matrix that are termed *cone matrix sheaths* are selectively associated with cone photoreceptor cell inner and outer segments. Chondroitin 6-sulfate, a major component of cone matrix sheaths,[55] is first present between

17 and 18 weeks of gestation and is solely associated with cone outer segments. Peanut agglutinin (PNA)–binding glycoconjugates, additional major structural components of cone matrix sheaths,[54,55,72,73] are present within the interphotoreceptor space at the time of its earliest formation. By 17 to 18 weeks of gestation, the interphotoreceptor matrix, which contains, peanut agglutinin–binding constituents, is visible as concentrated accumulations that is primarily associated with cone photoreceptor cells. It should be pointed out that the expression of these two major cone matrix sheath–associated constituents occurs at the time when rudimentary, outer segments first differentiate, approximately 10 weeks prior to the appearance of definitive photoreceptor disc membranes. Possibly cone matrix sheath–associated constituents may be necessary for the subsequent differentiation and survival of photoreceptor cell outer segments.

Retina–retinal pigmented epithelium–interphotoreceptor matrix: Morphology, composition, and function

As detailed above (see the previous section) the neural retina develops as a stratified epithelium, one basal surface bordering the vitreous cavity and the other apical surface in close association with the RPE. The cellular composition and organization of a mature retina is described in Chapter 5. Of most interest to this chapter is the scleral surface of the neural retina (figures 4.1 to 4.3). Microvillous extensions of Müller cells form junctional complexes with adjacent photoreceptor inner segments (known as the outer limiting membrane [see figure 4.3]) to seal the interphotoreceptor space lying between the neural retina and the RPE. The interphotoreceptor space is filled by a specialized extracellular matrix termed the interphotoreceptor matrix (figures 4.1 and 4.3). The apical surfaces of retinal pigmented epithelial cells contain numerous microvilli and are specialized for the phagocytosis of shed packets of photoreceptor outer segment membranes, one of a number of RPE cell activities that contribute to photoreceptor cell function.

RPE CELL CYTOLOGY AND FUNCTION The RPE has roles important to the maintenance of retinal, especially photoreceptor, cell function and homeostasis.[32]

The polygonal cells of the RPE form a simple (one cell layer thick) cuboidal epithelium with their basal surfaces attached to a basement membrane, which is part of a collagen-rich layer of extracellular matrix known as Bruch's membrane. Bruch's membrane separates the retinal pigmented epithelium from its primary vascular supply, the choroidal capillaries, which are the major source of nutrients for the outer retina; numerous basal infoldings of retinal pigmented epithelial cell plasma membranes facilitate nutrient and waste product exchange. The best characterized of the transport functions is retinol, which complexes with

opsin in photoreceptor cell outer segments and is absolutely necessary in the process of phototransduction. The RPE mediates the transport of retinol from the choroidal vasculature to the interphotoreceptor space by utilizing a number of retinoid-binding proteins as carriers.[17,18]

Laterally, RPE cell membranes are joined by intermediate (adhering) junctions, and between adjacent cells continuous bands of tight junctions prevent paracellular flow of large molecules to and from the subretinal space, thus contributing to the blood–retinal barrier (tightly sealed retinal vasculature also contributes significantly to this barrier).

Apically, RPE cells have numerous microvilli that project into the interphotoreceptor space and are closely associated with photoreceptor cell outer segments. This association facilitates another major function of the RPE cells, the phagocytosis and digestion of shed photoreceptor outer segment membrane produced by ongoing renewal of photoreceptor outer segments; phagosomes involved in the degradation of phagocytosed membrane are typical components of RPE cytoplasm. The dynamic relationship that exists between the RPE and photoreceptors during outer segment membrane turnover is well established.[20] The molecular mechanisms that regulate shedding and subsequent phagocytosis by the RPE have not been elucidated, although a receptor-mediated process involving both photoreceptors and retinal pigmented epithelium has been hypothesized.[15] Studies by McLaughlin and coworkers[95–97] have demonstrated a loss of certain lectin receptors in shed, unphagocytosed disc packets in the Royal College of Surgeons (RCS) rat (an animal that has a defect in the ability of the RPE to ingest shed disc), and this suggests that phagocytosis may involve a cell surface signal from the photoreceptor to the RPE. In other studies, RPE and outer segment membrane–associated molecules have been identified and are being characterized as potential participants in receptor-mediated recognition and/or phagocytosis. The sequence of morphological events that occurs during shedding and ingestion of outer segments has been thoroughly investigated in monkey and human retinas by transmission electron microscopy.[64,129,130,151] Cone photoreceptors are also known to shed their discs in a diurnal rhythm, the majority shedding their membranes at night, although species variations have been reported.

The apical surface membranes of RPE cells are also rich in Na+-K+ adenosine triphosphatase (ATPase) molecules that mediate ion fluxes and influence the transport of other molecules into and out of the subretinal space.[107] Abundant cytoplasmic pigment (melanin) granules are also present in retinal pigmented epithelial cells; these are also important to retinal function and serve to absorb scattered light.

Additionally, RPE cells are known to synthesize and secrete a number of proteins, glycoproteins, and proteoglycans that

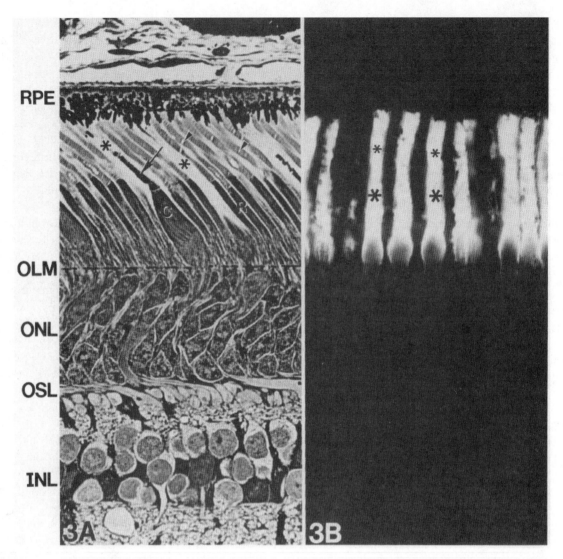

FIGURE 4.3 Light micrograph of a region of the section depicted in Figure 4.1 (left) and a fluorescence light micrograph (right) of a section of monkey retina that shows the distribution of peanut agglutinin–binding molecules in monkey retina. Peanut agglutinin–binding molecules in monkey and human retinas are specifically localized to domains of cone photoreceptor cell–associated interphotoreceptor matrix that have been termed cone matrix sheaths (asterisks). Chondroitin 6-sulfate containing proteoglycan and peanut agglutinin–binding glycoconjugates are major constituents of cone matrix sheaths (C = cone photoreceptor cell; R = rod photoreceptor cell; arrow, cone outer segment; arrowhead, rod outer segment; RPE = retinal pigmented epithelium; OLM = outer limiting membrane; ONL = outer nuclear layer; OSL = outer synaptic layer; INL = inner nuclear layer).

are part of the interphotoreceptor matrix.[4,5,14,41,131] The extent to which any of these interphotoreceptor matrix components are important to structural or functional interactions between retinal photoreceptors and the RPE is largely unknown. However, several recent studies suggest that as yet undefined factors secreted by RPE cells may be important in influencing retinal differentiation.[91,128,137] Additionally, it has been suggested that proteoglycans in the interphotoreceptor matrix, at least some of which are likely to be products of the RPE, may be important in retina–RPE adhesion.[56,58]

PHOTORECEPTOR CELL CYTOLOGY AND FUNCTION The highly polarized photoreceptor cells form the outermost layer of the neural retina (see figure 4.3A). Their cell bodies form the outer nuclear layer; their axonal processes extend basally to synapse with bipolar and horizontal cells in the outer synaptic layer. The scleral portions of photoreceptor cells, or outer segments (see figure 4.3A), are modified ciliary structures formed by elaborations of plasma membrane containing high concentrations of photosensitive, integral membrane molecules. The most abundant protein of rod outer segment disc membranes is the rod photopigment rhodopsin, a glycoprotein with a molecular weight of approximately 42 kilodaltons (kD) that is present with a packing density of approximately 30,000 molecules per μm^2. The carboxy terminus of rhodopsin is located in the interdiscal space, whereas the amino terminus projects into the intradiscal space. Another recently discovered outer segment membrane glycoprotein is the "rim" protein,[121] which has a molecular weight of 240 to 290 kD and is located along the edges of outer segment discs and incisures. Other proteins that have been identified in association with outer segment membranes include peripherin (33-kD dimer), glyceraldehyde-3-P-dehydrogenase (38 kD), a cyclic guanosine monophosphate gated channel protein (63 kD), and a spectrinlike protein (240 kD) (Molday, unpublished observations). Other molecular constituents located within photoreceptor outer segments participate in phototransduction. The adjacent inner segments, which contain mitochondria and the metabolic synthetic machinery responsible for the biosynthesis and transport of molecules for both the outer segment and axonal portions of the cell, extend into the interphotoreceptor space and are surrounded by the interphotoreceptor matrix. The photoreceptor inner segment membrances form junctional complexes with the surrounding glial elements of the retina, the Müller cells. These junctional complexes establish what has been termed the *outer limiting membrane* (see figure 4.1), a region thought to act as a molecular sieve[28] to partially seal the interphotoreceptor space from the neural retina.

Two types of photoreceptor cells, rods and cones, can be identified cytologically (see figures 4.1 and 4.3A). Subclasses of cone photoreceptors have been identified, each possessing different spectral sensitivities, and corresponding differences in the molecular nature of the photosensitive pigments concentrated in their outer segments.[102] The outer segments of rods and cones differ structurally; rod photoreceptor outer segments retain a relatively uniform diameter from apex to base, while cone photoreceptor outer segments are broader basally and taper toward their tips. In both cases, photoreceptor outer segments are formed by extensive folding of the photoreceptor cell membrane; in rods these "disc membranes" are pinched off and enclosed by the cell membrane.[20] In contrast to the case for rods, however, the structural relationship between vertebrate cone photoreceptor outer segment disc membranes and their enveloping plasma membrane remains uncertain, especially in primates. Conventional ultrastructural studies of nonmammalian species suggest that the majority of cone disc membranes remain continuous with the plasma membrane, and thus the intradiscal spaces are open to the interphotoreceptor space.[33,34,40,105,125] It has generally been assumed that most if not all of the discs in mammalian cones are also continuous with the plasma membrane, but many of the connections appear to be extremely small.[9,10,20,21,29] In several species, open intradiscal spaces are more easily visualized in the proximal than in the distal portions of cone outer segments.[33] Recent ultrastructural studies of monkey and human cone photoreceptors have identified novel regions of outer segments, termed *cone notches*, that demarcate a site of abrupt transition between cone photoreceptor discs that are open to the interphotoreceptor space and those that appear isolated. These results suggest that at least at some levels the gross organization of primate cone photoreceptor cell outer segment membranes may be more similar to that of rod photoreceptor cells. A number of investigators have shown that the fluorochrome Procion yellow selectively associates with cone outer segments in a variety of species, including primates.[36,37,82,83] These investigators have suggested that this staining may represent dye infiltration into open cone discs, although cone-specific binding of Procion yellow may be a result of preferential insult to cone membranes rather than a result of penetration into patent cone discs.

There also appear to be differences in the mechanism of membrane renewal in the outer segments of rod and cone photoreceptor cells. Rod cell outer segment discs are added basally and migrate as intact units toward the apical tip of the outer segment, where they are ultimately shed. This continuing assembly at the proximal end of the photoreceptor outer segment is balanced by continuing shedding of the distal tip of the outer segment such that the overall length of the outer segment remains constant. In contrast, cone photoreceptor cell outer segments renew more randomly and show no selective incorporation of amino acids into the basal region of the photoreceptor cell outer segment.[153,154] For both photoreceptor cell types, however, RPE cells appear to be responsible for the phagocytosis of shed outer segment membrane and clearance of the interphotoreceptor space. Cone photoreceptor cell inner segments are generally larger than those of rod photoreceptor cells and are densely packed with mitochondria. Cone photoreceptor cell bodies typically occupy the outermost layer (nearest the sclera) of the outer nuclear layer, with the remainder of the outer nuclear layer being composed of rod cell bodies.

Although rod and cone photoreceptor cells exhibit differences in their overall structure, function, and susceptibility to degeneration in various diseases, relatively little is known concerning the biochemical bases for these differences, especially with respect to cones. Our lack of knowledge pertaining to the molecular composition of cone photoreceptors is probably due to an inability to isolate these cells since they represent only a small percentage of the total population of photoreceptors in most species and since, until recently, few cone photoreceptor cell–specific probes have been available to aid investigators in this purification.

Significant new knowledge about the biochemical and morphological uniqueness of cone photoreceptor cells and their surrounding environment is emerging. For example, new information on compositional differences between rod and cone photoreceptor cells, including differences in the α-subunit of transducin,[53,89] cyclic guanosine monophosphate phosphodiesterase,[70] neurotransmitters and amino acid metabolism,[23,42,81,121] cytochrome oxidase activity, vitamin D–dependent calcium-binding protein,[122,144] disc rim protein,[108,109] bovine serum albumin–binding molecules, and carbonic anhydrase, have been documented. In addition, cone photoreceptors have been shown to accumulate selectively various sugars, including fucose by goldfish cone photoreceptor cells,[25,26] galactose by bovine cone photoreceptor cells,[77] and 2-deoxyglucose by dark-adapted primate cone photoreceptor cells.[126] Additional differences in the molecular composition of cone photoreceptor cells have been elucidated by monoclonal antibodies. Lemmon[88] and Szél and coworkers[133–136] have generated monoclonal antibodies that specifically label cone outer segments in a variety of species, and Bunt-Milam and coworkers have generated an antibody that binds to the outer segments of certain subclasses of cone photoreceptor cells in a number of species. Similarly, we have generated a monoclonal antibody that selectively labels cone but not rod photoreceptor cell plasma and disc membranes in pig, monkey, and human retinas. These probes should provide powerful tools with which to continue to establish the molecular bases for differences between rod and cone photoreceptor cells. More recently, molecular biological techniques have begun to provide some insights into compositional differences between rod and cone photoreceptor cells.[80,94,102,103,113,141]

MÜLLER CELL CYTOLOGY AND FUNCTION Müller cells are the primary glial elements of the retina. Unlike neurons of the retina, Müller cells span almost the entire width of the retina and extend radially from the inner limiting membrane at the vitreal surface to just beyond the level of the outer limiting membrane where they form junctional complexes with adjacent photoreceptor cells; their nuclei are located within the inner nuclear layer. The scleral surfaces of Müller cells border the interphotoreceptor space and extend numerous microvillous processes into it. Specific membrane-associated transport systems sequestered in these apical cell membranes are likely to be involved in controlling to some extent the composition of the interphotoreceptor matrix.[116] Müller cells may also participate in retinal carbohydrate metabolism by serving as a source of stored nutrients in the form of glycogen,[104] in the degradation of neurotransmitter levels,[120] and in the regulation of extracellular glutamine levels.[115] Maintenance of appropriate potassium levels in the retina by the active pumping of potassium ions into the vitreous also appears to be a major Müller cell function.[104]

INTERPHOTORECEPTOR MATRIX STRUCTURE AND FUNCTION As described above (see the section on embryological origins), the interphotoreceptor matrix is likely to play a major role in maintaining retinal function by mediating biochemical interactions between the retina, RPE, and choroidal vasculature. Ultrastructural studies of the inter-

photoreceptor matrix have confirmed the presence of amorphous extracellular substance within the interphotoreceptor space in a variety of species, including monkeys and humans.[48,117] Thick cuffs of amorphous material are observed to encapsulate most cone photoreceptor cell outer segments, in contrast to the finely granular material interspersed between adjacent rod photoreceptors.[48,72]

Early investigations identified the presence of anionic, carbohydrate-containing molecules in the interphotoreceptor matrix of a variety of species including monkeys and humans.[45–47,49,56,74,84,90,117,123,143,156] The observed susceptibility of some of these interphotoreceptor matrix components to specific enzyme treatments indicated that both glycoproteins and glycosaminoglycans are constituents. More recent studies employing lectin histochemistry have provided substantial additional information as to the nature of carbohydrate-containing molecules within the interphotoreceptor matrix.[16,54,73,76,78,97,118,138–140,148] One of the most striking contributions of these lectin-based studies has been the identification of microdomains of interphotoreceptor matrix glycoconjugates. These studies have demonstrated that interphotoreceptor matrix components are heterogeneously distributed and that the heterogeneities fall into two basic patterns, those showing apical-basal differences and those showing photoreceptor cell type–specific differences in composition. Wheat germ agglutinin–binding glycoconjugates in monkeys and humans are present within the interphotoreceptor matrix surrounding rod photoreceptors and are virtually absent in the interphotoreceptor matrix surrounding cone photoreceptor cells.[56,118] Additional evidence for compartmentalization of some molecules contained in the interphotoreceptor matrix has been provided by investigations of the distribution of PNA-binding molecules. PNA-binding molecules in monkey and human retinas are specifically localized to domains of cone photoreceptor cell–associated interphotoreceptor matrix. The existence of cone matrix sheaths in human retinas has been confirmed by histochemical staining with a cationic copper phthalocyanin dye, cuprolinic blue.[54,68,72,73,76,143]

The majority of studies directed toward biochemical characterization of the interphotoreceptor matrix have concentrated on its soluble rather than insoluble components.[14,61,62] Recently, however, investigations have focused on characterizing the aqueous, insoluble components of the interphotoreceptor matrix (figure 4.4). In higher vertebrate species, including monkeys and humans, these components appear to constitute a significant portion of the interphotoreceptor matrix as compared with soluble constituents.

The soluble fraction of the interphotoreceptor matrix from bovine eyes consists predominantly of protein and glycoprotein (98%) with some glycosaminoglycan (2%). The most prominent proteins identified by sodium dodecyl sulfate–polyacrylamide gel electrophoresis include bands of

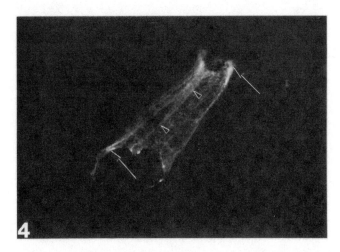

FIGURE 4.4 Fluorescence light micrograph depicting an isolated cone matrix sheath exposed to fluorescein-conjugated PNA. Cone matrix sheaths examined in this manner show a distinct substructure with numerous longitudinally orientated fibers extending the entire length of the sheath *(arrowheads)*. These longitudinal structures appear to be interconnected by a finer anastomosing fibrous network. In addition, longitudinal fibers appear to insert into distinct fibrous rings of similar dimension at both the proximal and distal ends of the sheath *(arrows)*.

47 kD and 140 kD.[4,5] Similar proteins have been identified in the interphotoreceptor matrix of human retinas.[1] The major soluble glycoprotein (140 kD) of the interphotoreceptor matrix is an interstitial retinol-binding protein.[27,30,110] In addition, a number of other soluble interphotoreceptor matrix proteins and glycoproteins have been identified; these include mucinlike glycoproteins,[2] a variety of enzymes,[3] a cyclic guanosine monophosphate–phosphodiesterase,[11] soluble antigen,[145] trophic factors (Adler and Hewitt, unpublished data), and a variety of serum-containing proteins, including immunoglobulins and albumin.[6,56] In addition, small–molecular weight, soluble glycosaminoglycans have been identified. These may be degradation products of larger interphotoreceptor proteoglycans.

More recent biochemical and immunocytochemical studies have confirmed that a large proportion of the interphotoreceptor matrix is composed of aqueous-insoluble glycoconjugates. These include proteoglycans which contain chondroitin 4-sulfate and chondroitin 6-sulfate.[55,111] Chondroitin 4-sulfate is distributed uniformly throughout the matrix, whereas chondroitin 6-sulfate proteoglycan is asociated specifically with cone matrix sheaths,[55] and may be a component of a larger proteoglycan intercalated within the cone photoreceptor cell plasma membrane. Based on high-performance liquid-size exclusion chromatography, the major constituent of cone matrix sheaths is resolved as a peak approximately 800 kD, which suggests that cone matrix sheaths are composed of extremely high molecule weight proteoglycans or proteoglycan aggregates. In addition to chondroitin 6-sulfate glycosaminoglycan, cone matrix sheath proteoglycans contain a significant quantity of O-linked oligosaccharides that bind PNA.

Relatively little is known about the function of most of the interphotoreceptor matrix constituents. Perhaps the only interphotoreceptor matrix molecules that have been characterized with respect to function are interstitial retinol-binding proteins and vitamin A. Preliminary studies in a number of laboratories[67,79,128,167,168] suggest that cone matrix sheath–associated constituents may indeed participate in retinal adhesion, since cone matrix sheaths retain their cellular attachments and become extremely elongated in experiments in which the retina is gently peeled from the pigmented epithelium immediately following enucleation. Intravitreal injection of xylosides (compounds that disrupt proteoglycan synthesis) results in cone matrix sheath disruption and localized retinal detachments.[87] Intravitreal or subretinal injections of chondroitinase or neuraminidase reduce adhesion by as much as 80% without affecting retinal function or histology.

It appears that rod photoreceptor cells are the primary cells involved in the synthesis of interstitial retinol-binding protein and its subsequent secretion into the interphotoreceptor matrix.[51,52,67,116] It has also been demonstrated that a number of interphotoreceptor matrix–containing constituents originate from the systemic vasculature and are transported into the interphotoreceptor space by the retinal pigmented epithelium.[61]

Pathologies affecting the RPE–photoreceptor–interphotoreceptor matrix complex

Pathologies affecting the RPE-photoreceptor-interphotoreceptor matrix interface have been reported in association with human disease and animal models. Such pathologies may be the direct result of abnormalities in either RPE or photoreceptor cells. Because of their close structural and functional relationships (see the previous section on structure and function of the interface), an abnormality in one of these cell types might be expected to influence the viability of the other. It can be speculated that this phenomenon would most often involve a primary abnormality in retinal pigmented epithelial cells that secondarily affects photoreceptor cells because of the numerous functions crucial to photoreceptor homeostasis that are performed by retinal pigmented epithelial cells. Such is the case for the RCS rat (see a later section), which exhibits a retinal pigmented epithelium–based pathology that indirectly results in photoreceptor cell death. Conversely, in a number of mutant mouse strains (see the later section on retinal-degenerative mice) the primary abnormalities are in photoreceptor cells themselves.

Our understanding of abnormalities affecting the RPE–photoreceptor interface comes largely from studies of animals, while less is known concerning the cellular bases of human retinal pathologies. Since a number of comprehensive reviews pertaining to animals exhibiting retinal degeneration have been published,[31] only a few specific examples are described below.

RPE-Based Pathologies

RCS rat The best characterized of retinal pigmented epithelium–based pathologies is that exhibited by the RCS rat.[19,22,38,98] This mutant strain of rat has a defect that affects the ability of retinal pigmented epithelial cells to phagocytose shed photoreceptor cell outer segment membrane. Photoreceptor cells develop apparently normally until about 18 days postnatally, but degenerate thereafter. As a result, the interphotoreceptor (subretinal) space becomes filled with membranous debris.[60,98] The recognition and binding of photoreceptor cell outer segments at the apical surfaces of RCS retinal pigmented epithelial cells may be normal, the defect specifically affecting phagocytosis. It has recently been shown[42a] that rod death can be prevented by various "sham operations" on the retina and especially by subretinal or intraretinal injection of basal fibroblast growth factor (bFGF). This is a constituent of the normal interphotoreceptor matrix (personal observations) and therefore the lack of specific trophic factors, derived from RPE, leads to the death of rods in the RCS rat.

Mucopolysaccharidosis VI Feline mucopolysaccharidosis VI (MPS VI) is an inherited disease affecting the lysosomal enzyme arylsulfatase B. Animals with this enzymatic defect exhibit large intracellular accumulations of dermatan sulfate owing to their inability to degrade this glycosaminoglycan.[58] This abnormality is systemically widespread but especially notable in cells of the retinal pigmented epithelium, which because of their highly phagocytic nature accumulate numerous membrane-bound inclusions containing poorly degraded glycosaminoglycans.[8] These inclusions are present at the time of birth of affected animals, increase in size and number with time, and ultimately result in massive hypertrophy of the retinal pigmented epithelium. This hypertrophy disrupts the normal orientation of adjacent photoreceptor outer segments but apparently does not result in photoreceptor cell death.[8] Retinal pigmented epithelial cells from cats with MPS VI thus appear to be capable of continued phagocytosis of shed photoreceptor cell outer segment membrane and physiological support of photoreceptor cells in spite of the fact that they have an important enzymatic defect and are severely hypertrophied.

Photoreceptor Cell–Based Pathologies

Retinal-degenerative mice A number of mutant mouse strains exhibiting inherited photoreceptor cell degeneration have been described. The best characterized of these are the *rd* (retinal degeneration[85,86]), *rds* (retinal degeneration slow[119,142]), and *pcd* (Purkinje cell degeneration[84,99]). Each of these mutants exhibits degeneration and death of photoreceptor cells, but with differing time courses. For example, almost all photoreceptor cells degenerate in homozygous *rd* mice by 2 months postnatally, while some viable photoreceptors remain in *rds* and *pcd* retinas as late as 1 year postnatally. In each of these mutants, the defect appears to be expressed in photoreceptor cells and leads directly to their death and degeneration. Specific biochemical defects have not been identified for any of these mutants; however, the *rd* strain develops abnormally high accumulations of cyclic guanosine monophosphate,[44] the result of an abnormality in the α subunit of the specific rod. Phosphodiesterase, which hydrolyses cyclic guanosine monophosphate in the matrix is greatly altered, but there are no known secondary changes in the RPE.[43,44]

Progressive rod-cone degeneration Miniature poodles exhibit an inherited disease, termed progressive rod-cone degeneration, that directly affects both rod and cone photoreceptor cells. This is a late-onset disease occurring after photoreceptor cells have fully differentiated in apparently normal fashion.[7] Later, individual rod outer segments become disordered, and die. Similar changes occur in cone outer segments, but slightly later than in rods. Ultimately, photoreceptor cell outer segments are completely lost, and degeneration of photoreceptor cell inner segments and cell bodies occurs. Late in the disease process, cells of the retinal pigmented epithelium are observed to become hypertrophied and may invade the remaining neural retina.

ACKNOWLEDGMENTS Portions of the research described herein were supported by grants from the National Eye Institute to G.S.H. (EY06463) and to L.V.J. (EY04741); by an unrestricted grant from Research to Prevent Blindness, Inc. (to the Bethesda Eye Institute); and by the Bethesda Eye Institute Resident Research Fund.

REFERENCES

1. Adler AJ, Evans CD: Some functional characteristics of purified bovine interphotoreceptor retinol-binding protein. *Invest Ophthalmol Vis Sci* 1985; 26:273–282.
2. Adler AJ, Klucznik KM: Proteins and glycoproteins of the bovine interphotoreceptor matrix: Composition and fractionation. *Exp Eye Res* 1982; 34:423–434.
3. Adler AJ, Martin KJ: Retinol-binding in bovine interphotoreceptor matrix. *Biochem Biophys Res Commun* 1983; 108: 1601–1608.
4. Adler AJ, Severin KM: Proteins of the bovine interphotoreceptor matrix. *Doc Ophthalmol Proc Ser* 1981; 25:25–40.
5. Adler AJ, Severin KM: Proteins of the bovine interphotoreceptor matrix: Tissues of origin. *Exp Eye Res* 1981; 32:755–769.

6. Adler AJ, Spenser SA, Heth CA, Schmidt SY: Comparison of protein in the interphotoreceptor matrix vertebrates. *Ophthalmol Res* 1988; 20:275–285.

7. Aguirre G, Alligood J, O'Brien P, Buyukmichi N: Pathogenesis of progressive rod-cone degeneration in miniature poodles. *Invest Ophthalmol Vis Sci* 1982; 23:610–630.

8. Aguirre G, Stramm L, Haskins M: Feline mucopolysaccharidosis VI: General ocular and pigment epithelial pathology. *Invest Ophthalmol Vis Sci* 1983; 24:991–1007.

9. Anderson DH, Fisher SK: The photoreceptors of diurnal squirrels: Outer segment structure, disc shedding and protein renewal. *J Ultrastruct Res* 1976; 55:119–141.

10. Anderson DH, Fisher SK, Steinberg RH: Mammalian cones: Disc shedding, phagocytosis, renewal. *Invest Ophthalmol Vis Sci* 1978; 17:117–133.

11. Barbehenn EK, Wiggert B, Lee L, Kapoor CL, Zonnenberg BA, Redmond TM, Passonneau JV, Chader GJ: Extracellular cGMP phosphodiesterase related to the rod outer segment phosphodiesterase isolated from bovine and monkey retinas. *Biochemistry* 1985; 24:1309–1316.

12. Barnstable CJ: A molecular view of vertebrate retinal development. *Mol Neurobiol* 1987; 1:9–45.

13. Bazan NG, Reddy TS, Redmond TM, Wiggert B, Chader GJ: Endogenous fatty acids are covalently and non-covalently bound to interphotoreceptor retinoid-binding protein in the monkey retina. *J Biol Chem* 1985; 260:13677–13680.

14. Berman ER: An overview of the biochemistry of the interphotoreceptor matrix, in Bridges CD, Adler AJ (eds): *The Interphotoreceptor Matrix in Health and Disease.* New York, Alan R. Liss, Inc, 1985, pp 47–64.

15. Besharse JC: The daily light-dark cycle and rhythmic metabolism in the photoreceptor–pigment epithelial complex. *Prog Retinal Res* 1982; 1:81–124.

16. Blanks JC, Johnson LV: Selective lectin binding of the developing mouse retina. *J Comp Neurol* 1983; 221:31–41.

17. Bok D: Retinal photoreceptor–pigment epithelium interactions. *Invest Ophthalmol Vis Sci* 1985; 26:1659–1694.

18. Bok D: Structure and function of the retina; pigment epithelium–photoreceptor complex, in Tso MOM (ed): *Retinal Diseases.* Philadelphia, JB Lippincott, 1988, pp 3–48.

19. Bok D, Hall MO: The role of the pigment epithelium in the etiology of inherited retinal dystrophy in the rat. *J Cell Biol* 1971; 49:664–682.

20. Borwein B: The retinal receptor: A description. In Enoch JM, Tobey FL (eds): *Vertebrate Photoreceptor Optics.* Springer Series in Optical Sciences, vol 23. Berlin, Springer-Verlag, 1981, pp 11–81.

21. Borwein B, Borwein D, Medeiros J, McGowan JW: The ultrastructure of monkey foveal photoreceptors, with special reference to the structure, shape, size, and spacing of the foveal cones. *Am J Anat* 1980; 159:125–146.

22. Bourne MC, Campbell DA, Tansley K: Hereditary degeneration of the rat retina. *Br J Ophthalmol* 1938; 22:613–623.

23. Brandon C, Lam DMK: L-Glutamic acid: A neurotransmitter candidate for cone photoreceptors in human and rat retinas. *Proc Natl Acad Sci USA* 1983; 80:5117–5121.

24. Breathnach AS, Wyllie LMA: Ultrastructure of the retinal pigment epithelium of the human fetus. *J Ultrastruct Res* 1966; 16:584–597.

25. Bunt AH, Klock IB: Fine structure and radioautography of retinal cone outer segments in goldfish and carp. *Invest Ophthalmol Vis Sci* 1980; 19:707–719.

26. Bunt AH, Saari JC: Fucosylated protein of retinal cone photoreceptor outer segments: Morphological and biochemical analyses. *J Cell Biol* 1982; 92:269–276.

27. Bunt-Milam AH, Saari JC: Immunocytochemical localization of two retinoid-binding proteins in vertebrate retina. *J Cell Biol* 1983; 97:703–712.

28. Bunt-Milam AH, Saari JC, Klock IB, Garwin GG: Zonuliae adherentes pore size in the external limiting membrane of the rabbit retina. *Invest Ophthalmol Vis Sci* 1985; 26:1377–1380.

29. Carter-Dawson LD, LaVail ML: Rods and cones in the mouse retina. I. Structural analysis using light and electron microscopy. *J Comp Neurol* 1979; 188:245–262.

30. Chader GJ: Interphotoreceptor retinoid-binding protein (IRBP): A model protein for molecular biological and clinically relevant studies. *Invest Ophthalmol Vis Sci* 1989; 30:7–22.

31. Chader GJ, Aguirre GD, Sanyal S: Studies on animal models of retinal degenerations, in Tso MOM (ed): *Retinal Diseases,* Philadelphia, JB Lippincott, 1988, pp 80–99.

32. Clark VM: The cell biology of the retinal pigment epithelium. In Adler R, Farber D (eds): *The Retina: A Model for Cell Biology,* part II, Orlando, Fla, Academic Press, Inc, 1986, pp 129–168.

33. Cohen AI: Further studies on the question of the patency of saccules in outer segments of vertebrate photoreceptors. *Vision Res* 1970; 10:445–453.

34. Cohen AI: New evidence supporting the linkage to extracellular space of outer segment saccules of frog cones but not rods. *J Cell Biol* 1968; 37:424–444.

35. Cohen AI: Rods and cones, in Fuortes MGF (ed): *Handbook of Sensory Physiology,* vol 7, no 2. Berlin, Springer-Verlag, 1972, p 63.

36. de Monasterio FM, McCrane EP, Newlander JK, Schein SJ: Density profile of blue-sensitive cones along the horizontal meridian of macaque retina. *Invest Ophthalmol Vis Sci* 1985; 26:289–302.

37. de Monasterio FM, Schein SJ, McCrane EP: Staining of blue-sensitive cones of the macaque retina by a fluorescent dye. *Science* 1981; 213:1278–1281.

38. Dowling JE, Sidman RL: Inherited retinal dystrophy in the rat. *J Cell Biol* 1962; 14:73–109.

39. Duke-Elder S, Cook C: Normal and abnormal development: Embryology. In Duke-Elder S (ed), *System of Ophthalmology,* vol 3, part I. London, Kimpton 1963.

40. Eckmiller MS: Cone outer segment morphogenesis: Taper change and distal invaginations. *J Cell Biol* 1987; 105: 2267–2277.

41. Edwards RB: Glycosamininoglycan synthesis by cultured human retinal pigmented epithelium from normal postmortem donors and a postmortem donor with retinitis pigmentosa. *Invest Ophthalmol Vis Sci* 1982; 23:435–446.

42. Ehinger B: [^{3}H]-D-aspartate accumulation in the retina of the pigeon, guinea pig and rabbit. *Exp Eye Res* 1981; 33:381–391.

42a. Faktorovich EG, Steinberg RH, Yasumura D, Matthes MT, LaVail MM: Photoreceptor degeneration in inherited retinal dystrophy delayed by basic fibroblast growth factor. *Nature* 1990; 347:83–86.

43. Farber DB, Lolley RN: Cyclic guanosine monophosphate: Elevation in degenerating photoreceptor cells of the C3H mouse retina. *Science* 1974; 186:449–451.

44. Farber DB, Shuster TA: Cyclic nucleotides in retinal function and degeneration, in Adler R, Farber D (eds): *The Retina: A Model for Cell Biology Studies.* New York, Academic Press, Inc, 1986, pp 239–296.

45. Feeney L: Synthesis of interphotoreceptor matrix. I. Autoradiography of ³H-fucose incorporation. *Invest Ophthalmol Vis Sci* 1973; 12:739–751.

46. Feeney L: The interphotoreceptor space. I. Postnatal ontogeny in mice and rats. *Dev Biol* 1973; 32:101–114.

47. Feeney L: The interphotoreceptor space. II. Histochemistry of the matrix. *Dev Biol* 1973; 32:115–128.

48. Feeney-Burns L: The interphotoreceptor matrix in health and disease. *Prog Clin Biol Res* 1985; 190:3–21.

49. Fine BS, Zimmerman LE: Observations on the rod and cone layer of the human retina. *Invest Ophthalmol Vis Sci* 1963; 2:446–459.

50. Fisher SK, Linberg KA: Intercellular junctions in the early human embryonic retina. *J Ultrastruct Res* 1975; 51:69–78.

51. Fong SL, Liou GI, Landers RA, Alvarez RA, Bridges CD: Purification and characterization of a retinol-binding glycoprotein synthesized and secreted by bovine neural retina. *J Biol Chem* 1984; 259:6534–6542.

52. Fong SL, Liou GI, Landers RA, Alvarez RA, Gonzalez-Fernandez F, Glazebrook PA, Lam DM, Bridges CD: The characterization, localization and biosynthesis of an interstitial retinol-binding glycoprotein in the human eye. *J Neurochem* 1984; 42:1667–1676.

53. Grunwald GB, Gierschik P, Nirenberg M, Spiegel A: Detection of α-transducin in retinal rods but not cones. *Science* 1986; 231:856–859.

54. Hageman GS, Johnson LV: Biochemical characterization of the major peanut agglutinin-binding glycoproteins in vertebrate retinae: A species comparison. *J Comp Neurol* 1986; 249:499–510, color plate 482–483.

55. Hageman GS, Johnson LV: Chondroitin 6-sulfate glycosaminoglycan is a major constituent of primate cone photoreceptor matrix sheaths. *Curr Eye Res* 1987; 6:639–646.

56. Hageman GS, Johnson LV: Structure, composition and function of the retinal interphotoreceptor matrix. *Prog Retinal Res*, in press.

57. Hall MO, Abrams T: Kinetic studies of rod outer segment binding and ingestion by cultured rat RPE cells. *Exp Eye Res* 1987; 45:907–922.

58. Haskins ME, Aguirre GD, Jezyk PF, Patterson DF: The pathology of the feline model of mucopolysaccharidosis VI. *Am J Pathol* 1980; 101:657–674.

59. Hendrickson AE, Yuodelis C: The morphological development of the human fovea. *Ophthalmology* 1984; 91:603–612.

60. Herron WL Jr, Riegel BW, Myers OE, Rubin ML: Retinal dystrophy in the rat: A pigment epithelial disease. *Invest Ophthalmol* 1969; 8:595–604.

61. Hewitt AT: Extracellular matrix molecules: Their importance in the structure and function of the retina. In Farber D, Adler R (eds): *The Retina: A Model For Cell Biology Studies* part II. London, Academic Press, Inc, 1986, pp 170–201.

62. Hewitt AT, Adler R: The retinal pigment epithelium and interphotoreceptor matrix: Structure and specialized function. In Ogden TE (ed): *Retina*, vol 1. St Louis, CV Mosby Co, 1989, pp 57–64.

63. Hilfer SR, Brady RC, Wang JW: Intracellular and extracellular changes during early ocular development in the chick embryo. In Hilfer SR, Sheffield JB (eds): *Ocular Size and Shape: Regulation During Development*. New York, Springer-Verlag NY, Inc, 1981, pp 47–78.

64. Hogan MJ, Wood I: Phagocytosis by pigment epithelium of human retinal cones. *Nature* 1974; 254:305–307.

65. Hollenberg MJ, Spira AW: Early development of the human retina. *Can J Ophthalmol* 1972; 7:472–491.

66. Hollenberg MJ, Spira AW: Human retinal development: Ultrastructure of the outer retina. *Am J Anat* 1973; 137:357–386.

67. Hollyfield JG, Fliesler SJ, Rayborn ME, Fong SL, Landers RA, Bridges CD: Synthesis and secretion of interstitial retinol-binding protein by the human retina. *Invest Ophthalmol Vis Sci* 1985; 26:58–67.

68. Hollyfield JG, Varner HH, Rayborn ME, et al: Retinal attachment to the pigment epithelium. *Retina* 1989; 9:59–68.

69. Hurley JB: Molecular properties of the cGMP cascade of vertebrate photoreceptors. *Annu Rev Physiol* 1987; 49:793–812.

70. Hurwitz RL, Bunt-Milam AH, Chang ML, Beavo JA: cGMP phosphodiesterase in rod and cone outer segments of the retina. *J Biol Chem* 1985; 260:568–573.

71. Johnson AT, Kretzer FL, Hittner HM, Glazebrook PA, Bridges CDB, Lam DM: Development of the subretinal space in the preterm human eye: Ultrastructural and immunocytochemical studies. *J Comp Neurol* 1985; 233:497–505.

72. Johnson LV, Hageman GS, Blanks JC: Domains of interphotoreceptor matrix ensheath cone photoreceptors in vertebrate retinae. *Invest Ophthalmol Vis Sci* 1986; 27:129–135.

73. Johnson LV, Hageman GS, Blanks JC: Restricted extracellular matrix domains ensheath cone photoreceptors in vertebrate retina, in Bridges CDB, Adler AJ (eds): *The Interphotoreceptor Matrix in Health and Disease*. New York, Alan R. Liss, Inc, 1985, pp 36–46.

74. Johnson NE: Distribution of acid mucopolysaccharides in normal and detached retinae. *Trans Ophthalmol Soc UK* 1977; 47:557–564.

75. Kageyama GH, Wong-Riley MTT: The histochemical localization of cytochrome oxidase in the retina and lateral geniculate nucleus of the ferret, cat, and monkey, with particular reference to retinal mosaics and on/off-center visual channels. *J Neurosci* 1984; 4:2445–2459.

76. Kawano K, Uehara F, Sameshima M, Ohba N: Binding sites of peanut agglutinin in mammalian retina. *Jpn J Ophthalmol* 1984; 28:205–214.

77. Keegan WA, McKechnie NM, Converse CA, Foulds WS: D-S³H-galactose incorporation in the bovine retina: Specific uptake and transport of the radiolabel in cones. *Exp Eye Res* 1985; 40:619–628.

78. Koide H, Suganuma T, Murata F, Ohba N: Ultrastructural localization of lectin receptors in the monkey retinal photoreceptors and pigment epithelium: Application of lectin-gold complexes on thin sections. *Exp Eye Res* 1986; 43:343–354.

79. Kozart DM: Anatomic correlates of the retina, in Duane TD (ed): *Clinical Ophthalmology*, vol 3. Philadelphia, JB Lippincott, 1988, pp 1–18.

80. Kuo CH, Yamagata K, Moyziz RK, Bitensky MW: Multiple opsin mRNA species in bovine retina. *Mol Brain Res* 1986; 1:251–260.

81. Lam DMK, Hollyfield JG: Localization of putative amino acid neurotransmitters in the human retina. *Exp Eye Res* 1980; 31:729–732.

82. Laties AM, Bok D, Liebman P: Procion yellow: A marker dye for outer segment disc patency and for rod renewal. *Exp Eye Res* 1976; 23:139–148.

83. Laties AM, Liebman PA: Cones of living amphibia eye: Selective staining. *Science* 1970; 168:1475–1477.

84. LaVail MM, Blanks JC, Mullen RJ: Retinal degeneration in the *pcd* cerebellar mutant mouse. I. Light microscopic and autoradiographic analysis. *J Comp Neurol* 1982, 212:217–230.

85. LaVail MM, Pinto LH, Yashamura D: The interphotoreceptor matrices in rats with inherited retinal dystrophy. *Invest Ophthalmol Vis Sci* 1977; 21:658–668.

86. LaVail MM, Sidman RL: C57BL/6J mice with inherited retinal degeneration. *Arch Ophthalmol* 1974; 91:394–400.

87. Lazarus HL, Hageman GS: Xyloside-induced perturbation of "cone matrix sheath" structure and composition *in vivo*. *Invest Ophthalmol Vis Sci* 1989; 30(suppl):490.

88. Lemmon V: A monoclonal antibody that binds to cones. *Invest Ophthalmol Vis Sci* 1986; 27:831–836.

89. Lerea CL, Somers DE, Hurley JB, Klock IB, Bunt-Milam AH: Identification of specific transducin α subunits in retinal rod and cone photoreceptors. *Science* 1986; 234:77–80.

90. Lillie RD: Histochemical studies on the retina. *Anat Rec* 1952; 112:477–495.

91. Liu L, Chen S-HG, Jiang L-Z, Hansmann G, Layer PG: The pigmented epithelium sustains cell growth and tissue differentiation of chicken retinal explants in vitro. *Exp Eye Res* 1988; 46:801–812.

92. Mann I: *The Development of the Human Eye*, ed 3, New York, Grune & Stratton, 1964.

93. McCrane EP, de Monasterio FM, Schein SJ, Caruso RC: Non-fluorescent dye staining of primate blue cones. *Invest Ophthalmol Vis Sci* 1983; 24:1449–1455.

94. McGinnis JF, Leveille PJ: A biomolecular approach to the study of the expression of specific genes in the retina. *J Neurosci Res* 1986; 16:157–165.

95. McLaughlin BJ, Boykins LG: Freeze-fracture study of photoreceptor outer segments and pigment epithelium in dystrophic and normal retinas. *J Comp Neurol* 1981; 199:555–567.

96. McLaughlin BJ, Boykins LG: Lectin cytochemistry and freeze-fracture study of phagocytosis in the rat retina. *J Comp Neurol* 1984; 223:77–87.

97. McLaughlin BJ, Wood JG: The localization of lectin binding sites on photoreceptor outer segments and pigment epithelium of dystrophic retinas. *Invest Ophthalmol Vis Sci* 1980; 19:728–742.

98. Mullen RJ, LaVail MM: Inherited retinal dystrophy: Primary defect in pigment epithelium determined with experimental rat chimeras. *Science* 1976; 192:799–801.

99. Mullen RJ, LaVail MM: Two new types of retinal degeneration in cerebellar mutant mice. *Nature* 1975; 258:528–530.

100. Mund ML, Rodrigues MM, Fine BS: Pigmentation in the developing eye. *Am J Ophthalmol* 1972; 73:167–182.

101. Murray RG, Jones AE, Murray A: Fine structure of photoreceptors in the owl monkey. *Anat Rec* 1973; 175:673–696.

102. Nathans J: Molecular biology of visual pigments. *Annu Rev Neurosci* 1987; 10:163–194.

103. Nathans J, Thomas D, Hogness DS: Molecular genetics of human color vision: The genes in coding blue, green, and red pigments. *Science* 1986; 232:193–202.

104. Newman EA: Membrane physiology of retinal glial (Müller) cells. *J Neurosci* 1985; 5:2225.

105. Nilsson SEG: The ultrastructure of the receptor outer segment in the retina of the leopard frog *(Rana pipiens)*. *J Ultrastruct Res* 1965; 12:207–231.

106. O'Rahilly R: The prenatal development of the human eye. *Exp Eye Res* 1975; 21:93–112.

107. Ostwald TJ, Steinberg RH: Localization of frog retinal pigment epithelium Na$^+$-K$^+$ ATPase. *Exp Eye Res* 1980; 31:351–360.

108. Papermaster DS, Reilly PM, Schneider BG: Cone lamellae and red and green rod outer segment discs contain a large intrinsic membrane protein on their margins: Ultrastructural immunocytochemical study of frog retinas. *Vision Res* 1982; 22:1417–1428.

109. Papermaster DS, Schneider BG, Zorn MA, Kraehenbuhl JP: Immunocytochemical localization of a large intrinsic membrane protein to the incisures and margins of frog and rod outer segment disks. *J Cell Biol* 1978; 78:415–425.

110. Pfeffer B, Wiggert B, Lee L, Zonnenberg B, Newsome D, Chader G: The presence of a soluble interphotoreceptor retinol-binding protein (IRBP) in the retinal interphotoreceptor space. *J Cell Physiol* 1983; 117:333–341.

111. Porrello K, Yasamura D, LaVail MM: Immunogold localization of chondroitin 6-sulfate in the interphotoreceptor matrix of normal and RCS rats. *Invest Ophthalmol Vis Sci* 1989; 30:638–651.

112. Pugh EN, Cobbs WH: Visual transduction in vertebrate rods and cones: A tale of two transmitters, calcium and cyclic GMP. *Vision Res* 1986; 26:1613–1643.

113. Reinke R, Krantz DE, Yen D, Zipursky SL: Chaoptin, a cell surface glycoprotein required for drosophila photoreceptor cell morphogenesis contains a repeat motif found in yeast and human. *Cell* 1988; 52:291–301.

114. Rhodes RH: A light microscopic study of the developing human neural retina. *Am J Anat* 1979; 154:195–210.

115. Riepe RE, Norenburg MD: Müller cell localization of glutamine synthetase in rat retina. *Nature* 1977; 268:654–655.

116. Rodrigues M, Hackett J, Wiggert B, Gery I, Spiegel A, Krishna G, Stein P, Chader G: Immunoelectron microscopic localization of photoreceptor-specific markers in the monkey retina. *Curr Eye Res* 1987; 6:369–380.

117. Röhlich P: The interphotoreceptor matrix: Electron microscopic and histochemical observations on the vertebrate retina. *Exp Eye Res* 1970; 10:80–96.

118. Sameshima M, Uehara F, Ohba N: Specialization of the interphotoreceptor matrices around cone and rod photoreceptor cells in the monkey retina, as revealed by lectin cytochemistry. *Exp Eye Res* 1987; 45:845–863.

119. Sanyal S, DiRuiter A, Hawkins RK: Development and degeneration of retina in *rds* mutant mice: Light microscopy. *J Comp Neurol* 1980; 194:193–207.

120. Sarthy PV: The uptake of [^{3}H]-gamma-aminobutyric acid by isolated glia (Müller) cells from the mouse retina. *J Neurosci Methods* 1982; 5:77–82.

121. Sarthy PV, Hendrickson AE, Wu JY: L-Glutamate: A neural transmitter candidate for cone photoreceptors in the monkey retina. *J Neurosci* 1986; 6:637–643.

122. Schreiner DS, Jandy SS, Lawson DEM: Target cells of vitamin D in the retina. *Acta Anat* 1985; 121:153–162.

123. Sidman RL: Histochemical studies on photoreceptor cells. *Ann NY Acad Sci* 1958; 74:182–195.

124. Sigelman J, Ozanicks V: Retina. In Duane TD, Jeagar (eds): *Biomedical Foundations of Ophthalmology*, vol 1. Philadelphia, JB Lippincott, 1988, pp 1–66.

125. Sjöstrand FS: Electron microscopy of the retina, in Smelser GK (ed): *The Structure of the Eye*, New York, Academic Press, Inc, 1961, pp 1–28.

126. Sperling HG, Harcombe ES, Johnson C: Stimulus-controlled labeling in the macque retina with H-2-D-deoxyglucose. In

Hollyfield JG (ed): *The Structure of the Eye*. New York, Elsevier Science Publishing Co, Inc, 1982, pp 55–60.

127. Spira AW, Hollenberg MJ: Human retinal development: Ultrastructure of the inner retinal layers. *Dev Biol* 1973; 31:1–21.

128. Spoerri PE, Ulshafer RJ, Ludwig HC, Allen CB, Kelley KC: Photoreceptor cell development in vitro: Influence of pigment epithelium conditioned medium on outer segment differentiation. *Eur J Cell Biol* 1988; 46:362.

129. Steinberg RH, Wood I: Pigment epithelium cell ensheathment of cone outer segments in the retina of the domestic cat. *Proc R Soc Lond [Biol]* 1974; 187:461–478.

130. Steinberg RH, Wood I, Hogan MJ: Pigment epithelial ensheathment and phagocytosis of extrafoveal cones in human retina. *Philos Trans R Soc Lond [Biol]* 1977; 277:459–474.

131. Stramm LE: Synthesis and secretion of glycosaminoglycans in cultured retinal pigment epithelium. *Invest Ophthalmol Vis Sci* 1987; 28:618–627.

132. Stryer L: The molecules of visual excitation. *Sci Am* 1987; 256:42–50.

133. Szél A, Röhlich P: Localization of visual pigment antigens to photoreceptor cells with different droplets in the chicken retina. *Acta Biol Hung* 1985; 36:319–324.

134. Szél A, Röhlich P, Govardovskii V: Immunocytochemical discrimination of visual pigments in the retinal photoreceptors of the nocturnal gecko *teratoscincus*. *Exp Eye Res* 1986; 43:895–904.

135. Szél A, Takacs L, Monostori E, Vigh-Teichmann I, Röhlich P: Heterogeneity of chicken photoreceptors as defined by hybridoma supernatants. *Cell Tissue Res* 1985; 240:735–741.

136. Szél A, Takacs L, Monostori E, Diamantstein T, Vigh-Teichmann I, Röhlich P: Monoclonal antibody-recognizing cone visual pigment. *Exp Eye Res* 1986; 43:871–883.

137. Tombran-Tink J, Johnson LV: Neuronal differentiation of retinoblastoma cells induced by medium conditioned by human RPE cells. *Invest Ophthalmol Vis Sci* 1989; 30:1700–1707.

138. Uehara F, Muramatsu T, Sameshima M, Kawano K, Koide H, Ohba N: Effects of neuraminidase on lectin binding sites in photoreceptor cells of monkey retina. *Jpn J Ophthalmol* 1985; 29:54–62.

139. Uehara F, Muramatsu T, Sameshima M, Ogata S, Ohba N: Identification of peanut agglutinin receptors in the monkey retina. *Exp Eye Res* 1983; 37:303–305.

140. Uehara F, Sameshima M, Muramatsu T, Ohba N: Localization of fluorescein-labeled lectin binding sites on photoreceptor cells of the monkey retina. *Exp Eye Res* 1983; 36:113–123.

141. Van Dop C, Medynski D, Sullivan K, Wu AM, Fung BK, Bourne HR: Partial cDNA sequence of the gamma subunit of transducin. *Biochem Biophys Res Commun* 1984; 124:250–255.

142. Van Nie R, Ivanyi D, Demant F: A new H-2–linked mutation, *rds*, causing retinal degeneration in the mouse. *Tissue Antigens* 1978; 12:106–108.

143. Varner HH, Rayborn ME, Osterfeld AM, Hollyfield JG: Localization of proteoglycan within the extracellular matrix sheath of cone photoreceptors. *Exp Eye Res* 1987; 44:633–642.

144. Verstappen A, Parmentier M, Chirnoaga M, Lawson DE, Pasteels JL, Pochet R: Vitamin D–dependent calcium binding protein immunoreactivity in human retina. *Ophthalmic Res* 1986; 18:209–214.

145. Wacker WB, Donoso LA, Kalsow CM, Yankeelor JA Jr, Organisciak DT: Experimental allergic uveitis. Isolation, characterization and localization of a soluble uveitopathogenic antigen from bovine retina. *J Immunol* 1977; 119:1949–1958.

146. Wang JW, Hilfer SR: The effect of inhibitors of glycoconjugate synthesis on optic cup formation in the chick embryo. *Dev Biol* 1982; 92:41–53.

147. Weidman TA: Fine structure of the developing retina. *Int Ophthalmol Clin* 1975; 15:65–84.

148. Wood JG, Besharse JC, Napier-Marshall L: Partial characterization of lectin-binding sites of retinal photoreceptor outer segments interphotoreceptor matrix. *J Comp Neurol* 1984; 28:299–307.

149. Yamada E, Ishikawa T: Some observations on the submicroscopic morphogenesis of the human retina, in Rohen J (ed): *The Structure of the Eye*. Stuttgart, West Germany, Schattaner, 1965, pp 5–16.

150. Yao XY, Marmor MF, Hageman GS: Interphotoreceptor matrix plays an important role in retinal adhesiveness. *Invest Ophthalmol Vis Sci* 1989; 30(suppl):240.

151. Yatsunami K, Khorana HG: GTPase of bovine rod outer segments: The amino acid sequence of the subunit as derived from the cDNA sequence. *Proc Natl Acad Sci USA* 1985; 82:4316–4320.

152. Young RW: An hypothesis to account for a basic distinction between rods and cones. *Vision Res* 1971; 49:303–318.

153. Young RW: The renewal of photoreceptor outer segments. *J Cell Biol* 1967; 33:61–72.

154. Young RW, Bok D: Participation of the retinal pigment epithelium in the rod outer segment renewal process. *J Cell Biol* 1969; 42:392–403.

155. Yuodelis C, Hendrickson A: A qualitative and quantitative analysis of the human fovea during development. *Vision Res* 1985; 26:847–855.

156. Zimmerman LE: Applications of histochemical methods for the demonstration of acid mucopolysaccharides to ophthalmic pathology. *Trans Am Acad Ophthalmol Otolaryngol* 1958; 62:697–703.

5 Membrane Mechanisms of the Retinal Pigment Epithelium

OLAF STRAUSS

The retinal pigment epithelium (RPE) interacts closely with photoreceptors, an activity that is essential to maintain excitability of photoreceptors. The RPE helps to control the environment of the subretinal space, supplies nutrients and retinal to the photoreceptors, phagocytoses shed photoreceptor outer segments in a renewal process, and secretes a variety of growth factors, helping to maintain the structural integrity of the retina. Some of these functions are coupled to ion fluxes across cell membranes of the RPE. Since movements of charges across the RPE can be monitored in the electroretinogram (ERG) and electro-oculogram (EOG), these methods provide insights into these RPE functions.

In this chapter, RPE functions involving ion fluxes across RPE cell membranes will be described. The first part will describe ion channels and transporters that are present in the RPE. In the second part, the interaction of ion channels and transporters will be put into models of RPE function.

RPE functions that involve the movements of ions across the cell membranes

The ultrastructure of the RPE is characteristic for a transporting epithelium,[2,11,61,62,81,82] and adjacent RPE cells form tight junctions and thus become organized into an apical and basolateral membrane with distinct and often separate functions. The RPE transports ions and metabolic end products from the retinal to the choroidal (vascular) side.[6,118] Ion transport serves to control the ion composition in the subretinal space, which is essential for the maintenance of photoreceptor excitability and also drives water transport across the RPE.[34,36,148] The removal of fluid from the subretinal space (volume transport) ensures that its volume is small and that photoreceptors and RPE are closely opposed and therefore can interact easily. In addition to transport of ions, the transport of metabolic end products involves the movements of charged molecules such as lactic acid.[35,36,148] Another RPE function that is coupled to movements of charges is the rapid, nearly instantaneous compensation for changes in ion composition in the subretinal space.[66,72,118] Stimulation of photoreceptors by light decreases the potassium concentration in the subretinal space. To compensate, the RPE releases potassium ions through the apical membrane into the subretinal space. Changing from light to dark increases the potassium concentration in the subretinal space, which is compensated by the absorption of potassium ions. Both the capability for epithelial transport and fast instantaneous compensation can be monitored by ERG or EOG measurements.

Membrane proteins involved in transporting ions

ION CHANNELS

The delayed rectifier Characterization: Delayed rectifier K^+ channels activate slowly in response to depolarization and repolarize the membrane potential back to the resting potential by developing increasing K^+ outward current amplitudes with increasing positive membrane voltages (outward rectification).[45,122,123,130,133,135,141] Whether the channels are located in either apical or basolateral membrane is unclear. The channels carrying such currents in RPE cells have been found to be mainly composed of Kv1.3 subunits,[123] of which four assemble a tetramer to form the K^+ conducting pore.

Function: The role of the delayed rectifier potassium channel for RPE function is not fully understood. The delayed rectifier is regulated by protein kinases and has an activation threshold comparable to that of voltage-dependent Ca^{2+} channels, i.e., they conduct after membrane voltage changes to potentials more positive than $-30\,mV$. RPE cells show a resting potential of approximately $-40\,mV$. The RPE cell membrane is maximally depolarized by $+10\,mV$ by changes from light to dark. Thus, it is unlikely that the delayed rectifier potassium channels contribute to ERG or EOG signals. It is likely that delayed rectifier represent a functional antagonist to voltage-dependent Ca^{2+} channels.

Inward rectifier Characterization: Inward rectifier channels are activated by hyperpolarization of the cell and display increasing inward currents with increasing negative membrane potentials.[45,46,64,65,113,115,117,122,130,135,136,141] Depolarization from very negative membrane potentials can lead to outwardly directed currents depending on electrochemical driving forces. The inward rectifier channels in mammalian RPE cells show mild inward rectification, decreased conductance when extracellular K^+ concentration was increased, and voltage-dependent inhibition by extracellular Na^+.[46,47,115,117] The channels are mainly composed of Kir7.1 subunits, which are located in the apical microvilli.[65,117]

Function: The inward rectifier provides a general potassium conductance and stabilizes the membrane potential. The location of Kir7.1 subunits in the apical processes imply additional functions. The ability to conduct potassium in both directions and sensitivity to extracellular potassium enable the inward rectifier to compensate for changes in subretinal K^+ concentration. Another important role might be the support of Na^+/K^+ ATPase activity.[117] The Kir7.1 subunits colocalize with Na^+/K^+ ATPase in the apical processes. The inward rectifier provides a K^+ conductance, which is open under all physiological conditions, that could recycle K^+ ions that have been transported into the cell by Na^+/K^+ ATPase. This cycling of K^+ ions over the apical membrane supports the ATPase activity in building Na^+ gradients, because inward rectifiers decrease the K^+ gradient. Thus, the inward rectifier plays an important role for the driving forces of epithelial transport. Since the c-wave of the ERG is based on changes in the apical K^+ conductance, it seems also likely that the inward rectifier is involved in this ERG signal.[46]

Ca²⁺-dependent K⁺ channels Characterization: Rises in intracellular free Ca^{2+} activate outwardly rectifying K^+ channels. RPE cells express large conductance Ca^{2+}-dependent K^+ channels[110,134] (maxi K or BK). Such maxi-K channels are caused to open by a rise in intracellular free Ca^{2+}, which occurs in response to activation of purinergic receptors.[110]

Function: The main function of maxi-K potassium channels is the modulation of epithelial transport. These channels can be activated by the Ca^{2+} second-messenger system. The subsequent hyperpolarization of the membrane potential changes the driving forces for ions over the cell membrane and can, for example, increase Cl^- secretion. This might be the basis for the effect of purinergic stimulation on epithelial transport.[110]

M-type currents Characterization: In bovine and human RPE cells, another outwardly rectifying K^+ channel with a different voltage dependence and sensitivity to K^+ channel blockers could be identified.[133] With its voltage dependence and insensitivity to Cs^+, this current resembles currents through M-type K^+ channels. The term *M channels* is shorthand for muscarinic channels, which are known to be silenced after a period of exposure to muscarinic agonists. However, such an effect could not be observed in RPE cells.

Function: Since M channels are active over a broad voltage range, M channels stabilize the membrane potential. Depolarization leads to activation of M channels. The corresponding increase in K^+ membrane conductance moves the membrane potential toward the equilibrium potential for K^+, which in turn hyperpolarizes the cell back toward the resting potential. A contribution to the c-wave of the ERG is likely but not proven.

Voltage-dependent Ca²⁺ channels: L-type channels Characterization: L-type Ca^{2+} channels are activated by relatively large depolarizing voltage changes. They are highly specific for Ca^{2+} ions.[85,86,107,114,120,121,127–129,138,140] Ca^{2+} channels are composed of several subunits, of which the largest one, the α- or Ca_V-subunit, forms the Ca^{2+}-conducting pore and determines such Ca^{2+} channel properties as voltage-dependence or sensitivity to Ca^{2+} channel blockers. Four different Ca_V subunits are known to represent L-type channels: $Ca_V1.1$—the skeletal subtype; $Ca_V1.2$—the cardiac subtype; $Ca_V1.3$—the neuroendocrine subtype; and $Ca_V1.4$—the retinal subtype. In the RPE, these channels were identified as the neuroendocrine subtype of L-type channels composed of $Ca_V1.3$ subunits.[107,120] The L-type channels are regulated by protein tyrosine kinase and protein kinase C.[85,121] In addition, L-type channels are activated during stimulation of the InsP3/Ca^{2+} second-messenger signaling cascade.[86]

Function: The function of these L-type channels is not fully understood. The neuroendocrine subtype of L-type channels is known to regulate secretion rates and can transduce voltage-dependent changes in gene expression. The RPE is known to secrete a variety of growth factors. Thus, it is likely that these Ca^{2+} channels regulate the secretion of growth factors. Since these Ca^{2+} channels are activated by depolarization of the membrane potential, L-type channels could contribute to signals of the EOG. This is most likely for the light peak that arises mainly from activation of basolateral Cl channels, which leads to depolarization of the basolateral cell membrane.

Nonspecific cation channels Characterization: So called nonspecific cation channels can conduct both Na^+ and K^+ ions. Nonspecific cation channels in the RPE are coupled to activation of purinergic receptors.[100,110,111] Stimulation of RPE cells by ATP leads to a G-protein-coupled activation of nonspecific cation channels.

Function: The function of these channels is not fully understood. Activation of Na^+ and K^+ conducting ion channels leads to depolarization. It is likely that these potential changes modulate driving forces for ions across the cell membranes and thus epithelial transport.

Chloride channels

Ca²⁺-dependent Cl channels Characterization: These Cl channels are activated by a rise in intracellular free Ca^{2+}, show outwardly rectifying currents, and can be blocked by stilbene derivatives such as DIDS.[124,126,139] The activation of these channels requires not only Ca^{2+} but also cofactors such as tyrosine kinases.[124,126]

Function: Activation of Ca^{2+}-activated Cl channels is coupled to activation of the InsP3/Ca^{2+} second-messenger system.[124,126] Activation of this second-messenger system requires a Ca^{2+} influx into the cell. The amount of inflowing Ca^{2+} is determined by electrochemical driving forces for Ca^{2+}. Activation of Ca^{2+}-dependent Cl channels hyperpolarizes the cell, leading to increase the driving force for Ca^{2+} into the cell and to larger rises in intracellular free Ca^{2+} acting as second messenger. On the other hand, activation of these Cl channels by the InsP3/Ca^{2+} second-messenger system can increase Cl$^-$ outflow and thus increase Cl$^-$ secretion.[112] The light peak originates in an increase in the Cl conductance in the basal membrane of the RPE.[27,28] In addition, this is ultimately caused by a transmitter, probably by a biogenic amine, which is released by the neuronal retina during light exposure.[26,29] Biogenic amines are known to stimulate the InsP3/Ca^{2+} second-messenger system.

Volume-activated Cl channels Characterization: This type of Cl channel is activated to counterbalance hypoosmotic swelling.[8,139] It seems that activation of this Cl channel does not require changes in intracellular Ca^{2+}.[8]

Function: The volume-activated Cl channels help to control the volume of RPE cells, which is important for the integrity of the epithelial barrier.

ClC-2 channel Characterization: RPE cells express ClC-2 Cl channels.[7] ClC (Chloride Channel) is a large family of Cl channels related to a Cl channel that has been isolated from the electric organ of the electric ray.[50] The voltage-dependent ClC-2 channels are inactive at the resting potential of RPE cells and open in response to hyperpolarization.[50] In addition, ClC-2 is activated in response to extracellular acidification. Knock-out of the ClC-2 chloride channel in a mouse model leads to retinal degeneration arising from absence of epithelial Cl transport by the RPE.[7]

Function: The retinal degeneration in the ClC-2 knockout mouse indicates that ClC-2 channels are essential for epithelial transport of Cl$^-$ across the RPE. The transport of Cl might be coupled to transport of lactic acid. This is made very likely by the finding that ClC-2 channels are very sensitive to changes in extracellular pH.[7] A failure of Cl and lactic acid transport by the RPE might be the cause for the retinal degeneration in the ClC-2 knock-out mouse model.

Ion Transporters
ATPases

Na$^+$/K$^+$-ATPase Characterization: Na$^+$/K$^+$-ATPase is able to transport Na$^+$ and K$^+$ against their concentration gradients.* Using the energy of ATP degradation, this enzyme

---

*9,10,13,15,33,39,49,63,84,96,103,105,106,108,109,116,142

transports Na$^+$ to the extracellular space and K$^+$ to the cytosol. These gradients can be used by the cell for Na$^+$-dependent transport mechanisms. The transport by the Na$^+$/K$^+$-ATPase is electrogenic. Na$^+$/K$^+$-ATPase transports 3 mol Na$^+$ to the extracellular space and 2 mol K$^+$ into the cell per mol of ATP consumed. This results in a transmembranal potential of approximately 10 mV. Na$^+$/K$^+$-ATPase in the RPE is located in the apical membrane.[33,39,81,96,97,103–105,131,142] This is a unique feature of the RPE. The location is achieved during ontogenesis from the first expression of this enzyme.

Function: Na$^+$/K$^+$-ATPase is the main energy source for epithelial transport by the RPE. This ensures a close interaction between RPE and neuronal retina. The adhesion forces between both tissues are dependent on the activity of Na$^+$/K$^+$-ATPase.

Ca^{2+}-ATPase Characterization: Ca^{2+}-ATPase uses metabolic energy to eliminate Ca^{2+} from intracellular space. This ATPase can transport Mg^{2+} and Ca^{2+} and was identified as the plasma membrane (Ca^{2+} + Mg^{2+})-ATPase (PMCA).[57]

Function: This transporter terminates rises in intracellular free Ca^{2+} that are acting as a second messenger.

Na$^+$/Ca^{2+} exchanger Characterization: Using the Na$^+$ gradient the Na$^+$/Ca^{2+} exchanger extrudes Ca^{2+} from intracellular space.[20,79]

Function: This transporter plays a role in the Ca^{2+} second-messenger system. Together with the Ca^{2+}-ATPase, the Na$^+$/Ca^{2+} exchanger terminates rises in intracellular free Ca^{2+} acting as a second messenger.

Na$^+$/HCO$_3^-$ cotransporter Characterization: Using the Na$^+$ gradient established by the Na$^+$/K$^+$-ATPase, the Na$^+$/HCO$_3^-$ cotransporter serves to transfer HCO$_3^-$ ions into the cell.[14,18,41,67–69,76] The transporter is located in the apical as well as basolateral membranes and can be inhibited by stilbene derivatives such as DIDS or SITS. The transport of Na$^+$ and HCO$_3^-$ is electrogenic. The cotransporter transports 1 Na$^+$ together with 2–3 HCO$_3^-$ ions.[1,51,67–69,87]

Function: The Na$^+$/HCO$_3^-$ cotransporter accumulates HCO$_3^-$ ions in the cytosol, which is a prerequisite for epithelial transport of HCO$_3^-$ and pH regulation.

Na$^+$/H$^+$ exchanger Characterization: The Na$^+$/H$^+$ exchanger is electroneutral and exchanges Na$^+$ ions against protons.[53,54,58,147] This amiloride-sensitive transporter is located in the apical membrane of the RPE.

Function: The ability of the Na$^+$/H$^+$ exchanger to use the Na$^+$ gradient to extrude protons from the cytosol gives this transporter a central role in the regulation of intracellular pH. Since accumulation of HCO$_3^-$ is coupled to the pH regulation, the Na$^+$/H$^+$ exchanger is involved in the transport of HCO$_3^-$.

Na⁺/K⁺/2 Cl⁻ cotransporter Characterization: The $Na^+/K^+/2 Cl^-$ transporter is located in the apical membrane of the RPE.[1,22,24,38,51,55,70,87] It is electroneutral and transports $2 Cl^-$ together with $1 Na^+$ and $1 K^+$. Exploiting the Na^+ gradient established by the Na^+/K^+-ATPase, the $Na^+/K^+/2 Cl^-$ cotransporter moves K^+ and Cl^- ions into the cell against the concentration gradients. The transporter can be inhibited by bumetanide.

Function: The $Na^+/K^+/2 Cl^-$ plays a central role in epithelial NaCl transport. It mediates the uptake Na^+, K^+, and Cl^- over the apical membrane.

Cl⁻/HCO₃⁻ exchanger Characterization: Located in the basolateral membrane, the Cl^-/HCO_3^- electroneutral exchanger exchanges Cl^- against HCO_3^-.[18,19,53,54,76,77] Since the exchanger transports HCO_3^- ions, it is involved in pH regulation. Intracellular alkalinization is compensated for by extrusion of HCO_3^- from the cytosol.[53,54] Intracellular acidification causes a reduction in the activity of the Cl^-/HCO_3^- exchanger. The Cl^-/HCO_3^- exchanger is sensitive to DIDS.

Function: The main function of the Cl^-/HCO_3^- exchanger is to provide an outflow pathway for HCO_3^- out of the cell over the basolateral membrane. This is used for epithelial transport of HCO_3^- and for intracellular pH regulation. Since extrusion of HCO_3^- is connected to uptake of Cl^-, the HCO_3^- transport decreases Cl^- secretion over the basolateral membrane.

Transporters for lactic acid Characterization: Several transporter systems that are capable of transporting lactic acid have been described in the RPE.[35,36,59,71,75,99,146,148] Two transporters belong to the monocarboxylate transporter family. MCT1 (monocarboxylate transporter 1) is located in the apical membrane, and MCT3 (monocarboxylate 3) is located in the basolateral membrane.[99,146] Both transporters function as lactate/H^+ cotransporters. In the apical membrane, a Na^+-dependent transporter for organic ions is also capable of transporting lactic acid. In addition to these transporters, an electrogenic Na^+-dependent lactate transporter, the Na/lac cotransporter, has been found in the basolateral membrane.[59] The monocarboxylate transporters are also able to transport water efficiently.[35]

Function: All transport systems mediate an epithelial transport of lactic acid and water from the subretinal space to the choroid.

RPE functions

Fast Capacitative Compensation for Changes in the Subretinal Space Activation of photoreceptors by light leads to changes of ion composition in the subretinal space.[25–28,30,31,83,87,94,95,118] To maintain the excitability of photoreceptors, these changes have to be compensated for. The RPE is able to compensate for these changes the moment they arise. This compensation has to occur very fast.

The origin is a change in the equilibrium potential across the apical membrane of RPE cells. Activation of photoreceptors by light leads to a shutdown of the dark current of the photoreceptors and a decrease in the potassium concentration in the subretinal space because the K^+ outward current from the inner segment counterbalancing the Na^+ inward current into the outer segment decreases and the Na^+/K^+-ATPase removes K^+ from subretinal space. The consequence is hyperpolarization[94,95] of the apical membrane and activation of inward rectifier K^+ channels.[46,115] This results in potassium outflow into the subretinal space.[72] The hyperpolarization also decreases the transport of Cl^-[3,19,31] because the decrease in the subretinal K^+ concentration decreases uptake of Cl^- by the $Na^+/K^+/2 Cl^-$ cotransporter. The subsequent decrease in the intracellular Cl^- and K^+ activity transduces changes in the apical transmembranal potential to a hyperpolarization of the basolateral membrane. A decrease in the intracellular K^+ concentration results also from K^+ outflow through hyperpolarization-activated inward rectifier channels because it can be prevented by application of the K^+ channel blocker Ba^{2+}.[32,44] Light-dependent changes in the photoreceptor activity also change the Na^+ concentration in the subretinal space. These changes are compensated for by uptake of Na^+ by the Na/H exchanger and by Na^+ release by the Na^+/K^+-ATPase.[37]

Epithelial Transport The RPE transports ions and water volume from the subretinal space to the choroid, especially when light adapted.[4–6,16–19,23,38,41,51,60,73,81,87–89,93,101,102,118,137] The transport of ions (see figure 5.1A) drives the transport of water. Since the RPE shows properties of a tight epithelium,[90] most of the water transports occurs via the transcellular route. Transcellular water transport occurs through aquaporins, water channels that are present in the apical and the basolateral membrane.[117] A smaller amount of water might be transported by monocarboxylate transporter, electroneutral Na^+/glucose cotransporter, $Na^+/K^+/2 Cl^-$ cotransporter, Cl^-/HCO_3^- exchanger or by Cl channels.[34] Since the transport of water is coupled to transport of ions, the transport of water occurs isotonically. This volume transport is essential and keeps the volume of the subretinal space very small, enabling a close interaction between RPE and photoreceptors. In disease, such as macular edema, in which this relationship breaks down, function is lost, and cell death may occur.

Epithelial transport is energized by the activity of the Na^+/K^+-ATPase in the apical membrane of the RPE.[13,39,43,49,96,97,104,105,132,145] The ATPase eliminates Na^+ from intracellular space and establishes a gradient for Na^+ into the cell. K^+ ions are transported into the cell and cycle over the apical membrane via K^+ channels.[32,44,109] This supports

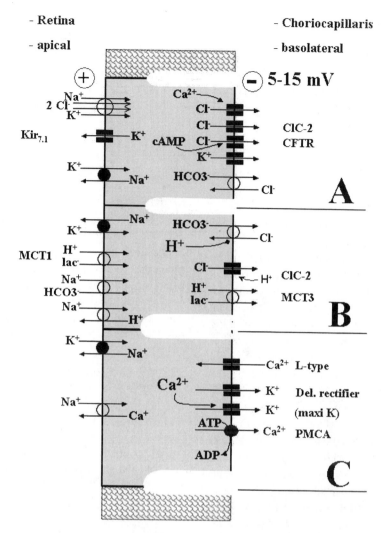

FIGURE 5.1 Simplified models of transepithelial transport and pH regulation. Transporters are drawn with open circles; ATPases are drawn with closed circles. Arrows indicate stimulation, and arrows ending with squares indicate inhibition. A (upper panel), Epithelial transport of ions across the RPE. Explanations see text. B (middle panel), Epithelial transport of lactic acid and pH regulation. C (lower panel), Simplified model of intracellular Ca^{2+} homeostasis.

the ATPase to build a Na^+ gradient because K^+ channels decrease the K^+ gradient.

Uptake of ions over the apical membrane is mediated by the $Na^+/K^+/2\ Cl^-$ cotransporter,[1,55,56,70] which uses the Na^+ gradient to transport K^+ and Cl^- into the cell while maintaining electroneutrality. Cl^- leaves the cell via Cl channels in the basolateral membrane.[25,30,70] These Cl channels can be Ca^{2+}-dependent Cl channels[124–126,139] or ClC-2 channels.[7] Cl^- is transported only via the transcellular pathway and represents the most important part of the epithelial transport by the RPE. This Cl^- transport results in a net retinal positive transepithelial potential of approximately 5–15 mV.[89,90]

K^+ ions leave the cells across basolateral membrane via K^+ channels.[87] It is not clear which type of K^+ channels mediate K^+ efflux. They could be Ca^{2+}-dependent K^+ channels[110,134] or M channels.[133] However, whether either or both of these channels are located in either apical or basolateral membranes (or both)

remains unknown. In addition, a part of the K^+ is transported via the paracellular pathway driven by the transepithelial potential.

A portion of the Na^+ is possibly transported via the paracellular pathway from the subretinal space to the choroid.[81,87,101] This transport is driven by the apical positive transepithelial potential.[51] The role of the paracellular Na^+ transport route is not clear. On one hand, the direction of transepithelial Na^+ fluxes is dependent on the transepithelial potential.[42,89] On the other hand, the RPE was classified as a tight epithelium, which means that paracellular resistance is approximately 10 times higher than transcellular resistance.[90] This would speak against an important role for paracellular Na^+ transport. The portion of the transcellularly transported Na^+ is not known, because the efflux pathway for Na^+ over the basolateral membrane is not clear. The mechanism could be the Na^+/HCO^- cotransporter, which uses the HCO_3^- gradient to extrude Na^+ from the cytosol.[58]

Uptake of HCO_3^- occurs over the apical membrane via the Na^+/HCO_3^- cotransporter,[41,67–69] and release of HCO_3^- to the basolateral site occurs via the Cl^-/HCO_3^- exchanger[18,19,53,54,77] and possibly by the basolateral Na^+/HCO_3^- cotransporter.[58] However, the release of HCO_3^- by the Cl^-/HCO_3^- exchanger decreases the efficiency of Cl^- secretion. This can be used as a resource to enhance Cl^- transport. Inhibition of carbonic anhydrase increases transepithelial Cl^- transport and supports the removal of volume in the treatment of macula edema.[12,21,80,119,143,144] This can be explained by the fact that the Cl^-/HCO_3^- exchanger is inhibited by intracellular acidification.[77] Inhibition of carbonic anhydrase leads to a decrease in the HCO_3^- concentration and to acidification.[52] In consequence, the Cl^-/HCO_3^- exchanger is inhibited and no longer counterbalances the effect of basolateral Cl channels. The result is an increase in Cl^- and volume transport from the subretinal space to the choroid.[18] Another mechanism to enhance fluid absorption might be the purinergic stimulation of RPE. Purinergic stimulation leads to enhancement of fluid absorption via activation of several types of ion channels.[78,92,98,110] Furthermore, epithelial transport can be stimulated by adrenergic stimulation and subsequent increase in intracellular free Ca^{2+} as second messenger.[112]

The transepithelial transport of volume varies with changes in illumination. The apical Na^+/HCO_3^- exchanger is voltage-dependent. Light-induced hyperpolarization of the apical membrane reduces transport activity and results in intracellular acidification. Intracellular acidification facilitates Cl^- transport and thus transport of water across the RPE. Although the physiological relevance of this adaptive mechanism is not clear, the occurrence of light-dependent transient volume changes in the subretinal space has been confirmed by in situ measurements.[40,74]

INTRACELLULAR Ca^{2+} SIGNALING Rises in intracellular free Ca^{2+} serve as a second messenger to regulate many cellular functions, such as phagocytosis, secretion, or gene expression (see figure 5.1C). L-type Ca^{2+} channels provide a major influx pathway for Ca^{2+} into the cell.[86] This influx is limited by voltage-dependent or Ca^{2+}-dependent K^+ channels. L-type channels are activated by depolarization. Delayed rectifier K^+ channels are activated in parallel[48,121–123,129,140,141] by depolarization, which leads to hyperpolarization and to deactivation of L-type channels. Increases in intracellular free Ca^{2+} activate Ca^{2+}-dependent K^+ channels, which also hyperpolarizes the cell and deactivates L-type Ca^{2+} channels. Increases in cytosolic free Ca^{2+} are terminated by Ca^{2+}-ATPase[57] and the Na^+/Ca^{2+}-exchanger.[20,79]

REGULATION OF INTRACELLULAR pH The interaction of the RPE and the photoreceptors includes the digestion of photoreceptor outer segments and the recycling retinal and fatty acids. In addition, the RPE transports lactic acid from subretinal space to the blood site. The high throughput of metabolites is based on an efficient pH regulation (see figure 5.1B). Intracellular acidification is compensated for by the Na^+/H^+ exchanger; intracellular alkalinization is recovered by the Cl^-/HCO_3^- exchanger.[53,54]

TRANSPORT OF LACTIC ACID The retina contains high amounts of lactic acid. The subretinal space shows a much lower concentration of lactic acid than the neuronal retina does. This is caused by the transport of lactic acid by the RPE.[35,36,71,75,146,148] Lactic acid is taken up by the RPE by a lactate/H^+ cotransporter (MCT1) and by the Na^+-dependent transporter for organic acids (see figure 5.1B). Lactic acid leaves the cell via MCT3 and the Na^+/lac^- exchanger in the basolateral membrane. Translocation of lactic acid is coupled to transport of protons. Thus, transport of lactic acid creates a need for pH regulation. This is enabled by the activity of the Cl^-/HCO_3^- exchanger and the Na^+/H^+ exchanger.[53,54] The proper function of the Cl^-/HCO_3^- exchanger requires a recycling pathway for Cl^-. This recycling pathway is provided by ClC-2 Cl channels, which are activated by extracellular acidification.[7]

REFERENCES

1. Adorante JS, Miller SS: Potassium-dependent volume regulation in retinal pigment epithelium is mediated by Na,K,Cl cotransport. *J Gen Physiol* 1990; 96(6):1153–1176.
2. Ban Y, Rizzolo LJ: Differential regulation of tight junction permeability during development of the retinal pigment epithelium. *Am J Physiol Cell Physiol* 2000; 279(3):C744–C750.
3. Bialek S, Joseph DP, Miller SS: The delayed basolateral membrane hyperpolarization of the bovine retinal pigment epithelium: mechanism of generation. *J Physiol* 1995; 484(1): 53–67.
4. Bialek S, Miller SS: K^+ and Cl^- transport mechanisms in bovine pigment epithelium that could modulate subretinal space volume and composition. *J Physiol* 1994; 475(3): 401–417.
5. Bialek S, Quong JN, Yu K, Miller SS: Nonsteroidal anti-inflammatory drugs alter chloride and fluid transport in bovine retinal pigment epithelium. *Am J Physiol* 1996; 270(4): C1175–C1189.
6. Bok D: The retinal pigment epithelium: a versatile partner in vision. *J Cell Sci Suppl* 1993; 17:189–195.
7. Bosl MR, Stein V, Hubner C, Zdebik AA, Jordt SE, Mukhopadhyay AK, Davidoff MS, Holstein AF, Jentsch TJ: Male germ cells and photoreceptors, both dependent on close cell-cell interactions, degenerate upon ClC-2 Cl^- channel disruption. *Embo J* 2001; 20(6):1289–1299.
8. Botchkin LM, Matthews G: Chloride current activated by swelling in retinal pigment epithelium cells. *Am J Physiol* 1993; 265(4):C1037–C1045.
9. Burke JM, McKay BS: In vitro aging of bovine and human retinal pigment epithelium: Number and activity of the Na/K ATPase pump. *Exp Eye Res* 1993; 57(1):51–57.

10. Burke JM, McKay BS, Jaffe GJ: Retinal pigment epithelial cells of the posterior pole have fewer Na/K adenosine triphosphatase pumps than peripheral cells. *Invest Ophthalmol Vis Sci* 1991; 32(7):2042–2046.

11. Caldwell RB, McLaughlin BJ: Redistribution of Na-K-ATPase in the dystrophic rat retinal pigment epithelium. *J Neurocytol* 1984; 13(6):895–910.

12. Chen JC, Fitzke FW, Bird AC: Long-term effect of acetazolamide in a patient with retinitis pigmentosa. *Invest Ophthalmol Vis Sci* 1990; 31(9):1914–1918.

13. Crider JY, Yorio T, Sharif NA, Griffin BW: The effects of elevated glucose on Na+/K+-ATPase of cultured bovine retinal pigment epithelial cells measured by a new nonradioactive rubidium uptake assay. *J Ocul Pharmacol Ther* 1997; 13(4):337–352.

14. Dawis S, Hofmann H, Niemeyer G: The electroretinogram, standing potential, and light peak of the perfused cat eye during acid-base changes. *Vision Res* 1985; 25(9):1163–1177.

15. Defoe DM, Ahmad A, Chen W, Hughes BA: Membrane polarity of the Na+-K+ pump in primary cultures of Xenopus retinal pigment epithelium. *Exp Eye Res* 1994; 59(5):587–596.

16. Dimattio J, Degnan KJ, Zadunaisky JA: A model for transepithelial ion transport across the isolated retinal pigment epithelium of the frog. *Exp Eye Res* 1983; 37(5):409–420.

17. Dornonville De La Cour M: Ion transport in the retinal pigment epithelium: A study with double barrelled ion-selective microelectrodes. *Acta Ophthalmol Suppl* 1993; 209:1–32.

18. Edelman JL, Lin H, Miller SS: Acidification stimulates chloride and fluid absorption across frog retinal pigment epithelium. *Am J Physiol* 1994; 266(4):C946–C956.

19. Edelman JL, Lin H, Miller SS: Potassium-induced chloride secretion across the frog retinal pigment epithelium. *Am J Physiol* 1994; 266(4):C957–C966.

20. Fijisawa K, Ye J, Zadunaisky JA: A Na+/Ca2+ exchange mechanism in apical membrane vesicles of the retinal pigment epithelium. *Curr Eye Res* 1993; 12(3):261–270.

21. Fishman GA, Gilbert LD, Fiscella RG, Kimura AE, Jampol LM: Acetazolamide for treatment of chronic macular edema in retinitis pigmentosa. *Arch Ophthalmol* 1989; 107(10): 1445–1452.

22. Frambach DA, Misfeldt DS: Furosemide-sensitive Cl transport in embryonic chicken retinal pigment epithelium. *Am J Physiol* 1983; 244(6):F679–F685.

23. Frambach DA, Valentine JL, Weiter JJ: Initial observations of rabbit retinal pigment epithelium-choroid-sclera preparations. *Invest Ophthalmol Vis Sci* 1988; 29(5):814–817.

24. Frambach DA, Valentine JL, Weiter JJ: Furosemide-sensitive Cl transport in bovine retinal pigment epithelium. *Invest Ophthalmol Vis Sci* 1989; 30(10):2271–2274.

25. Fujii S, Gallemore RP, Hughes BA, Steinberg RH: Direct evidence for a basolateral membrane Cl− conductance in toad retinal pigment epithelium. *Am J Physiol* 1992; 262(2): C374–C383.

26. Gallemore RP, Griff ER, Steinberg RH: Evidence in support of a photoreceptoral origin for the "light-peak substance." *Invest Ophthalmol Vis Sci* 1988; 29(4):566–571.

27. Gallemore RP, Steinberg RH: Effects of DIDS on the chick retinal pigment epithelium: I. Membrane potentials, apparent resistances, and mechanisms. *J Neurosci* 1989; 9(6):1968–1976.

28. Gallemore RP, Steinberg RH: Effects of DIDS on the chick retinal pigment epithelium: II. Mechanism of the light peak and other responses originating at the basal membrane. *J Neurosci* 1989; 9(6):1977–1984.

29. Gallemore RP, Steinberg RH: Effects of dopamine on the chick retinal pigment epithelium. Membrane potentials and light-evoked responses. *Invest Ophthalmol Vis Sci* 1990; 31(1):67–80.

30. Gallemore RP, Steinberg RH: Light-evoked modulation of basolateral membrane Cl− conductance in chick retinal pigment epithelium: The light peak and fast oscillation. *J Neurophysiol* 1993; 70(4):1669–1680.

31. Griff ER: Potassium-evoked responses from the retinal pigment epithelium of the toad Bufo marinus. *Exp Eye Res* 1991; 53(2):219–228.

32. Griff ER, Shirao Y, Steinberg RH: Ba2+ unmasks K+ modulation of the Na+-K+ pump in the frog retinal pigment epithelium. *J Gen Physiol* 1985; 86(6):853–876.

33. Gundersen D, Orlowski J, Rodriguez-Boulan E: Apical polarity of Na,K-ATPase in retinal pigment epithelium is linked to a reversal of the ankyrin-fodrin submembrane cytoskeleton. *J Cell Biol* 1991; 112(5):863–872.

34. Hamann S: Molecular mechanisms of water transport in the eye. *Int Rev Cytol* 2002; 215:395–431.

35. Hamann S, Kiilgard JF, La Cour M, Prause JU, Zeuthen T: Cotransport of H+, lactate, and H2O in porcine retinal pigment epithelial cells. *Exp Eye Res* 2003; 76:1–12.

36. Hamann S, La Cour M, Lui GM, Bundgaard M, Zeuthen T: Transport of protons and lactate in cultured human fetal retinal pigment epithelial cells. *Pflugers Arch* 2000; 440(1):84–92.

37. Hodson S, Armstrong I, Wigham C: Regulation of the retinal interphotoreceptor matrix Na by the retinal pigment epithelium during the light response. *Experientia* 1994; 50(5): 438–441.

38. Hu JG, Gallemore RP, Bok D, Frambach DA: Chloride transport in cultured fetal human retinal pigment epithelium. *Exp Eye Res* 1996; 62(4):443–448.

39. Hu JG, Gallemore RP, Bok D, Lee AY, Frambach DA: Localization of NaK ATPase on cultured human retinal pigment epithelium. *Invest Ophthalmol Vis Sci* 1994; 35(10):3582–3588.

40. Huang B, Karwoski CJ: Light-evoked expansion of subretinal space volume in the retina of the frog. *J Neurosci* 1992; 12:4243–4252.

41. Hughes BA, Adorante JS, Miller SS, Lin H: Apical electrogenic NaHCO3 cotransport: A mechanism for HCO3 absorption across the retinal pigment epithelium. *J Gen Physiol* 1989; 94(1):125–150.

42. Hughes BA, Miller SS, Machen TE: Effects of cyclic AMP on fluid absorption and ion transport across frog retinal pigment epithelium. Measurements in the open-circuit state. *J Gen Physiol* 1984; 83(6):875–899.

43. Hughes BA, Miller SS, Joseph DP, Edelman JL: cAMP stimulates the Na+-K+ pump in frog retinal pigment epithelium. *Am J Physiol* 1988; 254(1):C84–C98.

44. Hughes BA, Shaikh A, Ahmad A: Effects of Ba2+ and Cs+ on apical membrane K+ conductance in toad retinal pigment epithelium. *Am J Physiol* 1995; 268(5):C1164–C1172.

45. Hughes BA, Steinberg RH: Voltage-dependent currents in isolated cells of the frog retinal pigment epithelium. *J Physiol* 1990; 428:273–297.

46. Hughes BA, Takahira M: Inwardly rectifying K+ currents in isolated human retinal pigment epithelial cells. *Invest Ophthalmol Vis Sci* 1996; 37(6):1125–1139.

47. Hughes BA, Takahira M: ATP-dependent regulation of inwardly rectifying K+ current in bovine retinal pigment epithelial cells. *Am J Physiol* 1998; 275(5):C1372–C1383.

48. Hughes BA, Takahira M, Segawa Y: An outwardly rectifying K⁺ current active near resting potential in human retinal pigment epithelial cells. *Am J Physiol* 1995; 269(1):C179–C187.

49. Jaffe GJ, Burke JM, Geroski DH: Ouabain-sensitive Na⁺-K⁺ ATPase pumps in cultured human retinal pigment epithelium. *Exp Eye Res* 1989; 48(1):61–68.

50. Jentsch TJ, Stein V, Weinreich F, Zdebik AA: Molecular structure and physiological function of chloride channels. *Physiol Rev* 2002; 82(2):503–568.

51. Joseph DP, Miller SS: Apical and basal membrane ion transport mechanisms in bovine retinal pigment epithelium. *J Physiol* 1991; 435:439–463.

52. Kawasaki K, Mukoh S, Yonemura D, Fujii S, Segawa Y: Acetazolamide-induced changes of the membrane potentials of the retinal pigment epithelial cell. *Doc Ophthalmol* 1986; 63(4):375–381.

53. Keller SK, Jentsch TJ, Janicke I, Wiederholt M: Regulation of intracellular pH in cultured bovine retinal pigment epithelial cells. *Pflugers Arch* 1988; 411(1):47–52.

54. Keller SK, Jentsch TJ, Koch M, Wiederholt M: Interactions of pH and K⁺ conductance in cultured bovine retinal pigment epithelial cells. *Am J Physiol* 1986; 250(1):C124–C137.

55. Kennedy BG: Na⁺-K⁺-Cl⁻ cotransport in cultured cells derived from human retinal pigment epithelium. *Am J Physiol* 1990; 259(1):C29–C34.

56. Kennedy BG: Volume regulation in cultured cells derived from human retinal pigment epithelium. *Am J Physiol* 1994; 266(3 Pt 1):C676–C683.

57. Kennedy BG, Mangini NJ: Plasma membrane calcium-ATPase in cultured human retinal pigment epithelium. *Exp Eye Res* 1996; 63(5):547–556.

58. Kenyon E, Maminishkis A, Joseph DP, Miller SS: Apical and basolateral membrane mechanisms that regulate pHi in bovine retinal pigment epithelium. *Am J Physiol* 1997; 273(2):C456–C472.

59. Kenyon E, Yu K, La Cour M, Miller SS: Lactate transport mechanisms at apical and basolateral membranes of bovine retinal pigment epithelium. *Am J Physiol* 1994; 267(6):C1561–C1573.

60. Khatami M: Na⁺-linked active transport of ascorbate into cultured bovine retinal pigment epithelial cells: Heterologous inhibition by glucose. *Membr Biochem* 1987; 7(2):115–130.

61. Konari K, Sawada N, Zhong Y, Isomura H, Nakagawa T, Mori M: Development of the blood-retinal barrier in vitro: Formation of tight junctions as revealed by occludin and ZO-1 correlates with the barrier function of chick retinal pigment epithelial cells. *Exp Eye Res* 1995; 61(1):99–108.

62. Kniesel U, Wolburg H: Tight junction complexity in the retinal pigment epithelium of the chicken during development. *Neurosci Lett* 1993; 149(1):71–74.

63. Korte GE, Wanderman MC: Distribution of Na⁺ K⁺-ATPase in regenerating retinal pigment epithelium in the rabbit: A study by electron microscopic cytochemistry. *Exp Eye Res* 1993; 56(2):219–229.

64. Kusaka S, Horio Y, Fujita A, Matsushita K, Inanobe A, Gotow T, Uchiyama Y, Tano Y, Kurachi Y: Expression and polarized distribution of an inwardly rectifying K⁺ channel, Kir4.1, in rat retinal pigment epithelium. *J Physiol* 1999; 520(2):373–381.

65. Kusaka S, Inanobe A, Fujita A, Makino Y, Tanemoto M, Matsushita K, Tano Y, Kurachi Y: Functional Kir7.1 chan-nels localized at the root of apical processes in rat retinal pigment epithelium. *J Physiol* 2001; 531(1):27–36.

66. La Cour M: The retinal pigment epithelium controls the potassium activity in the subretinal space. *Acta Ophthalmol Suppl* 1985; 173:9–10.

67. La Cour M: Rheogenic sodium-bicarbonate co-transport across the retinal membrane of the frog retinal pigment epithelium. *J Physiol* 1989; 419:539–553.

68. La Cour M: pH homeostasis in the frog retina: the role of Na⁺:HCO₃⁻ co-transport in the retinal pigment epithelium. *Acta Ophthalmol (Copenh)* 1991; 69(4):496–504.

69. La Cour M: Kinetic properties and Na⁺ dependence of rheogenic Na⁽⁺⁾-HCO₃⁻ co-transport in frog retinal pigment epithelium. *J Physiol* 1991; 439:59–72.

70. La Cour M: Cl⁻ transport in frog retinal pigment epithelium. *Exp Eye Res* 1992; 54(6):921–931.

71. La Cour M, Lin H, Kenyon E, Miller SS: Lactate transport in freshly isolated human fetal retinal pigment epithelium. *Invest Ophthalmol Vis Sci* 1994; 35(2):434–442.

72. La Cour M, Lund-Andersen H, Zeuthen T: Potassium transport of the frog retinal pigment epithelium: autoregulation of potassium activity in the subretinal space. *J Physiol* 1986; 375:461–479.

73. Lasansky A, De Fisch FW: Potential, current, and ionic fluxes across the isolated retinal pigment epithelium and choriod. *J Gen Physiol* 1966; 49(5):913–924.

74. Li JD, Govardovskii VI, Steinberg RH: Light-dependent hydration of the space surrounding photoreceptors in the cat retina. *Vis Neurosci* 1994; 11:743–752.

75. Lin H, La Cour M, Andersen MV, Miller SS: Proton-lactate cotransport in the apical membrane of frog retinal pigment epithelium. *Exp Eye Res* 1994; 59(6):679–688.

76. Lin H, Miller SS: pHi regulation in frog retinal pigment epithelium: two apical membrane mechanisms. *Am J Physiol* 1991; 261(1):C132–C142.

77. Lin H, Miller SS: pHi-dependent Cl-HCO₃ exchange at the basolateral membrane of frog retinal pigment epithelium. *Am J Physiol* 1994; 266(4):C935–C945.

78. Maminishkis A, Jalickee S, Blaug SA, Rymer J, Yerxa BR, Peterson WM, Miller SS: The P2Y(2) receptor agonist INS37217 stimulates RPE fluid transport in vitro and retinal reattachment in rat. *Invest Ophthalmol Vis Sci* 2002; 43(11):3555–3566.

79. Mangini NJ, Haugh-Scheidt L, Valle JE, Cragoe EJ Jr, Ripps H, Kennedy BG: Sodium-calcium exchanger in cultured human retinal pigment epithelium. *Exp Eye Res* 1997; 65(6):821–834.

80. Marmor MF: Mechanisms of fluid accumulation in retinal edema. *Doc Ophthalmol* 1999; 97(3–4):239–249.

81. Marmorstein AD: The polarity of the retinal pigment epithelium. *Traffic* 2001; 2(12):867–872.

82. Marmorstein AD, Finnemann SC, Bonilha VL, Rodriguez-Boulan E: Morphogenesis of the retinal pigment epithelium: Toward understanding retinal degenerative diseases. *Ann N Y Acad Sci* 1998; 857:1–12.

83. Maruiwa F, Naoi N, Nakazaki S, Sawada A: Effects of bicarbonate ion on chick retinal pigment epithelium: membrane potentials and light-evoked responses. *Vision Res* 1999; 39(1):159–167.

84. McGrail KM, Sweadner KJ: Immunofluorescent localization of two different Na,K-ATPases in the rat retina and in identified dissociated retinal cells. *J Neurosci* 1986; 6(5):1272–1283.

85. Mergler S, Steinhausen K, Wiederholt M, Strauss O: Altered regulation of L-type channels by protein kinase C and protein tyrosine kinases as a pathophysiologic effect in retinal degeneration. *Faseb J* 1998; 12(12):1125–1134.

86. Mergler S, Strauss O: Stimulation of L-type Ca^{2+} channels by increase of intracellular InsP3 in rat retinal pigment epithelial cells. *Exp Eye Res* 2002; 74(1):29–40.

87. Miller SS, Edelman JL: Active ion transport pathways in the bovine retinal pigment epithelium. *J Physiol* 1990; 424:283–300.

88. Miller S, Farber D: Cyclic AMP modulation of ion transport across frog retinal pigment epithelium. Measurements in the short-circuit state. *J Gen Physiol* 1984; 83(6):853–874.

89. Miller SS, Steinberg RH: Active transport of ions across frog retinal pigment epithelium. *Exp Eye Res* 1977; 25(3):235–248.

90. Miller SS, Steinberg RH: Passive ionic properties of frog retinal pigment epithelium. *J Membr Biol* 1977; 36(4):337–372.

92. Mitchell CH: Release of ATP by a human retinal pigment epithelial cell line: Potential for autocrine stimulation through subretinal space. *J Physiol* 2001; 534(1):193–202.

93. Negi A, Marmor MF: The resorption of subretinal fluid after diffuse damage to the retinal pigment epithelium. *Invest Ophthalmol Vis Sci* 1983; 24(11):1475–1479.

94. Oakley B II: Potassium and the photoreceptor-dependent pigment epithelial hyperpolarization. *J Gen Physiol* 1977; 70(4):405–425.

95. Oakley B II, Steinberg RH, Miller SS, Nilsson SE: The in vitro frog pigment epithelial cell hyperpolarization in response to light. *Invest Ophthalmol Vis Sci* 1977; 16(8):771–774.

96. Okami T, Yamamoto A, Omori K, Takada T, Uyama M, Tashiro Y: Immunocytochemical localization of Na$^+$,K$^+$-ATPase in rat retinal pigment epithelial cells. *J Histochem Cytochem* 1990; 38(9):1267–1275.

97. Ostwald TJ, Steinberg RH: Localization of frog retinal pigment epithelium Na$^+$-K$^+$ ATPase. *Exp Eye Res* 1980; 31(3):351–360.

98. Peterson WM, Meggyesy C, Yu K, Miller SS: Extracellular ATP activates calcium signaling, ion, and fluid transport in retinal pigment epithelium. *J Neurosci* 1997; 17(7):2324–2337.

99. Philp NJ, Yoon H, Grollman EF: Monocarboxylate transporter MCT1 is located in the apical membrane and MCT3 in the basal membrane of rat RPE. *Am J Physiol* 1998; 274(6 Pt 2):R1824–R1828.

100. Poyer JF, Ryan JS, Kelly ME: G protein-mediated activation of a nonspecific cation current in cultured rat retinal pigment epithelial cells. *J Membr Biol* 1996; 153(1):13–26.

101. Quinn RH, Miller SS: Ion transport mechanisms in native human retinal pigment epithelium. *Invest Ophthalmol Vis Sci* 1992; 33(13):3513–3527.

102. Quinn RH, Quong JN, Miller SS: Adrenergic receptor activated ion transport in human fetal retinal pigment epithelium. *Invest Ophthalmol Vis Sci* 2001; 42(1):255–264.

103. Rizzolo LJ: The distribution of Na$^+$,K$^+$-ATPase in the retinal pigmented epithelium from chicken embryo is polarized in vivo but not in primary cell culture. *Exp Eye Res* 1990; 51(4):435–446.

104. Rizzolo LJ: Basement membrane stimulates the polarized distribution of integrins but not the Na,K-ATPase in the retinal pigment epithelium. *Cell Regul* 1991; 2(11):939–949.

105. Rizzolo LJ: Polarization of the Na$^+$, K$^+$-ATPase in epithelia derived from the neuroepithelium. *Int Rev Cytol* 1999; 185:195–235.

106. Rizzolo LJ, Zhou S: The distribution of Na$^+$,K$^+$-ATPase and 5A11 antigen in apical microvilli of the retinal pigment epithelium is unrelated to alpha-spectrin. *J Cell Sci* 1995; 108(11):3623–3633.

107. Rosenthal R, Thieme H, Strauss O: Fibroblast growth factor receptor 2 (FGFR2) in brain neurons and retinal pigment epithelial cells act via stimulation of neuroendocrine L-type channels (Ca(v)1.3). *Faseb J* 2001; 15(6):970–977.

108. Ruiz A, Bhat SP, Bok D: Characterization and quantification of full-length and truncated Na,K-ATPase alpha 1 and beta 1 RNA transcripts expressed in human retinal pigment epithelium. *Gene* 1995; 155(2):179–184.

109. Ruiz A, Bhat SP, Bok D: Expression and synthesis of the Na,K-ATPase beta 2 subunit in human retinal pigment epithelium. *Gene* 1996; 176(1–2):237–242.

110. Ryan JS, Baldridge WH, Kelly ME: Purinergic regulation of cation conductances and intracellular Ca^{2+} in cultured rat retinal pigment epithelial cells. *J Physiol* 1999; 520 (3):745–759.

111. Ryan JS, Kelly ME: Activation of a nonspecific cation current in rat cultured retinal pigment epithelial cells: involvement of a G(alpha i) subunit protein and the mitogen-activated protein kinase signalling pathway. *Br J Pharmacol* 1998; 124(6):1115–1122.

112. Rymer J, Miller SS, Edelman JL: Epinephrine-induced increases in [Ca^{2+}](in) and KCl-coupled fluid absorption in bovine RPE. *Invest Ophthalmol Vis Sci* 2001; 42(8):1921–1929.

113. Sakai H, Saito T: Development of voltage-dependent inward currents in dissociated newt retinal pigment epithelial cells in culture. *Neuroreport* 1994; 5(8):933–936.

114. Sakai H, Saito T: Na$^+$ and Ca^{2+} channel expression in cultured newt retinal pigment epithelial cells: comparison with neuronal types of ion channels. *J Neurobiol* 1997; 32(4):377–390.

115. Segawa Y, Hughes BA: Properties of the inwardly rectifying K$^+$ conductance in the toad retinal pigment epithelium. *J Physiol* 1994; 476(1):41–53.

116. Shimura M, Kakazu Y, Oshima Y, Tamai M, Akaike N: Na$^+$,K$^+$-ATPase activity in cultured bovine retinal pigment epithelium. *Invest Ophthalmol Vis Sci* 1999; 40(1):96–104.

117. Shimura M, Yuan Y, Chang JT, Zhang S, Campochiaro PA, Zack DJ, Hughes BA: Expression and permeation properties of the K$^+$ channel Kir7.1 in the retinal pigment epithelium. *J Physiol* 2001; 531(2):329–346.

117. Stamer WD, Bok D, Hu J, Jaffe GJ, McKay BS: Aquaporin-1 channels in human retinal pigment epithelium: Role in transepithelial water movement. *Invest Ophthalmol Vis Sci* 2003; 44:2803–2808.

118. Steinberg RH: Interactions between the retinal pigment epithelium and the neural retina. *Doc Ophthalmol* 1985; 60(4):327–446.

119. Steinmetz RL, Fitzke FW, Bird AC: Treatment of cystoid macular edema with acetazolamide in a patient with serpiginous choroidopathy. *Retina* 1991; 11(4):412–415.

120. Strauss O, Buss F, Rosenthal R, Fischer D, Mergler S, Stumpff F, Thieme H: Activation of neuroendocrine L-type channels (alpha1D subunits) in retinal pigment epithelial cells and brain neurons by pp60(c-src). *Biochem Biophys Res Commun* 2000; 270(3):806–810.

121. Strauss O, Mergler S, Wiederholt M: Regulation of L-type calcium channels by protein tyrosine kinase and protein kinase C in cultured rat and human retinal pigment epithelial cells. *Faseb J* 1997; 11(11):859–867.

122. Strauss O, Richard G, Wienrich M: Voltage-dependent potassium currents in cultured human retinal pigment epithelial cells. *Biochem Biophys Res Commun* 1993; 191(3):775–781.

123. Strauss O, Rosenthal R, Dey D, Beninde J, Wollmann G, Thieme H, Wiederholt M: Effects of protein kinase C on delayed rectifier K+ channel regulation by tyrosine kinase in rat retinal pigment epithelial cells. *Invest Ophthalmol Vis Sci* 2002; 43(5):1645–1654.

124. Strauss O, Steinhausen K, Mergler S, Stumpff F, Wiederholt M: Involvement of protein tyrosine kinase in the InsP3-induced activation of Ca2+-dependent Cl− currents in cultured cells of the rat retinal pigment epithelium. *J Membr Biol* 1999; 169(3):141–153.

125. Strauss O, Steinhausen K, Wienrich M, Wiederholt M: Activation of a Cl−-conductance by protein kinase-dependent phosphorylation in cultured rat retinal pigment epithelial cells. *Exp Eye Res* 1998; 66(1):35–42.

126. Strauss O, Wiederholt M, Wienrich M: Activation of Cl− currents in cultured rat retinal pigment epithelial cells by intracellular applications of inositol-1,4,5-triphosphate: Differences between rats with retinal dystrophy (RCS) and normal rats. *J Membr Biol* 1996; 151(2):189–200.

127. Strauss O, Wienrich M: Cultured retinal pigment epithelial cells from RCS rats express an increased calcium conductance compared with cells from non-dystrophic rats. *Pflugers Arch* 1993; 425(1–2):68–76.

128. Strauss O, Wienrich M: Extracellular matrix proteins as substrate modulate the pattern of calcium channel expression in cultured rat retinal pigment epithelial cells. *Pflugers Arch* 1994; 429(1):137–139.

129. Strauss O, Wienrich M: Ca2+-conductances in cultured rat retinal pigment epithelial cells. *J Cell Physiol* 1994; 160(1):89–96.

130. Strauss O, Weiser T, Wienrich M: Potassium currents in cultured cells of the rat retinal pigment epithelium. *Comp Biochem Physiol A Physiol* 1994; 109(4):975–983.

131. Sugasawa K, Deguchi J, Okami T, Yamamoto A, Omori K, Uyama M, Tashiro Y: Immunocytochemical analyses of distributions of Na, K-ATPase and GLUT1, insulin and transferrin receptors in the developing retinal pigment epithelial cells. *Cell Struct Funct* 1994; 19(1):21–28.

132. Suson JD, Burke JM: Modulation of sodium-potassium adenosine triphosphatase in cultured bovine retinal pigment epithelium by potassium. *Invest Ophthalmol Vis Sci* 1993; 34(3):694–698.

133. Takahira M, Hughes BA: Isolated bovine retinal pigment epithelial cells express delayed rectifier type and M-type K+ currents. *Am J Physiol* 1997; 273(3):C790–C803.

134. Tao Q, Kelly ME: Calcium-activated potassium current in cultured rabbit retinal pigment epithelial cells. *Curr Eye Res* 1996; 15(3):237–246.

135. Tao Q, Rafuse PE, Kelly ME: Potassium currents in cultured rabbit retinal pigment epithelial cells. *J Membr Biol* 1994; 141(2):123–138.

136. Thoreson WB, Chacko DM: Lysophosphatidic acid stimulates two ion currents in cultured human retinal pigment epithelial cells. *Exp Eye Res* 1997; 65(1):7–14.

137. Tsuboi S, Manabe R, Iizuka S: Aspects of electrolyte transport across isolated dog retinal pigment epithelium. *Am J Physiol* 1986; 250(5):F781–F784.

138. Ueda Y, Steinberg RH: Voltage-operated calcium channels in fresh and cultured rat retinal pigment epithelial cells. *Invest Ophthalmol Vis Sci* 1993; 34(12):3408–3418.

139. Ueda Y, Steinberg RH: Chloride currents in freshly isolated rat retinal pigment epithelial cells. *Exp Eye Res* 1994; 58(3):331–342.

140. Ueda Y, Steinberg RH: Dihydropyridine-sensitive calcium currents in freshly isolated human and monkey retinal pigment epithelial cells. *Invest Ophthalmol Vis Sci* 1995; 36(2):373–380.

141. Wen R, Lui GM, Steinberg RH: Whole-cell K+ currents in fresh and cultured cells of the human and monkey retinal pigment epithelium. *J Physiol* 1993; 465:121–147.

142. Wetzel RK, Arystarkhova E, Sweadner KJ: Cellular and subcellular specification of Na,K-ATPase alpha and beta isoforms in the postnatal development of mouse retina. *J Neurosci* 1999; 19(22):9878–9889.

143. Wolfensberger TJ: The role of carbonic anhydrase inhibitors in the management of macular edema. *Doc Ophthalmol* 1999; 97(3–4):387–397.

144. Wolfensberger TJ, Dmitriev AV, Govardovskii VI: Inhibition of membrane-bound carbonic anhydrase decreases subretinal pH and volume. *Doc Ophthalmol* 1999; 97(3–4):261–271.

145. Yokoyama T, Lin LR, Chakrapani B, Reddy VN: Hypertonic stress increases NaK ATPase, taurine, and myoinositol in human lens and retinal pigment epithelial cultures. *Invest Ophthalmol Vis Sci* 1993; 34(8):2512–2517.

146. Yoon H, Fanelli A, Grollman EF, Philp NJ: Identification of a unique monocarboxylate transporter (MCT3) in retinal pigment epithelium. *Biochem Biophys Res Commun* 1997; 234(1):90–94.

147. Zadunaisky JA, Kinne-Saffran E, Kinne R: A Na/H exchange mechanism in apical membrane vesicles of the retinal pigment epithelium. *Invest Ophthalmol Vis Sci* 1989; 30(11):2332–2340.

148. Zeuthen T, Hamann S, La Cour M: Cotransport of H+, lactate and H2O by membrane proteins in retinal pigment epithelium of bullfrog. *J Physiol* 1996; 497(Pt 1):3–17.

6 Functional Organization of the Retina

HELGA KOLB

THE RETINA IS A thin, filmy piece of brain tissue (in development, the retina arises as outpouching of the embryonic forebrain) that lines the inside of the eyeball (figure 6.1). It consists of millions of closely packed nerve cells arranged in layers with synaptic neuropil between the layers. The retina is the most important part of the eye, for it contains both the sensory neurons that are responsive to light and the first stages of image processing via intricate neural circuits. These circuits construct an electrical message concerning the visual scene that can be sent to the brain for further processing and visual perception. All this takes only a fraction of a second. Vision is truly a miracle of neural processing. If the retina is damaged or degenerates owing to disease, the brain centers cannot be stimulated, and the person or animal is blind.

The retina is organized the reverse of the way one might intuitively expect. The sensory cells, the photoreceptors, lie at the very back of the retina, and light rays have to pass all the way through the three layers of cells, two layers of neuropils, and the length of the photoreceptors themselves before finally finding pigment molecules to excite. The reason that the photoreceptors lie at the last level of the retina in terms of light reaching them (although we call it the first level of excitation) is that some of these important pigment-bearing membranes of the photoreceptor, known as outer segment disks, have to be in contact with the pigment epithelial layer of the eye (also brain-derived tissue). An amazing exchange of molecules has to take place between the photoreceptors and the pigment epithelium for vision to occur. The vital molecule retinal, or vitamin A, has to be passed from the pigment epithelium to the opsin molecule in the photoreceptor outer segment membranes to form the photoactive molecules in rods and cones. The vitamin A comes from the blood system, so the pigment epithelium has to be provided with a rich blood source via the choroid of the eye. Retinal lies embedded in the center of the opsin molecule, and only the complete rhodopsin molecule is reactive to photons of light (figure 6.2). A cis-trans isomerization occurs in each of the millions of rhodopsin molecules occurs on exposure to light rays, and the retinal molecule is shifted back to the pigment epithe-

lium in a different form and is there recycled to return to the opsin molecule to form new rhodopsin, ready for more photic activation. The pigment epithelium is usually a very black layer of cells owing to melanin granules contained in them (except in albino people or animals), and these pigment granules have a protective role in both absorbing stray photons that bypass the photoreceptor outer segments and masking the outer segments from too much constant light exposure. If the black retinal pigment epithelium layer and its necessary blood supply, the choroid, were to lie over photoreceptors at the front of the retina, not much light would penetrate at all to excite the photoreceptors and successive chains of neurons in the retina.

All vertebrate species have retinas that contain at least two types of photoreceptor. Simply put, rods are the photoreceptors for low-light vision, and cones are the photoreceptor type for daylight, bright-colored vision. Animal species have adapted their eyes and retinal design according to the environment in which they live. Most nonmammalian species have very well-developed cone types as their photoreceptors of choice. Most fish, frogs, turtles, and birds have very good color vision too because they have retinas that are designed to take advantage of daylight. When the time of the dinosaurs was over, possible owing to climate changes and extremely long times of darkness because the earth's atmosphere was covered with ash and dark clouds, tiny fur-covered nocturnal mammals evolved that were able to generate their own heat by well-designed blood supplies. The earliest mammals were almost certainly nocturnal and developed visual systems that were most sensitive to dim light conditions. Their visual systems were dependent on rod photoreceptor–dominated retinas. Rodents such as rats and mice today still have the early rod photoreceptor–driven retinal design. Their cones are small and slender and form only 3–5% of the photoreceptor numbers.

Most other mammals have a preponderance of rods in their retinas too, but often cones are organized in higher numbers in specialized areas of the retina to deal with aspects of their visual environment that are important for their survival. Most mammals have their eyes at the side of the head with very little binocular overlap and thus little depth perception. So most mammals have either totally unspecialized areas of retina that are nocturnal in design (rats and mice) or a partial binocularity for daylight vision with a focusing of the image to a central specialized area (area centralis) where cones and cone pathways predominate

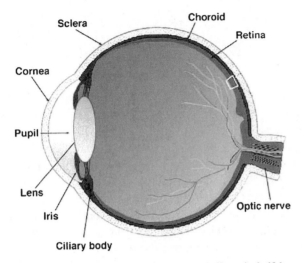

FIGURE 6.1   Schematic diagram of the eyeball cut in half longitudinally to show the various layers and structure of the human eye. The retina lines the back of the eye against the pigment epithelium and choroid. The blood supply to the retina radiates from the optic nerve; 3.5 mm temporal from the optic nerve lies the fovea which is the center of focus. The white box shows a section of retina enlarged and stained and redrawn in Figures 6.4 and 6.5.

(cats and dogs), or they have an elongated horizontal strip of specialized retina called a visual streak over which movement and fast actions of predators can be detected (rabbits, squirrels, and turtles). The ultimate in frontal projecting eyes and complete binocular overlap is achieved in some birds and primates. In these cases, the eyes are specialized for good daylight vision, color, and very fine detail discrimination. Thus, primates and raptor birds have a fovea and a foveate design of the retina.

Humans and monkeys have a retina that is specialized to have the cone-predominant daylight vision in the fovea and the rod-predominant vision for night-time sensitivity to poor lighting in the extrafoveal and peripheral parts of the retina (figure 6.3). We have what is called a duplex retina, and we can make good visual discriminations in all lighting conditions. Our retina has the ability to adapt to different lighting conditions, from using our rods at night to perceive the slightest glimmer of photons to our cones taking over in sunlight, allowing us to make color and the finest spatial discriminations. Three separate cone types in primates (red-sensitive, green-sensitive, and blue-sensitive) and two types in most mammals (green-sensitive and blue-sensitive) sense wavelength, allowing the visual system to detect color. We can see with our cone vision from gray dawn to the extreme dazzle condition of high noon with the sun burning down onto white sand. The daylight adaptation to brighter and brighter conditions takes place in the cone photoreceptors themselves initially and then by exclusive circuitry through the retina. Dark adaptation to lower and lower light

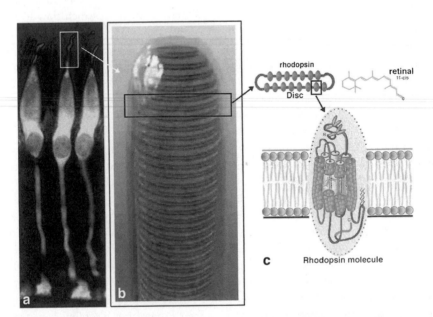

FIGURE 6.2   A, Cone photoreceptors of the monkey retina are stained by using a fluorescein-conjugated antibody to GCAP (guanylate cyclase activating protein) contained within them. B, The outer segments of the rods and cones (boxed area) are enlarged to show their interior structure of stacked doubled-over membrane disks. C, The disks contain thousands of rhodopsin molecules embedded in the lipid bilayers of the disks. Each rhodopsin molecule consists of seven transmembrane portions of the protein opsin surrounding the chromophore (11-*cis*-retinal).

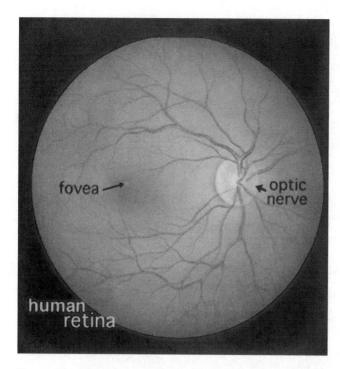

fovea →

← optic nerve

human retina

FIGURE 6.3   The human retina as seen by an ophthalmologist. The optic nerve head has an array of arteries and veins radiating from it to nourish every part of the retina. Toward the temporal side of the optic disk is the fovea, which is the center of vision and binocular overlap, specialized for high-acuity daylight vision using only cone photoreceptors.

conditions takes place in the rod photoreceptor–initiated neural circuitry through the retina. These tasks of the retina are placed on millions of nerve cells that are specifically connected into specialized neural chains that are able to influence the output of ganglion cells under constantly varying light stimuli.

The retina has four to six types of photoreceptor (dependent on species) in the photoreceptor layer, one to four types of horizontal cell and 11 types of bipolar cell in the second (inner) nuclear layer, 22 to 30 types of amacrine cell in the inner nuclear layer, and about 20 types of ganglion cells in the ganglion cell layer sending the visual messages to the brain through over a million optic nerve fibers. The photoreceptors synapse with bipolar and horizontal cell dendrites in the outer plexiform layer of neuropil, and the bipolar, amacrine, and ganglion cells talk to each other in the inner plexiform layer neuropil. To understand the shapes and sizes of the different cell types, we have had to use different staining techniques, from old-style Golgi silver staining employed originally over a hundred years ago by Ramon y Cajal to modern-day immunocytochemical or gene gun techniques. We have been able to understand how the different morphological cell types synapse on each other by examining the synaptic neuropil by electron microscopy to visualize the actual synapses. A great advance in our understanding came

with the electron microscope description of the retinal synapses by Dowling and Boycott in 1966. We could recognize different cell-specific synapses made by photoreceptor terminals on horizontal and bipolar cells and by bipolar cells on amacrine and ganglion cells. This arrangement of synapses has been extended now to include staining techniques to reveal gap (electrical) junctions and the neurotransmitter receptor molecules and neurotransmitter uptake transporters. So now we know that the neurotransmitter of the vertical pathways through the retina (photoreceptors, bipolar cells, and ganglion cells) is glutamate and the neurotransmitters of the laterally extending horizontal and amacrine cells are various excitatory and inhibitory amino acids, catecholamines, peptides, and nitric oxide (figures 6.4 and 6.5).

Electrophysiological investigations of the retina started 60 years ago. Studies of optic nerve discharges showed that indeed the optic nerve fibers could be stimulated to give traditional depolarizing spikes. However, the first recordings in the retina by Svaetichin in the 1950s showed very odd responses to light. The neurons of the outer retina (it was not immediately clear which cells were being recorded from) responded in a slow hyperpolarizing manner and not as depolarizing spikes. These "S potentials" are now known to originate with the photoreceptor and to be transmitted with relatively unchanged waveform to horizontal cells and one set of bipolar cell. The membrane hyperpolarization starts at light ON, follows the time course of the light flash, and then returns to the baseline value at light OFF. We now know that the photoreceptors, both rods and cones, release neurotransmitter during the dark, because under dark conditions, the membrane of the sensory neuron is in a depolarized state. Cyclic GMP–gated channels are open to sodium influx in the dark state. On light exposure, the rhodopsin molecules undergo their conformational change as mentioned above, and a resulting phototransduction cascade closes the membrane channels, sodium is kept out, and the membrane of the whole cell goes into a hyperpolarized state for as long as the light is present. The hyperpolarizing response can be recorded both in the outer segment of the photoreceptor by suction electrodes and in the cell body or synaptic region of the photoreceptor by sharp microelectrodes. The hyperpolarizing response of a cone has a small area over which it responds that is not much bigger than the diameter of the cone. This space over which the cone gives its response is known as its receptive field (figure 6.6).

Both rods and cones respond to light with the slow hyperpolarizing response described above, yet rods and cones report different image properties. Rod vision typically deals with a slow type of feature detection in which dim light against dark is detected. Cones deal with bright signals and can detect rapid light fluctuations. Cone system signals are

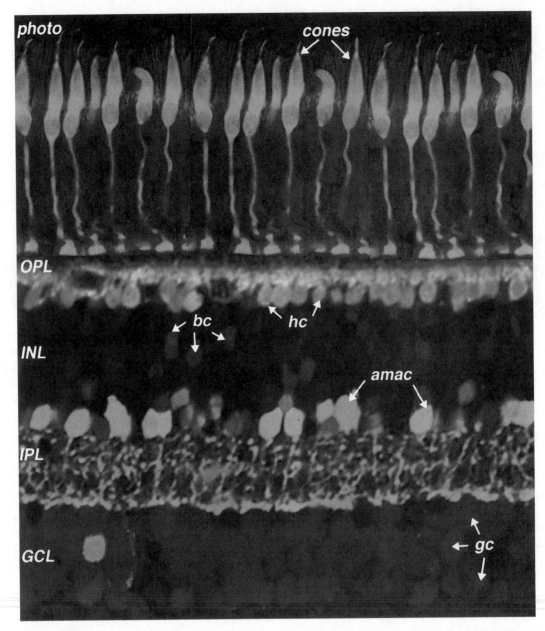

FIGURE 6.4 Immunostained monkey retina close to the fovea. Some neurons of each of the layers are immunolabeled with antibodies against GCAP (photoreceptors), calbindin (horizontal cells and some bipolar cells), calretinin (AII amacrine cells and two other varieties of amacrine cells), and parvalbumin (ganglion cells).

Photo, photoreceptor layer—rods and cones; OPL, outer plexiform layer; bc, bipolar cells; hc, horizontal cells; INL, inner nuclear layer; amac, amacrine cells; IPL, inner plexiform layer; GCL, ganglion cell layer; gc, ganglion cells. (See also color plate 1.)

revealed in forms of feature detection in which bright against dark (or vice versa) colors or edges are being detected. Thus, photoreceptors are the first neurons in the visual chain to decompose the image into separate parts. However, now the image has to be differentiated into further component elements. This happens at the first synapses of the visual pathway: the synapses between photoreceptors and bipolar cells. Here, different bipolar cell types selectively express different types of receptors for glutamate, allowing each bipolar type to respond to photoreceptor input in a different way. Some bipolar cells are tuned to faster and some to slower fluctuations in the visual signal. Electron microscopy shows that bipolar cell dendrites make different types of contact with the cone or rod synaptic region, either beneath the synaptic ribbon or at more distant basal contacts.

The types of bipolar cells that make the basal contacts express either rapidly desensitizing, rapidly resensitizing

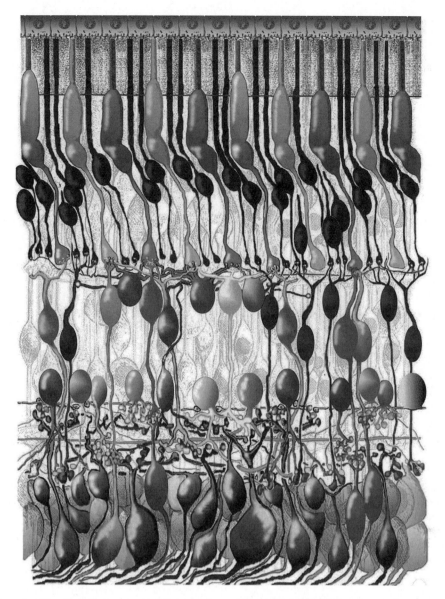

FIGURE 6.5   A drawing of a slice of the human retina showing all the nerve cells we currently understand on the basis of their shape, function, and neurocircuitry. The photoreceptors lie deep at the back of the retina against the pigment epithelial cells (top of drawing), and the ganglion cells lie at the superficial surface of the retina (bottom of drawing). Bipolar cells and horizontal and amacrine cells pack the middle of the retina with two plexiform layers dividing them, where synaptic interactions take place. (See also color plate 2.)

AMPA receptors or slowly resensitizing kainate receptors. Both of these types of receptor are excitatory and are called ionotropic glutamate receptors (iGluRs). But the most extraordinary difference between bipolar cells is that another, separate group of bipolar cells express inhibitory glutamate receptors. Inhibitory glutamate receptors known as metabotropic glutamate receptors (mGluRs) are unique to the vertebrate retinas. Typically, bipolar cells that make the central element, ribbon-related contacts with the photoreceptor synaptic terminal, use these inhibitory mGluRs. Together, these iGluR- and mGluR-expressing bipolar cells initiate a set of parallel visual pathways con-necting photoreceptors to ganglion cells, for shadow and for highlight detection. These are known as OFF (dark-on-light) and ON (light-on-dark) pathways, respectively (figure 6.7).

This parallel set of visual channels for ON and OFF qual-ities of the image are fundamental to our seeing. Our vision consists of the contrast of one image against a different background. For example, we read black letters against a white background, actually thereby using the OFF channels started in the retina. In the retina, the parallel bipolar chan-nels are maintained by segregated and parallel inputs to gan-glion cells. The architecture of the inner plexiform layer in fact becomes demarcated early in development for the

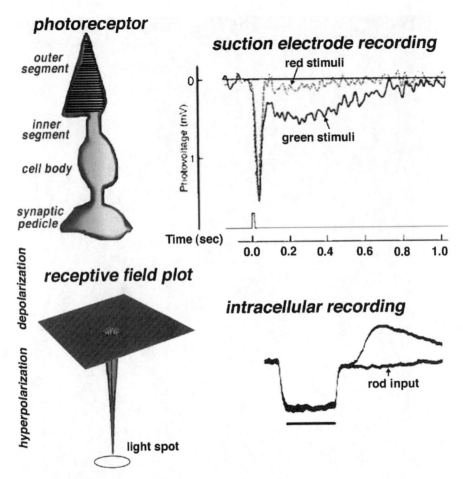

FIGURE 6.6 Physiological response of single cone photoreceptors. Suction electrodes record the response of the outer segment area. A brief light flash momentarily hyperpolarizes (by 1–2 millivolts) the cone cell's membrane. The intracellular response to a longer flash of light can be recorded in the cone cell body as a slow hyperpolarization (20 or more millivolts) that lasts as long as the light flash. Input from neighboring rods that are coupled to the cone by gap junctions can also be recorded in the cone response under certain stimulating conditions (rod input). The receptive field of a cone is very narrow and is a hyperpolarization (downward direction) of the cell's membrane potential.

segregation of synaptic input to parallel ON and OFF ganglion cell pathways. In the upper inner plexiform layer (called sublamina a), connections occur only between OFF iGluR-bearing bipolar cells and OFF ganglion cells; in the inner part of the inner plexiform layer (sublamina b), the ON mGluR-bearing bipolar cells contact solely ON ganglion cells (figure 6.8).

Thus, the parallel series of ganglion cells have been developed to receive those segregated bipolar inputs. This has happened particularly strikingly in the mammalian retina, where the same morphological type of ganglion cell has been split into two subtypes: one for the ON pathway and the other for the OFF pathway. In the cat retina, these are known as ON or OFF center alpha cells and ON or OFF center beta cells. In the human (primate), these ganglion cells are known as ON or OFF center P cells (because they project to the parvocellular layers of the lateral geniculate nucleus) and ON or OFF center M cells (because they project to the magnocellular layers of the lateral geniculate nucleus). The beta and P cells are for carrying ON and OFF views of the image to the cortex for fine detail discrimination, while the alpha and M cells inform on larger-sized, fast action ON and OFF images.

If the retina were simply to inform the brain concerning these opposite contrast images, one could imagine the resultant vision to be rather coarse-grained and blurry. How do we get our precise edges to the images and our ability to read and focus on the finest detail? This process of honing of the image and putting boundaries on it also starts in the retina and even at the first synaptic level. There are horizontal cells at the outer plexiform layer that are making their play at the ribbon synapse of the photoreceptor terminal. Here the horizontal cells receive their excitatory input from the photoreceptors; in actual fact in all species, the horizontal cells receive only input from cones. And they receive input from a lot of cones, so their collection area or receptive field is

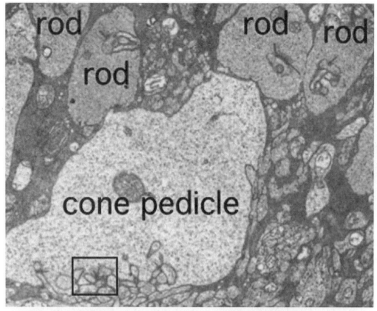

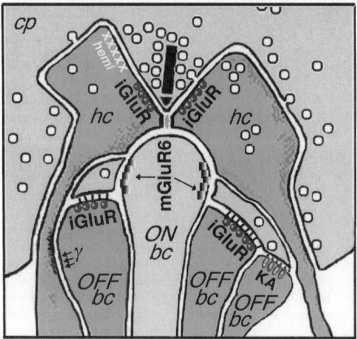

FIGURE 6.7 The photoreceptor endings (rod, cone pedicle) contact second-order neurons, with horizontal and bipolar cell dendrites, at specialized synapses. The detailed structure of the photoreceptor synapse (boxed area) can be understood only after electron microscopic investigations. The actual glutamate receptors that are known to be associated with each type of contact at the synaptic ribbon synapse (black bar) are indicated. Ionotropic glutamate receptors (iGluRs) are of two basic types, AMPA and kainate (KA), and are associated with excitatory fast transmission to OFF bipolar cells (OFF bc) and horizontal cells (hc). Metabotropic glutamate receptors (mGluR6) receptors are on ON bipolar cell dendrites (ON bc) and are associated with slow inhibitory transmission in which G proteins and second messengers are involved in transduction. Horizontal cell processes (hc) are thought to feed electrical information back to the cone synaptic area at hemi gap junctions (hemi, crosses) and to bipolar cell dendrites at GABA receptors (γ, arrows).

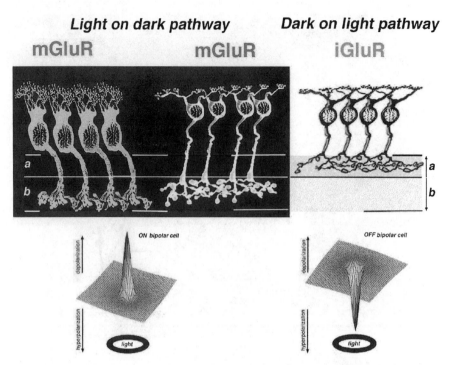

Light on dark pathway   **Dark on light pathway**

mGluR   mGluR   iGluR

FIGURE 6.8   The synaptic contact of the bipolar cell dendrites and the cone synaptic pedicle determines whether the signal carried by the bipolar cell stream is detecting light-on-dark (ON pathway) or dark-on-light (OFF pathway) to the ganglion cells. The former pathways are initiated at mGluRs and the latter at iGluRs with the cone synapse. The mGluR-containing bipolar cells send their axons to lower sublamina b of the inner plexiform layer, while the iGluR-containing bipolar cells have axons ending in upper sublamina a of the inner plexiform layer, thereby continuing segregation of the pathways into the connections with ganglion cells. The receptive fields of mGluR containing cells are ON center (depolarizing, upward-pointing response) with a surround inhibition that is OFF (hyperpolarizing, downward indentation). The receptive fields of iGluR bipolar cells is OFF center (hyperpolarizing, downward pointing) and has a surround of the opposite or ON polarity.

very large. Their collective input gives them a large hyperpolarizing slow potential response following the time course of the light ON. The size of their receptive field is very large, not only because of the large number of cones with their individual small receptive fields summating but also because horizontal cells are joined, one to another, at electrical junctions known as gap junctions. Thus, a whole sheet of cells have their membranes potential sitting at the same hyperpolarized level, and their response to light is consequently very large in area. [The receptive field is orders of magnitude large that that of a single cone and even that of the single bipolar cell, which receives input from a handful of cones and thus has a medium-size receptive field.] Remember that the bipolar cell receives either excitatory input and thus responds like the photoreceptor and horizontal cell and has a hyperpolarizing response (due to iGluRs) or gets an inhibitory input (due to mGluRs) and gives a depolarizing response to light.

So a single bipolar cells with its hyperpolarizing (OFF) or depolarizing (ON) light response would carry a fairly blurry, large-field response to its ganglion cell were it not for the horizontal cells adding an opponent surround that is spatially constrictive, puts an edge around the field, and gives the bipolar cell what is known as a center surround organization (figure 6.9). The bipolar center would be of one sign, i.e., either ON in the center, or OFF in the center, and the horizontal cell by a feedback mechanism adds an OFF or ON surround, respectively. There are two means by which the horizontal cell can add the opponent surround: either by synapsing, directly on the bipolar cell at a chemical synapse, which seems to occur in some species, or by feeding back information to the cone photoreceptor itself, and this information then feeds forward to the different varieties of bipolar cell making contact with that cone. Feedback to the cone itself is now thought to take place by a very novel electrical synapse consisting of half a gap junction. Hemi gap junctions are thought to change the ionic environment at the photoreceptor ribbon synapse and cause membrane changes in the cone photoreceptor and thence in the bipolar cell dendrite—a complicated circuit that still is a subject of hot debate in the retinal research community. Horizontal cell function in general has occupied many vision researchers for decades, and much is now known of the role of these cells in the organization of the visual message. Horizontal cells are influenced by more than photoreceptors that have input to them though. There is neuronal feedback from inner to

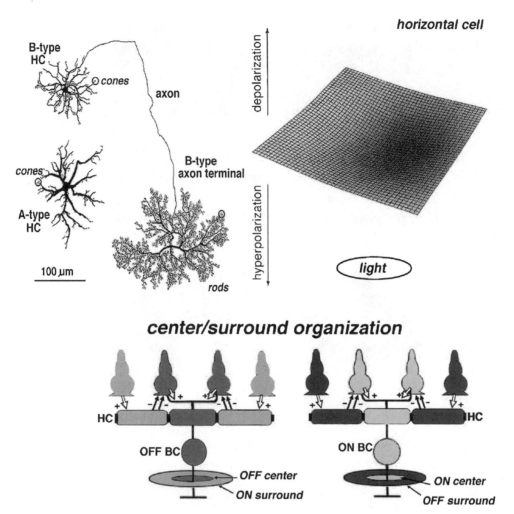

FIGURE 6.9 Cat retina (and most mammalian retinas) contains two morphological types of horizontal cell (A-type HC and B-type HC), but they serve the same purpose of interconnecting and modulating responses of photoreceptors and bipolar cells. Receptive fields of horizontal cells are very wide owing to electrical coupling between cells at gap junctions, so the spread of membrane poten-tial is hyperpolarizing (downward pointing) and large in extent. The model shows how horizontal cells feed back their wide field responses (black arrows, minus signs) to the cones to influence the bipolar cell response in the form of an inhibitory surround response to their OFF or ON center photoresponse.

outer plexiform layer influencing horizontal cell activity as well. These feedback signals are mostly chemical, coming from neuroactive substances such as dopamine, nitric oxide, and even retinoic acid. The end result is that horizontal cells modulate the photoreceptor signal under different lighting conditions in addition to shaping the receptive field of the bipolar cell response. In species in which color signals are carried by ganglion cells, the horizontal cells have a major influence on the bipolar cells, often making them color coded; again, this is all thought to take place through feedback circuits to the cones at the first synaptic level.

Now we have learned that the horizontal cell is responsible for adding the surround mechanism to the bipolar cell receptive field. This mechanism allows the two sets of cone bipolar cell channels (i.e., ON center and OFF center) to transmit their center-surround receptive field organization to the ganglion cells with which they synapse in the inner plexiform layer. The ON and OFF center ganglion cells thus have concentric receptive field organization that is often modeled as the sum of two Gaussian curves in a "Mexican hat" shape, where membrane potential and center size are the "peak" and the much wider surround of the opposite membrane potential direction is the wide "brim" of the hat (figure 6.10).

Recent research has shown that amacrine cell circuitry in the inner plexiform layer also adds information to the surround of the ganglion cell, possibly sharpening the boundary between center and surround even further than the horizontal cell input does. The pair of ON- and OFF-center, concentrically organized types of the P (beta) and M (alpha) ganglion cells are highly developed in retinas of mammals

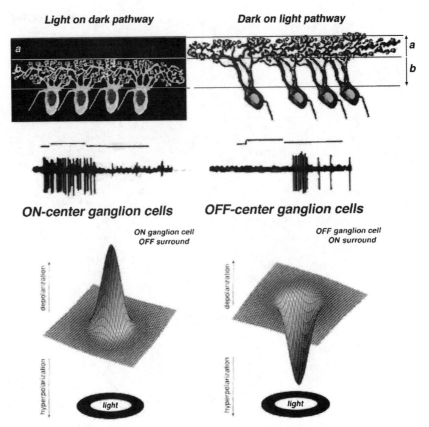

Light on dark pathway   **Dark on light pathway**

ON-center ganglion cells   **OFF-center ganglion cells**

ON ganglion cell
OFF surround

OFF ganglion cell
ON surround

FIGURE 6.10   Ganglion cells are morphologically similar but are split into two subtypes or paramorphic pairs in mammalian retinas. The types that branches in sublamina a of the inner plexiform layer receive input from iGluR-containing bipolar cells and transmit messages concerning dark on light (OFF responses). The subtypes of ganglion cell that branch in sublamina b of the inner plexiform layer receive input from mGluR-bearing bipolar cells and transmit a message concerning light on dark images (ON responses). The message that is transmitted to the brain is a burst of spikes when the light is present for ON center ganglion cells or a burst of spikes when the light terminates for OFF center ganglion cells (middle traces). Receptive fields are the "Mexican hat" shape with depolarizing membrane potentials (upward going) for ON center cells and hyperpolarizing (downward going) for OFF center cells. Both ON and OFF ganglion cells have large and strong inhibitory surrounds (downward or upward responses) in the "brim."

with area centrales or foveas. In the human retina, these two types of ganglion cell are extremely well developed and form the major output of the retina to the higher visual centers (figure 6.11). The ganglion cells of the fovea are the ultimate type of P cell. They are called midget ganglion cells because they have the minutest dendritic trees in a one-to-one connection with a single midget bipolar cell. The midget bipolar to midget ganglion cell channel carries information concerning a single cone to the brain. Because only a single cone is involved, we know that the center response of such midget bipolar and ganglion cells will be either ON or OFF center to red or green cone messages. As in the case of bipolar cells that collect from several cones (diffuse bipolar cells), midget bipolar cells come in the ON and OFF variety. Thus, from the center of our focus, the fovea, a dark on light (OFF) or light on dark (ON) message is sent to the brain for each cone. If there are 200,000 cones in the central fovea, then 400,000 midget ganglion cells are carrying their message to the brain. And the message carries both spatial and spectral informa-

tion of the finest resolution, because the message from each cone is both spectrally and spatially opponent.

Electrical recordings indicate that several varieties of ganglion cell do not appear to have the concentric organization of those described above, particularly in retinas with a nonfoveate organization. These would be in most nonmammalian species and in mammalian species that have a visual streak organization to their retinas. These latter species have a great deal more feature detection going on in the retina itself rather than postponing this finer honing of the visual message to the brain. Such species have really well developed directionally selective, motion selective edge detectors and dimming detectors already in their retinal ganglion cell responses. Also, it will be noted by the perceptive that blue cones have not been mentioned yet. The message concerning blue light is carried by a special pathway of bipolar cells to a bistratified ganglion cell type in the retina. For some reason, the blue cones are not part of the dual ON or OFF pair of midget bipolar/ganglion cell channels described

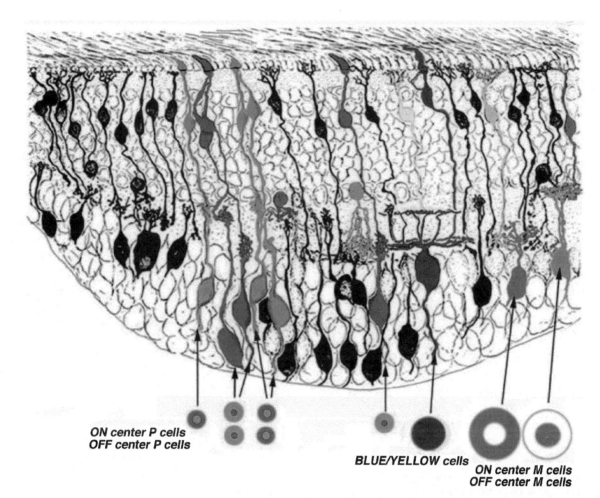

ON center P cells
OFF center P cells

BLUE/YELLOW cells

ON center M cells
OFF center M cells

FIGURE 6.11 A drawing, based on an original from Polyak (1941), showing the neurocircuitry of the fovea in the primate retina. Midget or P cell pathways consist of a single cone, two midget bipolar cells, and two midget ganglion cells. Because P cells carry information from only one cone, it will also be spectrally tuned. Red and green cones pass either ON center/OFF surround information or OFF center/ON surround information concerning which are both spectrally and spatially opponent (small red and green circles and rings). Blue cones have their own pathway through a dedicated blue ON center bipolar cell feeding to the lower dendrites of a bistratified blue/yellow ganglion cell type. The yellow message carried to the top tier of the bistratified ganglion cells dendrites comes from a diffuse bipolar cell (yellow) that contacts green and red cones. M ganglion cells of the fovea carry a message from diffuse ON center or OFF center bipolar cells (orange and brown bipolar cells) and form the parallel OFF and ON center, achromatic channels (gray and white circles and rings) concerned with movement and contrast to the brain. (See also color plate 3.)

above. The blue system is an older system in evolutionary terms. Blue cones are found in just about all species retinas. The absorption peak (428 nm) is very different from that of the red 563 nm and green 535 nm cones and so are the opsins. Color contrast between blue and the others is very strong. By contrast, the red and green are similar, and this recent evolutionary split permits fine color discrimination in the appropriate spectral regions. Even the red and green opsins are so similar in molecular design that we cannot yet make an antibody against each to separate them by immunohistochemical staining techniques. In mammals, blue and green cones are the common cone types. Color vision in most nonprimate mammals consists of contrasting blue (light on dark) against orange/green or dark shapes (dark on light) so the blue system has a more spread apart distribution and a convergent and divergent set of neural interactions. The blue system ganglion cell responds with a blue ON response and a large receptive field and gives a yellow OFF response in a spatially coextensive broad receptive field. In other words, one ganglion cell is carrying an opposite but superimposed message to the brain concerning blue and yellow—quite a different organization from the red and green midget systems!

To understand more about the organization of the ganglion cell receptive field, whether it be about concentric organization or direction and motion detection, we need to study the organization of the inner plexiform layer in detail. We need to find out what are the roles of those 22-plus different varieties of amacrine cell making their synaptic connections with 20 or more different types of ganglion cells here. Although it was clear from the time of Cajal's description in the nineteenth century that amacrine, ganglion, and bipolar cell dendrites and axons were organized into layers of intermeshing processes (Cajal divided the inner plexiform layer neuropil into five different strata of layering of processes), we could not immediately figure out what this meant and what sort of synapses were going on between the layered and opposed processes. Using the electron microscope, we began to unravel this neurocircuitry. We now know something of the input/output relationships of nine different types of bipolar cell, 14 different types of amacrine cell, and eight different types of ganglion cell, so we are halfway to the goal of understanding the neural interplay between all the nerve cells of the retina. In the neuropil of the inner plexiform layer with the higher magnification of the electron microscope, we can recognize bipolar cell axons by their containing a synaptic ribbon and the amacrine cells on their vesicle clusters at synaptic sites (figure 6.12).

Much has been learned of the types of neurochemicals that are contained within different amacrine cells and the organization of receptors at the different synapses. Glutamate receptors between bipolar cells and ganglion cells are both NMDA and AMPA types, and amacrine cells are about equally divided between those that use glycine and those that use GABA inhibitory neurotransmitters.

Glycinergic amacrine cells are typically small field. Their processes are usually full of appendages and lobules that are able to spread interactions vertically across several of the five strata in the inner plexiform layer. Glycinergic amacrine cells mostly make a lot of synapses between bipolar axons in either the OFF layer or the ON layer and feed forward synapses to ganglion cell dendrites and other bipolar and amacrine cells. Some glycinergic amacrine cells cross the two major OFF and ON sublaminae of the inner plexiform to provide interconnections between ON and OFF systems of bipolar and ganglion cells. The most famous of these small bilaminar, glycinergic amacrine cells is called the AII cell. The AII cell together with a wide-field GABAergic amacrine cell called A17 is pivotal in the connectivity of the rod pathways to ganglion cells and in the circuitry of rod or dim light vision in the mammalian retina. Both these "rod" amacrine cell types are not found in nonmammalian species or in mammalian species that are diurnal and contain very few rods in their retinas (squirrels, for example).

When we considered the ON and OFF channels and their separate connectivity through different receptor contacts at the cone synapses (mGluR- and iGluR-driven bipolar cells) and their spatial segregation to the ON and OFF ganglion cell types, we neglected to talk about the connections of the mGluR-driven rod bipolar cells. The reason is that, unlike the direct pipeline from cone to ganglion cell for the cone-driven ON or OFF channels, rod bipolar cells do not synapse with ganglion cells at all. These bipolar cells, and there is only one type that contains an mGluR receptor and hence

is an ON type, uses the glycinergic AII and the GABAergic A17 amacrine cells as intermediaries to get rod information to ganglion cells. The small field AII cell collects rod messages from a group of approximately 30 axon terminals in the ON sublamina of the inner plexiform layer and passes this rod sensitivity depolarizing message through a gap junction with ON cone bipolar cells to ON ganglion cells. At the same time, the AII passes rod information to the OFF system cone bipolars and ganglion cells via direct chemical inhibitory synapses at their lobular appendages in the OFF sublamina of the inner plexiform layer. The AII amacrine cell seems to have been developed in the rod-dominated parts of mammalian retinas as an afterthought to the original direct cone-to-ganglion cell architecture. The rod system has inserted the new amacrine cells to piggyback on the original cone system connections (figure 6.13).

At the same time, the A17 amacrine cell is also collecting rod messages from, in this case, thousands of rod bipolar axons to amplify and feed this information back into the AII to cone bipolar–ganglion cell route. How it does this is not completely understood yet, although we know this GABAergic wide-field amacrine type uses the novel GABAc (rho) receptor to feed back on rod bipolar axons, thus presumably influencing the whole state of the rod system. The rod pathway with its series of convergent and then divergent intermediary neurons in the retina is clearly well designed to collect and amplify on widely scattered vestiges of light in night and twilight vision. The rod pathways are solely ON system neural chains that is, designed to detect light on dark only.

GABA is commonly the neurotransmitter used by wide-field amacrine cells that stretch laterally across the inner plexiform layers for hundreds of microns and can interact with hundreds of bipolar cells and many ganglion cells. Such amacrine cells are usually stratified in one of the five different strata of the retina in beautifully organized mosaics of elegant meshworks of dendrites (figure 6.14).

Their synaptic interactions would be with other neurons branching in the same layer or stratum. Frequently, GABAergic amacrine cells with rather simple, sparsely branching dendritic trees connect to neighboring homologous amacrine cells by gap junctions, thus increasing their field of influence and speed of transmission of signals across large areas of retina. In many instances, wide-field GABAergic amacrine cells send out even farther-reaching axonlike processes to other layers of the inner plexiform or to the inner nuclear and outer plexiform layers and the blood vessels of the retina. Most GABAergic amacrine cells in the retina contain at least one other neuroactive substance besides GABA. The secondary neuroactive substance is usually acting as a neuromodulator rather than a fast neurotransmitter. The peptides substance P, somatostatin, vasointestinal peptide, and cholecystokinin have been associated with such amacrine cells, as have serotonin,

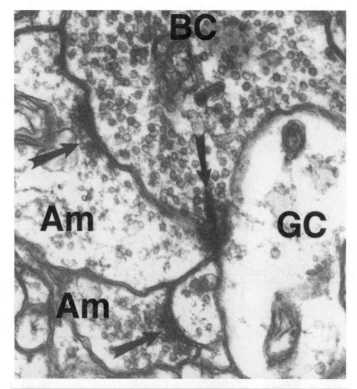

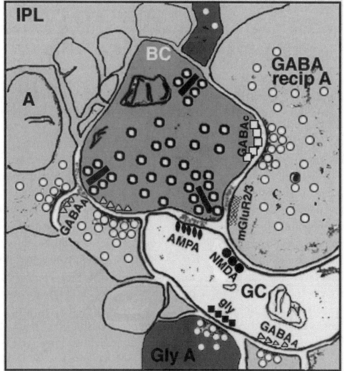

FIGURE 6.12 The synaptic connections of the different nerve cell types in the inner plexiform layer has to be studied by electron microscopy. Bipolar cells (BC) are detected by their containing a synaptic ribbon pointing to synaptic output sites, commonly consisting of a ganglion cell dendrite (GC) and an amacrine cell process (Am). Amacrine cells synapse on bipolar cells, other amacrine cells, and ganglion cells (clusters of vesicles at synaptic sites). The types of receptors for the neurotransmitter glutamate in bipolar cells and glycine and GABA in amacrine cells have now been described for such synaptic circuitry. For glutamate transmission, mGluRs and the iGluRs AMPA and NMDA are present on ganglion cell and amacrine cell dendrites. For amacrine cells, glycine receptors and GABA$_A$, GABA$_B$, and GABA$_C$ have been detected on bipolar, amacrine, and ganglion cell dendrites.

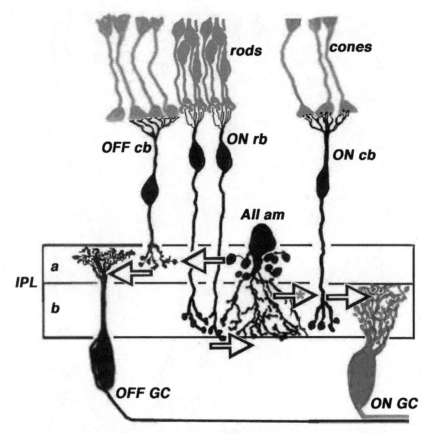

FIGURE 6.13 Summary of the rod pathways through the mammalian retina and how the AII amacrine cell piggybacks on the cone pathways because the rod bipolar cells do not have direct synapses on a ganglion cell of any type. The AII amacrine cell receives input from rod bipolar axons (ON rb) and passes that information to OFF cone bipolar (OFF cb) and OFF ganglion cells (OFF GC) at glycinenergic chemical synapses (large open arrows). The AII amacrine cells contacts ON cone bipolar cells (ON cb) at gap junctions (large arrow, asterisk), and the electrical message is passed to the ganglion cells that those cone bipolar cells contact (ON GC, large arrow).

dopamine, acetylcholine, and adenososine. Nitric oxide has been localized to certain wide-field amacrines as well. Peptidergic, nicotinic, and muscarinic receptors in addition to different varieties of GABA$_A$, GABA$_B$, and GABA$_C$ receptors have all been found on ganglion and bipolar cells, indicating that such neuroactive agents in amacrine cells are influencing the organization of the ganglion cell receptive field. Most of these neuromodulators are not released at conventional synapses, though, and their release is thought to influence neurons even at a distance by diffusion in a "paracrine" manner. We have discovered that frequently, the role of such neuromodulators in the retina is to influence the retinal circuitry under changing lighting conditions or even to stabilize activity to different times of day in the circadian clock.

Dopamine is released from a specialized amacrine cell on stimulation of the retina by intermittent light flashing. Dopamine influences horizontal cell activity by uncoupling the gap junctions between these cell types, thus reducing their effective receptive field sizes and consequent expression of surround size on bipolar cells. Dopamine also directly affects the glutamate receptor on horizontal cells so that the amplitude of the photoresponse is reduced under different light conditions. In the inner plexiform layer, dopamine is particularly effective on gap junctions again, but this time on the gap junctions that join the AII amacrine cell in large coupled networks in the dark state. Light causes dopamine release, which by diffusion to the lower inner plexiform neuropil affects the gap junctions between neighboring AII cell distal processes. This uncoupling of AIIs from their dark network makes the effective field of influence of the rod system amacrine cell much less significant in the light. Any large-field rod pathway interference in the direct cone pathways is thereby removed. Similarly, another wide-field amacrine cell branching in the center of the inner plexiform neuropil releases nitric oxide, which uncouples the AII cell and the ON cone bipolar cell system at that particularly gap junction (figure 6.15). Again this has an additive effect to that of dopamine of removing the rod system neurons from the cone system direct pipeline to ganglion cells, thereby helping to make the operative image in bright light conditions a high-contrast, high-acuity signal (figure 6.16).

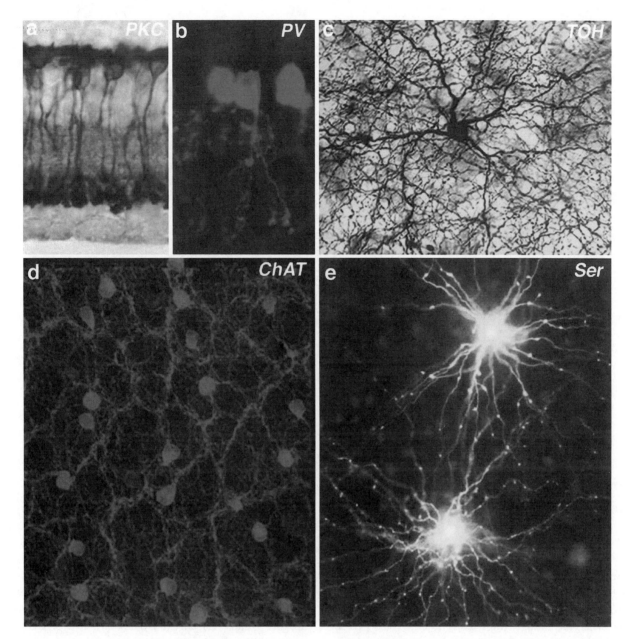

FIGURE 6.14 A, An immunostained image of rod bipolar cells immunostained with antibodies against protein kinase c (PKC). B, Small-field bistratified AII amacrine cells are immunostained with antibodies to parvalbumin (PV). C, Dopamine-containing cells are immunostained with antibodies to tyrosine hydroxylase (TOH) as seen in a flat mount of the retina. Thousands of dopamine cell processes cross each other and make a dense network of processes in the top part of the inner plexiform layer, to synapse on various cell types, among them the AII amacrine cell. D, Two mirror symmetric amacrine cell populations, known as starburst cells, are immunostained for their acetylcholine neurotransmitter (ChAT) and seen in flat mount of retina. One set of starburst cells sits in the ganglion cell layer, and the other sits in the amacrine cell layer. Their respective dendritic plexi run and synapse in sublamina b and sublamina a. Starburst amacrine cells are thought to influence ganglion cells to be able to transmit messages concerning direction of movement in the visual field. These cells are particularly well developed in animals with visual streaks in their retinas. E, A17 amacrine cells immunolabeled with antibodies to serotonin (Ser) and also to GABA. A17 cells connect rod bipolar axon terminals in reciprocal GABAc receptor–activated circuits across the entire retina. (E from Vaney DI: Many diverse types of retinal neurons show tracer coupling when injected with biocytin or Neurobiotin. *Vision Res* 1998; 38:1359–1369.) (See also color plate 4.)

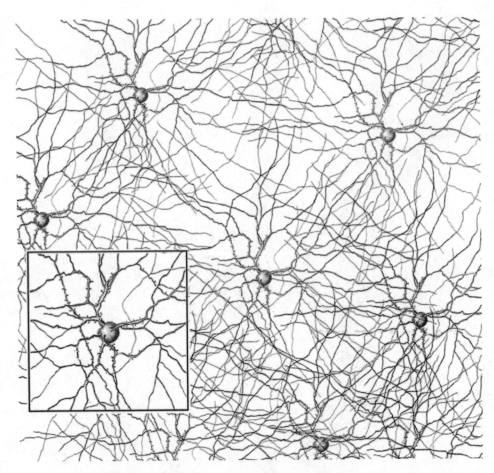

FIGURE 6.15   Nitric oxide–containing amacrine cells form a beautiful network of processes across the middle of the inner plexiform layer to influence various nerve cells penetrating this network and making synapses or gap junctions in this area of neuropil. The NO-containing amacrine cells also contain GABA as their conventional inhibitory chemical messenger.

So, as can be seen from the above broad sketch of retinal circuitry and modes of action of the nerve cells into systematically organized pathways, the retina is surprisingly more complex than was initially thought, and its function takes on an increasingly more active role in visual perception than was originally thought. Although we do not fully understand the neural code that is sent as trains of spikes through the ganglion cell axons to the central brain areas, we are coming close to understanding how consorts of ganglion cells respond differently to different aspects of the visual scene and how receptive fields of influence on particular ganglion cells are constructed. It seems that much construction of the visual image does take place in the retina itself, although the final consequence, "seeing," is indisputably done by the brain. Are we finished with the retina? Do we know all that we need to know to understand the first stages if vision, or are there more surprises on the horizon? Earlier surprises included finding that so much information transfer rested on electrical connections over standard chemical synapses. The major rod pathway is dependent in large part on electrical connections to get information through the retina. Some other fast-acting amacrine pathways also use direct access to ganglion cell at gap junctions. Neuromodulators and gases change the milieu of circuits of neurons but act from a far distance by diffusion rather than at closely apposed synapses. Again this is a new and surprising concept compared to our older view that all neural interactions took place at specialized isolated patches of membrane apposition known as synapses by packaged neurotransmitter substances. The most recent surprise has been the revelation of a new ganglion cell type in the retina that appears to be able to function as a giant photoreceptor itself and needs no rod or cone bipolar inputs to drive it. This ganglion cell's membrane contains photoactive molecules known as melanopsins, so this ganglion cell can respond to light in the absence of neural circuitry.

In conclusion, we have certainly come far in our understanding of the organization of this piece of the brain, the retina, in the last half century. However, we cannot rest on our laurels. We still undoubtedly have much more to learn about how the retina creates the first steps of our visual perception—"seeing."

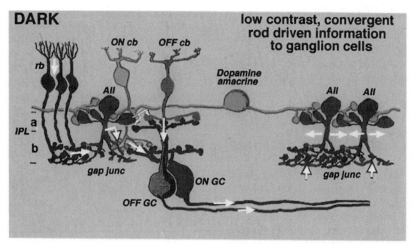

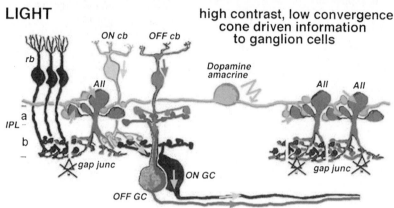

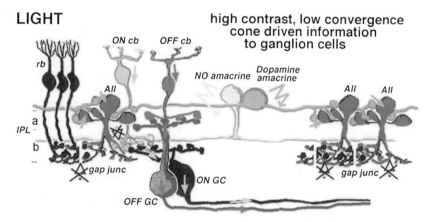

FIGURE 6.16   The retinal circuits that are thought to influence the ganglion cell message to the brain concerning low light vision and bright light vision. The AII amacrine cell is driven in the dark to pass messages to both ON and OFF center ganglion cells about very low light levels. The whole network of involved neurons is designed to be very wide-field and to collect every glimmer of light through convergence, divergence, and further convergence of information. Gap junctions between AII cells allows the spread of rod-driven messages over large areas of retina together with the A17 cells' convergent input (not shown in this figure). In the light,

the dopamine amacrine cell releases dopamine, and this uncouples the AII cell from its electrical network; thus, information through the cone bipolar to ganglion cell pathways is less convergent, narrower in field, with sharp edge contrast and concerned more with only bright, cone-initiated messages. At the same time, amacrine cells containing nitric oxide (NO) as a neurotransmitter release this nitric oxide to sever the gap junction between AII amacrine cells and ON cone bipolar cells, thus contributing to the high-contrast, narrow cone-driven messages reaching ganglion cells.

REFERENCES

1. Cajal SR: *The Structure of the Retina*, translated by SA Thorpe and M Glickstein. Springfield, Ill., Thomas, 1972 (1892).

2. Dowling JE: *The Retina: An Approachable Part of the Brain.* Cambridge, Mass., Belknap Press of Harvard U. Press, 1987.

3. Dowling JE, Boycott BB: Organization of the primate retina: Electron microscopy. *Proc R Soc* 1966; B166:80–111.

4. Hattar S, Liao H-W, Takao M, Berson DM, Yau K-W: Melanopsin-containing retinal ganglion cells: Architecture, projections, and intrinsic photosensitivity. *Science* 2002; 295:1065–1070.

5. Kolb H, Famiglietti EV: Rod and cone pathways in the inner plexiform layer of the cat retina. *Science* 1974; 186:47–49.

6. Kolb H, Nelson R, Ahnelt P, Cuenca N: Cellular organization of the vertebrate retina. In Kolb H, Ripps H, Wu S (eds): *Concepts and Challenges in Retinal Biology: A Tribute to John E. Dowling.* New York, Elsevier Press, 2001, pp 3–26.

7. Kolb H, Fernandez E, Nelson R: Webvision: The Organization of the Retina and Visual System. Available at: www.webvision.med.utah.edu.

8. Liebman PA, Parker KR, Dratz EA: The molecular mechanism of visual excitation and its relation to the structure and composition of the rod outer segment. *Ann Rev Physiol* 1987; 49:765–791.

9. Nelson R, Famiglietti EV, Kolb H: Intracellular staining reveals different levels of stratification for on-center and off-center ganglion cells in the cat retina. *J Neurophysiol* 1978; 41:427–483.

10. Polyak SL: *The Retina.* Chicago, University of Chicago Press, 1941.

11. Rodieck RW: *The First Steps in Seeing.* Sunderland, Mass., Sinauer Associates Inc., 1998.

12. Vaney DI: Many diverse types of retinal neurons show tracer coupling when injected with biocytin or Neurobiotin. *Neurosci Lett* 1991; 125:187–190.

13. Vardi N, Morigiwa K, Wang T-L, Shi Y-J, Sterling P: Neurochemistry of the mammalian cone "synaptic complex." *Vision Res* 1998; 38:1359–1369.

14. Wässle H: Glycine and GABA receptors in the mammalian retina. *Vision Res* 1998; 38:1411–1430.

7 Phototransduction and Photoreceptor Physiology

W. CLAY SMITH

Photoreceptors

Vision begins in the photoreceptors of the retina, where light energy is absorbed and converted to a neural response, a process known as phototransduction. In vertebrates, this process occurs in two classes of photoreceptors: rods and cones, which function in dim and bright light, respectively. Both rods and cones are polarized, having two biochemically and morphologically distinct compartments: the inner segment and the outer segment (figure 7.1).

The outer segment (OS) of photoreceptors is composed of a dense packing of disk-shaped membranes. In rods, these disks are pinched off from the plasma membrane. In cones, the disks form as invaginations of the plasma membrane, as in rods, but are not pinched off and maintain their continuity with the plasma membrane. These disks contain a very high concentration of the visual pigment rhodopsin, accounting for one third of the dry weight of the OS. In addition to rhodopsin, the OS are rich in proteins necessary for the visual transduction pathway as well as structural proteins responsible for maintaining the organization of the OS.

The inner segment contains the metabolic and synthetic machinery of the cell. The distal end of the inner segment, known as the ellipsoid, contains a dense packing of mitochondria. The mitochondria provide the substantial energy required by photoreceptors. For a dark-adapted rod, this requirement has been estimated at 90,000 ATP molecules per second per cell, ranking it as one of the most energetically demanding cells of the entire body. The proximal inner segment, known as the myoid, contains the synthetic machinery of the cell, including the endoplasmic reticulum and Golgi complex. Although responsible for providing all the photoreceptor components, the synthetic machinery is largely devoted to producing rhodopsin-containing vesicles to replace the disk membranes that are continuously phagocytosed at the distal end by the retinal pigmented epithelium.[91]

The inner and outer segments of rod and cone photoreceptors are connected by a narrow cilium through which must pass all components that travel between the segments (figure 7.2). The basic structure of the cilium is typical of nonmotile sensory cells, containing a "$9 \times 2 + 0$" arrange-

ment of microtubule doublets that extends from the basal body in the inner segment into the outer segment. The microtubule doublet composition is quickly lost within the proximal outer segment with the microtubules projecting as singlets into the distal outer segment, stopping short of the extreme distal tip.[13,31,69,82] This structure is collectively known as the axoneme and provides a cytoskeletal framework for structural support and for transporting molecules between the photoreceptor compartments using kinesin and dynein motors.[46,79,84,86] Microtubules are also abundant in the inner segment, functioning in the transport of macromolecular components from the endoplasmic reticulum and Golgi complex to the connecting cilium. The microtubules that form the axoneme contain acetylated tubulin and are thus more stable than the inner segment microtubules.[6,70] Microtubules also run the length of rod OS along the multiple incisures of the disks. These incisures are invaginations along the outer edge of the disks in rods and likely have a structural role. Interestingly, the number of incisures is quite variable between species, ranging from just one or a few invaginations in rodents and cows to several dozen in frogs and primates (summarized in Ref. 19).

In addition to microtubules, the photoreceptor cytoskeleton also utilizes microfilaments.[10,11,26,87] In the connecting cilium, these microfilaments have myosin VIIa associated with them, suggesting that they are not simply structural elements, but also function in moving cellular contents.[12,89] In addition to the connecting cilium, microfilaments are also found in calycal processes. These processes are fingerlike extensions of the inner segment that project around the basal portion of the OS. The calycal processes often align with the grooves formed by the multiple incisures in the OS disks.[87]

There are two broad classes of cargoes that move through the connecting cilium: biosynthetic cargo destined for the outer segment (for example, phospholipid membranes and visual pigment) and proteins that show substantial intersegmental redistribution in response to light. How some of these cargoes utilize the ciliary cytoskeleton is beginning to be revealed. Recent studies have shown that kinesin II is a motor protein that is located in the cilium[84] and is at least involved in the transport of opsin-containing vesicles to the outer

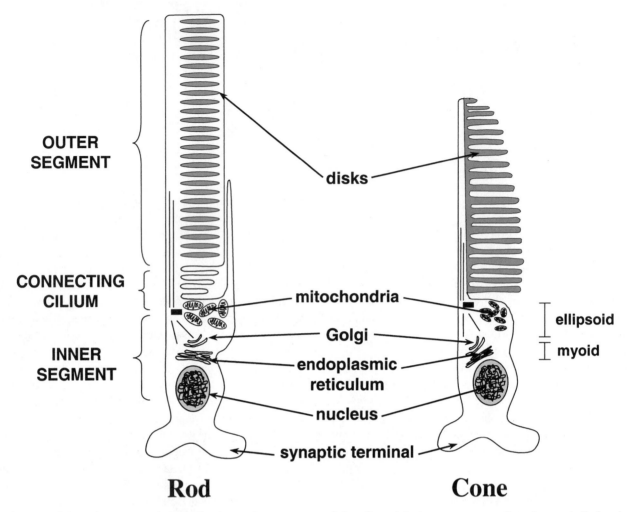

OUTER SEGMENT

CONNECTING CILIUM

INNER SEGMENT

disks

mitochondria

Golgi

endoplasmic reticulum

nucleus

synaptic terminal

ellipsoid

myoid

Rod

Cone

FIGURE 7.1 Schematic representation of rod and cone photoreceptors. The outer segments contain the phototransduction machinery of the cells, and the inner segments perform the metabolic functions of the cells. The two compartments are joined by the connecting cilia.

segment.[46,86] A similar role for myosin VIIa has also been demonstrated, although how the two motor proteins function together, whether in parallel or in series, is uncertain.[38,39,86,89] Additionally, an intraflagellar transport (IFT) particle has been identified in photoreceptor cilia, much like the IFT particles in the sensory cilia of *Caenorhabditis* and *Chlamydomonas*.[62] In these organisms, the IFT particle has been shown to transport cargo along the axoneme, moved by kinesin in the plus direction and transported by dynein in the minus direction. The presence of a homologous molecular "raft" in photoreceptors argues strongly for kinesin transport of protein/vesicle cargoes on the raft from the inner segment to the outer segment along the axoneme microtubules. Further, the ciliary localization of dynein 1b/2[62] suggests that the raft may also be used for retrograde transport to the inner segment. At this point, no specific cargoes have been associated with the IFT particle in photoreceptors.

Although the basic ciliary structure has been the subject of decades of study, new components of the cilium and new roles of ciliary elements continue to be identified. For example, RP1, RPGR, and RPGRIP are newly recognized proteins that localize to the cilia and appear to be involved in protein/vesicle transport through the cilium.[29,65] Further, an immunoscreen of retinal cDNA's using anti-axoneme-enriched antibodies identified several potentially new components of the connecting cilium.[71] Clearly, there is much work to be done before the photoreceptor cilium and cytoskeleton are fully understood. Importantly, defects in ciliary proteins can be a significant cause of retinal degeneration. For example, RP1 is a member of the doublecortin family of proteins, and defects in this protein lead to severe retinitis pigmentosa.[37] This relationship emphasizes the role that protein trafficking through the cilium plays in the health of photoreceptor cells.

Phototransduction

Much of what we know about visual biochemistry has been learned from the rod photoreceptors, owing to their relative abundance in vertebrate retinas as well as their relatively

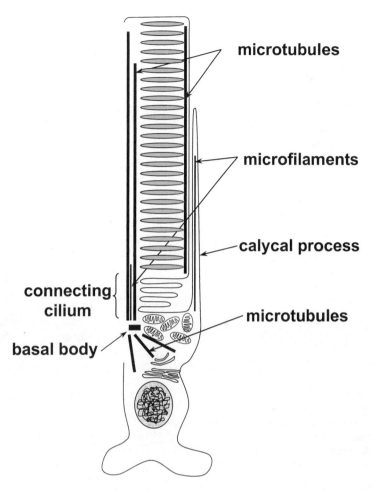

microtubules

microfilaments

calycal process

connecting cilium

microtubules

basal body

FIGURE 7.2   The cytoskeleton of photoreceptors is composed principally of microtubules and microfilaments. The axoneme in the connecting cilium is composed of nine microtubule doublets, typical of nonmotile sensory cilia, and project to nearly the distal end of the outer segment. Microfilaments are found in the connecting cilia as well. In the inner segment, microtubules form the molecular train tracks between the Golgi complex and the connecting cilium. (See also color plate 5.)

large size in comparison to cones. The details of the phototransduction cascade have largely been established in the last two decades in a wealth of publications. This chapter can in no way give proper tribute to all the studies that have contributed to the details of the cascade. Instead, the intention is to provide the reader with an overview to serve as a launching site for more in depth studies.

At its simplest, phototransduction is a G-protein-coupled receptor cascade, initiated by the visual pigment rhodopsin (figure 7.3). On absorbing light, rhodopsin undergoes a conformational change and becomes activated. This activated rhodopsin then activates the G-protein transducin, inducing an exchange of nucleotide and a release of inhibitory subunits. Activated transducin activates a phosphodiesterase that rapidly hydrolyzes cGMP. The resultant decrease in intracellular cGMP causes a closure of the cGMP-gated ion channels in the OS, resulting in a hyperpolarization of the membrane that is propagated as a nervous impulse through multiple neural layers to the visual cortex of the brain. The

following provides more details on each of these major steps in the visual transduction pathway.

RHODOPSIN

Activation   The initial steps of phototransduction in the visual organs of all animals studied to date are essentially the same: a retinaldehyde-based visual pigment absorbs light, becoming activated, which in turn then activates a heterotrimeric G-protein.

The visual pigment of rods, known as rhodopsin, is the prototypical member of the G-protein-coupled receptor family. This receptor family is responsible for transducing a host of signals across the cell membrane, including light, odors, and hormones. Like other GPCRs, rhodopsin's apoprotein (known as opsin) contains seven transmembrane-spanning domains. The recent crystal structure of rhodopsin shows there to be an additional eighth α-helix in the C-terminus of rhodopsin, lying parallel to the cytoplasmic membrane surface.[61]

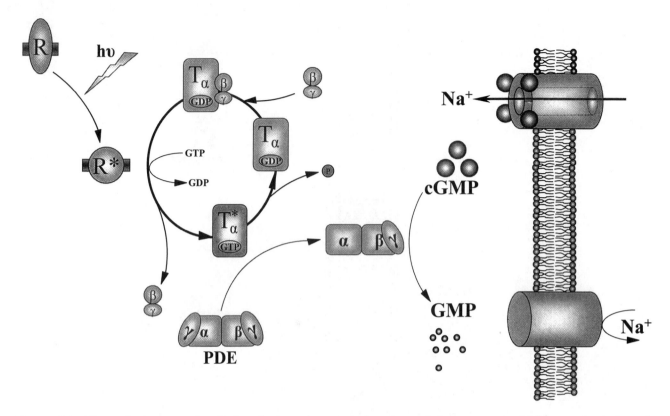

FIGURE 7.3 The activation cascade of the phototransduction pathway. Light is absorbed by rhodopsin (R). Photoactivated rhodopsin (R*) binds heterotrimeric transducin (T), catalyzing the exchange of GTP for GDP on the α-subunit.

Activated transducin removes an inhibitory subunit from the cGMP phosphodiesterase (PDE), which hydrolyzes cGMP to GMP. Reduction of cGMP causes the cyclic nucleotide-gated channels to close. (See also color plate 6.)

The light absorbing chromophore of rhodopsin, 11-*cis* retinaldehyde, is cross-linked to opsin via a Schiff-base on the ε-amino group of the lysine in the seventh membrane helix. Some animals use other retinaldehyde derivatives as the chromophore for their visual pigment, including 3-dehydroretinal (found in amphibians, fish, reptiles, and some invertebrates—crayfish and squid[16,33,78,80]), 3-hydroxyretinal (common in some species of insects[22,74]), and 4-hydroxyretinal (found in some squid[47]). The absorption maximum of the visual pigment is dictated by several factors, including the type of chromophore that is used, whether or not the Schiff base is protonated, and the particular amino acids that form the chromophore binding pocket. These factors combine to give a range of absorption maxima from 350 nm to 570 nm.

On absorption of light, the retinal chromophore isomerizes around the 11-*cis* bond, forming all-*trans* retinal. This change in configuration induces a conformational change in the surrounding opsin protein. As rhodopsin changes its conformation, it goes through several spectroscopically distinct intermediates, ultimately achieving the activated or "metarhodopsin" form of the visual pigment. It is this form of rhodopsin that then binds and activates transducin.

Inactivation Rhodopsin is inactivated in a multistep process, involving phosphorylation at its C-terminus, followed by binding of arrestin, until the all-*trans* chromophore is reduced to retinol and released from the opsin protein (figure 7.4). Metarhodopsin is first phosphorylated on its C-terminus by rhodopsin kinase, a member of the GPCR-kinase (GRK) family. Serine and threonine residues on the C-terminus of rhodopsin are targeted by rhodopsin kinase. Independent studies from several laboratories have shown that the different serines and threonines are phosphorylated in a preferential pattern in vitro. In bovine rhodopsin, this pattern starts with Ser-343 and then includes phosphorylations at Ser-338 and Ser-334. Studies of phosphorylation in vivo, also demonstrate that rhodopsin is multiply phosphorylated, although there is some disagreement about the extent to which multiple phosphorylation occurs (recently reviewed in Ref. 41).

Phosphorylation of metarhodopsin does not remove the visual pigment from the activation cascade, although it does diminish its affinity for transducin approximately sixfold.[21] Rapid quenching of rhodopsin is achieved only by the binding of arrestin. Arrestin was first identified as a 48-kDa retinal protein (by SDS-PAGE) involved in experimentally induced autoimmune uveitis[81] and was therefore called S-

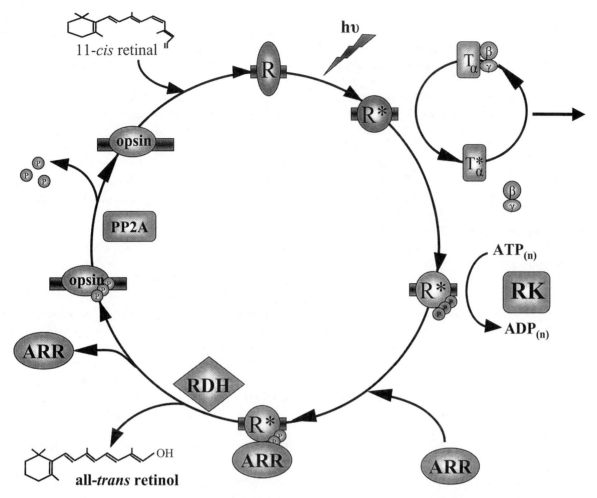

FIGURE 7.4 The rhodopsin cycle. Light is absorbed by rhodopsin (R), becoming photoactivated (R*). R* is phosphorylated on C-terminal serine and threonine residues by rhodopsin kinase (RK). Phosphorylated, photoactivated rhodopsin is bound by arrestin, blocking the ability of R*P to bind to transducin (T). Arrestin remains bound until the all-*trans* retinal chromophore is reduced by a retinal dehydrogenase (RDH) to all-*trans* retinol and released from the phospho-opsin. The phospho-opsin is dephosphorylated by protein phosphatase 2A (PP2A) and opsin regenerated back to rhodopsin by the binding a new 11-*cis* retinal molecule. (See also color plate 7.)

antigen. A role for arrestin in phototransduction was subsequently identified when arrestin was demonstrated to bind specifically to photoactivated and phosphorylated rhodopsin (R*P) and thus terminate rhodopsin's ability to activate transducin, presumably through steric interference with transducin.[36] Arrestin binds to the cytoplasmic surface of rhodopsin, utilizing a binding surface contributed by amino acids from intracellular loops 1–3.[67,68]

Arrestin requires rhodopsin to be both photoactivated and phosphorylated to bind with high affinity. Apparently, the recognition sequences for the activation state and phosphorylation state of rhodopsin involve separate mechanisms in arrestin, since the photoactivation and phosphorylation requirements can be separated, as has been demonstrated by using point mutations, serial truncations, and peptide mimics.[25,34,55,75] Interestingly, a naturally occurring splice variant of arrestin that is found in rod outer segments is a C-terminal truncation that results in an arrestin that can bind unphosphorylated metarhodopsin.[56,61,73,76] The bovine arrestin splice variant, known as p44, is formed from the use of an alternative exon in place of exon 16 that replaces the C-terminal 35 amino acids with a single alanine residue. Although its precise role in phototransduction inactivation has not been determined, the arrestin splice variant is hypothesized to inactivate rhodopsin under conditions of low photon flux.[66,72]

Arrestin remains bound to R*P until the all-*trans* retinal chromophore is reduced to all-*trans* retinol by a retinal dehydrogenase.[58,60] Reduction of the chromophore leads to its dissociation from the opsin apoprotein. The chromophore is then cycled out of the photoreceptors to the RPE, where it is processed by multiple enzymes in the visual cycle and recycled to 11-*cis* retinal. Phospho-opsin is dephosphorylated by a protein phosphatase 2A,[57] and then regenerated with 11-*cis* retinal to reform rhodopsin.

TRANSDUCIN

Activation Transducin is a heterotrimeric guanine nucleotide-binding protein. Although aqueous-soluble, transducin is modified by fatty acelyation, being myristoylated on its α-subunit, and farnesylated on its γ-subunit, giving it a propensity to associate with the membrane surface. Consequently, most transducin in a dark-adapted rod is membrane bound, associated with the rhodopsin-rich disk membranes.

In the inactive state, GDP is bound to transducin on the α-subunit, which is complexed with the β- and γ-subunits. On binding to the cytoplasmic surface loops of photoactivated rhodopsin (R*), the affinity of Tα for GDP is weakened, and the GDP dissociates. GTP then binds in the empty pocket, inducing a conformational change in Tα. This change in conformation leads to dissociation of Gα from both R* and Tβγ. The release of the βγ-subunits allows for a substantial repartitioning of Tα-GTP, with a large fraction moving into the cytoplasmic volume of the OS to activate the cGMP phosphodiesterase.[8] Release of Tα from R* allows R* to catalyze the activation of additional transducin molecules. Although this catalysis rate has been widely measured, an in situ estimation of this rate indicates that a single R* can catalyze the activation of 120 transducin molecules per second.[35] Details of transducin function in phototransduction have been recently reviewed.[2]

Inactivation Like rhodopsin, inactivation of transducin is precisely controlled. The effects of Tα* on PDE remain until GTP is hydrolyzed to GDP, at which point Gα dissociates from PDE, thus restoring PDE to its inactive state. Transducin has an endogenous GTPase activity that serves to self-limit the lifetime of Tα-GTP. However, this lifetime is approximately two orders of magnitude greater than the lifetime of the photoresponse when measured in vitro. Recent studies have reconciled the discrepancy, identifying a GTPase activating protein (GAP) in photoreceptors. This GAP, known as RGS9 (for ninth member of the regulators of G-protein signaling), acts allosterically on Tα-GTP, stabilizing a conformation in which hydrolysis of GTP is more favorable (reviewed in Ref. 15), and thus increasing GTP hydrolysis by 15–30-fold.

PHOSPHODIESTERASE

Activation The photoreceptor cGMP phosphodiesterase is a heterotetramer, composed of two highly homologous catalytic subunits (α and β) and two inhibitory subunits (γ).[3,17] Even when bound by its inhibitory subunits, PDE has a basal hydrolysis activity, converting cGMP to GMP. Binding of Tα-GTP to a single γ-subunit serves to activate one of the catalytic (α or β) subunits, increasing its catalytic activity by approximately 100-fold. The second catalytic subunit can be activated by a second Tα-GTP molecule binding to the other inhibitory γ-subunit, effectively doubling the phosphodiesterase activity of the holoenzyme. This increased activity is sufficient to deplete the local intracellular cGMP within 10 ms of PDE activation.

Inactivation Return of the PDE to its basal state requires the release of the γ-subunits from Gα-GTP. This occurs when GTP is hydrolyzed, thus reducing the affinity of Gα for PDEγ. As was described previously, this hydrolysis activity is significantly enhanced by RGS9. Exquisitely, RGS9 binding to Gα-GTP requires the inhibitory subunit of PDE, thus ensuring that transducin binds and activates PDE before its GTP is hydrolyzed.[27,42]

cGMP-GATED CHANNELS The cGMP-gated channels of rods are found in the plasma membrane, concentrated specifically in the OS and are responsible for the light-induced change in membrane potential.[20] These channels are a tetramer of two α-subunits and two β-subunits, each of which has a single cGMP-binding site (reviewed in Ref. 92). Consequently, the channel can exist in five different states with 0–4 cGMP molecules bound. To be open (the dark state), the channel must have three or four molecules of cGMP bound. Channels with 0–2 cGMP molecules are closed (the light state) to ionic conductance.

In the dark-adapted state, rod photoreceptors are partially depolarized, owing to the influx of Na^+ and Ca^{2+} ions through the open cGMP-gated channels (figure 7.5). Complete depolarization is prevented, and ionic balance is achieved by the action of an ion exchanger and an ion pump. In the OS, a sodium/calcium-potassium exchanger uses the sodium gradient to exchange Ca^{2+} and K^+ out of the photoreceptor.[9,14,90] The Na^+ balance is maintained by an ATP-requiring Na^+/K^+ pump that actively pumps sodium ions out of the rod.

In response to light, reduction of the local cGMP concentration by activated PDE causes the release of cGMP from the channel subunits, resulting in closure of the cGMP-gated channels. This closure blocks the influx of sodium and calcium ions that normally flow through the channel. Because the activity of the exchanger and pump are not altered, the photoreceptor is hyperpolarized by the action of the Na^+/K^+ pump, and local free Ca^{2+} is dramatically reduced by the Na^+/Ca^{2+} exchanger. The hyperpolarization of the membrane results in a reduction in the rate of glutamate release at the synaptic terminal of the rod. Depending on the type of cell to which the rod is attached, whether it is a horizontal cell or a rod bipolar ON or OFF cell, this reduction in glutamate signaling is propagated as either a hyperpolarization or a depolarization. Regardless, the photoreceptor has performed its function of converting a quantum of light energy into a neuronal potential that can be integrated by the visual cortex.

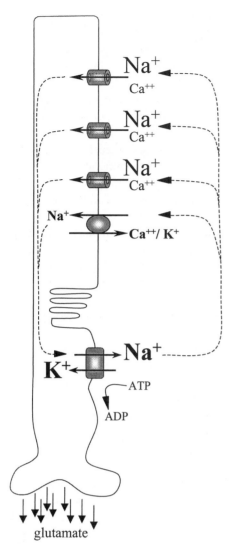

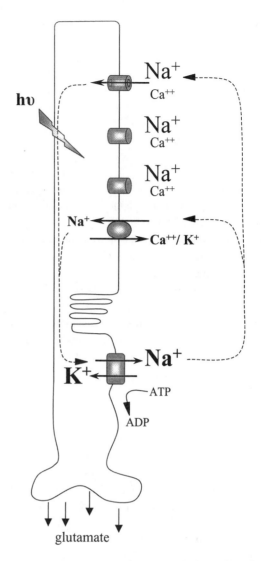

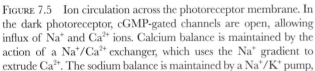

FIGURE 7.5   Ion circulation across the photoreceptor membrane. In the dark photoreceptor, cGMP-gated channels are open, allowing influx of Na^+ and Ca^{2+} ions. Calcium balance is maintained by the action of a Na^+/Ca^{2+} exchanger, which uses the Na^+ gradient to extrude Ca^{2+}. The sodium balance is maintained by a Na^+/K^+ pump, which uses ATP to return Na^+ against its ionic gradient. In response to light, one or more cGMP-gated channels are closed, resulting in a hyperpolarization of the cell membrane, since the Na^+/K^+ pump continues to operate. Membrane hyperpolarization causes a decrease in glutamate release from the synaptic terminal. (See also color plate 8.)

OTHER REGULATORY COMPONENTS   Guanylate cyclase (GC) is a membrane protein that is responsible for restoring cGMP levels. In the dark, GC converts GTP to cGMP at a rate that essentially offsets the catalysis rate of unactivated PDE. Consequently, restoration of cGMP following a light response and subsequent channel opening would occur slowly if there were no activation of the GC. Recently, a class of calcium-binding proteins was identified that regulate the activity of GC.[23,24] These guanylate cyclase–activating proteins (GCAP) are normally bound to GC when occupied by calcium in the dark photoreceptor (high calcium state). Channel closure, with its concomitant reduction of intracellular calcium, causes the release of Ca^{2+} from GCAP, which allows GCAP to dissociate from GC. The release of GCAP results in a tenfold increase in cat-alytic activity of GC, rapidly increasing the intracellular cGMP levels and restoring the cGMP-gated channels to the open state. Experiments using GCAP knock-out mice suggest that the effect of GCAP on GC is the only Ca^{2+}-sensitive feedback mechanism that affects the dim light or single photon response of the rod cell.[50]

Although the calcium-binding GCAPs are the primary point for calcium to impact the single photon response, several other components have been identified in rods that are influenced by calcium. Recoverin (also known as S-modulin) is a calcium-binding protein that has been shown to associate with rhodopsin kinase. At elevated Ca levels (dark state), recoverin binds rhodopsin kinase and reduces the kinase activity. As calcium is depleted (light state), calcium-free recoverin dissociates from rhodopsin kinase, increasing the rate at which RK phosphorylates rhodopsin.[18,32]

Calmodulin is another calcium-binding protein found in the OS. Calmodulin binds to the β-subunit of the cGMP-gated channel when occupied by calcium. Binding of calmodulin reduces the affinity of the channel for cGMP, forming a negative feedback loop.[30]

Phosducin is a 33-kDa protein that is phosphorylated through the protein kinase A pathway. This pathway is activated by calcium, which leads to phosphorylation of phosducin in the dark. When calcium levels drop in response to light, phosducin is dephosphorylated. This dephosphorylated phosducin can then bind the Tβγ dimer. Binding Tβγ reduces the pool available to Tα-GDP to regenerate the full trimeric complex, thus diminishing the potential of the photoreceptor to respond to light.[85]

Although the intersection of these calcium-sensitive components with the transduction pathway has been identified, their specific function in visual response has not been completely delineated. Most likely, these elements form part of the light-adaptation mechanism that regulates the visual response in background illumination.

Phototransduction in cones

Although much of what we know about the phototransduction pathway has been learned from rods, it is clear that cone photoreceptors function in a very similar manner. Most of the components identified in rods have a cone homologue, although in some cases, the same protein is utilized in both types of photoreceptors.[28] This being said, it is clear that cones are different from rods. Aside from the obvious differences in response to different light intensity ranges, cones are approximately 25–100 times less sensitive to light than rods are but have response kinetics that are two to four times faster than those of rods. The molecular explanation behind these differences in the two cell types has not been fully developed. However, recent use of cone-rich model animals and increasingly sensitive molecular tools has identified some of the biochemical differences. For example, cones contain a much higher concentration of RGS9, suggesting that GTPase acceleration may be involved in the faster response inactivation of cones.[96] Additional biochemical differences between rods and cones will undoubtedly create a more complete picture of the divergences in the transduction pathways that lead to the different response kinetics of rods and cones.

Relationship to electrical activity

The considerations above go a long way toward explaining the form, duration, and sensitivity of the electrical responses of rods and cones (figure 7.6).[4] The important features are that the responses to the flash of light long outlast the stimulus, even though the stimulus is weak. Under these circumstances, adaptation does not occur, and the rise of the response then reflects the rate of depletion of cGMP. However, almost immediately, adaptive mechanisms come into play (see the paragraphs on regulatory components above), so only the initial portion of the responses is unaffected.

The change in kinetics of the steps in the cascade could account for the differing temporal kinetics and sensitivities of rods' and cones' electrical signals. During the declining phase of the response to intense flashes, the system is desensitized, and the cGMP concentrations presumably rise, mostly as a result of the combined activity of guanylate cyclase, GCAP, and RGS9. Step stimuli activate all the regulatory mechanisms described above, and it is a combination of these that lead to the increment threshold function ($\Delta L/L = K$) (see chapter 37).

The photocurrents that are measured from single receptors represent a large gain between the energy of a photon and the energy released by R*. In darkness, small transient voltage changes ("bumps") can be recorded across photoreceptor membranes (figure 7.7).[5] These are presumably caused by thermal activation of molecules in the excitatory cascade. However, the entire sequence is rarely activated because rhodopsin is a very stable molecule. Therefore, these "thermal" bumps are in general much smaller than the signals caused by single photon events. In addition, these changes are "smoothed" at the receptor-bipolar synapse and receptor-receptor junctions, thus permitting the unambiguous detection of very weak signals. However, this elegant system demands the continuous use of energy, since every signal is a reduction of the dark current. Maintaining the dark current requires high activity in the ATP-requiring Na^+/K^+ pump and helps to explain why in mitochondrial diseases, the retina may be disproportionately affected.

Migration of proteins in photoreceptors

Phototransduction was described above as though it were a cascade that occurs in a static cell. In actuality, the photoreceptor is a dynamic structure with several proteins that dramatically change their localization between the inner and outer segments in response to light (figure 7.8). These include arrestin[1,7,40,43-45,48,49,51-54,63,64,83,88,94] and transducin.[48,51,64,77,83,94] In the dark-adapted retina, arrestin is principally distributed in the inner segment and quickly moves to the outer segment in response to light on a time scale of several minutes. Interestingly, the splice variant of arrestin does not appear to translocate, remaining in the ROS regardless of lighting conditions.[74] Arrestin migration has also been documented in cone photoreceptors.[93,95] In contrast to arrestin translocation, transducin is principally

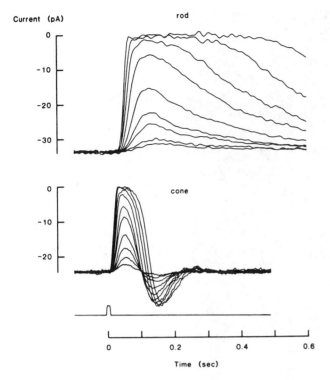

FIGURE 7.6 Reduction in circulating current through a monkey rod and a cone that is produced by light flashes. In the dark, there is an inward current through the outer segment membranes, and this current is reduced by light. The flash intensity was increased by a factor of about 2, ranging between 3 and 900 photoisomerizations in the rod and between 200 and 36,000 in the cone. Timing of the flash is shown in the lower panel. (Source: From Baylor DA.[5] Used by permission.)

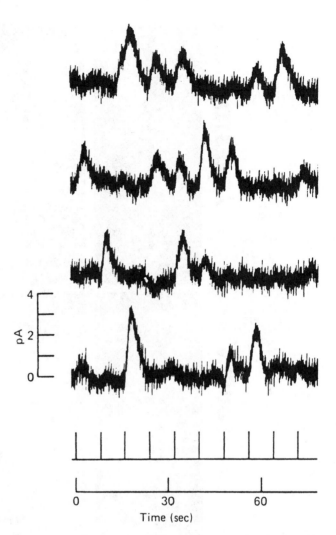

FIGURE 7.7 Fluctuations of the photocurrent of a single rod in response to dim light flashes. These records show that rods respond to single photons. Each row is part of that same continuous record. The timing of the flashes is shown in the trace. (Source: From Baylor DA, Lamb TD, Yau K-W.[4] Used by permission.)

localized to the outer segment in the dark, moving to the inner segment in response to light.

For arrestin, the localization in the dark-adapted rod seems somewhat counterintuitive, since one would expect arrestin to be principally localized to the outer segment, where it quenches photoactivated rhodopsin. The fact that this is not the case suggests that arrestin migration likely serves an additional role. Perhaps in the case of dim light (with few rhodopsin isomerizations), either the splice variant of arrestin performs the role of rhodopsin quenching as hypothesized previously,[58,66,72,74] or sufficient full-length arrestin is present in the outer segments for rhodopsin quenching but it is below immunocytochemical detection limits. However, in the case of brighter lights, perhaps arrestin/transducin translocation plays a role in rod desensitization. In this scenario, increased arrestin concentration in the illuminated ROS would effectively reduce the lifetime of R*P, and decreased transducin would decrease the coupling efficiency between R* and the cGMP PDE. A recent reinvestigation of transducin migration shows that transducin decline in the outer segment in response to light parallels the decline in rod signal amplification.[77] This result

suggests that protein translocation may be one of the underlying mechanisms for light adaptation, although all the results are only correlative at this juncture.

Mechanistic studies of protein translocation

Like the function of light-driven protein migration in photoreceptors, the mechanism that mobilizes the proteins has remained elusive. There are two broad categories that could account for the light-induced translocation of arrestin and other proteins between the inner segment and outer segment through the connecting cilium: passive migration along a diffusion gradient and active migration requiring a motor-driven process. The first mechanism appeared intuitive for arrestin, since light activation and phosphorylation of rhodopsin would provide a sink, removing free arrestin in

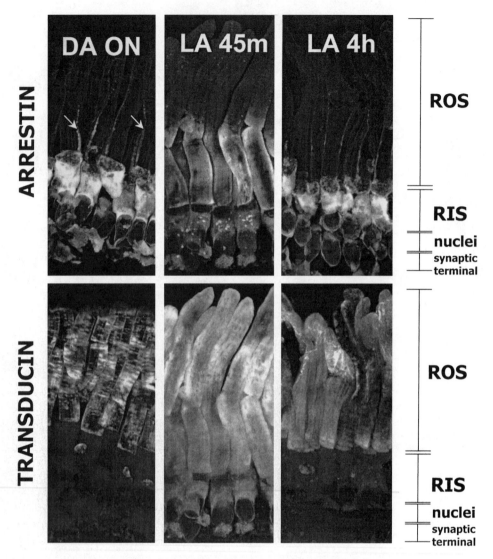

FIGURE 7.8   Translocation of photoreceptor proteins in response to light. In a dark-adapted *Xenopus* retina, arrestin (upper panels) immunolocalizes to the inner segments, axonemes (arrows), and synaptic terminals. Transducin (lower panels) immunolocalizes to the outer segments. In response to 45 minutes of adapting light, there is a massive translocation of the proteins, with arrestin moving to the outer segments and transducin moving to the inner segments. In *Xenopus*, if the frog is maintained in the adapting light for an extended period of time (>2 hours), the proteins translocate back to their respective cellular compartments. (See also color plate 9.)

the outer segment and drawing more arrestin in from the inner segment along a concentration gradient. However, studies using transgenic mice offer evidence that rhodopsin-driven diffusion is not the mechanism that mobilizes arrestin from the inner segment to the outer segment. In mice that are deficient for rhodopsin phosphorylation, either because they lack rhodopsin kinase or because the C-terminus of rhodopsin has been mutated to remove the phosphorylation sites, light-driven arrestin migration between the inner segment and outer segments occurs in a manner that is indistinguishable from that in wild-type mice.[51,94]

This evidence eliminates arrestin binding to R*P as the mechanism for arrestin's migration into the outer segment, suggesting that arrestin's migration is partially controlled by a motor-driven process. Support for this motor-driven hypothesis is provided by Marszalek et al.,[46] who showed that photoreceptors that are made deficient for kinesin-II by Cre-lox mutagenesis accumulate arrestin at the base of the cilium in the inner segment. The one potential caveat to this observation is that rhodopsin also accumulates at a similar site. Consequently, the misaccumulation of arrestin may simply reflect arrestin's binding affinity for rhodopsin rather than disrupted transportation of arrestin, especially since the mislocalized rhodopsin is at least partially phosphorylated.[86]

The light signal that initiates translocation is currently undefined. Mendez et al.[51] and Zhang et al.[94] have both shown that arrestin translocation occurs in the absence of phototransduction. In transducin knock-out mice (knock-out of the α-subunit), arrestin migrates normally in response to light. Interestingly, both arrestin distribution and transducin distribution are disrupted in the RPE65$^{-/-}$ mouse, with no evidence for light-driven translocation.[51] This result suggests that functional visual pigment may be required to promote arrestin and transducin migration.

Studies such as these highlight the fact that although we know much about photoreceptor physiology and biochemistry, many areas are incomplete and underdeveloped, and some are likely yet undiscovered.

REFERENCES

1. Agarwal N, Nir I, Papermaster DS: Loss of diurnal arrestin gene expression in rds mouse retinas. *Exp Eye Res* 1994; 58:1–8.

2. Arshavsky VY, Lamb TD, Pugh EN: G proteins and phototransduction. *Ann Rev Physiol* 2002; 64:153–187.

3. Baehr W, Devlin MJ, Applebury ML: Isolation and characterization of cGMP phosphodiesterase from bovine rod outer segments. *J Biolog Chem* 1979; 254:1169–1177.

4. Baylor DA, Lamb TD, Yau K-W: Responses of retinal rods to single photons. *J Physiol* 1979; 288:613–634.

5. Baylor DA: Photoreceptor signals and vision. Proctor lecture. *Invest Ophthalmol Vis Sci* 1987; 28:34–49.

6. Besharse JC, Horst CJ: The photoreceptor connecting cilium: A model for the transition zone. In Bloodgood RA (ed): *Ciliary and Flagellar Membranes.* New York, Plenum, 1990, pp 389–417.

7. Broekhuyse RM, Tolhuizen EFJ, Janssen APM, Winkens HJ: Light induced shift and binding of S-antigen in retinal rods. *Curr Eye Res* 1985; 4:613–618.

8. Bruckert F, Chabre M, Vuong MT: Light and GTP dependence of transducin solubility in retinal rods: Further analysis by near infra-red light scattering. *Eur Biophys J* 1988; 16:207–218.

9. Cervetto L, Lagnado L, Perry RJ, Robinson DW, McNaughton PA: Extrusion of calcium from rod outer segments is driven by both sodium and potassium gradients. *Nature* 1989; 337:740–743.

10. Chaitin MH, Bok D: Immunoferritin localization of actin in retinal photoreceptors. *Invest Ophthalmol Vis Sci* 1986; 27:1764–1767.

11. Chaitin MH, Carlsen RB, Samara GJ: Immunogold localization of actin in developing photoreceptor cilia of normal and rds mutant mice. *Exp Eye Res* 1988; 47:437–446.

12. Chaitin MH, Coelho N: Immunogold localization of myosin in the photoreceptor cilium. *Invest Ophthalmol Vis Sci* 1992; 33:3103–3108.

13. Cohen AI: Rods and cones. *Handbook of Sensory Physiology* 1972; VII/2:63–110.

14. Cook NJ, Kaupp UB: Solubilization, purification, and reconstitution of the sodium-calcium exchanger from bovine retinal rod outer segments. *J Biolog Chem* 1988; 263:11382–11388.

15. Cowan CW, He W, Wensel TG: RGS proteins: Lessons from the RGS9 subfamily. *Prog Nucleic Acid Res Molec Biol* 2000; 65:341–359.

16. Crescitelli F: The gecko visual pigment: The dark exchange of chromophore. *Vision Res* 1984; 24:1551–1553.

17. Deterre P, Bigay J, Forquet F, Robert M, Chabre M: cGMP phosphodiesterase of retinal rods is regulated by two inhibitory subunits. *Proc Natl Acad Sci USA* 1988; 85:2424–2428.

18. Dizhoor AM, Ray S, Kumar S, Niemi G, Spencer M, Brolley D, Walsh KA, Philipov PP, Hurley JB, Stryer L: Recoverin: A calcium sensitive activator of retinal rod guanylate cyclase. *Science* 1991; 251:915–918.

19. Eckmiller MS: Microtubules in a rod-specific cytoskeleton associated with outer segment incisures. *Visual Neurosci* 2000; 17:711–722.

20. Fesenko E, Kolesnikov S, Lyubarsky A: Induction by cyclic GMP of cationic conductances in plasma membrane of retinal rod outer segment. *Nature* 1985; 313:310–313.

21. Gibson SK, Parkes JH, Liebman PA: Phosphorylation modulates the affinity of light-activated rhodopsin for G protein and arrestin. *Biochemistry* 2000; 39:5738–5749.

22. Goldsmith TH, Marks BC, Bernard GD: Separation and identification of geometric isomers of 3-hydroxyretinoids and occurrence in the eyes of insects. *Vision Res* 1986; 26:1763–1769.

23. Gorczyca WA, Gray-Keller MP, Detwiler PB, Palczewski K: Purification and physiological evaluation of a guanylate cyclase activating protein from retinal rods. *Proc Natl Acad Sci USA* 1994; 91:4014–4018.

24. Gorczyca WA, Polans AS, Surgucheva IG, Baehr W, Palczewski K: Guanylyl cyclase activating protein: A calcium-sensitive regulator of phototransduction. *J Biol Chem* 1995; 270:22029–22036.

25. Gurevich VV, Benovic JL: Visual arrestin binding to rhodopsin: Diverse functional roles of positively charged residues within the phosphorylation-recognition region of arrestin. *J Biol Chem* 1995; 270:6010–6016.

26. Hale IL, Fisher SK, Matsumoto B: The actin network in the ciliary stalk of photoreceptors functions in the generation of new outer segment discs. *J Comp Neurol* 1996; 376:128–142.

27. He W, Lu L, Zhang X, El-Hodiri HM, Chen CK, Slep KC, Simon MI, Jamrich M, Wensel TG: Modules in the photoreceptor RGS9-1. Gbeta 5L GTPase-accelerating protein complex control effector coupling, GTPase acceleration, protein folding, and stability. *J Biolog Chem* 2000; 275:37093–37100.

28. Hisatomi O, Tokunaga F: Molecular evolution of proteins involved in vertebrate phototransduction. *Comp Biochem Physiol B-Biochem Mol Biol* 2002; 133:509–522.

29. Hong DH, Pawlyk BS, Sokolov M, Strissel KJ, Yang J, Tulloch B, Wright AF, Arshavsky VY, Li T: RPGR isoforms in photoreceptor connecting cilia and the transitional zone of motile cilia. *Invest Ophthalmol Vis Sci* 2003; 44:2413–2421.

30. Hsu Y-T, Molday RS: Modulation of the cGMP-gated channel of rod photoreceptor cells by calmodulin. *Nature* 1993; 361:76–79.

31. Kaplan MW, Iwata RT, Sears RC: Lengths of immunolabeled ciliary microtubules in frog photoreceptor outer segments. *Exp Eye Res* 1987; 44:623–632.

32. Kawamura S: Rhodopsin phosphorylation as a mechanism of cyclic GMP phosphodiesterase regulation by S-modulin. *Nature* 1993; 362:855–857.

33. Kito Y, Seki T, Suzuki T, Uchiyama I: 3-Dehydroretinal in the eye of a bioluminescent squid, Watasenia scintillans. *Vision Res* 1986; 26:275–279.

34. Krupnick JG, Gurevich VV, Schepers T, Hamm HE, Benovic JL: Arrestin-rhodopsin interaction: Multi-site binding delineated by peptide inhibition. *J Biol Chem* 1994; 269:3226–3232.

35. Leskov IB, Klenchin VA, Handy JW, Whitlock GG, Govardovskii VI, Bownds MD, Lamb TD, Pugh EN,

Arshavsky VY: The gain of rod phototransduction: Reconciliation of biochemical and electrophysiological measurements. *Neuron* 2000; 27:525–537.

36. Liebman PA, Pugh EN: The control of phosphodiesterase in rod disk membranes: Kinetics, possible mechanisms and significance for vision. *Vision Res* 1979; 19:375–380.

37. Liu Q, Zhou J, Daiger SP, Farber DB, Heckenlively JR, Smith JE, Sullivan LS, Zuo J, Milam AH, Pierce EA: Identification and subcellular localization of the RP1 protein in human and mouse photoreceptors. *Invest Ophthalmol Vis Sci* 2002; 43:22–32.

38. Liu X, Vansant G, Udovichenko IP, Wolfrum U, Williams DS: Myosin VIIa, the product of the Usher 1B syndrome gene, is concentrated in the connecting cilia of photoreceptor cells. *Cell Motil Cytoskel* 1997; 37:240–252.

39. Liu XR, Udovichenko IP, Brown SDM, Steel KP, Williams DS: Myosin VIIa participates in opsin transport through the photoreceptor cilium. *J Neurosci* 1999; 19:6267–6274.

40. Loeffler KU, Mangini NJ: Anti-arrestin immunoreactivity in the human retina: Difference between light- and dark-adaptation. *Current Eye Res* 1995; 14:1165–1168.

41. Maeda T, Imanishi Y, Palczewski K: Rhodopsin phosphorylation: 30 years later. *Prog Retin Eye Res* 2003; 22:417–434.

42. Makino ER, Handy JW, Li T, Arshavsky VY: The GTPase activating factor for transducin in rod photoreceptors is the complex between RGS9 and type 5 G protein beta subunit. *Proc Natl Acad Sci USA* 1999; 96:1947–1952.

43. Mangini NJ, Pepperberg DR: Localization of retinal "48K" (S-antigen) by electron microscopy. *Jpn J Ophthalmol* 1987; 31:207–217.

44. Mangini NJ, Pepperberg DR: Immunolocalization of 48K in rod photoreceptors. *Invest Opthalmol Vis Sci* 1988; 29:1221–1234.

45. Mangini NJ, Garner GL, Okajima TL, Donoso LA, Pepperberg DR: Effect of hydroxylamine on the subcellular distribution of arrestin (S-antigen) in rod photoreceptors. *Vis Neurosci* 1994; 11:561–568.

46. Marszalek JR, Liu XR, Roberts EA, Chui D, Marth JD, Williams DS, Goldstein LSB: Genetic evidence for selective transport of opsin and arrestin by kinesin-II in mammalian photoreceptors. *Cell* 2000; 102:175–187.

47. Matsui SSM, Uchiyama I, Sekiya N, Hiraki K, Yoshihara K, Kito Y: 4-Hydroxyretinal, a new visual pigment chromophore found in the bioluminescent squid, Watasenia scintillans. *Bioshim Biophys Acta* 1988; 966:370–374.

48. McGinnis JF, Whelan JP, Donoso LA: Transient, cyclic changes in mouse visual cell gene products during the light-dark cycle. *J Neurosci Res* 1992; 31:584–590.

49. McGinnis JF, Matsumoto B, Whelan JP, Cao W: Cytoskeleton participation in subcellular trafficking of signal transduction proteins in rod photoroecptor cells. *J Neurosci Res* 2002; 67:290–297.

50. Mendez A, Burns ME, Sokal I, Dizhoor AM, Baehr W, Chen J: Role of guanylate cyclase-activating proteins (GCAPs) in setting the flash sensitivity of rod photoreceptors. *Proc Natl Acad Sci USA* 2001; 98:9948–9953.

51. Mendez A, Lem J, Simon M, Chen J: Light-dependent translocation of arrestin in the absence of rhodopsin phosphorylation and transducin signaling. *J Neurosci* 2003; 23:3124–3129.

52. Mirshahi M, Thillaye B, Tarraf M, deKozak Y, Faure J-P: Light-induced changes in S-antigen (arrestin) localization in retinal photoreceptors: Differences between rods and cones and defective process in RCS rat retinal dystrophy. *Eur J Cell Biol* 1994; 63:61–67.

53. Nir I, Agarwal N: Arrestin mRNA expression, biosynthesis, and localization in degenerating photoreceptors of mutant rds mice retinas. *J Comp Neurol* 1991; 308:1–10.

54. Nir I, Ransom N: Ultrastructural analysis of arrestin distribution in mouse photoreceptors during dark/light cycle. *Exp Eye Res* 1993; 57:307–318.

55. Palczewski K, Hargrave PA, McDowell JH, Ingegritsen TS: The catalytic subunit of phophatase 2A dephosphorylates phosphoopsin. *Biochem* 1989; 28:415–419.

56. Palczewski K, McDowell JH, Jakes S, Ingebritsen TS, Hargrave PA: Regulation of rhodopsin dephosphorylation by arrestin. *J Biol Chem* 1989; 264:15770–15773.

57. Palczewski K, Buczylko J, Imami NR, McDowell JH, Hargrave PA: Role of the carboxyl-terminal region of arrestin in binding to phosphorylated rhodopsin. *J Biol Chem* 1991; 266:15334–15339.

58. Palczewski K, Buczylko J, Ohguro H, Annan RS, Carr SA, Crabb JW, Kaplan MW, Johnson RS, Walsh KA: Characterization of a truncated form of arrestin isolated from bovine rod outer segments. *Prot Sci* 1994; 3:314–324.

59. Palczewski K, Jager S, Buczylko J, Crouch RK, Bredberg DL, Hofmann KP, Asson-Batres MA, Saari JC: Rod outer segment retinol dehydrogenase: Substrate specificity and role in phototransduction. *Biochem* 1994; 33:13741–13750.

60. Palczewski K, Smith WC: Splice variants of arrestin. *Exp Eye Res* 1996; 63:599–602.

61. Palczewski K, Kumasaka T, Hori T, Behnke CA, Motoshima H, Fox BA, Le Trong I, Teller DC, Okada T, Stenkamp RE, Yamamoto M, Miyano M: Crystal structure of rhodopsin: A G protein-coupled receptor. *Science* 2000; 289:739–745.

62. Pazour GJ, Baker SA, Deane JA, Cole DG, Dickert BL, Rosenbaum JL, Witman GB, Besharse JC: The intraflagellar transport protein, IFT88, is essential for vertebrate photoreceptor assembly and maintenance. *J Cell Biol* 2002; 157:103–113.

63. Peterson JJ, Tam BM, Moritz OL, Shelamer CL, Dugger DR, McDowell JH, Hargrave PA, Papermaster DS, Smith WC: Arrestin migrates in photoreceptors in response to light: A study of arrestin localization using an arrestin-GFP fusion protein in transgenic frogs. *Experimental Eye Research* 2003; 76:553–563.

64. Philp NJ, Chang W, Long K: Light-stimulated protein movement in rod photoreceptor cells of the rat retina. *FEBS Lett* 1987; 225:127–132.

65. Pierce EA: Gene targeted and transgenic models of retinitis pigmentosa 1 (RP1). *Invest Ophthalmol Vis Sci Suppl* 2002; 43:1.

66. Pulvermuller A, Maretzi D, Rudnicka-Nawrot M, Smith WC, Palczewski K, Hofmann KP: Functional differences in the interaction of arrestin and its splice variant, p44, with rhodopsin. *Biochemistry* 1997; 36:9253–9260.

67. Raman D, Osawa S, Weiss ER: Binding of arrestin to cytoplasmic loop mutants of bovine rhodopsin. *Biochemistry* 1999; 38:5117–5123.

68. Raman D, Osawa S, Gurevich VV, Weiss ER: The interaction with the cytoplasmic loops of rhodopsin plays a crucial role in arrestin activation and binding. *J Neurochem* 2003; 84:1040–1050.

69. Roof D, Adamian M, Jacobs D, Hayes A: Cytoskeletal specializations at the rod photoreceptor distal tip. *J Comp Neurol* 1991; 305:289–303.

70. Sale WS, Besharse JC, Piperno G: Distribution of acetylated alpha-tubulin in retina and in vitro-assembled microtubules. *Cell Motil Cytoskel* 1988; 9:243–253.

71. Schmitt A, Wolfrum U: Identification of novel molecular components of the photoreceptor connecting cilium by immunoscreens. *Exp Eye Res* 2001; 73:837–849.

72. Schroder K, Pulvermuller A, Hofmann KP: Arrestin and its splice variant Arr(1–370A) (P-44): Mechanism and biological role of their interaction with rhodopsin. *J Biol Chem* 2002; 277:43987–43996.

73. Smith WC, Goldsmith TH: Phyletic aspects of the distribution of 3-hydroxyretinal in the class Insecta. *J Mol Evol* 1990; 30:72–84.

74. Smith WC, Milam AH, Dugger DR, Arendt A, Hargrave PA, Palczewski K: A splice variant of arrestin: Molecular cloning and localization in bovine retina. *J Biolog Chem* 1994; 269:15407–15410.

75. Smith WC: A splice variant of arrestin from human retina. *Exp Eye Res* 1996; 62:585–592.

76. Smith WC, McDowell JH, Dugger DR, Miller R, Arendt A, Popp MP, Hargrave PA: Identification of regions of arrestin that bind to rhodopsin. *Biochemistry* 1999; 38:2752–2761.

77. Sokolov M, Lyubarsky AL, Strissel KJ, Savchenko AB, Govardovskii VI, Pugh EN, Arshavsky VY: Massive light-driven translocation of transducin between the two major compartments of rod cells: A novel mechanism of light adaptation. *Neuron* 2002; 34:95–106.

78. Suzuki T, Makino-Tasaka M, Eguchi E: 3-Dehydroretinal (vitamin A2 aldehyde) in crayfish eye. *Vis Res* 1984; 24: 783–787.

79. Tai AW, Chuang J-Z, Bode C, Wolfrum U, Sung C-H: Rhodopsin's carboxy-terminal cytoplasmic tail acts as a membrane receptor for cytoplasmic dynein by binding to the dynein light chain Tctex-1. *Cell* 1999; 97:877–887.

80. Tsin ATC, Alvarez RA, Fong S-L, Bridges CDB: Use of high-performance liquid chromatography in the analysis of retinyl and 3,4-didehydroretinyl compounds in tissue extracts of bullfrog tadpoles and goldfish. *Vision Res* 1984; 24:1835–1840.

81. Wacker WB, Donoso LA, Kalsow CM, Yankeelov JAJ, Organisciak DT: Experimental allergic uveitis: Isolation, characterization, and localization of a soluble uveitopathogenic antigen from bovine retina. *J Immunol* 1977; 119:1949–1958.

82. Wen GY, Soifer D, Wisniewski HM: The doublet microtubules of rods of the rabbit retina. *Anat Embryol* 1982; 165:315–328.

83. Whelan JP, McGinnis JF: Light-dependent subcellular movement of photoreceptor proteins. *J Neurosci Res* 1988; 20:263–270.

84. Whitehead JL, Wang SY, Bost-Usinger L, Hoang E, Frazer KA, Burnside B: Photoreceptor localization of the KIF3A and KIF3B subunits of the heterotrimeric microtubule motor kinesin II in vertebrate retina. *Exp Eye Res* 1999; 69:491–503.

85. Willardson BM, Wilkins JF, Yoshida T, Bitensky MW: Regulation of phosducin phosphorylation in retinal rods by Ca^{2+}/calmodulin-dependent adenylyl cyclase. *Proc Natl Acad Sci USA* 1996; 93:1475–1479.

86. Williams DS: Transport to the photoreceptor outer segment by myosin VIIa and kinesin II. *Vision Res* 2002; 42:455–462.

87. Williams DS, Linberg DK, Vaughan DK, Fariss RN, Fisher SK: Disruption of microfilament organization and deregulation of disk membrane morphogenesis by cyotchalasin D in rod and cone photoreceptors. *J Comp Neurol* 1988; 272: 161–176.

88. Williams MA, Mangini NJ: Immunolocalization of arrestin (S-antigen) in rods of pearl mutant and wild-type mice. *Curr Eye Res* 1991; 10:457–462.

89. Wolfrum U, Schmitt A: Rhodopsin transport in the membrane of the connecting cilium of mammalian photoreceptor cells. *Cell Motil Cytoskel* 2000; 46:95–107.

90. Yau K-W, Nakatani K: Light-induced reduction of cytoplasmic free calcium in retinal rod outer segment. *Nature* 1985; 313:579–582.

91. Young RW: The renewal of photoreceptor cell outer segments. *J Cell Biol* 1967; 33:61–72.

92. Zagotta WN, Siegelbaum SA: Structure and function of cyclic nucleotide-gated channels. *Annu Rev Neurosci* 1996; 19:235–263.

93. Zhang HB, Cuenca N, Ivanova T, Church-Kopish J, Frederick JM, MacLeish PR, Baehr W: Identification and light-dependent translocation of a cone-specific antigen, cone arrestin, recognized by monoclonal antibody 7G6. *Invest Ophthalmol Vis Sci* 2003; 44:2858–2867.

94. Zhang HB, Huang W, Zhang HK, Zhu XM, Craft C, Baehr W, Chen CK: Light-dependent redistribution of visual arrestins and transducin subunits in mice with defective phototransduction. *Mol Vis* 2003; 9:231–237.

95. Zhang X, Wensel TG, Kraft TW: GTPase regulators and photoresponses in cones of the eastern chipmunk. *J Neurosci* 2003; 23:1287–1297.

96. Zhu X, Li A, Brown B, Weiss ER, Osawa S, Craft CM: Mouse cone arrestin expression pattern: Light induced translocation in cone photoreceptors. *Molec Vision* 2002; 8:462–471.

8 Synaptic Transmission: Sensitivity Control Mechanisms

GERTRUDE FALK AND RICHARD SHIELLS

OUR CURRENT understanding about how the signals that are generated in rods and cones are transmitted through the retina to the optic nerve has advanced rapidly in recent years. The basic principles were established from work using intracellular microelectrodes. More recent advances derive from using patch electrodes, which have the advantage of controlling the intracellular biochemistry and permitting more direct analysis of the properties of membrane ionic channels. Coupled with other novel techniques, such as imaging single neurons in retinal slices of both lower vertebrates and mammals, the advances that have been made in recent years have been striking. Furthermore, molecular biological approaches using mutant mice that lack specific receptors or channels have demonstrated the roles these play in signal transduction.

Transmitter release from rods and cones

Rod and cone photoreceptors respond to light with a graded hyperpolarization, which spreads without decrement to their presynaptic terminals. The rate of release of transmitter L-glutamate that is stored in synaptic vesicles at the terminal is controlled by the membrane potential. The hyperpolarization reduces transmitter release, changing the membrane potential of the postsynaptic horizontal and bipolar cells.

At virtually all synapses, transmitter release is dependent on intracellular Ca^{2+} levels, which increase on depolarization owing to the opening of voltage-dependent Ca^{2+} channels. Rods and cones are nonspiking neurons that release transmitter continuously when relatively depolarized in the dark (membrane potential: <40 mV). Hyperpolarization by light leads to a reduction in intracellular Ca^{2+} in the synaptic terminals. There is a high cooperativity in the action of Ca^{2+} on glutamate release such that, with changes in membrane potential, glutamate release changes exponentially. Recent estimates are that for a 6-mV rod hyperpolarization, there is a tenfold decrease in release, while a 12-mV light response reduces release by 100-fold. A 6-mV rod response represents the limit of the linear response range. The photoreceptor responses generate the initial part of the electroretinogram (ERG), the vitreal-negative a-wave.

The actions of glutamate are terminated by uptake mechanisms, which actively transport glutamate from the extra-cellular space into the surrounding cells. Rods and cones and bipolar, ganglion, and Müller cells all possess glutamate transporters. Blocking uptake has been shown to enhance the potency of exogenously applied glutamate and alter light response kinetics.

Rods and cones are electrically coupled via low-resistance gap junctions in lower vertebrates. There is, however, some question about the extent of coupling in mammals and primates. Coupling results in spatial averaging, and because current can spread to adjacent rods, the response to a single photon in the coupled network is much smaller than that in an isolated rod. However, because many rods converge onto horizontal and bipolar cells, the spread of the presynaptic signal over many terminals confers an advantage in the detection of nonuniform illumination. Biasing the rod and cone membrane potential in the depolarizing direction in the dark, so that they operate at the most sensitive part of the relation for transmitter release, optimizes the system for the detection of dim light signals.

Responses of horizontal and bipolar cells to light

Horizontal and bipolar cells are immediately postsynaptic to the photoreceptors. Mammalian horizontal cells, with the exception of those of rodents, can be divided into two types based on their morphology. Type A cells have a large soma with relatively thick dendrites radiating to form a circular receptive field, while type B cells have a smaller soma, densely branching fine dendrites and a fine long axon which terminates in an elaborate arborization. The dendrites of both types are postsynaptic exclusively to cones, while only the axon terminals are postsynaptic exclusively to rods. Rod and cone signals can be recorded from both types of horizontal cell, but this mixing is thought to result from electrical coupling between rods and cones rather than via transmission across the axon.

The light responses of rod horizontal cells consists of a graded hyperpolarization that is dependent on light intensity. Horizontal cells possess very large receptive fields because they are extensively electrically coupled via low-resistance gap junctions. Wide-field illumination evokes large horizontal cell responses, while focal illumination yields only very small responses because of electrical loading by the rest of the coupled network. In lower vertebrates, horizontal cells provide the antagonistic surround, which opposes the center response of bipolar cells. Horizontal cells are particularly suited for this because of their large-field characteristics. Horizontal cells make synaptic contact with bipolar cells and, by means of the inhibitory transmitter GABA, oppose the light-induced center response of bipolar cells.

The response to an annulus of light, concentric with the center of the bipolar cell's receptive field, is of opposite polarity to the center response. The antagonistic surround is abolished by procedures such as applying dopamine to horizontal cells, which removes their electrical coupling. Center surround antagonism is important for edge detection and in enhancing contrast sensitivity. It is much reduced in the dark-adapted retina, in part because transmission of the center bipolar cell response occurs at a much higher gain than the surround response mediated by the horizontal cells. In mammalian retina, rod bipolar cells do not exhibit any clear antagonistic surround input from horizontal cells. The center surround organization that is characteristic of ganglion cell receptive fields in the rod pathway is thought to be set up at the level of the inner plexiform layer (IPL) by inhibitory input from amacrine cells forming the antagonistic surround.

Retinal parallel processing

Mammalian rod bipolar cells depolarize in response to light that is absorbed within the center of their receptive field (ON center). Figure 8.1 shows the voltage responses of a bipolar cells in a pure rod retina to light flashes of varying intensity. Noteworthy is the very high sensitivity of response of rod bipolar cells in the dark-adapted retina, such that an easily recordable response without signal averaging was evident when only one out of ten rods would have absorbed a photon.

Cone bipolar cells are of two types: those that depolarize (ON center) and those that hyperpolarize (OFF center) in response to central illumination, so called because they provide excitatory or inhibitory inputs to amacrine or ganglion cells in response to light. The retina is thus organized into two parallel pathways: the ON pathway, which responds to a local increase in brightness, and the OFF pathway, which responds to a decrease in brightness. Such parallel processing enhances the contrast sensitivity of the eye. The ON and OFF bipolar cells make synaptic contact with amacrine and ganglion cells in different parts of the IPL. Figure 8.2 shows a rod ON bipolar cell injected with a fluorescent dye after its light responses had been recorded. The axon terminals of ON bipolar cells extend to the proximal part of the IPL, while the OFF bipolar cells make their synaptic contacts within the distal part of the IPL. Although there is only one type of mammalian rod bipolar cell, rod-

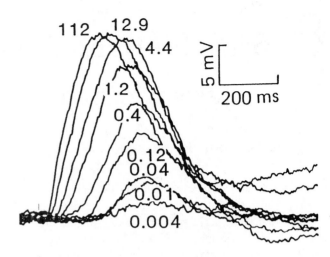

FIGURE 8.1 Voltage responses of a single dark-adapted rod bipolar cell to brief flashes of varying intensity recorded from the all-rod dogfish retina, using an intracellular microelectrode. Numbers by the records indicate the mean number of rhodopsin molecules bleached in each rod by the flash (timing indicated by the lowest trace). The slow time course of the response arises because recordings were obtained at low temperature, about 18°C. Note that depolarization is indicated as upward deflection. (Source: From Falk G.[4] Used by permission.)

driven ON and OFF responses can be recorded from ganglion cells because there is a special rod pathway via amacrine cells (discussed later in the chapter). In mammals, bipolar cells receiving exclusive input from rods are the depolarizing ON type, while cones drive both ON and OFF bipolar cells. However, recently, it has been shown that there is an additional pathway for rod signals: via cone OFF bipolar cells making direct synaptic contact with rods. The response to light that is selectively absorbed by the cones is much faster than the rod-elicited response in part because of more rapid cone phototransduction. The cone-driven response is also much less sensitive (per absorbed photon).

Glutamate receptors and conductance changes

Given that the presynaptic input to horizontal, OFF bipolar, and ON bipolar cells from photoreceptors is essentially identical, consisting of a light-induced reduction in glutamate release, how then are the center postsynaptic responses of opposing polarities generated? Quite simply, the polarity depends on the type of glutamate receptors that are expressed on the postsynaptic membrane of these second-order cells. The decrease in glutamate is sensed in OFF bipolar and horizontal cells by ionotropic glutamate receptors (iGluRs), which directly gate nonselective cation channels. Glutamate that is bound to these receptors opens the channels, so in the dark, the fraction of channels that are opened by the tonic release of glutamate is high, and these cells are relatively depolarized. Light suppresses glutamate

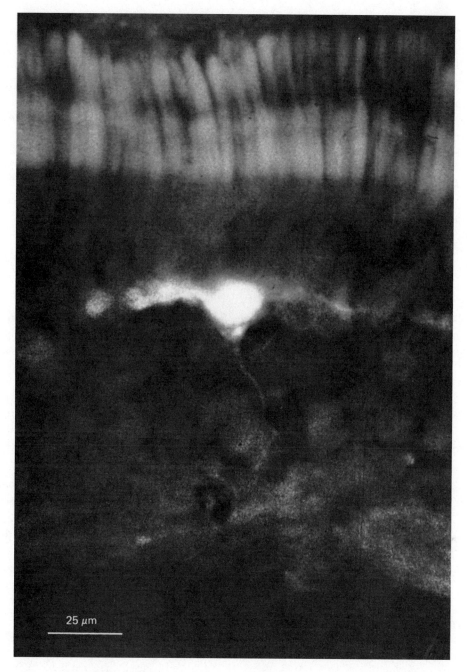

FIGURE 8.2 Radial section of a dogfish retina viewed in a fluorescence microscope. In the center of the field is a rod bipolar cell injected with the fluorescent dye in situ after recording light responses, as in Figure 8.1. In the upper part of the photomicrograph, the autofluorescent rod outer segments can be seen. The larger bipolar cell dendrites extending through the outer plexiform layer have filled with fluorescent dye. The fine axon of the bipolar cell can be traced deep into the inner plexiform layer, terminating as a bulbous knob (calibration bar 25 μm). The large size of the cell body enabled stable recordings to be made. (Source: From Ashmore JF, Falk G.[1] Used by permission.) (See also color plate 10.)

release, so the fraction of open channels is reduced, and the reduction in inward cationic current results in hyperpolarizing responses. So the polarity of the photoreceptor response is conserved in OFF bipolar and horizontal cells. On the other hand, rod ON bipolar cells express a unique metabotropic glutamate receptor (mGluR6) that is indirectly linked to postsynaptic cation channels by a biochemical cascade, leading to the control of concentration of the internal messenger, cyclic guanosine monophosphate (cGMP).

The cGMP cascade of the rod bipolar cell

Figure 8.3 illustrates the biochemical cascade linking the glutamate receptor mGluR6 via a GTP-binding protein (G-protein) to the hydrolysis of cGMP by phosphodiesterase (PDE). In the dark, when glutamate release from rod synaptic terminals is high, PDE activity is also high, and consequently, cGMP levels are low. A large proportion of cGMP-activated channels, permeable to cations (Na^+, K^+, and Ca^{2+}) in the dendritic membrane are therefore closed in the dark, so the bipolar cell is relatively hyperpolarized. On

the other hand, in the light, when glutamate release falls as a result of rod hyperpolarization, bipolar cell PDE activity is reduced, so cGMP levels rise, opening cGMP-activated channels, enabling a cation influx, thereby depolarizing the cell. Cyclic GMP is synthesized by guanylate cyclase, which in the bipolar cell is the type containing a heme group, activated by nitric oxide. The analogy of the rod bipolar cell cGMP cascade linked to the glutamate receptor with the rod phototransduction cascade linked to rhodopsin is illustrated in figure 8.4. However, the elements of the cascade are distinct from a molecular standpoint. It is likely that the blue cone ON bipolar cell also operates via a cGMP cascade, but evidence for the red and green mammalian ON pathway is less clear.

Synaptic gain and the light sensitivity of postsynaptic cells

High visual sensitivity depends not only on the high gain that is inherent in the process of phototransduction in rods, but also on amplification of photoreceptor signals by synaptic events. For synaptic transmission to rod horizontal and OFF bipolar cells, the voltage gain is 5–10, but for rod transmission to ON bipolar cells, it is at least 100 when dark-adapted. This difference is reflected in the much greater sensitivity of the rod ON bipolar cells to light such that an appreciable signal is generated when a photon is absorbed by only 1 out of 40 human rods making synaptic contact with the ON bipolar cell. Biophysical modeling of synaptic transmission from rods to ON bipolar cells has shown that such high amplification at this synapse is possible if the biochemical gain of the glutamate receptor–linked cGMP cascade underlying generation of their light responses is sufficiently high. More simply, the linking of single glutamate receptors to the control of a large number of cGMP-activated channels would provide for such large signal amplification, while the glutamate receptors of OFF bipolar or horizontal cells are constrained to the regulation of single channels.

A second factor in generating higher gain in the rod bipolar cell is purely electrical. Because most of the channels are closed in the dark by the action of glutamate, the voltage change produced in the ON bipolar cell by a given conductance change will be larger than would be the case if there were many channels open in the dark. The presence of open channels would otherwise shunt out the voltage produced by a given fall in transmitter concentration. The synapse with ON bipolar cells also behaves as a high-pass filter, which improves temporal resolution in the rod pathway. This is now thought to be due to a nonlinear positive feedback intracellular mechanism operating on the cGMP-sensitive channels to speed up the rising phase of their responses.

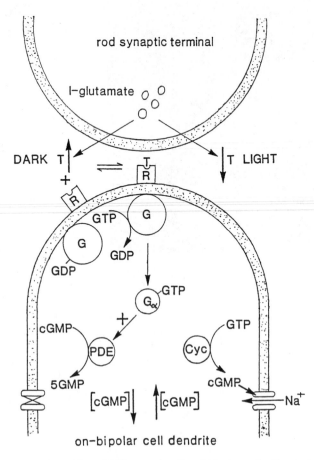

FIGURE 8.3 The cGMP cascade of rod bipolar cells. See text. (Source: Modified from Shiells RA, Falk G.[11])

PHOTOTRANSDUCTION   **SYNAPTIC-TRANSDUCTION**

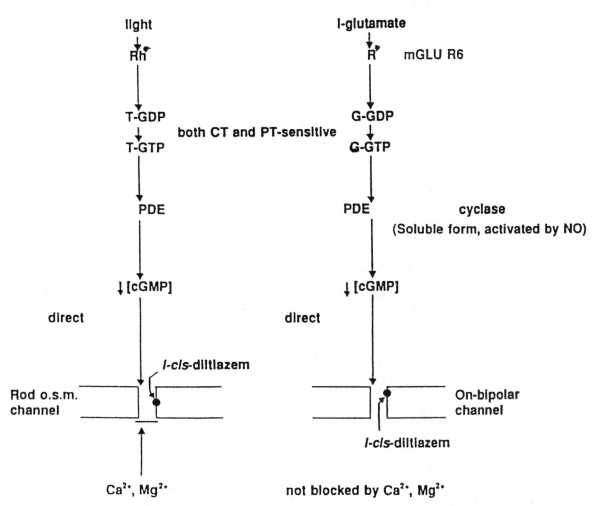

FIGURE 8.4   Comparison between phototransduction in rods and synaptic transduction in rod bipolar cells. Light-activated rhodopsin (Rh*) and the glutamate receptor that is bound to glutamate (R*) stand in an analogous role in activating a cell-specific G-protein, transducin (T) in rods and G_o in rod bipolar cells, leading to a fall in cGMP by the action of phosphodiesterase (PDE). Because these two cascades are in series and glutamate release depends on rod voltage, the effects of light on cGMP levels are opposite, hyperpolarizing rods and depolarizing the bipolar cell. The cGMP-sensitive channels are distinct. Rod channels are blocked by divalent cations, and both channels can be blocked by L-cis-diltiazem but at different blocking sites. (Source: From Shiells RA, Falk G.[13] Used by permission.)

Generation of the b-wave

The large gain in synaptic transmission from rods to ON bipolar cells accounts for the very large difference in the light required to elicit the a-wave of the ERG as compared with the scotopic b-wave. Figure 8.5A shows simultaneously recorded intracellular rod ON bipolar cell and b-wave responses to light, showing a clear correlation in time course. The correlation between the peak amplitudes of the bipolar cell voltage response and the isolated b-wave, extending over a range of 10^4 in light intensity, is shown in figure 8.5B. Because rod ON bipolar cells possess distinctly different glutamate receptors from OFF bipolar or horizontal cells, it is possible to selectively block their light responses with the mGluR6 agonist 2-amino-4-phosphonobutyrate (APB) experimentally, which results in a loss of the b-wave.

It was also shown that the DC component of the ERG arises from plateau rod bipolar cell responses to steps of light. A large part of the delay between the a- and the b-waves of the ERG arises because of the cGMP cascade of ON bipolar cells.

There have been two theories of how the rod bipolar cells generate the b-wave. One of these is that the b-wave is a result of the voltage drop in the extracellular medium as a result of radial current flow through the ON bipolar cell membrane. The second idea would attribute the radial current flow originating from Muller cells as a result of their depolarization by a rise in K^+ leaked from bipolar cells. A diffusional delay would be expected, and the close

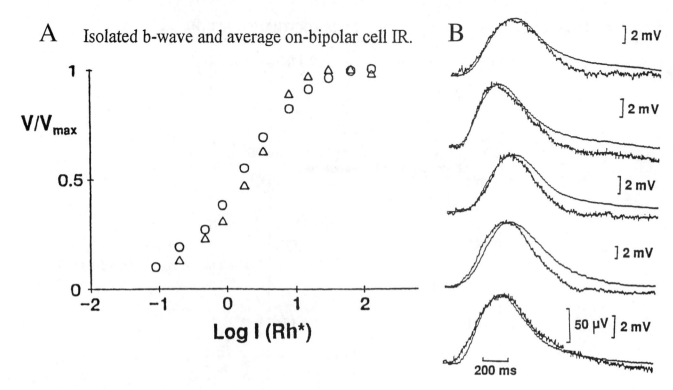

A Isolated b-wave and average on-bipolar cell IR.

B

FIGURE 8.5 Relationship between light-induced depolarization of rod bipolar cells and the b-wave. A, The normalized bipolar cell light responses as a function of log flash intensity compared with the simultaneously recorded b-waves. The amplitude of the b-waves at higher light intensities was corrected for the amplitude of the a-wave (PIII in Granit's terminology), determined after selectively blocking the b-wave. Rh* denotes the mean number of rhodopsin molecules per rod isomerised by the flash. B, The time course of five rod bipolar cell voltage responses to brief dim flashes isomerizing 1.8 Rh* compared with the simultaneously recorded b-waves (noisy traces), scaled to the same peak amplitudes. (Source: Modified from Shiells RA, Falk G,[15] 1999.)

agreement in time course of the rod bipolar cell response and the b-wave would tend to rule out a Muller cell origin. A further finding that the b-wave is unaffected by blocking Muller cell K channels also supports this conclusion.

Light adaptation

The gain in synaptic transmission from rods to ON bipolar cells is not fixed but decreases on exposure even to dim background light that is too weak to desensitize rods. Desensitization of rod ON bipolar cell light responses occurs on exposure to backgrounds that isomerize less than one rhodopsin molecule per rod per second (1 Rh**/s). Figure 8.6A shows a whole-cell voltage clamp recording from an ON bipolar cell in the dogfish all-rod retinal slice, with a Ca^{2+} buffer added to the intracellular patch pipette solution. The method allows the experimenter to alter the diffusible contents of a single cell and to measure ionic currents, which flow through ionic channels. The initial downward deflections are inward *current* responses (which underlie the cell's typical depolarizing voltage responses) to a range of flash intensities applied to determine the cell's intensity response relation in the dark. On exposure to a dim light step, the cell responded with a sustained inward

current, and the superimposed test flashes showed little reduction. Figure 8.6B shows the same experiment repeated on equilibration with a patch pipette solution containing no internal Ca^{2+} buffer. At the onset of the light step, there was a transient inward current that rapidly decayed, returning close to the dark level despite continued illumination. Test flash responses were suppressed for 30s by the dim background, then recovered to about half their initial flash sensitivity. At step offset, there was a small outward transient, followed by recovery of flash response sensitivity to control.

Figure 8.6C shows that a light step 10 times brighter than in figure 8.6B does not elicit a sustained response in the absence of Ca^{2+} buffering. Moreover, the desensitization that is induced by the background light is more profound, such that a bright flash (128 Rh*) superimposed on the background produces almost no response, whereas in the dark-adapted state, it would have yielded a maximum flash response. In contrast, a step of light even 10 times brighter than that in figure 8.6C elicits a sustained response (figure 8.6D) when intracellular Ca^{2+} was well buffered. Light of this intensity is sufficient to produce significant rod desensitization, which accounts for the diminished responses to the test flashes after the offset of the light step.

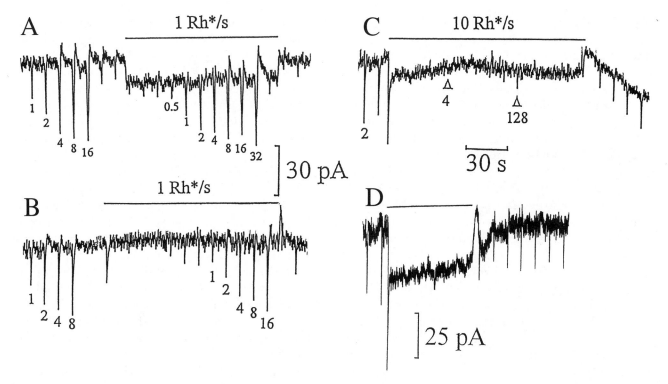

FIGURE 8.6 Ca²⁺ induces light adaptation in rod bipolar cells in a retinal slice. A, Current responses to a long step of light isomerizing 1 Rh*/s with a Ca²⁺ chelator filling the cell interior, with the cell voltage-clamped. Downward deflections are inward current responses to light. In the absence of the voltage clamp, the cell would have given depolarizing responses proportional to the current. The numbers below the responses indicate the intensity of test flashes in rhodopsin molecules isomerized per rod per flash. Note the sustained response during the light step and the absence of desensitization. B, The same protocol without Ca²⁺ chelator.

Note the brief transient response at onset of the light step rapidly decaying despite the continued presence of light. Sensitivity to superimposed flashes was reduced by a factor of 2–3. C, Responses to a brighter light step (10 Rh*/s) without Ca²⁺ chelator. Note the large initial response followed by a rapid decay and absence of sustained inward current during the light step. Test flashes (arrowheads) even 60 times higher than those used in the dark-adapted state produced almost no response. D, Responses to a step isomerizing 100 Rh*/s when Ca²⁺ is well buffered. (Source: Modified from Shiells RA, Falk G.[14])

These results indicate that Ca²⁺ enters the cGMP-activated channels when they are opened by light, and the rise in Ca²⁺ acts to desensitize the rod ON bipolar cell. Similar results have been obtained in mammalian retina. Subsequent work has shown that this action of Ca²⁺ is mediated by the enzyme Ca²⁺/calmodulin kinase II (CaMKII), which phosphorylates the cGMP-activated channels and reduces their conductance. This form of desensitization occurs only in the rod pathway. Cone bipolar cells in mammalian retina do not show this form of desensitization (with the possible exception of blue cone ON bipolar cells). This mechanism underlies network or postphotoreceptor adaptation in the retina, the reduction in synaptic gain extending the operating range of the rod pathway, which would otherwise saturate at relatively low light levels.

Signal pathways from bipolar cells

TRANSMITTER RELEASE FROM BIPOLAR CELLS   Like photoreceptors, bipolar cells also release glutamate as their transmitter. They make highly specialized ribbon and basal synaptic contacts with amacrine and ganglion cells. The presynaptic ribbon (also present in rods) is thought to line up synaptic vesicles for rapid release, which are then replenished from the vesicular pool. Bipolar cells possess both sustained and transient Ca²⁺ currents. These mechanisms participate in forming distinct phasic and tonic components in the transmitter release process, functioning to speed up the kinetics and increase synaptic gain on transmission to third-order cells.

POSTSYNAPTIC RESPONSES OF AMACRINE CELLS   Action potentials are generated only in the inner retina, in amacrine and ganglion cells. The synaptic input to amacrine cells from bipolar cells is mediated primarily by iGluRs, of which there are two principal types, termed NMDA and AMPA receptors. Many subtypes of amacrine cells have been classified, according to physiological (e.g., sustained—responding to a step of light with a maintained discharge—or transient—responding to a light step with transient changes in firing at light onset and offset), morphological (e.g., starburst), or pharmacological criteria (e.g., indoleamine accumulating cells (IACs)). Their principal function, rather like that of horizontal cells in the outer retina, is to mediate lateral interactions, particularly in the formation of the inhibitory surround of the ganglion cell receptive field. Gap junctions extensively couple these cells and their degree of coupling is highly dependent on their state of light- or dark-adaptation. Some amacrine cells release the inhibitory transmitter GABA to oppose the excitatory actions of glutamate released by ON or OFF bipolar cells. Amacrine cells make reciprocal synapses, which feed lateral information back onto bipolar cell synaptic terminals. It is thought that sustained amacrine cells possess predominantly NMDA-type glutamate receptors, while transient amacrine cell responses are mediated by rapidly desensitizing AMPA-type glutamate receptors.

In mammalian retina, rod bipolar cells make synaptic contact almost exclusively with IACs and AII amacrine cells, there being no direct contact with ganglion cells as in lower vertebrates. IACs show no antagonistic surround, while the AII cells have a highly developed surround formed via inhibitory drive from neighboring amacrine cells. In both the ON and OFF pathways, rod signals reach the ganglion cells from the amacrine cells via the synaptic terminals of the cone bipolar cells. Cone signals follow the much more direct route, ON and OFF cone bipolar cells driving ON and OFF ganglion cells directly. Low-resistance electrical junctions exist between the AII cells and the ON bipolar cell of the cone pathway, so the signal that is conveyed to the AII cell from the rod bipolar cell is in turn fed directly to the cone ON bipolar cell and then on to the ON ganglion cell. Rod signals reach OFF ganglion cells again via the AII cells, but here the signal is inverted via an inhibitory glycinergic synapse onto cone OFF bipolar cell synaptic terminals, which act to reduce glutamate release, forming an OFF response to light.

Very recently, the role of electrical gap junction synapses in transmission of rod signals in the mammalian retina has been demonstrated. Gap junctions are composed of intercellular channels that span the plasma membrane of adjacent cells, thereby coupling them with a low-resistance electrical pathway. In mice that lack expression of the protein connexin36, which is essential for gap junction formation in the retina, rod ON signals are not transmitted to the ON ganglion cells, while cone signals are transmitted normally. This is because, as is illustrated in figure 8.7, there are no direct synaptic contacts made between rod ON bipolar cells and ganglion cells. Instead, rod signals are relayed to ganglion cells via several indirect pathways, which are dependent on electrical coupling.

POSTSYNAPTIC RESPONSES OF GANGLION CELLS   Figure 8.8 shows the spike trains from a single ON center ganglion cell. As is typical for mammalian ganglion cells, there is a main-tained discharge in the dark, resulting from the spontaneous thermal isomerization of rhodopsin in the rods within the receptive field of the ganglion cell. Although rhodopsin is very stable, there is a small probability that one of the 10^8 rhodopsin molecules in each rod will spontaneously isomerize, leading to events identical to those resulting from the absorption of a single photon. As shown in figure 8.8A, the ON ganglion cell firing rate promptly increases when a small spot of light is centered within the receptive field. An annulus of light (figure 8.8B) suppresses the spontaneous discharge, and when the annulus is removed, there is a transient increase in the firing rate. Uniform illumination (figure 8.8C), which stimulates both the center and the surround, has a lesser effect on the firing rate. When the observations are repeated with OFF ganglion cells, the firing pattern is reversed. A small central spot of light inhibits firing, but at light offset, there is a brisk increase in firing. A bright annulus increases firing, which is then inhibited at the offset of the light. Uniform illumination again has much less effect on firing. Center surround characteristics are much reduced in the well-dark-adapted retina.

ON and OFF ganglion cells are further classified as sustained or transient. Some ganglion cells are directionally sensitive, responding only to light moving across their receptive field in a preferred direction and not responding to stationary light. Other cells act as simple motion detectors. Others function as edge detectors and have been termed ON-OFF cells, responding to both light onset and offset with bursts (or suppression) of action potentials. Many ganglion cells simply reflect the properties of the bipolar cells that are presynaptic to them; for instance, color-opponent receptive fields, developed at the bipolar cell level, can be observed in ganglion cells. However, a high degree of complexity in the integration of signals is introduced at the level of the IPL.

Retinal neurotransmitters

Most of the neurotransmitters that are found in the central nervous system are also found in the retina. Glutamate is perhaps the most predominant, being released by photoreceptors, bipolar cells, and probably some amacrine cells. Glutamate acts on ganglion cells to increase the visually evoked response of both ON- and OFF-sustained ganglion cells but not of transient cells. On the other hand, acetylcholine enhances the firing of transient ganglion cells and is released by ON and OFF amacrine cells that have a characteristic elaborate morphology: the starburst amacrine cells.

The inhibitory transmitters are γ-amino butyric acid (GABA) and glycine. Glycine and GABA$_A$ receptors open Cl channels and thus reduce the effect of excitatory transmitters that act on cationic channels. GABA is accumulated by horizontal cells in some species and mediates surround

Rod signaling pathways

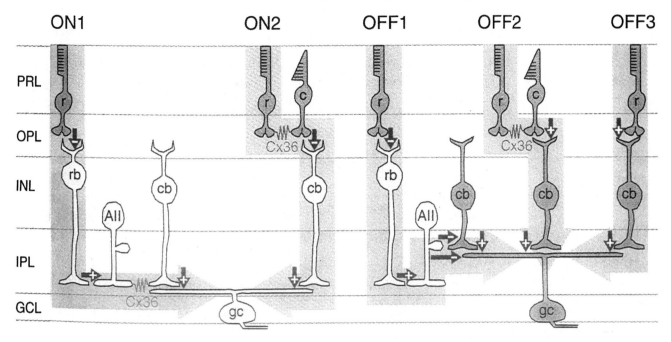

FIGURE 8.7 Mammalian retinal signaling pathways. On-pathways are shown in green, off-pathways in blue (and are labelled ON or OFF above). Synapses are shown by arrows with (+) indicating sign conserving and (−) sign indicating reversing. Dark gray cells hyperpolarize in response to light. Gap junctions are indicated in red.

Symbols: r, rod; c, cone; rb, rod bipolar cell; AII, amacrine cell; gc, ganglion cell; PRL photo-receptor layer; OPL, outer plexiform layer; INL, inner nuclear layer; GCL ganglion cell layer. Horizontal cells have been excluded from the diagram. (Source: Reproduced from Demb JB, Pugh EN.[3] Used by permission.) (See also color plate 11.)

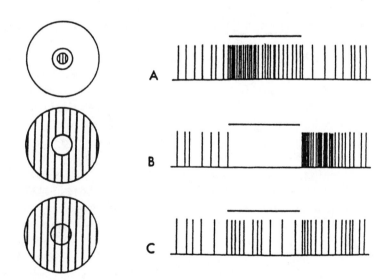

FIGURE 8.8 Center surround antagonism in an ON center retinal ganglion cell. The pattern of illumination of the receptive field is shown by the hatched area. A, The large initial increase in firing rate is followed by a slowing in the rate at light offset. B, The opposite occurs when only the surround is illuminated. C, Uniform illumination results in little change in firing rate. In an OFF center ganglion cell (not shown), the pattern of response is the reverse of the above: inhibition during central illumination and increased firing at light offset. Under scotopic conditions, there is little center surround antagonism. (From Kuffler S.W., *Invest. Ophthal.* 12, 1973. Used by permission.)

inhibition of bipolar cells. ON center ganglion cells receive inhibitory input from GABA-ergic amacrine cells, while OFF center ganglion cells receive inhibitory input from glycinergic amacrine cells.

Dopamine is released by some amacrine cells and interplexiform cells. This transmitter functions as a neuromodulator and is thought to elicit some of the receptive field changes that occur in horizontal and some amacrine cells with light adaptation. Dopamine acts on D_1-type receptors on horizontal cells to raise the intracellular level of the second-messenger cyclic AMP, which reduces the permeability of intercellular electrical gap junction connections. Light stimulates dopamine release, so horizontal cells show a reduction in receptive field size with light adaptation and, consequently, a decrease in the extent of surround antagonism of bipolar cell responses. Dopaminergic amacrine cells make extensive connections with AII amacrine cells. Dopamine reduces the light responses of rod bipolar cells and the b-wave. Many of the effects of dopamine are exerted at sites that are distant from the initial site of release. The dispersion of pigment granules of the pigment epithelium in the light is mediated by dopamine that is released more proximally in the retina.

Nitric oxide (NO) also functions as a neuromodulator in the retina. Most retinal neurons possess NO synthase, which is activated by a rise in intracellular Ca^{2+} with depolarization. NO activates the soluble form of guanylate cyclase, leading to a rise in intracellular cyclic GMP. NO enhances ON bipolar cell light responses and regulates gap junction permeability in horizontal and amacrine cells, elevated cyclic GMP acting to reduce receptive fields. NO also acts to increase local blood flow.

Further investigation will determine the role of other neurotransmitters, such as serotonin, adrenaline, substance P, and other peptides, in visual processing. There is also now evidence suggesting a role for neurotrophins such as insulin-stimulated growth factor in regulating rod sensitivity, while epidermal growth factor may be involved in regulating the function of cGMP-activated channels of rod bipolar cells[17]. The latter is particularly interesting in view of the autoimmune disease melanoma-associated retinopathy (MAR), which specifically involves the failure of ON bipolar cell responsivity.

Possible relevance to clinical states

We consider cases in which photoreceptor function is normal or nearly normal but vision and the b-wave of the ERG are abnormal.

INHERITED NIGHT-BLINDNESS   A patient with an absent or defective gene for the elements of the cGMP cascade linking the metabotropic glutamate receptor mGluR6 to the unique cGMP-activated membrane channel of the rod bipolar cell will be permanently night-blind (see figure 8.3). This glutamate receptor, mGluR6, occurs only in the ON bipolar cell; it is not expressed elsewhere in either the retina or the nervous system. On the other hand, the G-protein G_o is fairly ubiquitous, being found in other retinal neurons, the nervous system, and elsewhere, associated with some second-messenger systems. We found that incorporating an antibody raised to the C-terminal intracellular portion of mGluR6 into rod bipolar cells abolished their light responses. This result showed the importance of the linkage between the transmembrane glutamate receptor and the intracellular G-protein. Knock-out mice lacking the mGluR6 gene have no b-wave (similar to the b-wave deficiency in night-blind patients) but are not totally blind, since they avoid objects using visual cues.

The type of phosphodiesterase expressed in rod bipolar cells has not been identified, so little can be said about genetic defects at this site. Other possible defective sites in the cGMP cascade could be the membrane cGMP channel or the enzyme that generates cGMP: guanylate cyclase.

MELANOMA-ASSOCIATED RETINOPATHY (MAR)   MAR is an autoimmune disease in which some patients with cutaneous melanoma have a circulating antibody to the retinal ON bipolar cell. Scotopic vision of such patients may be severely affected, and their dark-adapted b-wave may be markedly reduced. Injection of immunoglobulin (IgG) from MAR patients into the vitreous of monkey eyes caused the loss of the b-wave within 3 hours. As a control, IgG from patients with cutaneous melanoma but without visual problems had no effect on the b-wave recorded from monkey eyes.

What the precise relationship is between cutaneous melanoma and defective bipolar cell signaling has not been obvious. Our recent work suggests a possible, if speculative, connection. We discovered an apparent involvement of epidermal growth factor (EGF) in regulating the sensitivity of the ON bipolar cell cGMP–activated channel. Possible targets of the antibody in MAR might be the EGF receptor or the protein tyrosine phosphatase that is known to be present in rod bipolar cell dendrites. The rod cGMP–activated channel, which differs from the bipolar cell cGMP channel (messenger RNA encoding the cone cGMP–activated channel has recently been identified in ON bipolar cells), is not affected in MAR. It is interesting to note that the sensitivity of the rod cGMP channel is also regulated by a growth factor, the insulinlike growth factor.

CONE DYSFUNCTION WITH MILD NYCTALOPIA   The ERG results on five patients with cone dysfunction and mild nyctalopia compared with normal are shown in figure 8.9. In these patients, flash sensitivity is lower, by 1 log unit, and the b-wave increases supralinearly with light intensity, becoming

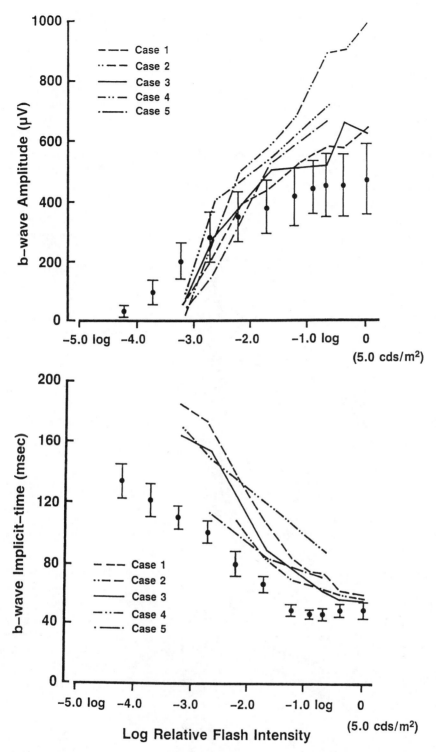

FIGURE 8.9   Dark-adapted amplitude and temporal characteristics of the b-wave as a function of flash intensity in five cone dystrophy patients with abnormal function of the rod pathway. Circles: normal values ± standard deviations. Note the shift of 1 log unit to increased threshold in patients, the supralinear increase in b-wave amplitude, supernormal b-waves at high light intensity, and increased implicit times. (Source: Reproduced with permission from Rosenberg T, Simonsen SE.[8])

supranormal at high light intensity. Normal subjects had a b-wave that increased linearly with light intensity, then rose less steeply before reaching maximum at high intensity. The rate of rise of the b-wave is slower, and its time to peak (implicit time) is markedly increased in these patients. A number of investigators have proposed that this condition arises from an abnormally high level of cGMP in the retina, with a number of different loci suggested.

Recent experimental results on the depolarizing rod bipolar cell, however, suggest that the abnormal b-wave and sensitivity results could be duplicated by an abnormally *low* level of ON bipolar cell cGMP. The current in response to light from a rod bipolar cell at low cGMP and that after the cGMP level was elevated by dim background light are shown in figure 8.10. At low cGMP, flash sensitivity was low, and responses rose supralinearly as the square of intensity. The rate of rise to peak of the flash responses was slow, and the peak was delayed. With an increase in cGMP level, flash sensitivity increased by 1 log unit, the responses became linear at low light levels and the time to peak decreased. The effect of background light could be reproduced by directly elevating intracellular cGMP by $20\,\mu M$. However, there was no difference in the maximum current elicited by bright light flashes.

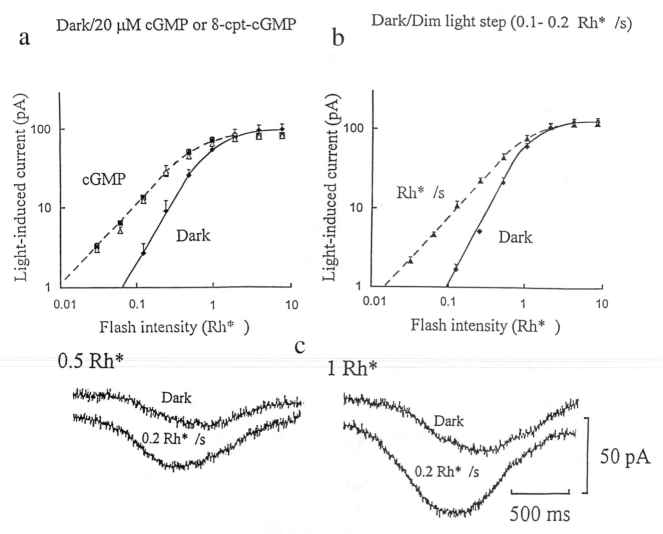

FIGURE 8.10 The potentiating effect on rod bipolar cell light responses of raising intracellular cGMP by dim background light or by intracellular addition. A, The effect of inclusion of cGMP ($20\,\mu M$) in the recording pipette. Current responses to brief flashes were measured from voltage-clamped rod bipolar cells. Circles indicate mean responses before diffusion of cGMP into the cells, triangles on equilibration with cGMP. Note that both response amplitude and flash intensity (Rh*, number of rhodopsins isomerized per rod) are plotted on log scales so that the slopes, close to unity and 2 for raised cGMP and control, respectively, show that with raised cGMP, responses increase linearly with light, while with low cGMP, they rise as the square of intensity. B, The effect of dim background light (0.1–0.2 Rh*/s) on responses to brief flashes. C, The speeding up of flash responses (and decrease in implicit time) by dim background light. (Source: From Shiells RA, Falk G.[17])

The latter result is not necessarily at variance with the observations of supernormal b-waves in patients with this cone dysfunction. The b-wave represents the voltage change across the retina as a result of current flow arising from the membrane voltage change of rod bipolar cells responding to light. The experiments described above represent the *current flow* through the cGMP-dependent channels under voltage clamp. This current would produce a voltage change whose magnitude would depend on the impedance of the bipolar cell. If the dark level of cGMP is low, there would be fewer open channels than normal and a higher impedance. Consequently, there would be a larger voltage response when all channels are opened by a bright flash. The situation is more complicated in b-wave recordings, but one would also expect a larger maximum b-wave response with low cGMP. Another factor is the delay between the a- and b-waves. With low cGMP, the response of the bipolar cell is delayed in comparison with normal and hence there is less interference between the a- and b-wave amplitudes. Another possible factor is the antagonism between the rod and cone pathways. It is known that rod signals decrease signals in the cone pathway. If this occurs normally, any such antagonism would not occur in the case of cone dystrophy.

There are several ways of testing whether the ERG results in patients arise as a result of a deficiency in rod bipolar cell cGMP levels. One way is to raise cGMP by testing in the presence of a very dim background light, too low to light adapt the retina, of the order of one to two rhodopsin molecules isomerized per rod per second. Another is to raise cGMP by stimulating the bipolar cell enzyme guanylate cyclase with NO. Rod guanylate cyclase, being a different type, would be unaffected. Agents that generate NO in vivo are amyl nitrite by inhalation or nitroglycerine sublingually. It is important to measure the b-wave over a wide range of light intensities, from very dim to bright flashes.

REFERENCES

1. Ashmore JF, Falk G: Responses of rod bipolar cells in the dark-adapted retina of the dogfish, *Scyliorhinus canicula. J Physiol (Lond)* 1980; 300:115–150.

2. Bloomfield SA, Dacheux RF: Rod vision: Pathways and processing in the mammalian retina. *Prog Ret Eye Res* 2001; 20:351–384.

3. Demb JB, Pugh EN: Connexin36 forms synapses essential for night vision. *Neuron* 2002; 336:551–553.

4. Falk G: Signal transmission from rods to bipolar and horizontal cells: A synthesis. *Prog Ret Res* 1989; 8:255–289.

5. Lei B, Bush RA, Milam AH, Sieving PA: Human melanoma-associated retinopathy (MAR) antibodies alter the retinal ON-response of the monkey ERG in vivo. *Invest Ophthal Vis Sci* 2000; 41:262–266.

6. Milam AH, Saari JC, Jacobson SG, et al: Autoantibodies against retinal bipolar cells in cutaneous melanoma-associated retinopathy. *Invest Ophthal Vis Sci* 1993; 34:91–100.

7. Nakajima Y, Iwakabe H, Akazawa C, et al: Molecular characterization of a novel retinal metabotropic glutamate receptor mGluR6 with a high agonist selectivity for L-2-amino-4-phosphonobutyrate. *J Biol Chem* 1993; 268:11868–11873.

8. Rosenberg T, Simonsen SE: Retinal cone dysfunction of supernormal rod ERG type. *Acta Ophthalmologica* 1993; 71:246–253.

9. Savchenko A, Kraft TW, Molokanova E, Kramer RH: Growth factors regulate phototduction in retinal rods by modulating cyclic nucleotide-gated channels through dephosphorylation of a specific tyrosine residue. *Proc Natl Acad Sci USA* 2001; 98:5880–5885.

10. Shiells RA, Falk G: Glutamate receptors of rod bipolar cells are linked to a cyclic GMP cascade via a G-protein. *Proc Roy Soc Lond* 1990; B 242:91–94.

11. Shiells RA, Falk G: Properties of the cGMP–activated channel of retinal on-bipolar cells. *Proc Roy Soc Lond* 1992; B 247:21–25.

12. Shiells RA, Falk G: Retinal on-bipolar cells contain a nitric oxide-sensitive guanylate cyclase. *Neuroreport* 1992; 3:845–848.

13. Shiells RA, Falk G: Signal transduction in retinal bipolar cells. *Prog Ret Eye Res* 1995; 14:223–247.

14. Shiells RA, Falk G: A rise in intracellular Ca^{2+} underlies light adaptation in dogfish retinal "on" bipolar cells. *J Physiol (Lond)* 1999; 514:343–350.

15. Shiells RA, Falk G: Contribution of rod, on-bipolar, and horizontal cell light responses to the ERG of dogfish retina. *Vis Neurosci* 1999; 16:503–511.

16. Shiells RA, Falk G: Activation of Ca^{2+}-calmodulin kinase II induces desensitization by background light in dogfish retinal "on" bipolar cells. *J Physiol (Lond)* 2000; 528:327–338.

17. Shiells RA, Falk G: Potentiation of "on" bipolar cell flash responses by dim background light and cGMP in dogfish retinal slices. *J Physiol (Lond)* 2002; 542:211–230.

18. Troy JB, Shou T: The receptive fields of cat retinal ganglion cells in physiological and pathological states: where we are after half a century of research. *Prog Ret Eye Res* 2002; 21:263–302.

9 Structure and Function of Retinal Synapses: Role of Cell Adhesion Molecules and Extracellular Matrix

WILLIAM J. BRUNKEN, THOMAS CLAUDEPIERRE, MARY K. MANGLAPUS, AND DALE D. HUNTER

RETINAL ORGANIZATION is deceptively simple; its simplicity and beauty have drawn many a researcher's attention. The relationship between structure and function has been explored since the time of the elegant work of Ramón y Cajal. Although over 100 years of study has unraveled many secrets, a complete understanding of retinal function eludes us.

Nevertheless, the basic principles of retinal organization and development are understood in greater detail than those of any other region of the central nervous system. The basic anatomy and physiology of the retina were discussed in the foregoing chapters of this edition (see chapters 6, 7, and 8; see also the Selected Readings). Two questions are the subject of this review:

1. What is the ultrastructural organization of the synaptic layers in the retina?

2. How do cell adhesion and extracellular matrix molecules contribute to the development of connectivity in the retina?

Basic organization of retinal synaptic layers

Anatomically, the retina is a club sandwich: three cellular layers with two interposing synaptic layers. The cell layer immediately adjacent to the vitreous humor is the ganglion cell layer, wherein the cell bodies (nucleus and perinuclear organelles) of most ganglion cells (and some amacrine cells) lie. The layer most distant from the vitreous humor, that is, the outermost layer, contains the cell bodies of the photoreceptors and is called the outer nuclear layer (ONL; the photoreceptor nuclei are the most prominent element in the light microscope). Between photoreceptors and ganglion cells are the second-order neurons (or interneurons) of the retina, whose cell bodies are collected together in the middle cell

layer, called the inner nuclear layer (INL); these are the bipolar cells, horizontal cells, and amacrine cells.

Connections between photoreceptors and retinal interneurons are confined to a discrete synaptic layer immediately vitreal (toward the vitreous humor) from the ONL in a plexus known as the outer plexiform layer (OPL). Connections between interneurons and ganglion cells are confined to a larger, more complex synaptic layer called the inner plexiform layer (IPL). Ramón y Cajal deduced from this organization that the information transfer in the retina was from photoreceptors to bipolar cells (one of the interneurons) to ganglion cells (see figure 9.1). Moreover, he understood implicitly that an understanding of retinal function would come about by unraveling the complex connections among cells in the IPL. He wrote, "in the inner plexiform layer, the multiplicity of the surfaces of contact or of the horizontal plexuses seems to be for the purpose of enabling a large number of distinct pathways to exist within a small area of the retina." Indeed, on the basis of his observations of the termination patterns of bipolar cells and ganglion cells, Ramón y Cajal divided the IPL into five layers. Since the advent of electrophysiological recordings, first extracellular, then a variety of intracellular, and now a large array of techniques, we have learned a vast amount about retinal connectivity and retinal processing.

One general principle is that there are, in mammalian retina, separate rod and cone pathways. Rod photoreceptors terminate within a discrete region of the OPL; cones terminate in another region adjacent to the INL. As was discussed in chapters 6 and 7, there are direct connections between rods and cones; nevertheless, the fundamental division of rod and cone signals predominates, and the retina can be described in this duplex fashion. Similarly in the IPL, rod and cone information at the first stage of processing is kept separate: Rods connect predominantly to a special bipolar cell that arborizes tightly in layer 5 of the IPL (adjacent to the ganglion cell layer). Here the so-called rod bipolar cell connects with a specialized amacrine cell, the AII or rod amacrine; the output of the AII amacrine cell is

---

This chapter is dedicated to the memory of our colleague and friend Grant W. Balkema (July 1, 1951–Nov 24, 2004), a pioneer in the understanding of photoreceptor structure and function.

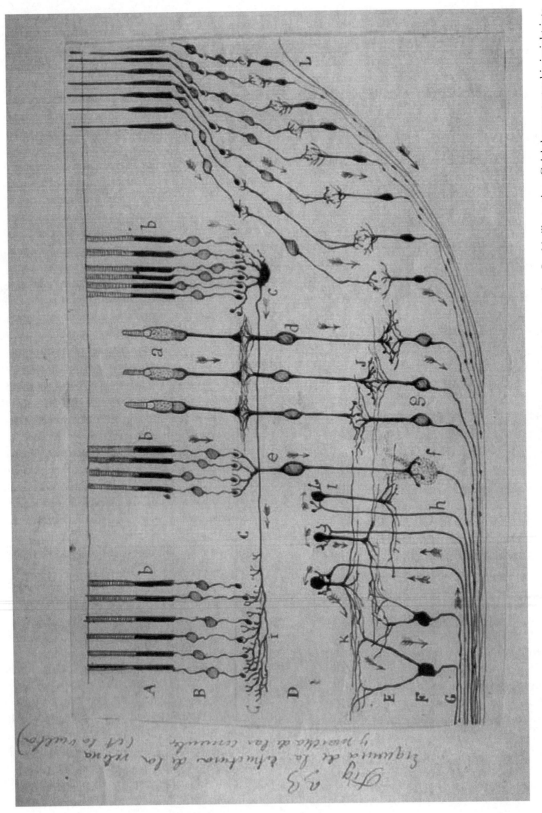

FIGURE 9.1 Santiago Ramón y Cajal's schematic drawing of the parafoveal region of the vertebrate retina. In this illustration, Cajal demonstrates his insight into the connectivity of the retina and the dynamic polarization of retinal neurons and consequently information transfer from photoreceptors to bipolar cells and ganglion cells. In addition to vertical organization, Cajal illustrates the lateral pathways. A, Inner and outer segments. B, Outer nuclear layer. C, Outer plexiform layer. D, Inner nuclear layer. E, Inner plexiform layer. F, Ganglion cell layer. G, Nerve fiber layer. b, rods; a, cones; c, horizontal cell; d, cone bipolar cell; e, rod bipolar cell; g, ganglion cell; h, centrifugal fiber. (Note: Not all suggestions implicit in this prescient drawing have been found correct. For example, rod bipolars do not make direct contact with ganglion cells—see text.) (Source: The original figure is in the collection of the Cajal Institute, CSIC, Madrid.) (See also color plate 12.)

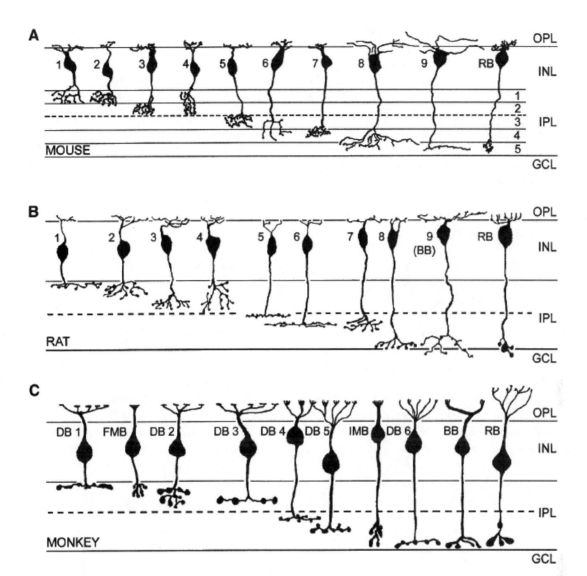

FIGURE 9.2 Summary diagram of bipolar types in the mammalian retina; rod bipolar cells (RB) end in layer 5 of the IPL, the innermost region and are all depolarizing in nature. In each species, a large number of cone bipolars cells are found; those terminating above the dashed line are hyperpolarizing, and those terminating below the dashed line are depolarizing. (Source Figure 8 from Ghosh KK et al.[26])

predominantly in layer 1 of the IPL. Cones connect to a large number of specialized cone bipolars cells; these terminate in layers 2, 3, and 4 of the IPL, where they connect with both ganglion and amacrine cells (figure 9.2).

The earliest recordings of retinal activity demonstrated that there were two fundamental ganglion cell types: those that respond to increments in light intensity (ON cells) and those that respond to decrements in light intensity (OFF cells). Underlying this duality of function is a fundamental anatomical division of the retina: ON cells receive information in layers 4 and 5 of the IPL, and OFF cells receive information in layers 1 and 2 (layer 3 contains processes of both types). This separation in the processing of incremental and decremental information is so fundamental to visual processing that it is maintained to the first levels in primary

visual cortex! Rod information and cone information are also separated, initially in the IPL. The rod bipolar cells, a single class, end in the deepest layer of the IPL, layer 5, where they synapse onto the AII amacrine. The AII or rod amacrine has output in deep layers of the IPL and in the upper layers of the IPL. So the IPL can be conceived as a bit of a rod sandwich.

So far, we have focused on a division in radial connectivity, that is between primary receptors (rods and cones) and second-order cells. There is another fundamental functional organization of the retina that needs to be appreciated: the tangential array of cells over the retinal surface. The retina is a convex spherical detector, much like a satellite dish. For any given cell type, there is a precise arrangement or mosaic of this cell type over the retinal surface. Homotypic cells

(cells of one type—for example, the AII rod amacrine or the dopamine amacrine cell) are arrayed following precise mathematical formulae; heterotypic cells (cholinergic amacrine cells and AII rod amacrine cell) are apparently arrayed independently. This arrangement was studied first in shark retina and independently in the mammalian retina. Wässle and colleagues developed the mathematical formulation that is still used today to analyze this aspect of retinal anatomy. Thus, one can describe, for example, the distribution of dopaminergic amacrine cells, type 9 cone bipolar cells, red cones, or any given subset of retinal ganglion cells. Further readings on the functional organization of the retina are given at the end of this chapter.

The mechanisms that guide these developmental processes (i.e., lamination and array formation) are not well understood and are just coming under study. On the other hand, the mechanisms that guide neurogenesis and retinal cell fate determination are understood at greater depth (see the Selected Readings for recent reviews and key papers). Retinal cell types are born in a characteristic order, with the generalization that cell types of the inner retina are generated first, followed by cell types in the outer retina. The mechanisms that control cell fate appear to be largely intrinsic to the progenitor cells; a series of transcription factors guide the orderly production of cell types, and there is a progressive restriction of the progenitor cell, limiting the types of neurons it makes late in development. A thorough discussion of this process cannot be undertaken here. (Suggested Readings in this area are listed at the end of the chapter.) The remainder of this chapter will focus on what we know and what we don't know about the processes of lamination in the retina and array formation.

Outer plexiform layer: a model for processing and synaptic organization

At the first synapse between photoreceptors (rods and cones) and second-order neurons (bipolar and horizontal cells), considerable processing is taking place. The divisions between low-light (rod) and high-light (cone) processing and between incremental (ON) and decremental (OFF) processing noted above begin at the OPL, the level of the bipolar cell. As was covered in chapters 7 and 8, photoreceptors release glutamate continuously in the dark; at light onset, they hyperpolarize and decrease glutamate release. The ON and OFF bipolar responses are generated by the expression of different subclasses of glutamate receptor. All depolarizing (ON) bipolar cells express mGluR6 receptors, whereas hyperpolarizing (OFF) bipolar cells use other glutamate receptors (see the Suggested Readings). Moreover, two types of photoreceptor-to-bipolar synapses are present in the outer retina: a flat contact, in which a bipolar cell merely touches the base of the photoreceptor, and an invaginating

synapse, in which the bipolar cell punches into the base of the photoreceptor (figure 9.3). In general, outside the primate fovea, all flat contacts are hyperpolarizing, and invaginating contacts are depolarizing. There are differences between the rod and cone synapses as well; for example, cones make contact with multiple types of bipolar cells (both ON and OFF), whereas rods in general make contact with only one type of bipolar cell.

Synaptic communication and signal processing therefore requires the recognition of synaptic partners (e.g., rod-to-rod bipolar; cone-to-cone bipolar) and the assembly of proper components (e.g., mGluR6, metabotropic, glutamate receptors at ON, invaginating synapses and other, ionotropic, glutamate receptors at OFF, flat synapses). Moreover, synaptic transmission is dependent on the proper alignment of presynaptic and postsynaptic elements.

On the presynaptic side of the photoreceptor synapse, the most prominent feature is the synaptic ribbon, a proteinaceous structure that is a docking site for synaptic vesicles. Although the function of the synaptic ribbon is not completely understood, it is thought to facilitate the rapid and continuous release of glutamate that occurs from the photoreceptor terminal. It is generally conceived of as a conveyor mechanism to deliver vesicles to the release site, but some evidence suggests that it may serve to allow for multivesicular fusion. Nonetheless, the ribbon specialization is found in photoreceptors, other sensory neurons that have a high-basal rate of release such as hair cells in the ear, and electrosensory neurons in fish. In addition to the obvious ribbon, other elements of the transmitter release cascade are present in the photoreceptor; these include a variety of calcium channels, both voltage gated and not, calcium transporters, and proteins that are associated with the fusion of vesicles and the plasma membrane.

Thus, considerable stable and precisely located cellular machinery is required for the process of chemical transmission from the presynaptic terminal. Partly because of this, the photoreceptor synapse has been thought to be stable and nonplastic, unlike many synapses in the central nervous system (CNS) that are plastic and capable of dynamic remodeling—that is, until recently. Two lines of evidence demonstrate that photoreceptor synapses are plastic: circadian changes in the photoreceptor terminal (the ribbon) have been identified, as has transmitter modulation of photoreceptor synaptic output.

On the postsynaptic side, the transmitter receptors must be juxtaposed to the release sites; in addition, other elements of the response cascade must be localized to the synaptic region. The molecular identities of these response cascade elements depend on the type of receptor: ionotropic (ion channel) or metabotropic (coupled to second-messenger systems). In the case of the former, voltage-gated ion channels are likely to be present; in the latter, the enzymes

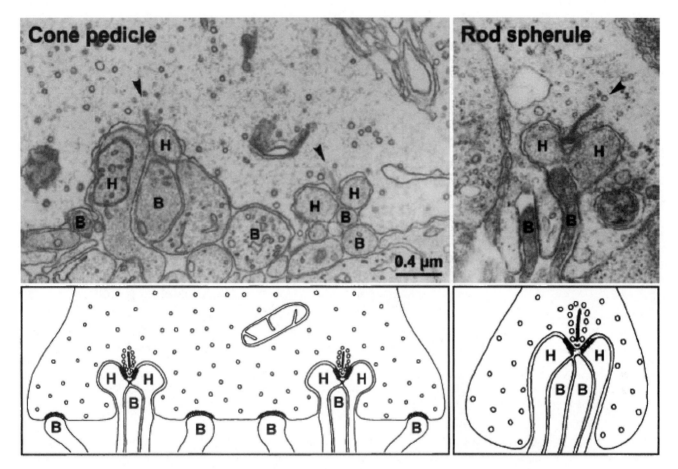

FIGURE 9.3   Below the representative electron micrographs of cone and rod terminals are cartoons of the idealized anatomy. In the cone terminal, two types of synapse are seen. Invaginating synapses are classically described with three postsynaptic elements: two horizontal cell processes (H) and one central bipolar process (B). More conventional synapses, or flat contacts, are seen between bipolar cells (B) and the cone. In the rod terminal, only the invaginating synapse is found, and the postsynaptic elements, consisting of two horizontal cells (H) and the process of two bipolar cells, are seen. The prominent presynaptic ribbon and its cluster of synaptic vesicles are seen in invaginating synapses. Bipolar cells making contact with photoreceptors at invaginating synapses are depolarizing (ON center) whereas those making contact at flat synapses are hyperpolarizing (OFF center). (Source: Figure 2 from Brandstätter JH, Hack I.[22])

associated with the particular second-messenger cascade will be present. Moreover, at all chemical synapses, transmitter action is terminated either by enzymatic degradation of the transmitter or clearing of the transmitter by high-affinity transport mechanisms. Transporters may be located on either side of the synapse; enzymatic degradation of transmitter generally takes place postsynaptically.

Synaptic transmission and signaling in the nervous system are critically dependent on the precise alignment of all these molecular species. Moreover, the presynaptic release mechanism must be in direct apposition to the postsynaptic response cascade. In the case of the photoreceptor terminal, where vesicular release is continuous and occurs at relatively high rates, there is also concomitant considerable membrane flux and turnover. Logic dictates that the presynaptic and postsynaptic cascades should be stabilized relative to each

other. That is, like boats in a marina, they should be tied up to a dock.

Molecular mechanisms of synaptic stabilization and development

What provides for this molecular stability? Cell-matrix and cell-cell adhesion are involved in various aspects of stabilizing macromolecular complexes and contributing to changes in cell shape and cell motility, as well as regulating cell proliferation and death. Recently, molecules involved in cell-matrix and cell-cell adhesion have also been implicated in the process of synapse formation (figures 9.4 and 9.5). For example, the cadherins and associated β-catenin, well known in the field of epithelial cell biology, are known to be present at synapses, as are, of course, the well-studied cell adhesion

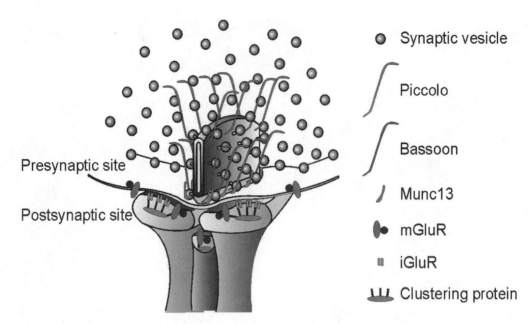

Presynaptic site

Postsynaptic site

- ● Synaptic vesicle
- ∫ Piccolo
- ∫ Bassoon
- ∫ Munc13
- ⦚ mGluR
- ▥ iGluR
- ⊔⊔⊔ Clustering protein

FIGURE 9.4   Diagrammatic scheme of the molecular organization of the photoreceptor synapse is shown. The ribbon (large, gray, saclike structure) is studded with synaptic vesicles; in association with the ribbon are cytomatrix molecules bassoon and piccolo; Munc13 is seen at the release site. Ribeye, not shown in this figure, labels the ribbon itself. Directly opponent to the release site are the molecules of the transmitter response cascade; these include both iontropic (IGluR) and metabotropic (mGluR) glutamate receptors and clustering molecules. Outside the release area, other molecules are expressed, including various cell adhesion molecules and, in the photoreceptor, glumate receptors. (Source: This figure was kindly supplied by Dr. J. H. Brandstätter for use in this chapter.) (See also color plate 13.)

molecules (CAM) and the like. New molecules have been shown recently to be present at CNS synapses, including synapses in the retina. One class of note is the nectins; these are members of the IgG superfamily but are Ca^{2+}-independent adhesion molecules. The nectins are coupled to the actin cytoskeleton via elements of the cytomatrix. They function, together with cadherins, in stabilizing synapse formation; initial apposition of presynaptic and postsynaptic cells are stabilized at an adherens junction, and then synaptic specializations take place at this point. This sequence of events involving nectins is most clearly understood at spine formation in the hippocampus, but other regions of the CNS, including the retina, express nectins, suggesting that nectins play similar roles throughout the CNS, including the retina.

Recently, a novel family of CAMs, sidekicks, have been shown to be important in lamination in the IPL. These molecules are homophilic binding molecules and are expressed by bipolar cells and ganglion cells; they are conceived to mediate recognition between presynaptic and postsynaptic target cells. Sidekicks appear to be important in setting up the division between ON and OFF in the IPL: Sidekick 1 is expressed in the ON sublamina, and sidekick 2 is expressed in the OFF sublamina. Sidekicks are differentially expressed in nonoverlapping subsets of presynaptic (bipolar and amacrine) and postsynaptic (ganglion) cells. In heterologous expression systems, sidekicks mediate cell-cell adhesion; in vivo, the overexpression of sidekicks in normally sidekick-negative cells redirects tagged dendrites to a sidekick-expressing sublamina. Together, these data suggest that sidekicks in specific and adhesion molecules in general are critical elements of the molecular mechanism of lamination in the IPL. Ongoing work in both the zebrafish and the mouse by the Wong laboratory demonstrates that lamination of amacrine cell dendrites requires the presence of retinal ganglion cell dendrites, suggesting that cell-cell recognition mechanisms are critical to the process.

Thus, a picture is emerging of CAM-mediated cell-cell interactions that guide the lamination and dendritic development in the IPL. However, in addition to cell adhesion molecules, components of the extracellular matrix are also critical in maintaining the structural integrity of synapses, including those of the retina. Components of the extracellular matrix and their receptors (including integrins) are crucial stabilizers at one of the most well-studied of synapses, the neuromuscular junction (NMJ). At the NMJ, the basement membranes of the components of the synapse, including the motor neuron, glial (Schwann) cell, and muscle contain a variety of fixed elements of the ECM that guide the formation and stabilization of the NMJ. Vital among these molecules are the laminins, heparan sulfate protoglycans (e.g., agrin), and others. These molecules interact with a variety of cell surface receptors, including integrins and components of the dystrophin complex.

CNS synapses lack obvious basement membranes. However, because integrin modulation of synaptic function

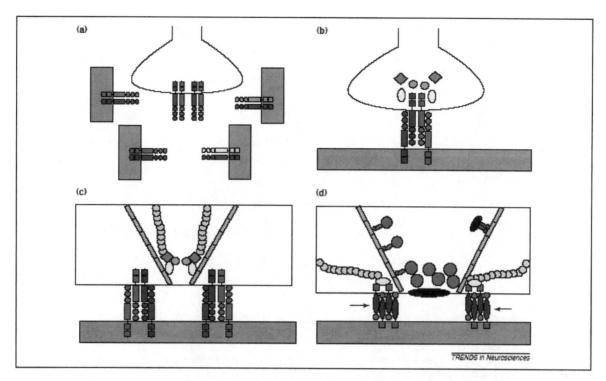

FIGURE 9.5 The process of target recognition and synapse formation is idealized in this cartoon. Presynaptic terminals express certain target recognition molecules on their leading processes; here, these are conceived of as homophilic binding molecules (such as CAM, nectins, or sidekicks). Target selection is based on the expression of homophilic partners on the postsynaptic (A to B transition); on binding to the postsynaptic receptor pair, a variety of proteins are recruited to the synapse (B, colored circles and diamonds); these elements produce a reorganization of the cytoskeleton (actin and microtubule, gray circles and rods, respectively) and assembly of the elements of the release mechanism, including the synaptic vesicle (green circles), and proteins of the release cascade (black ovals). Homophilic molecules and other molecules (arrows) are recruited to stabilize the synapse. (Source: Figure 2 from Ackley BD, Jin Y.[1]) (See also color plate 14.)

has been well documented, it is likely that extracellular matrix ligands for integrins exist at CNS synapses. One obvious candidate is the laminins. Laminins have been reported in the brain and retina for some time now, and a model has emerged for their distribution (figure 9.6). The classical basement membranes of the retina, Bruch's membrane and the inner limiting membrane, contain classical basement membrane components, including laminins, type IV collagens, and nidogen, a molecule that cross-couples laminin and collagen polymers. In addition, laminins without either collagen IV or nidogen are present in the synaptic layers of the retina. Biochemical isolation of laminins from synapse-enriched preparations (synaptosomes) supports anatomical evidence for the presence of laminins in the synaptic layers.

Genetic ablation of at least one laminin gene (Lamb2) produces marked synaptic defects in the OPL (figure 9.7). Electrophysiological data demonstrate that the b-wave of the ERG in Lamb2 null mice is greatly reduced; the a-wave, on the other hand, while slightly reduced, is statistically unaltered from the control animals. In addition to reduction in the amplitude of the b-wave, the intensity-response function

of the b-wave is altered. The normal sigmoidal curve, reflecting Michaelis-Menton kinetics, is replaced with a linear function. These data suggest that the transfer function of the photoreceptor to bipolar cell synapse is failing: The excitation-release mechanism is defective in these mutant mice. Anatomical inspection of the synapse revealed that the majority of photoreceptor synapses are malformed. In the normal mouse, as in human, the photoreceptor has multiple postsynaptic partners, usually two horizontal cells and a central bipolar cell, forming the classic triad. The output site is marked by an electron-dense structure: the ribbon. The ribbon is studded with synaptic vesicles; as was noted above, the function of the ribbon is a matter of some debate. Either it functions to transport vesicles to the release site or it acts as a common fusion site. In any case, the ribbon facilitates the high-frequency release of the photoreceptor. In the Lamb2 knock-out mouse, the ribbon synapse is disrupted: The presynaptic ribbon is released from the membrane, appearing to float in the cytoplasm, and the postsynaptic elements are disorganized.

The physiological defect in the laminin mutant mouse is similar to that seen in humans with Duchenne's muscular

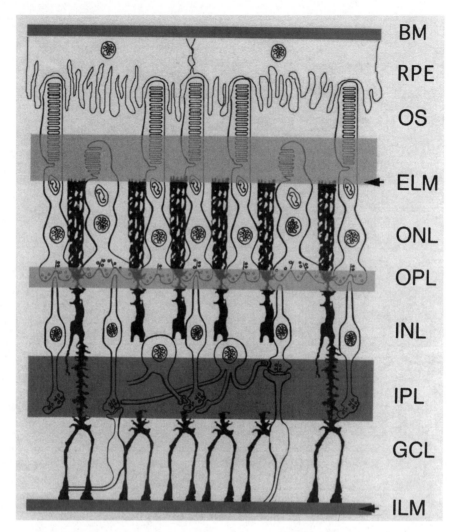

BM
RPE
OS
← ELM
ONL
OPL
INL
IPL
GCL
ILM

FIGURE 9.6 This cartoon illustrates the various cell adhesion compartments of the retina; two true basement membranes are illustrated (red): Bruch's (BM) and the inner limiting membrane (ILM). These basement membranes form the adhesion substrate for the basal side of the retinal pigmented epithelium (RPE) and the endfeet of the Müller cells (black cells). These are known to contain many elements of epithelial basement membranes, including collagen type IV, laminins (many), and nidogen. Cell adhesion molecules expressed here include integrins, CAMs, and cadherins. In green are the matrices surrounding the photoreceptor; these do not contain either collagen type IV or nidogen but do contain other critical ECM molecules, including laminins, usherin, crumbs, and various heparin sulfates. Receptor molecules in these compartments include various CAM such as sidekicks, integrins, and transmembrane collagens. Genetic disruptions of these molecules lead to photoreceptor dysmorphogenesis and degeneration. The blue indicates the matrix compartment in the IPL. The matrix components expressed here are not well established; on the other hand, some CAM molecules, such as sidekicks, are found here. The mechanisms that control lamination and dendrite elongation are just coming under study (see the papers from the Masland and Wong laboratories). (Source: This figure is taken from the authors' work; it was published in Libby RT et al.[15]) (See also color plate 15.)

dystrophy. That disease is caused by a mutation in the molecule dystrophin and results in night-blindness. Dystrophins are cytomatrix molecules, that is, molecules in the cytoplasm coupled to the cytoskeleton (actin and intermediate filaments and microtubules). In muscles, dystrophins are part of the mechanism by which the excitation cascade of the muscle is scaffolded in the plane of the membrane.

Putting these observations together suggests that the release machinery of the photoreceptor synapse may be anchored by attachment to the extracellular matrix. If such a coupling exists, then there need to be ligands in the ECM, transmembrane receptors, and scaffolding elements in the cytomatrix. A complementary observation supports this hypothesis. Bassoon is a presynaptic cytomatrix molecule that is found in both conventional and ribbon synapses. In photoreceptor ribbon synapses, bassoon is associated with the ribbon-anchoring point, the arciform density; targeted mutation of bassoon phenocopies some of the aspects of the Lamb2 knock-out (figure 9.8). For example, presynaptic ribbons float, and the b-wave is disrupted. However, there is

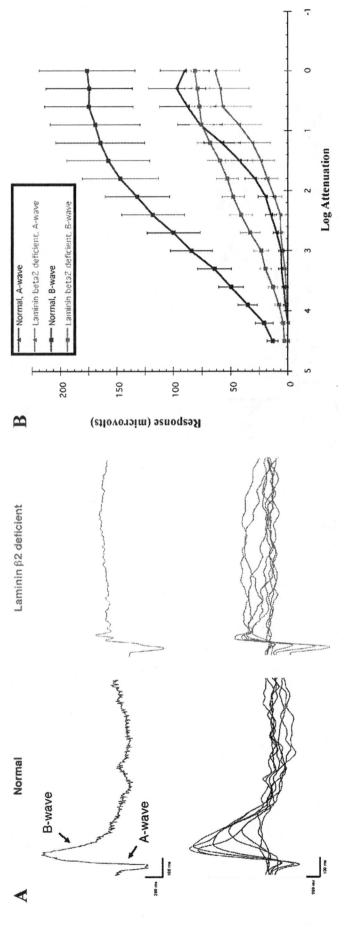

FIGURE 9.7 Laminin gene ablation results in the loss of photoreceptor-to-bipolar signaling. Mice in which a key laminin gene, the laminin β2 gene, was ablated by targeted mutagenesis have dysmorphic photoreceptors. The outer segments fail to form, and the synaptic structures are altered. In these mice, there is loss of the b-wave of the ERG. Wild-type (normal) and littermate homozygote nulls mice (laminin β2 deficient) mice are compared. A, Representative ERGs; a single flash intensity is shown above, and a whole intensity series is shown below. B, Response-intensity functions for both a-wave and b-waves. The mutant mice a-waves overlap those of the wild-type controls and are not significantly different. The b-waves from normal mice show a nice sigmoidal curve; the intensity-response function of the mutant mice is significantly decreased in amplitude, and the response-intensity function is linear. These data together suggest that the transfer function of the synapse is failing. The time to peak values for the b-wave were not affected. (Source: This figure is taken from the authors' work; it was published in Libby RT et al.[14])

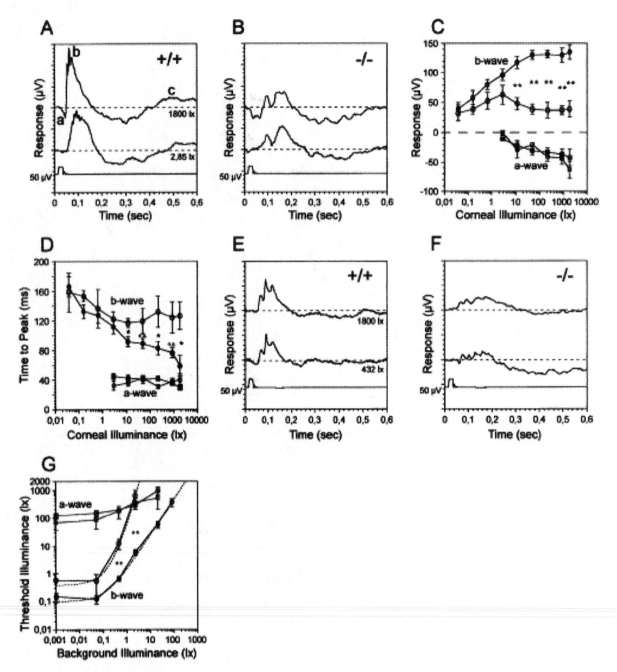

FIGURE 9.8   The genetic ablation of bassoon produces an anatomical and physiological phenotype similar to that of the laminin knockout. A shows normal ERGs and B shows responses from the mutant for 2 intensities of flash. The b-waves are reduced but the a-waves are not. In C, the voltage/intensity relation is shown, confirming that in the knockout mouse the b-wave only is affected. Graph D shows that the reduction in ERG voltage as background light intensity is increased affects the b-wave of the mutant, but not the a-wave. E and F show that photopic b-waves are also selectively affected. G results from a more elaborate experiment in which ERG thresholds were obtained as a function of background illumination. The a-wave threshold of normal and knockout mice are similar: over a large range of background intensities but the corresponding functions for the b-waves are very different. (Source: From Dick O et al.[7])

a more severe disruption in the organization of the bassoon knock-out retina, where extensive sprouting of neurons and ectopic synapses are formed. It is likely that bassoon is a critical component of the cytomatrix; together, the available data suggest that the release cascade of the photoreceptor is anchored to the ECM via transmembrane receptors that in turn are coupled to elements of the cytomatrix. What is the function of this coupling? The lipid turnover and additions and recycling of membrane make the presynaptic membrane as unstable as the tide levels, whereas the ECM is more stable. Thus, teleologically, this arrangement would provide stability to the molecular components of the release mechanism much like tying a boat to a dock.

The hypothesis that laminins in the ECM serve to anchor the apposition of transmitter release cascades on the presynaptic side of the synapse and the recipient cascade on the postsynaptic side has several predictions, including that there are receptors for the laminins in each side of the synapse and that the laminin receptors are scaffolded with elements of the transduction cascades. These questions are in active study in several laboratories at the present. Data from our laboratory demonstrate that one class of laminin receptors, a transmembrane form of collagen known as collagen XVII, is present in photoreceptors, colocalizes with laminin deposition, and binds laminins. Moreover, we have shown that dystonin, also known as BPAG1, a scaffolding molecule known to interact with collagen XVII, is present in photoreceptors and is enriched in synaptic regions. In addition, we and others are studying the distribution of another class of laminin receptor: the integrins; these receptors have long been implicated in a variety of retinal and CNS functions, including synaptic plasticity. In the retina, integrins have been shown to be important in guiding retinal development, promoting the adhesion and polarity of retinal pigmented epithelium, and the phagocytosis of photoreceptor outer segments. Interestingly, genetic ablation of several integrin genes results in dysgenic retinae that display disruptions in lamination, photoreceptor ectopia, and other abnormalities.

Within the clinical setting, it is worth noting that the molecules identified here, collagen XVII, dystonin (BPAG1), integrins, and laminins form a portion of the anchoring structure of the epidermis; that is the molecular mechanism for attachment of the basal layer of epidermal cells to the basement membrane and underlying hypodermis. Laminins are found on the basement membrane of the epithelium; collagen XVII and integrins ($\alpha 6 \beta 4$) form the transmembrane receptors; and BPAG1 part of the anchoring system for the hemidesmosome. Mutations of these genes in humans result in skin-blistering diseases called junctional epidermolysis bullosa (JEB); the severity of the phenotype depends on the gene that is affected (COL17, LAMx, etc.) and on the type of mutation (null, truncation, missense, etc.).

It may be that these patients also suffer considerable visual defects; extensive study of this hypothesis has not been undertaken, in part because the severity of disease in the JEB patients precludes some standard electroretinogram (ERG) methods. Nevertheless, the JEB data suggests a paradigm for understanding the genetics of ECM-cyotmatrix stabilization.

Other laminin receptors are likely to play a role in photoreceptor development and organization. Dystroglycan is another laminin receptor found in retina and CNS. It is the expression of a single gene from which two proteins are produced: α-dystroglycan and β-dystroglycan. The former is an extrinsic membrane protein, and the latter is a transmembrane protein; they remain associated under most circumstances. Several laboratories have shown that dystroglycan is expressed in the outer retina. There has been some controversy over the location of the dystroglycan (presynaptic or postsynaptic); recently, our laboratory has shown that β-dystroglycan colocalizes with several markers of rod bipolar cells in the retina, including αPKC and mGluR6. Moreover, conditional knock-outs of the dystroglycan gene result in disrupted brain and retina; in the retina, preliminary reports demonstrate that the ERG is disrupted in a similar fashion as in the LamB2 null mouse.

If the laminin hypothesis is valid, then in the laminin-null animal, we should observe rearrangements of the molecular components of the scaffolding apparatus. Our laboratory has recently shown that in the Lamb2-null animal, there is a misalignment of the release cascade (as measured by bassoon localization) and the recipient cascade (as measured by mGluR6 localization) (figure 9.9); these results support the hypothesis that laminins are critical to stabilizing photoreceptor synapses.

What couples the laminin receptor and transmitter receptors or elements of the release cascade on the postsynaptic side? Some progress in understanding this scaffolding has been made. On the postsynaptic side of the synapse, we have shown that in wild-type retina, mGluR6 and β-dystroglycan are associated with a cytomatrix molecule: dystrophin. In the Lamb2 knock-out animal, this association fails; specifically, mGluR6 and β-dystroglycan are no longer colocalized, and the colocalization of β-dystroglycan and mGluR6 is also disrupted. The dystrophin family is a strong candidate for the linker molecule.

Dystrophin was first described as a 427-kDa protein-sharing homology with the spectin family of membrane cytoskeletal protein; the full-length molecule is composed of four structural domains: an N-terminal domain actin-binding region with homology to α-actinin, a rod structure composed of 24 spectrinlike repeats, a cystein-rich domain with calcium-binding motives, and a C-terminal domain that interacts with a dystroglycan. These different domains gave to dystrophin the ability to bridge the cytoskeleton and

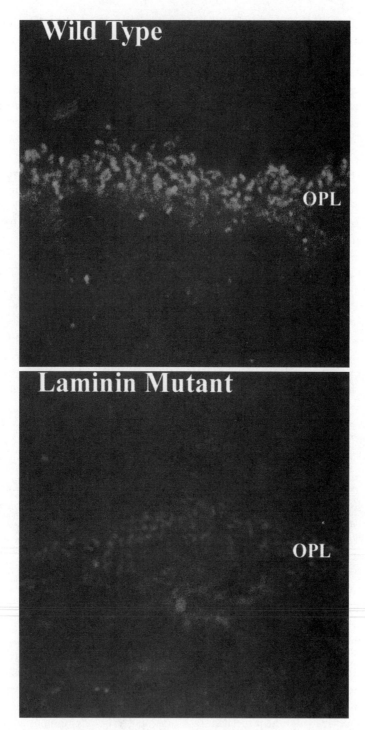

FIGURE 9.9   Laminin deletion results in a disruption of the transsynaptic molecular organization of the photoreceptor synapse. Immunohistochemical localization of the bassoon (red) and mGluR6 (blue) in wild-type retina demonstrates the normal arrangement of molecules. Bassoon, associated with the ribbon, is directly opponent to mGluR6, the transmitter receptor that is expressed in invaginating bipolar cells. In the laminin-mutant (β2 null) mouse, both molecules are expressed by mGluR6 is delocalized and not concentrated at the synapse. (Source: This is taken from the author's unpublished work.) (See also color plate 16.)

the extracellular matrix. In addition to the full-length isoforms of dystrophin, four internal promoters of the DMD gene control the expression of short products named in reference to their respective molecular weight: Dp260, Dp140, Dp116, and Dp71. Defective expression of the full-length molecule results in a Duchenne's muscular dystrophy. This is a fatal, X-linked disease; affected males suffer from a variety of retinal defects. Various isoforms of dystrophin have been identified in retina by molecular and biochemical methods; some controversy arose in the literature about whether dystrophin is expressed by the photoreceptor or the bipolar cell. Future experiments are needed to sort this issue out.

In muscle, the dystroglycan-dystrophin complex binds to laminins in the extracellular space and is thought to couple ion channels such as Ca^{2+} channels or synaptic receptors in functional domains. It may be that in retina, the dystrophin-dystroglycan complex is performing a similar function. Our laboratory has demonstrated that both dystrophin and dystroglycan colocalize with markers of the postsynaptic (bipolar) cell. Specifically, there is colocalization of mGluR6 and both dystrophin and dystroglycan. In the laminin knock-out animals, there is a profound rearrangement of these molecules.

Other scaffolding molecules are likely to emerge that link the ECM to the cytomatrix. Considerable progress has been made in understanding scaffolding of transmitter receptors; it is outside the scope of this chapter to discuss these in detail, and the readers is referred to recent papers in the area. Nevertheless, coupling of signaling cascades, either presynaptic or postsynaptic, is an area of intensive study. The continued development in the field combines genetic and proteomic approaches to the molecular anatomy of the synapse. Nevertheless, these recent studies identify at synapses (both peripheral and central) elements of the adhesion complexes in epithelial tissues (laminin, integrins, dystroglycan, cadherins, nectins, etc.); they suggest that similar molecular complexes are formed to stabilize synaptic structure. Moreover, the commonality of these molecular complexes has consequences for human disease. Genetic disruptions of many of these genes (laminin, integrin, cadherins) have both peripheral (epithelial) and central (CNS) defects.

ECM molecules are involved in other aspects of retinal structure and function. The laminin knock-out animals have defects in the outer segment formation. Moreover, two other molecules of great interest have been identified recently: usherin and crumbs. Both of these molecules contain laminin motifs in their domain structure, and mutations in either genes produce blinding illness in humans and dysmorphic photoreceptors in mice. Usherin is associated with Usher's syndrome, and crumbs are associated with one form of RP (RP12). Interestingly, usherin2 is widely expressed in epithelial tissues outside the retina. Another molecule, basigin or EMMPIRN, is a member of the IgG superfamily of molecules and is involved in cell-cell, cell-ECM interactions. It is expressed in the Müller cells and the photoreceptor; experimentally produced null mutations of this gene result in a failure of normal photoreceptor outer segment formation and retinal degeneration, as well as disruptions in the ERG. There is some evidence that suggests that EMMPIRN is an ECM, perhaps a laminin receptor. Retinoschisin is a recently described protein that is related to the discoidins, a family of transmembrane of secreted proteins that are involved in cell adhesion and bind to ECM components, particularly collagens. Retinoschisin I was identified by positional cloning of the gene that causes retinoschisis, a blinding illness typified by loss of b-wave function and loss of retinal integrity resulting in a splitting of the neural retina. Experimentally produced mutations in mice show defects that are similar, though not identical, to those that cause the human disease and have disruptions in the photoreceptor-to-bipolar transmission as well as structural tears at the OPL/INL border. To date, no binding partner or ligand for RS1 has been found.

Summary

Old questions turn new again with the advent of new technologies. The beautiful lamination of the retina, so elegantly studied by Ramón y Cajal, is again the subject of molecular research. Now the molecular anatomy and mechanisms of connectivity of the retina are under study. The molecules that promote lamination and synaptic specificity are not fully known, but they are likely to share homology with those molecules that mediate adhesion in nonneural tissues. Moreover, a complete understanding of the molecules that are involved in these processes may help us to design rescue and repair strategies for the retina.

ACKNOWLEDGMENTS   This work was supported by grants from the NIH, NS 39508 (WJB); EY12676 (WJB); R01EY12037 (DDH); and P30EY013078 (Tufts Center for Vision Research). We thank Germán Pinzon-Duarte for his reading of the manuscript.

SELECTED READINGS

SYNAPSE STRUCTURE AND FUNCTION

1. Ackley BD, Jin Y: Genetic analysis of synaptic target recognition and assembly. *Trends Neurosci* 2004; 27:540–547.
2. Balkema GW, Cusick K, Nguyen T-H: Diurnal variation in synaptic ribbon length and visual threshold. *Vis Neurosci* 2001; 18:789–797.
3. Blank M, Blake DJ, Kroger S: Molecular diversity of the dystrophin-like protein complex in the developing and adult avian retina. *Neurosci* 2002; 111:259–273.
4. Beggs HE, Schahin-Reed D, Zang K, Goebbels S, Nave K-A, Gorski J, Jones KR, Sretavan D, Reichardt LF: FAK deficiency in cells contributing to the basal lamina results in cortical abnormalities resembling congenital muscular dystrophies. *Neuron* 2003; 40:501–514.
5. Brandstätter JH, Dick O, Boeckers TM: The postsynaptic scaffold proteins ProSAP1/Shank2 and Homer1 are associated with glutamate receptor complexes at rat retinal synapses. *J Comp Neurol* 2004; 475:551–563.
6. Claudepierre T, Dalloz C, Mornet D, Matsumura K, Sahel J, Rendon A: Characterization of the intermolecular associations of the dystrophin-associated glycoprotein complex in retinal Müller glial cells. *J Cell Sci* 2000; 113:3409–3417.
7. Dick O, tom Dieck S, Altrock WD, Ammermüller J, Weiler R, Garner CC, Gundelfinger ED, Brandstätter JH: The

presynaptic active zone protein bassoon is essential for photoreceptor ribbon synapse formation in the retina. *Neuron* 2003; 37:775–786.

8. Fischer F, Kneussel M, Tintrup H, Haverkamp S, Rauen T, Betz H, Wässle H: Reduced synaptic clustering of GABA and glycine receptors in the retina of the gephyrin null mutant mouse. *J Comp Neurol* 2000; 427:634–648.

9. Holt M, Cooke A, Neef A, Lagnado L: High mobility of vesicles supports continuous exocytosis at a ribbon synapse. *Curr Biol* 2004; 14:173–183.

10. Parsons TD, Sterling P: Synaptic ribbon: Conveyor belt or safety belt? *Neuron* 2003; 37:379–382.

11. Schmitz F, Königstorfer A, Südhof TA: RIBEYE a component of synaptic ribbons: A protein's journey through evolution provides insight into synaptic ribbon function. *Neuron* 2000; 28:857–872.

12. Takai Y, Shimizu K, Ohtsuka T: The roles of cadherins and nectins in interneuronal synapse formation. *Curr Opin Neurobiol* 2003; 13:520–526.

ECM, RECEPTORS AND FUNCTION

13. Georges-Labouesse E, Mark M, Messaddeq N, Gansmuller A: Essential role of alpha 6 integrins in cortical and retinal lamination. *Curr Biol* 1998; 27:983–986.

14. Libby RT, Lavalle C, Balkema GW, Brunken WJ, Hunter DD: Disruption of laminin β2 chain production causes alterations in morphology and function in the CNS. *J Neurosci* 1999; 19:9399–9411.

15. Libby RT, Champliaud MF, Claudepierre T, Xu Y, Gibbons EP, Koch M, Burgeson RE, Hunter DD, Brunken WJ: Laminin expression in adult and developing retinae: Evidence of two novel CNS laminins. *J Neurosci* 2000; 20:6517–6528.

16. Moore SA, Saito F, Chen J, Michele DE, Henry MD, Messing A, Cohn RD, Ross-Barta SE, Westra S, Williamson RA, Hoshi T, Campbell KP: Deletion of brain dystroglycan recapitulates aspects of congenital muscular dystrophy. *Nature* 2002; 418:422–425.

17. Michele DE, Campbell KP: Dystrophin-glycoprotein complex: Post-translational processing and dystroglycan function. *J Biol Chem* 2003; 278:15457–15460.

18. Sasaki T, Fässler R, Hohenester E: Laminin: The crux of basement membrane assembly. *J Cell Biol* 2004; 164:959–963.

19. Yamagata M, Sanes JR, Weiner JA: Synaptic adhesion molecules. *Curr Opin Cell Biol* 2003; 15:621–632.

20. Yamagata M, Weiner JA, Sanes JR: Sidekicks: Synaptic adhesion molecules that promote lamina-specific connectivity in the retina. *Cell* 2002; 110:649–660.

21. Yurchenco PD, Amenta PS, Patton BL: Basement membrane assembly, stability and activities observed through a developmental lens. *Matrix Biol* 2004; 22:521–538.

RETINAL STRUCTURE AND DEVELOPMENT

22. Brandstätter JH, Hack I: Localization of glutamate receptors at a complex synapse: The mammalian photoreceptor synapse. *Cell Tissue Res* 2001; 303:1–14.

23. Cayouette M, Barres BA, Raff M: Importance of intrinsic mechanisms in cell fate decisions in the developing rat retina. *Neuron* 2003; 40:897–904.

24. Eglen SJ, Willshaw DJ: Influence of cell fate mechanisms upon retinal mosaic formation: A modelling study. *Development* 2002; 129:5399–5408.

25. Erdmann B, Kirsch F-P, Rathjen FG, More MI: N-cadherin is essential for retinal lamination in the zebrafish. *Dev Dyn* 2003; 226:570–577.

26. Ghosh KK, Bujan S, Haverkamp S, Feigenspan A, Wässle H: Types of bipolar cells in the mouse retina. *J Comp Neurol* 2004; 469:70–82.

27. Haverkamp S, Grünert U, Wässle H: The cone pedicle, a complex synapse in the retina. *Neuron* 2000; 27:85–95.

28. Kay JN, Roeser T, Mumm JS, Godinho L, Mrejeru A, Wong ROL, Baier H: Transient requirement for ganglion cells during assembly of retinal synaptic layers. *Development* 2004; 131:1331–1342.

29. Lin B, Wang SW, Masland RH: Report retinal ganglion cell type, size, and spacing can be specified independent of homotypic dendritic contacts. *Neuron* 2004; 43:475–485.

30. Livesey FJ, Cepko CL: Vertebrate neural cell-fate determination: lessons from the retina. *Nat Rev Neurosci* 2001; 2:109–119.

31. Malicki J: Cell fate decisions and patterning in the vertebrate retina: the importance of timing, asymmetry, polarity and waves. *Curr Opin Neurobiol* 2004; 14:15–21.

32. Marquardt T, Gruss P: Generating neuronal diversity in the retina: one for nearly all. *Trends Neurosci* 2002; 25:32–38.

33. Mumm JS, Godinho L, Morgan JL, Oakley DM, Schroeter EH, Wong ROL: Laminar circuit formation in the vertebrate retina. *Prog Brain Res* 2004; 147:155–169.

34. Rockhill RL, Daly FJ, MacNeil MA, Brown SP, Masland RH: The diversity of ganglion cells in a mammalian retina. *J Neurosci* 2002; 22:3831–3843.

35. Stell WK, Witkovsky P: Retinal structure in the smooth dogfish, Mustelus canis: General description and light microscopy of giant ganglion cells. *J Comp Neurol* 1973; 148:1–32.

36. Tian N, Copenhagen DR: Visual stimulation is required for refinement of ON and OFF pathways in postnatal retina. *Neuron* 2003; 39:85–96.

37. Wässle H, Riemann HJ: The mosaic of nerve cells in the mammalian retina. *Proc Royal Soc B* 1978; 200:441–461.

GENETIC MUTATIONS AND DYSFUNCTION

38. den Hollander AI, ten Brink JB, de Kok YJM, van Soest S, van den Born LI, van Driel MA, van de Pol DJR, Payne AM, Bhattacharya SS, Kellner U, Hoyng CB, Westerveld A, Brunner HG, Bleeker-Wagemakers EM, Deutman AF, Heckenlively JR, Cremers FPM, Bergen AAB: Mutations in a human homologue of *Drosophila crumbs* cause retinitis pigmentosa (RP12). *Nat Genet* 1999; 23:217–221.

39. Hori K, Katayama N, Kachi S, Kondo M, Kadomatsu K, Usukura J, Muramatsu T, Mori S, Miyake Y: Retinal dysfunction in basigin deficiency. *Invest Ophthalmol Vis Sci* 2000; 41:10 3128–3133.

40. Horie M, Kobayashi K, Takeda S, Nakamura Y, Lyons GE, Toda T: Isolation and characterization of the mouse ortholog of the Fukuyama-type congenital muscular dystrophy gene. *Genomics* 2002; 80:482–486.

41. Molday LL, Hicks D, Sauer CG, Weber BHF, Molday RS: Expression of X-linked retinoschisis protein RS1 in photoreceptor and bipolar cells. *Invest Ophthalmol Vis Sci* 2001; 42:816–825.

42. Ochrietor JD, Moroz TM, Kadomatsu K, Muramatsu T, Linser PA: Retinal degeneration following failed photorecep-

tor maturation in 5A11/basigin null mice. *Exp Eye Res* 2001; 72:467–477.

43. Pearsall N, Bhattacharya G, Wisecarver J, Adams J, Cosgrove D, Kimberling W: Usherin expression is highly conserved in mouse and human tissues. *Hear Res* 2002; 174:55–63.

44. Rivolta C, Sweklo EA, Berson EL, Dryja TP: Missense mutation in the USH2A gene: Association with recessive retinitis pigmentosa without hearing loss. *Am J Hum Genet* 2000; 66:1975–1978.

45. Takeda S, Kondo M, Sasaki J, Kurahashi H, Kano H, Arai K, Misaki K, Fukui T, Kobayashi K, Tachikawa M, Imamura M, Nakamura Y, Shimizu T, Murakami T, Sunada Y, Fujikado T, Matsumura K, Terashima T, Toda T: Fukutin is required for maintenance of muscle integrity, cortical histogenesis and normal eye development. *Hum Mol Genet* 2003; 12:1449–1459.

46. Weber BHF, Schrewe H, Molday LL, Gehrig A, White KL, Seeliger MW, Jaissle GB, Friedburg C, Tamm E, Molday RS: Inactivation of the murine X-linked juvenile retinoschisis gene, RS1H, suggests a role of retinoschisin in retinal cell layer organization and synaptic structure. *Proc Nat Acad Sci* 2002; 99:6222–6227.

10 Central Disorders of Vision in Humans

CHRISTOPHER A. GIRKIN

Introduction

Ophthalmologists tend to view the striate cortex as an afferent structure that receives visual information mostly from the lateral geniculate nucleus (LGN). Indeed, most of our efforts as ophthalmologists center on the preservation or restoration of these inputs into the visual cortex. However, a wide variety of visual disorders may occur from damage to the visual cortex and its occipitofugal connections with associative visual areas. These syndromes are often called *disorders of higher cortical function* and remind us that the striate cortex is not the end of the line but the beginning of a complex system of visual analysis that ultimately leads to global awareness of the visual environment.

CORTICAL VISUAL AREAS   Over the past 20 years, over 30 visual cortical areas have been isolated in macaque monkeys. These areas make up almost 50% of the entire cortical volume. Although the function of most of these areas is unclear, studies of the visual cortex in lower primates[25,100,105,109] and clinical correlation with cerebral lesions in patients,[51,80,102] along with electrophysiologic studies,[7,31] postmortem histologic examinations,[11,14] and functional imaging studies,[17,28,89,95,112] have identified several cortical areas that may have clinical importance in humans.

The visual cortex in the macaque was initially divided into six subregions named visual areas 1 through 6 (areas V1–V6). Area V1 is the primary visual cortex and corresponds to the striate cortex in both humans and lower primates. Areas V2–V6 are extensively interconnected visual areas that lie anterior to V1 and contain specialized maps of the visual field. Area V2 is immediately adjacent to area V1 in most primates, including humans. It corresponds to Brodmann's area 18 and was previously called the *parastriate cortex*.

Hubel and Wiesel initially believed that Brodmann's area 19, also called the *peristriate cortex* in humans, was composed entirely of the human homologue of V3,[29] but further studies indicated that the peristriate cortex is composed of two functionally distinct areas: areas V3 and V3A.[95]

Area V4 in the macaque lies in the lateral occipital lobe. While the caudal lingual and fusiform gyri within Brodmann's area 18 are involved in color processing in humans, whether or not it is homologous to area V4 in the macaque is controversial.[66] Area V5, also called area MT because of its location in the middle temporal gyrus of the owl monkey, is located in humans in the gyrus subangularis of the ventrolateral occipital lobe.

Area V6 in the macaque has no clear homologue in humans; however, an area associated with visuospatial processing in the posterior parietal cortex is the most likely candidate. Figure 10.1 illustrates the presumed location of several of the corresponding visual areas in humans. Only those cortical areas that are associated with distinct clinical syndromes will be discussed.

OCCIPITOFUGAL PATHWAYS   On the basis of numerous studies of lesions in humans,[19,22] functional imaging of normal subjects,[17] and experiments in monkeys,[100] it is clear that the information that is processed by the striate cortex and visual associative areas is projected through two occipitofugal pathways: a ventral occipitotemporal pathway and a dorsal occipitoparietal pathway (figure 10.2).[47] The ventral pathway, often called the "what" pathway, is involved in processing the physical attributes of a visual image that are important to the perception of color, shape, and pattern. These, in turn, are crucial for object identification and object-based attention.[101] The ventral pathway originates in V1 and projects through V2 and V4 to specific inferior temporal cortical areas, the angular gyrus, and limbic structures. It provides visual information to areas that are involved in visual identification, language processing, memory, and emotion.[91] Thus, a lesion in this pathway may cause a variety of associative defects, including visual alexia and anomia, visual agnosia, visual amnesia, and visual hypoemotionality.

The dorsal or "where" pathway, begins in V1 and projects through V2 and V3 to V5.[91,101] From V5, this pathway continues to additional areas in the parietal and superior temporal cortex.[90] These projections are involved in visuospatial analysis, in the localization of objects in visual space, and in modulation of visual guidance of movements toward these objects.[39,99] Thus, lesions of this pathway may cause a variety of visuospatial disorders such as Bálint's syndrome and hemispatial neglect. Although the ventral and dorsal pathways are clearly involved in the analysis of different

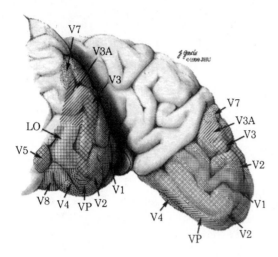

FIGURE 10.1 Posterior lateral view of the human visual cortex showing several of the visual associative areas. The cerebellum has been removed, and the hemispheres have been separated and displaced to display medial and lateral occipital regions. Area V1 corresponds to the primary of striate visual cortex. The other associative visual areas are discussed in the text except V7, V8, and LO (lateral occipital, which plays a role in object processing), because these areas have not been associated with distinct clinical syndromes.

aspects of the visual environment,[101] they are extensively interconnected laterally and in feedback and feedforward directions, indicating that the flow of perceptual processing does not necessarily proceed in a stepwise, hierarchic manner.[91] This "what" and "where" dichotomy of visual processing is an oversimplification of how these cortical areas function, but it serves as a useful framework in which to develop a clinical model of cortical visual processing. A number of specific syndromes in humans involving the central processing of visual information can be localized primarily to one of the six visual cortical areas or one of the two occipitofugal pathways and thus are of clinical value. These syndromes are summarized in table 10.1.

Syndromes associated with damage to the striate cortex (area V1)

ANTON SYNDROME Denial of blindness, or Anton syndrome, is an uncommon form of anosagnosia that usually follows extensive damage to the striate cortex.[4,69] Although Anton syndrome usually occurs with geniculostriate lesions, it can occur from any etiology, including blindness from prechiasmal disorders such as optic neuropathies and retinal detachment.

There are several theories regarding the etiology of Anton syndrome, but a definitive etiology remains elusive.[62]

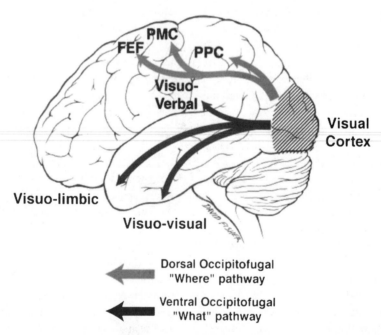

FIGURE 10.2 Parallel visual processing pathways in the human. The ventral or "what" pathway begins in the striate cortex (V1) and projects to the angular gyrus for language processing (visuo-verbal pathway), the inferior temporal lobe for object identification (visuo-visual pathway) and limbic structures (visuo-limbic pathway). The dorsal or "where" pathway begins in the striate cortex and projects to the posterior parietal cortex (PPC) and superior temporal cortex and is concerning with visuospatial analysis. This pathway continues forward to project to the premotor cortex (PMC) and the frontal eye fields (FEF) to convey visuospatial information used in the guidance of limb and eye movements.

Geschwind noted that patients with this condition often had altered emotional reactivity with a "coarse and shallow" affect similar to some patients with frontal lobe lesions. He attributed the denial of blindness to damage to higher cognitive centers.[62] Psychiatric denial may explain other cases.[54] Finally, lesions of the geniculostriate pathway that disrupt input to the visual cortex may also interfere with output from the visual cortex to areas that are involved in the conscious awareness of visual perception. In such cases, the striate cortex is unable to communicate the nature of the patient's visual loss to areas that are concerned with conscious awareness.[54]

BLINDSIGHT   Studies of visually guided behavior following removal of the striate cortex in monkeys demonstrate definite preservation of visual sensory function.[70] A similar phenomenon is thought to occur in humans who experience severe damage to one or both occipital lobes.[76] Weiskrantz coined the term *blindsight* to refer to this rudimentary level of visual processing that occurs below the level of visual awareness.[107] Over the past 20 years, the phenomenon of blindsight has been extensively studied in humans and lower primates. This entity encompasses a wide variety of visual-processing mechanisms, all occurring without conscious awareness.[93]

Higher levels of cortical processing have been evaluated in humans by both implicit processing, which measures induced responses to stimuli presented to the blind field,[64,75,98,106] and direct responses, including forced-choice experiments, saccadic localization tasks, and manual pointing to objects presented in the blind hemifield.[90] Using these techniques, researchers have shown that rare patients exhibit preservation of the ability to detect direction of motion,[64] wavelength,[92] target displacement,[9] stimulus presence,[107] orientation,[71] and object discrimination.[107] Behavior studies in monkeys and humans have demonstrated that this unconscious discrimination exhibits a learning effect, with increased accuracy with extensive training.[113] However, the potential use of blindsight in visual rehabilitation is controversial.[113]

Although much controversy still surrounds the existence of blindsight in humans and the pathways that are involved, the availability of improved functional imaging methods may help to resolve these conflicts in the future.

RIDDOCH PHENOMENON   Since George Riddoch's initial description of 10 patients with wounds to the occipital area who were able to perceive movements within their otherwise blind hemifield,[77] several studies of similar patients by other investigators have confirmed what has become known as *the Riddoch phenomenon*: preservation of motion perception in an otherwise complete scotoma.[68,111]

The etiology of the Riddoch phenomenon is not clear. It has been suggested that patients who exhibit this phenomenon have preserved islands of function within the striate cortex[77] or that extrastriate areas, area V5 in particular, may be involved through activation of subcortical pathways that bypass V1.[12,111] Alternatively, statokinetic dissociation may be related to lateral summation of moving images. It has been demonstrated in normal subjects that a kinetic target may be seen more readily in some areas of the visual field than nonmoving objects of the same intensity and size.[43] Variable degrees of dissociation of perception between moving and nonmoving stimuli have been demonstrated in normal subjects[36] and in patients with compression of the anterior visual pathways.[84,108]

Syndromes caused by damage to the parastriate and peristriate visual cortex (areas V2 and V3)

The effect of lesions of V2 and V3 in humans is unclear. Horton and Hoyt reported two patients with lesions that were thought to involve the superior parastriate and peristriate cortex.[51] Both patients had homonymous quadrantic visual field defects that respected the horizontal and vertical meridians. Of course, a congruous homonymous quadrantanopia is not specific to parastriate lesions; it not infrequently results from striate lesions as well.[65]

Syndromes caused by damage to the human color center (area V4)

PERCEPTION OF COLOR AND AREA V4   Unlike a camera, the visual system has the ability to compensate for the changing spectral components of a light source. Therefore, in most viewing situations, a red object will appear red regardless of the wavelength of light that illuminates it, even though the dominant spectral component that is reflected from the object may vary with lighting conditions. This effect is called *color constancy*. The visual system creates the concept of color by comparing areas of the visual field. Thus, a red object appears red not because it reflects long-wavelength light, but because it reflects relatively more long-wavelength light than do other objects within the visual field. Physiological experiments, along with lesion studies in macaques, have led some investigators to conclude that area V4 is the site of color constancy in lower primates.[110]

Although the localization of a color center in humans has been clearly identified,[63] whether or not this area is homologous to area V4 in monkeys and whether or not cerebral achromatopsia in humans is a defect of color constancy alone are currently unresolved issues.[15,50,56] Many authors use the term *human color center* interchangeably with the term *human V4*.[66] However, the complaints of patients with cerebral achromatopsia from damage to this region are not entirely explained by loss of color constancy.[80] In addition, extirpation of area V4 in the monkey does not lead to achromatopsia, for the animals retain the ability to discriminate and order hues despite clearly impaired form recognition.[37,86,87]

CEREBRAL ACHROMATOPSIA   Cerebral achromatopsia is an acquired defect in color perception that is caused by damage to the ventromedial visual cortex.[110] Affected patients describe a world that looks faded, gray, and washed out or completely devoid of color, like a black-and-white photograph. Unlike patients with congenital achromatopsia, patients with acquired cerebral achromatopsia show preserved trichromacy and intact cortical responses to chromatic visual evoked potentials (VEPs).[18] Thus, the chromatic pathways from the retina to the striate cortex are intact. Because of preserved function of wavelength-selective cells in the striate cortex, achromatopsic patients may still retain the ability to distinguish the border between two adjacent isoluminant colored patches[18] and may perform well on testing with pseudoisochromatic plates.[67]

Bilateral infarction in the posterior cerebral artery distribution is the most common etiology and is often due to vertebrobasilar ischemia.[59] Additional causes include metastatic tumors,[40] posterior cortical dementia,[33] and herpes simplex encephalitis.[49] Transient achromatopsia may occur with migraine,[61] focal seizures,[1] and vertebrobasilar insuffi-

ciency.[59] Cerebral achromatopsia is often associated with a superior homonymous visual field defect from damage to the inferior striate cortex.[23] In such cases, the residual inferior field on that side is achromatopsic. Bilateral lesions are required for a complete achromatopsia, whereas unilateral lesions produce hemiachromatopsia.

Three-dimensional magnetic resonance imaging (MRI) in patients with cerebral achromatopsia indicates that the critical lesion involves the middle third of the lingual gyrus or the white matter posterior to the tip of the lateral ventricle.[21] Zeki and coworkers used functional MRI (fMRI) to define the representation of the visual field in the human color center.[66] This study localized the color center to the lateral aspect of the collateral sulcus on the fusiform gyrus (figure 10.3). Additionally, these investigators described a retinotopic organization of the fusiform gyrus, the superior field being represented within the medial fusiform gyrus and the inferior field being located more laterally.

If achromatopsia were due solely to defective color constancy, then patients with the condition should not see the world as gray or desaturated but instead should experience dramatic fluctuations in color as environmental lighting conditions change. Since this is not the case, the defect in achromatopsia may involve more than just color constancy.

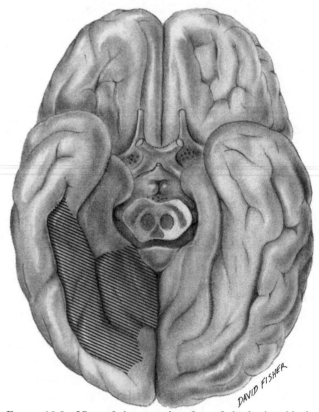

FIGURE 10.3   View of the ventral surface of the brain with the cerebellum removed. The posterior fusiform and lingual gyri, which contain the human color center, are highlighted.

Indeed, Rizzo et al. have hypothesized that color constancy, like lightness constancy, is generated by earlier visual associative areas.[82] Alternatively, lesions of the fusiform gyrus may disrupt white matter deep to the collateral sulcus and disconnect the striate and extrastriate areas from a more rostral color center, possibly an area that is homologous to a wavelength-selective inferior temporal area in monkeys that, when extirpated, produces a deficit similar to cerebral achromatopsia in humans.[18]

Syndromes caused by damage to area V5

NEUROPHYSIOLOGY OF MOTION PERCEPTION Functional imaging,[96,112] experiments using myelin, cytochrome oxidase, and monoclonal-antibody staining;[97] and cortical stimulation experiments suggest that the most likely location of area V5 in humans is the ventrolateral occipital gyrus, a key area that is involved in the perception of visual motion. However, the analysis of motion involves a complex system of several interrelated cortical areas that are involved in processing various components of motion perception and that may adapt to the loss of area V5.[32,96] This would explain the preservation of some aspects of visual motion perception in patients with akinetopsia (see below) and the rarity of this syndrome in humans.

AKINETOPSIA Akinetopsia is the loss of perception of visual motion with preservation of the perception of other modalities of vision, such as form, texture, and color. In 1983, Zihl et al. provided the first clearly described example of akinetopsia.[114] L.M., the patient described by these investigators, is one of only two patients who have been extensively studied. She developed bilateral cerebral infarctions involving the lateral occipital, middle temporal, and angular gyri, secondary to sagittal sinus thrombosis (figure 10.4). She

described moving objects as jumping from place to place. For example, when pouring tea, she observed that the liquid appeared frozen like a glacier, and she failed to perceive the tea rising in the cup. Additionally, subtle deficits in motion processing in the contralateral hemifield in patients with unilateral occipitoparietal lesions involving area V5 have also been described.[102] This "hemiakinetopsia" is often obscured by coexistent incomplete homonymous field defects.

The dorsal occipitofugal pathway and visuospatial processing in humans

NEUROANATOMY AND NEUROPHYSIOLOGY The dorsal or "where" pathway receives information primarily from area MT and, to a lesser extent, area V4.[101] This information is conveyed along the dorsal longitudinal fascicles to the posterior parietal cortex, frontal motor areas, and frontal eye fields (FEF). This pathway is concerned with spatial localization, visuomotor search and guidance, and visuospatial synthesis.[19] Lesions of the dorsal pathway produce visuomotor and attention deficits, in contrast to the visuoassociative deficits produced by ventral lesions.

The posterior parietal cortex is neither a purely sensory nor a purely motor area; rather, it combines characteristics of both. Thus, it serves as a junction between multimodal sensory input and motor output, linking the afferent and efferent arms of the visual pathways and providing the connection that encompasses the entire field of neuro-ophthalmology, from the eyes to the extraocular muscles.[2]

SYNDROMES OF THE DORSAL OCCIPITOFUGAL PATHWAY IN HUMANS
Bálint syndrome Bálint syndrome is classically defined as the combination of simultanagnosia, optic ataxia, and acquired oculomotor apraxia, also called *psychic paralysis of gaze*.[104] The

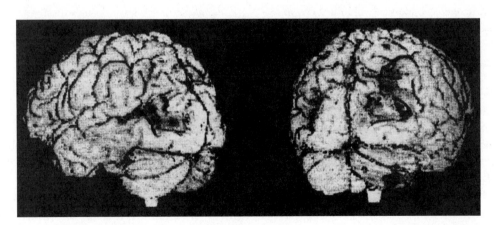

FIGURE 10.4 Three-dimensional magnetic resonance imaging reconstruction's of bilateral temporo-occipital lesions of a patient who developed akinetopsia associated with a sagittal sinus thrombosis. Left, View of the left posterior brain; Right, View of the right posterior brain. (Source: Used with permission from Shipp S, de Jong BM, Zihl J, et al. The brain activity related to residual motion vision in a patient with bilateral lesions of V5. *Brain* 117:1023–1038, 1994.)

components of Bálint syndrome are not closely bound together[73] and may occur in isolation or in association with other disorders of visuospatial perception. Therefore, this triad has no specific anatomically localizable correlate.[46,73] Most authors believe that the concept of Bálint syndrome as a specific clinical entity offers little to the scientific or clinical understanding of visuospatial processing and, although historically interesting, should be abandoned. We will therefore consider the specific components of this "syndrome" separately.

Patients with dorsal simultanagnosia can perceive whole shapes, but their perception of these shapes is limited to a single visual area because they are unable to shift visual attention. Patients with this condition therefore behave as if they are blind even though they have intact visual fields. Dorsal simultanagnosia, although clearly a visualspatial disorder of attention, is discussed in more detail below along with apperceptive agnosias and ventral simultanagnosia because of the clinical similarities among these conditions.

Optic ataxia is a disorder of visual guidance of movements in which visual inputs are disconnected from the motor systems.[74] Therefore, patients reach for targets within an intact field as if they were blind.[81] A complex sensorimotor network involves the posterior parietal lobe, motor areas, ventromedial cortical areas, and subcortical structures, such as the cerebellum, that modulate the control of visually guided limb movement.[78] Thus, a variety of lesions that affect this network can produce optic ataxia.[79] Lesions of superior parietal cortex are more likely to damage areas that are involved with limb guidance, whereas inferior parietal lesions are more likely to affect visual attention and thus produce neglect syndromes.[34,55]

Spasm of fixation or psychic paralysis of gaze is sometimes erroneously called *ocular motor apraxia*, thus adding to the confusion already surrounding this phenomenon. Spasm of fixation is characterized by loss of voluntary eye movements with persistence of fixation on a target. However, in contrast to true ocular motor apraxia, saccades are easily made to peripheral targets in the absence of a fixation target. Thus, a patient who is asked to fixate an object centrally and then move the eyes to a peripheral target cannot do so, whereas a patient who is not fixing on any object in particular can easily move the eyes to fixate a peripheral target when asked to do so.

The location of the lesion that causes spasm of fixation is obscure. The FEF is required for the release of fixation for voluntary saccades, and lesions of this region may prolong saccadic latency. Posterior parietal, middle temporal, and superior temporal areas mediate cortical maintenance of fixation by inhibition of attention shifts. Thus, damage to the FEF that spares these regions may prevent the release of fixation by disinhibiting the inhibitory effect of the substan-tia nigra pars reticulata on the superior colliculus, thus sppressing the generation of saccades.[53]

Hemispatial (hemifield) neglect Complex visual scenes constantly bombard the visual system. Because cognitive and motor activities are generally concerned with one object at a time, these elements of the visual scene must compete for the limited resources of focal attention.[5,13] Modulation of attention occurs at many levels in the visual system, even at the level of area V1.[58,103]

Numerous lines of evidence suggest that a complex network of cortical and subcortical areas primarily in the dorsal occipitofugal pathway is involved in the modulation of spatial attention. These include the superior colliculus, the posterior parietal cortex, the striatum, the pulvinar, and areas in the prefrontal cortex.[16] In particular, the posterior parietal cortex, the FEF, and the cingulate gyrus play key roles in spatial-based attention mechanisms. The posterior parietal cortex builds the sensory representation of extrapersonal space, the FEF plans and initiates exploratory movements, and the cingulate gyrus provides the motivational potential.[16]

Hemispatial neglect involves multiple sensory modalities, but visual extinction often is the most prominent feature. Affected patients see stimuli that are presented separately in either their right or their left hemifield but ignore stimuli in the left hemifield when both hemifields are stimulated simultaneously. Thus, any patient who appears to have a homonymous hemianopia when bilateral simultaneous stimulation confrontation testing is performed should undergo testing of each homonymous hemifield separately to determine whether the apparent field defect is real or the consequence of hemifield extinction. In patients with full visual fields, double simultaneous stimulation or testing line bisection is an excellent bedside examination technique to detect hemifield neglect.

Visual allesthesia Classic visual allesthesia is a disorder of visuospatial perception in which the retinotopic visual field is rotated, flipped, or even inverted (figure 10.5, center left and right sketches). This syndrome localizes to two seemingly diverse areas of the brain: the lateral medulla and the occipitoparietal area, usually on the right side. Although visual allesthesia is a common component of the lateral medullary syndrome of Wallenberg[83] and is usually due to infarction, a variety of disorders that affect the cerebral cortex can produce visual allesthesia, including infarction,[48] neoplasm, trauma, infection,[3] and multiple sclerosis.[88] Transient visual allesthesia can occur during seizures[72] and migraine attacks.[44]

Several theories have been proposed to explain visual allesthesia; however, an all-encompassing explanation remains elusive. Jacobs suggested that allesthesia may involve transcallosal transmission of the contralateral hemifield to the damaged parietal cortex, with retention of the image as a

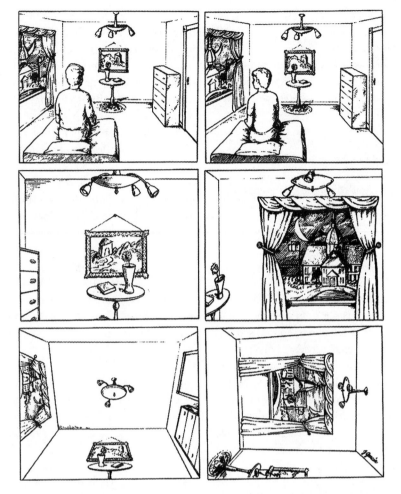

FIGURE 10.5   Illustrations on the left show the view and orientation looking forward. Illustrations on the right show the view and orientation looking to the left. The top left and right figures show a third person view of the patient's room indicating the head position and the orientation of the environment that would be seen by a normal person looking forward (left) and to the left (right). The center left and right figures illustrate the appearance of the environment that would be seen by a patient with classic visual allesthesia looking forward (center left) and to the left (center right). Note that there is transposition of the visual field. The bottom left and right figures illustrate the environmental rotation experienced by our patient in contrast to the visual field rotation in classic allesthesia. Note that the rotation in our patient is independent of head position. (Source: From Girkin CA, Perry JD, Miller NR.[38] Used by permission.)

palinoptic phenomenon.[52] Although this theory might explain the patient he described who had transposition of the visual field from left to right, it fails to explain the varieties of rotational or inverted allesthesia described by other patients.

Alternatively, visual allesthesia may be the result of a disorder of integration of visuospatial input. The causative lesion may disturb the integration of visual and otolithic inputs at the level of the medulla, as in Wallenberg syndrome, in which otolith inputs are interrupted directly, or at the site of integration in the posterior parietal cortex.[94]

Environmental rotation   Classic visual allesthesia is characterized by tilting or rotation of the visual field. However, some patients have a form of visual allesthesia in which the environment rather than the field is rotated. For example, we reported a patient who experienced transient episodes of static rotation of the visual environment following a ventriculoperitoneal shunt placed through the right occipitoparietal cortex for normal pressure hydrocephalus.[38] During each episode, the patient noted that the environment was rotated 90 degrees, independent of head position (figure 10.5, bottom left and right sketches). This visuospatial derangement abated 6 days after surgery. As was discussed above, the parietal lobe integrates visual information with vestibular and proprioceptive input to form an internal model of visual space that represent the "real position" of objects independent of head-centered coordinates. We believe that the phenomenon that our patient experienced resulted from a disorder of the "real position" system[35] in the posterior parietal lobe and was caused by irritation from the shunt.

The ventral occipitofugal pathway in humans

NEUROANATOMY AND NEUROPHYSIOLOGY

The ventral occipitofugal or "what" pathway is conducted mainly through the inferior longitudinal fascicles. Lesions of this pathway were initially divided into three types of disconnection syndromes:

1. Visual-visual disconnection that isolates visual inputs from the inferior temporal areas, producing an agnosia.

2. Visual-verbal disconnection that isolates the language centers in the dominant angular gyrus from visual input, producing alexia and anomia.

3. Visual-limbic disconnection that isolates visual inputs from the amygdala and hippocampus, producing deficits in visual memory and emotion.[26]

Although this disconnection theory was helpful in developing a general categorization scheme for these defects, it is inadequate in that it assumes that visual perception, semantic understanding, and memory are all processed in a staged, modular fashion. This separation is not distinct, and patients seldom display completely isolated manifestations of these syndromes. For example, visual-verbal defects may occur in combination with visual-visual defects, and disorders that were previously categorized as visual-verbal disconnections, such as pure alexia, are now considered by some authors as subtypes of visual agnosia (see below).

LESIONS OF THE VENTRAL OCCIPITOFUGAL PATHWAY IN HUMANS

Visual-visual disconnection Visual information processed in area V4 projects anteriorly to the temporal cortex, where it is integrated with stored memory templates.[6] Lesions of this pathway may cause true visual agnosia, that is, unimodal deficits in object knowledge.[30] In contrast to object anomia, patients with pure visual agnosia cannot provide the name or the associative features of an object, thus indicating a defect in recognition, not just in naming. Neuropsychologists generally divide the agnosias into two groups: apperceptive agnosia and associative agnosia.

The term *apperceptive agnosia* has been applied to patients with impaired object recognition due to perceptual difficulties in which elementary visual function remains intact. Perception involves the integration of visual information to form an internal image of an object. Thus, patients may have good visual acuity, color vision, and brightness discrimination but still be unable to perceive an object because of an inability to integrate incoming visual information. These patients often have visual field defects, but their perceptual deficit cannot be explained by their field loss. They perceive their visual environment in a piecemeal fashion, being unable to integrate multiple characteristics of a visual scene into a global perception. Although patients with apperceptive agnosia might exhibit behavior that is superficially similar to the behavior of patients with associative agnosia, the underlying deficit in apperceptive agnosia, when interpreted in the narrowest sense, applies only to patients who exhibit a disorder in which only focal contour is perceived.

Patients with true associative agnosia have intact perception and can draw and match objects but are unable visually to identify objects or categories of objects. Tactile recognition and auditory recognition are intact in these patients. This condition is most often caused by lesions that damage the ventral posterior cortex bilaterally and disturb occipitotemporal interactions responsible for correlation of visual perception to memory centers involved in object recognition.[20]

Agnosias may be generalized or restricted to specific classes of objects. Prosopagnosia and pure alexia (see the next section, "Visual-verbal disconnection") are specific subtypes of agnosia restricted to individual categories of visual objects.

Patients with prosopagnosia have impaired ability to recognize familiar faces or to learn new faces, often relying on nonfacial clues such as posture or voice to distinguish friends, colleagues, and family from strangers.[20] They are usually but not universally aware of this deficit. The retained ability to identify people by nonfacial cues differentiates this disorder from person-specific amnesia, which has been reported in patients with lesions of the temporal poles and presumably renders the personal identity nodes inaccessible.[45] Patients with prosopagnosia usually can match faces and distinguish among unfamiliar faces, and some can accurately judge age, sex, and emotional expression from facial information, indicating that perception of some facial information is intact.[24] However, performance of these tasks is often abnormal, indicating some degree of perceptual disturbance.[24]

Generalized object agnosia refers to agnosias that extend to include a wide variety of classes of objects. The causative lesions and associated findings in generalized object agnosia are similar to those of prosopagnosia.[57] That agnosias may be specific to a variety of classes of objects has led many researchers to assume that object recognition is achieved in a modular fashion, with specific areas in the brain that are responsible for recognition of various classes of objects.[20] However, it is more likely that these class-specific agnosia result from differences in the way in which different types of stimuli are processed in the brain.

Visual-verbal disconnection A visual-verbal disconnection produces difficulties in naming objects despite intact object recognition. These deficits must be distinguished from agnosia, in which identification of objects is defective (see above).[60] Three main syndromes of visual-verbal disconnec-

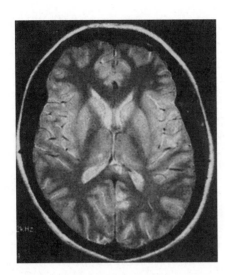

FIGURE 10.6 T2-weighted magnetic resonance image through the splenium of the corpus callosum of a patient who developed alexia without agraphia following hypovolemic shock. A well-defined infarction involving the splenium is evident.

tion have been described in humans: pure alexia (alexia without agraphia), color anomia, and object anomia (optic aphasia).

Patients with pure alexia can write and converse normally; however, they have profound difficulties reading, even words that they have just written. Because identification of lexical stimuli is intact by other sensory modalities, patients with pure alexia might be able to identify words by tracing. The degree of deficit is variable. Most patients exhibit slow, letter-by-letter reading; others are completely unable to identify words, letters, or symbols.[8] Many cases of pure alexia are overlooked or wrongly attributed to the hemianopic defects that are frequently seen in these patients.

The dominant parietal cortex is involved in the evaluation of lexical symbols. The most common lesions associated with this deficit damage the left striate cortex and the splenium of the corpus collosum (figure 10.6), although lesions that damage the left LGN and splenium can also cause this syndrome.[19] Affected patients usually have a right homonymous hemianopia. Thus, no visual information is transmitted from the left striate cortex to the ipsilateral (dominant) angular gyrus. In addition, although their right (nondominant) striate cortex is intact, information from this region cannot be transmitted to the dominant angular gyrus because of the associated damage to the splenium of the corpus callosum, through which this information is normally conducted.[41] Lesions in the left subangular white matter may also cause pure alexia by isolating incoming information at a more distal level.[42] Patients with such lesions may or may not have a hemianopic defect depending on whether or not the optic radiations are also involved. In cases with hemianopia, the alexia is caused not by the visual field defect but rather by disruption of visual inputs to higher-order linguistic centers.

Although there are cases in which color is disproportionately affected, most cases of color anomia are part of a more general visual-verbal defect with coexistent pure alexia.[85] Patients with color anomia can match colors and therefore do not have achromatopsia or an agnostic deficit. Their semantic recall of color is intact, and they are thus able to recall accurately the color of known objects (e.g., the color of a banana or an apple).

Object anomia (optic aphasia) is characterized by a generalized defect in visual naming. Affected patients are unable to recall the name of objects presented visually, although their recall based on tactile and auditory input is preserved. Object matching and recognition are also intact. Such patients may be able to describe the characteristics of an object and its purpose, but they cannot provide the name of the object solely on the basis of visual information. Often deficits in object identification are also present, making the separation between agnosia and aphasia difficult. The anatomic bases for color anomia, pure alexia, and object anomia are not entirely clear but probably represent variations in the disruption of visual information reaching the angular gyrus.

Visual-limbic disconnection The sensory-limbic system plays a critical role in processing the emotional impact of sensory stimuli and in reinforcing certain aspects of multimodal sensory memory traces that are emotionally relevant through reciprocal circuits involving the temporal lobe.[27] Thus, lesions of the limbic system may cause multimodal amnestic disorders that impair recall of the recent past and an inability to establish new memories. Lesions that disconnect visual input to this system may cause a modality-specific deficit. Two such disorders associated with lesions that disrupt visual axons projecting to the ventromedial temporal lobe are visual amnesia and visual hypoemotionality. These syndromes are rarely reported because object agnosia or prosopagnosia often mask their presence.

Closing remarks

As investigators uncover the complexities of the higher visual system, a greater understanding of these clinical syndromes will emerge. A familiarity with these syndromes will enable the ophthalmologist to identify patients who have these disorders and perform appropriate testing. Additionally, the study of higher cortical disorders may provide insight into the mechanisms of visual awareness and the global sense of the perception of our environment. Understanding this crucial function of the mind will be an integral step in forming a global theory of consciousness.

REFERENCES

1. Aldrich MS, Vanderzant CW, Alessi AG, Abou-Khalil B, Sackellares JC: Ictal cortical blindness with permanent visual loss. *Epilepsia* 1989; 30:116–120.

2. Andersen RA: Multimodal integration for the representation of space in the posterior parietal cortex. *Philos Trans R Soc Lond B Biol Sci* 1997; 352:1421–1428.

3. Ardila A, Botero M, Gomez J: Palinopsia and visual allesthesia. *Int J Neurosci* 1987; 32:775–782.

4. Argenta PA, Morgan MA: Cortical blindness and Anton syndrome in a patient with obstetric hemorrhage. *Obstet Gynecol* 1998; 91:810–812.

5. Barrett AM, Beversdorf DQ, Crucian GP, Heilman KM: Neglect after right hemisphere stroke: a smaller floodlight for distributed attention [see comments]. *Neurology* 1998; 51:972–978.

6. Beason-Held LL, Purpura KP, Van Meter JW, et al: PET reveals occipitotemporal pathway activation during elementary form perception in humans. *Vis Neurosci* 1998; 15:503–510.

7. Beckers G, Zeki S: The consequences of inactivating areas V1 and V5 on visual motion perception. *Brain* 1995; 118:49–60.

8. Binder JR, Mohr JP: The topography of callosal reading pathways: A case-control analysis. *Brain* 1992; 115:1807–1826.

9. Blythe IM, Bromley JM, Kennard C, Ruddock KH: Visual discrimination of target displacement remains after damage to the striate cortex in humans. *Nature* 1986; 320:619–621.

10. Blythe IM, Kennard C, Ruddock KH: Residual vision in patients with retrogeniculate lesions of the visual pathways. *Brain* 1987; 110:887–905.

11. Burkhalter A, Bernardo KL: Organization of corticocortical connections in human visual cortex. *Proc Natl Acad Sci USA* 1989; 86:1071–1075.

12. Celesia GG, Bushnell D, Toleikis SC, Brigell MG: Cortical blindness and residual vision: Is the "second" visual system in humans capable of more than rudimentary visual perception? *Neurology* 1991; 41:862–869.

13. Chelazzi L: Neural mechanisms for stimulus selection in cortical areas of the macaque subserving object vision. *Behav Brain Res* 1995; 71:125–134.

14. Clarke S, Miklossy J: Occipital cortex in man: organization of callosal connections, related myelo- and cytoarchitecture, and putative boundaries of functional visual areas. *J Comp Neurol* 1990; 298:188–214.

15. Clarke S, Walsh V, Schoppig A, Assal G, Cowey A: Colour constancy impairments in patients with lesions of the prestriate cortex. *Exp Brain Res* 1998; 123:154–158.

16. Colby CL: The neuroanatomy and neurophysiology of attention. *J Child Neurol* 1991; 6:S90–118.

17. Courtney SM, Ungerleider LG: What fMRI has taught us about human vision. *Curr Opin Neurobiol* 1997; 7:554–561.

18. Cowey A, Heywood CA: There's more to colour than meets the eye. *Behav Brain Res* 1995; 71:89–100.

19. Damasio AR, Damasio H: The anatomic basis of pure alexia. *Neurology* 1983; 33:1573–1583.

20. Damasio AR, Damasio H, Van Hoesen GW: Prosopagnosia: Anatomic basis and behavioral mechanisms. *Neurology* 1982; 32:331–341.

21. Damasio H, Frank R: Three-dimensional in vivo mapping of brain lesions in humans. *Arch Neurol* 1992; 49:137–143.

22. Damasio AR, McKee J, Damasio H: Determinants of performance in color anomia. *Brain Lang* 1979; 7:74–85.

23. Damasio A, Yamada T, Damasio H, Corbett J, McKee J: Central achromatopsia: behavioral, anatomic, and physiologic aspects. *Neurology* 1980; 30:1064–1071.

24. De Haan EH, Young A, Newcombe F: Faces interfere with name classification in a prosopagnosic patient. *Cortex* 1987; 23:309–316.

25. Desimone R, Schein SJ: Visual properties of neurons in area V4 of the macaque: sensitivity to stimulus form. *J Neurophysiol* 1987; 57:835–868.

26. Desimone R, Schein SJ, Moran J, Ungerleider LG: Contour, color and shape analysis beyond the striate cortex. *Vision Res* 1985; 25:441–452.

27. Drew WG, Weet CR, De Rossett SE, Batt JR: Effects of hippocampal brain damage on auditory and visual recent memory: comparison with marijuana-intoxicated subjects. *Biol Psychiatry* 1980; 15:841–858.

28. Engel SA, Rumelhart DE, Wandell BA, et al: fMRI of human visual cortex [letter] [published erratum appears in Nature 1994 Jul 14;370(6485):106]. *Nature* 1994; 369:525.

29. Essen DC, Zeki SM: The topographic organization of rhesus monkey prestriate cortex. *J Physiol (Lond)* 1978; 277:193–226.

30. Farah MJ: Agnosia. *Curr Opin Neurobiol* 1992; 2:162–164.

31. ffytche DH, Guy CN, Zeki S: The parallel visual motion inputs into areas V1 and V5 of human cerebral cortex. *Brain* 1995; 118:1375–1394.

32. Felleman DJ, Van Essen DC: Distributed hierarchical processing in the primate cerebral cortex. *Cereb Cortex* 1991; 1:1–47.

33. Freedman L, Costa L: Pure alexia and right hemiachromatopsia in posterior dementia. *J Neurol Neurosurg Psychiatry* 1992; 55:500–502.

34. Friedrich FJ, Egly R, Rafal RD, Beck D: Spatial attention deficits in humans: a comparison of superior parietal and temporal-parietal junction lesions. *Neuropsychology* 1998; 12:193–207.

35. Galletti C, Battaglini PP, Fattori P: Eye position influence on the parieto-occipital area PO (V6) of the macaque monkey. *Eur J Neurosci* 1995; 7:2486–2501.

36. Gandolfo E: Stato-kinetic dissociation in subjects with normal and abnormal visual fields. *Eur J Ophthalmol* 1996; 6:408-414.

37. Ghose GM, Ts'o DY: Form processing modules in primate area V4. *J Neurophysiol* 1997; 77:2191–2196.

38. Girkin CA, Perry JD, Miller NR: Visual environmental rotation: A novel disorder of visiuospatial integration. *J Neuroophthalmol* 1999; 19:13–16.

39. Goldberg ME, Segraves MA: Visuospatial and motor attention in the monkey. *Neuropsychologia* 1987; 25:107–118.

40. Green GJ, Lessell S: Acquired cerebral dyschromatopsia. *Arch Ophthalmol* 1977; 95:121–128.

41. Greenblatt SH: Alexia without agraphia or hemianopsia: Anatomical analysis of an autopsied case. *Brain* 1973; 96:307–316.

42. Greenblatt SH: Subangular alexia without agraphia or hemianopsia. *Brain Lang* 1976; 3:229–245.

43. Greve EL: Single and multiple stimulus static perimetry in glaucoma: The two phases of perimetry. Thesis. *Doc Ophthalmol* 1973; 36:1–355.

44. Hachinski VC, Porchawka J, Steele JC: Visual symptoms in the migraine syndrome. *Neurology* 1973; 23:570–579.

45. Hanley JR, Pearson NA, Young AW: Impaired memory for new visual forms. *Brain* 1990; 113:1131–1148.

46. Hausser CO, Robert F, Giard N: Balint's syndrome. *Can J Neurol Sci* 1980; 7:157–161.

47. Haxby JV, Grady CL, Horwitz B, et al: Dissociation of object and spatial visual processing pathways in human extrastriate cortex. *Proc Natl Acad Sci USA* 1991; 88:1621–1625.

48. Heo K, Kim SJ, Kim JH, Kim OK, Cho HK: Flase lateralization of seizure perceived by a patient with infarction of the right parietal lobe who showed the neglect syndrome. *Epilepsia* 1997; 38:122–123.

49. Heywood CA, Cowey A, Newcombe F: On the role of parvocellular (P) and magnocellular (M) pathways in cerebral achromatopsia. *Brain* 1994; 117:245–254.

50. Heywood CA, Gadotti A, Cowey A: Cortical area V4 and its role in the perception of color. *J Neurosci* 1992; 12:4056–4065.

51. Horton JC, Hoyt WF: Quadrantic visual field defects: A hallmark of lesions in extrastriate (V2/V3) cortex. *Brain* 1991; 114:1703–1718.

52. Jacobs L: Visual allesthesia. *Neurology* 1980; 30:1059–1063.

53. Johnston JL, Sharpe JA, Morrow MJ. Spasm of fixation: A quantitative study. *J Neurol Sci* 1992; 107:166–171.

54. Joseph R: Confabulation and delusional denial: Frontal lobe and lateralized influences. *J Clin Psychol* 1986; 42:507–520.

55. Karnath HO: Spatial orientation and the representation of space with parietal lobe lesions. *Philos Trans R Soc Lond B Biol Sci* 1997; 352:1411–1419.

56. Kennard C, Lawden M, Morland AB, Ruddock KH: Colour identification and colour constancy are impaired in a patient with incomplete achromatopsia associated with prestriate cortical lesions. *Proc R Soc Lond B Biol Sci* 1995; 260:169–175.

57. Kertesz A: Visual agnosia: The dual deficit of perception and recognition. *Cortex* 1979; 15:403–419.

58. Knierim JJ, van Essen DC: Neuronal responses to static texture patterns in area V1 of the alert macaque monkey. *J Neurophysiol* 1992; 67:961–980.

59. Lapresle J, Metreau R, Annabi A: Transient achromatopsia in vertebrobasilar insufficiency. *J Neurol* 1977; 215:155–158.

60. Larrabee GJ, Levin HS, Huff FJ, Kay MC, Guinto FC Jr: Visual agnosia contrasted with visual-verbal disconnection. *Neuropsychologia* 1985; 23:1–12.

61. Lawden MC, Cleland PG: Achromatopsia in the aura of migraine. *J Neurol Neurosurg Psychiatry* 1993; 56:708–709.

62. Lessel S: Higher disorders of visual function: Negative phenomena. In Glaser J, Smith J (eds): *Neuro-ophthalmology*. 8 vol. St. Louis, Mosby, 1975, pp 3–4.

63. Lueck CJ, Zeki S, Friston KJ, et al: The colour centre in the cerebral cortex of man. *Nature* 1989; 340:386–389.

64. Marcel AJ: Blindsight and shape perception: Deficit of visual consciousness or of visual function? *Brain* 1998; 121:1565–1588.

65. McFadzean RM, Hadley DM: Homonymous quadrantanopia respecting the horizontal meridian: A feature of striate and extrastriate cortical disease. *Neurology* 1997; 49:1741–1746.

66. McKeefry DJ, Zeki S: The position and topography of the human colour centre as revealed by functional magnetic resonance imaging. *Brain* 1997; 120:2229–2242.

67. Meadows JC: Disturbed perception of colours associated with localized cerebral lesions. *Brain* 1974; 97:615–632.

68. Mestre DR, Brouchon M, Ceccaldi M, Poncet M: Perception of optical flow in cortical blindness: a case report. *Neuropsychologia* 1992; 30:783–795.

69. Misra M, Rath S, Mohanty AB: Anton syndrome and cortical blindness due to bilateral occipital infarction. *Indian J Ophthalmol* 1989; 37:196.

70. Mohler CW, Wurtz RH: Role of striate cortex and superior colliculus in visual guidance of saccadic eye movements in monkeys. *J Neurophysiol* 1977; 40:74–94.

71. Morland AB, Ogilvie JA, Ruddock KH, Wright JR: Orientation discrimination is impaired in the absence of the striate cortical contribution to human vision. *Proc R Soc Lond B Biol Sci* 1996; 263:633–640.

72. Nakajima M, Yasue M, Kaito N, Kamikubo T, Sakai H: [A case of visual allesthesia]. *No To Shinkei* 1991; 43:1081–1085.

73. Ogren MP, Mateer CA, Wyler AR: Alterations in visually related eye movements following left pulvinar damage in man. *Neuropsychologia* 1984; 22:187–196.

74. Perenin MT, Vighetto A: Optic ataxia: A specific disruption in visuomotor mechanisms. I. Different aspects of the deficit in reaching for objects. *Brain* 1988; 111:643–674.

75. Poppel E: Long-range colour-generating interactions across the retina. *Nature* 1986; 320:523–525.

76. Poppel E, Held R, Frost D: Leter: Residual visual function after brain wounds involving the central visual pathways in man. *Nature* 1973; 243:295–296.

77. Riddock G: Dissociation of visual perceptions due to occipital injuries, with especial reference to appreciation of movement. *Brain* 1917:15–57.

78. Rizzo M, Butler A, Darling W: Sensorimotor transformation inpatients with lateral cerebellar damage. *Soc Neurosci Abstr* 1995:415.

79. Rizzo M, Darling W, Damasio H: Disorders of reaching with lesions of the posterior cerebral hemisphere. *Soc Neurosci Abstr* 1995:269.

80. Rizzo M, Nawrot M, Blake R, Damasio A: A human visual disorder resembling area V4 dysfunction in the monkey [see comments]. *Neurology* 1992; 42:1175–1180.

81. Rizzo M, Rotella D, Darling W: Troubled reaching after right occipito-temporal damage. *Neuropsychologia* 1992; 30:711–722.

82. Rizzo M, Smith V, Pokorny J, Damasio AR: Color perception profiles in central achromatopsia. *Neurology* 1993; 43:955–1001.

83. Ropper AH: Illusion of tilting of the visual environment: Report of five cases. *J Clin Neuroophthalmol* 1983; 3:147–151.

84. Safran AB, Glaser JS: Statokinetic dissociation in lesions of the anterior visual pathways: A reappraisal of the Riddoch phenomenon. *Arch Ophthalmol* 1980; 98:291–295.

85. Sakata H, Taira M, Murata A, Mine S: Neural mechanisms of visual guidance of hand action in the parietal cortex of the monkey. *Cereb Cortex* 1995; 5:429–438.

86. Schiller PH: The effects of V4 and middle temporal (MT) area lesions on visual performance in the rhesus monkey. *Vis Neurosci* 1993; 10:717–746.

87. Schiller PH: Effect of lesions in visual cortical area V4 on the recognition of transformed objects. *Nature* 1995; 376:342–344.

88. Seigel AM: Inverted vision in MS [letter]. *Neurology* 1988; 38:1335.

89. Sereno MI, Dale AM, Reppas JB, et al: Borders of multiple visual areas in humans revealed by functional magnetic resonance imaging [see comments]. *Science* 1995; 268:889–893.

90. Shipp S, Blanton M, Zeki S: A visuo-somatomotor pathway through superior parietal cortex in the macaque monkey:

Cortical connections of areas V6 and V6A. *Eur J Neurosci* 1998; 10:3171–3193.

91. Shipp S, Zeki S: Segregation of pathways leading from area V2 to areas V4 and V5 of macaque monkey visual cortex. *Nature* 1985; 315:322–325.

92. Stoerig P, Cowey A: Wavelength discrimination in blindsight. *Brain* 1992; 115:425–444.

93. Stoerig P, Cowey A: Blindsight in man and monkey. *Brain* 1997; 120:535–559.

94. Tiliket C, Ventre-Dominey J, Vighetto A, Grochowicki M: Room tilt illusion: A central otolith dysfunction. *Arch Neurol* 1996; 53:1259–1264.

95. Tootell RB, Mendola JD, Hadjikhani NK, et al: Functional analysis of V3A and related areas in human visual cortex. *J Neurosci* 1997; 17:7060–7078.

96. Tootell RB, Reppas JB, Kwong KK, et al: Functional analysis of human MT and related visual cortical areas using magnetic resonance imaging. *J Neurosci* 1995; 15:3215–3230.

97. Tootell RB, Taylor JB: Anatomical evidence for MT and additional cortical visual areas in humans. *Cereb Cortex* 1995; 5:39–55.

98. Torjussen T: Residual function in cortically blind hemifields. *Scand J Psychol* 1976; 17:320–323.

99. Ungerleider LG, Brody BA: Extrapersonal spatial orientation: The role of posterior parietal, anterior frontal, and inferotemporal cortex. *Exp Neurol* 1977; 56:265–280.

100. Ungerleider LG, Desimone R: Cortical connections of visual area MT in the macaque. *J Comp Neurol* 1986; 248:190–222.

101. Ungerleider LG, Mishkin M: Two cortical visual systems. In Ingle DJ, Goodale MA, Mansfield RJW (eds): *Analysis of Visual Behaviour.* Cambridge, MIT Press, 1982, pp 549–586.

102. Vaina LM: Selective impairment of visual motion interpretation following lesions of the right occipito-parietal area in humans. *Biol Cybern* 1989; 61:347–359.

103. Vuilleumier P, Landis T: Illusory contours and spatial neglect. *Neuroreport* 1998; 9:2481–2484.

104. Wang MY, Chen L: [The Balint syndrome]. *Chung Hua Shen Ching Ching Shen Ko Tsa Chih* 1989; 22:84–85, 126.

105. Watanabe M: [Visual information processing from the retina to the prefrontal cortex]. *Shinrigaku Kenkyu* 1986; 56:365–378.

106. Weiskrantz L: The Ferrier lecture, 1989. Outlooks for blindsight: Explicit methodologies for implicit processes. *Proc R Soc Lond B Biol Sci* 1990; 239:247–278.

107. Weiskrantz L, Warrington EK, Sanders MD, Marshall J: Visual capacity in the hemianopic field following a restricted occipital ablation. *Brain* 1974; 97:709–728.

108. Zappia RJ, Enoch JM, Stamper R, Winkelman JZ, Gay AJ: The Riddoch phenomenon revealed in non-occipital lobe lesions. *Br J Ophthalmol* 1971; 55:416–420.

109. Zeki SM: Representation of central visual fields in prestriate cortex of monkey. *Brain Res* 1969; 14:271–291.

110. Zeki S: A century of cerebral achromatopsia. *Brain* 1990; 113:1721–1777.

111. Zeki S, Ffytche DH: The Riddoch syndrome: Insights into the neurobiology of conscious vision. *Brain* 1998; 121:25–45.

112. Zeki S, Watson JD, Lueck CJ, Friston KJ, Kennard C, Frackowiak RS: A direct demonstration of functional specialization in human visual cortex. *J Neurosci* 1991; 11:641–649.

113. Zihl J: "Blindsight": Improvement of visually guided eye movements by systematic practice in patients with cerebral blindness. *Neuropsychologia* 1980; 18:71–77.

114. Zihl J, von Cramon D, Mai N: Selective disturbance of movement vision after bilateral brain damage. *Brain* 1983; 106:313–340.

III ORIGINS OF SLOW ELECTROPHYSIOLOGICAL COMPONENTS

11 Origin and Significance of the Electro-Oculogram

GEOFFREY B. ARDEN

Discovery and the first analyses

The potential voltage difference that occurs between the cornea and the fundus was discovered by Du Bois Reymond in 1849.[23] He showed that it persisted for long periods in the isolated eye. In 1878, Kühne and Steiner[56] and de Haas[21] measured the voltages after successively removing the cornea, iris, lens, vitreous, and retina. Only when the retinal pigmented epithelium (RPE) had been damaged did the potential vanish, and this localized the source of the current production. Although illumination was known to affect the potential recorded between cornea and fundus,[44] the capillary electrometers that were used in early work were not sufficiently sensitive or stable to analyze the changes in detail. With the advent of electronic amplification, condenser coupling prevented recording the changes caused by light. It was not until the 1940s that Noell[76] was able to employ stable d.c. recording systems and follow the slow changes; he related the c-wave of the electroretinogram (ERG) to the later and still slower responses. He used poisons that selectively damaged the RPE, as demonstrated by histological changes. He found that azide acting on the RPE increased the "standing potential" and the c-wave of the ERG, while iodate, which damaged the RPE selectively, not only caused a fall in the standing potential, but also reduced the azide increase and reduced the c-wave. Faster changes caused by illumination, that is, other components of the electroretinogram, were less affected.

Development of current fields round the eyes

The RPE consists of a layer of cells connected by tight junctions, so the resistance across the layer (the paracellular resistance) is quite high. Therefore, voltage developed across the RPE implies that at its origin, current will flow at each point normally to the surface, and the return paths are through the paracellular resistance. Because the RPE follows the curvature of the globe, the current flow at each point can be split (formally) into three vectors. One is in the optic axis, and two are at other axes at right angles to it, pointing medially or vertically. At the fundus, nearly all the current flows in the radial vector (in the optic axis). At other positions, there will be current vectors flowing in the optic axis, and vectors in the lateral, medial, superior, and inferior directions will also be developed. Because of the approximately hemispherical shape of the eye, nonradial current vectors will approximately cancel. For example, in the nasal part of the RPE, there will be a temporally directed vector, which will cancel with the nasally directed vector from the temporal part of the RPE. Hence, the net current flow will be due to the vector in the optic axis and appears to be a dipole in the optic axis, with the cornea positive and the fundus negative. This explains the name given to the potential recorded across the eye: the corneofundal potential. The current flowing from such a dipole will spread symmetrically in all directions about the optic axis. Therefore, as the eye moves, the voltages that are recorded between relatively distant skin electrodes will vary with the angle of rotation of the eye. This is shown in figure 11.1, which illustrates how the magnitude of the responses to fixed eye movements can be used to measure the magnitude of the current produce by the RPE. This property of the EOG voltage led to attempts to use it for eye movement recordings. However, difficulties were found in calibrating such a system because the apparent magnitude of the dipole was not constant.[12,25,53,73,95,96] It became apparent that one of the factors modifying the voltage was light. The first complete description of the human light-dark sequence was due to Kris,[55] but an analysis of the nature of the response and the recognition of its clinical utility are usually attributed to Arden[2-5] (figure 11.1), who showed that a small reduction in light intensity provoked a decrease in voltage, the dark trough, which was not related to the preceding light level, although the change from dark to light caused a transient rise of voltage (the light peak), the magnitude of which was linearly related to the logarithm of retinal illumination.

The full picture of the d.c. ERG

The full sequence of the voltage changes is shown in figure 11.2. The electroretinographic a- and b-waves occur in about 0.2 s; following this, there is a slower c-wave. These responses are considered in chapters that deal with the electroretinogram. Following this sequence, there is a slow

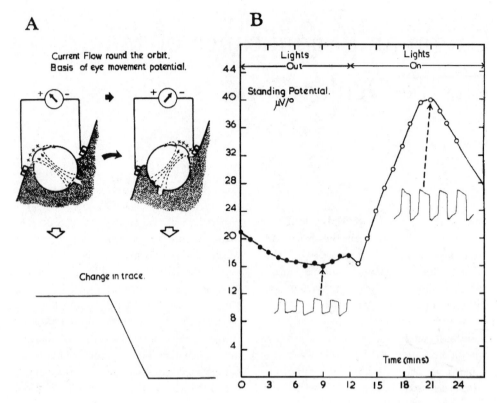

A

Current Flow round the orbit.
Basis of eye movement potential.

Change in trace.

B

FIGURE 11.1 Diagram to show how eye movements elicit an eye movement potential (A) and how the eye movement potential varies in time and with light and darkness in a standard clinical EOG (B). The ratio of minimum to maximum voltage (arrows) is an indicator of RPE function. (Source: Modified from Arden GB,

Barrada A, Kelsey JH: A new clinical test of retinal function based upon the standing potential of the eye. *Br J Opthalmol* 1962; 46:449–467; and Arden GB, Kelsey JH: Changes produced by light in the standing potential of the human eye. *J Physiol* 1962; 161:189–204.)

cornea-negative swing, the after-negativity, followed by a second c-wave and then a still slower and larger increase of voltage, the *light rise*. These changes have been observed in a number of different mammals. There are species differences. In humans, even though light continues, this increase in the corneofundal potential is not maintained but after a peak at 8 minutes sinks to a trough level at 27 minutes. If a light-adapted eye is placed in darkness, the potential falls to a level that is nearly identical to the lowest level reached at the 22 to 24-minute trough. Following this trough, in light or in darkness, further slow rhythmic changes in voltage are seen that may persist for 2 hours or more. The negativity following the c-wave and the slower voltage changes (the dark trough, the light peak, and the light trough) are treated in this chapter as parts of the electro-oculogram.[70]

Membrane mechanisms of the EOG

Since the original description of the human electro-oculogram, work in animals, isolated eyes, and isolated RPE preparations has resulted in a great deal of information about the nature of the ionic channels, cotransporters, and pumps in the apical and basal surfaces of the RPE and how

these are related to the electro-oculogram and to ion and to water movement across the RPE. The pumps in the photoreceptors that maintain the "dark current" slow down in light, but the sodium entry into the outer limbs is reduced more rapidly (see chapters 6 to 8). Therefore, in light, the photoreceptors lose sodium to and gain potassium from the subretinal fluid. The potassium concentration $[K^+]_{out}$ of the subretinal fluid decreases. The voltage across the apical surface of the RPE is determined in large part by the potassium channels and is related to the ratio $[K^+]_{out}/[K^+]_{in}$. Thus, following illumination, the potential across the apical membrane of the RPE temporarily increases, producing a c-wave. (A smaller opposing voltage also occurs across the Müller cell junction in the outer limiting membrane.) This voltage change has the exact timing of the reduction in potassium concentration.[90] Following this, the fast trough of the EOG develops. The mechanism whereby this occurs is thought to be also indirectly caused by the reduction in potassium in the subretinal fluid described above. This reduces the activity of the apical membrane Na, K, 2 Cl cotransporter (see chapter 5). Consequently, intracellular RPE chloride activity decreases. The membrane potential of the basal surface of the RPE is largely controlled by the ratio

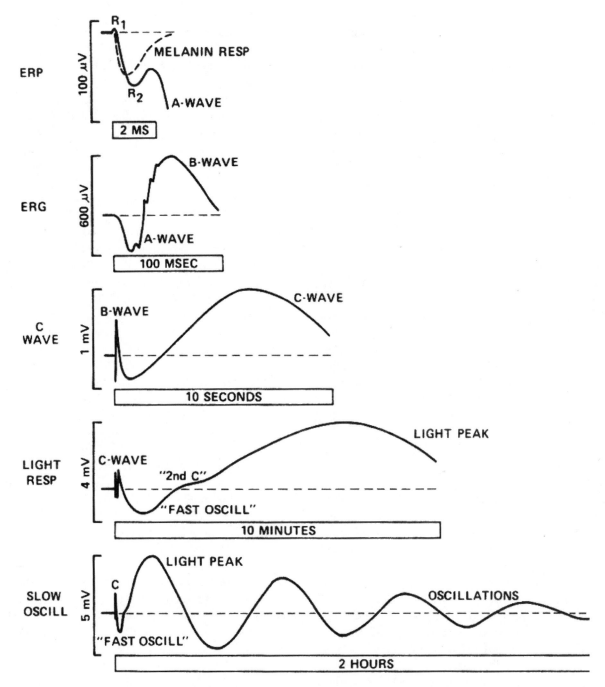

FIGURE 11.2 Time scale of the different electrical voltages produced by retina and RPE, from the most rapid and brief (above) to the slowest (lower). (Source: Modified from Marmor MF, Lurie M: Light induced responses of the retinal pigment epithelium. In Zinn K, Marmor MF (eds): *The Retinal Pigment Epithelium.* Cambridge, MA, Harvard University Press, 1979, pp 226–244.)

of internal to external chloride concentrations, and as a result of the change in activity of the cotransporter, the basal surface of the RPE hyperpolarizes, reducing the transepithelial potential and causing a reduction in the EOG. (The nature of the chloride channels that are involved is discussed below.) The mechanisms mentioned above are an oversimplification because a variety of channels and pumps and cotransporters in the apical membrane contribute to maintaining the constancy of the ionic composition of the subretinal fluid, and there are increases in apical chloride conductances, which tend to depolarize the apical membrane and may contribute to the reduction in the TEP. The after-negativity is of clinical interest because the voltage changes in humans form the basis of another electrooculographic test, the "fast oscillation" (see below).

The slower rise in the transepithelial potential in animal preparations is related to the light rise in the human EOG. It is caused by a depolarization of the basal membrane of the RPE, so the net difference between apical and basal membrane voltages increases. This slow rise must be produced by a second messenger within the cytosol of the RPE. Therefore, for the light rise, the entire sequence must be that the retina liberates a light substance that, binding to receptors in the apical membrane of the RPE, liberates an internal second messenger. The second messenger causes the increase in basal chloride conductance. The most notable contributions are by Steinberg, Miller, Oakley, and other collaborators.[13,27,29–31,33,35,47,49,64,65,77] The nature of the second messenger has not yet been identified. The light substance must diffuse through the subretinal space to reach the RPE. It must be liberated in the outer retina, presumably mostly by photoreceptors, because the action of the light substance is limited. Only when relatively large regions of retina are illuminated does the messenger cause any local change in basal conductance. Presumably with small spots of light, the light substance diffuses from its point of origin so rapidly that the concentration at the RPE does not rise. The receptors on the apical RPE membrane that are satisfied by the light substance are unknown. However, a variety of substances—epinephrine, dopamine, and melatonin—have been shown to indirectly affect the basal chloride conductance.[26] They are presumably related to the two major pathways[20,22,32] that cause the liberation of intracellular second messengers. How these second messengers interact with the basal chloride conductance is unknown, but recent work on alcohol suggests that some intermediate mechanism in the RPE determines the time course of the increase in the TEP.

In animal experiments, two classes of basal RPE membrane chloride conductance can be distinguished. The slow change in voltage that corresponds to the light rise does not occur if the posterior surface of the RPE is exposed to 4,4′-diisoethylcyanostilbene-2,2′disulphonate (DIDS), which inhibits changes in the chloride conductance of a particular type of chloride channel, one that is activated by a Ca^{2+} inward current and related to inositol-1,4,5-triphosphate, Ca^{2+}, and tyrosine kinase mechanisms[92,93] (see chapter 5). The second type of chloride channel is cAMP-sensitive and is determined by the cystic fibrosis transmembrane conductance regulator protein; this is affected, and the fast oscillation is suppressed in such patients with cystic fibrosis, but the light peak remains normal.[13,26,47,49,65,77] How this finding is related to the proposed ionic cause of the fast oscillation has not been explained.

Activation of the second-messenger system involves a generation of Ca^{2+} influx into the cell. The amount of inflowing Ca^{2+} is determined by electrochemical driving forces for Ca^{2+}. Activation of Ca^{2+}-dependent chloride channels hyperpolarizes the cell, leading to increase the driving force for Ca^{2+} into the cell and to larger rises in intracellular free Ca^{2+} as second messenger.[92] While this system can be implicated in chloride transport and other secretory mechanisms, including volume transport from retina to choroid, and regulation of pH, the interactions of RPE membrane mechanisms are complex and help to maintain homeostasis. Changes in the EOG voltage have not been shown to be associated with visual function, and in conditions in which the EOG response to light is abnormal, visual function may be unimpaired, so over several minutes, changes in the composition of the subretinal fluid do not seem to affect the signals that are produced by rods.

Physiological characteristics and pharmacology

The pharmacology of the d.c. potential, its relation to neurotransmitters, and its reliance on changes in metabolism have been investigated by several authors. The slow light peak is extremely sensitive to anoxia,[54,63,66,91] as is shown in figure 11.3, in distinction to the earlier neuronal ERG components, and this was early noted in clinic cases in which retinal blood flow was reduced.[3–5,78] Small changes in pH and pCO_2 also dramatically reduce the slow potentials. In view of the complex acid-base regulatory systems that have been described, it is not surprising that carbon dioxide and acidification exert differential affects.[18,75]

Acetazolamide[51,67] and changes in osmolarity[52,68] cause a slow reduction in the EOG voltages, and these findings are the basis on which clinical tests have been developed (see below). In addition, the potentials are influenced by biogenic amines and other substances.[14,19,48] In particular, the RPE is extremely sensitive to epinephrine in nanomolar concentration,[62] suggesting that there are specific receptors on the apical RPE surface for this substance. Although this is interesting in the search for the "light substance," no recent work has progressed to its conclusive identification. Recently, it has been shown that ethyl alcohol affects the human corneo-

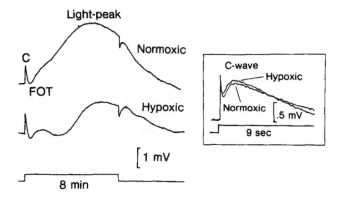

FIGURE 11.3 The light peak (on the left) is greatly reduced by hypoxia, while the electrical responses of the retina, the c-wave labeled, on the left, and the b and c-waves (inset at a faster time scale) are relatively unaffected. (Source: Modified from Gallemore R, Griff E, Steinberg RH: Evidence in support of a photoreceptoral origin for the "light peak substance." *Invest Ophthalmol Vis Sci* 1988; 29:566–571; and Linsenmeier RA, Steinberg RH: Mechanisms of hypoxic effects on the cat DC electroretinogram. *Invest Ophthalmol Vis Sci* 1986; 27:1385–1394.)

fundal potential,[6,7,9,86,105] also at very low dosage. Nonsteroidal anti-inflamatory drugs alter the TEP in isolated preparations,[14] and in doses higher than clinically advisable, they also affect the human EOG (Arden, unpublished).

Clinical tests utilizing the RPE potential

TECHNICAL DETAILS An ISCEV standard appended to this book gives recommendations for standard clinical tests.

The eye movement potential is easily recorded with skin electrodes placed one on either side of the eye (see chapter 19 for comments on electrodes). The voltage varies considerably depending on how close the electrodes are placed to the eye, but 12–30 μV per degree is usual. Rapid saccadic eye movements may be made over 30°, so the voltage change that is recorded for such eye movements is ~1 mV. This relatively large signal makes the EOG test technically undemanding. Eye movements greater than 30° are not desirable because they tend to be carried out in two jumps and determination of the voltage is difficult or impossible. Horizontal eye movements should be made because otherwise, artifactual voltages associated with lid elevation may also be recorded. Direct recording of the d.c. voltage between the two electrodes is possible, but changes in polarization of the electrodes and slow changes in skin potentials occur, and interpretation of such slow voltage changes without eye movement is impossible in clinical conditions. With a.c.-coupled amplifiers recording eye movement voltages, any type of surface electrode can be used, including disposable silver–silver chloride pads or gold cup electrodes. It is desirable to lightly abrade the skin on which the electrodes are

placed to reduce contact resistance below 5000 ohms. The epidermal layers at the lateral fornix are very delicate. The eye movements can be made in any way that is convenient. Some workers have advocated that the subject be given two (red) fixation points and asked to look left and right between them at any convenient rate. Other workers expose only one fixation point at a time and alternate the fixation points at a suitable rate, which should be constant throughout the test. (Various subjects are most comfortable between one and two eye movements per second.) More elaborate schemes have been proposed. For example, a number of closely spaced fixation points have been used, lit sequentially, and the subject is asked to follow the moving spot. The fixation points are so spaced that the angle of gaze varies sinusoidally with time. The amplitude of the voltage change can be determined precisely by a suitable software package (Fourier analyzer). In the author's experience, the simplest method is preferable.

TECHNICAL DIFFICULTIES Technical problems are very rare with the EOG. In a very few cases, patients may find it difficult to make standard eye movements. These include cases of ophthalmoplegia or nystagmus (muscle paralyses, Parkinsonism, myasthenia). In certain of these cases, the patient may attempt to compensate by moving the head, not the eye. Such problems can usually be overcome by providing a solid, comfortable head rest and encouraging the patient to relax the neck muscles.

When the patient is first instructed how to do the test, the tester should always observe the patient to make sure that satisfactory eye movements are made. In addition, some patients' saccades may undershoot or overshoot, giving spuriously large or small responses. These can be dealt with by averaging (see below) if the subject's eye movements remain constant throughout the test period. One condition in which this may not be the case is when there is local central or peripheral disease that makes it difficult for the patient to visualize the fixation points. They may be easy to see in darkness but become invisible against a brightly illuminated background. When dedicated illuminators are used, a larger opaque black area should surround the fixation points. In some patients with very poor vision, it may be necessary to make extreme eye movements if the fixation targets cannot be seen. It has been suggested that in such cases, constant eye movements can be made with the aid of proprioception. The patient can be seated in a chair with arms, on which the elbows can rest, and the forearms are placed vertically. The patient is encouraged to move his or her eyes toward the position of one thumb and then toward the other.

Finally, if the eye movements displace the electrodes, an artifactual voltage can be recorded. These rapid deflections at the beginning or ending of saccades are easily seen (see the ISCEV standard) but should be absent in clinical circumstances with an ordinarily competent electrode technique. They may be disturbing when passive rotations of the eye are induced to obtain EOGs in small animals. With blocking capacitors in the input amplifier giving a time constant (high-pass filter) of 0.3 s, alternating saccades give a sawtooth response. Measurement of the peak-to-peak amplitude of the sawtooth is easy, and many software packages allow horizontal cursors to be adjusted through the average peak or trough voltages, disregarding any artifactual voltage or incomplete movements that may occur.

All subjects can continue making eye movements for about 10 s, at 1-minute intervals, without fatigue or discomfort. The record derived from such recordings is completely suitable for experimental work. In clinical situations, it is common either to make records at 2-minute intervals or to make only a few measurements (e.g., with totally blind patients). The aim is to determine the lowest level to which the voltage sinks in darkness (the dark trough) and the peak in subsequent illumination (the light peak). For further detail, consult the ISCEV standard. The magnitude of the ratio of these voltages gives an index of the change in RPE voltage, which is the result of the test. However, it is desirable to provide more detail, and various schemes have been proposed to provide standard traces without the need for measurement and graph drawing. Often, records are made on a very slow chart recorder (or its virtual equivalent) so that the individual eye movements merge; the average excursion during the 10 seconds or so of eye movement during each minute can be visualized as a thick line, and a graph of 20 or more consecutive lines shows the slow change in waveform.

In clinical tests, it is important to specify the degree of dark adaptation and the intensity of the subsequent light adaptation. Some workers advocate a prolonged pretest period during which, in constant dim illumination, the voltage becomes steady. This is desirable but adds to the duration of the test and is not commonly employed. After this, the subject is put in complete darkness for 10–12 minutes. This is sufficient time to produce a dark trough. The time in the dark should be fixed, because when the light is turned on, there is a relationship between the dark period and the size of the subsequent rise. Although the maximum rise is not achieved with less than 22 minutes of dark adaptation, the development of the light rise is much faster and approximately exponential, relating to the regeneration of rhodopsin, and after 12 minutes, the subsequent rise is greater than 90% maximal.[5] The response is derived from the entire retina, and therefore a Ganzfeld illumination with white light is required. Ganzfeld bowls are recommended, but (especially in view of the eye movements) ad hoc large-field viewing (e.g., diffusely and evenly illuminated white walls floor and ceiling) may suffice. It is important to adjust illumination to compensate for individual variation and individual change in pupil size with illumination. Two alternatives are available. If a very bright light is to be used, then saturated responses are obtained, and changes in pupillary diameter compensate for any change in illumination. Alternatively, the pupils may be dilated and the illumination may be reduced to obtain a standard retinal illumination.

Even though much information is available from various manufacturers, it is desirable to establish clinic normal values of the light peak/dark trough ratio. For most centers, the mean value will be 2.2 (220%), and the lower limit of normal will be 1.8. There is some evidence that very large values (more than 3) are indicative of abnormality.

"CLASSIC EOG" DESCRIPTION The patient is prepared in dim lighting. The test begins with a reduction of light intensity to zero. After 12 minutes, the full illumination is turned on. Recording continues for more than 8 minutes, until the light peak is past. Measurements are made of the dark trough voltage, the light peak voltage, and the time to the peak, which should not be greater than 9 minutes.

"FAST OSCILLATION" DESCRIPTION The patients makes nearly continuous eye movements (at a reduced rate or for the last 15 s of every minute). The illumination is turned on and off every 60 s. Six or more cycles are recorded (figure 11.4). Measurements are taken of eye movement voltages in the last 10 s of recording in each minute, and average values of dark and light voltages are computed.

VARIANTS: STEADY STATE The patient is maintained in dim illumination until the voltage appears to be constant. The full light intensity is turned on until a light peak and subsequent trough can be seen. The baseline and light peak voltage are measured, as is the time to the light peak. The later light trough voltage and time of light trough are not usually measured in this form of the test.

Nonphotic responses

HYPEROSMOLARITY, ACETAZOLAMIDE, AND BICARBONATE TESTS In these tests, after a period of recording during which a stable baseline is established, a chemical is infused intravenously. It is advisable to set up a venous line before the test begins and to incorporate a two-way tap in the line so that normal saline can be infused during the pretest period and the change in infusion can be made without the subject's knowledge. Otherwise, changes of recorded voltage due to anxiety may affect the test.

Recording continues until the decrease in the voltage reaches a lower level. With acetazolamide[51,57] and bicarbonate,[28,83,84] the infusion causes a reduction in EOG voltage until a trough is reached after 8–10 minutes (figure 11.5). With hyperosmolar solutions, a rather slower fall occurs.[28,68,69] Following the trough, the potential may increase slightly if the infusion continues.

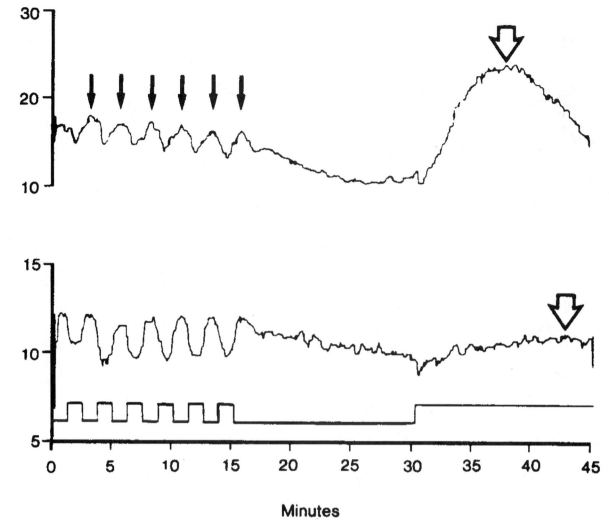
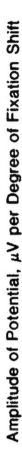

FIGURE 11.4 Recordings of the fast oscillation and the light rise of the EOG, in the normal (top), and in a patient with Best's disease (bottom). The smaller solid arrows point to the FO's (note that light causes a decrease in voltage). The open broad arrows point to the peak of the light rise, which in Best's in nearly absent. (Source: Modified from Weleber RG: Fast and slow oscillations of the electro-oculogram in Best's macular degeneration and retinitis pigmentosa. *Arch Ophthalmol* 1989; 107:530–537.)

The quantity of acetazolamide that is recommended is 8–10 mg/kg, given by slow intravenous infusion in a period of 1 minute. Hyperosmolar solutions that are used consist of 0.9% normal saline with 25% weight/volume (w/v) mannose added or 15% mannose plus 10% fructose (1400 mOsmolar). The aim is to increase tissue osmolality by 15–20 mOsm. In the bicarbonate test, 0.9% saline, to which sodium bicarbonate 7% w/v has been added, is infused at the rate of 0.83 mg/kg per minute. Alcohol can also be infused intravenously (see below). In the author's experiments, 4 g, 10% volume/volume (v/v) in 0.9% saline, can be given in a period of 25 seconds. The use of several agents can be combined in a sequence to reduce the number of tests.[28,36,37,59,68,80,85,104]

MECHANISMS AND USEFULNESS During the hyperosmolarity trough, the light rise is abolished. However, following admin-istration of acetazolamide, the light rise is unaffected (figure 11.6), so the two tests must provoke different retinal-RPE mechanisms.[37,69] Although experimental work on isolated epithelia has indicated that the hyperpolarization of the basal membrane may account for the decrease in voltage associated with these agents, the precise mode of action is unknown, so any abnormality that is detected is merely phe-nomenological. The light EOG test depends on the integrity of the retina, the subretinal space, and the retinal pigment epithelium, and is thus affected by a wide range of patho-logical processes. The recorded current is generated by large regions of the retina/RPE and is often normal when localized lesions develop.[37] These factors decrease the value of the test. It was hoped that the sensitivity of the test to widespread pathologies could make it useful as a screening test, but other clinical methods (e.g., fundoscopy, angiogra-phy, electroretinography, and field testing) provide more

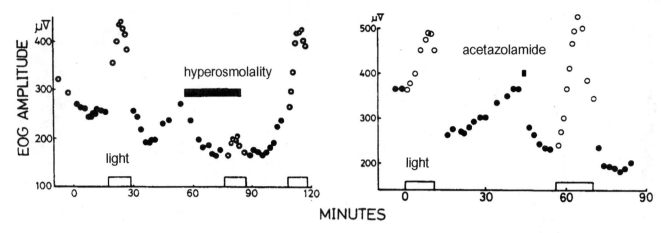

FIGURE 11.5 The reductions in the EOG voltage caused by hyperosmolality and acetazolamide. The light peak is unaffected by these agents. (Source: Modified from Kawasaki K, Yonemura D, Madachi-Yamamoto S: Hyperosmolarity response of ocular standing potential as a clinical test for retinal pigment epithelial activity. *Doc Ophthalmol* 1984; 58:375–384.

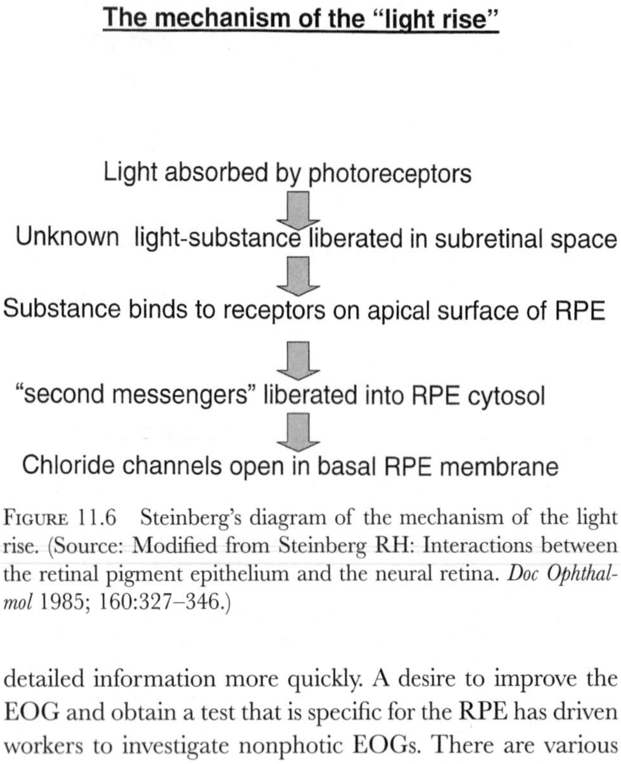

The mechanism of the "light rise"

Light absorbed by photoreceptors

⇩

Unknown light-substance liberated in subretinal space

⇩

Substance binds to receptors on apical surface of RPE

⇩

"second messengers" liberated into RPE cytosol

⇩

Chloride channels open in basal RPE membrane

FIGURE 11.6 Steinberg's diagram of the mechanism of the light rise. (Source: Modified from Steinberg RH: Interactions between the retinal pigment epithelium and the neural retina. *Doc Ophthalmol* 1985; 160:327–346.)

detailed information more quickly. A desire to improve the EOG and obtain a test that is specific for the RPE has driven workers to investigate nonphotic EOGs. There are various reported differences between the light EOG and the chemically induced changes. Some are of interest in terms of pathology. In Best's disease, the light-EOG is "flat," but the acetazolamide response continues normally[37,68,104] (see figure 11.4). Since acetazolamide affects carbonic anhydrase in the RPE and can enter via the choroidal circulation, this lends some support to the mechanism that has been proposed for the light EOG. It has been found in small series that the abnormality that is shown by these agents may be more severe in cases of retinal degenerations (particularly X-linked heterozygotes of RP)[59] than is the case for the ERG

or the light rise. In AMD, the acetazolamide response continues normally until choroidal neovascularization appears.[80] However, in advanced cases of RP, the acetazolamide response is often normal.[28]

The alcohol EOG

In animal experiments and in humans, a rise in the d.c. level occurs after giving alcohol.[6,86] Unlike the other agents that are used to produce nonphotic EOGs, alcohol can be given by mouth. It also has important differences from the results with the chemically provoked changes described above. Only recently has there been a comparison of the nature and time course of the changes caused by light and the change caused by alcohol. After allowing for the time taken for alcohol to pass from the gullet to the capillaries, both light and alcohol appear to provoke exactly the same complex prolonged voltage changes (within the limit of the experimental precision). The first peak, the first trough, and the second peak are all so similar (given the equivalent doses of both agents) that it seems that the responses to both agents must be caused in the same manner and by the same mechanisms; see below (figure 11.7). For low doses, the responses of light and alcohol sum. For high doses, light and alcohol occlude, that is, when both agents are given, the response is only very slightly bigger than when each is given alone. The dose-response curve for the "peak" and "trough" alcohol responses are quite different. The latter requires approximately 20 times less alcohol than the peak. The quantity of alcohol required to produce minimal changes in the EOG is very small indeed: about 12 mg/kg taken orally in a 7% v/v solution. When alcohol is taken by mouth, the blood level rises slowly for about 15 minutes, but the RPE voltage changes are determined by the blood levels in the first few

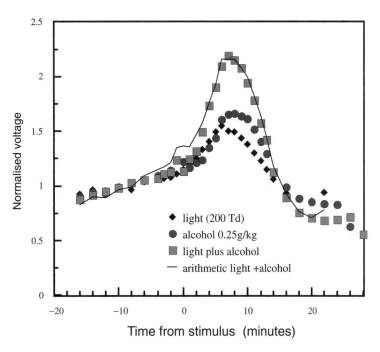

FIGURE 11.7   Addition of responses to weak light and small amounts of alcohol. The responses to both agents sum. (Source: Modified from Arden GB, Wolf JE: The human electro-oculogram: Interaction of light and alcohol. *Invest Ophthalmol Vis Sci* 2000; 41:2722–2729.)

minutes. A standard dose that produces acceptable voltage changes is 220 mg/kg, 20% v/v. With this, the peak blood level never exceeds 80 mg/100 ml, and by the end of the test, it is less than 40 mg/100 ml, a level that is widely considered to be lower than that which reduces motor efficiency and judgment. The effective minimal blood alcohol concentration that causes any voltage change is too small to be measurable with standard tests. This suggests that there is an amplifier between the RPE mechanisms that generate the voltage changes and the mechanisms that detect the changes in the alcohol composition of the tissues. Alcohol is known to act on a variety of tissues, including the central nervous system, and a number of biochemical pathways have been described. Very few experiments on the physiological effects of alcohol have employed such low doses as those that appear effective in the eye. There is at present no proof that the isolated RPE responds to alcohol.

MODELING   In the absence of information about mechanisms, attempts have been made to construct mathematical models that would describe the time course of the EOG changes.[45,97] These treat the changes as a damped oscillation. In view of the descriptions above, which indicate that the early rise and the subsequent fall are produced by different mechanisms, it would be expected that the models would be complex; in fact, a number of free parameters have to be introduced before the model predictions correspond to experimental observations.

INFERENCES FROM HUMAN WORK: DETERMINANTS OF SIZE AND DURATION   Many experiments on human EOGs yield interesting results, but without experimental recordings on isolated tissues, the interpretation has to be the simplest mechanism possible, and there is no guarantee that this is in fact the case. The EOG appears to be dose dependent: There is an approximate linear relationship between the logarithm of retinal illumination and the magnitude of the light peak that extends over 3.5 decadic units. More recently, the same has been observed of the dose dependency of the response to alcohol. A simple explanation is that the "light substance" is liberated in quantities that are related to the light absorptions in photoreceptors and the magnitude of the effect of light or alcohol is governed by the law of mass action. However, there is no proof of this, and the magnitude of the (very similar) voltage response to alcohol is not related to the instantaneous concentration of alcohol in the blood. It is natural to consider that alcohol may liberate the "light rise substance" but this is not so, because the effects of light and alcohol do not interact as they must do if that were to be the case. Figure 11.8 shows that when illumination is increased during the alcohol rise, the voltage produced by light simply sums with the voltage change produced by alcohol. However, for each agent by itself, there is a pronounced effect of prior stimulation. A prior (low) illumination level suppresses the response to a large step increase of illumination (figure 11.9). In addition, the presence of a low concentration of alcohol in the blood prevents

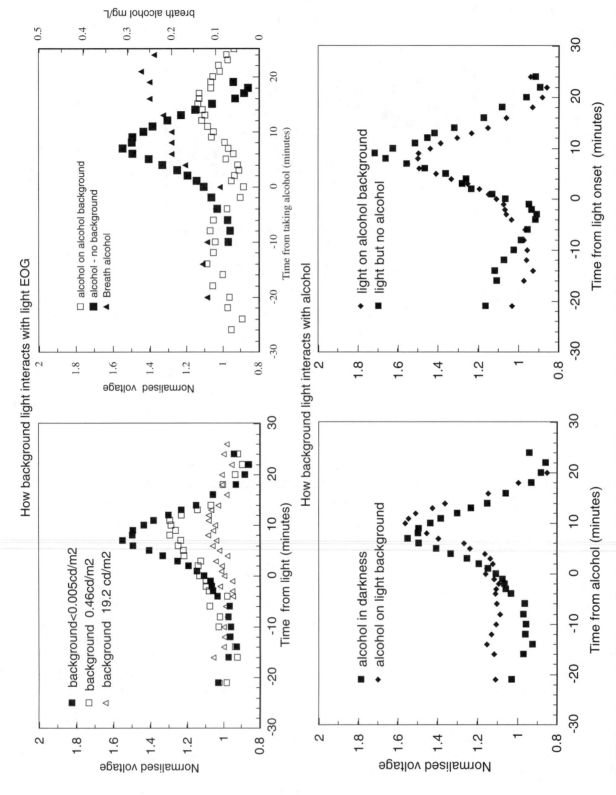

FIGURE 11.8   Weak backgrounds of light greatly reduce the light rise (top left), but the amplitude of the alcohol response is the same in light and in darkness (bottom left). Therefore alcohol cannot act by causing the production of the light rise substance. The boxes on the right show the comparative experiments: the alcohol response is greatly reduced if at the time of ingestion there is any alcohol in the bloodstream, but the response amplitude is the same in darkness and in light.

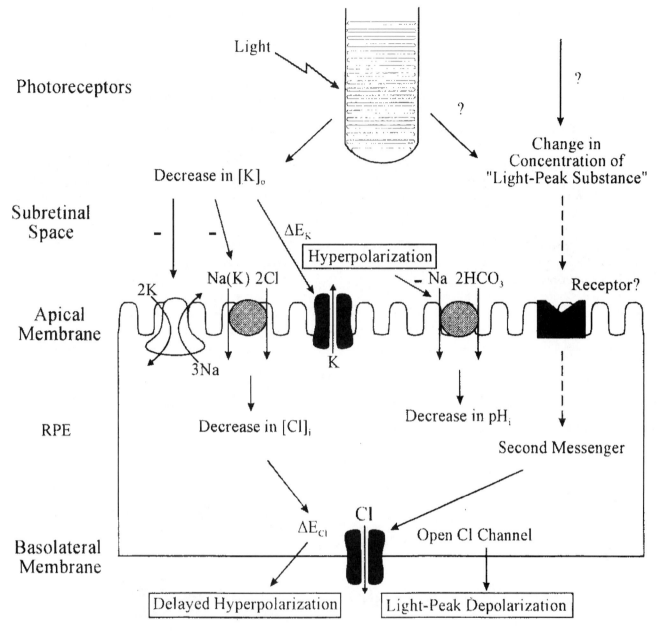

FIGURE 11.9 RPE mechanisms involved in the production of the EOG. For further information see text. Compare to figure 11.6. Alcohol must operate on the internal second messenger in the RPE.

the development of an alcohol rise. However, the alcohol response is scarcely affected by illumination, and the light response is scarcely affected by established blood alcohol concentrations. The time course of the production of the "light rise substance" is unknown, but the very similar prolonged responses that are produced by alcohol can be mimicked by the brief injection of a bolus of alcohol, which rapidly disappears from the circulation. The simplest way of accounting for these findings is that the mechanism that causes the change in potential of the RPE (in this case, the depolarization of the basolateral surface) is a slow intracel-lular generator within the RPE cells, and a trigger mechanism activates the generator. Extracellular change (of the light substance or alcohol) operates the trigger mechanisms, which then rapidly become desensitized. The triggers release two types of second messengers that activate the generator. A mechanism on the RPE apical surface is apparently a receptor for epinephrine, at nanomolar concentration.[49] No such receptor has been demonstrated for alcohol, which is also apparently active at less than micromolar concentration in the RPE or retina.

Clinical utility of EOGs

Although the EOG is a simple test to carry out, all EOGs are lengthy tests, and this limits their clinical utility. Furthermore, while the light EOG is abnormal in a number of conditions (e.g., retinal degenerations, retinal vasculopathies) in which the retina is abnormal, as determined by inspection or electroretinography, these findings do not add to diagnostic efficiency or reveal much about the underlying pathophysiology, because the light rise originates in the retina. The main exception is in Best's disease and its variants, in which the EOG light rise is absent or very much reduced. This occurs in the absence of severe visual or ERG defects and is therefore pathognomonic. The diagnosis of this condition demands carrying out an EOG. The simplest explanation for the abnormality is that in Best's disease, there is a barrier between retina and apical RPE that prevents the penetration of the "light substance" to the apical RPE receptors. The fast oscillation response, which is caused directly by a change in the subretinal potassium concentration, can still affect the RPE.[68] Alcohol responses are present in Best's disease (though maybe delayed), but the alcohol can penetrate from the choroid.

The development of a clinical test involving alcohol raises the possibility of extending the value of electro-oculography. So far, it has been shown that the alcohol response is absent in all cases of retinitis pigmentosa, including (at least some) heterozygotes for X-linked RP (Arden and Wolf, unpublished) (figure 11.10). Since ERGs and fundal appearances in such people are often very nearly normal and very rarely seriously depressed, the results shown in figure 11.10 may be of significant use, especially where genetic screens may not be available. It may also have some bearing on pathogenesis. Patch-clamp studies show that L-type calcium channels in the RPE (see chapter 5) are abnormal in at least one rat dystrophy, carrying three times the normal current. The relationships of conductance to protein tyrosine kinase and protein kinase C agonists and blockers are also abnormal, suggesting additional calcium channels. The importance of the calcium channel is that it is concerned both in phagocytosis and in $[Ca^{2+}]_{in}$ regulation and thus the operation the second messenger systems that open the chloride channels

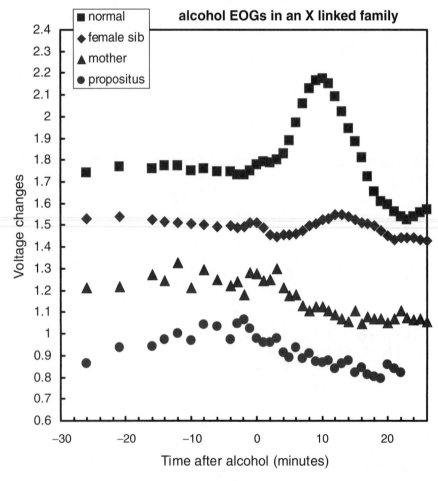

FIGURE 11.10   Alcohol EOGs in X-linked RP. The response is absent in the propositus, but his mother and sister, although having almost normal retinal function, have grossly abnormal alcohol EOGs.

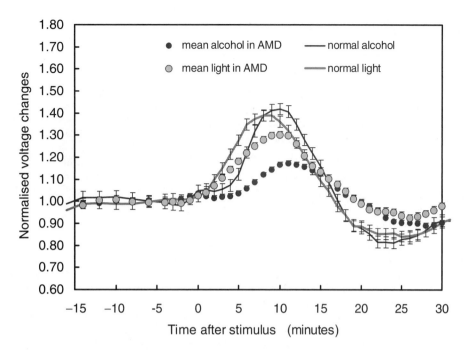

FIGURE 11.11 EOGs evoked by light and by alcohol in normal subjects, and by age-matched patients with age-related macular degeneration. The standard errors are shown for every data point. Those for the patients are as small as the symbols. Note that although the RPE responses are all abnormal the alcohol EOG is clearly more affected. (Source: Modified from Arden GB, Wolf JE: Differential effects of light and alcohol on the electro-oculographic responses of patients with age-related macular disease. *Invest Ophthalmol Vis Sci* 2003 44:3226–3332.)

in the basal surface of the RPE. This finding suggests that an alteration in RPE function occurs in retinal degenerations and may contribute to them.[72,94,101] The alcohol EOG is also abnormal in age-related maculopathy, whereas the light EOG test is much less affected[8] (see figure 11.11). (However, see Ref. 103.) Hyperosmolarity EOGs also show abnormality in choroidal neovascular disease but not in AMD without neovascularization.[85] It has been suggested that the alcohol abnormality in ARM may be the result of a barrier between the RPE and the choroid that prevents entry of alcohol to the sites where it can affect the RPE. This may be of significance in the pathology of ARM but has little diagnostic possibility, even though early cases of ARM show reduction and delay in the alcohol peak, unless there is a direct and simple relationship between the degree of alcohol EOG abnormality and the severity of ARM.

Clinical findings of general interest in the last 10 years

Apart from the matters discussed above, 273 papers on the EOG have been published since 1993, according to Medline. Most of these relate to findings in series of patients with varying pathologies, in which the EOG was part of a battery of diagnostic tests given to all patients. There are, however, some current issues relating to the EOG.

Vigabatrin retinopathy has been reported to cause a considerable change to the EOG in many patients, and this is taken as evidence that this drug can alter RPE function.[11,16,39–42] The frequency of abnormality is greater than that of the ERG and is much less in patients on Vigabatrin who do not have field defects. If field defects reverse, the EOG abnormality may remain. However, cases have been reported with normal EOGs, and the value of carrying out EOGs in patients under treatment remains undetermined.

It has been reported that malignant melanomata of the posterior uveal tract cause abnormalities in the EOG,[15] and in a large multicenter study, this finding was claimed to be of use in distinguishing between naevi, other forms of retinal detachment, and metastasis into the eye.[88–89] However, malignant choroidal melanomata have been observed with normal EOGs.[71] The EOG has been reported as abnormal in cases of Desferrioxamine toxicity,[38] which is not surprising in view of the effect in reducing the rate of dark adaptation.[1] However, other methods of assessing toxicity have been reported.[10,17] A number of authors have emphasized the utility of the EOG in experimental studies involving the genotyping of various retinal degenerations (especially the carrier states of these conditions), from retinitis pigmentosa, Usher's syndrome, Best's disease, helicoidal peripapillary chorioretinal degeneration, neuronal ceroid lipofuscinosis, senior syndrome, choroideremia, and butterfly dystrophy. Abnormalities have been reported in multiple evanescent white dot syndrome and in immunodeficiency syndromes.[24,34,36,43,46,50,57,60,74,79–82,89,100,102] It has been reported that in some cases of pigmentary disturbance or in degenerations with symptoms occurring delayed to late in life, EOG disturbances are more frequent and profound than are ERG disturbances.[24] It has been shown that the fast oscillation is abnormal (although the ordinary light-evoked EOG is unaffected) in patients with cystic fibrosis and determined abnormalities in the CFTR, a cAMP-dependent membrane chloride channel.[58] Finally, it has been reported that the EOG was abnormal in a person who had been struck by lightning.[61]

REFERENCES

1. Arden GB: Desferrioxamine administered intravenously by infusion causes a reduction in the electroretinogram in rabbits anaesthetized with urethane. *Hum Toxicol* 1986; 5:229–236.

2. Arden GB, Barrada A: An analysis of the electrooculograms of a series of normal subjects. *Br J Ophthalmol* 1962; 46:468–482.

3. Arden GB, Barrada A, Kelsey JH: A new clinical test of retinal function based upon the standing potential of the eye. *Br J Ophthalmol* 1962; 46:449–467.

4. Arden GB, Kelsey JH: Changes produced by light in the standing potential of the human eye. *J Physiol* 1962; 161:189–204.

5. Arden GB, Kelsey JH: Some observations on the relationship between the standing potential of the human eye and the bleaching and regeneration of visual purple. *J Physiol* 1962; 161:205–226.

6. Arden GB, Wolf JE: The human electro-oculogram: Interaction of light and alcohol. *Invest Ophthalmol Vis Sci* 2000; 41:2722–2729.

7. Arden GB, Wolf JE: The electro-oculographic responses to alcohol and light in a series of patients with retinitis pigmentosa. *Invest Ophthalmol Visl Sci* 2000; 41:2730–2734.

8. Arden GB, Wolf JE: Differential effects of light and alcohol on the electro-oculographic responses of patients with age-related macular disease. *Invest Ophthalmol Vis Sci* 2003 44:3226–3332.

9. Arden GB, Wolf JE, Singbartl F, Berninger TE, Rudolph G, Kampik A: Effect of alcohol and light on the retinal pigment epithelium of normal subjects and patients with retinal dystrophies. *Br J Ophthalmol* 2000; 84:881–883.

10. Arden GB, Wonke B, Kennedy C, Huehns ER: Ocular changes in patients undergoing long-term desferrioxamine treatment. *Br J Ophthalmol* 1984; 68:873–877.

11. Arndt CF, Derambure P, Defoort-Dhellemmes S, Hache JC: Outer retinal dysfunction in patients treated with vigabatrin. *Neurology* 1999 12; 52:1201–1205.

12. Aserinsky E: Effect of illumination and sleep on the amplitude of the electrooculogram. *Arch Opthalmol* 1955; 53:542–546.

13. Bialek S, Joseph DP, Miller SS: The delayed basolateral membrane hyperpolarization of the bovine retinal pigment epithelium: mechanism of generation. *J Physiol* 1995; 484:53–67.

14. Bialek S, Quong JN, Yu K, Miller SS: Nonsteroidal anti-inflammatory drugs alter chloride and fluid transport in bovine retinal pigment epithelium. *Am J Physiol* 1996; 270:C1175–1189.

15. Brink HM, Pinckers AJ, Verbeek AM: The electro-oculogram in uveal melanoma: A prospective study. *Doc Ophthalmol* 1990; 75:329–334.

16. Coupland SG, Zackon DH, Leonard BC, Ross TM: Vigabatrin effect on inner retinal function. *Ophthalmology* 2001; 108:1493–1496; discussion 1497–1498.

17. Davies SC, Marcus RE, Hungerford JL, Miller MH, Arden GB, Huehns ER: Ocular toxicity of high-dose intravenous desferrioxamine. *Lancet* 1983; 23;2(#8343):181–184.

18. Dawis S, Hoffman H, Niemeyer G: The electroretinogram, standing potential and light peak of the perfused cat eye during acid–base changes. *Vision Res* 1985; 25:1163–1177.

19. Dawis SM, Neimeyer G: Dopamine influences the light peak in the perfused mammalian eye. *Invest Ophthalmol Vis Sci* 1984; 27:330–335.

20. De Camilli P, Emr SD, McPherson PS, Novick P: Phosphoinositides as regulators in membrane traffic. *Science* 1996; 271:1533–1539.

21. De Haas HK: Lichtprikkelsen retinastroomen in hun quantitatief Verbund. (dissertation), University of Leiden, 1903. Quoted by Kohlrausch A Electriches Erscheinungen in Auge. In *Handbuch der normalen und pathologischen Physiologie*. Vol 12. Berlin, Springer Verlag, 1931, pp 1394–1426.

22. Delmas P, Brown DA: Junctional signaling microdomains: bridging the gap between the neuronal cell surface and Ca^{2+} stores. *Neuron* 2002; 36:787–790.

23. Du Bois Reymond E: *Untersuchungen über dei thierische Electricität*. Vol II. Berlin, Reimer Ged, 1849.

24. Eysteinsson T, Jonasson F, Jonsson V, Bird AC: Helicoidal peripapillary chorioretinal degeneration: Electrophysiology and psychophysics in 17 patients. *Br J Ophthalmol* 1998; 82:280–285.

25. Francois J, Verriest G, De Rouck A: Modification of the amplitude of the human electrooculogram by light and dark adaptation. *Brit J Ophthalmol* 1955; 39:398–408.

26. Gallemore RP, Hughes BA, Miller SS: Light induced responses in the retinal pigment epithelium. In Marmor MF, Wolfensberger TJ (eds): *The Retinal Pigment Epithelium*. OUP, 1998, pp 175–198.

27. Gallemore R, Griff E, Steinberg RH: Evidence in support of a photoreceptoral origin for the "light peak substance." *Invest Ophthalmol Vis Sci* 1988; 29:566–571.

28. Gallemore RP, Maruiwa F, Marmor MF: Clinical electrophysiology of the retinal pigment epithelium. In Marmor MF, Wolfensburger TJ (eds): *The Retinal Pigment Epithelium*. OUP, 1998, pp 199–223.

29. Gallemore R, Steinberg RH: Effect of DIDS on the chick retinal pigment epithelium: I. Membrane potentials apparent resistance and mechanisms. *J Neurosci* 1989; 9:1968–1976.

30. Gallemore R, Steinberg RH: The light peak of the DC ERG is associated with an increase in Cl⁻ conductance in chick RPE. *Invest Ophthalmol Vis Sci* 1991; 32:837.

31. Gallemore R, Steinberg RH: Light-evoked modulation of basolateral Cl⁻ conductance in chick retinal pigment epithelium: The light peak and fast oscillation. *J Neurophysiol* 1993; 70:1656–1668.

32. Goni FM, Alonso A: Structure and functional properties of diacylglycerols in membranes. *Prog Lipid Res* 1999; 38:1–48.

33. Griff E, Steinberg RH: Origin of the Light Peak: In vitro study of Gekko gecko. *J Physiol (Lond)* 1982; 331:637–652.

34. Greenstein VC, Seiple W, Liebmann J, Ritch R: Retinal pigment epithelial dysfunction in patients with pigment dis-

person syndrome: Implications for the theory of pathogenesis. *Arch Ophthalmol* 2001; 119:1291–1295.

35. Griff E, Steinberg RH: Changes in apical $[K^+]_o$ produce delayed basal membrane responses of the retinal pigment epithelium in the gekko. *J Gen Physiol* 1984; 83:193–211.

36. Gupta LY, Marmor MF: Sequential recordings of photic and nonphotic electro-oculographic responses in patients with extensive extramacular drusen. *Doc Ophthalmol* 1994; 88:46–55.

37. Gupta LY, Marmor MF: Electrophysiology of the retinal pigment epithelium in central serous chorioretinopathy. *Doc Ophthalmol* 1995–1996; 91:101–107.

38. Haimovici R, D'Amico DJ, Gragoudas ES, Sokol S: The expanded clinical spectrum of deferoxamine retinopathy. *Ophthalmology* 2002; 109:164–171.

39. Harding GF, Robertson K, Spencer EL, Holliday I: Vigabatrin: Its effect on the electrophysiology of vision. *Doc Ophthalmol* 2002; 104:213–229.

40. Harding GF, Wild JM, Robertson KA, Lawden MC, Betts TA, Barber C, Barnes PM: Electro-oculography, electroretinography, visual evoked potentials, and multifocal electroretinography in patients with vigabatrin-attributed visual field constriction. *Epilepsia* 2000; 41:1420–1431.

41. Harding GF, Wild JM, Robertson KA, Rietbrock S, Martinez C: Separating the retinal electrophysiologic effects of vigabatrin: treatment versus field loss. *Neurology* 2000; 55:347–352.

42. Hardus P, Verduin WM, Berendschot TT, Kamermans M, Postma G, Stilma JS, van Veelen CW: The value of electrophysiology results in patients with epilepsy and vigabatrin associated visual field loss. *Acta Ophthalmol Scand* 2001; 79:169–174.

43. Harrison JM, van Heuven WA: Retinal pigment epithelial dysfunction in human immunodeficiency virus-infected patients with cytomegalovirus retinitis. *Ophthalmology* 1999; 106:790–797.

44. Himstedt F, Nagel WA: Fest.d. Univ Freiburg z 50jahr.Reg-Jubil. SR. Kgl Hocheit dl.l Grosshertzogs Freidrich von Baden. 1092, pp 262–263. Quoted by Kohlrausch A Electriches Erscheinungen in Auge. In *Handbuch der normalen und pathologischen Physiologie*. Vol 12. Berlin, Springer Verlag, 1931, pp 1394–1426.

45. Homer LD, Kolder HEJW: Mathematical model of oscillations of the human corneoretinal potential. *Pflug Arch* 1966; 287:197–202.

46. Jarc-Vidmar M, Popovic P, Hawlina M, Brecelj J: Pattern ERG and psychophysical functions in Best's disease. *Doc Ophthalmol* 2001; 103:47–61.

47. Joseph D, Miller S: Apical and basal membrane ion transport mechanisms in bovine retinal pigment epithelium. *J Physiol (Lond)* 1991; 435:439–463.

48. Joseph D, Miller S: Alpha-1-adrenergic modulation of K and Cl transport in bovine retinal pigment epithelium. *J Gen Physiol* 1991; 99:269–301.

49. Joseph D, Miller S: Alpha-1-Adrenergic modulation of K and Cl transport in bovine retinal pigment epithelium. *J Gen Physiol* 1992; 99:263–290.

50. Jurklies B, Weismann M, Kellner U, Zrenner E, Bornfeld N: Clinical findings in autosomal recessive syndrome of blue cone hypersensitivity. *Ophthalmologe* 2001; 98:285–293.

51. Kawasaki K, Mukoh S, Yonemura D, Fujii S, Segawa Y: Acetazolamide-induced changes in the membrane potentials of the retinal pigment epithelium. *Doc Ophthalmol* 1986; 63:375–381.

52. Kawasaki K, Yonemura D, Madachi-Yamamoto S: Hyperosmolarity response of ocular standing potential as a clinical test for retinal pigment epithelial activity. *Doc Ophthalmol* 1984; 58:375–384.

53. Kolder H: Spontane und experimentelle Anderungen des Bestandspotenzials der menschlichen Auges. *Pflugers Arch Gesamt Physiol* 1959; 268:258–272.

54. Kreinbuhl B, Neimeyer G: Standing potential and c-wave during changes in pO_2 and flow in the perfused cat's eye. *Doc Ophthalmol* 1985; 60:353–360.

55. Kris C: Corneo-fundal potential variations during light and dark adaptation. *Nature* 1958; 182:1027–1028.

56. Kuhne W, Steiner J: Über electrische Vorgange im Sehorgane. *Untersuch der Universität Heidelberg* 1881; 4:64–160.

57. Lafaut BA, Loeys B, Leroy BP, Spileers W, De Laey JJ, Kestelyn P: Clinical and electrophysiological findings in autosomal dominant vitreoretinochoroidopathy: report of a new pedigree. *Graefes Arch Clin Exp Ophthalmol* 2001; 239:575–582.

58. Lara WC, Jordan BL, Hope GM, Dawson WW, Foster RA, Kaushal S: Fast oscillation of the electro-oculogram in cystic fibrosis. 2003; ARVO abst.

59. Leon JA, Arden GB, Bird AC: The standing potential in Best's macular dystrophy: Baseline and drug induced responses. *Invest Ophthalmol Vis Sci* 1990; 31 (supp):497.

60. Lim JI, Kokame GT, Douglas JP: Multiple evanescent white dot syndrome in older patients. *Am J Ophthalmol* 1999; 127:725–728.

61. Lin CJ, Yang CH, Yang CM, Chang KP: Abnormal electroretinogram and abnormal electrooculogram after lightning-induced ocular injury. *Am J Ophthalmol* 2002; 133:578–579.

62. Lin H, Miller S: Apical epinephrine modulates $[Ca^{2+}]_I$ in bovine retinal pigment epithelium. *Invest Ophthalmol Vis Sci* 1991; 32:371.

63. Linsenmeier R, Smith VC, Pokorny J: The light rise of the electrooculogram during hypoxia. *Clin Vis Sci* 1987; 2:111–116.

64. Linsenmeier R, Steinberg RH: Origin and sensitivity of the light peak in the intact cat eye. *J Physiol* 1982; 331:653–673.

65. Linsenmeier R, Steinberg RH: Delayed basal hyperpolarisation of the cat retinal pigment epithelium and its relation to the fast oscillation of the DC ERG. *J Gen Physiol* 1984; 83:213–232.

66. Linsenmeier RA, Steinberg RH: Mechanisms of hypoxic effects on the cat DC electroretinogram. *Invest Ophthalmol Vis Sci* 1986; 27:1385–1394.

67. Madachi-Yamamoto S, Yonemura D, Kawasaki K: Diamox response of ocular standing potential as a clinical test for retinal pigment epithelial activity. *Acta Soc Ophthalmol Jpn* 1984; 88:1267–1272.

68. Madachi-Yamamoto S, Yonemura D, Kawasaki K: Hyperosmolarity response of ocular standing potential as a clinical test for retinal pigment epithelial activity. *Doc Ophthalmol* 1984; 57:153–162.

69. Marmor MF: Clinical electrophysiologic tests for evaluating the retinal pigment epithelium. In Zingirian M, Piccolino FC (eds): *The Retinal Pigment Epithelium*. Amsterdam, Kugler and Gherdini, pp 9–15.

70. Marmor MF, Lurie M: Light induced responses of the retinal pigment epithelium. In Zinn K, Marmor MF (eds): *The Retinal Pigment Epithelium*. Cambridge, MA, Harvard University Press, 1979, pp 226–244.

71. McCormick SA, Gentile RC, Odom JV, Farber M: Normal electro-oculograms in two patients with malignant melanoma of the choroid. *Doc Ophthalmol* 1996–1997; 92:167–172.

72. Mergler S, Steinhausen K, Wiederholt M Strauss O: Altered regulation of L-type channels by protein kinase C and protein tyrosine kinases as a pathophysiologic effect in retinal degenerations. *FASEB J* 1998; 12:1125–1134.

73. Miles WR: Modification of the human eye potential by dark and light adaptation. *Science* 1940; 91:456.

74. Miyake Y, Horiguchi M, Suzuki S, Kondo M, Tanikawa A: Electrophysiological findings in patients with Oguchi's disease. *Jpn J Ophthalmol* 1996; 40:511–519.

75. Niemeyer G, Steinberg RH: Differential effects of pCO_2 and pH on the ERG and light peak of the perfused cat's eye. *Vision Res* 1984; 24:275–280.

76. Noell W: Studies on the electrophysiology and metabolism of the retina. USAF School of Aviation Medicine Project 21-1201-0004 Randolph Field, Texas 1953.

77. Oakley B II, Steinberg R: Effect of maintained illumination on the $[K^+]_o$ in the subretinal space of the frog retina. *Vision Res* 1982; 22:767–773.

78. Papakostopoulis D, Bloom PA, Grey RH, Dean Hart JC: The electrooculogram in central vein occlusion. *Br J Ophthalmol* 1992; 76:515–519.

79. Pinckers A, Cuypers MH, Aandekerk AL: The EOG in Best's disease and dominant cystoid macular dystrophy (DCMD). *Ophthalmic Genet* 1996; 17:103–108.

80. Pinckers A, van Aarem A, Brink H: The electro-oculogram in heterozygote carriers of Usher syndrome, retinitis pigmentosa, neuronal ceroid lipofuscinosis, senior syndrome and choroideremia. *Ophthalmic Genet* 1994; 15:25–30.

81. Ponjavic V, Eksandh L, Andreasson S, Sjostrom K, Bakall B, Ingvast S, Wadelius C, Ehinger B: Clinical expression of Best's vitelliform macular dystrophy in Swedish families with mutations in the bestrophin gene. *Ophthalmic Genet* 1999; 20:251–257.

82. Seddon JM, Afshari MA, Sharma S, Bernstein PS, Chong S, Hutchinson A, Petrukhin K, Allikmets R: Assessment of mutations in the Best macular dystrophy (VMD2) gene in patients with adult-onset foveomacular vitelliform dystrophy, age-related maculopathy, and bull's-eye maculopathy. *Ophthalmology* 2001; 108:2060–2067.

83. Segawa Y: Electrical response of the retinal pigment epithelium to sodium bicarbonate: I. Experimental studies in animals. *J Juzen Med Soc* 1987; 96:1008–1021.

84. Segawa Y: Electrical response of the retinal pigment epithelium to sodium bicarbonate: II. Clinical use for electrophysiological evaluation of the retinal pigment epithelium activity experimental studies in animals. *J Juzen Med Soc* 1987; 96:1022–1041.

85. Shirao Y, Ushimura S, Kawasaki K: Differentiation of neovascular maculopathies by nonphotic electrooculogram responses. *Jpn J Ophthalmol* 1997; 41:174–179.

86. Skoog KO, Textorius O, Nilsson S-E: Effects of ethyl alcohol on the directly recorded standing potential of the human eye. *Acta Ophthalmol* 1975; 53:710–720.

87. Spadea L, Bianco G, Magni R, Rinaldi G, Ponte F, Brancato R, Ravalico G, Balestrazzi E: Electro-oculographic abnor-mality in eyes with uveal melanoma. *Eur J Ophthalmol* 2002; 12:419–423.

88. Spadea L, D'Amico M, Dragani T, Balestrazzi E: Electro-oculographic changes after local excision of uveal melanoma. *Doc Ophthalmol* 1994; 86:239–245.

89. Stavrou P, Good PA, Broadhurst EJ, Bundey S, Fielder AR, Crews SJ: ERG and EOG abnormalities in carriers of X-linked retinitis pigmentosa. *Eye* 1996; 10:581–589.

90. Steinberg RH: Interactions between the retinal pigment epithelium and the neural retina. *Doc Ophthalmol* 1985; 160:327–346.

91. Steinberg RH: Monitoring communication between photoreceptors and pigment epithelial cells: Effects of "mild" systemic hypoxia. *Invest Ophthalmol Vis Sci* 1987; 281:1888–1904.

92. Strauss O, Steinhausen K, Mergler S, Stumpff F, Wiederholt M: Involvement of protein tyrosine kinase in the InsP3-induced activation of Ca^{2+}-dependent Cl^- currents in cultured cells of the rat retinal pigment epithelium. *J Membr Biol* 1999; 169:141–153.

93. Strauss O, Wiederholt M, Wienrich M: Activation of Cl^- currents in cultured rat retinal pigment epithelial cells by intracellular applications of inositol-1,4,5-triphosphate: Differences between rats with retinal dystrophy (RCS) and normal rats. *J Membr Biol* 1996; 151:189–200.

94. Strauss OW, Wienrich M: Ca^{2+} conductances in rat retinal pigment epithelial cells. *J Cell Physiol* 1994; 160:80–96.

95. Taumer R, Hennig J, Pernice D: The ocular dipole: A damped oscillator stimulated by the speed of change of illumination. *Vision Res* 1974; 14:637–645.

96. Taumer R, Kapp H, Hennig J, Rohde N: A first electrical analog model of the ODM-oscillations. *Doc Ophthalmol Proc Ser*

97. Ten Doesschate G, Ten Doesschate I: *Ophthalmologica* 1956; 132:308–320.

98. Taumer R, Rohde N, Pernice D: The slow oscillation of the retinal potential: A biochemical feedback stimulated by the activity of rods and cones. *Bibl Ophthalmol* 1976; 85:40–56.

99. Textorius O, Nilsson SEG, Andersson B-F: Effects of intravitreal perfusion with dopamine in different concentrations on the DC electroretinogram and the standing potential of the albino rabbit eye. *Doc Ophthalmol* 1989; 73:149–162.

100. Theischen M, Schilling H, Steinhorst UH: EOG in adult vitelliform macular degeneration, butterfly-shaped pattern dystrophy and Best disease. *Ophthalmologe* 1997; 94:230–233.

101. Ueda Y, Steinberg RH: Voltage-operated calcium channels in fresh and cultured rat retinal pigment epithelial cells. *Invest Ophthalmol Vis Sci* 1993; 60:3408–3418.

102. Walter P, Brunner R, Heimann K: Atypical presentations of Best's vitelliform macular degeneration: clinical findings in seven cases. *Ger J Ophthalmol* 1994; 3:440–444.

103. Walter P, Widder RA, Luke C, Konigsfeld P, Brunner R: Electrophysiological abnormalities in age-related macular degeneration. *Graefes Arch Clin Exp Ophthalmol* 1999; 237:962–968.

104. Weleber RG: Fast and slow oscillations of the electro-oculogram in Best's macular degeneration and retinitis pigmentosa. *Arch Ophthalmol* 1989; 107:530–537.

105. Wolf JE, Arden GB: Two components of the human alcohol electro-oculogram. *Doc Opthalmol* 2004; 109:123–130.

12 Origins of the Electroretinogram

LAURA J. FRISHMAN

Introduction

The electrical response of the eye to a flash of light that can be recorded at the cornea is generated by radial currents that arise either directly from retinal neurons or as a result of the effect on retinal glia of changes in extracellular potassium concentration ($[K^+]_o$) brought about by the activity of these neurons. This response, the electroretinogram (ERG) (figure 12.1), is an excellent tool for studying retinal function in both the clinic and the laboratory because it can be recorded easily and noninvasively with a corneal electrode in intact subjects under physiological or nearly physiological (anesthetized) conditions. However, it is a gross potential that reflects the activity of all of the cells in the retina. For the ERG to be an effective tool in assessing normal and pathological retinal activity, it is important that the contributions of the various retinal cells be well characterized.

This chapter will survey the current state of knowledge regarding the origins of better-known and more recently described waves of the ERG. There is an increasing literature on the origins of ERG in a primate model (macaque monkey) whose retina is very similar to that of humans (see figure 12.1), so work in primates will be highlighted wherever possible. Current and previous work based on other mammalian species and lower vertebrates that is critical to an understanding of the origins of the ERG will also be included. In some cases, new information based on genetically manipulated murine models will be described as well.

GENERAL PRINCIPLES Extracellular potentials such as the ERG (and visual evoked potential [VEP] of the cortex) arise because localized conductance changes in the membranes of active cells give rise to inward or outward currents that also flow in the extracellular space (ECS) and give rise to extracellular potential gradients. The extracellular current through the conductive medium surrounding a cell whose activation has given rise to a local source or sink is principally directed toward the relatively less activated parts of the cell. Thus, if the neurons are arranged in an orderly fashion so that the extracellular currents of many synchronously activated cells flow in the same direction, the resulting extracellular potential changes, called *field potentials*, may be large enough to be recorded at a distance. In the retina, all neurons generate light-evoked currents, and in principle, all must contribute to the retinal field potentials. However,

depending on various factors, the contribution from a certain type of cell could be undetectable or could dominate the recording.

Orientation of cells and pattern of extracellular flow One factor that affects a cell's contribution to the ERG is its orientation in the retina. Because it is the radial component of the extracellular current that gives rise to the radial potential differences that are sensed in the commonly recorded transretinal ERG, radially oriented retinal neurons (photoreceptors, bipolar cells) and glial cells (Müller cells and retinal pigment epithelial [RPE] cells) should make larger contributions to the ERG than cells that are oriented more irregularly or tangentially (e.g., horizontal and amacrine cells). Current enters the ECS at one retinal depth (the current source), and it returns into the cell at another depth (the current sink), creating a current dipole. Most of the extracellular current flowing from source to sink traverses the ECS within the retina, but a small fraction travels extraretinally, through vitreous humor, extraocular tissues, sclera, choroid, the high resistance of the pigment epithelium, and back into the neural retina. ERG polarity and amplitude are critically dependent on where the active and reference electrodes are placed in this circuit. A common placement for the active electrode in noninvasive studies is the cornea, but for studying origins of the waves, the electrode may be positioned anywhere in the path, in particular at different depths in the retina. The reference electrode can also be positioned anywhere in the path but is often either retrobulbar (in invasive studies) or remote from the eye (e.g., on the temple) in clinical applications. If a remote reference electrode is used, its exact position is of little consequence except for the possibility of contamination of the recorded retinal signal by other sources.

Factors determining the relative magnitude of electrical signals in the ERG Other factors that are important in determining the magnitude of the contribution to the ERG of particular cell types include stimulus conditions such as stimulus energy, stimulus wavelength (spectrum), background illumination (that determines adaptation level of the retina), duration and spatial extent of the stimulus, and location of the stimulus within the visual field, as these stimulus parameters have different effects on the responses of the different cells. For example, the relative contributions of various neuronal

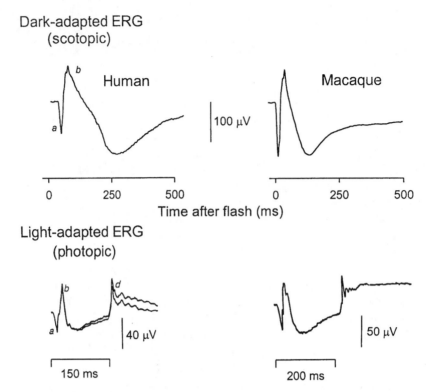

Dark-adapted ERG (scotopic)

Human · Macaque

100 µV

Time after flash (ms)

Light-adapted ERG (photopic)

40 µV · 50 µV

150 ms · 200 ms

FIGURE 12.1 Dark- and light-adapted flash ERGs of human subjects and macaque monkeys. Top, Dark-adapted (scotopic) ERGs in response to brief high-energy flashes from darkness occurring at time zero for a normal human subject (left) and a macaque monkey (right). The stimulus energy was ~400 sc td.s. (Source: Adapted from Robson JG, Frishman LJ.[193] Used by permission.) Bottom, Light-adapted (photopic) flash ERGs in response to longer-duration flashes on a rod-saturating background for a normal human subject (left) and a macaque monkey (right). For the human subject, the stimulus were 150 ms white ganzfeld flashes of 4.0 log ph td presented on a steady background of 3.3 log sc td. For the macaque, the same stimulus was used, but the flashes were 200 ms. (Source: Adapted from Sieving PA, Murayama K, Naarendorp F.[209] Used by permission.)

types are quite different under dark-adapted (scotopic) and light-adapted (photopic) conditions when rod and cone pathways, respectively, are involved in generation of the responses (see figure 12.1). Spatially extended diffuse stimuli, that is, full-field flashes that fill the retina, are commonly used to elicit the major waves of the ERG from photoreceptors and bipolar cells. The ERG contributions from these cells generally increase with the area of the retina that is stimulated as the number of cells, and hence the total extracellular current, is increased. On the other hand, contributions of ganglion cells (and other postreceptoral cells with antagonistic regions within their receptive fields) to the full-field flash ERG will be limited by the strength of surround antagonism, particularly late in the response and for long-duration stimulation. For photopic ERGs, particularly from trichromats such as the macaque monkey and human, stimulus wavelength also affects contributions from cells whose responses are dependent on spectral antagonism.[48]

Spatial buffering of [K+]$_o$ The contributions of Müller cells and RPE cells to the ERG are more delayed than neuronal responses because the responses of these cells depend on relatively slow changes in [K+]$_o$. These cells integrate the stimulus for longer durations than retinal neurons; hence, the amplitude of their responses will grow more than those of neurons when the stimulus duration is lengthened.

As was indicated above, Müller cells and RPE cells are radially oriented in the retina. Spatial buffering of [K+]$_o$ by the glial cells is an important mechanism for generation of the radial currents that underlie several ERG components or subcomponents, such as c-wave and slow PIII, scotopic threshold response (STR), M-wave, photopic negative response (PhNR), the tail of the b-wave. An overview of [K+]$_o$ spatial buffering in Müller cells will be presented here. (Details of K+ movement across RPE cells can be found in chapter 5 and in the section of this chapter on components from distal retina.)

The function of [K+]$_o$ spatial buffering is to minimize the changes in local [K+]$_o$ that occur as a consequence of neuronal activity, so the electrochemical gradients across cell membranes that are necessary for normal activity are maintained. Membrane depolarization leads to release (leak) of K+ from neurons, causing [K+]$_o$ to be elevated, particularly in the synaptic layers of the retina (figure 12.2); membrane hyperpolarization leads to a reduction in $[K^+]_o$ as the leak conductance is reduced, but the Na^+-K^+ ATPase in the membrane continues to pump K^+ into the cell. K^+ from the extracellular space enters the Müller cells and is carried radially as an intracellular (spatial buffer) current to regions of lower $[K^+]_o$. Thus, a current loop is set up: The current inside the Müller cell is carried by K^+, and to complete the circuit, the extracellular return current is carried by the dominant extracellular ions, Na^+ and Cl^-. The rate of flow of K^+ current through the glia is dependent on the establishment of a K^+ concentration gradient. Because $[K^+]_o$ changes are dependent on the integral of K^+ flow rate into the extracellular space, ERG components that reflect this glial current will be slowed relative to ERGs that reflect the (K^+) currents around neurons. This slowing would be equivalent to low-pass filtering of the neuronal signal.

The electrical properties of the Müller cell membrane are important for the creation of spatial buffer currents. The cell membrane is selectively permeable to K^+,[34,151] but the K^+ conductance is not distributed uniformly over the cell surface. Instead, it is very concentrated in the vicinity of extracellular sinks (i.e., the vitreous body, subretinal space, and blood vessels). The regional distribution creates "K^+ siphoning" from synaptic areas where $[K^+]_o$ is high to those sinks where K conductance is high.[152,157,160,189] Recent work in mice has shown a differential regional distribution of the inward-rectifying K^+ (Kir) channels that are involved in spatial buffering. As is indicated in figure 12.2, strongly inward-rectifying Kir 2.1 channels are present in the synaptic layers (small arrows on the left) where K^+ is removed for the ECS, whereas weakly inward-rectifying Kir 4.1 channels at the sinks are bidirectional conductance (bidirectional arrows), thus allowing the K^+ to leave the Müller cell.[114]

Approaches for Determining the Origins of the Electroretinogram Several different approaches, described briefly below, have been used over the years to

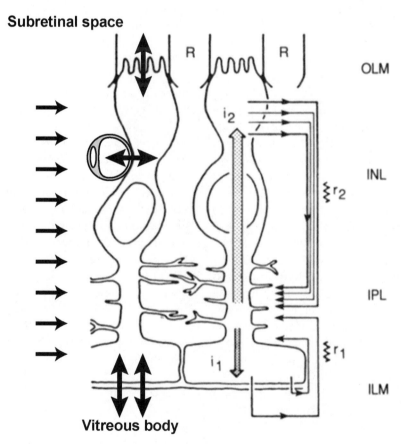

FIGURE 12.2   Model of K^+-induced flow of current through Müller cells and extracellular space. The Müller cell currents (gray arrows) are K^+ currents induced by K^+ increases in the IPL or decreases in the subretinal space (SRS), the return currents in the extracellular space are carried by Na^+ and Cl^- ions. K^+ enters the Müller cell via strongly rectifying Kir 2.1 channels in and around the synaptic layers (short arrows on the left) and weakly rectifying Kir 4.1 channels near the vitreous body, blood vessels, and the subretinal space (bidirectional arrows on the left). (Source: Adapted from Frishman LJ, Steinberg RH,[59] and from Kofuji P, et al.[114] Used by permission.)

determine the neuronal origins and cellular mechanisms of generation of the ERG.

Intraretinal depth recordings A microelectrode positioned somewhere in the retinal extracellular space records a field potential termed the local or intraretinal ERG.[20] When activated by a local stimulus, the recorded potential will reflect the electrical activity of the cells that are in the immediate vicinity of the microelectrode. However, when full-field diffuse flashes are used, currents can be sufficiently large that a corneal ERG will occur simultaneously with the local ERG. Large potentials of similar time course to the corneal ERG components at a particular retinal depth can be used to infer the cells of origin.

Although intraretinal studies have been useful, there are some problems associated with this sort of analysis: First, field potentials may spread over long distances and superimpose in space and time, making it difficult to determine whether a change in amplitude of one locally recorded potential is intrinsic to that component or is due to some other component. Second, retinal resistivity varies between and within retinal layers.[100,174] Thus, currents passing through layers of different resistance will set up complex voltage distributions. Both of these problems will occur in the intact eye when a scleral reference is used: The local signal recorded with a microelectrode will be contaminated with the diffuse ERG, owing to the high resistance of the RPE and sclera.[221]

Current source density (CSD) or source-sink analysis provides a solution to these difficulties; potential gradients are measured and analyzed, taking radial resistance into account to obtain direct estimates of radial current.[52] The result is a spatiotemporal profile of relatively well-localized current sources and sinks, and this profile can be compared with known features of retinal structure and physiology. When properly performed, CSD analysis can provide powerful evidence regarding the origins of ERG components (e.g., for the bipolar cell origin of the b-wave[106,252]).

When an ERG component is thought to depend on K^+ spatial buffer currents in glial cells, intraretinal depth recordings with ion-selective microelectrodes can be used to locate the retinal layer(s) where neuronally induced changes of $[K^+]_o$ are largest and most similar in time course to the component of interest.[40,60,101,166] Application of barium (Ba^{2+}) to block the Kir channels on glia cells have shown that ERG components that are dependent on the currents disappear but the neuronally induced $[K^+]_o$ changes remain, at least in the short term, after the blocker is applied.

Correlation with single-cell recordings Correlation with single-cell electrophysiology also can be useful in determining the origins of particular ERG components. Correlations are most straightforward when the light-evoked currents from a single type of cell are the primary determinant of an ERG component, as is the case for rod photoreceptors and the photocurrents that generate the scotopic a-wave[179] or rod bipolar cells and the scotopic b-wave in mammals.[191,194] Correlation also is useful if a specific response property is evident, such as light-evoked oscillations recorded in amacrine cells as a possible source of the oscillatory potentials in the ERG.[196] However, when currents from several cell types contribute to a field potential, the exact relationship between field potential waveform and cellular responses may be complex.[94]

Pharmacological dissection The use of pharmacological agents that have specific effects on cellular functions has been particularly productive in determining origins of ERG components. In Granit's classical pharmacological dissection study of the dark-adapted ERG of the cat, he found that various components disappeared sequentially during induction of ether anesthesia.[74] He called the components *processes* and numbered them in the order in which they disappeared: PI, the positive c-wave, was first to go; then PII, the positive b-wave, disappeared; and finally, PIII the negative a-wave disappeared. These processes correspond roughly to RPE, bipolar, and photoreceptor cell contributions to the ERG, respectively. The terms PII and PIII are still commonly used today.

In recent years, much has been learned about retinal microcircuitry and at cellular and molecular levels about retinal neurotransmitters (their identity, release mechanisms, and receptors), signal transduction cascades, ion channels, and other cellular proteins. This knowledge has allowed better use of pharmacological tools in isolating ERG components and in interpreting experimental observations. For example, specific knowledge about glutamatergic transmission in the retina and application of agonists and antagonists has provided many of the insights that we now have into origins of the major waves of the primate ERG.[26,195,209] Use of the voltage-gated Na^+ channel blocker tetrodotoxin (TTX) has made it possible to identify ERG components resulting from the Na^+-dependent spiking activity of retinal cells.

Site-specific lesions/pathology or targeted mutations Removal of a cell type or types or circuits allows assessment of the role of their contributions to the ERG. A specific cell type can be lesioned (e.g., retinal ganglion cells as a consequence of optic nerve section)[129] or lost owing to pathological changes (e.g., ganglion cells in glaucoma) or genetically determined degenerations (e.g., cone dystrophy). Cellular functions, such as light responses or synaptic transmission, can be abnormal or eliminated owing to inherited or acquired conditions or specifically altered by genetic manipulation, most commonly in murine models.

Modeling of cellular responses and ERG components As our knowledge of the function of particular retinal cell types has improved, it has been possible to develop quantitative models that accurately predict the light responses of those cells and to apply those models to analysis of the ERG. For example, models based on suction electrode recordings from single photoreceptor outer segments can be used to predict the leading edge of the a-wave,[13,88,89] and extended to predict the leading edge of the scotopic b-wave. Models of stimulus response relations of photoreceptors and cells at more proximal stages of processing also can be used to analyze amplitude-versus-energy curves obtained from recordings of ERG to a range of stimulus intensities into components related to different cell types.[54,199]

OVERVIEW This chapter will review current knowledge of the cellular origins and mechanisms of generation of the various ERG components, progressing from distal to proximal retina: from RPE to optic nerve head. At the end of the chapter, some retinal extracellular potentials that are not generated by light will be described.

Components arising in the distal retina: Slow PIII, c-wave, fast oscillation trough and light peak

After the onset of steady illumination, the relatively fast a- and b-waves are followed by the c-wave and then by a series of even slower responses that includes a negative deflection (the fast oscillation trough [FOT]) and a large slow positive deflection (the light peak). Clinically, these slower responses are usually recorded by electro-oculography (EOG), but direct-current electroretinography (d.c.-ERG) has been used experimentally in humans and animal preparations.[163,222]

The origins of the c-wave, the FOT, and the light peak of the d.c.-ERG involve ion concentration changes in the sub-retinal space that in turn produce membrane responses in the cells that border this space, particularly the Müller and RPE cells. These responses are relatively slow and overlap in time, so the Müller and/or RPE subcomponent voltages sum to produce the recorded d.c.-ERG component. These subcomponent voltages can be recorded in animal models by positioning a microelectrode in the subretinal space (figure 12.3).

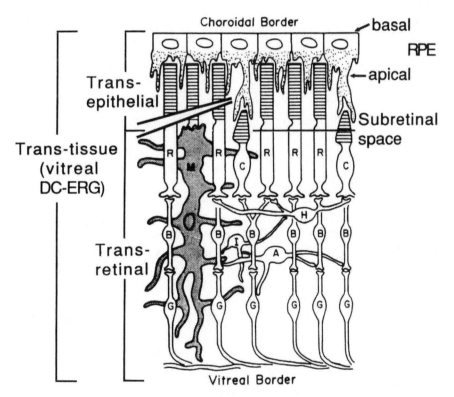

FIGURE 12.3 Schematic of a retina showing standard electrode placements. The RPE, photoreceptors (R = rods, C = cones), and Müller cells (M) send processes into the subretinal space. A microelectrode can be positioned in this space; and with reference electrodes behind the eye and in the vitreous, simultaneous recordings can be made of the RPE subcomponent (as a change in the transepithelial potential, TEP) and the neural retinal subcomponent (as a change in the transretinal potential). A vitreal ERG is recorded between the vitreous and the choroid. Micro-electrodes can also be positioned intracellularly (not shown) to record photoreceptor, Müller, and/or RPE membrane potential changes. For the RPE, there are two electrically separated membranes: The apical membrane faces the subretinal space (SRS), and the basal membrane faces the choroid. (Source: Adapted from Farber D, Adler R: Issues and questions in cell biology of the retina. In Adler R, Farber D (eds): *The Retina: A Model for Cell Biology Studies*, part I. Orlando, Fla, Academic Press, Inc, 1986.)

c-Wave The c-wave, a corneal positive potential that follows the b-wave, is the sum of two major subcomponent voltages. These voltages have been examined in mammals, birds, reptiles, and amphibians, and the mechanisms of origin are well understood. The accepted model is that a corneal negative subcomponent is generated by the neural retina and a cornea-positive subcomponent with a similar latency and time course is generated by the RPE. In most species, the RPE subcomponent is larger, so the resulting c-wave is cornea-positive. The amplitude of the c-wave reflects primarily the *difference* in the amplitudes of the two subcomponents, and if the subcomponents are equal, the c-wave will be absent, as it is in the recording in macaque retina shown in figure 12.6B.[235] This is likely the case in those species (and possibly for some individuals within a species) in which the c-wave is small, one example being the cone-dominated retina of the turtle.[134]

Evidence for two c-wave subcomponents comes from several types of experiments. Using a pharmacological approach in the rabbit, Noell[164] showed that the intravenous injection of sodium iodate, which poisoned primarily the RPE, abolished the corneal-positive c-wave and left a corneal-negative potential. In in vitro preparations, a c-wave can be recorded only if the RPE is intact; if the RPE is removed (isolated retina), a corneal-negative response with a similar time course is recorded.[214] Intraretinal microelectrode recordings in the cat, rabbit,[49] monkey,[233] chick,[65] gecko,[76] and frog have confirmed the existence of the two subcomponents in both intact and in vitro preparations. An example of such recordings is shown in figure 12.4. The component from the neural retina is commonly termed *slow PIII*.

There is strong evidence that both of the c-wave subcomponents are responses to the light-evoked decrease in extracellular potassium concentration $[K^+]_o$ that occurs in the subretinal space. Measurements of $[K^+]_o$ in the subretinal space (subretinal or distal $[K^+]_o$) have been made in intact and in vitro preparations from several species; the time course of the $[K^+]_o$ decrease was found to be similar to the c-wave and to each of its subcomponents.[125,167] Blocking K^+ conductance with various agents abolishes both slow PIII[12,30] and the cornea-positive RPE c-wave.[75,92]

Müller cell contribution (slow PIII) The cornea-negative PIII component of Granit can be separated into a fast component (the receptor photocurrent as reflected by the leading edge of the a-wave) and a slower component: slow PIII. Intraretinal recording at various depths[251] and current source density analysis[49] suggested that slow PIII was generated by a cell that spanned the neural retina. The persistence of slow PIII after aspartate treatment to block postreceptoral neuronal responses suggested a Müller cell origin.[250] Additional support for a Müller cell origin is the

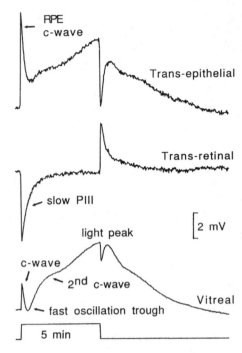

FIGURE 12.4 Subretinal recordings from the intact cat eye. The vitreal, transretinal, and transepithelial potentials were recorded simultaneously in response to a 5-minute period of illumination. At this slow time scale, the a- and b-waves cannot be seen Müller in the vitreal ERG a c-wave is followed by a fast oscillation trough and then by a prominent light peak; the shoulder on the rising phase of the light peak is the second c-wave. The intraretinal recordings show that the c-wave has two subcomponents. The initial increase in the transepithelial recording is the large corneal-positive RPE component; the initial decrease in the transretinal recording is slow PIII. For the light peak, only an RPE component is found. (Source: From Steinberg RH, Linsenmeier RA, Griff ER.[222] Used by permission.)

long integration time, for example, up to 40s in the carp.[250]

The present understanding of the origin of slow PIII is that the light-evoked reduction in subretinal $[K^+]_o$ decrease passively hyperpolarizes the distal end of the Müller cells, and this sets up a transretinal K^+ spatial buffer current due to the elongated geometry of the cells (reviewed by Newman[156]) and the distribution of inward-rectifying K^+ channels (Kir).[114,115] The current drop across the extracellular resistance produces the slow PIII voltage.[49,103,250,261] In support of the Müller cell hypothesis, Karwoski and Proenza[103] recorded a slow hyperpolarization in *Necturus* Müller cells; later, Dick et al. demonstrated in tiger salamander and rabbit retina[40,41] (figure 12.5) that the time course of the Müller cell hyperpolarization was similar both to the $[K^+]_o$ decrease and slow PIII. Also consistent with the Müller cell hypothesis is the suppression of slow PIII by Ba^{2+} because Ba^{2+} blocks all Müller cell K^+ conductances[155] while having little effect on the light-evoked K^+ decrease.[30,58–60] Perhaps most convincing is recent work showing that genetic

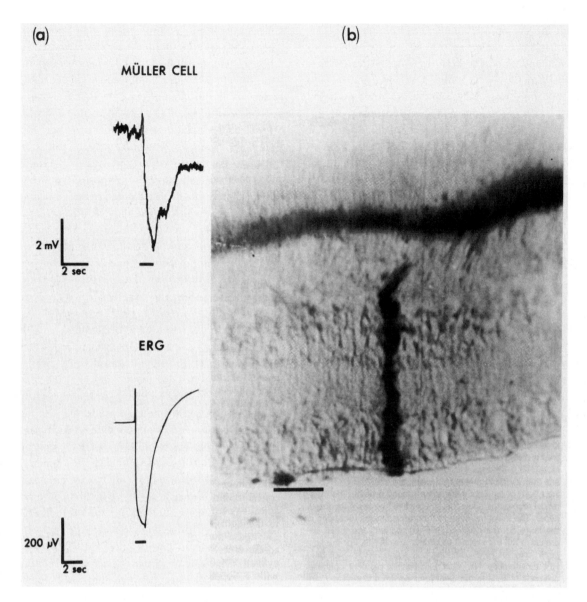

(a)

MÜLLER CELL

2 mV

2 sec

ERG

200 µV

2 sec

(b)

FIGURE 12.5 Origin of slow PIII. A, Intracellularly recorded Müller cell response (upper trace) and simultaneously recorded ERG (lower trace) from a superfused rabbit eyecup. The duration of the diffuse white light stimulus is indicated by the horizontal bars. The light response consists of a transient depolarization followed by a sustained hyperpolarization. The ERG shows a positive b-wave followed by a sustained negative PIII component. B, The HRP-stained Müller cell from which the intracellular recording in A was obtained (calibration bar: 25 mm). (Source: From Dick E, Miller RF, Bloomfield S.[41] Used by permission.)

inactivation in mice of the dominant Kir channel (Kir 4.1 subunit) in Müller cells removes slow PIII.[115]

The spatial buffering hypothesis presented above predicts that the K^+ spatial buffer current should lead to a reaccumulation of subretinal $[K^+]_o$. Shimazaki and Oakley[204] described a $[K^+]_o$ reaccumulation that occurs with maintained illumination in detail, but they conclude that it is caused primarily by a slowing of the Na^+-K^+ pump of the photoreceptor. However, subretinal $[K^+]_o$ during maintained illumination will eventually be subject to other factors; with a duration of illumination of at least 38 s in cat[121] or 85 s in frog,[93] subretinal $[K^+]_o$ will be reduced by light-dependent hydration (volume increase) of subretinal space.

Distal versus proximal PIII Intraretinal depth recordings in isolated retina preparations from a number of species have identified a PIII component whose origin is more proximal than that of slow PIII; it was observed in frog and turtle retinas,[145] as well as in fish,[50] cat, rat,[176] and rabbit.[80] In rabbit retina, it was found to be aspartate-sensitive, separating it from the distally generated slow PIII and indicating a post-receptoral origin. This component, termed *proximal PIII*,[145] has been difficult to study in isolation from other proximal field potentials, and its origins have been ascribed to various neurons of the INL as well as to spatial buffer currents in Müller cells. These spatial buffer currents would resemble the slow PIII currents but would be due to a neuronally induced increase in $[K^+]_o$ in proximal retina rather than a photoreceptor-dependent decrease in distal retina (see figure 12.2). The term is not commonly used now that Müller cell–mediated responses reflecting $[K^+]_o$ changes in proximal retina, such as the M-wave and STR, have been described.[57,104]

Pigment epithelial component The RPE c-wave, a corneal-positive potential recorded across the RPE, results from an increase in the RPE's transepithielial potential (TEP). The RPE has two membranes, apical and basal, and a trans-epithelial potential exists because the membranes are electrically separated by the high resistance of tight junctions that encircle RPE cells (the R membrane).[15] The potentials across the apical (V_{ap}) and basal (V_{ba}) membranes differ, and this difference is equal to the TEP. In every species that has been studied, the apical membrane is more hyperpolarized than is the basal membrane, so the TEP in the dark is corneal-positive. For example, if $V_{ap} = -90$ mV and $V_{ba} = -75$ mV, the TEP will be $V_{ba} - V_{ap}$ or $+15$ mV. The TEP is a major component of the standing potential of the eye.

During the c-wave, the TEP increases (becomes more positive). Intracellular RPE recordings from both intact and in vitro preparations[223] have shown that the increase in TEP is generated by a hyperpolarization of the RPE apical membrane. The amplitude of the RPE c-wave, however, is not equal to the apical hyperpolarization because there is some passive current shunting between the apical and basal surfaces (the two membranes are only partially separated). This basal voltage subtracts from the apical voltage and makes the recorded TEP smaller. Thus, the RPE c-wave amplitude depends on the responses of both the apical and basal membranes. Experimental work (and theoretical predictions) shows, for example, that a decrease in basal membrane resistance (see the later section on interactions between distal ERG components) decreases the passive basal response and therefore increases the RPE (and corneal) c-wave.

Recordings with double-barreled K^+-selective micro-electrodes, where one barrel measures intraretinal voltages and the other measures $[K^+]$, show that the RPE c-wave and the apical hyperpolarization have a time course similar to that of the light-evoked, subretinal $[K^+]_o$ decrease. The apical membrane has a large relative potassium conductance.[139] In the frog, Oakley[166] compared light-evoked responses from a retina-RPE preparation with K^+-evoked responses from an isolated RPE preparation (where only K^+ in the apical bath in solution was altered). He showed that the RPE c-wave was due solely to the $[K^+]_o$ decrease. Experiments using Ba^{2+} and ouabain, an inhibitor of the Na^+-K^+ pump, have shown that a decrease in $[K^+]_o$, in addition to increasing the K^+-equilibrium potential and hyperpolarizing the apical membrane, also slows the electrogenic apical Na^+-K^+ pump[140] and produces a small apical depolarization in the RPE cells of a range of species, including frog,[75] bovine,[98] and human retinas.[83] This indicates that at least two apical mechanisms contribute to the RPE c-wave.

The findings presented above show that the c-wave reflects responses of both Müller and RPE cells to a light-evoked $[K^+]_o$ decrease. Since the amplitude of the vitreal c-wave is the difference between these two components, a change in the $[K^+]_o$ response should alter both components, and the c-wave amplitude may change little. On the other hand, if only one of the components is altered, the percent change in the amplitude of the vitreal c-wave will be greater than the percent change in that component.

With longer periods of illumination, subretinal K^+ starts to reaccumulate, and this causes both the RPE c-wave and slow PIII to recover from their peaks. In the frog, the time course of this recovery is quite similar to that of the K^+ reaccumulation.[168] In response to maintained illumination, $[K^+]_o$ fell to a minimum value and then began to recover, reaching a steady state approximately 10 minutes after light onset. In the frog, the TEP of the RPE TEP followed $[K^+]_o$ during this entire time period, whereas in other species, the recovery toward the dark-adapted baseline is greater than is predicted by the K^+ reaccumulation (see below).

THE FAST OSCILLATION TROUGH (FOT) The FOT (usually measured by EOG) is a change in the corneoretinal poten-

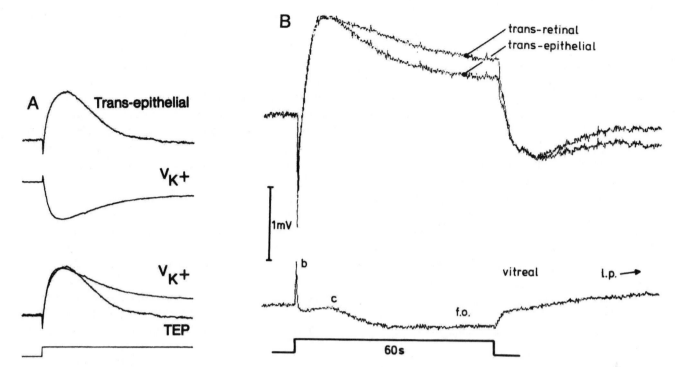

FIGURE 12.6 Intraretinal recordings during the fast-oscillation trough. A, Simultaneous recordings of the TEP and the potassium change (V_K) in an in vitro gecko retina-RPE-choroid preparation in response to a 3-minute period of white light illumination. The potassium response has been inverted and scaled to the peak of the TEP recording so that the two recordings can be compared. The TEP decrease from its peak is greater than is predicted by the change in V_K. (Source: Adapted from Griff ER, Steinberg RH.[76]) B, Simulta-neous recordings of the vitreal, transretinal, and transepithelial potentials in the macaque in response to a 60-second stimulus. The transretinal potential was inverted and superimposed on the transepithelial recording. The TEP decreases from its peak more than the transretinal potential does. It was coincidental that the two recordings had equal amplitudes. Since the vitreal ERG is the sum of the two subcomponent voltages, the vitreal c-wave is very small in this example. (Source: From van Norren D, Heynen H.[235] Used by permission.)

tial, decreasing in light and increasing in dark in synchrony with an alternating light/dark stimulus. In this section, we examine the responses evoked by maintained illumination that corresponds to the EOG decrease (trough) that Van Norren and Heynen[235] termed the *FOT*. This decrease in potential follows the c-wave peak (figure 12.6B), and if a light peak is evoked by the stimulus (see the next section), the FOT appears as a dip between the c-wave and the light peak (figure 12.4).

The FOT has subcomponents that originate in both the neural retina and the RPE. One subcomponent involves the recovery of Müller and RPE cells from their peak polarizations as $[K^+]_o$ reaccumulates. However, in many species, including mammals, birds, and reptiles, the recovery of both slow PIII and the RPE c-wave (TEP) from their peaks is greater than is predicted by the reaccumulation of subretinal $[K^+]_o$ (figure 12.6A). The deviation is greatest for the RPE component such that it recovers more toward the dark-adapted level than does transretinal slow PIII (figure 12.6B). As discussed by Steinberg et al.,[222] this extra decrease in TEP produces much of the corneal-negative potential during the FOT.

Intracellular RPE recordings in cat, gecko, chick, and bovine RPE show that this extra TEP decrease is generated by a hyperpolarization that originates at the RPE basal membrane. This basal hyperpolarization is passively shunted to the apical membrane, where it overrides the apically generated depolarization that should occur as $[K^+]_o$ reaccumulates. Thus, light produces, first, a hyperpolarization generated at the apical membrane that *increases* the TEP and, second, a hyperpolarization generated at the basal membrane that *decreases* TEP. Since the basal hyperpolarization follows the apical hyperpolarization, it has been called *delayed basal hyperpolarization*.[76] Experiments in isolated RPE preparations[76] suggested that the light-evoked $[K^+]_o$ decrease in the subretinal space of an intact retina is sufficient to produce both the c-wave and the FOT. A maintained decrease in $[K^+]_o$ in the apical bath first hyperpolarized the apical membrane so that the TEP increased (analogous to the RPE c-wave) and subsequently hyperpolarized the basal membrane so that the TEP decreases back toward the baseline. In these experiments, the only "stimulus" was a step decrease in $[K^+]_o$ with no reaccumulation.

The ionic mechanisms that underlie the basal membrane hyperpolarization have been clarified by Miller and colleagues, who described the important role of intracellular chloride activity (and basolateral Cl^- conductance[11,97]) in generating this response. On the basis of studies in isolated bovine RPE-choroid preparations (for a review, see Gallemore et al.[64]), they proposed that a light-evoked decrease in subretinal $[K^+]_o$ slows Cl^- uptake by the $Na^+, K^+, 2Cl^-$ transporter in the RPE apical membrane, which reduces intracellular Cl^- activity. In turn, the reduced Cl^- activity altered the Cl^- equilibrium across the basolateral membrane Cl^- channels, which produced a basal hyperpolarization. Importantly, they observed that the delayed basolateral membrane hyperpolarization was greatly reduced either by apical bumetanide, an $Na^+, K^+, 2Cl^-$ cotransport blocker, or by basal 4,4'-diisothiocyanostilbene-2, 2'-disulfonate (DIDS), a Cl^- channel blocker. The importance of Cl^- activity and conductance for generation of the fast oscillation in situ was confirmed in recordings in the chick retina RPE-choroid preparation as illustrated in figure 12.7.[67]

More recently, studies by Miller and coworkers in intact sheets of RPE choroid from human fetal eyes have distinguished two different types of Cl^- channels on the basal membrane (see figure 12.7): a DIDS-inhibitable Ca^{2+}-sensitive Cl^- channel and a cAMP-dependent channel that is inhibited by DIDS and by 5-nitro-2-(3)phenylpropylamino benzoate (NPPB), which identifies it as a cystic fibrosis transmembrane regulator (CFTR) channel (see Quinn et al.[184] for a review). In CF patients, the FOT but not the light peak (see below) was reduced, implicating CFTR in generation of the FOT.

THE LIGHT PEAK   In mammals, birds, and reptiles, maintained illumination causes a slow increase in the standing potential that is called the *light peak*,[109] and this can also be recorded as a slow oscillation of the EOG. Intraretinal recordings in the cat,[124] monkey,[233] chick,[63] and gecko[77] show that this corneal-positive potential comes exclusively from the RPE as an increase in the TEP (see figure 12.4). Intracellular RPE recordings show that the TEP increase is generated by

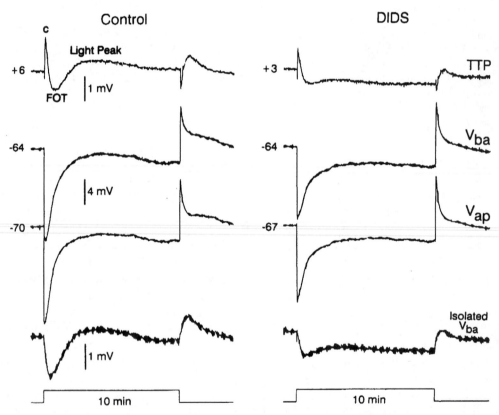

FIGURE 12.7   Intracellular recording of the DC-ERG in the chick retina RPE-choroid preparation. Responses are shown to 10-minute steps of diffuse illumination before and 20 minutes after perfusion of the basal membrane with 500 μM DIDS. The intracellular d.c. ERG consists of the c-wave hyperpolarization of V_{ap} ($V_{ba}h$ also hyperpolarizes), the delayed basal membrane hyperpolarization of the FOT, and, last, the slow basal depolarization of the light peak. Basal membrane voltage changes are clearest in the isolated V_{ba} responses obtained by scaling and subtracting the apical response from the basal response. In DIDS, the delayed basal hyperpolarization and the light-peak depolarization were suppressed. (Source: From Gallemore RP, Steinberg RH: *Invest Ophthalmol Vis Sci* 1995; 36:113–112. Used by permission.)

a slow depolarization of the RPE basal membrane, with strong evidence that the depolarization is due to an increase in chloride conductance (T_{CL}) of the basal membrane. In chick, this increase in Cl⁻ conductance during the light peak was an average of 55%, and the light peak was suppressed by DIDS. Furthermore, the reversal potential for the conductance increase during the light peak was equal to the Cl⁻ equilibrium potential. More recent work in human fetal RPE cell sheets (figure 12.8) is consistent with the channels involved in generation of the light peak being DIDS-inhibitable Ca^{2+}-sensitive Cl⁻ channels on the basal membrane.

Although the light peak voltage comes from the basal membrane of the RPE, an initial event occurs in the neural retina that triggers, first, a change in the concentration of an as yet unidentified "light peak substance," which then affects the basal membrane via a second-messenger system. Since the light peak persists following treatments to block synaptic transmission to postreceptoral cells,[63] photoreceptor activity alone probably modulates the concentration of the light peak substance. The sensitivity of the light peak to levels of hypoxia that do not affect the ERG b-wave[123] also suggests a photoreceptor origin. While both experimental and clinical studies have suggested that the inner retina may also contribute,[72,122,127] the perturbations used in these studies could also have affected the photoreceptors and/or RPE directly.

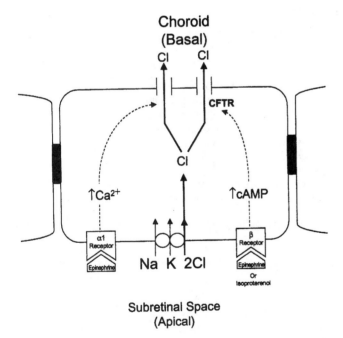

Choroid
(Basal)

Subretinal Space
(Apical)

FIGURE 12.8 Model of the human RPE showing identified membrane mechanisms and putative second messengers that contribute to the adrenergic responses. The apical membrane contains both α_1 and β adrenergic receptors. Activation of either receptor type by epinephrine opens depolarizing conductances at the basolateral membrane. (Source: From Quinn RH, Quong JN, Miller SS.[184] Used by permission.)

The identities of the "light peak substance" and the intracellular second messenger(s) involved in producing the light peak have been the subject of many investigations. Although dopamine suppresses the light peak in the perfused cat eye,[36] careful studies in chick have indicated that it cannot be the "light peak substance."[66] Epinephrine via its binding to adrenergic receptors on the apical membrane also has been proposed as a candidate[98] and has been disputed.[64] More recent work indicates that a role for adrenergic agents binding to alpha-1-adrenergic receptors, is likely.[184] In human fetal RPE, intracellular Ca^{2+} activity elevated by activation of alpha-1 receptors affects a DIDS-sensitive Cl⁻ conductance on the basal membrane that probably underlies the light peak depolarization.[184] A role for pH in the regulation of the Cl⁻ channels is possible as well.[47]

As a second-messenger candidate, cAMP, has been thoroughly studied, but opposite effects on chloride conductance in the basal membrane in different species have been observed (see Gallemore et al.[64] for a review), and as described above and illustrated in figure 12.7, cAMP is the likely second messenger involved in the FOT rather than the light peak.

INTERACTION BETWEEN DISTAL ELECTRORETINOGRAPHIC COMPONENTS The amplitude of the c-wave undergoes significant variation during the rise and fall of the light peak.[124] When repetitive flashes that elicit both c-waves and a light peak are used, intraretinal recordings have shown that the increase in the c-wave during the light peak originates from the RPE component. Intracellular recordings reveal that the RPE c-wave increases as a result of a decrease in the resistance of the RPE basal membrane. A similar increase in c-wave amplitude has also been observed with systemic mild hypoxia[123,161] and intravenous azide injections,[126,164] both of which also decrease RPE basal membrane resistance. It would not be surprising to find a similar effect in diseases that affect the RPE.

Nikara et al.[162] described an ERG wave in the cat that he called the *second c-wave*. This consists of a shoulder on the rising phase of the light peak (see figure 12.4). Detailed analysis of the subcomponents arising in the neural retina and RPE show that this shoulder probably does not represent a discrete subcomponent.[125] Rather, it results from the interaction between the end of the delayed basal hyperpolarization, the initiation of the light peak, and the maintained K⁺-dependent hyperpolarization of the apical membrane.

Origins of the a-wave

The ERG response to a flash of light measured at the cornea is the sum of positive and negative component potentials that originate from different stages of retinal processing and

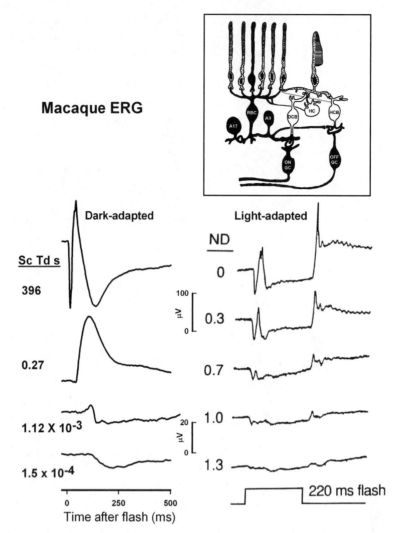

Macaque ERG

Dark-adapted   Light-adapted

ND

Sc Td s

396   0

100 μV 0

0.27   0.3

0.7

1.12 X 10⁻³   1.0

20 μV 0

1.5 x 10⁻⁴   1.3

0   250   500

Time after flash (ms)

220 ms flash

FIGURE 12.9 Dark- and light-adapted ERGs of the macaque retina. Left, Dark-adapted full-field ERGs of anesthetized macaque monkeys were measured in response to brief (<5 ms) flashes from darkness generated by computer-controlled light-emitting diodes (LEDs). Responses were recorded differentially between DTL fibers on the two eyes. Flash strength increased over a 6 log unit range. Responses to the weakest stimuli were rod-driven (scotopic), whereas responses for the strongest stimuli were mixed rod-cone responses. (Source: From Robson JG, Frishman LJ.[193]) Right, Light-adapted full-field ERGs of anesthetized macaques were measured by using Burian Allen electrodes. Stimulus strength was controlled with neutral density (ND) filters. Stimulus strength increased over a 1.3 log unit range to a maximum at 0 ND of 4.0 log ph.td for 220 ms flashes. Responses were cone-driven (photopic); stimuli were presented on a steady rod-saturating background of 3.3 log sc-td. (Source: From Sieving PA, Murayama K, Naarendorp F.[209] Used by permission.) The inset shows a simplified schematic of rod and cone pathways in the mammalian retina.

overlap in time. This section will focus on the origins of the cornea-negative a-wave, which is mainly associated with the photoreceptors, but also has postreceptoral contributions, primarily from the OFF pathway. Figure 12.9 shows dark- and light-adapted flash ERGs of the macaque monkey, which is a good animal model for studying the origins of the human response, as illustrated in figure 12.1.

The dark-adapted a-wave is the initial negative wave that occurs in response to strong stimuli from darkness (figure 12.9, top left), and it is primarily rod-driven (i.e., scotopic). The light-adapted a-wave is the initial negative wave in

response to a stimulus presented on an adapting background (right), and when the background is rod-saturating, the a-wave is cone-driven (photopic). Under both dark- and light-adapted conditions, the a-wave is truncated by the rise of the b-wave, the prominent positive-going component of the ERG, which originates primarily from ON bipolar cells. The slow negative wave in the dark-adapted ERG in response to the weakest stimuli (bottom of figure 12.9) is a relatively small component, called the *scotopic threshold response* (STR), which can be distinguished pharmacologically from the a-wave and is related to inner retinal (amacrine and/or gan-

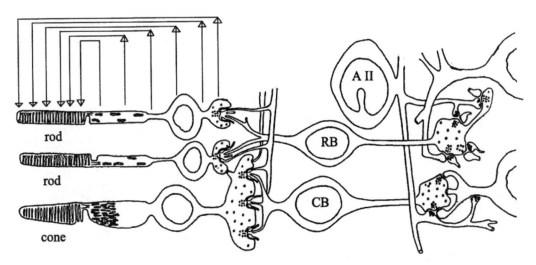

Figure 12.10 Schematic of a longitudinal section of the mammalian retina illustrating how circulating currents in the photoreceptor layer create an extracellular field potential, in which the vitreal side of the retina has a more positive potential than the scleral side. A high-intensity flash will suppress the circulating current around the photoreceptor, leading to a vitreal or corneal response that is negative in relation to the resting preflash baseline. (Source: From Pugh EN Jr, Falsini B, Lyubarsky A.[183] Used by permission.)

glion cell activity.[207,243] Under light-adapted conditions, for longer duration stimuli, another positive potential, the d-wave, occurs at light offset. The d-wave reflects the transient depolarization of hyperpolarizing cone bipolar cells in combination with the positive-going termination of the cone photoreceptor response (see the inset in figure 12.9, which shows a schematic diagram of the mammalian retina). The origins these postreceptoral components will be described more fully in later sections.

EARLY STUDIES SHOW THAT THE a-WAVE REFLECTS THE ROD AND CONE RECEPTOR PHOTOCURRENT   The a-wave (Granit's PIII) that is produced in response to a long duration stimulus has long been associated with the photoreceptors.[17,19,20,60,73,74,84,85,180] In early intraretinal studies using microelectrodes, the a-wave was observed in isolated amphibian retina preparations in which the RPE was absent, and this established its origin in the neural part of the retina.[29,227] In intraretinal depth studies in cat, it was found to be largest in the vicinity of the photoreceptors.[20]

The case for a receptoral origin for PIII was strengthened by microelectrode recordings in macaque monkey retina with the inner retinal circulation clamped to suppress activity of retina proximal to the photoreceptors.[17,18] Clamping the circulation removed the b-wave and revealed a later, more slowly recovering portion of PIII. This slow potential was named the *late receptor potential*, rod or cone, depending on the stimulus conditions.[17] The late receptor potential, slower for rods than for cones, is now considered to reflect the recovery stage of the receptor photoresponse and to be

a part of (fast) PIII. The origins of an even slower photoreceptor-related negative potential, slow PIII, were addressed in the previous section.

In current source density (CSD) analyses of the isolated rat retina, Penn and Hagins[179,180] demonstrated the suppressing effect of light on the circulating (dark) current of the photoreceptors and proposed that this suppression was seen in the ERG as the a-wave (Granit's PIII). Figure 12.10 provides a schematic of the photoreceptor layer current reproduced from a review by Pugh et al.[183] The figure shows that in the dark, cation channels (Na^+, Ca^{2+}, and Mg^{2+}) in the receptor outer segment (ROS) are open, current flows into the ROS (a current sink with respect to the extracellular space), and K^+ leaks out of the inner segment (a current source), creating dipole current. This dipole current produces a corneal (and vitreal) potential that is positive with respect to the scleral side of the retina. Suppression of the dark current reduces the corneal positive potential, creating the negative-going a-wave. Consistent with this view, as illustrated in figure 12.11, intraretinal recordings and CSD analyses in the intact macaque retina have localized current sources and sinks for a local potential, corresponding to the a-wave, to the distal third of the retina.

Hood and Birch[88,89] sought to directly relate the time course of the leading edge of the ERG a-wave to the leading edge of the photoreceptor response to light. In doing so, they hoped to improve the utility of the ERG a-wave for studying photoreceptor function in normal and diseased human retinas. They demonstrated that both the linear and nonlinear (i.e., saturating) behavior of the leading edge of the a-

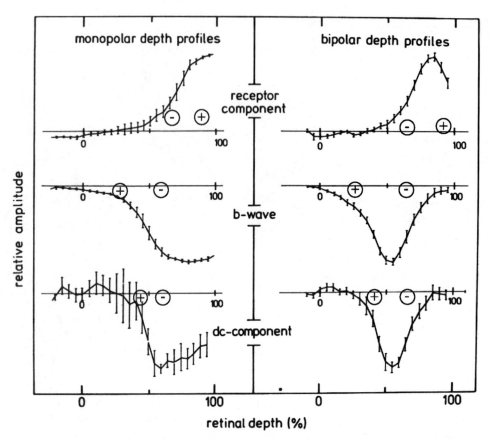

Figure 12.11 Depth profiles and CSD results in anesthetized macaque monkey retina for the a-wave, the b-wave, and the d.c. component of the b-wave. Left, Monopolar depth profiles using an intraretinal microelectrode referenced to the forehead. Right, bipolar depth profiles using a coaxial electrode with a distance of 25 mm between the tips to measure field potential amplitudes at the peak time of the receptor component, the b-wave, and the d.c. component of the macaque light-adapted ERG. The plus and minus signs indicate the current sources and sinks, respectively, for the components as calculated from current source density analyses based on the coaxial electrode recordings and resistance measurements. The a-wave source and sink are in the distal quarter of the retina. The b-wave and the d.c. component have similar source-sink distributions, with a large sink near the outer nuclear layer and a distributed source extending to the vitreal surface of the retina. Plots represent means of 26 penetrations. (Source: From Heynen H, van Norren D.[85] Used by permission.)

wave in the human ERG can be predicted by a model of photoreceptor function derived from in vitro suction electrode recordings of currents around the outer segments of primate rod photoreceptors.[10] Subsequently, a simplified kinetic model of the leading edge of the photoreceptor response (in vitro current recordings) that took the stages of the biochemical phototransduction cascade into account was developed by Lamb and Pugh.[118] This model was shown to predict the leading edge of the human a-wave generated by strong stimuli,[13] and it has been used extensively in studies of human photoreceptor function. A detailed description of the use of such models in analyzing photoreceptor behavior appears in chapter 35.

PHARMACOLOGICAL DISSECTION STUDIES REVEAL POSTRECEP-TORAL CONTRIBUTIONS TO THE a-WAVE   In his now classical pharmacologic dissection study of the ERG, Granit[25] isolated a potential that he named *PIII* by induction of ether anesthesia in vivo in the cat. PIII was more resistant to the effects of ether than the contributions to the ERG that came either from the RPE or postreceptoral neurons. In subsequent in vitro studies of the isolated frog retina, sodium (L) aspartate in the perfusate was found to eliminate all postreceptoral responses, and to isolate PIII.[214] Aspartate, in the L-isomer form, is now known to be an agonist for glutamate, the neurotransmitter that is released both by photoreceptors and bipolar cells in all vertebrate retinas. In high concentrations (e.g., more than ~40 mM), aspartate renders light-evoked glutamate release from photoreceptors (and bipolar cells) ineffective in synaptic transfer of signals.[214] Transmission from photoreceptors to bipolar cells, and hence the b-wave, also can be blocked with the D isomer of aspartate.[249] D-Aspartate blocks glutamate transporters, causing signal transfer to postreceptoral neurons to be blocked owing to accumulation of excess glutamate in the extracellular space.

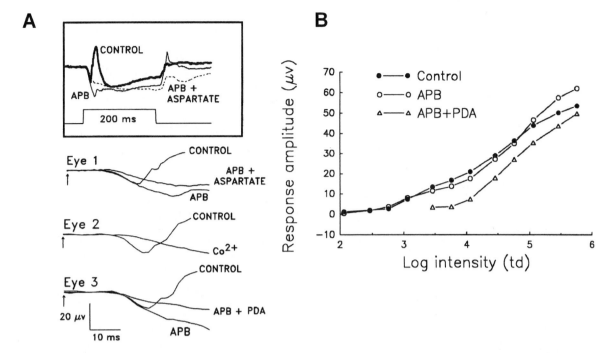

A

B

FIGURE 12.12 Postreceptoral contributions to the a-wave of the macaque ERG. A, Comparison of the effects of APB (1-mm vitreal concentration) and APB+PDA (5 mM) with those of aspartate (50 mM) and cobalt (10 mm CO^{2+}) on the photopic ERG a-wave of three different eyes of two anesthetized monkeys. The inset at the top shows the response of eye #1 to the 200-ms stimulus of 3.76 log td (2.01 log cd/m²) on a steady background of 3.3 log td (1.55 cd/m²). The a-waves for eyes 1, 2, and 3 were all in response to the same stimulus. For this stimulus, most of the small a-wave (10 μV) that was elicited was postreceptoral in origin. In the clinic, the a-wave that is elicited by brief flashes often is larger, 20 μV or more, and therefore also will include several microvolts of photoreceptor contribution,

as shown in part B. B, Stimulus response function (V log I plot) of the photopic a-wave of the macaque measured a times corresponding to the a-wave peak in the control responses (solid circles). Amplitudes after APB (open circles) and after APB + PDA (triangles) were measured at the same latency as the trough of the control a-waves measured at the same stimulus intensity. The points are connected by solid lines. In this figure, as in part A, APB had no effect on the a-wave amplitude. In contrast, PDA reduced the amplitude, and the postreceptoral contribution was maximally between 10 and 15 μV, about 50% of a 20-μV a-wave but less than 25% of a saturated a-wave of about 65 μV. (Source: From Bush RA, Sieving PA.[26] Used by permission.)

Our understanding of the origins of the light-adapted (photopic) a-wave, as well as other waves of the macaque photopic ERG, was greatly advanced by studies of Sieving and colleagues in which they used more specific glutamate agonists and antagonists than asparate to dissect the retinal circuits.[26,27,116,209] They made intravitreal injections of L-2-amino-4-phosphonobutyric acid (termed APB or AP4), a mGluR6 receptor agonist, to block metabotropic transmission and hence to eliminate light-evoked responses of depolarizing (ON) bipolar cells and thus more proximal ON pathway contributions as well.[215] Cis-2,3-piperidine dicarboxylic acid (PDA) or kynurenic acid (KYN) was injected to block major ionotropic glutamate receptors in the retina (a-amino-3-hydroxy-5-methyl-4-isoxazolepropionic acid [AMPA] and kainate [KA] receptors).[216] Complete blockade of these receptors eliminated signal transmission to hyperpolarizing (OFF) bipolar cells and horizontal cells, as well as to amacrine and ganglion cells in both ON and OFF pathways. The results of such experiments are illustrated in figure 12.12A for responses to fairly weak stimuli presented

on a rod-suppressing background; functions relating a-wave amplitude and stimulus intensity over a wider range of stimulus strengths in the same study are shown in figure 12.12B. The a-wave was reduced in amplitude by PDA (and KYN, not shown) but not by APB alone. Figure 12.12A also shows that PDA had an effect similar to that of aspartate or to cobalt (Co^{2+}). Co^{2+} blocks the voltage-gated Ca^{2+} channels that are essential for vesicular release of glutamate at synapses, and hence neurotransmission to postrecepetoral neurons, to occur.

When the effects of PDA versus APB on the photopic a-wave amplitude were evaluated over a wide range of stimulus strengths, PDA-sensitive postreceptoral neurons, rather than cone photoreceptors or APB-sensitive contributions from ON bipolar and ON pathway neurons, were found to generate the leading edge of the a-wave for the first 1.5 log units of flash intensity that generated a measurable response (figure 12.12B). The postreceptoral contributions contributed 10–15 μV to the response over much of its range, causing the proportion of the response that was of

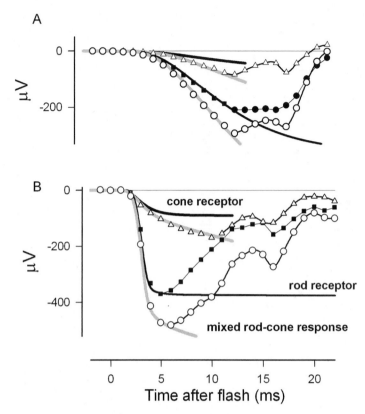

A

B

cone receptor

rod receptor

mixed rod-cone response

Time after flash (ms)

FIGURE 12.13 Dark-adapted ERG of a macaque showing the mixed rod-cone a-wave and separate components measured (symbols) and modeled (solid lines fit to the leading edge of the a-wave) for two stimulus strengths. A, Responses of an anesthetized macaque are shown to a brief blue LED flash of 188 sc td.s (57 ph td.s). B, Responses are shown to a xenon white flash of 59,000 sc td.s (34,000 ph td.s). In both parts, the largest response (open circles) is the entire mixed rod-cone a-wave; the solid line restricted to the leading edge shows the modeled mixed rod/cone response. The second largest response is the (isolated) rod-driven response (solid circles); the solid line through the leading edge is the modeled rod postreceptoral origin. The second-to-smallest response (open triangles) is the (isolated) cone-driven response, including the postreceptoral contribution; the solid line through the leading edge shows the modeled cone-driven response. The smallest is the modeled cone photoreceptor contribution, based on post-PDA findings for the cone-driven response. Given the animal's 8.5-mm pupil, the stimulus for part A was about $1\,cd\,m^{-2}\,s$, that is, about 10 times less intense (for cones) than ISCEV standard flash of $10\,cd\,m^{-2}\,s$, whereas the stimulus for part B is about 600 times stronger. (Source: From Robson JG, Saszik S, Ahmed J, Frishman LJ.[195] Used by permission.)

postreceptoral origin to decline from about 50% when the response was $20\,\mu V$, a common size in clinical recordings, to about 25% when the a-wave was saturated.

More recent studies indicate that under stimulus conditions similar to those used by Sieving and colleagues, the photopic a-wave in the macaque also will be reduced, almost as much as by PDA, by injection of the glutamate agonist NMDA (N-methyl-D-aspartate) (Frishman, unpublished observations). NMDA selectively activates NMDA receptors, which are ionotropic glutamate receptors found on amacrine and retinal ganglion cells, and in doing so, depolarizes the cells so that their activity is no longer altered by light stimulation. Under some stimulus conditions, blockade of Na^+-dependent action potentials of inner retinal neurons (amacrine and ganglion cells) by tetrodotoxin (TTX) will also reduce the photopic a-wave.[185,239]

Postreceptoral contributions to the dark-adapted a-wave have also been demonstrated in monkey[95,193,195] as well as in human[53,90,91,177] and cat ERGs.[191,192] Stimuli that are just strong enough to elicit an a-wave will be dominated by rod signals, but a strong flash from darkness will elicit a mixed rod-cone ERG like the one illustrated in figure 12.13 for one monkey. Therefore, it is necessary to separate the rod-driven and cone-driven contributions to responses to strong stimuli from darkness in investigating relative contributions from the different receptor systems and their postreceptoral pathways to the ERG.

The rod-driven response can be extracted by subtracting the isolated cone-driven response to the same stimulus from the mixed rod-cone response. The isolated cone-driven responses in figure 12.13 (triangles) were obtained by briefly suppressing the rod response with an adapting flash and then measuring response to the original test stimulus presented a few hundred milliseconds (300 ms) after offset of the adapting flash. Cone-driven responses in primates will recover to full amplitude within about 300 ms, whereas the rod

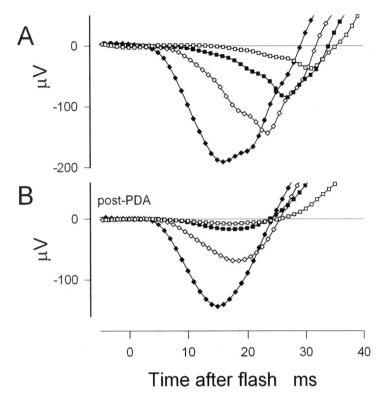

FIGURE 12.14 Postreceptoral contribution to rod-driven dark-adapted macaque ERG. Rod-driven responses from an anesthetized macaque were obtained after subtracting isolated cone-driven response from the mixed rod-cone ERG. Rod-driven responses are shown to a range of stimulus energies (15.8–509 sc td.s) before (A) and after (B) intravitreal injection of PDA (4 mM). (Source: From Robson JG, Saszik S, Ahmed J, Frishman LJ.[195] Used by permission.)

responses will take at least a second, making it possible to isolate the cone-driven response.[195]

The effect of intravitreal PDA on the rod-isolated a-wave of the macaque is shown in figure 12.14 for a range of stimulus strengths. Most of the leading edge of the a-wave in response to the weakest stimulus was eliminated (top trace of figure 12.14), and much of the a-wave occurring later than about 15 ms after the flash was removed in response to stronger stimuli (lower traces); this was true for even stronger stimuli that saturate the response (e.g., figure 12.13B). It is important to note that PDA blocks signal transmission not only to hyperpolarizing bipolar and horizontal cells, but also to inner retinal amacrine and ganglion cells. Results in the presence of NMDA, which is used to selectively suppress inner retinal responses, were similar in both monkey and cat dark-adapted ERG to those after PDA, indicating an inner retinal origin for most of the rod-driven contributions (data not shown). APB did not reduce the a-wave, indicating that the effects of NMDA on the a-wave were due to suppression of inner retinal OFF, rather than ON, circuitry.

For comparison, the effects of PDA on isolated dark-adapted cone-driven responses are shown in figure 12.15. As was found in previously described studies by Bush and Sieving,[26] for the light-adapted cone-driven ERG, PDA reduced the amplitude of the a-wave of the dark-adapted cone-driven response as well. (The light-adapted cone-driven ERG for the same animal was similar to the dark-adapted response, but the PDA-sensitive portion was slightly smaller in the light-adapted response.) Figure 12.15 also shows that PDA-sensitive postreceptoral contributions were present at much earlier times (starting around 5 ms after the flash) for the cone-driven response than for the rod driven responses where they appeared around 15 ms after the flash (see figure 12.14).

The time course of the photoreceptor response The leading edge of the a-wave is the only visible portion of the photoreceptor response in the normal ERG. To see the whole time course of the photoreceptor response directly, it is necessary to eliminate the postreceptoral contributions, as was done by Bush and Sieving[26] for the photopic ERG in figure 12.12A, for example. However, such a manipulation is invasive and will not eliminate the photoreceptor-dependent, glia-mediated slow PIII or the c-wave, should they be present. Another approach to use is the paired flash technique developed by Pepperberg and colleagues[181] to derive, in vivo, the photoreceptor response. The approach is described in detail in chapter 37. The full time course of the derived photoreceptor response is shown for three different stimulus strengths for a macaque monkey in figure 12.16. The

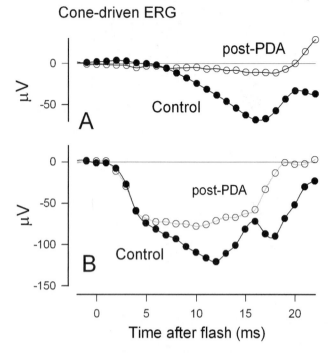

Cone-driven ERG

FIGURE 12.15 Postreceptoral contributions to cone-driven dark-adapted macaque ERG. Dark-adapted cone-driven responses from an anesthetized macaque obtained in response to a stimulus of ~15,000 ph td.s applied 300 ms after a 1-second rod-saturating adapting light (2500 sc td) was turned off. Results after intravitreal injection of PDA are denoted by the solid symbols. (Source: From Robson JG, Saszik S, Ahmed J, Frishman LJ.[195] Used by permission.)

derived photoreceptor response is similar in time course to current recordings from isolated rod photoreceptors outer segments in the macaque,[10] although it reaches its peak a little earlier in vivo than in vitro. This figure shows that the photoreceptor response is quite large at its peak time even when the leading edge cannot be seen. More generally, the figure nicely illustrates the overlapping nature of the ERG components from different stages of retinal processing.

Origins of the b-wave

The largest component of the diffuse flash ERG is the cornea-positive b-wave, initially identified in the dark-adapted ERG of the cat as PII by Granit.[25] There is general consensus that the b-wave is related primarily to the activity of depolarizing (ON) bipolar cells.[79,112,191,224] Although influences on the b-wave of third-order neurons has been reported both in cold-blooded animals[6] and mammals,[43] this section will focus on the major generator(s). Until recently, the relative contributions from transmembrane currents of the bipolar cells versus spatial buffer currents of Müller cells (caused by K+ outflow from the bipolar cells) have remained unresolved. Although there is experimental support for a

Müller cell contribution (as reviewed below), there is now strong evidence that the b-wave (at least the scotopic ERG of mammalian retinas) to a large extent directly reflects bipolar cell currents, the contribution from Müller cells being smaller than was previously thought.[106,191,194,252]

The issue of how the b-wave is generated has long occupied the efforts of retinal physiologists. Early work determined that the b-wave was generated by the neural retina, proximal to the photoreceptors. Application of compounds that block synaptic transmission, for example, Mg^{2+}, Co^{2+}, and Na^{2+}-aspartate, abolished the b-wave but left photoreceptor responses intact.[45,62,204] Occlusion of the central retinal artery in primates, which supplies oxygen to the neural retina proximal to the photoreceptors, also abolished the b-wave but spared photoreceptor responses.[18]

Identification of the exact cell(s) in the postreceptoral neural retina that generate the b-wave has been a more difficult task. Early evidence from intraretinal depth recordings of local ERGs made with microelectrodes[3] (figure 12.17) demonstrated that the intraretinal b-wave was negative-going with a negative peak amplitude in the distal retina near the outer plexiform layer (OPL), and the largest change in its amplitude occurred across the inner nuclear layer (INL).[3,19,20,226,228] These results suggested that the b-wave was generated by current flowing through a radially oriented cell that acted as a dipole. Bipolar cells, which are the only radially oriented neurons that span the INL, were thus implicated. However, it was noted early on that Müller cells also are radially oriented, and they span the entire width of the neural retina, from the inner limiting membrane (ILM) to past the outer limiting membrane (OLM).[49,138] On the basis of studies described below, it was suggested that Müller cells are a likely generator of the b-wave (reviewed by Newman[152]) (figure 12.18).

MÜLLER CELL HYPOTHESIS

Current source density analysis and intracellular recordings Faber[49] computed CSD profiles for the b-wave from intraretinal ERG recordings in rabbit retina and found a current sink near the OPL and a current source extending from the sink all the way to the vitreal surface. He reasoned that this source-sink pattern must arise from current flow through Müller cells. A CSD analysis of the b-wave (and the a-wave; see figure 12.11) in the intact monkey eye[85] yielded results similar to those in rabbits.

In CSD analyses of b-wave generation in frog retina, Newman[149,150] provided greater detail. He found that the frog b-wave was generated principally by two current sinks located near the IPL and OPL and by a large current source at the ILM (figure 12.17). He estimated that 65% of the transretinal b-wave response in the frog was generated by the OPL current sink, which had a more transient time course than the IPL sink.

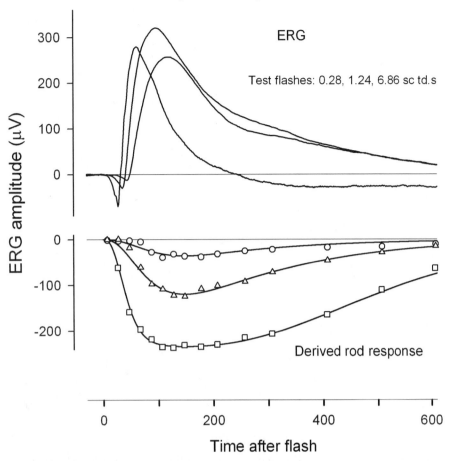

Dark-adapted macaque

ERG

Test flashes: 0.28, 1.24, 6.86 sc td.s

Derived rod response

Time after flash

FIGURE 12.16 Dark-adapted ERG response of the anesthetized macaque monkey to three different test stimulus strengths (0.28, 1.24, and 6.86 sc td.s) and the derived rod photoreceptor response for each test stimulus. The photoreceptor response was derived by using the paired flash approach of Pepperberg et al.,[180] as is described in chapter 37, and the model lines used modifications of equations from Robson et al.[28] (Source: Unpublished observations: Frishman LJ, Robson JG.)

The Müller cell hypothesis also received support from the work of Miller and Dowling,[138] who monitored the intracellular responses of Müller cells of the mud puppy retina during b-wave generation (figure 12.19). They found that the Müller cell and b-wave responses had similar latencies, time courses (under certain conditions), and responses to flickering stimuli. Both had a dynamic range of approximately five decades, much larger than the one and one half to two decade dynamic range of some retinal neurons.

Both Faber[49] and Miller and Dowling[138] suggested that current flow through Müller cells was generated by light-evoked variations in extracellular K^+ concentration ($[K^+]_o$). They proposed that a light-evoked increase in $[K^+]_o$ in the distal neural retina would lead to an influx of K^+ into Müller cells in this retinal region. This K^+ influx would depolarize Müller cells and drive an equal amount of K^+ out from more proximal regions of the cell. The return current flowing through extracellular space from proximal to distal retina would generate a vitreal-positive transretinal (and corneal)

potential: the b-wave (see figure 12.18 and the introduction to this chapter).

Measurements of changes in light-evoked $[K^+]_o$ Measurements of light-evoked $[K^+]_o$ made with K^+-selective microelectrodes lent support to the Müller cell model. Oakley and Green[167] and Karwoski and coworkers[100,103] (figure 12.20) demonstrated a large, sustained $[K^+]_o$ increases in the IPL of the amphibian retina at the onset and offset of a light stimulus. $[K^+]_o$ measurements in skate,[110] amphibian,[39,40,100,107,111,245] and rabbit[57] retinas identified a second, more transient, $[K^+]_o$ increase in the OPL at light onset (figure 12.20).

The source of the distal light-evoked $[K^+]_o$ increase was believed to be depolarizing bipolar cells, which are only cells with dendrites in the OPL that depolarize and thus release K^+ on light stimulation.[41] L-APB (or AP4), the glutamate analogue that binds to glutamate (mGluR6) receptors on depolarizing (ON) bipolar cells,[215] abolishes the b-wave in amphibian and mammalian retinas, including those of

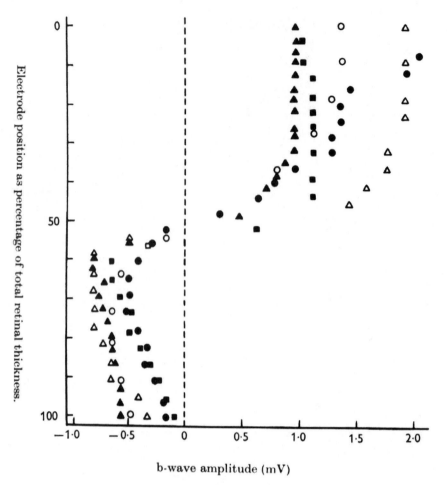

FIGURE 12.17 Amplitude of the b-wave recorded with an intraretinal electrode in the intact cat eye. B-wave amplitude is plotted as a function of retinal depth, with 0% corresponding to the inner limiting membrane (INL) and 100% to the retinal pigment epithelium. The b-wave response reaches its maximal negative amplitude in the outer plexiform layer (OPL)

and undergoes its greatest change in amplitude in the INL. Data are from five separate electrode penetrations (indicated by different symbols). The vitreous humor was replaced by a nonconducting oil, and responses were referenced to an electrode in the mouth. (Source: From Arden GB, Brown KT.[3] Used by permission.)

primates,[58,112,133,224] as well as the ON-response of Müller cells.[260] (For teleost retinas, however, at least some ON bipolar cells have another mechanism for depolarization in response to light.[33,197])

The larger, more prolonged IPL $[K^+]_o$ increase is believed to result from amacrine and ganglion cell depolarization,[41,59,60,104,203] although bipolar cells may contribute.[60,224] This proximal $[K^+]_o$ increase is now understood to contribute primarily to Müller cell–mediated ERG components of proximal retinal origin, that is, M-wave and STR (see later sections of this chapter).

As was described in the introduction to this chapter, the selective permeability of Müller cell membrane to K^+ and the nonuniform distribution of K^+ conductances (see figure 12.2), creates the opportunity for K^+ siphoning from synaptic layers of the retina to the regions of lower $[K^+]_o$. In species with avascular retinas, including fish,[154] amphibians,[15,152,153,157] and rabbits,[153,188] the Müller cell endfoot ad-

jacent to the vitreous humor has a much larger K^+ conductance than do other regions of the cell, as is shown in Newman's[153] study of enzymatically isolated Müller cells subjected to puffs of K^+ (figure 12.21). Because much of the endfoot conductance is only weakly rectifying (essentially bidirectional; see figure 12.2), K^+ entering the Müller cell via strongly inward rectifying channels in synaptic regions will exit predominately from the endfoot.[114,115] In species with avascular retinas, a $[K^+]_o$ increase in the OPL will establish a current loop that extends all the way to the vitreal surface (see figure 12.18). A $[K^+]_o$ increase in the IPL will contribute to the same current loop, creating a vitreal-positive proximally generated potential (M-wave) in addition to the bipolar cell–dependent b-wave.[39]

In species with vascularized retinas such as the mouse and monkey, K^+ conductance is high at the endfoot but is greatest in the INL, near the capillaries. In cat retina, K^+ conductance is greatest distally near the subretinal space (figure

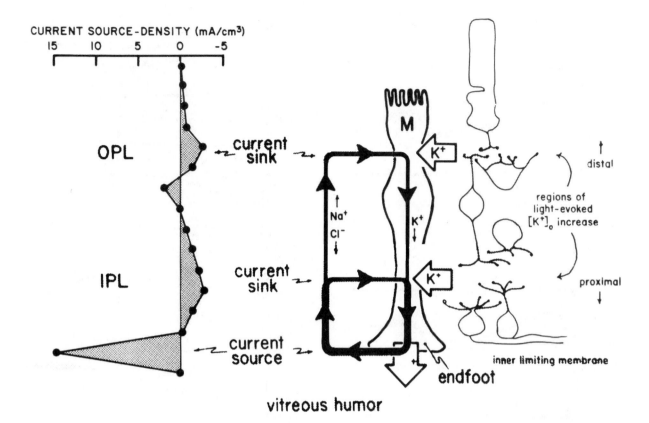

FIGURE 12.18 CSD profile and the Müller cell-K⁺ hypothesis of b-wave generation. Left, CSD profile of the b-wave. Data are from a single penetration of the frog retina (eyecup preparation). The b-wave in this species is generated by current sinks in IPL and OPL and by a large current source at the ILM. Right, summary of the Müller cell K⁺ hypothesis of b-wave generation. Light-evoked K⁺ increases in the IPL and OPL generate an influx of K⁺ into Müller cells in these retinal layers (open arrows). This current influx is balanced by a current efflux from the cell endfoot, which has high K⁺ conductance. The return current flow through extracellular space (solid lines) generates the b-wave (M, Müller cell; OPL, outer plexiform layer; INL, inner nuclear layer). (Source: From Newman EA.[152] Used by permission.)

12.21). In these species, the Müller cell current that arises as a consequence of a proximal K⁺ increase is likely to contribute to a distally directed current loop and to produce a corneal-negative potential (e.g., the negative STR[58,59]).

Newman and Odette[159] produced a quantitative model and computer simulations for the frog b-wave that supported the K⁺ Müller cell hypothesis. However, the model and CSD analysis on which it was based (figure 12.18), predicted a distal $[K^+]_o$ increase substantially greater than that observed in ion-selective electrode measurements.[169] This raised the possibility that the b-wave is not entirely generated by distal K⁺ affecting Müller cells. Other evidence described just below provided stronger evidence that much of the b-wave is directly due to bipolar cell currents.

THE ON BIPOLAR CELL AS THE GENERATOR OF THE b-WAVE
Experiments using Ba²⁺ pointed to a bipolar cell generator of the b-wave. Ba²⁺ effectively blocks inward-rectifying K⁺ channels (Kir) in Müller cells[155] and therefore should abolish ERG components generated by K⁺ current flow through Müller cells. Ba²⁺ has been shown to block slow PIII[12] as well

as other responses associated with Müller cell currents: the M-wave[60,101,252] and the STR.[58] However, Ba²⁺ was far less effective in blocking the b-wave.[31,58,105,248,252]

Even more definitive evidence came from the use of Ba²⁺ in combination with CSD studies in frogs[252] and later in rabbits.[106] As is illustrated in figure 12.22A, Xu and Karwoski[252] measured depth profiles of ERGs before and after application of Ba²⁺. Ba²⁺ removed the proximal negative-going responses at light onset and offset corresponding to the M-wave, but the negative-going responses in more distal retina that formed the b-wave remained. Xu and Karwoski also made local tissue resistance measurements under both conditions so that they could calculated sources and sinks for the frog b-wave based on microelectrode recordings. As is shown in figure 12.22B, in the presence of Ba²⁺, at least two thirds of the OPL sink was retained, and the IPL source involved in generating the b-wave was enhanced. Only the proximal sink-source activity associated with the M-wave was removed. These results indicated that the major b-wave generator is the bipolar cell itself rather than the Müller cell.

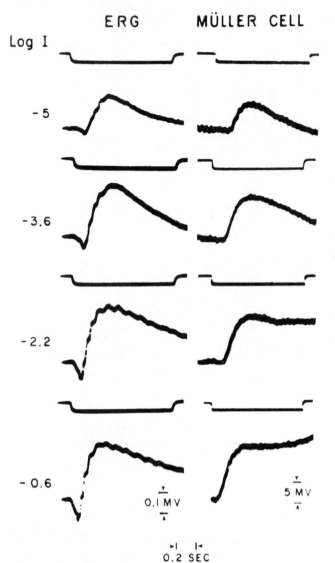

FIGURE 12.19 Intracellular Müller cell responses (right column) and the ERG (left column) recorded from the mud puppy (eyecup preparation). Both the negative a-wave and the larger, positive b-wave are seen in the ERG records. The time course of the Müller cell responses resemble those of the b-wave, particularly at the lower stimulus intensities (−5 and −3.6). Stimulus intensity is given to the left of the traces. (Source: From Miller RF, Dowling JE.[138] Used by permission.)

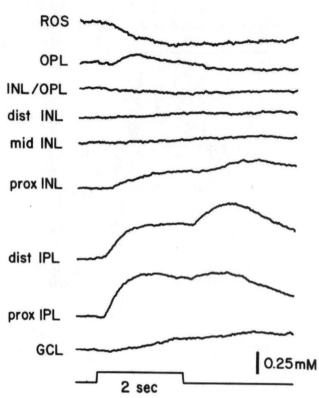

FIGURE 12.20 Light-evoked variations in $[K^+]_o$ recorded at different depths in the frog retina (retinal slice preparation). Increases in $[K^+]_o$ are maximal within the inner plexiform (IPL) and the outer plexiform (OPL) layers. The $[K^+]_o$ increase in the IPL has both ON and OFF components. The $[K^+]_o$ increase in the OPL occurs only at stimulus ON and is more transient. (Source: From Karwoski CJ, Newman EA, Shimazaki H, Proenza LM: *Gen Physiol* 1985; 86:189–213. Used by permission.)

DARK-ADAPTED, ROD-DRIVEN b-WAVE Experiments in which the PII component of the scotopic ERG was pharmacologically isolated from other ERG components also have lent support to the idea that bipolar cell current contributes directly to b-wave. In the mammalian retina, the scotopic ERG response to weak stimuli will reflect activity of elements of the sensitive rod circuit, such as the STR (see figure 12.9). With inner retinal contributions from the amacrine and ganglion cells pharmacologically suppressed, the isolated b-wave (PII) should reflect the rod bipolar cell

contribution, either directly as the bipolar cell current or via K^+ currents in Müller cells resulting from the depolarization of the bipolar cell and the release of K^+. Figure 12.23A shows pharmacologically isolated PII from four normal mouse retinas in response to a very weak stimulus; an intravitreal injection of the inhibitory neurotransmitter γ-aminobutyric acid (GABA) was used to suppress inner retinal activity.[194,199] The isolated PII responses have been superimposed on an average of several patch electrode current recordings in a mouse retinal slice preparation of responses of rod bipolar cells to a stimulus of similar effect on the rods. The time courses of the ERG and single-cell current are remarkably similar. The similarity of the time course supports the view that the isolated PII reflects rod bipolar cell activity. If Müller cell currents generated the PII response to this stimulus in mouse retina, the signal would be expected to be delayed, owing to the time necessary for accumulation of K^+ ions in the extracellular space. A similarity in time course of the intracellular and extracellular recordings was shown even more directly by Sheills and Falk, who compared

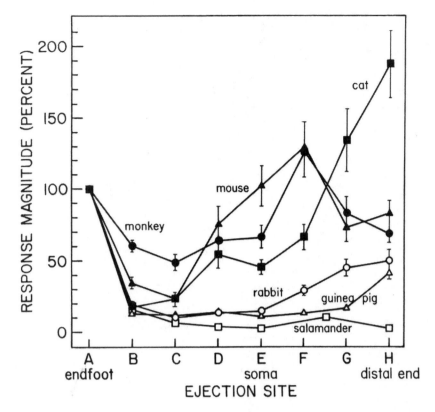

FIGURE 12.21   Distribution of K⁺ conductance over the surface of enzymatically dissociated Müller cells. The magnitude of cell depolarizations in response to focal K⁺ ejections are plotted as a function of ejection location along the cell surface. Responses are normalized to response magnitude at the endfoot. In species with avascular retinas (salamander, rabbit, guinea pig), K⁺ conductance is largest at the endfoot. In vascularized species, conductance is largest near the cell soma (mouse, monkey) or at the distal end of the cell (cat). (Source: From Newman EA.[153] Used by permission.)

intracellular recordings from rod bipolar cells and extracellular recordings of the ERG b-wave in dogfish retina.[202]

Pharmacologically isolated PII in the cat (figure 12.23B) (in this case, using NMDA to suppress inner retinal responses; see the figure legend) revealed a response similar to that in mouse in its rising phase, but the response showed a slower recovery to baseline. The cat PII response to a brief flash can be analyzed into a fast component and a slow component that is a low-pass-filtered version of the fast component, and these are shown by the lines in the figure. Intravitreal Ba^{2+} was used to test the hypothesis that the fast component is the direct bipolar cell contribution and the slow component is the K⁺ current in the Müller cell. The inset to the figure shows that Ba^{2+} eliminated a slow portion of the response that was very similar in time course to the modeled slow component. This suggests that bipolar cell current dominates the leading edge of PII in the cat ERG and that the Müller cell current contributes at later times. Pharmacologic isolation of macaque PII showed a similar waveform to that in cat (not shown). It is interesting to note that although the amplitude of the slower component (in response to a brief flash) was lower than that of the faster one, the area under the two curves was similar. With longer stimulus durations, such as those used in early studies of the b-wave origins, the contribution to the ERG of the two sources would be about equal.[193]

CONE-DRIVEN b-WAVE   The scotopic ERG response to weak stimuli is predominantly rod-driven. When strong stimuli are presented from darkness, cone signals also contribute to the response (e.g., figure 12.12). This mixed rod cone b-wave was as first described by Motokawa and Mita[144] for the human ERG. A sharp positive peak was observed to occur prior to the more prolonged major portion of the b-wave in response to intense flashes from darkness. The sharp peak due to cone signals, called the x-wave (or b1), could be distinguished from the slower rod response (b2) by its sensitivity to long-wavelength stimuli.[1,2,144]

The photopic ERG is more commonly measured in the presence of a rod-suppressing background. The depth profile of the rod b-wave measured under dark-adapted conditions and the cone b-wave measured under light-adapted conditions are similar in cat[207,208] and monkey retinas,[85] suggesting a similar origin for the two responses, but in the case of the photopic ERG, depolarizing cone rather than rod bipolar cells would be involved in generation of the response.

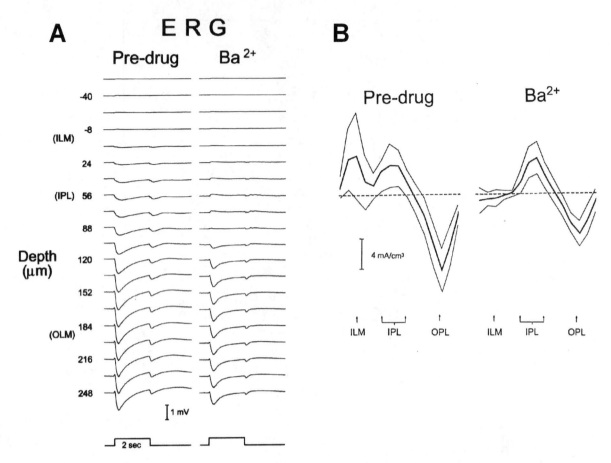

A

ERG

Pre-drug   Ba²⁺

-40

(ILM)   -8

24

(IPL) 56

88

Depth (μm)   120

152

(OLM) 184

216

248

1 mV

2 sec

B

Pre-drug   Ba²⁺

4 mA/cm³

ILM   IPL   OPL   ILM   IPL   OPL

FIGURE 12.22 Effects of Ba^{2+} on the b-wave in the frog retina: Depth profiles and CSD analyses. A, Depth profiles: The electrode was advanced to the RPE and then withdrawn in 16-mM steps (left). Then the electrode was advanced again, and Ba^{2+} (100 mM) was applied for about 10 minutes until responses were stable, and the withdrawal series was repeated. The retinal surface was at 0 mm retinal depth. Note the reversal of the signal in proximal retina after Ba^{2+} consistent with the presence of a dipole current generating the b-wave with a sink in the OLM and a source in the IPL. B, CSDs calculated at the time of the b-wave peak in the OPL: Mean (+/−) CSD profiles were obtained before Ba^{2+} (predrug) and during Ba^{2+}. The sink in IPL and the source at the ILM that generate the M-wave were eliminated by Ba^{2+}. The findings show that the Ba^{2+}-resistant OPL sink and IPL source generated a large portion of the b-wave. The sink in IPL and the source at the ILM that generate the M-wave were eliminated by Ba^{2+}. (Source: From Xu X, Karwoski CJ.[252] Used by permission.)

The origins of the photopic b-wave of the macaque retina were studied by Sieving and collaborators using glutamate analogues in the same series of experiments as those described in the previous section, in which the a-wave was examined. Figure 12.24 (from Bush and Sieving[26]) shows, on the right, the macaque photopic ERG response to long-duration flashes, before and after APB was injected intravitreally (eye 1, left). APB removed the transient b-wave, supporting an origin of this response in depolarizing bipolar cells. However, when PDA was injected first in another eye (eye 2, right), to remove the OFF pathway (and horizontal cell inhibitory feedback), a much larger and more sustained b-wave was revealed. These findings indicate that transient nature of the peak of the cone b-wave in control recordings was due to truncation of a more prolonged depolarizing bipolar cell response. The truncation under control condi-

tions was due either to addition of PDA-sensitive OFF pathways' response of opposite polarity in the ERG (a push-pull effect[209]) or to inhibition via PDA-sensitive horizontal cell feedback onto cones of ON bipolar cell signals. The isolated photoreceptor response that remained after all postreceptoral activity was eliminated by APB followed by PDA (or PDA followed by APB) was similar for the two eyes.

d.c. COMPONENT OF THE b-WAVE   The b-wave is only one of the two positive ERG components that Granit[74] called PII. The other, which has been studied only in mammals, is a sensitive steady potential termed the *d.c. component*.[18,20] The d.c. component continues at reduced amplitude after the transient response (the b-wave) and then decays at stimulus offset. As shown in a series of ERG records from the intact

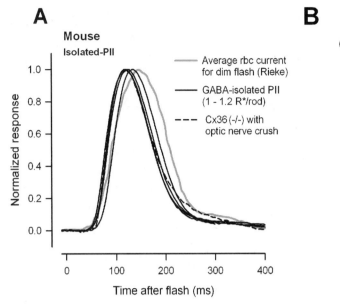

A

Mouse
Isolated-PII

Legend:
— Average rbc current for dim flash (Rieke)
— GABA-isolated PII (1 - 1.2 R*/rod)
--- Cx36 (-/-) with optic nerve crush

Normalized response (y-axis): 0.0, 0.2, 0.4, 0.6, 0.8, 1.0
Time after flash (ms) (x-axis): 0, 100, 200, 300, 400

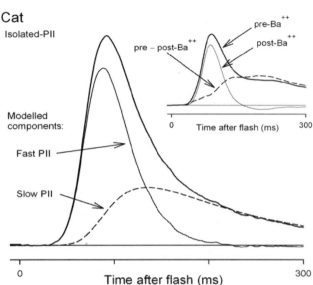

B

Cat
Isolated-PII

Modelled components:
Fast PII
Slow PII

Inset labels: pre-Ba++, pre – post-Ba++, post-Ba++

Time after flash (ms): 0, 300

FIGURE 12.23 Pharmacologically isolated PII in mouse and cat ERG. A, Mouse PII, isolated using intravitreally inected GABA compared with an average of several patch electrode current recordings from rod bipolar cells in a mouse retinal slice preparation (Courtesy of F. Rieke); the time courses are remarkable similar. (Source: From Robson JG, Maeda H, Saszik S, Frishman LJ.[194] Used by permission.) B, Pharmacologically isolated cat PII (by inner retinal blockade). The response has been analyzed into a fast component, proposed to be a direct reflection of the postsynaptic current, and a slow component that is a low-pass-filtered version of the faster com-

ponent, believed to be the Müller-cell response, contributing mainly to the tail of the response. Identification of the Müller-cell component is corroborated by the observation (shown in the inset) that intravitreal injection of Ba^{2+} to block K^+ channels in Müller cells removes a similar part of the total PII response. Note that if stronger stimuli were used, to see the bipolar cell response alone, it would be necessary also to remove the underlying negative (photoreceptor) PIII signal, which can be done by subtracting the APB-sensitive component. (Source: From Robson JG, Frishman LJ[193] and unpublished observations of Frishman LJ, Robson JG. Used by permission.)

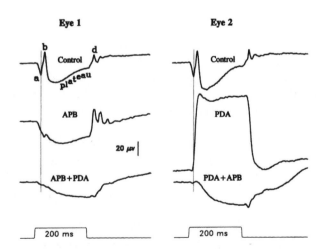

Eye 1 — Control, APB, APB+PDA (labels: b, d, a, plateau)
Eye 2 — Control, PDA, PDA+APB
20 µv
200 ms

FIGURE 12.24 Effects of APB and PDA on the light-adapted photopic ERG of two monkey eyes. Drugs were given sequentially, APB followed by PDA for eye 1, and PDA followed by APB for eye 2. The vertical line shows the time of the a-wave trough in the control response. The 200-ms stimulus was 3.76 logtd (2.01 logcd/m²) on a steady rod-saturating background of 3.3 logtd (1.55 cd/m²). (Source: From Bush RA, Sieving PA.[26] Used by permission.)

cat eye (figure 12.25), the d.c. component is the most sensitive positive component in the figure. It is only about 1.5 log units less sensitive than the very sensitive negative, scotopic threshold response (STR). For stronger stimuli, PII dominates the ERG, and above 7.1 log q deg⁻² s⁻¹, it peaks to form the b-wave. The d.c. component has a similar depth distribution to the b-wave in cats[207,208] and monkeys,[19] and in a CSD analysis performed in monkeys, it also had a similar source-sink distribution to the b-wave (see figure 12.3[85]). However, experiments in cats[19,219] showed that d.c. component was separable from the b-wave because (1) it was unaffected by low doses of intravitreal lidocaine whereas the b-wave was removed, (2) the d.c. component summed over a smaller area than the b-wave, and (3) the d.c. component was relatively less suppressed by light-adaptation than the b-wave. In fact, in the monkey, the d.c. component was more easily detected in the light-adapted retina, and it was under light-adapted conditions that depth and CSD analyses[84,85] (shown in figure 12.3) were performed. It is still unresolved whether the b-wave and d.c.-components have separate neuronal origins.

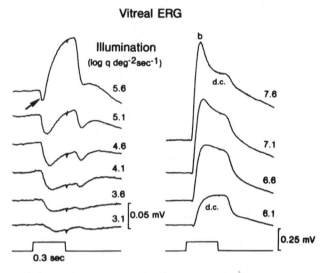

Vitreal ERG

FIGURE 12.25 Dark-adapted ERG recorded from an intact cat eye with an electrode in the vitreous humor. Responses are to diffuse stimuli of increasing illumination. The b-wave (b) is indicated at $7.6 \log q \deg^2 s^{-1}$. The dc component (d.c.) of the PII-dominated ERG is seen clearly in records 6.1, 6.6, and 7.1. An arrow marks where the STR (truncated by the d.c. component) resembles the a-wave. (Source: From Sieving PA, Frishman LJ. Steinberg RH.[207] Used by permission.)

Origins of the d-wave

The d-wave is a positive-going deflection in the ERG at light offset that is a characteristic of the photopic ERG. The d-wave of the primate (human and macaque) photopic ERG can be seen in figure 12.1 and again for the macaque in figures 12.9, 12.12A, and 12.24. Although positive d-waves have been described in the scotopic ERG of some species, they are probably not "true" d-waves that, as described below, include a strong contribution from the depolarizing response at light offset of hyperpolarizing (OFF) cone bipolar cells. For example, in amphibians, Tomita et al.[229] argued that the rod-specific positive "d-wave" has a long latency and is probably the e-wave rather than the d-wave (see the later section on the e-wave). In cats, Granit[74] described a d-wave in the predominantly rod-driven ERG, but an analysis by Brown[17] showed that this "d-wave" occurred only in response to the offset of very intense and long-duration stimuli. For these stimuli, the decay of the rod receptor potential appeared as a small positive deflection that followed, at light offset, the negative-going offset of PII.[17]

Although the d-wave is present in responses of vertebrates from amphibians to mammals, it has received less study than the prominent components at light onset (a- and b-waves). In part, this may be because the d-wave is small in mixed retinas that have more rods than cones. In animals in which the d-wave is prominent, researchers have traditionally pre-

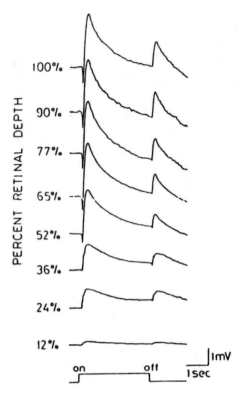

FIGURE 12.26 Depth series recordings of ERGs in isolated frog retina. The b- and d-waves are recorded at all depths, whereas the a-wave is seen only in the receptor layer and the distal part of the inner nuclear layer. The d-wave is relatively sharp at the depths where the a-wave is present, which is compatible with the OFF response of the late receptor potential contributing to the d-wave. More proximally, where the d-wave is slower, the receptor contribution may be less, and other postreceptoral contributions may be more important. (Source: From Yanagida I, Koshimizu M, Kawasaki K.[254] Used by permission.)

sented light flashes rather than dark flashes, and to see the d-wave as a separate event, the duration of the flash must be extended. Nevertheless, there is information regarding its origin, originally from cold-blooded species and more recently from pharmacological dissection experiments in macaques.[26,209]

In cold-blooded species, the d-wave is positive-going when recorded at the cornea or in the vitreous and negative-going when recorded intraretinally in the distal half of the retina (figure 12.26), which is consistent with the d-wave including a prominent photoreceptor OFF-response. The positive photoreceptor OFF response has also been in frog and mud puppy transretinal recordings[224,255] after pharmacological blockade of postreceptoral neural activity. However, results from these later studies, as well as others in amphibians, agree that cells that are postsynaptic to the photoreceptors also make a major contribution to the d-wave.[6,252,253]

CSD analyses by Xu and Karwoski[253] using dark flashes to evoke spatiotemporal profiles of the d-wave in frog retina

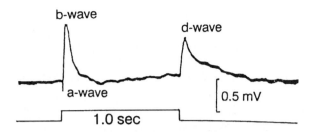

FIGURE 12.27 ERG from the all-cone retina of the squirrel. Recordings were made under light-adapted conditions between a contact lens electrode on the cornea and an electrode on the forehead. (Source: From Arden GB, Tansley K: *J Physiol* 1955; 127:592–602.)

clearly demonstrated a strong contribution from OFF bipolar cells to the d-wave. In this study, the largest d-wave current was similar to the b-wave current found in previous work of the same investigators[252] (see figure 12.22A). The d-wave had a sink at the outer plexiform layer (OPL sink) and a source at the inner plexiform layer (IPL source). As was found for the b-wave, the d-wave current was relatively insensitive to Ba^{2+} suggesting that it arose directly from OFF bipolar cells rather than from K^+ buffer currents in Müller cells. A contribution of K^+ buffer currents in amphibian to the d-wave has been suggested,[224] and contributions to the d-wave from inner retinal neurons, amacrine cells, or ganglion cells also have been reported.[6]

In mammals, the d-wave is very prominent in the all-cone retina of the ground squirrel (figure 12.27); in the monkey retina with its mixture of rods and cones, the d-wave is not quite as prominent but is still easily identified (e.g., figure 12.24). Intraretinal analysis of the monkey d-wave indicated that it represents a combination of the rapid offset of the cone late receptor potential (which is positive going), followed by the negative-going offset of PII component.[16] The distinctive fast offset of the cone receptor potential was viewed clearly by using long-wavelength stimuli under photopic conditions in the monkey after clamping of the retinal circulation to isolate the photoreceptors[17,246] and was seen in excised human retina in the presence of aspartate.[257]

Although the early work on primate ERG cited above did not identify the hyperpolarizing (OFF) bipolar cell as a major contributor to the d-wave, more recent work by Sieving and colleagues has clearly demonstrated that it is an important element of the response.[26,209] In experiments described in previous sections (e.g., figure 12.24), PDA, which blocks responses of OFF bipolar cells, reduced or, when a large b-wave was present, eliminated the d-wave at light offset. The effect of PDA was not replicated by blockade of inner retinal cells by NMDA, which also would have been affected by the PDA, confirming the role of the OFF bipolar cells themselves. PDA also will eliminate a small positive wave that occurs in the falling phase of the b-wave, or

just after it, in the brief flash ERG in monkeys and humans, called the *i-wave*. This wave also is not eliminated by blockade of inner retinal cells.[185]

In summary, the corneal d-wave in primates is largely produced by the depolarization of OFF bipolar cells and the positive-going offset of the late receptor potential. It is further shaped by the negative-going offset of PII. In contrast to cold-blooded species, for primates (and other mammals not presented here), there is little evidence for a positive-going d-wave component that originates in the proximal retina, either directly by neurons or indirectly by K^+ spatial buffering.

Origins of the photopic fast flicker ERG

Traditionally, the human (or macaque) photopic ERG response to fast-flickering stimuli (nominally 30-Hz flicker) was thought to reflect primarily the response of the cone photoreceptors. However, pharmacological dissection studies by Bush and Sieving[27] have shown that most of the response that would be seen clinically with a full-field stimulus is generated postreceptorally. Evidence for the photoreceptor hypothesis in primates came mainly from intraretinal recording studies in monkey fovea by Baron and Boynton[8] and Baron et al.[9] Baron and Boynton[8] found that pharmacological isolation of the cone photoreceptor response by Na^+ aspartate did not alter the phase of the locally recorded photopic fast flicker response. From this observation, they proposed that the fast flicker response reflects cone photoreceptor potentials. This proposal was supported by a subsequent component analysis that indicated independence of the flicker response from inner retinal contributions.[9]

Bush and Sieving[27] used the glutamate analogues APB and PDA to selectively remove postreceptoral ON- and OFF-pathway response as had been done in studies of the origins of the a-, b-, and d-waves described earlier in this chapter (see figures 12.12 and 12.24). Figure 12.28A illustrates the contributions of the OFF pathway after the ON pathway and hence the b-wave was eliminated by APB. Flicker was still present, but the peak was delayed, reflecting the residual contribution of the d-wave. When both APB and PDA were used (figure 12.28B), the flicker response was practically eliminated, similar to the effect of aspartate in their hands (not shown). From experiments of this type, Bush and Sieving concluded that postreceptoral cells that normally produce the b- and d-waves are strong contributors to the photopic fast flicker response. Further experiments on macaques have more thoroughly investigated the interaction of the ON and OFF pathways in the photopic flicker responses over a wide range of temporal frequencies and stimulus conditions[116] and have demonstrated small inner retinal contributions to the response, particularly to the second harmonic component.[239]

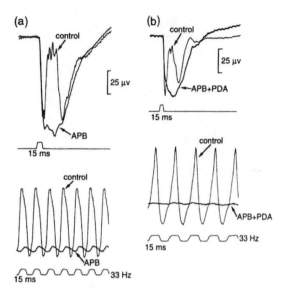

FIGURE 12.28 Postreceptoral origin of the photopic fast flicker ERG of the macaque monkey. Photopic ERG responses to strong (5.8 log Td) stimulus on a rod-saturating steady background of 3.3 log Td recorded before and after (a) APB in one monkey and (b) APB + PDA in another monkey. APB eliminated the b-wave and greatly reduced the flicker response, leaving a delayed response from OFF postreceptoral cells. It had little effect on the a-wave. (b) APB + PDA reduced the a-wave and the OFF response slightly, but most of the leading edge of the a-wave was present. The drugs further reduced the flicker from that observed with APB alone, so very little response was left. (Source: From Bush RA, Sieving PA.[27] Used by permission.)

Origins of the e-wave

The e-wave is a delayed field potential produced at light offset (i.e., a delayed OFF response) that was first recorded in the frog retina[205] and has since been observed in the tadpole,[35] mud puppy (C. J. Karwoski, unpublished observations), and trout.[44] It has been noted in proximal retinal recordings to occur at long latency in amphibia (2 to 60 s following stimulus offset) and has been recorded transretinally only rarely, for example, in frog retina.[158] Because delayed-OFF neuronal responses have been reported in the cat,[220] the e-wave may be present in mammals as well.

The e-wave is present only in dark-adapted retinas, indicating that it is rod-driven; in fact, Tomita et al.[229] have argued that the e-wave is essentially the scotopic version of the d-wave. In response to very intense light flashes, rod photoreceptors generate a large hyperpolarization that returns back to baseline very slowly (rod aftereffect).[220] Karwoski and Newman[102] proposed that this delayed decay of the rod response causes delayed responses in proximal retina cells that are involved in generating the e-wave. They have presented evidence that the e-wave arises, at least in part, from Müller cell spatial buffer currents induced by K+ released by proximal retinal neurons.

Proximal negative response

The proximal negative response (PNR) is a light-evoked field potential that can be recorded in the inner retina. It was named and most fully described by Burkhardt,[23,24] although recordings similar to it had been reported by a few groups since the pioneering studies of Tomita and colleagues[230,231] on the "intraretinal action potential." The PNR consists of a sharp, negative-going transient at the onset and again at the offset of a small light spot (figure 12.29). The spot must be centered precisely on the microelectrode tip. Annular and diffuse illumination elicits complex waveforms that are sometimes dominated instead by positive-going potentials.[24,172] The PNR can be recorded in all vertebrate retinas, including the cat[208] and primates.[172]

Dye-marking studies in birds and amphibians showed that the PNR is maximal in the IPL.[82,99,105] Several lines of evidence suggest that the PNR in amphibians arises from proximal ON/OFF neurons,[105] probably amacrine cells[24] rather than ganglion cells. This proposal is supported by the presence of a normal PNR in rabbit in which ganglion cell degeneration had been induced by optic nerve section (R. F. Miller, D. A. Burkhardt, and R. Dacheux, unpublished observations). The PNR in primates and cats[208] may arise from ON and OFF (amacrine) cells, because these retinas contain relatively few ON/OFF neurons.

In retinas in which an M-wave (see the later section on the M-wave) can be recorded in proximal retina (e.g., amphibians and cats), the PNR is thought to be the fast neuronally generated portion of the response, while the M-wave is the result of spatial buffer currents in Müller cells due to release into the extracellular space of K+ by proximal neurons (see figure 12.2).[60,105]

A PNR contribution to the transretinally recorded ERG is uncertain and necessarily small because the PNR, which is best developed intraretinally in response to a small spot, will be shunted through adjacent low-resistance regions of the retina that are not activated by the light, resulting in little potential drop in the vitreous.

Origins of the m-wave

Like the proximal negative response (PNR), the M-wave is a light-evoked field potential that can be recorded in the proximal retina. It was named and most fully described in studies of amphibians by Karwoski and Proenza,[103,104] although possibly related responses have been reported by several groups since the studies of Arden and Brown[3] and Byzov.[28] The M-wave consists of a slow, negative-going response at both light onset and offset to a small, well-centered spot (figure 12.29). Annular and diffuse illumination elicits complex waveforms in intraretinal recordings, sometimes dominated by the b-wave. The M-wave has also been described in the cat,[57,60,208]

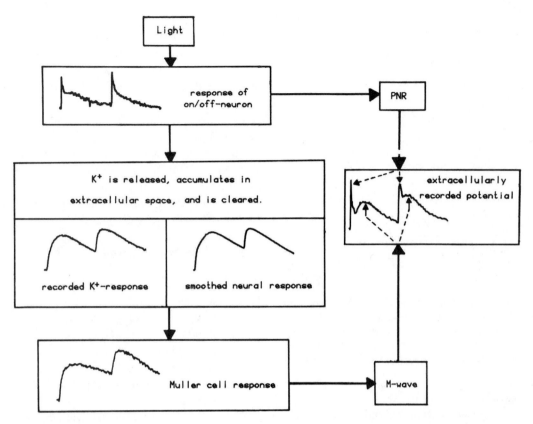

FIGURE 12.29   Summary of events underlying generation of the PNR and M-wave in the proximal retina of the mud puppy. A well-centered small-diameter light stimulus evokes depolarizing responses in ON-OFF neurons (top) whose extracellular currents generate the PNR. The PNR is seen in the extracellularly recorded potential to the right as initial, sharp voltage transients at light onset and offset (negative is up in the extracellular potential). The neurons also release K+, which accumulates in extracellular space and, in turn, depolarizes the Müller cells (bottom). Müller cell spatial buffer currents generate the M-wave, which is seen to the right as slower negative transients at light onset and offset. (Source: From Karwoski CJ, Proenza LM.[104] Used by permission.)

as shown in figures 12.30 and 12.31, and it may be a general feature in the vertebrate retina.

Because the M-wave has maximum amplitude at the same depth as the PNR,[99] it is likely that it originates from events in the IPL. In amphibians, the time course and stimulus dependence of the M-wave are similar to those of intracellular Müller cell responses as well as to light-evoked increases in $[K^+]_o$ in the IPL.[99,103] These similarities are summarized in the model of M-wave generation schematized in figure 12.29: Light evokes responses in proximal neurons, the neurons release K+, and this increase in $[K^+]_o$ generates spatial buffer currents in Müller cells. The model explains most intraretinal features of the M-wave, including its negative polarity. Figure 12.30 shows that certain key features of this model also hold for the M-wave in the cat.[57,60,208] The model receives additional support from experiments in amphibians[101,102] with the K+ channel blocker Ba^{2+}. That has only minor effects on light-evoked neural activity. The light-evoked increase in $[K^+]_o$ in the proximal retina is also little changed by Ba^{2+}, but it blocks Müller cell K+ conductance, K+ spatial buffering by Müller cells, and the M-wave.[98a,101]

In the cat retina in figure 12.31,[60] Ba^{2+} can be seen to eliminate the M-wave but the light-evoked $[K^+]_o$ increases in the proximal retina are still present, indicating that light-evoked neuronal activity was also present. The proximal $[K^+]_o$ increases were larger in the presence of Ba^{2+}, but the more distal increases were absent, consistent with blockade by Ba^{2+} of spatial buffer currents that normally would carry the K+ away from proximal retina to distal retina where $[K^+]_o$ was lower.

The M-wave contribution to the normal transretinal ERG in amphibians is positive-going[107] because, as was explained in the section on the b-wave (see figure 12.21), in the avascular retina of amphibian, spatial buffer currents in Müller cells flow mainly toward the vitreal endfoot, which produces a positive wave in the vitreous. In the cat, with its vascular retina, the M-wave response to small spots may contribute a small negative-going potential to the flash ERG, but any such contribution is small[208] because the local response to a spot would make only a small contribution to the ERG.

The contribution of the M-wave to the ERG may be greater when periodic stimuli such as grating patterns that

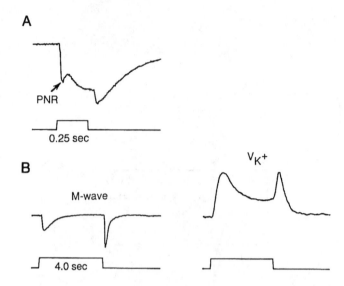

FIGURE 12.30 The PNR, M-wave, and light-evoked increases in extracelluar potassium concentration ($[K^+]_o$) recorded in the proximal retina of the cat. A, Recording of the M-wave with an unusually large initial transient following stimulus onset that has the appearance of the PNR in cold-blooded animals (arrow) (flash diameter: 0.8 degree; background illumination: $9.7 \log q \deg^{-2} s^{-1}$; flash illumination: $10.8 \log q \deg^{-2} s^{-1}$). (Source: Adapted from Sieving PA, Frishman LJ, Steinberg RH.[208]) B, M-wave and V_{K+} recorded simultaneously with a double-barreled K^+-selective microelectrode. The maximum K^+ increase was about 0.18 mM for the ON response. Other details are similar to those in A. (Source: Adapted from Frishman LJ, Sieving PA, Steinberg RH.[57])

stimulate large regions of retina are used. Sieving and Steinberg[211] showed that the M-wave is tuned to a spot diameter similar to the bar width of the optimal spatial frequency for the intraretinal pattern ERG in the cat and suggested that the M-wave may also contribute to the pattern ERG recorded at the cornea.

In contrast to the PNR (and M-wave), negative-going responses from proximal retina to full-field stimulation are present in the light-adapted and dark-adapted corneal ERG of several species, including cats, monkeys, and humans.[207,221,237,241] These responses, called the *photopic negative response* (PhNR), and *scotopic threshold response* (STR), respectively, will be described in the next sections.

Origins of the photopic negative response

The photopic negative response (PhNR) is a negative-going wave that occurs following the b-wave and again after the d-wave in response to a long flash. It is particularly easy to see in responses to red flashes on blue backgrounds in monkeys,[241] humans,[240,241] and cats.[237] The PhNR of the normal macaque ERG is shown in figures 12.32 and 12.33 in the left-hand column for long duration (top) and brief flashes (bottom).

Several lines of experimental evidence indicate that the PhNR originates from the spiking activity of retinal ganglion cells and their axons in these species. As shown in figure 12.32,[241] in monkeys (and cats), the response is eliminated by intravitreal TTX, which blocks Na^+-dependent action potentials that occur in all ganglion cells and some amacrine cells. In monkeys with laser-induced experimental

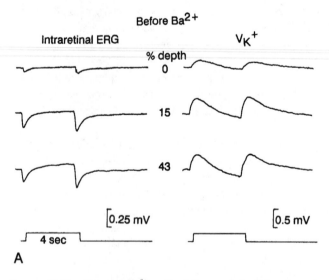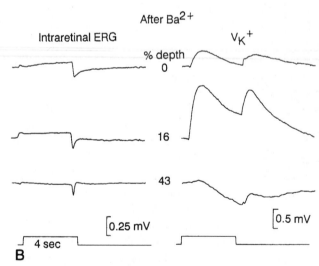

FIGURE 12.31 Effect of Ba^{2+} on the M-wave of the light-adapted cat retina. Effect of Ba^{2+} ($BaCl^{2+}$, 3 mM) on the depth distribution of field potentials and $[K^+]_o$ changes in light-adapted retina. Recordings were made before (A) and 30–60 minutes after (B) Ba^{2+} was injected intravitreally. The stimulus was a small spot (0.8 degree in diameter), steady background illumination was $10.5 \log q \deg^{-2} s^{-1}$, flash illumination was $11.6 \log q \deg^{-2} s^{-1}$. (Source: Adapted from Frishman LJ, Yamamoto F, Bogucka J, Steinberg RH.[60])

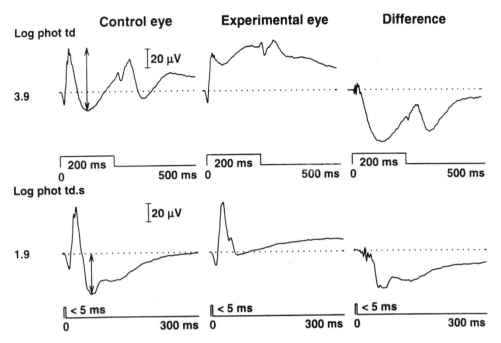

FIGURE 12.32 Photopic full-field flash ERG responses to long (upper row) and brief (lower row) red flashes on a rod-saturating blue background (3.7 log sc td) from the control (left) and experimental (middle) eye of a monkey with laser-induced experimental glaucoma in the "experimental" eye and the difference between the control and experimental records (right). The arrows mark the amplitude of the PhNR. The MD (static perimetry, C24-2 full threshold program) for the experimental eye was −2.65 dB. (Source: Adapted from Viswanathan S, Frishman LJ, Robson JG, et al.[241])

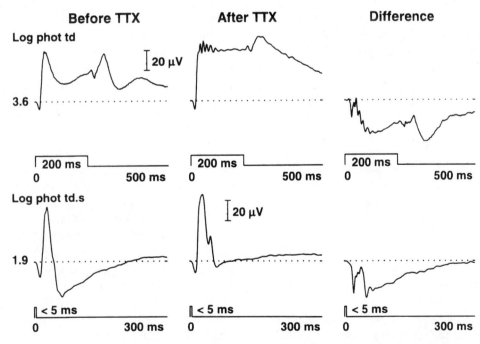

FIGURE 12.33 Photopic full-field flash ERG responses to long (upper row) and brief (lower row) red flashes on a rod-saturating blue background (3.7 log sc td) from a monkey eye before (left) and after (middle) intravitreal injection of TTX (6 mM) in the same eye and the difference (right). (Source: Adapted from Viswanathan S, Frishman LJ, Robson JG, et al.[241])

glaucoma, a pathological condition that destroys ganglion cells, the PhNR is reduced or eliminated, strongly implicating ganglion cell spiking activity in its generation (figure 12.33[241]). In intraretinal microelectrode recordings in cats, local signals of the same time course as the PhNR were largest in and around the optic nerve head.[237] The PhNR was disrupted in cats by Ba^{2+}, indicating glial (perhaps astrocytes in the nerve head) involvement in mediating generation of the response.[237]

RELATION TO THE PATTERN ERG The pattern ERG (PERG) has been the most common noninvasive measure of ganglion cell activity. The negative N_{95} wave in the transient PERG that is maximal about 95 ms after each contrast reversal of the stimulus pattern, is often reduced in glaucomatous eyes. Because the PhNR has an implicit time similar to that of the N_{95} and is likely to originate from ganglion cells, Viswanathan et al.[238] compared effects of experimental glaucoma and effects of TTX on the two responses in macaques and found similar effects on both, indicating common retinal origins. Furthermore, the PERG waveform for a given stimulation frequency (e.g., 2 or 8 Hz) could be simulated adequately by adding the ERGs at onset and offset of a uniform field, mainly due to the presence of the PhNR. Given that the two responses have similar origins, the PhNR has some advantages over the PERG as a clinical indicator of ganglion cell dysfunction. With appropriate stimulus conditions, the PhNR is a larger response, does not require refractive correction, and will be less affected by opacities in the ocular media than the PERG.

THE PhNR IN HUMANS AND RODENTS The PhNR is significantly reduced in human patients with primary open angle glaucoma,[32,46,240] anterior ischemic optic neuropathy,[185] and other optic nerve neuropathies,[69] consistent with an origin in ganglion cells or their axons in humans. In rats and mice, however, the response might not be completely ganglion cell–related, although it is dependent on TTX-sensitive spiking activity of inner retinal neurons.[21,128,141]

WAVELENGTH OF THE STIMULUS Most studies of the PhNR in monkeys have used a red flash on a rod-saturating blue background.[51,241] However, in humans, in addition to the red flash,[240] stimuli have included a 12° × 12° white field on a computer monitor,[32] full-field white flashes on a white background,[69] and use of a silent substitution technique to isolate S-cone ERG.[46] Monochromatic full field stimuli (red or blue) will produce a more distinguishable PhNR than will a broadband stimulus because the response to the broadband stimulus includes another long negative wave (compare figure 12.09, right panel, with figures 12.32 or 12.33) in addition to the PhNR (N. Rangaswamy, B. Dingle, and L. Frishman, unpublished observations).

Origins of the scotopic threshold response

For very weak flashes from darkness, near psychophysical threshold in humans,[54,210] a small postreceptoral potential of opposite polarity to the b-wave dominates the ERG. It has been observed in the ERG of several mammals, including humans,[54,210] such as cats, monkeys, rats, mice,[25,199,207,212] and probably sheep.[113] This negative-going response, which is more sensitive than PII (or PIII) and saturates at a lower light level than either component, was named the *scotopic threshold response (STR)* by Sieving et al.,[207] because of its sensitivity in intraretinal recording studies. As shown in figure 12.25 for the cat, the negative STR at stimulus onset dominates the dark-adapted diffuse flash ERG at intensities of 3.1 to 4.6 log q deg^{-2} s^{-1}. It grows in amplitude for the first 1.5 log units of stimulus strength, and then the (d.c.) component of PII, emerges. For stronger stimuli (e.g., 7.6 log q deg^{-2} s^{-1}) the b-wave dominates the response. The negative STR is distinct from the scotopic a-wave, although it can appear as a pseudo a-wave in the ERG (e.g., the arrow at 5.6 in figure 12.25). Aspartate, which isolates photoreceptor responses,[214] removes this STR but not the photoreceptor-dominated a-wave, showing that the STR originates postreceptorally.[243] The STR appears in the ERG in response to stimuli that are much weaker than those that elicit the a-wave (or b-wave; see below) because convergence of the rod signal in the retinal circuitry increases the gain of responses generated by neurons in the inner retina.

The STR was initially shown to be generated more proximally than PII, in the intraretinal depth analysis[207] to be described in more detail below, and subsequently, using pharmacological agents to suppress inner retinal responses proximal to bipolar cells (GABA, glycine, or NMDA[146,147,191,199]). These agents removed the STR but not the b-wave. In contrast, APB eliminated both the b-wave and STR. Because generation of the scotopic b-wave depends on the glutamatergic transmission from rods to depolarizing rod bipolar cells that is blocked by APB,[191] this indicates that the STR must depend on activation of rod bipolar cells. Because it is generated more proximally than the scotopic b-wave, it is believed to reflect activity of the amacrine (perhaps AII amacrine cells) and ganglion cell portion of the sensitive rod circuit that is specialized for handling quantal events (see the retinal schematic in the inset in figure 12.9).[58,59,147,199,207]

Since the initial description of the negative-going STR, it has become clear that there is an equally sensitive positive potential in the scotopic ERG of the species for which the negative-going response has been described. This wave has been called the *positive STR* (pSTR).[54,147,199] Because the pSTR is small and of opposite polarity to the nSTR, it can easily be cancelled out in the ERG. Such an instance can be seen in the dark-adapted macaque ERG shown in figure

12.9. The delay of the onset of nSTR for the weakest stimulus is due to the presence of a sensitive positive wave that is slightly larger than the negative wave at early times. In response to a stimulus about 1 log unit more intense (just above), the pSTR rides on the emerging PII as an early positive potential.

A linear model of the contributions of pSTR, nSTR, and PII for the dark-adapted cat ERG response to weak stimuli that has a small pSTR is shown in figure 12.34. It assumes that each ERG component initially rises in proportion to the stimulus strength and then saturates in a characteristic manner, as has been demonstrated in single-cell recordings in mammalian retinas.[6,10] Only with the inclusion of a small pSTR does the model accurately predict the whole ERG at a given time in the response after a weak stimulus. The model was fit in figure 12.34 to responses measured at 140 ms after a brief full-field flash (<5 ms), which was the

peak of the nSTR in the cat scotopic ERG. Similar modeling has been published for mouse[199] and human ERG.[54] The origins of the pSTR have not been investigated intraretinally, but studies have shown that the pharmacological agents listed above that suppress inner retinal responses and the nSTR will eliminate the pSTR as well.[147,199] For example, NMDA eliminated the nSTR and pSTR for responses such as those seen for the two weakest stimuli in figure 12.9.

Establishing the STR as a Separate Response from Proximal Retina

Depth distribution Intraretinal depth analysis in the cat initially showed that the nSTR originates in the proximal retina.[207] Responses recorded at increasing retinal depths to very low-intensity stimulus spots or diffuse stimuli were maximal around 17% retinal depth at the border between the ganglion cell layer and IPL. As is shown in figure 12.35, the retinal response recorded in proximal retina was negative-going for the duration of the stimulus when stimuli of durations less than 300 ms were used and returned slowly to baseline after light offset.

The STR recorded in proximal retina can be distinguished from the M-wave of the light-adapted retina[208] in the following ways: (1) It is rod- rather than a cone-dominated, (2) it lacks the prominent OFF response of the

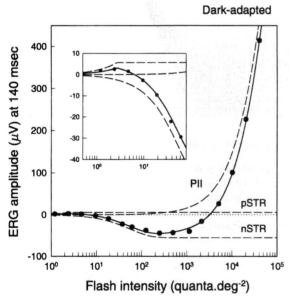

FIGURE 12.34 Amplitude of cat dark-adapted ERG responses measured 140 ms after a brief flash at the maximum negativity of the nSTR. Dashed lines show model curves for the pSTR, nSTR, and PII. Explicitly, the pSTR rises as a linear function that saturates abruptly at V_{max}, while the exponential saturation of the nSTR is defined by

$$V = V_{max} (1 - \exp(-I/I_0))$$

where V_{max} is the maximum saturated amplitude, and I_0 is the intensity for an amplitude of $(1 - 1/e)V_{max}$, while the hyperbolic relation used for PII is defined by

$$V = V_{max} I/(I + I_0)$$

where V_{max} has the same meaning but I_0 is the intensity at which the amplitude is $V_{max}/2$. The inset shows the pSTR and nSTR at the lowest light levels that were used. (1 q deg^{-2} is equivalent to ~-7.5 log sc cd m^{-2} s). (Source: Adapted from Frishman LJ, Robson JG: In Archer et al., *Adaptive Mechanisms in the Ecology of Vision*, London/Kluver, Chapman and Hall Ltd. (eds): 1999, pp 383–412.)

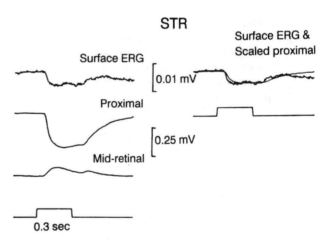

FIGURE 12.35 The STR dominates intraretinal recordings and the ERG at low stimulus intensities below the threshold for PII. Left, the top trace is the surface ERG recorded about 25 mm from the retinal surface, and the bottom two traces are recordings of the STR in the proximal retina (about 6% retinal depth) and the inverted STR around 50% retinal depth. Right, the scaled STR recorded in the proximal retina is superimposed on the surface ERG to show the similarity of the responses. For the surface ERG, a microelectrode was referenced to a wire in the vitreous to reduce the effects of stray light. This minimized contributions to the ERG of retinal regions distant from the recording site of the intraretinal signals (spot size, 9.9 degrees; spot illumination, 4.8 log q deg^{-2} s^{-1}). (Source: Adapted from Sieving PA, Frishman LJ, Steinberg RH.[207])

M-wave, and (3) it sums over a large retinal area and does not show the selectivity for small spots that is characteristic of the M-wave. Because it sums over a large retinal ERG, unlike the M-wave, the STR can be recorded in the vitreal (and corneal) ERG. The similarity of the onset times and time course of the proximal retinal STR and the negative potential in the cat ERG is shown in figure 12.35. It was possible to match the threshold negative response in the ERG by scaling the STR from proximal retina (offline on the computer) at its recorded negative polarity.

For stronger stimuli, PII (d.c. component and b-wave) was maximal near 50% retinal depth around the INL, as is well documented.[19] For stimuli that are too weak to elicit PII, the STR reversed polarity in midretina (figure 12.35) and became a positive-going signal in the midretina and distal retina. This reversal suggests a source proximal to, and a sink distal to, the reversal point, which was confirmed by current source density analysis.[213] For stronger stimuli, the reversed STR signals in midretina and distal retina were replaced by PII, which then dominated the ERG.

Sensitivity of the STR The plot in figure 12.36 shows peak amplitudes, as a function of stimulus intensity, of the nega-

tive responses in the proximal retina, where the STR was maximal, and in the midretina, where PII was maximal. The plot shows that the first measurable response for the STR (solid symbols) occurred for stimuli about 1.5 log units weaker than the first measurable response for PII (open symbols) in the same four cats. The STR also saturated at a lower intensity, around $5.8 \log q \deg^{-2} s^{-1}$ in the plot, which was about 2.4 log units lower than saturation of the rod b-wave in the cat.

Studies of the relative sensitivities of the STR and PII based on corneal ERGs of other species show that sensitivity of the STR is similar across species in terms of the luminance (about $6.6 \log sc \, cd. \, s. \, m^{-2}$),[199] even though the size of their eyes and pupils and their retinal photoreceptor distributions differ. In all species that were studied, the nSTR was more sensitive than PII.[56,147,199]

A K⁺-MÜLLER CELL MECHANISM FOR GENERATION OF THE STR The STR, like the M-wave, is associated with Müller cell responses to $[K^+]_o$ released by proximal retinal neurons.[58,59] Frishman and Steinberg[59] measured light-dependent changes in $[K^+]_o$ in cat retina and identified a proximal increase in $[K^+]_o$ with obvious functional similarities to the STR: The dynamic range from "threshold" to saturation of the increase in $[K^+]_o$ in the proximal retina was similar to that of the field potentials (figure 12.37), and the

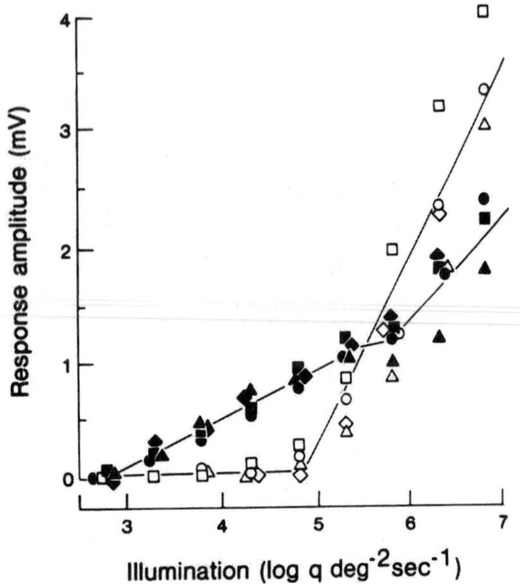

FIGURE 12.36 Amplitudes of dark-adapted responses in the proximal retina (solid symbols) and in the midretina (open symbols) as a function of stimulus illumination. Measurements were made in the proximal retinas of four cats in which the STR was maximal and in the midretinas of the same four cats in which PII was maximal. In the midretina, measurements were made from negative-going responses only, and they were made at the peak of the responses, which means that the d.c. component of PII was measured at low intensities and the b-wave was measured at high intensities. (Source: From Sieving PA, Frishman LJ, Steinberg RH.[207] Used by permission.)

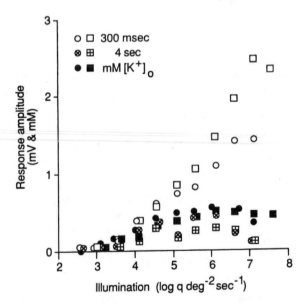

FIGURE 12.37 Amplitude of dark-adapted responses in the proximal retina and the light-evoked increase in $[K^+]_o$. Measurements were made with double-barreled K⁺-sensitive microelectrodes in the proximal retina where the STR was maximal. The plot includes amplitudes of the proximal responses at 300 ms after stimulus onset (open symbols) and 4.0 s after stimulus onset (crossed symbols). $[K^+]_o$ was measured at the peak of the response. Measurements were made in two cats. (Source: From Frishman LJ, Steinberg RH.[59] Used by permission.)

retinal depth maxima for the light-evoked increases in $[K^+]_o$ coincided with that of the STR field potentials. Comparisons of the latency and rise time of the $[K^+]_o$ increases with the kinetics of the field potentials were limited by the slow rise time of the K^+ electrode. Therefore, it was not possible to determine whether an initial portion of the response was directly neuronal in origin, corresponding to the PNR. At later times in the response, the $[K^+]_o$ increase in proximal retina was more sustained than the local field potentials, and the vitreal ERG contained a slow negative response that matched the duration of the proximal $[K^+]_o$ increase.

A causative role for the $[K^+]_o$ increase in generating the negative STR was supported by the finding that Ba^{2+}, a Kir channel conductance blocker, eliminated the proximal field potential in the cat and the negative potentials in the ERG but did not initially eliminate the light-evoked increase in $[K^+]_o$. The negative polarity of STR in the vitreous suggests a strong K^+ current directed toward the distal retina in the cat Müller cell (similar to the M-wave and PIII current; see figure 12.2). The distribution of K^+ conductivity in the cat Müller cell is consistent with a distally directed current because the cat, with its vascularized retina, has a Müller cell with high K^+ conductances at both ends (figure 12.21), that at the distal end being higher than the proximal end.[154] As illustrated for the effects of Ba^{2+} on the cat M-wave in figure 12.31, Ba^{2+} treatment of the dark-adapted retina also appeared to block K^+ siphoning by the Müller cells. Whereas the proximal $[K^+]_o$ increase remained intact, the distal $[K^+]_o$ increase was eliminated by Ba^{2+}, supporting the idea that the K^+ released in the proximal retina was normally carried (siphoned) to the distal retina via the Müller cell.[58,59]

NEURONAL ORIGINS OF THE STR   Although we do not know the exact neurons that are involved in generation of the nSTR and pSTR, we have some insights. Whether the neuronal contribution (via glia in the case of the nSTR) is dominated by amacrine or ganglion cells can be species-dependent. In monkeys, it is likely that the nSTR arises predominantly from ganglion cells. It was eliminated in eyes in which all the ganglion cells were eliminated as a consequence of laser-induced ocular hypertension[55] as well as by TTX intravitreally injected to block spiking activity of those neurons. In contrast, in cats and humans[206] as well as in mice and rats,[21,200] the response may be more amacrine cell–based and not totally reliant on spiking activity of either amacrine or ganglion cells. Following degeneration of ganglion cells due to optic nerve section or atrophy, the nSTR was reduced, not eliminated. TTX was partially effective in removing it in the animal studies.

In contrast to the nSTR, the pSTR, which is quite prominent in rats and mice, does appear to originate from gan-

glion cells. It was removed both by ganglion cell degeneration and by blockade of spiking activity.[21,200]

A characteristic of Müller/glial-mediated responses in the ERG is their slow time course. Glial mediation of the STR has been demonstrated only in cat, but the time course of the STR is slow in other species as well. The glial mediation of the nSTR may explain the similarity of its time course and amplitude across species regardless of which particular classes of local neurons produces the light-evoked changes in $[K^+]_o$ that generate the response in proximal retina. The relative contribution from different neuronal classes might depend on the density of the population of particular classes as well as their local relationship to the retinal glial. For example, the mouse retina[96] has a lower peak ganglion cell density than does the monkey retina,[182,244] and this might cause the proximally generated ERG to be more amacrine cell–related.

Origins of oscillatory potentials

The oscillatory potentials (OPs) of the ERG consist of a series of high-frequency, low-amplitude wavelets superimposed on the b-wave that occur in response to a strong stimulus. OPs are present under light- and dark-adapted conditions, with contributions from both rod and cone systems.[178] The number of OPs that are induced by a flash of light varies between four and about ten, depending on species and stimulus conditions; the frequency of the resulting OPs varies as well. Figure 12.38 shows the photopic flash ERG of a macaque monkey (top); at least five OPs at frequency of about 150 Hz can be seen by filtering the response to extract the high-frequency signals. In contrast, frequency of the OPs in intraretinal recordings in the frog retina was only about 20 Hz in figure 12.39.[255] There is consensus from experiments in amphibians and mammals, reviewed briefly below, that OPs are generated in proximal retina. Three major questions regarding their origins are as follows:

1. Do all of the OPs have the same origin?
2. Which cells generate the OPs?
3. What mechanisms are involved in generating the OPs?

DO ALL THE OPs HAVE THE SAME ORIGIN?   In amphibians, the various OPs do not all have the same origin. Depth profiles such as the one illustrated in figure 12.39 from isolated frog retina, have shown that the earlier OPs in the response arise near the IPL, while the later OPs arise more distally, perhaps within the INL. The finding that the various OPs are differentially sensitive to pharmacological agents also supports different origins for the potentials. Studies by Wachmeister and colleagues[242] in mud puppy retina, where OPs occur at about 15–30 Hz, found that the earlier OPs are depressed by GABA antagonists, the dopamine antagonist haloperidol, β-alanine, and substance P. The later OPs are

Monkey full-field flash ERG

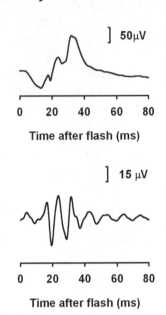

] 50 μV

Time after flash (ms)

] 15 μV

Time after flash (ms)

FIGURE 12.38 Full-field flash photopic ERG of a macaque monkey (top) and the OPs extracted from these records. Filtering was between 90 and 300 Hz for OPs that occurred between 100 and 200 Hz. The stimulus was a xenon flash presented on a rod-saturating blue background. (Source: Adapted from Rangaswamy N, Hood DC, Frishman LJ.[187] Used by permission).

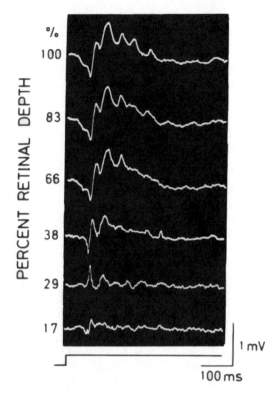

FIGURE 12.39 Depth profile of OPs of an isolated frog retina. The intraretinal electrode was introduced from the receptor side, and the reference electrode was placed on the vitreal side. The depth of the electrode tip within the retina is indicated relative to the vitreal surface (0%) and the receptor surface (100%). When the electrode was in the receptor layer (at 100% and 83% depths), five OPs could be identified. As the electrode was advanced proximally, the OPs with longer peak latencies disappeared. (Source: From Yanagida T, Koshimizi M, Kawasaki K, et al.[255] Used by permission.)

depressed by the glycine antagonist strychnine and by ethanol.

In primates, early intraretinal studies using stimuli that would elicit responses from both rod and cone systems did not find differences in the depth profiles of the various OPs.[86,171] However, these studies were not combined with use of pharmacological agents (other than TTX, which did not block OPs[171]). However, considering the complexity of inner retinal circuitry, the similarity in depth profiles does not necessarily mean that the same neurons were involved in all cases. For example, in the photopic flash ERG response to brief stimuli, the major OPs are APB-sensitive,[187] indicating an origin in the ON pathways, but later ones, particularly when the stimulus duration is increased, are not, indicating an origin in the OFF pathway. Such a difference could show up as a difference in depth of maximal response in recordings in the IPL, as ON pathway synapses occur more proximally than OFF pathway synapses.

WHICH CELLS GENERATE THE OPs? The observations described above indicate that proximal neurons are important for generating OPs. Early clinical and experimental evidence showed that the OPs are postreceptoral in origin. They are suppressed in cases of occlusion of the central retinal artery[259] and experimental occlusion of the central

retinal artery in monkey.[118] OPs (but not receptor signals) also are abolished in excised human retina by application of aspartate or glutamate to block photoreceptor synaptic transmission.[257] Pigment epithelial cells can be excluded as generators of the OPs as well. No rhythmic wavelets were observed in light-evoked responses from these cells,[223] and OPs are clearly observed in the isolated retina detached from the RPE (see figure 12.39).

Most work indicates that OPs originate in the vicinity of the IPL. Across species, the depth profiles that have been measured provide evidence for this layer of origin,[171] and a current source density analysis in primate also points to the IPL.[86] As was described above for amphibians, application of pharmacological agents that block inner retinal activity remove OPs in mammals as well. For example, glycine, an inhibitory neurotransmitter that is localized to the IPL, selectively suppresses OPs in vivo (rabbit[117]) and in vitro (rabbit,[256,258] human[256]), and this suppression is antagonized by strychnine.[256,258] GABA (as well as glycine) also eliminates

OPs in photopic ERG of monkeys, as does PDA.[187] On the other hand, genetic deletion of the main GABA receptor in the IPL, the GABA$_C$ receptor, enhances the OPs[135] in GABA$_C$ (−/−) mice compared to wild-type mice.

The role of retinal ganglion cells in the generation of OPs has been controversial. Under some stimulus conditions, OPs remain normal in cases of long-standing optic nerve atrophy[259] and after optic nerve section in rabbit,[247] conditions that should result in ganglion cell degeneration. On the other hand, in Ogden's studies, optic nerve section in primates resulted in ganglion cell degeneration and disappearance of the OPs,[171] and antidromic stimulation of the primate optic nerve resulted in a reduction in OP amplitude.[171] Furthermore, in the primate photopic ERG that was elicited by using a slow sequence multifocal paradigm, both TTX[187] and experimental glaucoma[186] removed or reduced OPs. It is possible in primates that high-frequency OPs under fully photopic conditions reflect activity in ganglion cell axons and the manifestation of an optic nerve head component of the ERG,[225] whereas under conditions in which rod signals are also involved,[55,171] the ganglion cell contribution is less prominent.

WHAT MECHANISMS ARE INVOLVED IN GENERATING OPs?
Neuronal interaction/inhibitory feedback circuits Two mechanisms are commonly thought to be involved in generating OPs: neuronal interactions/feedback circuits and the intrinsic membrane properties of the cells. The case for the inhibitory feedback mechanism is supported by involvement of neurotransmitter receptors for GABA and glycine, which are prominent in feedback circuits in the inner retina. Gap junctions between inner retinal neurons also are involved. When Connexin 36, which forms gap junctions between both amacrine cells and ganglion cells of the inner retina, is knocked out,[78] OPs are reduced.[201] A feedback model has recently been proposed to account for the high-frequency oscillatory, or "rhythmic," activity that has been observed in mammalian ganglion cell recordings.[5,218] On the basis of tracer coupling patterns in anatomical studies, Kenyon et al.[108] proposed a circuit that includes negative feedback coming from axon-bearing amacrine cells that are excited via electrical synapses with neighboring ganglion cells. These authors also allow that membrane properties of the wide-field (spiking) amacrine cells could be involved.

OPs in intracellular responses from neurons In retinal intracellular recordings from many different species, high-frequency oscillations have rarely been observed in the responses of more distal neurons: rods, cones, horizontal cells, and bipolar cells. Dark oscillations have been described in rods and horizontal cells,[165] but these are abolished by light onset. A slight "ringing" is sometimes observed at the peak of the ON responses of these cells, but it had only two to three cycles at most, its duration was short, and its amplitude was small. For one depolarizing and one hyperpolarizing bipolar cell in the turtle retina, Marchiafava and Torre showed one to two oscillations at about 20 Hz.[130]

Oscillations in intracellularly recorded responses of interplexiform cells that are radially oriented and feedback from IPL to OPL have been reported in only two studies. Hashimoto et al.[81] showed a response from one depolarizing cell with three to four oscillations occurring at about 40 Hz in the dace retina. In the mud puppy, R. F. Miller (personal communication) found the responses to be much slower.

In contrast to the other cell types, there are numerous accounts of oscillations in amacrine cell responses, particularly from studies of turtles and fish retina. The oscillations from depolarizing sustained-ON amacrine cells[42,131,232] were studied intensively by Naka's laboratory[196] (see figure 12.40). Oscillations in these cells could number more than ten, and they arose at a frequency of 30–50 Hz, which is similar to the frequency of OPs in the carp ERG (40 Hz[5]). Depolarizing ON/OFF amacrine cells show oscillations at the same frequency, but their appearance is less reliable.[42,130,131,196,232] Finally, hyperpolarizing amacrine cells do not show oscillations at light onset,[42,196] but they may contribute to OPs at light offset.[196]

Recently, studies of isolated wide-field amacrine cells from white bass retina have provided strong evidence for the

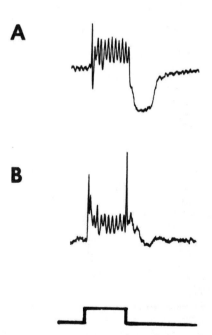

FIGURE 12.40 Light-evoked intracellular responses that include oscillatory potentials, recorded from amacrine cells in a catfish retina. A, Sustained-ON, or type N, neuron. Oscillations are regularly present during light onset. B, Transient ON/OFF, or type C, neuron. Only some type C neurons (including this one) exhibited oscillations (stimulus duration: 0.5 s). (Source: From Sakai H, Naka K-I.[196] Used by permission.)

involvement of intrinsic membrane mechanisms in generating high-frequency OPs.[236] Single GABAergic wide-field ACs were shown to generate oscillatory membrane potentials (OMPs) in response to extrinsic depolarization. The OMPs increased in frequency as depolarization was increased, reaching more than 100 Hz for strong depolarization (see figure 12.41). Analysis of the mechanism of generation of the OMPs in these isolated cells indicated that the oscillations arose from "a complex interplay between voltage-dependent calcium currents and voltage- and calcium-dependent potassium currents."[236] Such oscillations may be the source of the oscillations that have been reported in some ganglion cells.

SUMMARY There is consensus that high-frequency OPs originate from the inner retina and evidence, mainly from amphibian, that all the OPs in a given series do not always arise from the same cells. The exact cellular origin and mechanism of generation may depend on species and stimulus conditions. There is evidence for involvement of feedback circuitry, as well as the intrinsic membrane mechanisms of amacrine cells.

Retinal extracellular potential responses not evoked by light

POTENTIALS EVOKED BY OPTIC NERVE STIMULATION The contribution of ganglion cells and inner retina to the ERG has been explored by activating the cells via electrical stimulation of the optic nerve. Ogden and Brown[170,173] stimulated the optic nerve in primates and found a retinal field potential with a maximum positive amplitude in the IPL and a smaller negativity in the ganglion cell layer. This response, termed the *P-wave*, was also observed in primates by Gouras,[71] but he found a reversal point in the IPL and the largest positivity in the INL. A similar response profile was found by Miller et al.[137] in the mud puppy.

The origin of the intraretinal P-wave is uncertain. Gouras[71] suggested that the P-wave in monkey arises directly from antidromically activated ganglion cell spikes. Another possibility is that it results from activation of inner retinal neurons via efferent fibers in the optic nerve,[173] but this would occur only in the species in which retinal efferent innervation has been clearly demonstrated. Other investigators have suggested a role for Müller cell spatial buffering of K+ released by ganglion cells[137] or that activity of retinal neurons that are postsynaptic to ganglion cells.[170,197] Other mechanisms may also exist by which activity in ganglion cell axons may induce responses elsewhere in the retina, such as "blue arcs."[16] It is possible that multiple mechanisms contribute to the P-wave, and the size of the contribution of any particular mechanism may depend on the species and experimental methodology. There is also disagreement as to whether the P-wave can be recorded transretinally. Early studies in primates failed to find such a contribution, but a substantial negativity in the vitreous was seen in the mud puppy.[137] Given the recent association of the PhNR and the STR with ganglion cells in primates,[55,241] it is possible that these potentials and the P-wave have common origins.

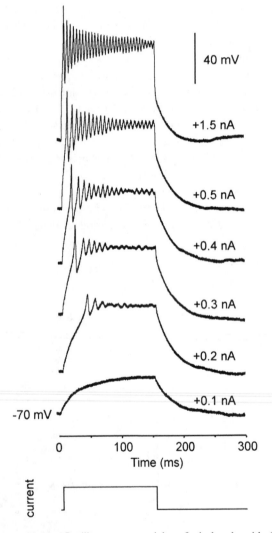

FIGURE 12.41 Oscillatory potentials of isolated wide-field amacrine cells in the white bass retina. Oscillatory membrane potentials (OMPs) were elicited by depolarizing current steps of increasing amplitude obtained in whole-cell recordings from isolated amacrine cells that were maintained in culture. The duration and frequency of the OMPs increased with depolarization. Voltage traces are shifted vertically for visibility. Bottom, Application of depolarizing pulse. The magnitude of depolarizing current is indicated with each trace. Holding potential was −70 mV. (Source: From Vigh J, Solessio E, Morgans CW, Lasater EM.[236] Used by permission.)

SPREADING DEPRESSION The phenomenon of spreading depression (SD), first described by Leaõ[120] in cerebral cortex, consists of a slowly propagating and transient depression of neural activity, and it is associated with a number of physiological events, including a large, local field potential. Gouras[70] described SD in amphibian retinas, and it has since been observed in the retinas of many species, including mammals.[136,190] The retina in which SD has been studied most extensively is the chick retina (for a review, see Martins-Ferreira et al.[132]), in which the phenomenon is pronounced and prominent intrinsic optical signals accompany the SD.[38]

The field potential associated with retinal SD has a maximum amplitude in the proximal retina, possibly at the inner limiting membrane.[142] Within the proximal retina, this potential is negative-going, but the transretinally recorded SD potential can be predominantly negative or positive, depending on the species.[61] SD is also associated with a large increase in $[K^+]_o$ in the IPL, and there is evidence to suggest that SD potentials are related to the spatial buffering of this increased $[K^+]_o$ by glial cells.[142,143,175] Propagation of SD also depends on intercellular coupling through gap junctions; SD waves in chick retina were blocked by common inhibitors of gap junctions in the retina.[148]

The frequency of occurrence of retinal SD can be increased by injury to a retinal region,[70] mechanical stimulation of the retina,[37] anoxia,[70] application of high concentrations of K^+ ions[87] or low concentrations of Cl^- ions,[142,143,175] application of the excitatory amino acids glutamate or aspartate,[142,143] light offset,[190] and antidromic stimulation of the optic nerve.[142,143]

Because of the large number of pathological conditions that facilitate or initiate SDs, it seems reasonable to assume that SD will sometimes be associated with disorders of the eye or retina in humans. Two difficulties in observing the SDs in humans are that (1) the retinal SD may be a transient event, and so the clinician must be recording an ERG or looking in the eye for the color change of the retina associated with SD[234] at the appropriate time, and (2) it is not certain whether a local retinal SD could be detected by noninvasive electroretinography.

In the brain, there is evidence that SD is involved in migraine headaches and other neurological disorders,[68,119] and SD can occur in conjunction with stereotaxic surgery.[22] Somjen and Aitkin[217] have suggested that SD be considered a transient and propagating type of cortical depression that is initiated at one point, while another type of depression is diffuse and nonpropagating. The latter would possibly include depressions arising during transient cerebral hypoxia (due to asphyxia or to brief failure of cerebral circulation) and during concussions. Events related to either category of cortical depressions (spreading and diffuse) could also occur in the retina.

ACKNOWLEDGMENT I am grateful to Chester Karwoski, Ed Griff, and Eric Newman for the first edition of this chapter, which forms the basis for the present one, and to John G. Robson for helpful discussions and suggestions.

REFERENCES

1. Adrian ED: Electrical responses of the human eye. *J Physiol (Lond)* 1945; 104:84–104.
2. Adrian ED: Rod and cone components in the electric response of the eye. *J Physiol (Lond)* 1946; 105:24–37.
3. Arden GB, Brown KT: Some properties of components of the cat electroretinogram revealed by local recording under oil. *J Physiol (Lond)* 1965; 176:429–461.
4. Ariel M, Daw NW, Rader RK: Rhythmicity in rabbit retinal ganglion cell responses. *Vision Res* 1983; 23:1485–1493.
5. Asano T: Adaptive properties of the b-wave and the PIII in the perfused isolated carp retina. *Jpn J Physiol* 1977; 27:701–716.
6. Awatramani G, Wang J, Slaughter MM: Amacrine and ganglion cell contributions to the electroretinogram in amphibian retina. *Vis Neurosci* 2001; 18:147–156.
7. Barlow HB, Levick WR, Yoon M: Responses to single quanta of light in retinal ganglion cells of the cat. *Vision Res* 1971; 11 (suppl 3):87–102.
8. Baron WS, Boynton RM: Response of primate cones to sinusoidally flickering homochromatic stimuli. *J Physiol* 1975; 246:311–331.
9. Baron WS, Boynton RM, Hammon RW: Component analysis of the foveal local electroretinogram elicited with sinusoidal flicker. *Vision Res* 1979; 19:479–490.
10. Baylor DA, Nunn BJ, Schnapf JL: The photocurrent, noise and spectral sensitivity of rods of the monkey *Macaca Fascicularis. J Physiol* 1984; 357:575–607.
11. Bialek S, Joseph DP, Miller SS: The delayed basolateral membrane hyperpolarization of the bovine retinal pigment epithelium: Mechanism of generation. *J Physiol* 1995; 484:53–67.
12. Bolnick DA, Walter AE, Sillman A: Barium suppresses slow PIII in perfused bullfrog retina. *Vision Res* 1979; 19:1117–1119.
13. Breton ME, Schueller AW, Lamb TD, Pugh EN Jr: Analysis of ERG a-wave amplification and kinetics in terms of the G-protein cascade of phototransduction. *Invest Ophthalmol & Vis Sci* 1994; 35:295–309.
14. Brew H, Gray PTA, Mobbs P, Attwell D: Endfeet of retinal glial cells have higher densities of ion channels that mediate K^+ buffering. *Nature* 1986; 324:466–468.
15. Brindley GS, Hamasaki DI: The properties and nature of the R membrane of the frog's eye. *J Physiol* 1963; 599–600.
16. Brindley CS: *Physiology of the Retina and Visual Pathway.* London, Edward Arnold Publishers, Ltd., 1970.
17. Brown KT: The electroretinogram: Its components and their origin. *Vision Res* 1968; 8:633–677.
18. Brown KT, Watanabe K, Murakami M: The early and late receptor potentials of monkey cones and rods. *Cold Spring Harb Symp Quant Biol* 1965; 30:457–482.
19. Brown KT, Wiesel TN: Localization of the origins of electroretinogram components by intraretinal recording in the intact cat eye. *J Physiol (Lond)* 1961; 158:257–280.
20. Brown KT, Wiesel TN: Analysis of the intraretinal electroretinogram in the intact cat eye. *J Physiol (Lond)* 1961; 158:229–256.

21. Bui BV, Fortune B: Ganglion cell contributions to the rat full-field electroretinogram. *J Physiol* 2004; 555:153–173.

22. Bures J, Buresova O, Krivanek J: The meaning and significance of Leaõs spreading depression. *An Acad Bras Cienc* 1984; 56:385–400.

23. Burkhardt DA: Distinction between a proximal negative response and the local b-wave in the retina. *Nature* 1969; 221:879–880.

24. Burkhardt DA: Proximal negative response of frog retina. *I Neurophysiol* 1970; 33:405–420.

25. Bush R, Reme CE: Chronic lithium treatment induces reversible and irreversible changes in the rat ERG in vivo. *Clin Vis Sci* 1992; 5:393–401.

26. Bush RA, Sieving PA: A proximal retinal component in the primate photopic ERG a-wave. *Invest Ophthalmol Vis Sci* 1994; 35:635–645.

27. Bush RA, Sieving PA: Inner retinal contributions to the primate photopic fast flicker electroretinogram. *J Opt Soc Am A* 1996; 13:557–565.

28. Byzov AL: Functional properties of different cells in the retina of cold-blooded vertebrates. *Cold Spring Harb Symp Quant Biol* 1965; 30:547–558.

29. Byzov KA: Analysis of the distribution of potentials and currents within retina on light stimulation: I. Activity of the bipolars of two types. *Biophysics* 1959; 4:46–59.

30. Byzov KA, Dmitriev AV, Skatchkov SN: Extracellular potassium and its light-induced changes in the frog retina. *Sechenoz Physiol J USSR* 1984; 70:1381–1387.

31. Coleman PA, Carras PL, Miller RF: Barium reverses the transretinal potassium gradient of the amphibian retina. *Neurosci Res* 1987; 80:61–65.

32. Colotto A, Falsini B, Salgarello T, Iarossi G, Galan ME, Scullica L: Photopic negative response of the human ERG: Losses associated with glaucomatous damage. *Invest Ophthalmol Vis Sci* 2000; 41:2205–2211.

33. Connaughton VP, Nelson R: Axonal stratification patterns and glutamate-gated conductance mechanisms in zebrafish retinal bipolar cells. *J Physiol* 2000; 524:135–146.

34. Conner JD, Detwiler PB, Sarthy PV: Ionic and electrophysiological properties of retinal Müller (glia) cells of the turtle. *J Physiol* 1985; 362:79–92.

35. Crescitelli F: The c-wave and inhibition in the developing retina of the frog. *Vision Res* 1970; 10:1077–1091.

36. Dawis SM, Niemeyer G: Dopamine influences the light peak in the perfused mammalian eye. *Invest Ophthalmol Vis Sci* 1986; 27:330–335.

37. DeAzeredo FAM, Martins-Ferreira H: Changes in fluid compartments and ionic composition in the isolated chick retina during SD. *Neurochem Res* 1979; 4:99–107.

38. deLima VMF, Hanke W: Excitation waves in central grey matter: The retinal spreading depression. *Prog Ret Eye Res* 1997; 16:657–690.

39. Dick E, Miller RE: Light-evoked potassium activity in mudpuppy retina: Its relationship to the b-wave of the electroretinogram. *Brain Res* 1978; 154:388–394.

40. Dick E, Miller RE: Extracellular K⁺ activity changes related to electroretinogram components: I. Amphibian (I-type) retinas. *J Gen Physiol* 1985; 85:885–909.

41. Dick E, Miller RE, Bloomfield S: Extracellular K⁺ activity changes related to electroretinogram components: II. Rabbit (E-type) retinas. *J Gen Physiol* 1985; 85:911–931.

42. Djamgoz NIBA: Common features of light-evoked amacrine cell responses in vertebrate retina. *Neurosci Lett* 1986; 71:187–191.

43. Dong CJ, Hare WA: Contribution to the kinetics and amplitude of the electroretinogram b-wave by third-order retinal neurons in the rabbit retina. *Vision Res* 2000; 40:579–589.

44. Douglas RH: Visual Adaptation and Spectral Sensitivity in Rainbow Trout (Ph.D. dissertation). University of Stirling, England, 1980.

45. Dowling JE, Ripps H: Adaptation in skate photoreceptors. *J Gen Physiol* 1972; 60:698–719.

46. Drasdo N, Aldebasi YH, Chiti Z, Mortlock KE, Morgan JE, North RV: The s-cone PHNR and pattern ERG in primary open angle glaucoma. *Invest Ophthalmol Vis Sci* 2001; 42:1266–1272.

47. Edelman JL, Lin H, Miller SS: Acidification stimulates chloride and fluid absorption across frog retinal pigment epithelium. *Am J Physiol* 1994; 266:C946–C956.

48. Evers HU, Gouras P: Three cone mechanisms in the primate electroretinogram: Two with, one without off-center bipolar responses. *Vision Res* 1986; 26:245–254.

49. Faber DS: Analysis of Slow Transretinal Potentials in Response to Light (Ph.D. thesis), University of New York, Buffalo, 1969.

50. Falk C, Shiells RA: Do horizontal cell responses contribute to the electroretinogram (ERG) in dogfish? *J Physiol* 1986; 381:113.

51. Fortune B, Bui BV, Cull G, Wang L, Cioffi GA: Inter-ocular and inter-session reliability of the electroretinogram photopic negative response (PhNR) in non-human primates. *Exp Eye Res* 2004; 78:83–93.

52. Freeman JA, Nicholson C: Experimental optimization of current source-density technique for anuran cerebellum. *J Neurophysiol* 1975; 38:369–382.

53. Friedburg C, Allen CP, Mason PJ, Lamb TD: Contribution of cone photoreceptors and post-receptoral mechanisms to the human photopic electroretinogram. *J Physiol* 2004; 556:819–834.

54. Frishman LJ, Reddy MG, Robson JG: Effects of background ground light on the human dark-adapted ERG and psychophysical threshold. *J Opt Soc Am A* 1996; 13:601–612.

55. Frishman LJ, Shen F, Du L, Robson JG, Harwerth RS, Smith III EL, Carter-Dawson L, Crawford MLJ. Scotopic ERG of macaque monkey after ganglion cell loss due to experimental glaucoma. *Invest Ophthalmol Vis Sci* 1996; 37:125–141.

56. Frishman LJ, Sieving PA: Evidence for two sites of adaptation affecting the dark-adapted ERG of cats and primates. *Vision Res* 1995; 35:435–442.

57. Frishman LJ, Sieving PA, Steinberg RH: Contributions to the electroretinogram of currents originating in proximal retina. *Vis Neurosci* 1988; 1:307–315.

58. Frishman LJ, Steinberg RH: Intraretinal analysis of the threshold dark-adapted ERG of cat retina. *J Neurophysiol* 1989; 61:1221–1232.

59. Frishman LJ, Steinberg RH: Light-evoked changes in [K⁺]ₒ in proximal portion of the dark-adapted cat retina. *J Neurophysiol* 1989; 61:1233–1243.

60. Frishman LJ, Yamamoto F, Bogucka J, Steinberg RH: Light-evoked changes in [K⁺]ₒ in proximal portion of light-adapted cat retina. *J Neurophysiol* 1992; 67:1201–1212.

61. Fujimoto M, Tomita T: Relationship between the electroretinogram (ERG) and the proximal negative response (PNR). *Jpn J Physiol* 1980; 30:377–392.

62. Furakawa I, Hanawa I: Effects of some common cations on electroretinogram of the toad. *Jpn J Physiol* 1955; 5:289–300.

63. Gallemore RP, Griff ER, Steinberg RH: Evidence in support of a photoreceptoral origin for the "light-peak substance." *Invest Ophthalmol Vis Sci* 1988; 29:566–571.

64. Gallemore RP, Hughes BA, Miller SS: Light-induced responses of the retinal pigment epithelium. In Marmor MF, Wolfensberger TJ (eds): *The Retinal Pigment Epithelium.* New York, Oxford University Press, 1998, pp 175–198.

65. Gallemore RP, Steinberg RH: Effects of DIDS on the chick retinal pigment epithelium: II. Mechanism of the light peak and other responses originating at the basal membrane. *J Neurosci* 1989; 9:1977–1984.

66. Gallemore RP, Steinberg RH: Effects of dopamine on the chick retinal pigment epithelium. Membrane potentials and light-evoked responses. *Invest Ophthalmol Vis Sci* 1990; 31:67–80.

67. Gallemore RP, Steinberg RH: Light-evoked modulation of basolateral membrane Cl$^-$ conductance in chick retinal pigment epithelium: The light peak and fast oscillation. *J Neurophysiol* 1993; 70:1669–1680.

68. Gorji A: Spreading depression: A review of the clinical relevance. *Brain Res Rev* 2001; 38:33–60.

69. Gotoh Y, Machida S, Tazawa Y: Selective loss of photopic negative response in patients with optic nerve atrophy. *Arch Ophthalmol* 2004; 122:341–346.

70. Gouras P: Electric activity of toad retina. *Am J Ophthalmol* 1958; 46:59–70.

71. Gouras P: Antidromic responses of orthodromically identified ganglion cells in monkey retina. *J Physiol* 1969; 240:407–419.

72. Gouras P, Carr RE: Light induced DC responses of monkey retina before and after central retinal artery interruption. *Invest Ophthamol Vis Sci* 1965; 4:310–317.

73. Granit R: Sensory Mechanisms of the Retina. London, Oxford University Press, 1947.

74. Granit R: The components of the retinal action potential in mammals and their relation to the discharge in the optic nerve. *J Physiol* 1933; 77:207–239.

75. Griff ER, Shirao V, Steinberg RH: Ba^{2+} unmasks K$^+$ modulation of the Na$^+$-K$^+$ pump in the frog retinal pigment epithelium. *J Gen Physiol* 1985; 86:853–876.

76. Griff ER, Steinberg RH: Changes in apical [K$^+$] produce delayed basal membrane responses of the retinal pigment epithelium in the gecko. *J Gen Physiol* 1984; 83:193–211.

77. Griff ER, Steinberg RH: Origin of the light peak: In vitro study of Gekko gekko. *J Physiol (Lond)* 1982; 33:637–652.

78. Guldenagel M, Ammermuller J, Feigenspan A, Teubner B, Degen J, Sohl G, Willecke K, Weiler R: Visual transmission deficits in mice with targeted disruption of the gap junction gene connexin 36. *J Neurosci* 2001; 21:6036–6044.

79. Gurevich L, Slaughter MM: Comparison of the waveforms of the ON bipolar neuron and the b-wave of the electroretinogram. *Vision Res* 1993; 33:2431–2435.

80. Hanitzsch R: Intraretinal isolation of PIII subcomponents in the isolated rabbit retina after treatment with sodium aspartate. *Vision Res* 1973; 13:2093–2102.

81. Hashimoto Y, Abe M, Inokuchi M: Identification of the interplexiform cell in the dace retina by dye-injection method. *Brain Res* 1980; 197:331–340.

82. Hayes BP, Holden AL: Depth-marking the proximal negative response in the pigeon retina. *J Comp Neurol* 1978; 180:193–202.

83. Hernandez EV, Hu JG, Frambach DA, Gallemore RP: Potassium conductances in cultured bovine and human retinal pigment epithelium. *Invest Ophthalmol Vis Sci* 1995; 36:113–122.

84. Heynen H, van Norren D: Origin of the electroretinogram in the intact macaque eye: I. Principal component analysis. *Vision Res* 1985; 25:697–707.

85. Heynen H, van Norren D: Origin of the electroretinogram in the intact macaque eye: II. Current source-density analysis. *Vision Res* 1985; 25:709–715.

86. Heynen H, Wachtmeister L, van Norren D: Origin of the oscillatory potentials in the primate retina. *Vision Res* 1985; 25:1365–1374.

87. Higashida H, Sakakihara M, Mitarai G: Spreading depression in isolated carp retina. *Brain Res* 1977; 120:67–83.

88. Hood DC, Birch DG: The *a*-wave of the human electroretinogram and rod receptor function. *Invest Ophthal & Vis Sci* 1990; 31:2070–2081.

89. Hood DC, Birch DG: A quantitative measure of the electrical activity of human rod photoreceptors using electroretinography. *Vis Neurosci* 1990a; 5:379–387.

90. Hood DC, Birch DG: Human cone receptor activity: The leading edge of the *a*-wave and models of receptor activity. *Vis Neurosci* 1993; 10:857–871.

91. Hood DC, Birch DG: Phototransduction in human cones measured using the *a*-wave of the ERG. *Vision Res* 1995; 35:2801–2810.

92. Hu KG, Marmor ME: Selective actions of barium on the c-wave and slow negative potential of the rabbit eye. *Vision Res* 1984; 24:1153–1156.

93. Huang B, Karwoski CJ: Light-evoked expansion of subretinal space volume in the retina of the frog. *J Neurosci* 1992; 12:4243–4252.

94. Hubbard JI, Lhinas R, Quastel DMJ: *Electrophysiological Analysis of Synaptic Transmission.* Baltimore, Williams & Wilkins, 1969.

95. Jamison JA, Bush RA, Lei B, Sieving PA: Characterization of the rod photoresponse isolated from the dark-adapted primate ERG. *Vis Neurosci* 2001; 18:445–455.

96. Jeon CJ, Strettoi E, Masland RH: The major cell populations of the mouse retina. *J Neurosci* 1998; 18:8936–8946.

97. Joseph DP, Miller SS: Apical and basal membrane ion transport mechanisms in bovine retinal pigment epithelium. *J Physiol* 1991; 435:439–463.

98. Joseph DP, Miller SS: Alpha-1-adrenergic modulation of K and Cl transport in bovine retinal epithelium. *J Gen Physiol* 1992; 99:263–290.

98a. Karwoski CJ, Coles JA, Lu H-K, Huang B: Current-evoked transcellular K$^+$ flux in frog retina. *J Neurophysiol* 1989; 61:939–952.

99. Karwoski CJ, Criswell MH, Proenza LM: Laminar separation of light-evoked K$^+$-flux and field potentials in frog retina. *Invest Ophthalmol Vis Sci* 1978; 17:678–682.

100. Karwoski CJ, Frambach DA, Proenza LM: Laminar profile of resistivity in frog retina. *J Neurophysiol* 1985; 54:1607–1619.

101. Karwoski CJ, Lu H-K, Newman EA: Spatial buffering of light-evoked potassium increases by retinal Müller (glial) cells. *Science* 1989; 244:578–580.

102. Karwoski CJ, Newman EA: Generation of the c-wave of the electroretinogram in the frog retina. *Vision Res* 1988; 28:1095–1105.

103. Karwoski CJ, Proenza LM: Relationship between Müller cell responses, a local transretinal potential, and potassium flux. *J Neurophysiol* 1977; 40:244–259.

104. Karwoski CJ, Proenza LM: Neurons, potassium, and glia in proximal retina of *Necturus. J Gen Physiol* 1980; 75:141–162.

105. Karwoski CJ, Proenza LM: Spatio-temporal variables in the relationship of neuronal activity to potassium and glial responses. *Vision Res* 1981; 21:1713–1718.

106. Karwoski CJ, Xu X: Current source-density analysis of light-evoked field potentials in rabbit retina. *Vis Neurosci* 1999;16:369–377.

107. Katz BJ, Wen R, Zheng JB, Xu ZA: Oakley B II: M-wave of the toad electroretinogram. *J Neurophysiol* 1991; 66:1927–1940.

108. Kenyon GT, Moore B, Jeffs J, Denning KS, Stephens GJ, Travis BJ, George JS, Theiler J, Marshak DW: A model of high-frequency oscillatory potentials in retinal ganglion cells. *Vis Neurosci* 2003; 20:465–480.

109. Kikawada N: Variations in the corneo-retinal standing potential of the vertebrate eye during light and dark adaptation. *Jpn J Physiol* 1968; 18:687–702.

110. Kline RP, Ripps H, Dowling JE: Generation of b-wave currents in the skate retina. *Proc Natl Acad Sci USA* 1978; 75:5727–5731.

111. Kline RP, Ripps H, Dowling JE: Light-induced potassium fluxes in the skate retina. *Neurosci* 1985; 14:225–235.

112. Knapp AC, Schiller PH: The contribution of on-bipolar cells to the electroretinogram of rabbits amid monkeys: A study using 2-amino-4-phosphonobutyrate (APB). *Vision Res* 1984; 24:1841–1846.

113. Knave B, Moller A, Perrson H: A component analysis of the electroretinogram. *Vision Res* 1972; 12:1669–1684.

114. Kofuji P, Biedermann B, Siddharthan V, Raap M, Landiev I, Milenkovic I, Thomzig A, Veh RW, Bringmann A, Reichenbach A: Kir potassium channel subunit expression in retinal glial cells: Implications for spatial potassium buffering. *Glia* 2002; 39:292–303.

115. Kofuji P, Ceelen P, Zahs KR, Surbeck LW, Lester HA, Newman EA: Genetic inactivation of an inwardly rectifying potassium channel (Kir4.1 subunit) in mice: Phenotypic impact in retina. *J Neurosci* 2000; 20:5733–5740.

116. Kondo M, Sieving PA: Post-photoreceptoral activity dominates primate photopic 32-Hz ERG for sine-, square-, and pulsed stimuli. *Invest Ophthalmol Vis Sci* 2002; 43:2500–2507.

117. Korol S, Leuenherger PM, Englert U, Babel J: In vivo effects of glycine on retinal ultrastructure and averaged electroretinogram. *Brain Res* 1975; 97:235–251.

118. Lamb TD, Pugh EN: A quantitative account of the activation steps involved in phototransduction in amphibian photoreceptors. *J Physiol* 1992; 449:719–758.

119. Lauritzen M: Cortical spreading depression in migraine. *Cephalalgia* 2001; 21:757–760.

120. Leaõ AAP. Spreading depression of activity in the cerebral cortex. *J Neurophysiol* 1944; 7:359–390.

121. Li JD, Govardovskii VI, Steinberg RH: Light-dependent hydration of the space surrounding photoreceptors in the cat retina. *Vis Neurosci* 1994; 11:743–752.

122. Lieberman HR: Origin of tile Ocular Light-Modulated Standing Potentials in Cat (Ph.D. thesis). University of Florida, 1977.

123. Linsenmeier RA, Mines AH, Steinberg RH: Effects of hypoxia and hypercapnia on the light peak and elec-troretinogram of the cat. *Invest Ophthalmol Vis Sci* 1983; 24:37–46.

124. Linsenmeier RA, Steinberg RH: Origin and sensitivity of the light peak of the intact cat eye. *J Physiol (Lond)* 1982; 331:653–673.

125. Linsenmeier RA, Steinberg RH: Delayed basal hyperpolarization of cat retinal pigment epithelium and its relation to the fast oscillation of the DC electroretinogram. *J Gen Physiol* 1984; 83:213–232.

126. Linsenmeier RA, Steinberg RH: Mechanisms of azide induced increases in the c-wave and standing potential of the intact cat eye. *Vision Res* 1987; 27:1–8.

127. Madachi-Yamamoto S: Abolition of the light rise by aspartate. *Soc Ophthalmol Jpn* 1980; 84:607–616.

128. Maeda H, Saszik SM, Frishman LJ: Postreceptoral Contributions to the a-wave of the photopic flash ERG of the mouse retina. *Invest ARVO Abstr* 2003; #1891.

129. Maffei L, Fiorentini A: Electroretinographic responses to alternating gratings before and after section of the optic nerve. *Science* 1981; 211:953–955.

130. Marchiafava FL, Torre V: The responses of amacrine cells to light and intracellularly applied currents. *J Physiol* 1978; 276:103–125.

131. Marchiafava FL, Weiler R: The photoresponses of structurally identified amacrine cells in the turtle retina. *Proc R Soc Lond* 1982; 214:403–415.

132. Martins-Ferreira H, Nedergaard M, Nicholson C: Perspectives on spreading depression. *Brain Res Rev* 2000; 32:215–234.

133. Massey SC, Redburn DA, Crawford MLJ: The effects of 2-amino-4-phosphonobutyric acid (APB) on the ERG and ganglion cell discharge of rabbit retina. *Vision Res* 1983; 23:1607–1613.

134. Matsuura T, Miller WH, Tomita T: Cone specific c wave in the turtle retina. *Vision Res* 1978; 18:767–775.

135. McCall MA, Lukasiewicz PD, Gregg RG, Peachey NS: Elimination of the rho1 subunit abolishes GABA(C) receptor expression and alters visual processing in the mouse retina. *J Neurosci* 2002; 22:4163–4174.

136. Miller RF, Dacheux R: Chloride-sensitive receptive field mechanisms in the isolated retina-eyecup of the rabbit. *Brain Res* 1975; 90:329–334.

137. Miller RF, Dacheux R, Proenza LM: Müller cell depolarization evoked by antidromic optic nerve stimulation. *Brain Res* 1977; 121:162–166.

138. Miller RF, Dowling JE: Intracellular responses of the Müller (glial) cells of mudpuppy retina: Their relation to b-wave of the electroretinogram. *J Neurophysiol* 1970; 33:323–341.

139. Miller SS, Steinberg RH: Passive ionic properties of frog retinal pigment epithelium. *J Membr Biol* 1977; 36:337–372.

140. Miller SS, Steinberg RH, Oakley B II: The electrogenic sodium pump of frog retinal pigment epithelium. *J Membr Biol* 1978; 44:259–279.

141. Mojumder DK, Frishman LJ: Effects of blocking spiking activity on the flash ERG of the rat are dependent upon background illumination. *ARVO Abstr* 2004; #812.

142. Mori S, Miller WH, Tomita T: Microelectrode study of spreading depression (SD) in frog retina: General observations of field potentials associated with SD. *Jpn J Physiol* 1977; 26:203–217.

143. Mori S, Miller WH, Tomita T: Microelectrode study of spreading depression (SD) in frog retina: Müller cell activity and [K+] during SD. *Jpn J Physiol* 1977; 26:219–233.

144. Motokawa K, Mita T: Uher eimie einfachiere umiter-suchungsniethode umid Eigenschaften der aktiomisstrome der netzhaut des menschiemi. *Tohoku I Exp Med* 1942; 42:114–133.

145. Murakami M, Kaneko A: Differentiation of PIII subcomponents in cold-blooded vertebrate retinas. *Vision Res* 1966; 6:627–636.

146. Naarendorp F, Sato Y, Cajdric A, Hubbard NP: Absolute and relative sensitivity of the scotopic system of rat: Electroretinography and behavior. *Vis Neurosci* 2001; 18:641–656.

147. Naarendorp F, Sieving PA: The scotopic threshold response of the cat ERG is suppressed selectively by GABA and glycine. *Vision Res* 1991; 31:1–15.

148. Nedergaard M, Cooper AJL, Goldman SA: Gap-junctions are required for the propagation of spreading depression. *J Neurobiol* 1995; 28:433–444.

149. Newman EA: b-Wave currents in the frog retina. *Vision Res* 1979; 19:227–234.

150. Newman EA: Current source-density analysis of the b-wave of frog retina. *J Neurophysiol* 1980; 43:1355–1366.

151. Newman EA: Membrane physiology of retinal glia (Müller) cells. *J Neurosci* 1985; 5:2225–2239.

152. Newman EA: Regulation of extracellular potassium by glial cells in the retina. *Trends Neurosci* 1985; 8:156–159.

153. Newman EA: Distribution of potassium conductance in amphibian Müller (glial) cells: A comparative study. *J Neurosci* 1987; 7:2423–2432.

154. Newman EA: Potassium conductance in Müller cells of fish. *Glia* 1988; 1:275–281.

155. Newman EA: Potassium conductance block by barium in amphibian Müller cells. *Brain Res* 1989; 498:308–314.

156. Newman EA: Müller cells and the retinal pigment epithelium. In Albert DM, Jakobiec RA (eds): *Principles and Practice of Ophthalmology.* Philadelphia, Saunders, 2000, pp 1762–1785.

157. Newman EA, Frambach DA, Odette LL: Control of extracellular potassium levels by retinal glial cell K+ siphoning. *Science* 1984; 225:1174–1175.

158. Newman EA, Lettvin JY: Relation of the c-wave to ganglion cell activity and rod responses in the frog. *Vision Res* 1978; 18:1181–1188.

159. Newman EA, Odette LL: Model of electroretinogram b-wave generation: A test of the K+ hypothesis. *J Neurophysiol* 1984; 51:164–182.

160. Newman EA, Reichenbach A: The Müller cell: A functional element of the retina. *Trends Neurosci* 1996; 19:307–317.

161. Niemeyer C, Nagahara K, Dernant E: Effects of changes in arterial Po_2 and Pco_2 on the ERG in the cat. *Invest Ophthalmol Vis Sci* 1982; 23:678–683.

162. Nikara T, Sato S, Takamatsu T, Sato R, Mita T: A new wave (2nd c-wave) on corneoretinal potential. *Experimentia* 1976; 32:594–596.

163. Nilsson SEG, Andersson BE, Corneal DC: Recordings of slow ocular potential changes such as the ERG c-wave and the light peak in clinical work: Equipment and examples of results. *Doc Ophthalmol* 1988; 68:313–325.

164. Noell WK: Studies on the Electrophysiology and the Metabolism of the Retina. USAF SAM Project No 21-2101-004, Randolph Field, Texas, 1953, pp 1–122.

165. Normann RA, Pochohradsky J: Oscillations in rod and horizontal cell membrane potential: Evidence for feed-hack to rods in the vertebrate retina. *J Physiol* 1976; 261:15–29.

166. Oakley B II: Potassium and the photoreceptor-dependent pigment epithelial hyperpolarization. *J Gen Physiol* 1977; 70:405–425.

167. Oakley B II, Green DC: Correlation of light-induced changes in retinal extracellular potassium concentration with the c-wave of the electroretinogram. *J Neurophysiol* 1976; 39:1117–1133.

168. Oakley B II, Steinberg RH: Effects of maintained illumination upon $[K^+]_o$ in the subretinal space of the frog retina. *Vision Res* 1982; 22:767–773.

169. Odette LL, Newman EA: Model of potassium dynamics in the central nervous system. *Glia* 1988; 1:198–210.

170. Ogden TE: Intraretinal slow potentials evoked by brain stimulation in the primate. *J Neurophysiol* 1966; 29:898–908.

171. Ogden TE: The oscillatory waves of the primate electroretinogram. *Vision Res* 1973; 13:797–807.

172. Ogden TE: The proximal negative response of the primate retina. *Vision Res* 1973; 13:797–807.

173. Ogden TE, Brown KT: Intraretinal responses of the cynamolgus monkey to electrical stimulation of the optic nerve and retina. *J Neurophysiol Jpn* 1964; 27:682–705.

174. Ogden TE, Ito H: Avian retina: II. An evaluation of retinal electrical anisotropy. *J Neurophysiol* 1971; 34:367–373.

175. Olsen JS, Miller RE: Spontaneous slow potentials and spreading depression in amphibian retina. *J Neurophysiol* 1977; 40:752–767.

176. Paulter EL, Murikami M, Nosaki H: Differentiation of PIII subcomponents in isolated mammalian retinas. *Vision Res* 1968; 8:489–491.

177. Paupoo AA, Mahroo OA, Friedburg C, Lamb TD: Human cone photoreceptor responses measured by the electroretinogram [correction of electoretinogram] a-wave during and after exposure to intense illumination. *J Physiol* 2000; 529:469–482.

178. Peachey NS, Alexander KR, Fishman GA: Rod and cone system contributions to oscillatory potentials: An explanation for the conditioning flash effect. *Vision Res* 1987; 27:859–866.

179. Penn RD, Hagins WA: Signal transmission along retinal rods and the origin of the electroretinographic a-wave. *Nature* 1969; 223:201–204.

180. Penn RD, Hagins WA: Kinetics of the photocurrent of retinal rods. *Biophys J* 1972; 12:1073–1094.

181. Pepperberg DR, Birch DG, Hood DC: Photoresponses of human rods in vivo derived from paired-flash electroretinograms. *Vis Neurosci* 1997; 14:73–82.

182. Perry VH, Cowey A: The ganglion cell and cone distributions in the monkey's retina: Implications for central magnification factors. *Vision Res* 1985; 25:1795–1810.

183. Pugh EN Jr, Falsini B, Lyubarsky A: The origin of the major rod- and cone-driven components of the rodent electroretinogram and the effects of age and light-rearing history on the magnitude of these components. In Williams TP, Thistle AB (eds): *Photostasis and Related Phenomena.* New York, Plenum Press, 1998, pp 93–128.

184. Quinn RH, Quong JN, Miller SS: Adrenergic receptor activated ion transport in human fetal retinal pigment epithelium. *Invest Ophthalmol Vis Sci* 2001; 42:255–264.

185. Rangaswamy N, Dorotheo EU, Ang RA, Schiffman JS, Bahrani HM, Frishman LJ: Photopic ERGs in patients with optic neuropathies: Comparison with primate ERGs after pharmacologic blockade of inner retina. *Invest Ophthalmol Vis Sci* 2004; 45:3827–3837.

186. Rangaswamy NV, Harwerth RS, Saszik SM, Maeda H, Frishman LJ: Frequency analysis of OPs in the slow-sequence MfERG in primates: Comparison of experimental glaucoma and pharmacological inner retinal blockade. *ARVO Abstract* 2003; #2702.

187. Rangaswamy N, Hood DC, Frishman LJ: Regional variation in local contributions to the photopic flash ERG revealed using the slow-sequence mfERG. *Invest Ophthalmol Vis Sci* 2003; 44:3233–3247.

188. Reichenhach A, Eherhardt W: Cytotopographical specialization of enzymatically isolated rabbit retinal Müller (glial) cells: K^+ conductivity of the cell membrane. *Glia* 1988; 1:191–197.

189. Reichenbach A, Henke A, Eberhardt W, Reichelt W, Dettmer D: K^+ ion regulation in retina. *Can J Physiol Pharmacol* 1992; 70 (suppl):S239–S247. Review

190. Ripps H, Mehaffey L, Siegel IM: "Rapid regeneration" in the cat retina. *J Gen Physiol* 1981; 77:335–346.

191. Robson JG, Frishman LJ: Response linearity and kinetics of the cat retina: The bipolar-cell component of the dark-adapted electroretinogram. *Vis Neurosci* 1995; 12:837–850.

192. Robson JG, Frishman LJ: Photoreceptor and bipolar-cell contributions to the cat electroretinogram: A kinetic model for the early part of the flash response. *J Opt Soc Am* 1996; A.13:613–622.

193. Robson JG, Frishman LJ: Dissecting the dark-adapted electroretinogram. *Doc Ophthalmol* 1998–1999; 95:187–215.

194. Robson JG, Maeda H, Saszik S, Frishman LJ: In vivo studies of signaling in rod pathways using the electroretinogram. *Vision Res* 2004; 44:3253–3268.

195. Robson JG, Saszik SM, Ahmed J, Frishman LJ: Rod and cone contributions to the *a*-wave of the electroretinogram of the dark-adapted macaque. *J Physiol (Lond)* 2003; 547:509–530.

196. Sakai H, Naka K-I: Neuron network in catfish retina: 1968–1987. *Prog Ret Res* 1988; 7:149–208.

197. Sakai HM, Naka K-I, Dowling JE: Ganglion cell dendrites are presynaptic in catfish retina. *Nature* 1986; 319:495–497.

198. Saszik S, Alexander A, Lawrence T, Bilotta J: APB differentially affects the cone contributions to the zebrafish ERG. *Vis Neurosci* 2002; 19:521–529.

199. Saszik S, Frishman LJ, Robson JG: The scotopic threshold response of the dark-adapted electroretinogram of the mouse. *J Physiol (Lond)* 2002; 543.3:899–916.

200. Saszik S, Robson JG, Frishman LJ: Contributions of spiking and non-spiking inner retinal neurons to the scotopic ERG of the mouse. *Invest Ophthalmol Vis Sci* 2002; 43 (suppl):1817.

201. Seeliger MW, Saszik S, Mayser H, Frishman LJ, Hormuzdi S, Biel M, Humphries P, Willecke K, Monyer H, Weiler R: Connexin 36-dependent retinal function in mice with specific rod or cone photoreceptor input. *ARVO Abstract* 2003; #1827.

202. Shiells RA, Falk G: Contribution of rod, on-bipolar, and horizontal cell light responses to the ERG of dogfish retina. *Vis Neurosci* 1999; 16:503–511.

203. Shimazaki H, Karwoski CJ, Proenza LM: Aspartate induced dissociation of proximal from distal retinal activity in the mudpuppy. *Vision Res* 1984; 24:587–595.

204. Shimazaki H, Oakley B II: Reaccumulation of $[K^+]_o$ in the toad retina during maintained illumination. *J Gen Physiol* 1984; 84:475–504.

205. Sickel W, Crescitelli F: Delayed electrical responses from the isolated frog retina. *Pflugers Arch Ges Physiol* 1967; 297:266–269.

206. Sieving PA: Retinal ganglion cell loss does not abolish the scotopic threshold response (STR) of the cat and human ERG. *Clin Vis Sci* 1991; 2:149–158.

207. Sieving PA, Frishman LJ, Steinberg RH: Scotopic threshold response of proximal retina in cat. *J Neurophysiol* 1986; 56:1049–1061.

208. Sieving PA, Frishman LJ, Steinberg RH: M-wave of proximal retina in cat. *J Neurophysiol* 1986; 56:1039–1048.

209. Sieving PA, Murayama K, Naarendorp F: Push-pull model of the primate photopic electroretinogram: A role for hyperpolarizing neurons in shaping the b-wave. *Vis Neurosci* 1994; 11:519–532.

210. Sieving PA, Nino C: Human scotopic threshold response. *Invest Ophthalmol Vis Sci* 1988; 29:1608–1614.

211. Sieving PA, Steinberg RH: Contribution from proximal retina to intraretinal pattern-ERG: The m-wave. *Invest Ophthalmol Vis Sci* 1985; 26:1642–1647.

212. Sieving PA, Wakabayashi K: Comparison of rod threshold ERG from monkey, cat and human. *Clin Vis Sci* 1991; 6:171–179.

213. Sieving PA, Wakabayashi K, Lemon WJ: Current source density analysis of the cat scotopic threshold response. *Invest Ophthalmol Vis Sci* 1988; 29 (suppl):103.

214. Sillman AJ, Ito H, Tomita T: Studies on the mass receptor potential of the isolated frog retina: 1. General properties of the response. *Vision Res* 1969; 9:1435–1442.

215. Slaughter MM, Miller RF: 2-Amino-4-phosphonobutyric acid: A new pharmacological tool for retina research. *Science* 1981; 211:182–185.

216. Slaughter MM, Miller RF: The role of excitatory amino acid transmitters in the mudpuppy retina: An analysis with kainic acid and N-methyl aspartate. *J Neurosci* 1983; 3:1701–1711.

217. Somjen GG, Aitkin PG: The ionic and metabolic responses associated with neuronal depression of *Leaõs* type in cerebral cortex and in hippocampal formation. *An Acad Bras Cienc* 1984; 56:495–504.

218. Steinberg RH: Oscillatory activity in the optic tract of cat and light adaptation. *J Neurophysiol* 1966; 29:139–156.

219. Steinberg RH: Comparison of the intraretinal b-wave and d.c. component in the area centralis of cat retina. *Vision Res* 1969; 9:317–331.

220. Steinberg RH: High-intensity effects on slow potentials and ganglion cell activity in the area centralis of cat retina. *Vision Res* 1969; 9:333–350.

221. Steinberg R, Frishman LJ, Sieving PA: Negative components of the electroretinogram from proximal retina and photoreceptor. In Osborne NN, Chader GJ (eds): *Progress in Retinal Research*. Oxford, UK: Permagon, 1991; 10:121–160.

222. Steinberg RH, Linsenmeier RA, Griff ER: Retinal pigment epithelial cell contributions to the electroretinogram and electrooculogram. In Osborne NN, Chader GJ (eds): *Progress in Retinal Research*. New York, Pergamon Press, 1985; 4:33–66.

223. Steinberg RH, Schmidt R, Brown KT: Intracellular responses to light from the cat retinal pigment epithelium: Origin of the electroretinogram c-wave. *Nature* 1970; 227:728–730.

224. Stockton RA, Slaughter MM: The b-wave of the electroretinogram: A reflection of ON bipolar cell activity. *J Gen Physiol* 1989; 93:101–122.

225. Sutter EE, Bearse MA Jr: The optic nerve head component of the human ERG. *Vision Res* 1999; 39:419–436.

226. Tomita T: Studies on the intraretinal action potential: Part I. Relation between the localization of micropipette in the

retina and the shape of the intraretinal action potential. *Jpn J Physiol* 1950; 1:110–117.

227. Tomita T: Study on electrical activities in the retina with penetrating microelectrodes. *Proc XXI Int Cong Physiol (Symposium and Special Lectures)* 1959; 245–248.

228. Tomita T, Funaishi A: Studies on intraretinal action potential with low-resistance microelectrode. *J Neurophysiol* 1952; 15:75–84.

229. Tomita T, Matsuura T, Fujimoto M, Miller WH: The electroretinographic c- and d-waves with special reference to the receptor potential. Presented at the 16th ISCEV Symposium, Morioka, Japan, 1978, pp 15–25.

230. Tomita T, Mizuno H, Ida T: Studies on the intraretinal action potential: Part III. Intraretinal negative potential as compared with b-wave in the ERG. *Jpn J Physiol* 1952; 2:171–176.

231. Tomita T, Torihama Y: Further study on the intraretinal action potentials and on the site of ERG generation. *Jpn J Physiol* 1956; 6:118–136.

232. Toyoda J-I, Hashimoto H, Ohtsu K: Bipolar-amacrine transmission in the carp retina. *Vision Res* 1973; 13:295–307.

233. Valeton JM, van Norren D: Intraretinal recordings of slow electrical responses to steady illumination in monkey: Isolation of receptor responses and the origin of the light peak. *Vision Res* 1982; 22:393–399.

234. Van Harreveld A: Visual concomitants of retinal spreading depression. *An Acad Bras Cienc* 1984; 56:519–524.

235. van Norren D, Heynen H: Origin of the fast oscillation in the electroretinogram of the macaque. *Vision Res* 1986; 26:569–575.

236. Vigh J, Solessio E, Morgans CW, Lasater EM: Ionic mechanisms mediating oscillatory membrane potentials in wide-field retinal amacrine cells. *J Neurophysiol* 2003; 90:431–443.

237. Viswanathan S, Frishman LJ: Evidence that negative potentials in the photopic ERGs of cats and primates depend upon spiking activity of retinal ganglion cell axons. *Soc Neurosci Abstr* 1997; 23:1024.

238. Viswanathan S, Frishman LJ, Robson JG: The uniform field and pattern ERG in macaques with experimental glaucoma: Removal of spiking activity. *Invest Ophthalmol Vis Sci* 2000; 41:2797–2810.

239. Viswanathan S, Frishman LJ, Robson JG: Inner-retinal contributions to the photopic flicker electroretinogram of macaques. *Doc Ophthalmol Special Issue: Animal Models in Clinical Electrophysiology of Vision* 2002; 105:223–242.

240. Viswanathan S, Frishman LJ, Robson JG, Walters JW: The photopic negative response of the flash electroretinogram in primary open angle glaucoma. *Invest Ophthalmol Vis Sci* 2001; 42:514–522.

241. Viswanathan S, Frishman LJ, Robson JG, et al: The photopic negative response of the macaque ERG is reduced by experimental glaucoma. *Invest Ophthalmol Vis Sci* 1999; 40:124–136.

242. Wachtmeister L: Oscillatory potentials in the retina: What do they reveal. *Prog Retinal Eye Res* 1998; 17:485–521.

243. Wakabayashi K, Gieser J, Sieving PA: Aspartate isolates the STR from the a-wave of cat and monkey. *Invest Ophthalmol Vis Sci* 1988; 29:1615–1622.

244. Wassle H, Grunert U, Rohrenbeck J, Boycott BB: Retinal ganglion cell density and cortical magnification factor in the primate. *Vision Res* 1990; 30:897–911.

245. Wen R, Oakley B II: K(+)-evoked Müller cell depolarization generates b-wave of electroretinogram in toad retina. *Proc Natl Acad Sci USA* 1990; 87:2117–2121.

246. Whitten DN, Brown KT: The time course of late receptor potentials from monkey cones and rods. *Vision Res* 1973; 13:107–135.

247. Winkler BS: Analysis of the rabbit's electroretinogram following unilateral transection of the optic nerve. *Exp Eye Res* 1972; 13:227–235.

248. Winkler BS, Gum KB: Slow PIII and b-wave have different ionic dependences. *Invest Ophthalmol Vis Sci* 1981; 20:183.

249. Winkler BS, Kapousta-Bruneau N, Arnold MJ, Green DG: Effects of inhibiting glutamine synthetase and blocking glutamate uptake on b-wave generation in the isolated rat retina. *Vis Neurosci* 1999; 16:345–353.

250. Witkovsky P, Dudek FE, Ripps H: Slow PIII component of the carp electroretinogram. *J Gen Physiol* 1975; 65:119–134.

251. Witkovsky P, Nelson J, Ripps H: Action spectra and adaptation properties of carp photoreceptors. *J Gen Physiol* 1973; 61:401–423.

252. Xu X, Karwoski CJ: Current source density analysis of retinal field potentials: II. Pharmacological analysis of the b-wave and M-wave. *J Neurophysiol* 1994; 72:96–105.

253. Xu X, Karwoski CJ: Current source density analysis of the electroretinographic d wave of frog retina. *J Neurophysiol* 1995; 73:2459–2469.

254. Yanagida T, Koshimizu M, Kawasaki K, Yonemura D: Microelectrode depth study of electroretinographic b- and d-waves in frog retina. *Jpn J Ophthalmol* 1986; 20:298–305.

255. Yanagida T, Koshimizu M, Kawasaki K, Yonemura D: Microelectrode depth study of the electroretinographic oscillatory potentials in the frog retina. *Doc Ophthalmol* 1988; 7:355–361.

256. Yonemura D, Kawasaki K: New approaches to ophthalmic electrodiagnosis by retinal oscillators' potential, drug-induced responses from retinal pigment epithelium and cone potential. *Doc Ophthalmol* 1979; 48:163–222.

257. Yonemura D, Kawasaki K, Shibata N, Tanahe J: The electroretinographic PIII component of the human excised retina. *Jpn J Ophthalmol* 1974; 18:322–333.

258. Yonemura D, Kawasaki K, Yanagida T, Tanabe J, Kawaguchi H, Nakata Y: Effects of γ-amino acids on oscillatory activities of the light-evoked potentials in the retina and visual pathways. Proceedings. 16th ISCEV Symposium, Morioka, 1978.

259. Yonemura D, Tsuzuki K, Aoki T: Clinical importance of the oscillatory potential in the human ERG. *Acta Ophthalmol Suppl* 1962; 70:115–122.

260. Zimmerman RP, Corfman TP: A comparison of the effects of isomers of alpha-aminoadipic acid and 2-amino-4-phosphonobutyric acid on the light response of the Müller glial cell and the electroretinogram. *Neurosci* 1984; 12:77–84.

261. Zuckerman R: Ionic analysis of photoreceptor currents. *J Physiol* 1973; 235:333.

13 The Origin of the Pattern Electroretinogram

MICHAEL BACH AND MICHAEL B. HOFFMANN

THE MASS RESPONSE from the retina (the electroretinogram, or ERG) that is evoked by pattern stimulation is called the pattern electroretinogram (PERG). Riggs and coworkers[47] were the first to record a PERG after they had successfully devised a local stimulus without stray light artifacts. Interestingly, they did not yet know that the generators for PERG and luminance ERG differ and did not call it PERG. While the luminance ERG is evoked by changes in stimulus luminance, the PERG is evoked by changes of stimulus contrast (in sign or magnitude). The PERG is therefore a retinal response (figure 13.1) that is evoked in the absence of a net change of stimulus luminance. This property has profound implications for the generators of the responses, which are mainly the retinal ganglion cells, as we will see in this chapter. Consequently, the PERG is a valuable diagnostic tool to examine diseases that are associated with a loss of ganglion cell activity as described in chapters 12 and 77. The ISCEV has developed a standard[6] with the aim to make PERG recordings comparable worldwide across laboratories while still allowing extension into any new fruitful direction. For an earlier comprehensive review of the physiological basis of the PERG, see Zrenner.[59]

The difference between luminance and pattern stimulation or: What does this "second harmonic" thing mean anyway?

Pattern stimulation without any change in net luminance (space-averaged luminance) is of particular interest because it helps to isolate nonlinear response properties, while linear responses will cancel out. This would be only of theoretical interest if it did not help in isolating a contribution to the retinal response, which otherwise, because of its small size, would be totally swamped by the luminance response. As illustrated in figure 13.2, the cancellation of any linear response component depends critically on two constraints. First, during pattern reversal, exactly half the retinal area covered by the stimulus has to be exposed to a light stimulus patch, while the other half has to be exposed to a dark stimulus patch. Second, the responses to these two stimuli have to be proportional to the local luminance step both in magnitude and in sign, as empirically confirmed for a large

proportion of the response (see figure 13.3).[5] A pattern-reversal stimulus will then elicit responses from dark and bright patches that are of the same magnitude but have a different sign. When "seen" from a corneal electrode, which averages across the entire retina, these linear responses will cancel out. Remarkably, any imbalance between the two responses will not cancel out and will therefore be revealed with pattern stimulation, as is schematically depicted in figure 13.2 and illustrated with real data in figure 13.3. The imbalance of the two responses is due to nonlinear properties of the underlying neural substrate such as a response with a strong ON component, but no OFF component, or a generator with very rapid adaptation[13,15,49] or a response from the interaction of neighboring bright and dark regions. It is, as was pointed out above, mandatory that equal retinal extents are stimulated with dark and bright patches; otherwise, linear response components will cancel out. Therefore, certain symmetry constraints have to be fulfilled while other aspects of the spatial stimulus arrangement are not relevant. Proper and improper stimulus patterns are illustrated in figure 1patt3.4. The stimulus has to be composed of an equal number of bright and dark patches, and these have to be symmetrically arranged with respect to the fovea to take account of the receptor density gradient across the retina. These conditions are automatically met by balanced pattern-reversal stimuli (figures 13.4A–13.4G are fine; figures 13.4I–13.4L are not balanced). Pattern onset/offset (figure 13.4H) is also a possibility because equal regions become bright and dark. It should be noted, however, that the local temporal contrast change can never exceed 50% with onset/offset stimulation; for reversal stimulation, it can be 100%. Furthermore, it is mandatory that the average luminance of the gray field is the same as that of the patterned field. This needs very careful calibration of the stimulation system (e.g., a CRT monitor[9,16]) and can be next to impossible for high contrasts.

We have now understood why the net luminance must not change to isolate the nonlinear response components. But why does this response occur at the second harmonic of the stimulation frequency? Let us first assume luminance modulation with a homogenous screen: For 0.5 s, it is dark; then for 0.5 s, it becomes bright; and so on. This corresponds to a temporal frequency of 1 Hz. The response will be

Definition. The PERG is

... short for "Pattern ERG" (which, in turn, is short for "Pattern Electroretinogram")

... the electrical signal

  —recorded from the cornea (with appropriate electrodes)

  —in response to visual pattern stimulation with constant mean luminance

  —and averaged over many (≈ 100) repetitions because of its small size relative to other sources such as eye movement and myogenic artifacts.

The typical PERG Stimulus

  Checkerboard pattern, check size 0.8°, contrast reversal ≤4 rev/s (transient), ≥8 rev/s (steady state), mean luminance ≈50 cd/m² , high contrast, >90%

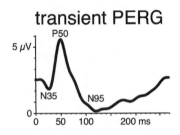

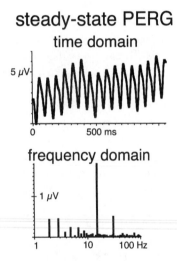

FIGURE 13.1   Top, The transient PERG with three major deflections (n35, p55, and N95). Bottom, The sinusoidally shaped steady-state PERG with corresponding Fourier spectrum.

dominated by the receptors and occur at the temporal frequency of the stimulus, which is 1 Hz (figure 13.2). Now let us envisage a patterned screen, a checkerboard pattern that reverses with the same temporal sequence: The top left square is dark for 0.5 s and will then become bright for 0.5 s, and so on. Clearly, the stimulation frequency still is 1 Hz, but the responses appear at 2 Hz! Why? When the top left square becomes bright, we will see a (local!) ON response from its area and some response from mechanisms that are sensitive to changes in its border contrast. When this square becomes dark, its neighbor becomes bright, and the same mechanisms

apply. So the local generators will not be identical but will be shifted to the neighbor square, but the same type of generator will respond. When results are superimposed to result in a global response, this occurs at every change of the stimulus and thus at twice the stimulus frequency. This is what is referred to when one says that the PERG is the second harmonic response. Since the response occurs at double the frequency of the stimulation frequency, it is misleading to give the stimulation rate in hertz and the term *reversal per second*, or *rev/s*, or *rps* must be used. For onset stimulation, as opposed to reversal stimulation, the frequency doubling does not occur, because there is no symmetry between the two stimulus states (patterned = ON, and homogenous gray = OFF).

Can we pinpoint the generator of the PERG?

Talking about the origin of the PERG implies that the PERG itself is one entity with a common origin of all its excursions, regardless of stimulus parameters such as check size, temporal frequency, or contrast. As we will see, this implication is indeed largely justified and will certainly do for a first approximation: The generators of the PERG clearly differ from those of the luminance ERG or the EOG. A more refined view will be developed later.

Various techniques have been employed to identify the generator of the PERG:

1. Physical source localization with microelectrode recordings. This identifies the retinal layer with the largest signal.

2. A knock-out of the generator with a corresponding loss of the PERG. This can be examined either in pathophysiological conditions or after pharmacological intervention.

3. The assessment of the parameter dependencies of the electrophysiological responses. These ought to mirror the physiological properties of their generators; for example, ganglion cells show lateral inhibition and should therefore cause low spatial frequency attenuation in the PERG.

All of these approaches have been tried, and each has some particular advantages and shortcomings. After various detours (e.g., using intricate stimulus modulation techniques),[46] a fairly consistent picture has formed.

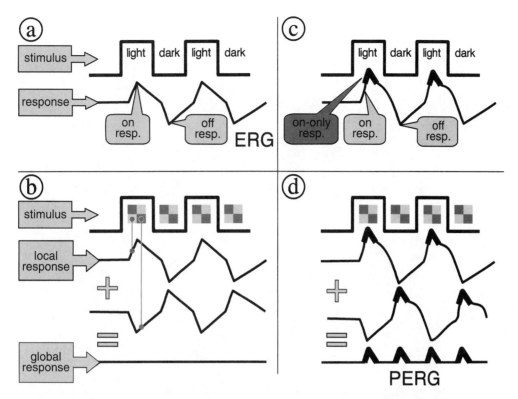

FIGURE 13.2   From luminance stimuli to pattern stimuli, from ERG to PERG. Local luminance ERGs (A) cancel each other in the absence of a nonlinear response (B). A response nonlinearity (C), such as greater ON than OFF responses, is isolated by the pattern ERG (D).

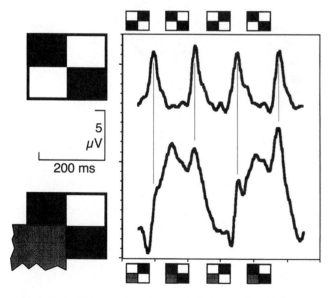

FIGURE 13.3   Effects of luminance imbalance. Top, Fully symmetric stimulus with very large check size, reversing four times, resulting in four PERG responses (with some overlap of N95 and succeeding N35). Bottom, Covering one quarter of the screen, and thus one check, results in a luminance response at every second reversal.

Physical source localization

We have seen that change of net stimulus luminance will result in a luminance ERG at the stimulus fundamental frequency. If we use a pattern stimulus with no net change of stimulus luminance, we obtain a pattern ERG response at the second harmonic of the stimulation frequency. The underlying mechanism of this response change is the cancellation of the local luminance ERG, which leaves the nonlinear components of the response. This happens because the corneal ERG electrode integrates across the local responses from the entire retinal area that is stimulated. However, if we record the local ERG with a microelectrode right at the retinal level, we should be able to obtain a local luminance ERG with the main response at the stimulus fundamental frequency. This is exactly what Sieving and Steinberg[51] were able to demonstrate in cats (figure 13.5): At a distinct retinal location, they recorded a luminance ERG at the stimulus fundamental frequency. They then varied the spatial cycle of the stimulus and obtained local ERGs for an entire spatial grating cycle. An integration across these local ERGs leads to a cancellation of the linear components and, as a consequence, yielded a response at the second harmonic of the stimulus frequency. The integration of local luminance responses therefore yielded a response that resembled a PERG recorded with a corneal electrode. In the next step,

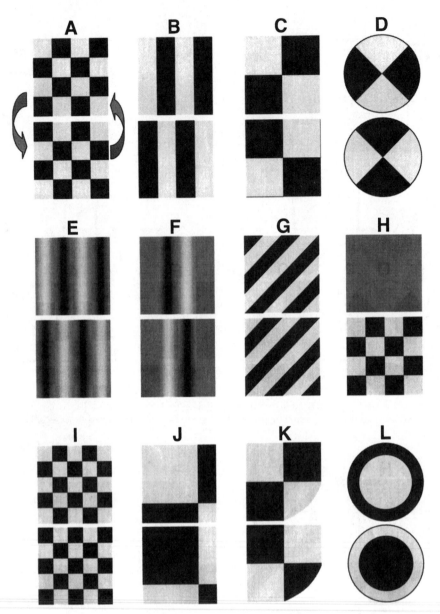

FIGURE 13.4 Proper and improper stimulus patterns. Patterns A through G are inherently symmetric and fine. Configuration (H) corresponds to pattern onset and requires good display calibration to avoid net luminance changes. Pattern I has an unequal number of light and dark checks. Pattern J has uneven areas for light and dark checks. Pattern K may arise through spectacle artifacts, resulting in similar luminance changes as for pattern J. Pattern L, when calibrated for cone density, may evoke an undiluted PERG even if space-average luminance changes (an academic case, clearly, but worth a thought).

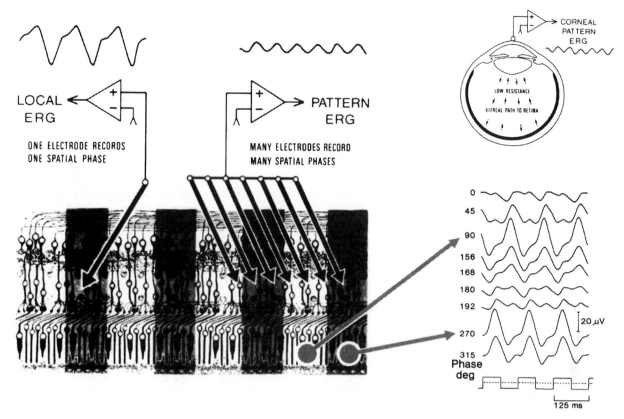

FIGURE 13.5 From local responses to the global PERG: microelectrode recordings from an acute cat preparation. A grating stimulus is depicted schematically. The left derivation shows local responses, dominated by the luminance response within the center of a grating stripe. Positioning this electrode at various positions in the grating cycle changes the polarity (extremes at 90° and 270°) with nearly PERG-like intermediate positions (at 0° and 180°). Averaging across these positions (center) mimics the situation of a corneal electrode. The luminance responses cancel, leaving the nonlinearities: the PERG. (After Sieving PA, Steinberg RH.[51])

Sieving and Steinberg[51] aimed to locate the generator of the PERG and moved the electrode gradually from proximal to distal retina. Current source density analysis revealed different generators for luminance and pattern ERG, namely, the distal and the proximal retina, respectively. In primates, Baker et al.[11] were able to locate the generators of ERG and PERG at retinal locations similar to those determined by Sieving and Steinberg.[51] They concluded that the PERG is generated in the proximal 30% of the retina, corresponding to the ganglion cell layer, inner plexiform layer, and inner nuclear layer (figure 13.6). Thus, synaptic and dendritic currents of ganglion, amacrine, and bipolar cells in these layers are potential candidates for generation of the PERG. However, the available spatial resolution of this technique is not sufficient to distinguish between these alternatives.

Knock-out of ganglion cells or their activity

Ganglion cells can be lost through atrophy, both in human disease and in animals by experimental intervention, or their activity can be pharmacologically suppressed. With regard

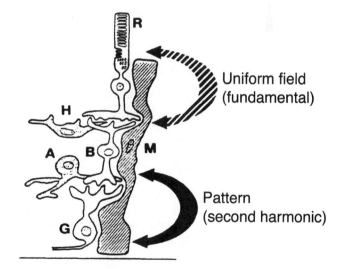

FIGURE 13.6 Schematic generator sites as derived from current source density analysis. The pattern response originates in the ganglion cell layer. (From Baker CL, Jr, Hess RR, Olsen BT, Zrenner E.[11])

to the first possibility, Groneberg and Teping[24] were the first to demonstrate a dissociation of ERG and PERG changes in (secondary) optic atrophy in humans. In the next year, Maffei and Fiorentini[41] reported a complete loss of the PERG in cats four months after optic nerve section, while the luminance ERG remained unchanged. In connection with careful histological analysis,[35] they related this PERG loss to the specific degeneration of retinal ganglion cells, which is a consequence of the section of the optic nerve, and discussed the far-reaching consequences of this finding. Similar findings have been reported in primates (monkeys[42] and humans[5,25,50]) (figures 13.7 and 13.8). These findings suggest that ganglion cell activity is reflected by the PERG of cats and primates. It should be noted that this relationship does not necessarily hold across species. The PERG of pigeons, for example, is not affected by optic nerve section and the subsequent degeneration of the retinal ganglion cells.[10]

Most studies on patients with unilateral (secondary) optic nerve atrophy report a reduction of PERG amplitudes down to about 30% (27% in Bach et al.[5]) (see also figure 13.8) compared to the normal fellow eye. Consequently, we find a severe but incomplete loss of the PERG after ganglion cell atrophy. This prompts the question of the origin of the residual PERG. To tackle this issue, we need to take a closer look

at the single components that we can discern in the transient PERG. It is dominated by an early positivity, P50, and a later negativity, the N95 (see figure 13.9 for nomenclature). Ganglion cell degeneration can affect both components to a variable degree[5,25] (see figures 13.7 and 13.8), but there is evidence that a loss of N95 is typical of optic nerve diseases. (See figure 13.10 for a 30-year-old female with dominant optic atrophy. The P50 is only mildly reduced, the N95 is lost, and there was no VEP response left.[34]) A preferential P50 reduction is associated with macular degeneration.[32,33] This supports the notion that N95 is generated by ganglion cells, but it questions whether the ganglion cells are the sole generator of P50. Here, the pharmacological approach has been able to provide valuable evidence in nonhuman primates.[36,56] Tetrodotoxin (TTX) blocks the voltage-gated Na⁺ channels.[43,44] Thus, it will suppress ganglion spikes but also some amacrine activity. After TTX application, the N95 component is completely gone, while P50 is only weakly affected[56] (figure 13.11). This indicates that there is a nonspiking contribution to P50. Another feature seen in figure 13.11 is the markedly differing shape between the monkey PERG and the human PERG: In the normal recording, the monkey N95 is about three times as large as the P50, while in humans, the N95 negativity is about 75% of the P50

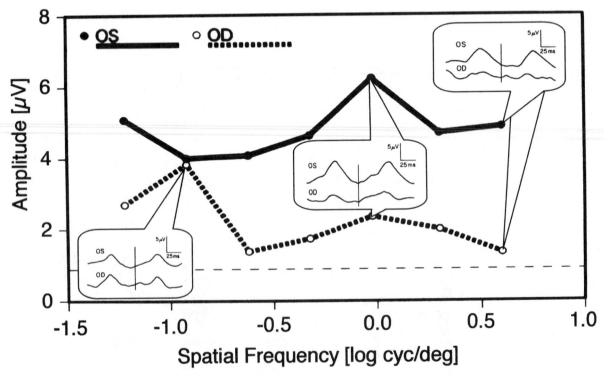

FIGURE 13.7 PERG in a case of unilateral total optic atrophy. PERG amplitude (ordinate, as derived from the inset traces) versus check size (quantified as dominant spatial frequency, large checks left). Apart from the unavoidable noise, the PERG from the atrophic eye is markedly reduced. (Modified from Harrison JM, O'Connor PS, Young RSL, et al.[25])

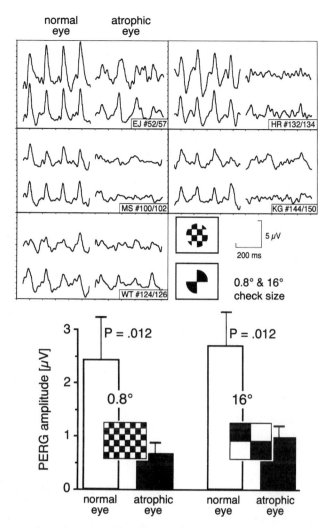

FIGURE 13.8 PERG in five cases of unilateral total optic atrophy. Top, Replicated recordings from the normal (left) and atrophic eye (right), respectively. Responses are reduced in the atrophic eye with a wide interindividual variability. Bottom,

positivity (figure 13.9). This underlines the strong species dependence of the PERG and cautions us about extrapolating from animal models to humans.

Grand mean amplitudes from Fourier analyses of the traces above. Responses to 0.8° and 16° check size are strongly reduced, with a slightly smaller effect for 16°. (Data from Bach M, Gerling J, Geiger K.[5])

A novel hypothesis on P50/N95 origin

We would like to offer a hypothesis that integrates the above somewhat bewildering findings: The P50 is generated within the ganglion cells but reflects the EPSPs/IPSPs, that is, "prespiking," activity or, in other words, the input into the ganglion cells. The N95 is also generated by the ganglion cells but reflects the ganglion cells' spiking activity. Because of the complicated interaction of distal dendritic activity with the differential distribution of excitatory and inhibitory synapses and their consequence at the axon hillock, they might easily differ with respect to their electrical mass activity seen from outside the ganglion cells. The hypothesis

would reconcile the preferential affection of the N95 by optic nerve diseases with the additional loss of the P50 with ganglion cell loss or preganglionic lesions. We have developed this hypothesis while writing this chapter, and the reader might view it as a proxy, successfully integrating the current understanding but awaiting experimental challenge.

Experimental tests might be difficult to devise because of the strong species differences previously mentioned.

Evidence from check size dependence (tuning), erroneously presumed to directly reflect lateral inhibition

Up to here, we have seen that ganglion cell activity is the main generator of the PERG. One should therefore expect the parameter dependence of the PERG to reflect the physiological properties of these neurons. The receptive fields of ganglion cells are structured into ON and OFF regions that

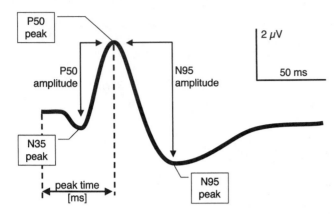

FIGURE 13.9 Peaks and components of the transient PERG. To clarify nomenclature, this figure helps to discern between peaks and amplitudes (e.g., P50 amplitude versus P50 peak). The components P50 and N95 are named after polarity and peak time.

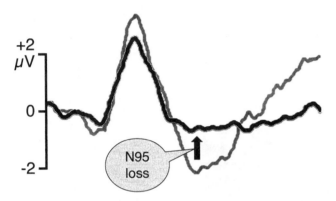

FIGURE 13.10 N95 loss. These traces demonstrate a complete N95 loss and a moderate P50 reduction. (Modified from figure 15 of Holder GE;[34] the thinner gray trace is from a normal subject).

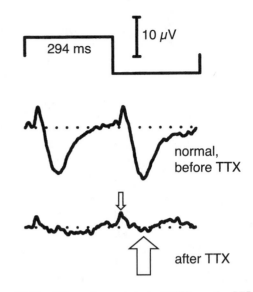

FIGURE 13.11 Effect of tetrodotoxin (TTX) on the PERG of a monkey (modified from Viswanathan et al.[56]). The top trace depicts stimulus polarity, indicating two reversals. The center trace shows the baseline PERG. The bottom trace shows the PERG after TTX application. TTX blocks the voltage-activated Na^+ channel and thus the action potentials. It affects mainly the N95 (reduced to 23%) and moderately the P50 (reduced to 60%). Note the large N95 trough in contrast to human PERGs (figures 13.9 and 13.10).

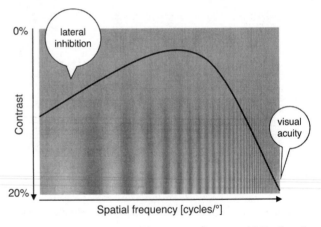

FIGURE 13.12 The normal human contrast sensitivity function (CSF), slightly schematized. The background is an Arden grating with increasing spatial frequency to the right and decreasing contrast to the top. The superimposed CSF curve depicts the upper end of visibility of the grating stimulus (the exact value depends on observer distance and possible rendering artifacts for the high spatial frequencies). The attenuation of the CSF for low spatial frequencies is due to lateral inhibition; the attenuation for high spatial frequencies is due to optics and neural sampling and determines the visual acuity.

are integrated in ganglion cell output. This is well known as *lateral inhibition*[26] and probably serves to compress data for efficient transfer along the optic nerve, as local changes of luminance are encoded rather than simply the luminance itself. When grating stimuli with different spatial frequencies are presented to such receptive fields, a band-pass-like tuning curve will result. This tuning curve probably underlies the band-pass nature of the psychophysical contrast sensitivity function,[18] which is demonstrated in figure 13.12, a variation of the Arden grating.[2] The high-spatial-frequency drop is caused by the optical transfer characteristics of the eye[19] and the finite receptor sampling density,[20] both of which also limit visual acuity. The low-spatial-frequency attenuation is governed by the maximal receptive field size combined with lateral inhibition, probably giving rise to phenomena such as the Hermann grid illusion.[3,12]

On the basis of these ideas, it was assumed that the PERG should mirror the low-spatial-frequency attenuation (LSFA) of the ganglion cells. Implicitly, this was transferred to check

size, equating LSFA with amplitude attenuation for large check sizes. A bewilderingly large number of papers have addressed this issue, and the emerging picture seems equally bewildering. To find our way through the jungle, let us clearly discern between data and interpretation.

Some data first: Relatively strong LSFA is found with stimuli that are sinusoidal in space,[31] pattern onset rather than reversal, low contrast (20%[40]), high temporal frequency (>10 rps), and low luminance.[39] Any deviation from these parameters will lead to a flatter tuning curve with little or no LSFA (too many references to cite; see, e.g., Bach and Holder[7]) (see also figure 13.13).

The retinal stimulus, namely, its contrast, depends on optics, especially for high spatial frequencies. Any conclusions based on the effects of decreasing check size assume that the optical imaging is optimal within the physiological limits (for an overview, see Bach and Mathieu[8]). This implies correct refraction for the stimulus distance and an electrode that does not impair optical quality (e.g., gold foil or DTL,[1,4,21,53] loop,[27] or other kinds with appropriate optical properties). And, of course, the electrodes need to be applied in an appropriate and consistent manner to achieve good reproducibility.[45]

How can we interpret the dependence (and independence) of the PERG on check size? Equating lateral inhibition with LSFA with check size tuning curves is flawed for three distinct reasons:

1. For intermediate and small checks (2°–0.1°), not only check size decreases, but also the retinal contrast[23,54] because of the optical low-pass properties of the eye.[17,37]

2. Checkerboards, when Fourier analyzed, contain a wide spectrum of spatial frequencies (see figure 15.10); therefore, large checks (e.g., >2°) still have strong harmonics that can excite small receptive fields. Yang et al.[57] analyzed this quan-

titatively and found that the Fourier spectrum of checks combined with the normal LSFA actually predicts a flat tuning curve for check sizes above 2°. Consequently, the absence of LSFA does not necessarily imply the absence of lateral inhibition.

3. It is rarely realized that the ganglion cells also respond well to spatially unstructured modulation, that is, flicker. This has two reasons: The ON and OFF regions of the receptive field are not necessarily of equal weight, so there is some luminance encoded as well; and the temporal properties of center and surround are not equal—usually the center properties are faster (e.g., Benardete and Kaplan[14]). Thus, a full-field (or at least larger-than-receptive field) ON stimulus will usually evoke a larger response than an OFF stimulus in ON ganglion cells.

We conclude for check size tuning that for the typical PERG stimulus with high-contrast transient reversal, the tuning curve (amplitude versus check size) will result in a marked decline of amplitude when check size becomes smaller than ≈0.8°; this is caused by optics and by the declining number of correspondingly small receptive fields. When check size exceeds ≈1°, there is only a shallow decline (LSFA, only ≈10%) even up to very large check sizes of 16°. As was indicated above, for checkerboard stimuli, this small LSFA does not indicate missing lateral inhibition. The following stimulus modifications will increase LSFA: sinusoidal profile in space and time,[31] higher temporal frequency (>≈10 rev/s), and pattern onset rather than pattern reversal.

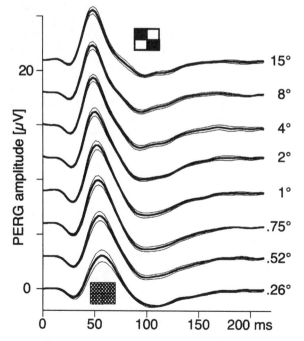

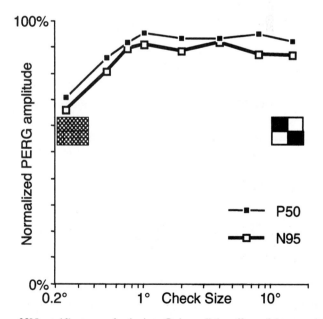

FIGURE 13.13   Check size tuning of the PERG. Left, Grand mean traces ± SEM for seven subjects at seven different check sizes. Right, Relative amplitude (normalized to the N95 at 1°) versus check size. Only a slight effect of low spatial frequency attenuation is apparent. (Data from Bach ME and Holder GE.[7])

Open questions

Many constraints force us to leave a number of alleys unexplored. However, we would at least like to mention one bewildering finding with respect to the contrast transfer function of the PERG, which does not follow from the generator model developed above: It was well established by Thompson and Drasdo[52] that the PERG amplitude depends fairly linearly on stimulus contrast, which is in striking contrast to the VEP (figure 13.14). The Pα ganglion cells feed the magno stream. The magnocellular system has a strongly saturating contrast transfer function[38,55] and dominates at higher temporal frequencies.[22] Thus one would have expected that the PERG contrast function has a more saturating characteristic in the steady-state region. However, Zapf and Bach[58] found the opposite: At 10 rev/s and higher, the contrast function has an accelerating characteristic; for instance, using 21 rev/s and 50% contrast the PERG amplitude is only at 20% of full contrast amplitude. This is unexpected, strong, confirmed in another laboratory, and so far inexplicable.

Finally, at least briefly, we would like to raise the aspect of contrast dynamics. Most considerations above assumed constant physiological properties with respect to time. However, it is known that contrast gain control and/or contrast adaptation takes place on various time scales from milliseconds to minutes.[15,28,30,48] It may well be the case that the physiological PERG properties are largely determined by very rapid adaptation processes (which show up, for instance, in the higher kernels of the mfERG). Furthermore, slower adaptation processes can also have a sizable effect (20% PERG reduction after 10 minutes of high-contrast adaptation[29]). All of these effects are likely altered by pathophysiological conditions, so currently unexplored effects could exist here.

Conclusion

As a rule of thumb, the PERG is generated by the retinal ganglion cells. To avoid contamination with signals from the outer retina, a pattern with full luminance symmetry on the retina is required. The extent of the pattern allows a degree of local resolution (i.e., to isolate macular function). The PERG consists of two major components: the P50 and N95 components, named after polarity and peak time. The P50 component may represent the input activity in the ganglion cells, while the N95 component represents their spiking output activity. With increasingly large checks, the amplitude stays fairly constant above 1° of check size, and the PERG is still generated by the ganglion cells.

While mechanisms and locations of PERG generation were topics of heated discussions 15 years ago, the field has matured into a wide consensus yielding a tool that can reliably address and answer appropriate questions from basic research and clinical situations.

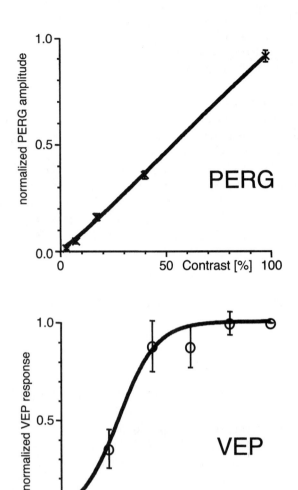

FIGURE 13.14   Contrast transfer function of the PERG (top, linear contrast scale) and VEP (bottom, logarithmic contrast scale). The PERG shows a linear contrast dependence, and the VEP shows early saturation (even on a log scale; the difference would be even more striking if the VEP were also plotted versus a linear contrast scale). Also note the lower intraindividual variability of the PERG, as evident from the smaller SEM antennas (individually normalized to 100% contrast). (Based on data published in Heinrich TS and Bach M.[28])

REFERENCES

1. Arden GB, Carter RM, Hogg C, Siegel IM, Margolis S: A gold foil electrode: Extending the horizons for clinical electroretinography. *Invest Ophthalmol Vis Sci* 1979; 18:421–426.
2. Arden GB, Jacobson JJ: A simple grating test for contrast sensitivity: Preliminary results indicate value in screening for glaucoma. *Invest Ophthalmol Vis Sci* 1978; 17:23–32.
3. Bach M: Some optical illusions and visual phenomena. 1997. <http://www.michaelbach.de/ot/> (14.05.2003)
4. Bach M: Preparation and montage of DTL-electrodes. 1998. <http://www.ukl.uni-freiburg.de/aug/mit/bach/ops/dtl/> (09.02.2001)

5. Bach M, Gerling J, Geiger K: Optic atrophy reduces the pattern-electroretinogram for both fine and coarse stimulus patterns. *Clin Vision Sci* 1992; 7:327–333.
6. Bach M, Hawlina M, Holder GE, Marmor MF, Meigen T, Vaegan, Miyake Y: Standard for pattern electroretinography. *Doc Ophthalmol* 2000; 101:11–18.
7. Bach M, Holder GE: Check size tuning of the pattern-ERG: A reappraisal. *Doc Ophthalmol* 1996; 92:193–202.
8. Bach M, Mathieu M: Different effect of dioptric defocus vs. light scatter on the pattern electroretinogram (PERG). *Doc Ophthalmol* 2004; 108:99–106.
9. Bach M, Meigen T, Strasburger H: Raster-scan cathode-ray tubes for vision research: Limits of resolution in space, time and intensity, and some solutions. *Spatial Vision* 1997; 10:403–414.
10. Bagnoli P, Porciatti V, Francesconi W, Barsellotti R: Pigeon pattern electroretinogram: A response unaffected by chronic section of the optic nerve. *Exp Brain Res* 1984; 55:253–262.
11. Baker CL Jr, Hess RR, Olsen BT, Zrenner E: Current source density analysis of linear and non-linear components of the primate electroretinogram. *J Physiol* 1988; 407:155–176.
12. Baumgartner G: Indirekte Größenbesti mmung der rezeptiven Felder der Retina beim Menschen mittels der Hermannschen Gittertäuschung. *Pflügers Arch ges Physiol* 1960; 272:21–22.
13. Benardete EA, Kaplan E: The dynamics of primate M retinal ganglion cells. *Vis Neurosci* 1999; 16:355–368.
14. Benardete EA, Kaplan E: Dynamics of primate P retinal ganglion cells: Responses to chromatic and achromatic stimuli. *J Physiol* 1999; 519 (Pt 3):775–790.
15. Benardete EA, Kaplan E, Knight BW: Contrast gain control in the primate retina: P cells are not x-like, some M cells are. *Vis Neurosci* 1992; 8:483–486.
16. Brigell M, Bach M, Barber C, Kawasaki K, Kooijman A: Guidelines for calibration of stimulus and recording parameters used in clinical electrophysiology of vision. *Doc Ophthalmol* 1998; 95:1–14.
17. Campbell FW, Gubisch RW: Optical quality of the human eye. *J Physiol* 1966; 186:558–578.
18. Campbell FW, Robson JG: Application of Fourier analysis to the visibility of gratings. *J Physiol* 1968; 197:551–566.
19. Charman WN: Wavefront aberration of the eye: A review. *Optom Vis Sci* 1991; 68:574–583.
20. Curcio CA, Sloan KR, Kalina RE, Hendrickson AE: Human photoreceptor topography. *J Comp Neurol* 1990; 292:497–523.
21. Dawson WW, Trick GL, Litzkow CA: Improved electrode for electroretinography. *Invest Ophthalmol Vis Sci* 1979; 18:988–991.
22. Derrington AM, Lennie P: Spatial and temporal contrast sensitivities of neurones in lateral geniculate nucleus of macaque. *J Physiol* 1984; 357:219–240.
23. Drasdo N, Thompson DA, Thompson CM, Edwards L: Complementary components and local variations of the pattern electroretinogram. *Invest Ophthalmol Vis Sci* 1987; 28:158–162.
24. Groneberg A, Teping C: Topodiagnostik von Sehstörungen durch Ableitung retinaler und kortikaler Antworten auf Umkehr-Kontrastmuster. *Ber Dtsch Ophthalmol Ges* 1980; 77:409–415.
25. Harrison JM, O'Connor PS, Young RSL, Kincaid M, Bentley R: The pattern ERG in man following surgical resection of the optic nerve. *Invest Ophthalmol Vis Sci* 1987; 28:492–499.
26. Hartline HK, Wagner HG, Ratliff F: Inhibition in the eye of limulus. *J Gen Physiol* 1956; 39:651–673.
27. Hawlina M, Konec B: New noncorneal HK-loop electrode for clinical electroretinography. *Doc Ophthalmol* 1992; 81:253–259.
28. Heinrich TS, Bach M: Contrast adaptation in human retina and cortex. *Invest Ophthalmol Vis Sci* 2001; 42:2721–2727.
29. Heinrich TS, Bach M: Contrast adaptation in retinal and cortical evoked potentials: No adaptation to low spatial frequencies. *Vis Neurosci* 2002; 19:645–650.
30. Heinrich TS, Bach M: Contrast adaptation: Paradoxical effects when the temporal frequencies of adaptation and test differ. *Vis Neurosci* 2002; 19:421–426.
31. Hess RF, Baker CL: Human pattern-evoked electroretinogram. *J Neurophysiol* 1984; 51:939–951.
32. Holder GE: The pattern electroretinogram in anterior visual pathway dysfunction and its relationship to the pattern visual evoked potential: A personal clinical review of 743 eyes. *Eye* 1997; 11 (Pt 6):924–934.
33. Holder GE: The pattern electroretinogram. In Fishman GA, Birch DG, Holder GE, Brigell MG (eds): *Electrophysiologic Testing in Disorders of the Retina, Optic Nerve and Visual Pathway*. American Academy of Ophthalmology, 2001, pp 197–235.
34. Holder GE: Pattern electroretinography (PERG) and an integrated approach to visual pathway diagnosis. *Prog Retin Eye Res* 2001; 20:531–561.
35. Holländer H, Bisti S, Maffei L, Hebel R: Electroretinographic responses and retrograde changes of retinal morphology after intracranial optic nerve section: A quantit. analysis in the cat. *Exp Brain Res* 1984; 55:483–493.
36. Hood DC, Frishman LJ, Viswanathan S, Robson JG, Ahmed J: Evidence for a ganglion cell contribution to the primate electroretinogram (ERG): Effects of TTX on the multifocal ERG in macaque. *Vis Neurosci* 1999; 16:411–416.
37. Jennings JA, Charman WN: An analytical approximation for the modulation transfer function of the eye. *Br J Physiol Opt* 1974; 29:64–72.
38. Kaplan E, Shapley RM: X and Y cells in the lateral geniculated nucleus of macaque monkeys. *J Physiol* 1982; 330:125–143.
39. Korth M: Human fast retinal potentials and the spatial properties of a visual stimulus. *Vision Res* 1981; 21:627–630.
40. Korth M, Rix R: Changes in spatial selectivity of pattern-ERG components with stimulus contrast. *Graefes Arch Clin Exp Ophthalmol* 1985; 223:23–28.
41. Maffei L, Fiorentini A: Electroretinographic responses to alternating gratings before and after section of the optic nerve. *Science* 1981; 211:953–954.
42. Maffei L, Fiorentini A, Bisti S, Holländer H: Pattern ERG in the monkey after section of the optic nerve. *Exp Brain Res* 1985; 59:423–425.
43. Menger N, Wässle H: Morphological and physiological properties of the A17 amacrine cell of the rat retina. *Vis Neurosci* 2000; 17:769–780.
44. Miller RF, Stenback K, Henderson D, Sikora M: How voltage-gated ion channels alter the functional properties of ganglion and amacrine cell dendrites. *Arch Ital Biol* 2002; 140:347–359.
45. Otto T, Bach M: Re-test variability and diurnal effects in the pattern electroretinogram (PERG). *Doc Ophthalmol* 1997; 92:311–323.
46. Riemslag FC, Ringo JL, Spekreijse H, Verduyn Lunel HF: The luminance origin of the pattern electroretinogram in man. *J Physiol* 1985; 363:191–209.
47. Riggs LA, Johnson EP, Schick AML: Electrical responses of the human eye to moving stimulus patterns. *Science* 1964; 144:567.

48. Shapley RM, Victor JD: The effect of contrast on the transfer properties of cat retinal ganglion cells. *J Physiol* 1978; 285:275–298.

49. Shapley RM, Victor JD: How the contrast gain control modifies the frequency responses of cat retinal ganglion cells. *J Physiol* 1981; 318:161–179.

50. Sherman J: Simultaneous pattern-reversal electroretinograms and visual evoked potentials in diseases of the macula and optic nerve. *Ann N Y Acad Sci* 1982; 388:214–226.

51. Sieving PA, Steinberg RH: Proximal retinal contributions to the intraretinal 8-Hz pattern ERG of cat. *J Neurophysiol* 1987; 57:104–120.

52. Thompson D, Drasdo N: The effect of stimulus contrast on the latency and amplitude of the pattern electroretinogram. *Vision Res* 1989; 29:309–313.

53. Thompson DA, Drasdo N: An improved method for using the DTL fibre in electroretinography. *Ophthal Physiol Opt* 1987; 7:315–319.

54. Thompson DA, Drasdo N: The origins of luminance and pattern responses of the pattern electroretinogram. *Int J Psychophysiol* 1994; 16:219–227.

55. Tootell RBH, Hamilton SL, Switkes E: Functional anatomy of macaque striate cortex: IV. Contrast and magno-parvo streams. *J Neurosci* 1988; 8:1593–1609.

56. Viswanathan S, Frishman LJ, Robson JG: The uniform field and pattern ERG in macaques with experimental glaucoma: Removal of spiking activity. *Invest Ophthalmol Vis Sci* 2000; 41:2797–2810.

57. Yang J, Reeves A, Bearse MA Jr: Spatial linearity of the pattern electroretinogram. *J Opt Soc Am A* 1991; 8:1666–1673.

58. Zapf HR, Bach M: The contrast characteristic of the pattern electroretinogram depends on temporal frequency. *Graefes Arch Clin Exp Ophthalmol* 1999; 237:93–99.

59. Zrenner E: Physiological basis of the pattern electroretinogram. *Progr Retin Res* 1989; 9:427–464.

14 The Multifocal Electroretinographic and Visual Evoked Potential Techniques

DONALD C. HOOD

Introduction

The electroretinogram (ERG) and the visual evoked potential (VEP) are massed electrical potentials, the result of the summed electrical activity of the cells of the retina (ERG) and the cells in the occipital cortex (VEP). ERGs and VEPs have been recorded in both the clinic and the laboratory to study the normal and abnormal activity of the retina and visual pathways. Chapters 12 and 15 describe the basis of the ERG and VEP, and the standard clinic tests are described in chapter 20. However, it is often desirable to study the local electrical activity of the retina or optic nerve. Conventional ERG and VEP tests involve stimuli that stimulate relatively large areas of the retina and therefore do not easily lend themselves to the study of localized activity. With the multifocal ERG and VEP techniques,[40,43] local ERG or VEP responses can be recorded simultaneously from many regions of the visual field. This chapter provides an introduction to these techniques.

The multifocal ERG

The multifocal ERG (mfERG) technique, although relatively new, is widely used to diagnose and study retinal diseases (see Hood[11] and the special issue of *Documenta Ophthalmologica*, vol. 100, 2000, for a review). While the mfERG is a powerful clinical tool, it is also a useful way to study the local physiology of the normal retina.

RECORDING mfERGs   The display contains an array of hexagons, typically either 61 or 103 (figures 14.1A and 14.1B). The hexagons are scaled so as to produce local responses of approximately equal amplitude in control subjects.[43] During the recording, the display appears to flicker because each hexagon goes through a pseudo-random sequence of black-and-white presentations. In the case of the most commonly used software (VERIS from EDI, San Mateo, CA), this sequence is called an M-sequence. (See Sutter[40] for details.)

A single continuous ERG record is obtained (figure 14.1C, bottom) with the same electrodes and amplifiers that are employed for standard full-field ERG recording. For technical details, see the ISCEV guidelines.[35] The mfERG responses are derived from the single continuous ERG record. Sample records are shown in figure 14.1D. The mfERG responses are derived as the first-order kernels of the cross-correlation between the stimulation sequence and the continuously recorded ERG. The responses in figure 14.1D are positioned so that they do not overlap; the scaling is not linear. (Notice the iso-degree circles in figures 14.1B and 14.1D.) For further details, see Hood,[11] Hood et al.,[19] Keating et al.,[30] Marmor et al.,[35] Sutter,[40,41] and Sutter and Tran.[43]

HOW DOES THE mfERG COMPARE TO THE FULL-FIELD ERG?   As typically recorded, the mfERG is a cone-driven response from the central 20° to 30° (radius) of the retina. The rods do not contribute to the mfERG except under very unusual circumstances.[23,45] The sum of all the mfERG responses in figure 14.1D is shown in figure 14.2A. The standard mfERG shows an initial negative component (N1), a positive component (P1), and a second negative component (N2) (figure 14.2A). The waveform of the mfERG differs from that of the conventional, full-field, flash ERG (see figure 14.2B).[11,22] These differences are not due to differences in the cutoffs of the amplifier, as can be seen in figure 14.2C. Rather, the differences in waveform between the mfERG and the full-field ERG are due to both different methods of light stimulation and different methods of deriving the responses.[22] Unlike the full-field ERG, the mfERG is a mathematical extraction. In spite of these differences, N1 of the human mfERG is composed of the same components as the a-wave of the full-field ERG, and P1 is composed of the same components as the positive waves (b-wave and OPs).[22]

When the rate of stimulation of the multifocal sequence is slowed, the waveform of the human mfERG more closely resembles the waveform of the full-field ERG.[22] With the slower sequence, considerable variation exists in the waveform of the mfERG as a function of retinal location.[22,36] Figure 14.3 shows how the waveforms of the human mfERG, obtained with both the fast (0F) sequence and the slow (7F) sequence, vary with retinal location. The 7F sequence has a minimum of seven blank frames (93 ms) between flashes. It is clear from figure 14.3 that the full-field ERG must consist of the sum of local responses that vary

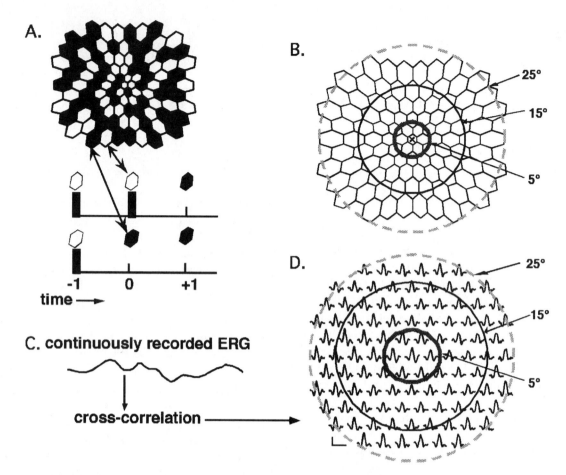

FIGURE 14.1 A, The mfERG display as it might appear at any moment in time and examples of the sequence of events at two locations. B, A schematic showing the mfERG display. C, A schematic of the continuous ERG signal. D, mfERG responses, which are the first-order correlations between the ERG signal (C) and the light sequence (A) of each hexagon. (Source: Modified from a figure in Hood DC.[11])

in waveform with eccentricity. Recently, the cellular contributions to these local variations have been examined with pharmacological techniques.[13,36] (See also chapter 15.)

THE mfERG AND THE ACTIVITY OF THE OUTER RETINA The standard mfERG is shaped largely by bipolar cell activity with smaller contributions from the photoreceptor and inner retinal (e.g., amacrine and ganglion) cells (see Hare and Ton[8] and Hood et al.[13] and chapter 15). For the standard mfERG paradigm, the inner retina makes a relatively small contribution to the waveform.[15] The standard mfERG, like the standard full-field ERG, provides a measure of the health of the outer retina (i.e., cone photoreceptors and bipolar cells).

THE mfERG AND RETINAL DISEASES The most common clinical use of the mfERG is to establish that a disease has an outer retinal origin. Deciding whether a visual field defect is due to damage to the outer retina (i.e., receptors and bipolar cells) or to damage of the ganglion cells or optic nerve is a common clinical problem. Typically, the issue can be settled with a fundus exam, an angiogram, and/or a full-field ERG. If one or more of these tests are abnormal, then the site of the problem is assumed to be in the outer retina. However, under some conditions, the results of these tests can be normal when damage to the outer retina is present. Figure 14.4B shows the mfERG responses from a patient who had a 1-year history of difficulty reading. The sensitivity of her visual field was depressed centrally in both eyes. Figure 14.4A shows the affected areas in the form of probability plots from the Humphrey 24-2 field test. The symbols code the significance of the field loss, which ranged from 5% (four dots) to 0.5% (black square). Her visual acuity was 20/25-2 and 20/60-1 for the right eye and left eye, respectively. Both her fundus exam and her full-field standard ERG were normal. The mfERG (figure 14.4B), however, established that the problem was in the outer retina. The central 5° (the disc) evokes the upper response in 14.4C, the 5° to 15° annulus the central response in C (thin continuous line), and the 15° to 25° degree region evokes the response indicated by gray interrupted lines. The mfERGs resemble those previously reported for patients with Stargardt disease in that they showed reduced amplitudes accompanied by only a modest increase in implicit time.[33]

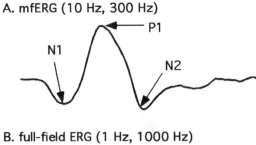

A. mfERG (10 Hz, 300 Hz)

N1 P1 N2

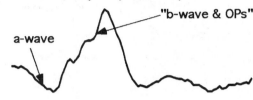

B. full-field ERG (1 Hz, 1000 Hz)

a-wave "b-wave & OPs"

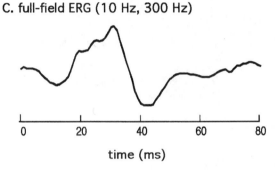

C. full-field ERG (10 Hz, 300 Hz)

0   20   40   60   80

time (ms)

FIGURE 14.2   A, The sum of all 103 responses in figure 14.1D. B, A full-field ERG elicited with about the same flash intensity and recorded with the typically employed amplifier cutoffs. C, A full-field ERG elicited with about the same flash intensity but recorded with the same amplifier cutoffs used in the case of the mfERG in panel A. (Source: Reprinted with permission from Hood DC.[11])

THE mfERG WAVEFORM AND SITES/MECHANISMS OF RETINAL DISEASES   The sites and/or mechanisms of a disease process can often be inferred from the specific pattern of amplitude and/or implicit time abnormalities. Since the standard mfERG is largely a bipolar response,[8,13] a disease process that substantially decreases the mfERG amplitude must be acting at, or before, the bipolar cell. Furthermore, a large delay in the timing of the mfERG is associated with damage to the receptors/outer plexiform layer.[10,11,17] Figure 14.5 shows the visual field (figure 14.5A) and the mfERG responses for a patient with retinitis pigmentosa (figure 14.5B). The responses from the central regions have normal timing. However, the responses from the peripheral regions show large delays in areas corresponding to those where the sensitivity of the visual field is depressed. The abnormal timing can be seen more easily in figure 14.5C, where the average responses are shown for three regions. Although retinitis pigmentosa (RP) is a disease of the receptors, the retina can still produce large, but delayed, responses in some

patients. Since the mfERG is generated largely by the bipolar cells, the site of the defect in these patients must be before the bipolar cells respond. It has been speculated that these delays are due to an abnormal adaptation process secondary to damage in the outer plexiform layer (see Hood[11] for a discussion). Various cytological and biochemical abnormalities have been reported in the outer plexiform layer of patients with RP,[4,34] including GABA-reactive and glycine-reactive processes from amacrine cells that extend as far as the external limiting membrane.[4]

SUMMARY OF THE mfERG   The mfERG is a powerful clinical tool for detecting local retinal abnormalities. The relationship of the mfERG to the activity of the retinal cells[8,13,36] is reasonably well understood, and we are beginning to associate various pathological processes with changes in the mfERG waveform.[11] Furthermore, when the sequence of stimulation is slowed, the mfERG resembles the full-field ERG.[22] This provides a tool for studying the local characteristics of the normal retina as well as the abnormal retina.

The multifocal VEP

The visual evoked potential (VEP), a gross electrical potential generated by the cells in the occipital cortex, has been recorded in the clinic and the laboratory for many years. With the multifocal VEP (mfVEP) technique, introduced by Baseler, Sutter, and colleagues,[1,2] VEP responses can be recorded simultaneously from many regions of the visual field.

RECORDING THE mfVEP   The same electrodes and amplifiers that are used for conventional VEP recordings are used in recording the mfVEP. However, the display, the method of stimulation, and the analysis of the raw records differ.

Most of the mfVEPs that have been published thus far have been recorded with pattern reversal stimulation using the display in figure 14.6A, first introduced by Baseler, Sutter, and colleagues.[1,2] The display contains 60 sectors, approximately scaled, based on cortical magnification. Each sector contains 16 checks: 8 black and 8 white.

The VEP (EEG) is recorded with electrodes placed over the occipital region. There is currently no agreement regarding standard placement for the electrodes. All mfVEP recordings include at least one midline placement of electrodes with so-called bipolar recording. That is, two electrodes, one serving as the active electrode and the other as a reference, are referred to a third electrode, the ground, on the forehead or the ear. It is not uncommon to record more than one channel.[14,26,31] For example, Hood and colleagues[14,26] use three active electrodes, one placed 4 cm above the inion and two placed 4 cm lateral to the inion on each side. Every active electrode is referenced to the inion,

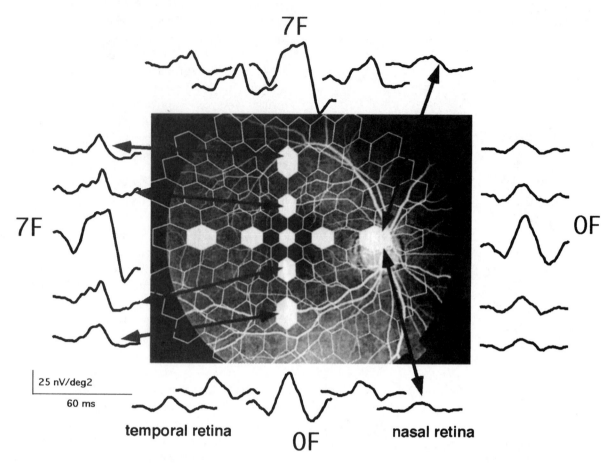

7F

7F

0F

0F

25 nV/deg2

60 ms

temporal retina

nasal retina

FIGURE 14.3 The mfERGs for a slow (7F) sequence and a standard (0F) sequence are shown for different retinal locations to illustrate the variation in waveform across the retina. (Source: Reprinted with permission from Hood DC.[11])

providing three channels of recording. This effectively provides six channels of records because with software the recordings that would result from three additional channels can be derived (see figure 14.6B). The best responses, defined in terms of a signal-to-noise ratio from all six channels, can be used for analysis.

Figure 14.6C shows mean mfVEP responses from 30 normal subjects. The display was viewed with one eye at a time. Each of the individual mfVEP responses in the array is derived via a correlation between the stimulation sequence of a particular sector and the overall, single, continuous VEP recording. The mfVEP responses are usually displayed as an array, as shown in figure 14.6C, in which the responses are positioned arbitrarily so that they do not overlap. The spatial scale for this array is not linear, as the iso-degree circles indicate. For example, there are 12 responses within the central 2.6° (5.2° in diameter).

INTERSUBJECT VARIABILITY As is the case of the conventional VEP, the waveform of the mfVEP differs among normal subjects. This intersubject variability is due to individual differences in the location and folding of the visual cortex.[14,25] As corresponding points in the visual field are represented in the same location in the primary visual cortex (V1), the responses from the two eyes of the same individual are nearly identical. This can be seen in the averaged data in figure 14.6C. Unilateral damage can be detected relatively easily with interocular comparisons of mfVEP responses.

INTRASUBJECT VARIABILITY Within a subject, there are at least five variations in waveform that are of interest. First, in general, the responses from the upper field are of opposite polarity compared to those from the lower field.[2,39] Second, the responses from the nasal retina are slightly faster than those from the temporal retina.[14,26] There is a small interocular latency difference of about 4 to 5 ms across the midline. The left eye response leads to the left of fixation, and the right eye leads in the right of fixation, as can be seen in the insets in figure 14.6C. For corresponding points, the ganglion cells in the temporal retina are farther from the optic disc compared to the cells in the nasal retina. The action

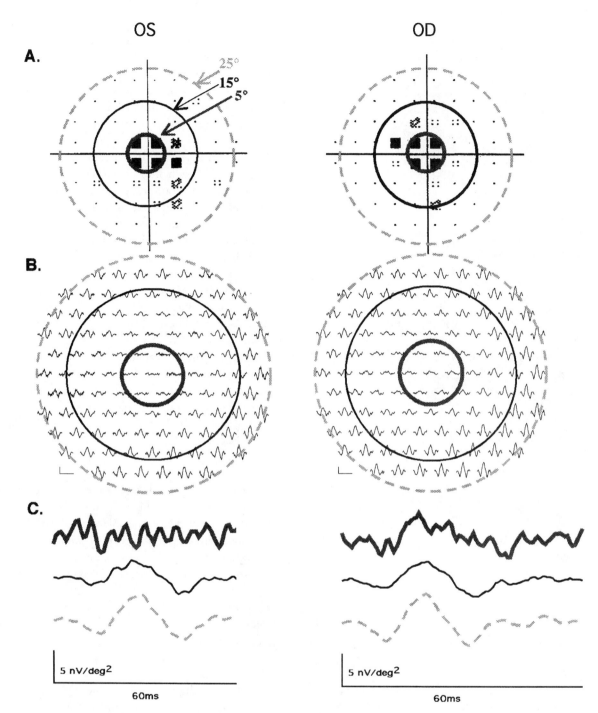

FIGURE 14.4 A, The OS (left panel) and OD (right panel) 24-2 Humphrey visual fields (total deviation probability plots) of a patient with central visual loss. B, The OS (left panel) and OD (right panel) mfERG responses for this patient. The vertical and horizontal calibration bars indicate 100 nV and 60 ms, respectively. Bold dark gray, thin black, and dashed light gray circles indicate radii of 5°, 15°, and 25°, respectively. C, The OS (left panel) and OD (right panel) mfERG responses, expressed as response density, for the area within 5° (dark gray), between 5° and 15° (black), and between 15° and 25° (light gray). (Source: Modified from a figure in Hood DC, Greenstcin VC, Odel JG, et al.[19])

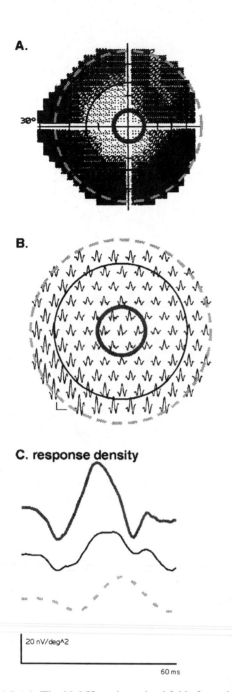

A.

30°

B.

C. response density

20 nV/deg^2

60 ms

FIGURE 14.5   A, The 30-2 Humphrey visual field of a patient with retinitis pigmentosa. B, The mfERG responses for this patient. C, The mfERG average responses, expressed as response density for the area within 5° (dark gray), between 5° and 15° (black), and between 15° and 25° (light gray). (Source: Modified from a figure in Hood DC.[12])

potentials from the ganglion cells in the temporal retina travel farther to the optic disc than do the action potentials from corresponding points on the nasal retina. The difference in the conduction time along these unmyelinated axons is of the right order of magnitude to account for the small interocular latency difference.[42]

The responses that are shown as insets in figure 14.6C illustrate a third intrasubject difference. On average, just above the horizontal meridian, the responses from the temporal retina are slightly larger than those from the nasal retina.[7] Hood and Greenstein[14] speculated that this amplitude difference reflected the small nasotemporal difference in sensitivity (approximately 1 dB or less) that is measured with perimetry.[3,9]

A fourth intrasubject variation is shown in the ellipses in figure 14.6C. Although there is considerable intersubject variability, responses from just above the horizontal meridian are larger in most individuals than are responses from just below the meridian.[14] It has been suggested that, on average, the horizontal meridian falls below the bend in the calcarine fissure rather than at the bend, as is commonly assumed.[14,46]

Finally, the waveform of the responses along the vertical meridian differs from the waveform of the other responses.[14,25,31,32,46] This finding argues that there must be more than one source of the mfVEP signal.[14,46] The region of V1 devoted to the vertical meridian is typically outside of the calcarine fissure on the medial surface of the cortex and adjacent to V2.[18] This has led to the suggestion that extrastriate regions may contribute more to the responses near the vertical meridian. However, a second source in V1 cannot be ruled out.[14,46]

DETECTING SPATIALLY LOCALIZED DAMAGE TO THE GANGLION CELLS OR OPTIC NERVE   Glaucoma, optic atrophy, ischemic optic neuropathy, and multiple sclerosis are among the diseases that can produce spatially localized damage to the ganglion cells and optic nerve. A number of studies have shown that these defects can be detected with the mfVEP and compared to visual defects measured with static, automated perimetry.[6,7,14,16,21,25,26,28,29,31,47] For reviews of this work, see Hood,[12] Hood and Greenstein,[14] and Hood et al.[20]

From the point of view of clinical neuroscience, two findings are of particular interest. First, the local changes in the mfVEP signal appear, to a first approximation, to be linearly related to local changes in behaviorally measured sensitivity.[14,16] This suggests that both the mfVEP signal and behavioral sensitivity are linearly related to the number of ganglion cells that are lost. This surprisingly simple relationship is consistent with a recent model relating behavioral changes to hypothetical losses in ganglion cells.[44]

Second, the results from patients with optic neuritis suggest that the effects of local demyelinization can be studied.[21,29] One of the earliest signs of multiple sclerosis (MS) is optic neuritis. Optic neuritis is a clinical syndrome characterized by an acute, unilateral loss of vision that partially recovers within three months. In fact, it is not uncommon for visual acuity to return to normal and for patients to

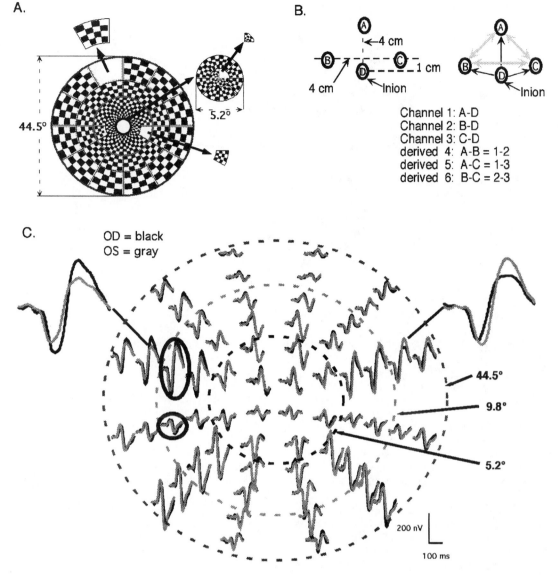

FIGURE 14.6 A, The display employed for the mfVEP recordings. B, The electrode locations employed for the mfVEP recordings. C, The averaged mfVEP responses for 30 normal control subjects. (Source: Modified from figures in Hood DC.[12])

have reasonably normal visual fields after recovery. The mfVEPs from such a patient are shown in figure 14.7. The patient noticed a "film" in the peripheral vision of her left eye, but her visual fields and visual acuity were normal. In addition, the conventional VEP was normal. An MRI scan confirmed a diagnosis of MS. The mfVEP records in figure 14.7 show that the responses from the two eyes are the same in most of the field. However, in some regions the response from the left eye is markedly delayed in comparison to the right (see inset). The mfVEP appears to be detecting local demyelinization due to MS.[21,29]

mfVEP SUMMARY The mfVEP technology allows for spatially localized VEP responses to be recorded from the occipital cortex. The mfVEP responses appear to be dominated by a component that is generated in the primary visual cortex (a.k.a. area 17 or V1).[5,14,39,46] While the clinical utility of the mfVEP has already been demonstrated, applications to basic neuroscience are only beginning to be explored.[24,38]

ACKNOWLEDGMENTS This work was supported in part by grants EY-02115 from the National Eye Institute.

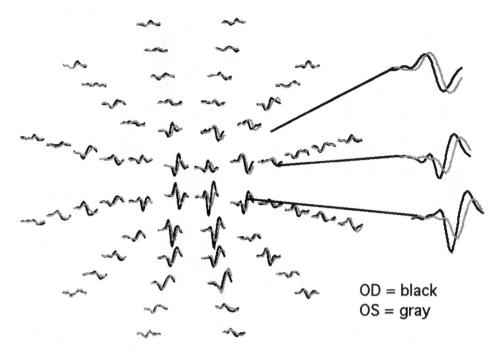

OD = black
OS = gray

FIGURE 14.7   The mfVEPs from both the left (gray) and right (black) eyes of a patient with multiple sclerosis.

REFERENCES

1. Baseler HA, Sutter EE: M and P components of the VEP and their visual field distribution. *Vision Res* 1997; 37:675–690.

2. Baseler HA, Sutter EE, Klein SA, Carney T: The topography of visual evoked response properties across the visual field. *Electroencephalogr Clin Neurophysiol* 1994; 90:65–81.

3. Brenton RS, Phelps CD: The normal visual field on the Humphrey field analyzer. *Ophthalmologica* 1986; 193:56–74.

4. Fariss RN, Li ZY, Milam AH: Abnormalities in rod photoreceptors, amacrine cells, and horizontal cells in human retinas with retinitis pigmentosa. *Am J Ophthalmol* 2000; 129:215–223.

5. Fortune B, Hood DC: Conventional pattern-reversal VEPs are not equivalent to summed multifocal VEPs. *Invest Ophthalmol Vis Sci* 2003; 44:1364–1375.

6. Goldberg I, Graham SL, Klistorner AI: Multifocal objective perimetry in the detection of glaucomatous field loss. *Am J Ophthalmol* 2002; 133:29–39.

7. Graham SL, Klistorner AI, Grigg JR, Billson FA: Objective VEP perimetry in glaucoma: Asymmetry analysis to identify early deficits. *J Glaucoma* 2000; 9:10–19.

8. Hare WA, Ton H: Effects of APB, PDA, and TTX on ERG responses recorded using both multifocal and conventional methods in monkey: Effects of APB, PDA, and TTX on monkey ERG responses. *Doc Ophthalmol* 2002; 105:189–222.

9. Heijl A, Lindgren G, Olsson J: Normal variability of static perimetric threshold values across the central visual field. *Arch Ophthalmol* 1987; 105:1544–1549.

10. Holopigian K, Seiple W, Greenstein VC, Hood DC, Carr RE: Local cone and rod system function in progressive cone dystrophy. *Invest Ophthalmol Vis Sci* 2002; 43:2364–2373.

11. Hood DC: Assessing retinal function with the multifocal technique. *Prog Retin Eye Res* 2000; 19:607–646.

12. Hood DC: Electrophysiological imaging of retinal and optic nerve damage: The multifocal technique. *Ophthalmol Clin N Am* 2003; 17:69–88.

13. Hood DC, Frishman LJ, Saszik S, Viswanathan S: Retinal origins of the primate multifocal ERG: Implications for the human response. *Invest Ophthalmol Vis Sci* 2002; 43:1673–1685.

14. Hood DC, Greenstein VC: The multifocal VEP and ganglion cell damage: Applications and limitations for the study of glaucoma. *Prog Retin Eye Res* 2003; 22:201–251.

15. Hood DC, Greenstein VC, Holopigian K, et al: An attempt to detect glaucomatous damage to the inner retina with the multifocal ERG. *Invest Ophthalmol Vis Sci* 2000; 41:1570–1579.

16. Hood DC, Greenstein VC, Odel JG, et al: Visual field defects and multifocal visual evoked potentials: Evidence of a linear relationship. *Arch Ophthalmol* 2002; 120:1672–1681.

17. Hood DC, Holopigian K, Seiple W, Greenstein V, Li J, Sutter EE, Carr RE: Assessment of local retinal function in patients with retinitis pigmentosa using the multi-focal ERG technique. *Vision Res* 1998; 38:163–180.

18. Horton JC, Hoyt WF: The representation of the visual field in human striate cortex: A revision of the classic Holmes map. *Arch Ophthalmol* 1991; 109:816–824.

19. Hood D, Odel JG, Chen CS, Winn BJ: The multifocal electroretinogram (ERG): Applications and limitations in neuro-ophthalmology. *J Neuroophthalmol* 2003; 23:225–235.

20. Hood D, Odel JG, Winn BJ: The multifocal visual evoked potential (VEP): Applications and limitations in neuro-ophthalmology. *J Neuroophthalmol* 2003; 23:279–289.

21. Hood DC, Odel JG, Zhang X: Tracking the recovery of local optic nerve function after optic neuritis: A multifocal VEP study. *Invest Ophthalmol Vis Sci* 2000; 41:4032–4038.

22. Hood DC, Seiple W, Holopigian K, Greenstein V: A comparison of the components of the multifocal and full-field ERGs. *Vis Neurosci* 1997; 14:533–544.

23. Hood DC, Wladis EJ, Shady S, Holopigian K, Li J, Seiple W: Multifocal rod electroretinograms. *Invest Ophthalmol Vis Sci* 1998; 39:1152–1162.

24. Hood DC, Yu AL, Zhang X, Albrecht J, Jagle H, Sharpe LT: The multifocal visual evoked potential and cone isolating stimuli: Implications for L- to M-cone ratios and normalization. *J Vis* 2002; 2:178–189.

25. Hood DC, Zhang X: Multifocal ERG and VEP responses and visual fields: Comparing disease-related changes. *Doc Ophthalmol* 2000; 100:115–137.

26. Hood DC, Zhang X, Greenstein VC, et al: An interocular comparison of the multifocal VEP: A possible technique for detecting local damage to the optic nerve. *Invest Ophthalmol Vis Sci* 2000; 41:1580–1587.

27. Hood DC, Zhang X, Hong JE, Chen CS: Quantifying the benefits of additional channels of multifocal VEP recording. *Doc Ophthalmol* 2002; 104:303–320.

28. Hood DC, Zhang X, Winn BJ: Detecting glaucomatous damage with multifocal visual evoked potentials: How can a monocular test work? *J Glaucoma* 2003; 12:3–15.

29. Kardon RH, Givre SJ, Wall M, Hood D: Comparison of threshold and multifocal-VEP perimetry in recovered optic neuritis. In Wall and Wills (eds): *Perimetry Update 2000: Proceedings of the XVII International Perimetric Society Meeting Sept. 6–9, 2000.* Wills, New York, Kugler, 2001, pp 19–28.

30. Keating D, Parks S, Evans A: Technical aspects of multifocal ERG recording. *Doc Ophthalmol* 2000; 100:77–98.

31. Klistorner A, Graham SL: Objective perimetry in glaucoma. *Ophthalmology* 2000; 107:2283–2299.

32. Klistorner AI, Graham SL, Grigg JR, Billson FA: Multifocal topographic visual evoked potential: Improving objective detection of local visual field defects. *Invest Ophthalmol Vis Sci* 1998; 39:937–950.

33. Kretschmann U, Seeliger MW, Ruether K, Usui T, Apfelstedt-Sylla E, Zrenner E: Multifocal electroretinography in patients with Stargardt's macular dystrophy. *Br J Ophthalmol* 1998; 82:267–275.

34. Li ZY, Kljavin IJ, Milam AH: Rod photoreceptor neurite sprouting in retinitis pigmentosa. *J Neurosci* 1995; 15:5429–5438.

35. Marmor MF, Hood D, Keating D, Kondo M, Miyake Y: Guidelines for basic multifocal electroretinography (mfERG). *Doc Ophthalmol* 2003; 106:105–115.

36. Rangaswamy NV, Hood DC, Frishman LJ: Regional variations in the local contributions to the primate photopic flash ERG revealed using the slow-sequence mfERG. *Invest Ophthalmol Vis Sci* 2003; 44:3233–3247.

37. Seeliger M, Kretschmann U, Apfelstedt-Sylla E, Ruther K, Zrenner E: Multifocal electroretinography in retinitis pigmentosa. *Am J Ophthalmol* 1998; 125:214–226.

38. Seiple W, Clemens C, Greenstein VC, Holopigian K, Zhang X: The spatial distribution of selective attention assessed using the multifocal visual evoked potential. *Vision Res* 2002; 42:1513–1521.

39. Slotnick SD, Klein SA, Carney T, et al: Using multi-stimulus VEP source localization to obtain a retinotopic map of human primary visual cortex. *Clin Neurophysiol* 1999; 110:1793–1800.

40. Sutter EE: The fast m-transform: A fast computation of cross-correlations with binary m-sequences. *Soc Ind Appl Math* 1991; 20:686–694.

41. Sutter EE: The interpretation of multifocal binary kernels. *Doc Ophthalmol* 2000; 100:49–75.

42. Sutter EE, Bearse MA: The optic nerve head component of the human ERG. *Vision Res* 1999; 39:419–436.

43. Sutter EE, Tran D: The field topography of ERG components in man: I. The photopic luminance response. *Vision Res* 1992; 32:433–446.

44. Swanson WH, Dul MW, Pan F: Relating ganglion cell loss to perimetric defects: A neural model. *Invest Ophthalmol Vis Sci* 2005; 46:235–240.

45. Wu S, Sutter EE: A topographic study of oscillatory potentials in man. *Vis Neurosci* 1995; 12:1013–1025.

46. Zhang X, Hood DC: A principal component analysis of multifocal pattern reversal VEP. *J Vision* 2004; 4:32–43.

47. Zhang X, Hood DC, Chen CS, Hong JE: A signal-to-noise analysis of multifocal VEP responses: An objective definition for poor records. *Doc Ophthalmol* 2002; 104:287–302.

15 Origin of the Visual Evoked Potentials

MANFRED FAHLE AND MICHAEL BACH

Introduction

Nearly 50 years ago, it became possible to study in some detail the electrical activity of the brain by recording evoked potentials.[22] This chapter begins by describing the growth of this discipline and then summarizes how the evoked potentials originate from activity transmitted from the retina to the visual cortex and what aspects of cortical function they demonstrate. This gives the framework against which clinical tests may be developed and enables an appreciation of their value in clinical diagnosis. The different modalities that are used to evoke cortical potentials as well as the important parameters that are involved are discussed. The different types of evoked potentials are described, and the concept of VEP latency is discussed. More technical issues of recording and analysis are also covered.

BASIC DEFINITION   The acronym *VEP* stands for "visual evoked potential." Some authors use the term *visual evoked response* (VER) instead, some the term *VECP*. Auditory evoked potentials (AEPs) and somatosensory evoked potentials represent the analogous phenomena as evoked through auditory or somatosensory stimuli, usually touch. Together, these potentials form the family of (cortical) evoked potentials (EPs). The VEP represents the response of the visual cortex to stimuli presented in (the middle of) the visual field. For the cortical response to the stimulation to be evaluated, it has to be separated from the activities of the brain that are unrelated to the stimulation, as recorded in the spontaneous electroencephalogram (EEG).

The EEG-based signal: Neuronal responses to extrinsic and intrinsic activation   The signal that is recorded on the scalp reflects activity related to both external stimulation and intrinsic activity in the neuronal networks of the brain. Using direct visualization of cortical activity by means of optical recording in animals, Arieli et al.[6] demonstrated that intrinsic activity has a larger influence on cortical activity patterns than external stimuli have, even in primary visual cortex. Therefore, it is not surprising that the response to external stimulation is often rather small in comparison to the "noise" caused by intrinsic activity, and averaging over several stimulus presentations is required (see "Signal averaging" and "Temporal summation" for details).

Potentials are recorded from the scalp   To record the cortical activity, electrodes are attached to the intact scalp, and the changes of electrical potentials over the (visual) cortex are recorded after strong amplification and appropriate filtering to remove external noise. Electrodal impedance below 5 kOhms and closest possible match in impedance between electrodes minimize interference from external sources. Optimal signal quality (highest ratio between signal and noise) is especially important given the extremely small potential differences recorded over the scalp. Their amplitudes are generally around $10\,\mu V$ (i.e., around 1/100,000th of a volt). Furthermore, the VEP is small in comparison to the EEG in which it is buried, with a signal-to-noise ratio that is typically around 1/10.

For VEP recordings, the electrodes are positioned at defined locations over the occipital skull that overlie the parts of the cortex that receive the input from the retina via the thalamus. The electrode positions are named according to a system adopted from EEG recordings, the most important electrode sites for visually evoked potentials being called O1, Oz, and O2 (from left to right). For details, see "Electrode positions" below.

Different types of visual stimulation elicit (different types of) VEPs   Not surprisingly, the visual cortex responds to a wide variety of different visual stimuli, since this is what it was made for. But to record the VEP, one often wants to stimulate the cortex as strongly as possible. From animal research (e.g., Hubel and Wiesel[43]), it is known that neurons in the cortex, unlike photoreceptors, are not strongly activated by stimuli that are homogeneous over space (and time). Hence, to produce a strong response, the stimulus has to be structured in either space or time or both. In line with this argument, the most common stimuli for VEPs are short flashes or else the appearance or contrast reversal of a visual pattern. Additional newer methods aim to investigate brain responses that are specific for stimulus color, motion, or depth and thus require specific types of stimuli as described in the section below on stimulus modalities.

Signal averaging over many stimulus presentations   As was mentioned above, the potentials that are evoked over the skull by means of visual stimulation are minute and usually smaller than the ongoing cortical activity, unrelated to the stimulation. Hence, the stimulus has to be repeated over and over again, usually about 100 times. A computer records the electrode potentials for a defined period of time, starting anew with each stimulus presentation. At the end of a recording, around 100 traces have been obtained from each electrode. In these traces, the cortical response to the stimulus will always occur at the same time after the stimulus presentation, say, 100 ms after the presentation, which is called the *response latency*. The spontaneous brain activity, on the other hand, will by definition be unrelated to the stimulus. Hence, in writing all traces in subsequent lines of a large monitor, starting each trace at the left border, there will always be a tendency of the trace to bend, say, upwards around a latency around 100 ms. At all shorter times, if only spontaneous activity is present, there will be no clear tendency of the traces to be either positive or negative. Now, by averaging over all traces separately for each latency, the amplitude of the spontaneous fluctuations will decrease (since a positivity in one trace will be averaged with a negativity in another trace). The amplitude of the VEP, on the other hand, will stay constant, and hence, the VEP will become clearer due to a reduction of the noise (by the square root of the number of presentations). Thus, after 100 repetitions, noise could be reduced tenfold, and after 1000 repetitions, more than 30-fold.

VEPs mirror the function of the visual pathway up to the (primary) visual cortex   Obviously, for a VEP to arise, the stimulus has to reach the retina, be detected by the photoreceptors, be transmitted via the optic nerve and optic tract to the thalamus (lateral geniculate nucleus) and further via the optic radiation. Any disturbance or defect anywhere in this chain of events may change the form and/or latency of the response recorded by the electrodes above the (primary) visual cortex. Hence, the VEP certainly mirrors the function of the visual system up to the primary cortex. It is less clear to what extent "higher" visual processing areas contribute to the VEP, and this contribution certainly depends on the type of stimulus that is employed. (For details, see "Stimulus modalities" and "The multifocal VEP" below.)

History: Early Work
Discovery of the EEG and the relationship between EEG and brain activation   Brazier[16] compiled a number of excellent treatises on the history of the EEG. Here, we will mention only a few highlights of this history. In 1808, the French Academy refused to admit Gall, who had proposed the concept of localization of mental functions in the cortex, on the grounds that the cortex has nothing to do with thinking. In 1875, Caton published observations of spontaneous and evoked electrical activity at the exposed cortex of rabbits and monkeys. Finally, in 1924, psychiatrist Berger recorded the first human EEG from the intact skull. In 1929, Berger[14]

published the first report on the human EEG, describing and defining the alpha and beta rhythms (figure 15.1) he had recorded, and soon the electroencephalogram (EEG) was under intensive study. The alpha waves were especially well developed in recordings over the occipital cortex, and they reduced considerably in amplitude when the eyes were opened. The electrical storms that were recorded in epilepsies and the demonstration that, in many cases, they originated from focal regions underneath the scalp were of considerable interest, as were the changes that were seen in other cases of brain damage and during sleep. The rhythmic activity was recognized, and it was deduced that waves of electrical activity spread with a relatively slow velocity over large areas of the scalp. There was much speculation about how this finding related to the actual function of neurons or how it could explain the way in which the brain carried out its normal activity.

Initially, there were reservations in the scientific community as to the significance of these new and most remarkable findings. Even Berger's own observations cast doubt on the idea that these brain potentials were associated with the mind. In a mentally relaxed state with eyes closed, the EEG amplitude proved very large, showing mainly alpha waves with a dominant frequency of around 10 Hz. With mental activity, such as arithmetic calculation, the EEG amplitudes decreased markedly. Although it took considerable time, it finally became clear that mental activity corresponded with several ongoing forms of desynchronized cortical activity with consequently lower mass potentials.[1] Grey Walter[76] subsequently was the first to localize a brain tumor by means of EEG recordings.

Evolution of cortical evoked responses: The flash response   A series of flashes (from a stroboscope) can evoke a series of occipital waves that are synchronized with each flash. This procedure was named *photic driving* and became an integral part of the EEG examination. The photically driven waves were no larger in most people than the spontaneous EEG waves, and the morphology of the response could not be studied at first. At long last, it was appreciated that the waves were linked in time to the stimulus, whereas the ongoing brain activity was not, and hence superimposition of many records of the response to individual flashes could provide an estimate of the response waveform. The first efforts were made manually, by the use of repeated exposure photography, or by mechanical devices. Only when averaging by electronic means became available were the evoked responses properly visualized. The memory capacity of the first equipment dictated the possible precision of measurement, and the equipment available to EEG clinics limited the types of stimuli to be displayed. Thus, potentials evoked by stroboscopic flashes were first studied.[20] This was unfortunate because the retinal illumination used was very high, and its localization on the

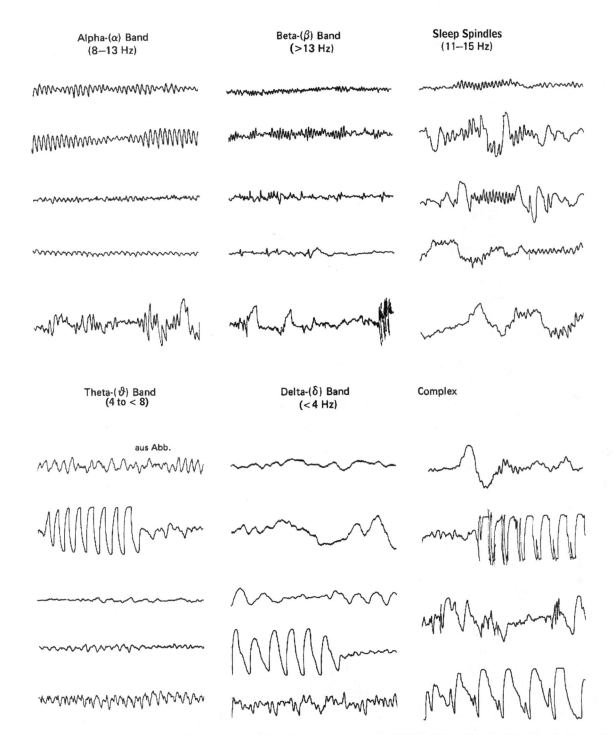

Alpha-(α) Band
(8–13 Hz)

Beta-(β) Band
(>13 Hz)

Sleep Spindles
(11–15 Hz)

Theta-(ϑ) Band
(4 to < 8)

aus Abb.

Delta-(δ) Band
(< 4 Hz)

Complex

FIGURE 15.1 Different rhythms of the EEG as first described by Berger.[14] (Source: Birbaumer N, Schmidt RF: Das Elektroenzephalogram [EEG], 1990/1991. In *Biologische Psychologie*, Berlin, Springer-Verlag, 1991.)

retina haphazard. In addition, clinically usable stroboscopes had diffusers placed between the light source and the subject's eye. Some of these diffusers were ribbed, so the subject, focusing on the screen, saw a variable but detailed image. The first reports of the nature of the flash-evoked responses were therefore very variable, and one center's "normative" data were entirely different from another's.

Gradually, a few principles were recognized. The occipital activity that correlated with visual performance could not begin at the moment of the stimulus onset. The major events occurred between 70 and 250 ms after the stimulus onset. However, following the initial events, delayed responses occurred even after more than 300 ms, which were related to the subject's expectancy of another, repetitive stimulus.[77] Although such events are not of practical significance in clinical visual electrophysiology, there exists a large literature on them. These and other evoked potential results and techniques were extensively reviewed by Regan.[64] It was realized that the physiology of the retina and the experience of psychophysicists were of importance in designing experiments on evoked potentials. Single cells in the visual cortex respond to bars and edges with more vigorous discharges than to diffuse illumination, suggesting the use of structured rather than homogeneous visual stimuli to evoke VEPs. Temporal aspects of vision[70] were being investigated, and the concept of spatial frequency was introduced into psychophysics,[26] opening the door to acuity testing. Analogous experiments were performed on the human evoked potentials.[63,72]

Evolution of cortical evoked responses: Contrast and pattern reversal
The first outcome was that larger and often simpler responses were obtained, either by using patterns appearing (and disappearing) abruptly[45] or by presenting a pattern that changed in contrast (contrast reversal) using refined optical techniques[71] or electronic means on a TV screen.[3,4] Cortical potentials evoked by such techniques are still today the most commonly (indeed almost universally) employed under clinical circumstances because of various attractive features. The first finding was that the electrical activity was greatest over the midline near the occiput, implying that visual cortex was predominantly involved. The second was that the response amplitude decreased greatly when there was an uncorrected refractive error.[18,65,70] The blurred pattern was far less apt to activate the cells in (primary) visual cortex that are sensitive to sharp border-contrast.[64] In the usual stimulus, a checkerboard, it was found that for squares subtending less than 40 minutes, the response fell greatly with refractive error, while for larger squares, this decrease was less pronounced. The concept of luminance versus pattern evoked potentials was hence introduced.

With standard electrode positioning of about 2 cm above the inion, the waveform that was elicited by patterned stimuli was simple, consisting of a small surface-negative wave peaking about 75 ms, followed by a larger surface-positive wave peaking at 100 ms (P100). This complex appeared to be unitary and very uniform, but later components were much more variable. The timing of the peak varied somewhat with the contrast of the stimulus and with the time required to present an image. (This was at first limited to television frame rate.) The usual practice is to initiate contrast reversals at 500- or 250-ms intervals and to neglect later portions of the response.

Origins of EEG potentials and transmission to scalp

SPATIAL SUMMATION: CORTICAL (SYNAPTIC) ACTIVITY PRODUCES DIPOLES What types of sources generate the EEG, and where are they? This important issue has received surprisingly little attention and is currently not an active research topic. The current understanding may be summarized as follows[24,49,56]: Those dipoles oriented (near) perpendicular to the cortical surface produce net potentials. Cortices running parallel (and closest) to the skull generally produce the largest potentials on the skull. Subcortical structures such as the thalamus and basal ganglia are generally too remote to influence electrodes on the skull. Dipoles that are oriented in an oblique angle to the surface will usually produce smaller dipoles. But depending on the direction of the cortex relative to the skull, they may, in some instances, produce larger potentials at certain positions on the surface of the skull than do those dipoles that are oriented perpendicular to the skull at the same cortical position. Moreover, visual as well as other types of stimulation will generally evoke not just one but a certain number of cortical dipoles that superimpose to produce the potentials recorded on the surface of the skull. Because of this superposition of different sources, it is not mathematically possible to infer from the potential distribution on the skull the exact distribution of sources within the cortex. Still, by recording simultaneously from many electrodes and using sophisticated software, certain inferences about cortical dipoles can be drawn. (See "Number of electrodes and multielectrode recordings" below.)

Experiments to determine the intracortical activity that gives rise to evoked potentials have been performed. As was expected, the inhibitory postsynaptic potentials (IPSPs) and excitatory postsynaptic potentials (EPSPs) of large cells are the generators, but except in conditioned recordings from awake primates, it has been difficult to relate clinical waveforms to known cell types in the cortex.[62] However, studies on binocular interaction show that both the N75 and P100 waves of the potential evoked by contrast reversals increase when both eyes receive an input.[28]

TEMPORAL SUMMATION: SIMULTANEOUS ACTIVATION OF LARGE NEURONAL POPULATIONS CAN BE RECORDED ON THE SKULL

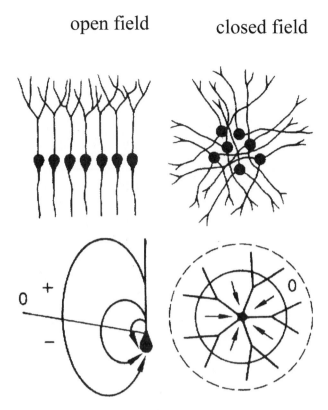

open field   closed field

FIGURE 15.2   EEG as a mass potential, the net outcome of a large number of dipoles superimposing over space and time. *Left,* Regular arrangement of neurons produces directed dipole. *Right,* Concentration of cell bodies produces circular field. (Source: Stöhr M: Physiologie und Pathophysiologie der Impulsleitung. In *Evozierte Potentiale.* Berlin, Springer, 1996.)

The EEG is a mass phenomenon, the net outcome of a great number of electrical processes adding or subtracting in space and time (figure 15.2). For a measurable scalp potential to occur, a degree of synchrony between a large number of sources is required. These sources are not the action potentials (spikes) themselves. The spikes are too brief and the probability is too low for sufficient synchronization to add up. More likely candidates are the EPSPs and IPSPs, which can add up to a sizable scalp potential with their longer time constants and larger current loops. Probably, the EEG is dominated by postsynaptic potentials in the large pyramidal cells (figure 15.3), because only currents in their elongated axial dendrites will build up sufficiently large uncompensated current loops. Over cortical areas that exhibit a convex fold (gyri) corresponding to a cortex running parallel to the skull, the following rule of thumb holds for neurons that are oriented at right angles to the cortical surface. There, IPSPs generate scalp surface positivity, while EPSPs generate negativity.[56] EPSPs from thalamic input (arriving in layer IVc) evoke surface negativity, and intracortical input arriving in layer II/III evokes surface positivity.[52] However, given our incomplete understanding as well as the complexities of cortical topology, it is best not to draw too specific conclusions from the EEG polarity. Hence, the VEP is the summation of a large number of cortical EPSPs and IPSPs, not of the action potentials themselves.

LOCALIZING THE CORTICAL AREAS PRODUCING SCALP POTENTIALS   As was indicated above, it is very difficult to discriminate between activation of different cortical areas using surface electrodes. Pattern appearance EPs are complex, and while the earliest positive portion CI (see figure 15.4) arising from the calcarine region (V1) peaks at ~90 ms and inverts across the horizontal meridian, there are further overlapping components. All work except the most recent appears to have underestimated the difficulties in assigning locations to the various components of the evoked potential. A large number of closely spaced electrodes are required,[45] and one must use small-subtense stimuli in each quadrant of the visual field to obtain even an approximation to the true complexity. Several attempts to describe these sources have been made, but the one that is illustrated is the most recent and comprehensive. Figure 15.5 shows the responses obtained for upper and lower quadrants of the left visual field in such an experiment. The separate waves are identified, and it is instructive to examine the figure closely to see how the EP changes with electrode position. (Note that the P1 component corresponds to Jeffreys's CII, but these responses are presented negative upward.) The earliest component CI from central electrodes (e.g., in the POz in figure 15.5) inverts across the horizontal meridian, while other waves do not. The timing of secondary peaks varies (e.g., N150 at PO4). Complexities such as this imply that the response has several principal components, shown diagrammatically in figure 15.6. When the actual locations of the electrodes in the montage are determined very precisely, software can be employed that localizes the sources of the principal components within the skull. The assumption is that these are relatively small dipoles, and figure 15.7 gives an example.

The location of the various gyri can be determined by functional magnetic resonance imaging (fMRI) and applied to the same data. Figure 15.8 shows the localization of the dipole that indicates calcarine activity in the same subject, for stimuli in each of the four quadrants of an individual subject, superimposed on a diagram of the location of the calcarine fissure as obtained from fMRI. The agreement between the results of the two methods is impressive. Figure 15.9 shows a distorted topographic view of the fMRI image of the cortical surface. The regions of activity shown in the fMRI are indicated in color, along with the corresponding localization of the electrophysiological component dipoles. The distortion is necessary to display all successive visual areas, as outlined and labeled in the figure.[27]

The VEP component named CI arises from V1. The early VEP component P1 peaking about 10 ms later than CI

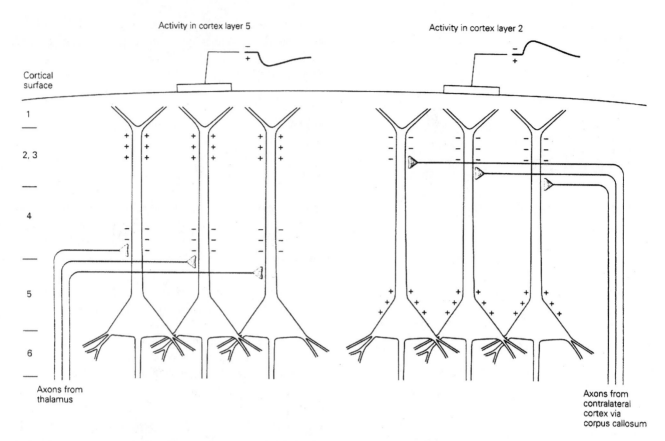

FIGURE 15.3 The EEG as the product of postsynaptic potentials in large pyramidal cells of cortex produced by either thalamic (left) or cortical (right) inputs. (From Westbrook GL, Kandel ER, Schwartz JE, Jessel TM (eds): *Principles of Neural Science*, 4th ed. New York, McGraw-Hill, 2000.)

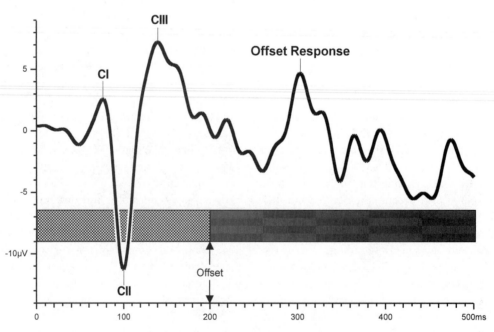

FIGURE 15.4 The VEPs caused by pattern onset (at time 0) and pattern offset (200 ms).

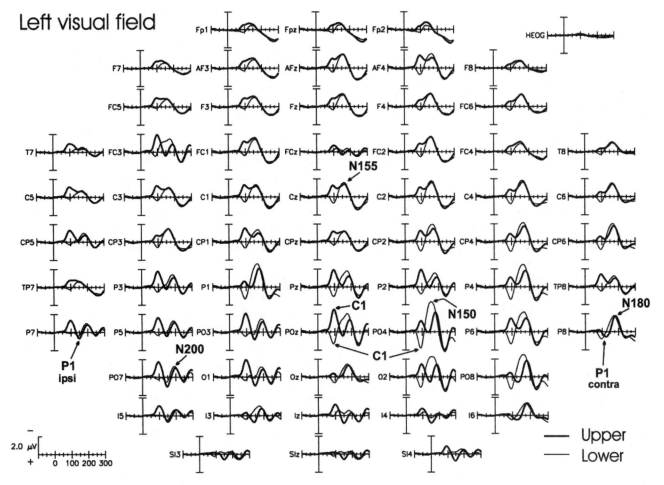

FIGURE 15.5 Evoked potentials to checkerboard stimulation placed in upper and lower quadrants of the left visual field. Sixty-two channels are recorded from closely spaced electrodes. Note how near Oz, the early responses invert across the horizontal meridian, while later components do not. Note that in this figure, unlike many in this book, positivity of the surface electrode is rendered as a *downward* deflection. (Source: DiRusso F, Martinez A, Sereno MI, et al: Cortical sources of the early components of the visual evoked potential. *Human Brain Mapp* 2002; 15(2):95–111.)

probably arises from V2 and V3. Owing to the position of areas V2 and V3, this component P1 does not invert across the horizontal meridian, unlike the potentials generated by V1. A further positive wave, late P1, peaking at ~140 ms seems to arise from V4 and the fusiform area. Finally, the later component N155 originates more from regions in the parietal cortex. There are still slower negative waves, characterized by their approximate peak times, N180 and N200.[27] The early responses to color contrast are larger than those to achromatic stimuli, suggesting that the slower parvocellular system generates these responses. Very large responses have been reported with stimuli in which there is a chromatic change only. (See chapter 47.)

THE THALAMUS AS THE MOST IMPORTANT PACEMAKER ENSURING SYNCHRONOUS CORTICAL ACTIVATION The sense organs supply the brain with a huge number of signals about the outer world. The optic nerve alone, with a spatial resolution of more than a million fibers, a temporal resolution

50 Hz or more, and a good luminance resolution (of, say, 8 bits), supplies an information content of $10^6 \times 50 \times 256$, equaling around 25 billion bits per second (2.5×10^{10}). This is clearly too much information for the human brain to handle, given its limited processing speed (around 100 Hz at maximum). Hence, relevant signals have to be selected for cortical processing while less important ones have to be suppressed, discarded, or dealt with by subcortical structures in an automatic way. Thus, not all retinal stimulation seems to affect the cortex. An important relay station on the way to the cortex is the thalamus, more specifically—for visual information—its posterior part, called the *lateral geniculate nucleus* (LGN). The thalamus is sometimes called "the gate to consciousness" because many signals seem to be filtered out there before reaching the cortex (and thus, finally, conscious processing). The exact nature of these filtering and suppression mechanisms is still poorly understood. One hypothesis states that failure to synchronize inputs may lead to cortical suppression and/or failure of awareness for the respective stimuli.

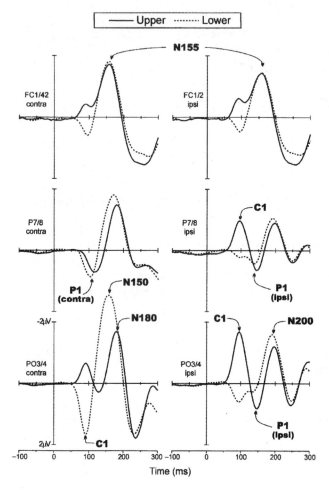

FIGURE 15.6 Analysis of the principal components of the EPs for several electrode positions, derived from figure 15.5. Note that in this figure, unlike many in this book, positivity of the surface electrode is rendered as a *downward* deflection. (Source: DiRusso F, Martinez A, Sereno MI, et al: Cortical sources of the early components of the visual evoked potential. *Human Brain Mapp* 2002; 15(2):95–111.)

The thalamus may shortly buffer the signals that are coming in from the sense organs and transmit to the cortex only the apparently important ones in the form of synchronous bursts. These bursts activate large numbers of cortical neurons at approximately the same time, thus producing large dipoles that can be recorded on the skull. The synchronization of inputs to the cortex is especially pronounced during sleep, leading to slow potentials (often below 10 Hz) with amplitudes that are larger than those usually recorded during the awake state. It is thought that these large potentials are based on rhythmic activity in the thalamus, probably due to an opening of Ca^{2+} channels in the hyperpolarized state of neurons only. The opening of Ca^{2+} channels leads to a depolarization of thalamic neurons, thus closing the charge-dependent channels, causing a renewed hyperpolarization of the membrane potential. This internal

oscillating activity obviously blocks, at least to a certain degree, sensory input from activating cortical areas. In a similar way, periodic changes of smaller amplitude may rhythmically create and close a window of excitability for sensory inputs to activate cortical neurons, thus synchronizing the arrival of sensory inputs in cortical neurons.

ALTERNATIVE METHODS TO RECORD BRAIN ACTIVITY INCLUDE MEG, PET, AND fMRI The EPs that are predominantly discussed in this chapter are not the only way to record the activity of the living brain through the intact skull. There are a number of additional methods based on different physical parameters of the nervous system. The first one to be presented here is the MEG, short for Magneto-Encephalo-Gram. This method records the magnetic rather than the electric potentials produced by cortical EPSPs and IPSPs. All electric currents produce magnetic fields, so recordings of the EEG and MEG refer ultimately to the same underlying cortical events. However, there are important differences between the two methods and the results they supply. First, the magnetic field runs perpendicular to the electric field. Hence, those cortical areas that run perpendicular to the skull and that produce the largest VEPs will contribute far less to the MEG, while those in the foldings of the sulci will generally produce small VEP amplitudes but larger MEGs. A second difference, which is a clear advantage of the MEG, is that magnetic fields are less distorted by the inhomogeneous conductance of brain tissues, liquor, and skull than the electric fields are. A third difference, this one a disadvantage, is that the MEG is much more expensive to record because it requires ultra-low-temperature sensors to be employed.

A second type of method is based on monitoring changes of brain activity through changes in metabolism (SPECT, PET) or by changes in local blood flow as indicated by O_2 concentration in tissues (fMRI). In SPECT (single photon emission computed tomography) and PET (positron emitting tomography), radioactive substances are injected into the bloodstream, and their distribution in the body is monitored. These radioactive substances decay at different speeds. For fast-decaying isotopes with half-life times of tens of minutes, which give best spatial resolution, as are often used in the PET, a nearby cyclotron is required, making this type of investigation expensive in addition to slightly hazardous for health. Radioactive sugars are employed to detect increases in local cortical activity while observers perceive specific (visual) stimuli. SPECT has a clearly lower spatial resolution and is used mostly to search for tumors in patients.

Functional magnetic resonance imaging (fMRI) uses modulations of strong magnetic fields rather than radioactivity and poses no known health risks to most patients. It monitors the changes of blood flow by measuring the amount of oxygen-laden hemoglobin locally in the brain under different stimulus conditions. The underlying assumption is that more

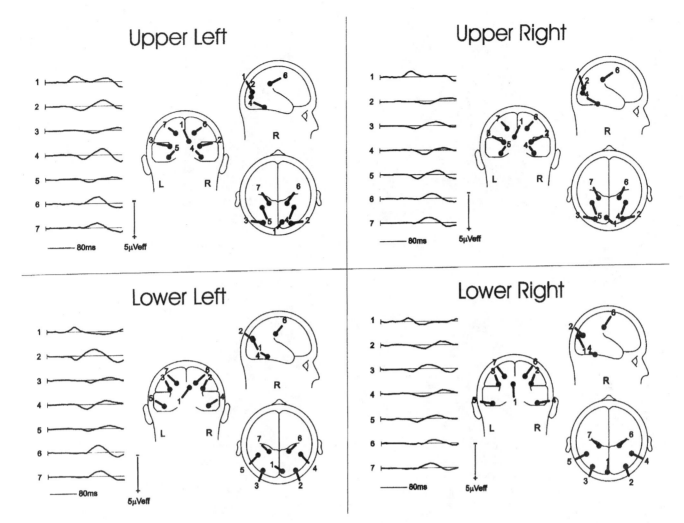

FIGURE 15.7   Applying dipole analysis to the separate components of figure 15.6. There are seven dipoles, and the EP waveforms of each are shown next to the representations of the brain, for each visual field quadrant separately. (Source: DiRusso F, Martinez A, Sereno MI, et al: Cortical sources of the early components of the visual evoked potential. *Human Brain Mapp* 2002; 15(2):95–111.)

active neurons need a larger oxygen supply, and hence, the local blood supply has to be increased. This method has an excellent spatial resolution, on the order of a few millimeters, but a much poorer temporal resolution than EEG and MEG have, and so far it is not used routinely in clinical practice.

Stimulation techniques: Modalities and parameters

STIMULUS MODALITIES

Modulation in space   The visual cortex is far less interested in homogeneous stimuli than the photoreceptors are. Its neurons respond to contours but hardly to homogeneous, static areas—unlike the retinal photoreceptors, as was mentioned above.[46] Hence, contours are better suited to evoke a large VEP than homogeneous fields are. Basically, two types of spatially structured fields are generally used to evoke cortical potentials by visual stimulation, with either a one-dimensional or a two-dimensional structure. One-dimensional stimuli consist of gratings that are usually defined by differences in luminance or color. The transitions between the dark and bright stripes (or between the two colors) can be either abrupt, in the form of a square wave, or else in the form of a sinusoid, that is, as a smooth transition. The latter form contains only a single spatial frequency (see "Modulation of spatial frequency" later), which is seen as an advantage by some. Two-dimensional stimuli consist most often of checkerboards (figure 15.10) and sometimes of radially structured dartboards that accommodate the fact that visual resolution decreases fast toward the periphery of the visual field (with little gain in VEP amplitude[67]). Checkerboards, on the other hand, are easily programmed and pose fewer problems with aliasing of oblique lines (their apparent "raggedness"). In the spatial frequency domain, they contain many different spatial frequencies. This may be an advantage because it tests the system in a wider range of

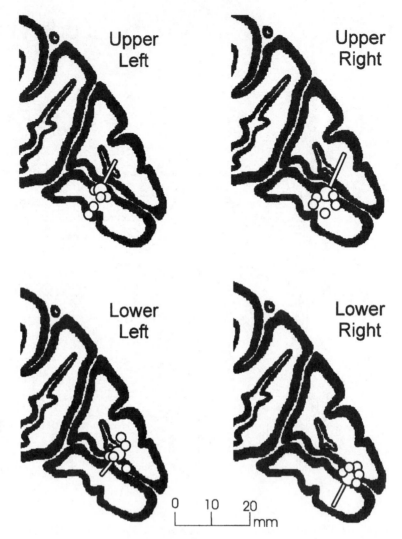

FIGURE 15.8 Diagram of MRI outlines of the calcarine sulcus, showing the position of the V1 dipole (large circle) and its major vector superimposed. Note that the upper field stimulus is located to the lower lip of the calcarine, and the lower field is (approximately) located to the upper lip. (Source: DiRusso F, Martinez A, Sereno MI, et al: Cortical sources of the early components of the visual evoked potential. *Human Brain Mapp* 2002; 15(2):95–111.)

input values. Interestingly, most dominant with these stimuli are spatial frequencies at the 45-degree direction (assuming a square checkerboard), as can be seen when employing a blurred version of a checkerboard. The dominant frequency can be calculated as follows.

Let d be the width = height of one checkerboard square. The diagonal of one square is the longest spatial period p. Thus, invoking Pythagoras, $p = \sqrt{2} \cdot d$. Since frequency is the inverse of the period, we arrive at

$$F_{\text{dominant}} = \frac{1}{\sqrt{2} \cdot d} = \frac{\sqrt{2}}{2 \cdot d}.$$

To give an example, for a check size of $0.5° = 30$ arcmin, the dominant spatial frequency is 1.4 c.p.d. The next higher frequency would be three times this value (4.2 c.p.d.), since symmetric square wave modulation does not contain any odd harmonics.

Modulation in time   To optimally stimulate neurons in the visual cortex and to produce a defined start of the stimulus (a prerequisite to separate the VEP from the background noise; see preceding "Signal averaging over many stimulus presentations"), stimuli have to be modulated in time. The easiest stimulus to produce is a flash of light (see "The normal flash VEP", following), but this is a suboptimal stimulus for several reasons, which were discussed in the preceding subsection. A better stimulus consists of the appearance and subsequent disappearance of a structured stimulus such as the checkerboards mentioned previously. (For details, see "The EPs to

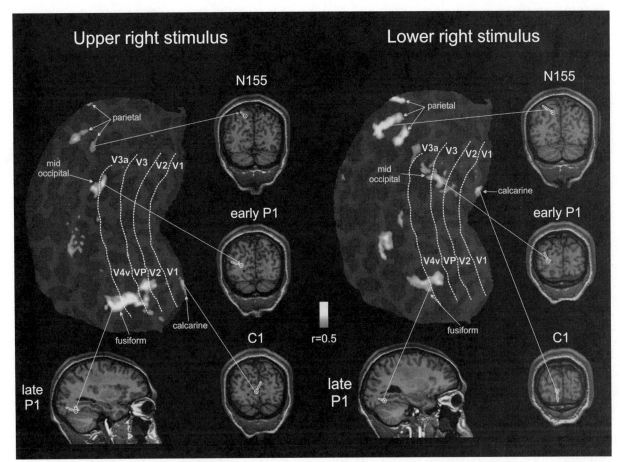

FIGURE 15.9 This figure shows agreement between imaging and electrophysiological techniques in placing cortical activities. The large "unfolded" fMRI images of the cortical surface show areas of activity caused by two visual stimuli, and the locations of the differing electrical dipoles are translated to the MRI image. The outlines of V1–V4 and the location of fusiform and parietal cortex are indicated. (Source: DiRusso F, Martinez A, Sereno MI, et al: Cortical sources of the early components of the visual evoked potential. *Human Brain Mapp* 2002; 15(2):95–111.)

appearance/disappearance" later.) Instead of these stimuli defined by appearance and disappearance, others can be used that are defined by contrast reversal. (See "The EPs to pattern reversal" later) While the appearance of a stimulus means that new contours are presented, contrast reversal means that the direction of contrast in spatially stable contours reverses. For example, changing all dark squares of a checkerboard to bright ones and vice versa reverses the direction of contrast at all the borders between bright and dark squares.

From the earliest recordings, stimuli have been employed in which the blank screen converts to a pattern containing contrasting edges in various forms. It is important that such a stimulus not alter the overall luminance of the display, and many commercial stimulator systems are unable to achieve this. When true "appearance stimuli" are produced, an entirely different waveform of EP emerges. The responses to appearance stimuli are usually labeled C0, CI, CII, and CIII.[45] Even though the same checkerboard pattern is generated, its subjective appearance is quite different from that of a pattern reversal: There is no impression of motion, and a typical motion detector model, such as the Reichardt detector,[37] does not respond to a pattern-onset stimulus. If each pattern is displayed very briefly (e.g., during just a single frame of a high–speed monitor), the image appears gray because contrast is integrated over a considerable period (20–30 ms), during most of which the screen is effectively blank owing to the fast decay of the monitor's phosphor.

Modulation in time and space: Motion Moving stimuli combine changes in time with changes over space (e.g., Clarke[21]). Technological development as well as intriguing findings rejuvenated this field. For example, Müller and Göpfert[57] showed that very low-contrast motion evokes a motion VEP, linking it to the magnocellular system. Initially, there was a controversy over what type of potential to expect from pure motion stimulation. It turns out that pure motion stimuli can indeed produce visual evoked potentials. However, their appearance depends critically on the duty cycle of stimula-

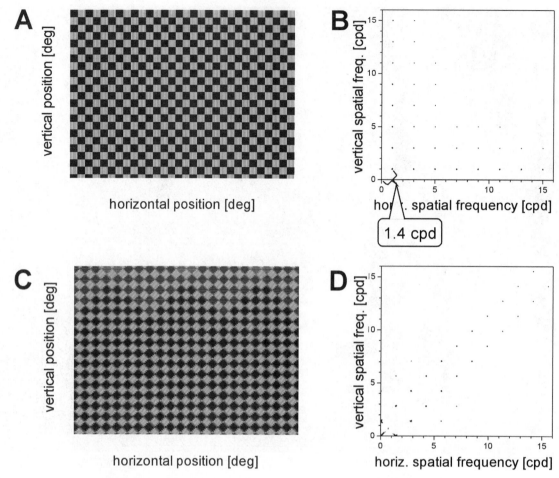

FIGURE 15.10 Fourier components of a checkerboard (Bach, unpublished calculations). On the left, a normal checkerboard with 0.5-degree square checks is seen at the top (A), and the same pattern rotated by 45 degrees is seen at the bottom (C); on the right are the corresponding Fourier spectra (magnitude only, B and D). In the spectrum, only isolated dots are seen because a regular pattern contains only discrete frequencies. The lowest (and dominant) spatial frequency is at horizontal = vertical = 1 cpd; thus, the distance from the origin corresponds to $\sqrt{2} \approx 1.4$ cpd. The higher harmonics decrease rapidly in amplitude; here, the size of the dots corresponds to the root of magnitude to make them more visible. Obviously, a wide range of spatial frequencies are contained in a checkerboard pattern, but none of the horizontal or vertical frequencies. The spectrum (D) of the rotated checkerboard (C) does contain horizontal and vertical spatial frequencies, as can be seen by slightly blurring (= spatial-frequency low-pass) pattern C. The slight scatter around the spatial frequency peaks is due to aliasing effects resulting from rotating a square on a rectangular pixel raster.

tion, that is, on the percentage of time during which the stimulus moves as opposed to being stationary. Because the visual system strongly adapts to motion, the stimulus must be stationary between trials for considerably longer than it moves during each trial to avoid such adaptation processes distorting the results.[13] A typical motion-evoked potential and its change with duty cycle are presented later in the chapter. Retinal potentials can also be evoked by motion, but these responses are probably from non-directionally sensitive detectors (e.g., flicker detectors) and therefore are not veridical motion responses.[8]

Modulation in color space Not only changes in luminance but also changes in color can evoke cortical sum potentials, for example, by presenting a grating or checkerboard that is defined purely by differences in color or by reversing or otherwise changing its color. (For an example, see the subsection entitled "EPs to chromatic stimuli" later in the chapter. For further details, see chapter 47.)

Modulation in depth Changing the binocular disparities between stimuli presented to the two eyes changes their apparent depth, that is, their distance from the observer. It could be shown that motion in depth produces VEPs in addition to those evoked by pure motion without any change in apparent depth. A simple demonstration consists of moving the dots in both eyes in vertical but opposite directions. This does not change disparity and hence produces no apparent change in depth. Moving the dots again in opposite directions in both eyes, but this time both in the horizontal direction, will produce an apparent shift in depth, resulting in an additional depth-specific VEP component when compared to the VEP that is elicited by vertical motion.

Modulation of spatial frequency　It is clear that a regular, periodic grating can be described by the width of its stripes. Two stripes, one dark and one bright, define the width of one period of this grating. The number of periods per degree of visual angle defines the spatial frequency of this grating. For example, a grating consisting of dark bars of 0.25-degree width and bright bars of the same width has a period length of 0.5 degree and a spatial frequency of 2 periods per degree. Often, the expression *cycles per degree* is used rather than *periods per degree*. Gratings, and stimuli in general, with high spatial frequencies stimulate neurons with small receptive fields, while the majority of neurons with large receptive fields cannot resolve the small lines of the gratings and are unable to discriminate such a grating from a homogeneous field. Gratings with low spatial frequencies will appeal to neurons with large receptive fields, while when neurons with small receptive fields are stimulated by a sinusoidal grating of low spatial frequency, the slow increase or decrease of luminance taking place within their small receptive field will not be an effective stimulus. It turns out that neurons with medium-sized receptive fields are the most sensitive to the difference in luminance between the bright versus dark stripes of a grating (and indeed any pattern). This is to say that these neurons require the least contrast for activation. Moreover, these neurons produce the largest VEP responses to appearance or contrast-reversing stimuli, while both coarser and finer gratings (and other patterns)

produce smaller VEP amplitudes. For high spatial frequencies, the properties of the eye's optics markedly reduce retinal contrast, contributing to the decline in amplitude and the increase in latency. Gratings that are too fine to be resolved will not evoke a VEP when reversing their contrast. This fact forms the basis for assessing visual acuity in babies and patients who are unable to cooperate. (See "Uses of the Flash VEP" and following sections.)

Figure-ground segregation and the VEP　Some cortical cells respond not to low-level features of the retinal image such as luminance contrast, color, motion, depth, or spatial frequency but to more complex features, such as the form of contours or figures. In an early stage of figure-ground discrimination, the visual system has to combine the local contour elements that together define a figure. Such activity produces an evoked potential. Presenting a stimulus consisting of line elements with random orientations such as in figure 15.11A and comparing the results with those evoked by another stimulus that contains the same line elements but arranged in a way to mark, say, a circle (figure 15.11B) yield significantly different VEPs. Thus, the VEP reflects the recognition of a figure. Figures may also be defined by differences in texture. Stimuli consisting of segregated elements, forming a checkerboard, consistently evoke potentials that differ significantly from the potentials that are evoked by random, nonsegregated presentation of the same elements, for elements defined by luminance, color, motion, texture, orientation, or depth.[9–12,33,50] Hence, the most widely used clinical VEP employing a checkerboard stimulus is based both on local differences of luminance and on the segregation between different parts of the stimulus. It is still under debate whether different types of segregation stimuli

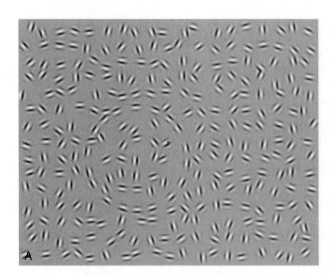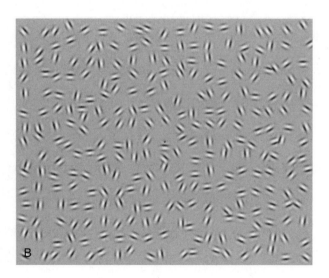

FIGURE 15.11　A, A contour defined by good continuation of line orientations. B, Randomized arrangement of the same elements as in A.

such as color-, luminance-, and motion-defined checkerboards all stimulate the same "master" map or are detected in partly different cortical structures.[11,31]

STIMULUS PARAMETERS   At the time of writing, a new document has been published[58] after prolonged consultations in the International Society for Clinical Electrophysiology of Vision (ISCEV). The basis for this standard rests on the uses that are envisaged for such a test and on the types of patients who are referred to the clinic. Work in pediatrics, in which the question is whether visual maturation is proceeding normally, evidently has quite different requirements (see Thompson and Drasdo,[74] as well as chapters 23 and 52) from the investigation of older children or adults, in which the common reason for referral is unexplained loss of vision. Procedures for incorporating EP testing with other electrophysiological procedures are described in other chapters (see chapters 36, 49, 56, and 79).

Field size   Not all retinal positions are equally represented in the (primary) visual cortex. Visual resolution falls steeply from the fovea to the periphery, and the same is true for the density of retinal ganglion cells. The size of cortical projections of any given area in the visual field is roughly proportional to the number of ganglion cells that are sampling this area of visual field. The so-called magnification factor indicates the size of cortical representations as a function of position in the visual field.[25,29,68] As a direct consequence, the representation of the central 10-degree radius represents more than half of the overall cortical representation of the visual world and dominates the VEP.[42] A stimulus diameter of 15 degrees will therefore suffice to elicit VEPs of near maximal amplitude.

Check size   Optimal amplitudes require the optimal stimulus size, as we saw in the last section. But what is the optimal check size? Given the varying resolution of the retinal areas that a stimulus of size 15 degrees covers, optimal check size differs between the center and the periphery of the area that is stimulated. One measure to compensate for this inhomogeneous nature of the receiving parts of the retina is to use as stimuli "dartboards" whose element size increases with increasing distance from the center (see above). But in addition, patients' visual resolution varies, sometimes dramatically, from one to the next. To yield good results, at least two sizes of checkerboard elements should be used sequentially in every patient, for example, element side lengths of both 0.25 degree and 1 degree; this helps, for instance, to distinguish between optical and neural problems: Neural problems, such as demyelination of the optic nerve, tend to influence results for all check sizes while optical problems will have less impact on coarser checkerboards than on finer ones.

Luminance   Of course, stimuli have to be bright enough for observers to perceive them. This statement might not be as unnecessary as it appears because some patients may require higher stimulus luminances than others owing to disturbances of the optic media or retinal disorders. In any case, stimulus luminance should be in the upper realm of the range possible for raster monitors, around $75\,cd/m^2$. Standardization of stimulus luminance (and contrast) is mandatory, since the transfer time of retinal photoreceptors depends on stimulus luminance.[7] Therefore, the stimulus luminance should be checked at regular intervals—monitors age![17] Latency between stimulus onset and the occurrence of discernible potential changes in the evoked response is one of the main parameters used in the evaluation of EPs. Using an insufficient stimulus intensity will distort the results, mimicking a delayed transmission of the stimulus. The good news is that the luminance dependence of VEP potentials as well as retinal photoreceptors is most pronounced for low luminances, approaching an asymptote for luminances above around $50\,cd/m^2$ (see figure 12 in Bach et al.[7]). To ensure optimal comparability between the results of different laboratories, the flash intensity should be normalized. Therefore, and for practical reasons, use of the ERG standard flash to evoke flash VEPs is strongly recommended.

Contrast   The common pattern-reversal stimulus with checks subtending about 40–50 minutes of arc at the pupil is used with a high contrast. Experiments in which the contrast is reduced show that the response saturates at about 20% contrast.

When check size is reduced with a high-contrast stimulus, the response diminishes, and attempts have been made to graph response amplitude as a function of check size and to determine whether extrapolation to zero voltage gives a check size commensurate with other measures of visual acuity. In general, there is a correlation with the result of this extrapolation, but the correlation is not as close as one would wish (see the section entitled "Uses of the Flash VEP"). Decrease in contrast below 35% increases the peak time of the VEP. Such slowing of the response also occurs in retinopathies. In these cases, the delay occurs in the retina, either in photoreceptors or in bipolar and amacrine processing. Hence, both luminance and contrast can have a distinct influence on the latency of VEPs. Use of stimuli at moderately high contrasts above around 60% is recommended.

Temporal frequency   The visual cortex responds more strongly to changing stimuli than to homogeneous stationary ones, as we saw above. So stimuli for VEP recordings may not just change in time to mark an onset on which to trigger the averaging but may be presented at higher frequencies. But let's start with the standard presentation of single stimuli. The rate of repetition should not exceed two reversals per second (rps) to allow a sufficient interval for the currents produced by the visual cortex to return to baseline. This will minimize any interactions between the responses to successful stimuli. Longer intervals would unnecessarily extend the time required for the test. The same holds true for flash stimulation: The repetition rate should be below 2 Hz. For appearance/disappearance stimuli, we recommend presenting the stimulus for 200-ms periods, each followed by a 400-ms pause.

Stimuli may also be presented at much higher frequencies or reverse at much higher frequencies, a stimulation type that is called *steady state*. In that case, the cortical responses to the individual stimuli superimpose and are no longer typical for single stimulation (see figure 5.12). Hence, simple averaging of the stimuli will lead to distorted results. In principle, two ways to evaluate the EPs are possible under these circumstances. First, a temporal Fourier analysis is performed. The Fourier analysis can be thought of as a large number of filters each transmitting a single temporal frequency. Hence, the Fourier analysis indicates the signal amplitude for each temporal frequency. The amplitude for the frequency corresponding to the stimulus repetition rate immediately indicates the signal strength of this stimulus. The second way to obtain the cortical response to a single stimulus from repetitive superimposed responses is based on a mathematical technique called *deconvolution analysis*. Basically, it supposes that the interactions between subsequent stimulations superimpose in a linear way. Then it is possible to subtract the late part of a response to one stimulus from the early part of the response to the next stimulus (see next section).

The multifocal VEP If later portions of the EP are recorded or the response is generated by cortical regions outside the striate cortex (V1), the situation becomes more complex, but this will not be the case in most clinical situations. Many attempts have been made to measure visual fields with the EP. However, it was shown early that most of the evoked response comes from the cortex connected to the central 3 degrees of the visual field (see "Field size" previously) and the convolutions of the visual cortex are quite variable; hence, the early work was largely unsuccessful. Recently, this idea of objective visual field testing has been revived by using multifocal techniques (see chapter 21). The multifocal technique presents a temporal pattern of stimulus that is unique and identifiable to each of a number of different adjacent retinal areas. The response (in the cortex) is identified by a cross-correlation technique, and the signal strength can be calculated separately for different visual field positions. The concept of perimetry by means of EPs, so to speak, is quite exciting, but a number of technical problems have so far limited its application in clinical practice (see chapter 26).

One of the main problems is the convoluted cortical folding and the small amplitude for peripheral stimulation, a problem that is far less present for multifocal ERGs.

Stimulation: Physiological targeting and response(s) to adequate stimulation

DIFFERENT TYPES OF EVOKED POTENTIALS Various more complex stimuli have been employed to evoke VEPs. Pattern appearance and disappearance EPs have been investigated with long exposures,[73] and the EPs that are generated by motion detection as distinct from appearance/disappearance have been distinguished.[54] Binocular interactions have also proved to be of interest, and good methods exist for controlled investigations of such features.[28] The mechanisms that detect coherent motion and moving objects formed by random dots evoke their own characteristic EPs. The relationship between auditory and visual stimulation has been investigated as well as how the spatial characteristics of combined visual and auditory stimuli are reflected in occipital EPs, indicating that part of the initial occipital complex is related to the subject's consciousness.[51,66] All these findings raise the possibility that EPs could be used for a variety of neurological and perceptual investigations in clinical conditions, but such recordings will not be routine for some time.

The responses to contrast-reversing achromatic stimuli are larger than those for chromatic stimuli. In the case of checkerboard stimuli, the contrast reversals can lead to the subjective impression that the squares of the stimulus "stream" across the screen as though they were moving. These observations are (weak) evidence that cells of the magnocellular pathway may primarily contribute to the generation of the EP, since this pathway is specialized for motion detection. In addition, the relationship between stimulus contrast and EP amplitude is very nonlinear, again compatible with M-pathway activation. Isoluminant color-defined checkerboards, on the other hand, should stimulate predominantly the parvocellular pathway, since the magnocellular stream is nearly color-blind.

The normal flash VEP Short flashes of bright light are able to strongly influence EEG activity, as was mentioned earlier, for example, in "photic driving." The flash VEP is useful to examine whether there is any cortical reaction to illumination of the retina, especially in patients who are unable to cooperate, since refraction and fixation problems are minimized. Today, the flash stimulus is not considered the first choice to evoke VEPs, since spatially structured stimuli evoke potentials that are much more consistent between subjects, allow the stimulation of restricted parts of the visual field (e.g., half-field), and are less disturbing for the patient. An example for a VEP evoked by flash stimuli of different intensities is shown in figure 15.12B.

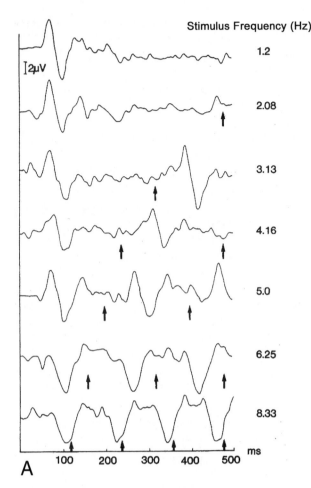

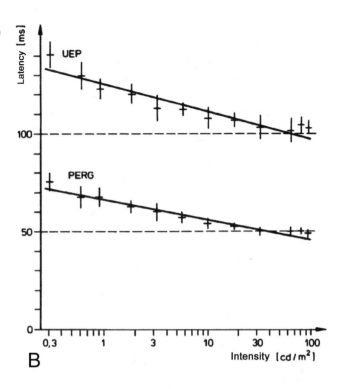

FIGURE 15.12 A, Dependence of VEP amplitude and latency on stimulus frequency. B, Dependence of VEP and pattern ERG on stimulus luminance. VEP latency decreases with increasing luminance (A, "the brighter, the faster"). This is due to retinal origin, as shown by the nearly parallel luminance dependence of the PERG (B). Above $\approx 100\,\mathrm{cd/m^2}$, the decline begins to be arrested.

(Source: A, from Altenmüller E, Ruether K, Dichgans J: Visuell evozierte Potentiale (VEP) und Elektroretinogramm (ERG). In *Evozierte Potentiale*. Berlin, Springer, 1996, pp 289–409. B, Modified after Bach M, Bühler B, Röver J: Die Abhängigkeit der visuell evozierten Potentiale von der Leuchtdichte: Konsequenzen für die Elektrodiagnostik. *Fortschr Ophthalmol* 1986; 83:532–534.)

The EPs to appearance/disappearance By and large, the VEPs that are evoked by the appearance of a structured stimulus or else by its disappearance resemble those evoked by the contrast reversal of the same type of stimulus. In both types of stimuli, it is important to ensure that the overall luminance of the stimulus stays constant, in order not to include a small "flash stimulus" into the pattern reversal. While this condition is easily met by the contrast-reversal stimuli, in which the luminances of the bright and dark elements are exchanged (as long as the number of dark elements equals the number of bright elements), the problem is more difficult in the case of appearing or disappearing stimuli. Obviously, the background luminance from which these stimuli appear or into which they disappear cannot correspond to the luminance of either the dark or bright elements but must be in between. A straightforward solution is to use the arithmetic mean of the luminances of the dark and bright ele-

ments. However, given the logarithmic gradient for human luminance perception, it may be more adequate to use the geometric mean.

Pattern-onset stimuli produce potentials with markedly higher interindividual variability than pattern-reversal stimuli do. Thus, they are preferred only in special situations such as diagnosis of albinism, for patients with nystagmus,[40] and for assessment of visual acuity. An example for a VEP evoked by a disappearing stimulus is presented in figure 15.13.

The EPs to pattern reversal The pattern-reversal stimulus is very widely employed, partly because the technique of generating the pattern is simple but also because the response is simple and is stable within and between subjects. The major positive component is generated in V1, and the time to peak of the major surface positive response (P100) varies very little

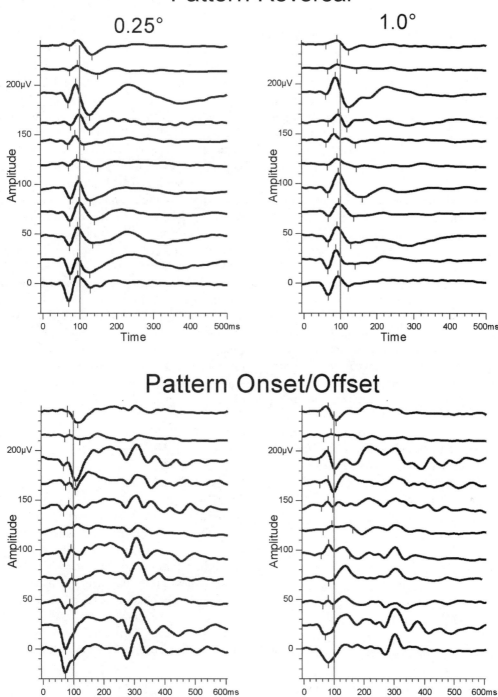

FIGURE 15.13 Examples of VEPs evoked by contrast reversal versus onset/offset. Recordings from 11 visually normal subjects, average of stimulation of the two eyes. Top, Pattern reversal (2 rev/s). Bottom, pattern onset/offset (200 ms ON, 413 ms OFF). Left, 0.25-degree check size. Right, 1.0-degree check size. The upper response in each of the four panels is from a stimulus limited to the central macula. The other responses are from a checkerboard that stimulated a much larger retinal area. For the bottom two traces of the pattern reversal panels, the stimulus frequency was 8 Hz. The wide variability between subjects is clearly seen and is obviously much more expressed for onset as compared to reversal (the corresponding traces in the top and bottom graphs correspond to identical subjects). Variability occurs both in absolute amplitude and in shape (e.g., the relative size of the peak troughs, N70/P100/N160). Changing the check size has less influence. (Source: From Altenmüller E, Ruether K, Dichgans J: Visuell evozierte Potentiale (VEP) und Elektroretinogramm (ERG). In *Evozierte Potentiale*. Berlin, Springer, 1996, pp 289–409.)

from person to person. Even minor damage to the neural pathway is frequently associated with increases in the peak time of this P100 potential. Contrary to the flash stimulus, the patterned stimulus allows hemifield stimulation, which usually will activate only the contralateral visual cortex. (The only exception is albino patients, who show a sizable anomalous projection of the nasal hemiretinae to the ipsilateral visual cortex.) With small field stimuli consisting of small checks, half-field stimulation produces larger VEP amplitudes on the contralateral occipital skull. However, large field stimuli with large checkerboard elements evoke a paradoxical lateralization on the ipsilateral skull. The explanation is based on the geometry of the primary visual cortex, which is folded in the calcarine fissure, close to the midline between the two hemispheres. The dipole resulting from activation of the primary visual cortex hence can point to the contralateral side, depending on the type of stimulation. Figure 15.14 presents some examples.

The EPs to moving stimuli Motion onset or offset of a structured stimulus can evoke a VEP, as outlined above ("Modulation in time and space: Motion"). Motion offset typically results only in a very small response. An example for a VEP evoked by motion onset is shown in figure 15.15A. The stimulus was a dartboard, which began an expanding motion at time zero for 200 ms, then rested for 1300 ms, and underwent a contracting motion for 200 ms followed by another stationary phase of 1300 ms. As a major response structure, a negativity at 160 ms after motion onset is seen. Motion is a more complicated stimulus than flash/pattern onset/reversal, and the stimulus paradigm described above avoids two major problems with motion stimuli:

1. Eye movement artifacts: Motion onset of any extended field typically evokes optokinetic nystagmus, which is not easily suppressed but is avoided by radially symmetric motion.

2. Motion adaptation: This phenomenon, well known from the motion aftereffect (a demonstration can be found at <www.michaelbach.de/mae.html>), is amazingly strong in motion VEPs. It can even lead to a (seeming) polarity reversal of the N160 (figure 15.15B, after Bach and Ullrich[13]). Since the adaptation time constant (about 3 s) is shorter than the recovery time constant (two to three times as long), even when the stimulus moves only half of the time, the subject is typically driven into 70–80% of motion adaptation.[39]

EPs to chromatic stimuli VEPs to chromatic stimuli are dominated by a negativity when the colors are fully equiluminant, that is, when the elements differ only in hue while having identical luminances (identical intensities for the normal human visual system). It is usually not possible to completely adjust the luminances of two colors in a way to ensure equiluminance in both the fovea and the (near)

periphery of the retina, but the remaining luminance contrast would be too low to elicit proper EPs given careful calibration of the monitor.

LATENCY OF VEPs: MORE THAN JUST TRANSMISSION TIMES OF RETINA, OPTIC NERVE, AND OPTIC TRACT   Several factors contribute to the latency between stimulus onset and the appearance of the large potentials that are usually used to evaluate the VEP in clinical practice. The first factor is transformation of electromagnetic waves by means of photochemical processes to neuronal potentials and eventually action potentials in the retinal ganglion cells. Depending on stimulus intensity, retinal photoreceptors require about 1–3 ms under optimal conditions to catch enough photons to produce a generator potential of sufficient size to be transmitted to the bipolar cells and to generate action potentials in ganglion cells. Retinal potentials in the electroretinogram (ERG) start a few milliseconds after a flash stimulus and peak (negatively) around 10–20 ms after stimulus onset. The first action potentials arise around 20–30 ms after stimulus onset in the retinal ganglion cells. Subsequently, the action potentials travel via the optic nerve and optic tract to the lateral geniculate nucleus, are transmitted to the neurons forming the optic radiation, and arrive at the visual cortex probably around 50 ms after stimulus onset. Indeed, the first changes of cortical activity are recorded after about 50 ms.[32] This delay fits rather well with the delay caused by retinal processing plus the conduction time of optic nerve, optic tract, and optic radiation. Moreover, reaction times to presentation of a flash stimulus decrease by about 40 ms in monkeys if the flash is substituted by a local stimulation of the visual cortex.[55] Given these latencies, it is surprising that the so-called early potentials of the VEP have latencies on the order of 100 ms, especially the P100. Hence, the latency of these large potentials does not reflect just the transmission time of signals arriving at the retina and traveling to the primary visual cortex. Quite to the contrary, the latency of these large early potentials is higher by about a factor of two than the pure transmission time. The reason for this massive additional delay is unclear at present. One possible explanation is that the visual cortex has to elaborate, by means of sequential processing, the information supplied by the retina before a strong and synchronous excitation of a sufficient number of neurons results. (See, for example, Palm[60] for a neuronal network model of visual cortex showing peak activity at 100 ms.) An alternative explanation would suppose that only after top-down feedback arrives at the primary visual cortex are the neurons there sufficiently synchronized to produce potentials with amplitudes such as that of the P100.

INFLUENCE OF THE COGNITIVE SET
Attention, arousal, and expectancy The discharge rate of single neurons at all stages of cortical signal processing can be

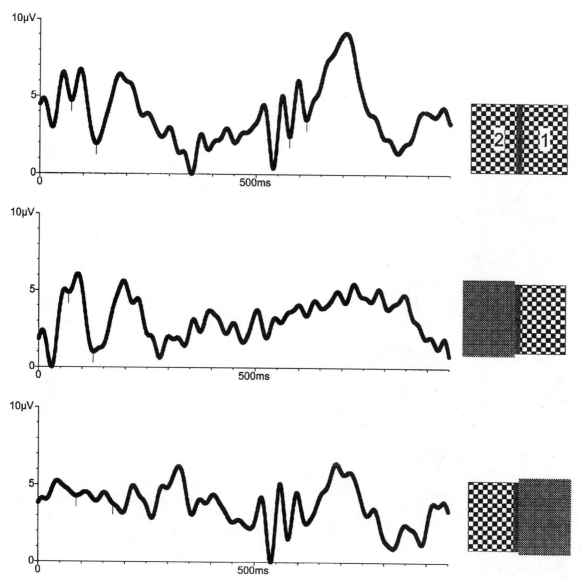

FIGURE 15.14 Examples of paradoxical lateralization with half-field stimulation. The stimulus was a checkerboard divided by a 1-degree-wide gray strip, which reversed at time zero on the right side and at 500 ms on the left side (indicated by the numbers on the small checkerboard insets; this is one of the stimulus paradigms in EP2000). This is a stimulus paradigm further explained at www.michaelbach.de/ep2000.html. The top trace was recorded from O1 (left hemisphere), the center trace from Oz, and the bottom trace from O2. In the top trace, the downward structure around 100 ms is small, the one around 600 ms is large, and the reverse holds for the bottom trace. This is contrary to what would be expected if the O1 response were dominated by activity in the right visual field. (The correctness of the stimulus was checked with cardboard partially covering the screen.)

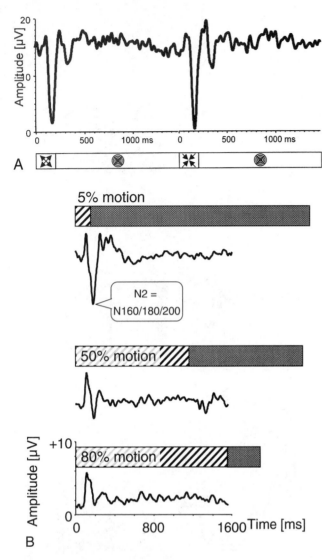

FIGURE 15.15 Examples of a VEP evoked by motion onset. Motion VEP evoked by (A) expanding (left) and contracting (right) a dartboard pattern (Molnar and Bach, unpublished data). The major response structure is a negativity at 160 ms after motion onset. Motion direction cannot be deduced from the potentials (but by selective adaptation, it could be[8]). The slight difference in amplitude between expansion and contraction is not significant. B, Effect of the duty cycle (% of motion versus total time) on the motion VEP. The hatched part in the horizontal bars represents the time where the stimulus pattern (here: sinusoidal gratings) moves; the gray part represents the stationary epoch. With a 5% duty cycle (top), there is a marked negativity (N2 or N160/N180), which decreases at 50% and vanishes at 80%, where the high duty cycle has caused strong motion adaptation.

modified by top-down signals reflecting the top-down influences that are commonly attributed to factors such as attention and arousal. While arousal denotes the general level of activation in the central nervous system, *attention* is a far more specific structure, reflecting the result of a focused direction of "processing power" to a specific portion of the visual field or to a specific feature of a (visual) stimulus.[53,61,75] Most studies employing flash VEPs demonstrate a small decrease in VEP amplitude with decreasing attention but constant latency.[36] Components of the VEP with larger latencies, above around 200 ms, depend more strongly on attentional influences and stimulus novelty.[23] With pattern-induced VEPs, the influence of the attentional factor is principally larger, not least because decreasing attention may lead to nonoptimal accommodation and fixation, leading to smaller amplitudes of the VEP. Latencies seem to be rather uninfluenced. We recommend limiting individual takes to 3–5 minutes at maximum to minimize the influence of fatigue and decreasing attention.

Preparation, motivation, and emotion Motivational and emotional factors influence predominantly the later portions of evoked potentials, at latencies beyond 200–300 ms, but even the early parts of the EPs may be influenced to a small degree. The P300 is especially sensitive to information regarding penalties or rewards. Motivational instructions increased the amplitude of the P300 evoked by an auditory stimulus, while its latency decreased nonsignificantly.[19] The P300 over the occipitotemporal and frontotemporal cortex is sensitive to reward magnitude but insensitive to its valence (penalty or reward),[47] while the error-related negativity, or feedback negativity, is sensitive to stimulus valence while not rewarding magnitude.[41,79] Both unpleasant and pleasant visual stimuli of low arousal content evoke widespread transient frontal steady-state VEPs over both sides.[48]

Derivation, electrode positions, equipment, and procedures

ELECTRODES

Electrode positions A difficult problem arose in experiments to determine the best electrode positioning around the occiput, the most suitable size of the stimulated part of the visual field, and the part of the field to be excited. Even the polarity of the response could invert with variation in stimulus size and electrode position.[34] The reason was soon shown to be the convolutions of the visual cortex in the calcarine fissure, as was mentioned above. The depth of the fissure represents a segment of retina that is approximately on the horizontal axis, or meridian. The superior surface of the fissure, facing downward, is connected to the upper part of the retina; that is, it represents the lower visual field. The lower lip of the fissure, which is opposed to the upper lip, is activated from the upper visual field. Recording above and below the horizontal axis evokes similar currents, but they flow normally to the cortical surface, and therefore, when monitored by surface electrodes that are somewhat remote, the voltage reverses when a small stimulus crosses the horizontal meridian. For this reason, the response becomes more stereotyped, and the interobserver variation is reduced if the stimulus field is large (10 degrees or more, despite most of the response originating from the visual field within 3 degrees of the fovea). However, for particular purposes, this might not be the best way to detect abnormalities.

The question of the "ideal" electrode position previously led to considerable debate. For a start, it must be realized that there is no absolute zero for potentials and that only potential differences are meaningful. Electrophysiology measures the potential at any point on the scalp and compares this to a hopefully inactive reference. Inactive or indifferent electrode positions on the body are only approximations to zero. An EEG channel represents the voltage difference between the two inputs of its differential input amplifiers connected to two electrodes.

Thus, the electrode positions (the montage) should be ruled not by dogmatic beliefs but rather by the specific experimental or clinical question. Typically, one wants to link the electrode position to an underlying cortical area. Here, the International 10/20 System[44] has proven useful: Standard easily detectable bony landmarks on the head (nasion and inion as front-back measures and the vertex and the preauricular points for lateral measures) serve as references. The electrodes are positioned at relative distances of 10% or 20% between these landmarks—hence the name *10/20 System*. This technique takes varying head size into account and has been shown to correlate with underlying brain morphology.

The current ISCEV VEP standard[58] suggests for prechiasmal diseases the use of a single channel, recording from Oz versus Fz. Because chiasmal and retrochiasmal diseases may be missed by using a single channel, it is useful in neuroophthalmological settings to add to this at least two lateral active electrodes.[58]

Problems of electrode placement Cortical potentials are generated as though from the ends of a dipole occupying the thickness of the cortex. Thus, for a large field, the signal is generated by equivalent dipoles tangential to the electrode over a considerable region of activated cortex, and the polarity, waveform, and response in general are less dependent on precise electrode placement. However, the maximum voltage is recorded between an occipital electrode and a remote electrode over the opposing hemisphere. When the occipital pole is stimulated by a small central target, the equivalent dipole is radial and is therefore maximal at the electrode directly above it. However, the voltage and even the polarity of the response are sensitive to electrode placement. To overcome

these problems, a large target is usually recommended for clinical VEPs.[35,59] In practice, placement of a single electrode at the midoccipital point (Oz in the International 10–20 System) can present a problem (figure 15.16). The position of Oz is determined by dividing in half the circumference of the head. It has been shown[44] that this location may be either on the midline or over either of the cerebral cortices, reflecting the amount of lateral shift or skew of the cerebral hemispheres. For any individual, therefore, Oz may be actually located on the midline, over the right visual cortex, or over the left visual cortex. Oz is hence placed in the worst position to record the response from all but the smallest visual targets. It will not be possible to know whether the potential generated by a small target is derived from the whole stimulus or from the part in the right or in the left visual field.

In addition, a single electrode placed on the midline should record the sum of the potentials from right and left visual cortices at the occiput. Unfortunately, this summing process is not simple, and an absence of evoked activity of one side of the cortex will still result in an apparently normal response. Equally, an asynchrony between the two visual cortices will result in apparent waves or "beats" that do not actually exist in each individual cortex. Such a complication will, of course, affect the apparent latency of the main peak.

It should also be remembered that the Oz-Fz potential depends not just on the potential at Oz, but also on the potential at the apparently inactive remote reference Fz. Many studies have shown that Fz is not inactive but has a strong negative potential concurrent with the positive potential at Oz.[38]

It is an established fact in electrophysiology that with two recording electrodes on the scalp, it is impossible to attribute the signal to either electrode. All forms of multichannel recording utilize a common reference form of VEP recording. With more than one channel, activity from the reference can be deduced because it is common between the two channels. With even more channels, the more precise potential gradient at the active electrodes can be plotted.[30] The only other method of locating potential peaks is using bipolar recording in which a chain of electrodes is connected in a bipolar manner.[35]

Number of electrodes and multielectrode recordings The number of electrodes that are employed in (clinical) studies varies from 2 to 128. For early evoked potentials, two may suffice. For clinical EEG interpretation, 12–16 channels are routinely used. For mapping and source derivation, 16 would be considered too few. Previously, there was debate whether a bipolar derivation (difference between equivalent positions on the two hemispheres) or a "linked-ear" reference or else an "average reference" is more advantageous. With current equipment, the debate has become nearly irrelevant, as any

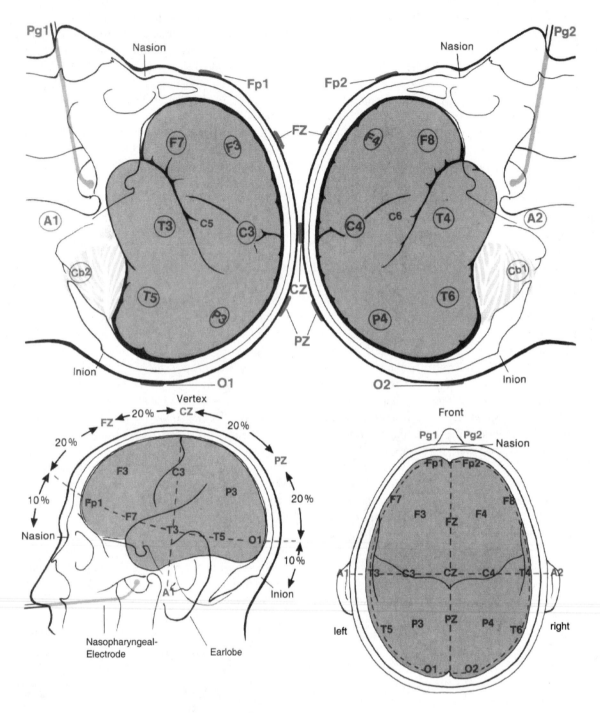

FIGURE 15.16   The 10/20 System of electrode placements for EEG recordings. (Source: Birbaumer N, Schmidt RF: Das Elektroenzephalogramm [EEG], 1990/1991. In *Biologische Psychologie*, Berlin, Springer-Verlag, 1991.)

montage can be simulated by appropriate postprocessing. The main requirement is that the electrode(s) used for reference be noise-free and preferably carry little activity; a popular choice is the average (not galvanic linkage!) of A1 and A2.[58] In a bipolar montage, an epileptic focus may be most evident.

AMPLIFIER CHARACTERISTICS Clinical electrophysiology is mainly concerned with the transient, or fast, responses of the visual cortex to visual stimuli. However, apart from these fast transient stimuli, far slower responses occur as responses to visual stimuli. Recording these stimulus responses requires d.c. amplifiers that are able to faithfully represent slow changes in signals and hence do not suffer from relatively fast drifts of amplification. Amplifiers that are used in clinical practice, on the other hand, usually remove in the filter module both slow and very fast changes of electrode potentials, a property that is called *band-pass characteristic*. These amplifier/filter combinations usually allow signals to pass (and to be amplified) that have frequencies between 1 and 100 Hz.

FILTERING, SAMPLING, AND UNDERSAMPLING The output signal of the amplifier has to be filtered to remove, to the greatest extent possible, all noise in the electrode signal that is unrelated to the signals to be detected. As was mentioned above, a common range of temporal frequencies to be recorded (while all others are removed or at least attenuated) is the one between 1 and 100 Hz. In case of such a filter, the signal has to be sampled at least about 300 times per second to ensure that more than two samples are collected by the computer during each cycle of the highest frequency present in the signal. Only if these conditions of the so-called sampling theorem[69] are met can the computer reliably reconstruct the original signal. If, on the other hand, the signal is sampled less than twice the highest frequency present in the signal, so-called undersampling may occur, distorting the signal that the computer reconstructs from the individual data points.

EYE POSITION CONTROL Given the strong decline of visual resolution toward the periphery of the visual field, it is important that fixation be in the center of the stimulus during all types of visual stimulation. Fixation may be controlled by means of two electrodes glued to both sides of the eyeballs, thus recording the vector, that is, the direction of the eye's dipole that is created by the electrical properties of the retina and pigment epithelium. Movements of the eye will produce changes in the direction in space of this dipole and hence changes in the potential recorded at the electrodes on both sides of the eye. Other methods to control fixation include monitoring of the patient's eye position by the investigator, either directly, via a mirror, or via a video camera plus monitor; presenting a number in the center of the screen, to be reported by the subject; or giving the subjects a laser pointer and having them point it to the center of the screen. Recently, video-based eye tracking devices have become widely available that analyze and record eye position continuously and automatically.

SYNCHRONIZATION OF THE STIMULUS MONITOR There are a number of options to define the start of a stimulus on a raster (TV) monitor. One possibility is to use the start of the scan, that is, the point in time when the new image starts to be displayed. But given the limited speed of raster monitors, it takes some time for the scan of the electron path to reach the middle of the monitor, where the observer fixates. Hence, it appears to be more logical to use the presentation time of the new stimulus at the center of gaze as the synchronization time rather than the start of scan. In some equipment (e.g., Veris), the local screen timing is taken into account for latency calculations for the multifocal ERG and VEP. For standard VEP (monofocal), at this time, most researchers still use the start of the scan as zero time reference (an exception is EP2000, Freiburg Evoked Potentials; see <www.michaelbach.de/ep2000.html>). There is currently a strong trend toward LCD monitors. While their switching times have improved (currently as low as 4 ms, which is fine), there is a sizable problem, because it is not currently possible to synchronize the monitor's[1] screen update with the computer's screen update. Thus the ensuing marked latency jitter of ±16 ms makes them currently unsuitable for electrophysiological stimulation.

Analysis techniques

LATENCY An important parameter of all evoked potentials is the latency, that is, the time between stimulus onset and clearly recognizable potentials in the averaged cortical sum potential. In visually evoked potentials, the first large, well-defined potential is the so-called P100, though there are earlier potentials, as was explained previously ("Latency of VEPs"). Thus, the term *latency* is misleading. "Peak time" would be more appropriate, but as of now, the term *latency* is used pervasively. The letter "P" in the P100 stands for positive deflection, and the number "100" stands for a latency around 100 ms. The latency is usually measured between the start of the raster scan on the monitor for the first presentation of the stimulus (see "Synchronization of the stimulus monitor" above) and the highest positive peak in the EP occurring between around 80 and 130 or 140 ms after stimulus onset. Low-contrast stimuli usually lead to higher latencies than high-contrast stimuli do, and several disorders, especially inflammation of the optic nerve (often as part of multiple sclerosis; see "Optic nerve dysfunction"), lead to significant delays of P100 latency, typically by more than 15–25 ms.

AMPLITUDE   The most pronounced early potential, the P100 mentioned above, is characterized not only by its latency, but also by its amplitude. The amplitude can be measured in different ways; most often, a baseline is produced by drawing a line between the lowest potentials, that is, the most negative parts of the EP just before (latency around 75 ms: N75) and just after the P100 (latency around 140 ms: N140; figure 15.17). The vertical distance between the peak of the P100 and this line corresponds to the amplitude of the P100. It depends on a large number of parameters, such as the exact geometry of the stimulus; its size, contrast, luminance, and speed; and the subject tested. Under optimal conditions, the amplitude of the P100 is up to 20–25 μV, but it is usually much lower, typical values being between 5 and 12 μV.

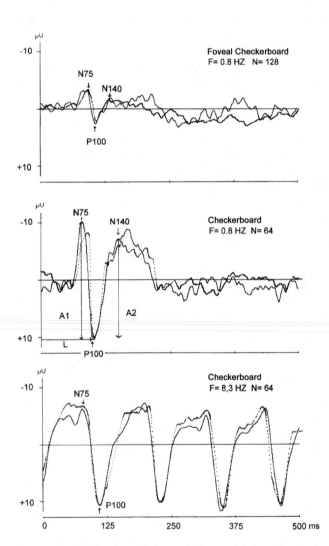

FIGURE 15.17   The form of the evoked potential depends greatly on the spatial and temporal properties of the stimulus, as illustrated above by three examples. Note that in this figure, unlike many in this book, positivity of the surface is rendered as a *downward* deflection.

FORM   The typical form of a visually evoked potential can be seen in figures 15.12, 15.13, 15.14, 15.15, and especially 15.17. After a small variable positivity with a latency around 50 ms after stimulus onset and a relatively small negativity thereafter, the typical EP features a large P100 followed by a distinct negativity, N170. As is to be expected from the information given above, the exact form of the VEP differs significantly between subjects and between different stimuli, while the general form shown in figures 15.12, 15.13, 15.14, 15.15, and especially 15.17 is usually preserved in all healthy observers.

FREQUENCY CONTENTS (FOURIER ANALYSIS)   As was mentioned earlier ("Modulation of spatial frequency"), stimuli can differ in the spatial frequency contents. For example, fine gratings contain higher spatial frequencies than coarse gratings do. The frequency contents of stimuli can be calculated by means of Fourier analysis. For gratings with a sinusoidal variation of luminance over space, the frequency content is rather straightforward: They contain only a single spatial frequency, defined as the reciprocal of their spatial period, that is, the distance between two subsequent peaks or troughs of the luminance distribution.

LAPLACIAN DERIVATION   It should be remembered that all EPs are voltage differences between the skin near the visual cortex and another, more remote location, usually in the midline near the frontal cortex or by (linked) earlobes. (There are many variations.) Current flowing in one visual cortex flows out of the calcarine fissure, and the return current pathway covers a larger area and is complex. It is commonly assumed that the early waves of the VEP represent activity only of the primary cortical areas, and refined experiments provide considerable evidence for this view (though see below). Thus, if a single scalp electrode is symmetrically surrounded by a number of other similar electrodes and all are connected to the same common reference, the average response of the surrounding electrodes will be less than the response of the central electrode if and only if the response is generated in the cortex beneath the central electrode. This technique is sometimes referred to as recording a Laplacian derivation, and in practice, four surround electrodes are sufficient.[64] The waveform of the Laplacian is essentially similar to that of a single electrode but indicates sources (i.e., additional current) or sinks (loss of current) within the array rather than a potential difference. However, with single occipital electrodes, it is not possible to be sure in all cases that the recording point always bears the same relationship to the underlying brain in each individual. Consequently, the waveforms that are recorded can vary with the stimulus parameters and the site of the recording electrodes. Such factors were responsible for what was called "paradoxical localization."[15] Binocular stimulation of one visual hemifield should produce early activity in only one cortex; for example, the right hemifield produces activity in the left visual cortex only. A contralateral pathway from the right nasal retina and an ipsilateral pathway from the left temporal retina meet at the chiasm. The response from a series of electrodes placed across the back of the head should reflect this. However, an early "paradoxical" result showed that the response to right hemifield stimulation appeared to come from the right cortex. It was found that this does not occur if the area of retina that is stimulated is small and/or if the square size is small and the contrast is less than maximal. The reason is that small subtense fields and small squares are resolvable only by the smaller area of *retina* near the fovea and excite cortex at the occipital pole, so the size and position of the active cortex are reduced.

Applications: Turning knowledge about basic physiology into clinical tests

Quite a number of different tests exist. The reasons for such a diversified approach are evident in the collections of acronyms that are used to describe clinical tests (VEP, VER, VCEP, etc.) and the number of different clinical protocols that have been advocated, each linked to different forms of stimulation. Here, we will give a short overview of a number of applications that evolved mainly from insights into the basic physiology of the visual system. More details are to be found in other chapters of this book (e.g., chapters 14, 23, 24, 36, 49, 51, and 52).

POOR VISUAL ACUITY: MEDIA OPACITIES AND RETINAL DYSFUNCTIONS   Media opacities will decrease the contrast of the retinal image and introduce blur. As a result, the potentials that are evoked by fine gratings and checkerboards consisting of small squares are decreased in a more pronounced manner than for coarser stimuli. Juvenile macular degenerations and optic neuropathies of various sorts can lead to loss of visual acuity before fundoscopy becomes abnormal. Under these circumstances, delays in the time to peak of the EP can be revealing, and recording an abnormal pattern electroretinogram (PERG) or multifocal ERG (mfERG) localizes the abnormality. Of course, the VEP, especially for fine stimuli, can be pathological as a result of age-related macular dystrophies, but these are better diagnosed morphologically. Recently, we[78] found a significant decrease in VEP amplitudes for a fine checkerboard in a patient whose retina appeared normal after a macular edema but who suffered from reduced visual acuity (Fahle et al., unpublished results).

OPTIC NERVE DYSFUNCTION, SUCH AS DEMYELINATION, ISCHEMIA, COMPRESSION, AND INFLAMMATION   This finding

leads to another difficulty: the possible influence of other intracerebral lesions on the EP. It is not possible to record a single-channel VEP and be sure that such pathologies are excluded. Chiasmal abnormalities can be detected by techniques described for analysis of albinism (chapter 25). Lateral displacements of the hemisphere(s) as a result of space-occupying lesions can be detected by multiple-electrode techniques. Asymmetries in both the amplitude and timing of occipital-temporal current flows can be detected. Such recordings cannot be carried out with the minimal two-channel ERG equipment that is sometimes purchased for office use but require multiunit recordings and appropriate software.

CHIASMAL (AND RETROCHIASMAL) DYSFUNCTION   Disorders of the chiasma and/or the optic tract as well as the optic radiation lead to changes similar to those that occur with the corresponding disorders of the optic nerve, with one important difference: The EPs that are elicited through both eyes will be changed in a similar way, making a diagnosis more difficult because a comparison between the potentials of both eyes with one serving as the normal control is impossible. As was mentioned above, chiasmal abnormalities can be diagnosed by specific techniques described in the chapter on albinism (see chapter 25).

OBJECTIVE ASSESSMENT OF VISUAL ACUITY   One common cause of referral is "hysteria" in a broader sense, or "functional visual loss." This can occur, for example, as a result of stress (at home or school) in children. Typically, there are no clinical findings, but this does not rule out juvenile macular degeneration. The EP is an important diagnostic test in these cases. If appearance VEPs are recorded and a response can be seen to the finest stimuli, relatively normal visual acuity must be present at the cortical level even if the history and the sight test chart suggest otherwise[2] (figure 15.18). Children who present at an electrophysiological department have already seen various medical and paramedical personnel and have had repeated eye tests, and one factor reinforcing the complaint is parental anxiety. The authors have found it useful to show the parent the screen that evokes a minimal appearance EP, taking care that the parent is placed slightly behind the child, that is, farther from the screen. The parent, who usually cannot resolve the pattern at all, thus receives a graphic illustration that the child's vision is not impaired. This is the only time when recording EPs can cure a condition! With practice, it is possible to detect mild abnormalities (e.g., anisometropic amblyopia) and still be certain that the slightly reduced VA shown by EP recording does not correspond to the previous test with an ordinary optotype. Other important diagnoses in children are developmental amblyopias, albinism, and S-cone syndromes. In all these cases, the presenting symptom may be reduced visual acuity,

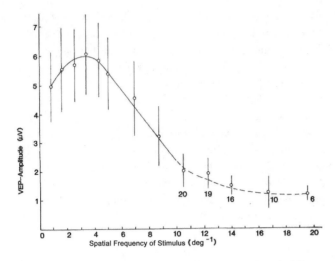

FIGURE 15.18 Acuity estimate by means of VEPs of different element sizes. (Source: From Altenmüller E, Ruether K, Dichgans J: Visuell evozierte Potentiale (VEP) und Elektroretinogramm (ERG). In *Evozierte Potentiale*. Berlin, Springer, 1996, pp 289–409.)

and a VEP may be requested. These are dealt with in other chapters.

In adults, functional losses of vision are often related to malingering or insurance claims, and the clinic must take great care that the person who is being tested has not developed a strategy to hoodwink the tester. Eyes may be closed during the test, or the image may be deliberately defocused. To avoid such spurious results, the EPs may be recorded with paralyzed accommodation, and proper refractive compensation, and precisely placed artificial pupils. It is helpful if the patient is under continuous closed-circuit television surveillance. In addition, active defocusing of pattern appearance cannot be performed by naïve subjects, since this is an entirely natural stimulus, whereas it is relatively easy to defocus a reversing stimulus. It is of use to project a colored isoluminant image (e.g., an animation) together with an achromatic flashed stimulus for evoking the EP. Of course, the ability to see properly depends on higher levels of the visual system than V1 and V2 (it has been shown that late activity in V1 is related to attention and perception).[5,51,66] Therefore, in reporting on functional loss, one should emphasize the level at which the normal response has been recorded. Recent work has demonstrated that part of the EP that is recorded from the primary cortex reflects the percept experienced by the subject. In the future, it might be possible (e.g., by the use of reverse correlation techniques; see chapters 25 and 32) to test psychological functions.

Note that the pattern VEP is usually abnormal in macular dysfunction. Inversely, a latency increase of the VEP does not necessarily imply optic nerve affection.

In summary, by changing the spatial frequency of the stimulus and registration of the amplitude of the visual evoked response, it is, in principle, possible to assess the patient's visual acuity, although the results are often not as clear as one would expect and are subject to a number of artifacts. However, as is described in detail in chapter 52, certain modifications, such as the sweep VEP with rapidly changing element sizes, may improve the validity of the method and lead to a more general use of this method in clinical practice.

USES OF THE FLASH VEP   Cortical neurons respond to the onset (and offset) of diffuse light stimulation quite vigorously, though somewhat less than they do to strongly structured stimuli such as luminance-modulated gratings or checkerboards. Hence, the flash VEP is not usually used anymore in most clinical settings. However, as is outlined below, it has a number of applications under special circumstances. (See also the sections that follow.)

Poor patient compliance   Patients are sometimes unable to fixate steadily on a monitor, often owing to physical problems or limitations, such as nystagmus, muscular problems, or general weakness. Patients who are suffering from functional disorders may also fail to fixate properly. In these cases, the flash VEP may be a better choice, since the interior of the eyeball will reflect a large amount of light and hence ensure that the fovea and parafovea are stimulated even during imperfect fixation.

Babies and infants   Babies and infants may be considered a special case of patients with poor compliance. While it is certainly possible to record VEPs from small children and infants, even newborns, and assess visual acuity, other babies will fail to fixate. For the same reasons as are outlined above, a flash VEP will be preferable to a pattern VEP in these cases.

Coma or reduced level of consciousness   Patients may suffer from a reduced level of consciousness or even coma, for example, after head trauma. Especially if there is no pupil response, the function of the optic nerve can be assessed by means of a flash VEP even in comatose patients. Such an assessment may, for example, guide the surgeon regarding whether or not to embark on a decompression of the optic nerve after bleeding or a fracture of the orbit.

ACKNOWLEDGMENTS   We are extremely grateful to Geoffrey Arden for contributions to the text regarding (not only) the history of the field.

REFERENCES

1. Adrian ED, Matthews BHC: The Berger rhythm: Potential changes from the occipital lobes in man. *Brain* 1934; 57:355–385.

2. Arden GB: An overview of the uses and abuses of electrodiagnosis in ophthalmology. *Int J Psychophysiol* 1994; 16:113–119.

3. Arden GB, Faulkner D: A versatile pattern generator based on television techniques for evoked potential generation. In JE Desmedt (ed): *The Evoked Potentials*. New York, Oxford University Press, 1977.

4. Arden GB, Gunduz K, Perry S: Colour vision testing with a computer graphics system. *Clin Vis Sci* 1988; 2:303–320.

5. Arden GB, Wolf JE, Messiter C: Electrical activity in visual cortex associated with combined auditory and visual stimulation in temporal sequences known to be associated with a visual illusion. *Vision Res* 2003; 43:2469–2478.

6. Arieli A, Sterkin A, Grinvald A, Aertsen A: Dynamics of ongoing activity: Explanation of the large variability in evoked cortical responses. *Science* 1996; 273:1868–1871.

7. Bach M, Bühler B, Röver J: Die Abhängigkeit der visuell evozierten Potentiale von der Leuchtdichte: Konsequenzen für die Elektrodiagnostik. *Fortschr Ophthalmol* 1986; 83:532–534.

8. Bach M, Hoffmann MB: Visual motion detection in man is governed by non-retinal mechanisms. *Vision Res* 2000; 40:2379–2385.

9. Bach M, Meigen T: Electrophysiological correlates of texture-segmentation in human observers. *Invest Ophthalmol Vis Sci (ARVO Suppl)* 1990; 31:104 (#515).

10. Bach M, Meigen T: Electrophysiological correlates of texture segregation in the human visual evoked potential. *Vision Res* 1992; 32(3):417–424.

11. Bach M, Meigen T: Similar electrophysiological correlates of texture segregation induced by luminance, orientation, motion and stereo. *Vision Res* 1997; 37(11):1409–1414.

12. Bach M, Meigen T: Do's and don'ts in Fourier analysis of steady-state potentials. *Doc Ophthalmol* 1999; 99(1):69–82.

13. Bach M, Ullrich D: Motion adaptation governs the shape of motion-evoked cortical potentials (motion VEP). *Vision Res* 1994; 34:1541–1547.

14. Berger H: Über das Elektroenkephalogramm des Menschen. *Arch Psych Nervenkrankheit* 1929; 87:527–570.

15. Blumhardt LD, Halliday AM: Hemisphere contributions of the composition of the pattern-evoked waveform. *Exp Brain Res* 1979; 36:53–69.

16. Brazier MAB: *A History of the Electrical Activity of the Brain*. London, Pitman, 1961.

17. Brigell M, Bach M, Barber C, Moskowitz A, Robson J: Guidelines for calibration of stimulus and recording parameters used in clinical electrophysiology of vision. *Doc Ophthalmol* 2003; 107:185–193.

18. Campbell FW, Maffei L: Electrophysiological evidence for the existence of orientation and size detectors in the human visual system. *J Physiol* 1970; 207:635–652.

19. Carrillo-de-la-Pena MT, Cadaveira F: The effect of motivational instructions on P300 amplitude. *Neurophysiol Clin* 2000; 30(4):232–239.

20. Ciganek L: The EEG response (evoked potential) to light stimulus in man. *Electroencephalogr Clin Neurophysiol* 1969; 13:165–172.

21. Clarke PG: Visual evoked potentials to sudden reversal of the motion of a pattern. *Brain Res* 1972; 36:453–458.

22. Cobb WA, Dawson GD: The latency and form in man of the occipital potentials evoked by bright flashes. *J Physiol* 1960; 152:108–122.

23. Courchesne E, Hillyard SA, Galambos R: Stimulus novelty, task relevance and the visual evoked potential in man. *Electroencephalogr Clin Neurophysiol* 1975; 39:131–143.

24. Creutzfeld OD, Kuhnt U: The visual evoked potential: Physiological, developmental and clinical aspects. *Electroencephalogr Clin Neurophysiol* 1967; 26 (suppl):29–41.

25. Daniel PM, Whitteridge D: The representation of the visual field on the cerebral cortex in monkeys. *J Physiol (Paris)* 1961; 159:203–221.

26. De Lange H: Research into the dynamic nature of the human fovea cortex system with intermittent and modulated light. *J Opt Soc Amer* 1958; 48:777–784.

27. Di Russo F, Martinez A, Sereno MI, Pitzalls S, Hillyard SA: Cortical sources of the early components of the visual evoked potential. *Human Brain Mapping* 2002; 15:96–111.

28. di Summa A, Polo A, Tinazzi M, Zanette G, Bertolasi L, Biongiovanni LG, Fiaschi A: Binocular interaction in normal vision: Studies by pattern reversal visual evoked potentials (PR-VEPs). *Ital J Neurol Sci* 1997; 18:81–86.

29. Drasdo N: The neural representation of visual space. *Nature* 1977; 266:554–556.

30. Drasdo N, Furlong P: Coordinate systems for evoked potential topography. *Electroencephalogr Clin Neurophysiol* 1988; 71:469–473.

31. Fahle M, Quenzer T, Braun C, Spang K: Feature-specific electrophysiological correlates of texture segregation. *Vision Res* 2003; 43:7–19.

32. Fahle M, Skrandies W: An electrophysiological correlate of perceptual learning in humans. *German J Ophthalmol* 1994; 3:427–432.

33. Fahle M, Spang K: Heterogeneity of brain responses to identical stimuli. *Int Rev Sociol* 2003; 13:507–532.

34. Halliday AM, Michael WF: Changes in the pattern-evoked responses in man associated with the vertical and horizontal meridians of the visual field. *J Physiol* 1970; 208:499–513.

35. Harding GFA, Smith GS, Smith PA: The effect of various stimulus parameters on the lateralisation of the visual evoked potential. In Barber C (ed): *Evoked Potentials*. Lancaster, MTP Press, 1980, pp 213–218.

36. Harter MR, Salmon LE: Intra-modality selective attention and evoked cortical potentials to randomly presented patterns. *Electroencephalogr Clin Neurophysiol* 1972; 32:605–613.

37. Hassenstein B, Reichardt W: Systemtheoretische Analyse der Zeit-, Reihenfolgen- und Vorzeichenauswertung bei der Bewegungsperzeption des Rüsselkäfers Chlorophanus. *Z Naturforsch* 1956; 11b:513–523.

38. Hobley AJ, Harding GF: The topography of the P1 component of the flash visual evoked response. *Doc Ophthalmol* 1989; 73:119–125.

39. Hoffmann M, Dorn T, Bach M: Time course of motion adaptation: Motion onset visual evoked potentials and subjective estimates. *Vision Res* 1999; 39:437–444.

40. Hoffmann MB, Seufert P, Bach M: Simulated nystagmus suppresses pattern-reversal but not pattern-onset visual evoked potentials. *Clin Neurophys* 2004; 115:3659–3665.

41. Holroyd CB, Larsen JT, Cohen JD: Context dependence of the event-related brain potential associated with reward and punishment. *Psychophysiology* 2004; 41(2):245–253.

42. Horton JC, Hoyt WF: The representation of the visual field in human striate cortex: A revision of the classic Holmes map. *Arch Ophthalmol* 1991; 109(6):816–824.

43. Hubel DH, Wiesel T: Functional architecture of macaque monkey visual cortex. *Proc R Soc Lond B Biol Sci* 1977; 198:1–59.

44. Jasper HH: The ten-twenty electrode system of the international federation. *EEG Clin Neurophysiol* 1958; 10:271–275.

45. Jeffreys DA: Separable components of human evoked responses to spatially patterned visual fields. *EEG Clin Neurophysiol* 1968; 24:596.

46. Kayama Y, Riso RR, Bartlett JR, Doty RW: Luxotonic responses of units in macaque striate cortex. *J Neurophysiol* 1979; 42:1495–1517.

47. Keil A, Gruber T, Müller MM, Moratti S, Stolarova M, Bradley MM, Lang PJ: Early modulation of visual perception by emotional arousal: Evidence from steady-state visual evoked brain potentials. *Cognit Affect Behav Neurosci* 2003; 3(3):195–206.

48. Kemp AH, Gray MA, Eide P, Silberstein RB, Nathan PJ: Steady-state visually evoked potential topography during processing of emotional valence in healthy subjects. *Neuroimage* 2002; 17(4):1684–1692.

49. Kiloh LG, McComas AJ, Osselton JW: *Clinical Electroencephalography*. London, Butterworths, 1972.

50. Lamme VAF, Van Dijk BW, Spekreijse H: Texture segregation is processed by primary visual cortex in man and monkey: Evidence from VEP experiments. *Vision Res* 1992; 32:797–807.

51. Lamme VA, Zipser K, Spekreijse H: Figure–ground activity in primary visual cortex is suppressed by anaesthesia. *Proc Natl Acad Sci U S A* 1998; 95:3263–3268.

52. Martin JH: The collective electrical behavior of cortical neurons: The electroencephalogram and the mechanisms of epilepsy. In Kandel ER, Schwartz JH, Jessel TM (eds): *Principles of Neural Science*. New York, Elsevier, 1991, pp 777–791.

53. Maunsell JH: Neuronal representations of cognitive state: Reward or attention? *Trends Cogn Sci* 2004; 8(6):261–265.

54. Maurer JP, Bach M: Isolating motion responses in visual evoked potentials by preadapting flicker–sensitive mechanisms. *Exp Brain Res* 2003; 151:536–541.

55. Miller JM, Glickstein M: Neural circuits involved in visuomotor reaction time in monkeys. *J Neurophysiol* 1967; 30:399–414.

56. Mitzdorf U: Properties of cortical generators of event-related potentials. *Pharmacopsychiatry* 1994; 27(2):49–51.

57. Müller R, Göpfert E: The influence of grating contrast on the human cortical potential evoked by motion. *Acta Neurobiol Exp* 1988; 48:239–249.

58. Nunez PL, Katznelson RD: Electric Fields of the Brain: The Neurophysics of the EEG. New York and Oxford, Oxford University Press, 1981.

59. Odom JV, Bach M, Barber C, Brigell M, Marmor MF, Tormene AP, Holder GE, Vaegan: Visual evoked potentials standard. *Doc Ophthalmol* 2004; 108:115–123.

60. Palm G: *Neural Assemblies: An Alternative Approach to Artificial Intelligence*. Berlin, Springer-Verlag, 1982.

61. Pessoa L, Kastner S, Ungerleider LG: Neuroimaging studies of attention: From modulation of sensory processing to top-down control. *J Neurosci* 2003; 23(10):3990–3998.

62. Raizada RDS, Grossberg S: Toward a theory of the laminar architecture of the cerebral cortex: Computational clues from the visual system. *Cereb Cortex* 2003; 13:100–113.

63. Regan D: Some characteristics of average and steady state responses evoked by modulated light. *Electroencephalogr Clin Neurophysiol* 1966; 20:238–248.

64. Regan D: *Human Brain Electrophysiology*. New York, Elsevier, 1989, Section 1.2.7 pp 16–21, 672; Section 2.6.8 pp 429–435.

65. Regan D, Richards W: Brightness and contrast evoked potentials. *J Opt Soc Amer* 1973; 66:606–611.

66. Roelfsema PR, Spekreijse H: The representation of erroneously perceived stimuli in the primary visual cortex. *Neuron* 2001; 31:853–863.

67. Röver J, Bach M: Visual evoked potentials to various check patterns. *Doc Ophthalmol* 1985; 59:143–147.

68. Schwartz EL: A quantitative model of the functional architecture of human striate cortex with application to visual illusion and cortical texture analysis. *Biol Cybern* 1980; 37:63–76.

69. Shannon CE: A mathematical theory of communication. *Bell Syst Tech* 1948; 27:623–656.

70. Sokol S: Measurement of infant visual acuities from pattern reversal evoked potentials. *Vision Res* 1978; 18:33–41.

71. Spekreijse H: Analysis of EEG responses in man, thesis. University of Amsterdam, 1966.

72. Spekreijse H, van der Tweel LH: Linearisation of evoked responses to sine wave modulated light by noise. *Nature* 1965; 205:913.

73. Spekreijse H, van der Tweel LH, Zuidema TH: The contrast evoked responses in man. *Vision Res* 1973; 13:1577–1601.

74. Thompson DA, Drasdo N: Clinical experience with preferential looking acuity tests in infants and young children. *Ophthalmic Physiol Opt* 1988; 12(2):225–228.

75. Treue S, Maunsell JH: Effects of attention on the processing of motion in macaque middle temporal and medial superior temporal visual cortical areas. *J Neurosci* 1999; 19(17):7591–7602.

76. Walter WG: The location of the cerebral tumours by electroencephalography. *Lancet* 1936; 2:305–312.

77. Walter WG, Cooper R, Aldridge VJ, McCallum WC, Winter AL: Contingent negative variation; an electrical sign of sensory-motor association and expectancy in the human brain. *Nature* 1964; 203:380–384.

78. Wolf ME, Mavrer JP, Bach M: VEP-based acuity assessment in normal vision, artificially degraded vision, and in patients with eye diseases. *Invest Ophthalmol Vis Sci* 2005; 46(5665):B868.

79. Yeung N, Sanfey AG: Independent coding of reward magnitude and valence in the human brain. *J Neurosci* 2004; 24(28):6258–6264.

IV EQUIPMENT

16 Data Acquisition Systems for Electrodiagnostic Testing

CHRIS HOGG AND STEVEN NUSINOWITZ

Data-recording systems

Equipment for performing visual electrodiagnostic testing of the visual system is described in this chapter. In acquiring information for this chapter, a limited survey was sent to a number of those performing electrodiagnostic testing in the clinic and laboratory to determine what equipment was being used for testing. On the basis of the responses to this survey, a broad array of equipment descriptions and sources has been collected. What was surprising was the lack of consensus about equipment for both clinical and laboratory applications. This chapter is intended as a starting resource for those who are interested in either purchasing a commercial system or designing and building their own.

A significant number of respondents to the survey indicated that their laboratories use systems that were designed and built in their own laboratories for their own specific purposes and that undergo modification as required. The need for self-built systems, it was reported, stemmed from finding that commercial systems were inadequate for the specific purposes of the laboratory or did not allow sufficient flexibility for experimental work. The cooperation between systems designers and clinical/research laboratories has led to a rapid improvement in the quality and design of commercial electrodiagnostic systems. As a result, these stand-alone systems have increasingly found their way into testing laboratories, particularly in clinical electrodiagnostic services, where they seem to dominate. However, research-oriented facilities continue to use their own systems. In acquiring a recording system, therefore, the main message that was derived from the survey seemed to be "know what you want to do with the system, and make sure that the system has enough flexibility to meet the needs of the laboratory for the expected life of the equipment."

COMPONENTS OF DATA ACQUISITION SYSTEMS Modern recording systems for use in clinical visual electrophysiology laboratories generally follow a standard format, be they for routine clinical work or more complex research applications. They are almost inevitably built around a personal computer (Macintosh or Windows), although in some cases, this may not be apparent on casual examination.

This equipment configuration is defined largely by the problems inherent in the task.

In simple instrumentation terms, the task or objective is to record small signals in an environment that is far from ideal. These signals generated from the various structures of the visual system fall within the range of 10 nV to 1000 µV in terms of amplitude and 0.1–300 Hz for frequency. As a signal generator, the patient is not ideal, having a low signal-to-noise ratio and no direct connection points to the system under investigation. The recording environment is also noisy electrically and becomes increasingly degraded with the proliferation of electronic equipment. Instrumentation systems are designed in part to circumvent these problems.

The main stages of a typical system are described (figure 16.1), along with some of the specific problems associated with each stage.

SYSTEM OVERVIEW The first component is the stimulator, commonly either a Ganzfeld bowl or a pattern stimulator, which provides a controlled light source that may be synchronized with the data acquisition components. These units are dealt with in more detail elsewhere.

Regardless of which stimulus source is used, it is essential that it is calibrated correctly and that the calibration is repeated at suitable intervals. If this is not done, there can be no certainty that variations from the norm are due to the patient and not to changes in stimulus parameters. Most visual stimulators (including monitors, simple xenon flashes, or LCD screens) cannot be assumed to be stable. All responses are sensitive to variations in stimulus parameters, many in a nonlinear fashion. Therefore, without precise definition of the stimulus, uncertainty relating to the responses that are produced is inevitable. For details of stimulus calibration, refer to the ISCEV guidelines.[1]

THE PATIENT In some tests, the patient must remain immobile in the same position for extended intervals, and care should be taken to ensure that the patient is not only correctly positioned for delivery of the stimulus, but also in a comfortable position that can be maintained for the duration of the examination. Incorrect positioning of the patient will mean that the stimulus varies between patients and with

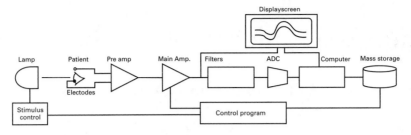

FIGURE 16.1   System overview.

time in the same patient. In addition, the quality of the recorded signals will deteriorate. A patient who is comfortable, relaxed, and well supported will generate much lower levels of artifact.

ELECTRODES   The electrodes through which signals are recorded are, superficially at least, the simplest piece of equipment in the chain. They generally consist of a piece of metal or other conductive material attached to a length of wire with a plug on the other end. This piece of equipment, frequently dismissed so briefly, is the most critical link in the chain after the patient. Any lack of care in the maintenance or attachment of the electrodes will render any data recorded at best suspect and at worst misleading and is by far the most common cause of obtaining poor results.

Although the complex electrochemistry involved in the electrode-patient interface is beyond the scope of this article, whichever of the numerous types of electrodes used for visual electrophysiology are selected for a specific application, the importance of rigorous standards of care in the application and maintenance of electrodes cannot be overstressed. The importance of good electrode application technique cannot be overstressed. If this stage of preparation is not carried out to the highest possible technical standards, then the best equipment available will not give good reliable results. The same can be said of the care and maintenance of electrodes. (See chapter 17.)

AMPLIFIERS   An amplifier is simply a device for increasing the level of a signal (figure 16.2). To cover the range of visual evoked potentials that are normally investigated, a gain ranging from 1000 to 100,000 times is required. Electrophysiology amplifiers have a high input impedance and low output impedance. Although the input impedance is high, it is not infinite, and therefore, it will draw current from the signal source. The amplifiers used in visual electrophysiological applications are differential or balanced input devices. These differ from the more common type of amplifier in that they have two signal inputs rather than one. The first is the active input, while the second is the reference, and the voltage difference between these two is amplified.

In the single-ended amplifier, the signal between ground and the input is amplified; this is adequate in an environment in which the noise signal is of such a low level that it may be neglected. In a biological setting, the noise signal, that is, any signal other than that which one wishes to record, is one or more orders of magnitude greater than the signal to be recorded, so the single-ended amplifier is of little practical use.

The differential amplifier amplifies the difference in signals between its two inputs. Any common mode signal, that is, a signal occurring equally at both inputs, is rejected. This common mode signal will, for example, by virtue of the relative distance of its source from the recording site, appear with identical amplitudes at both inputs to the amplifier and therefore will not be amplified, as would the true signal. The ability of an amplifier to reject common mode signals is known as the common mode rejection ratio (CMRR). Modern amplifiers will have a CMRR of >100 dB. However, this is for idealized inputs, in which the electrode impedances are equal and near zero. In real conditions, CMRR can drop significantly.

It is generally the case that a small (d.c.) offset voltage will exist between a pair of electrodes, whatever the materials used, and small offset voltages will be present within the input stages of an amplifier. These signals, once amplified, represent a significant proportion of the amplifier's dynamic range. (The dynamic range of an amplifier is the maximum input voltage that can be applied to the inputs at a given gain setting without overdriving the amplifier. If the amplifier is overdriven, the signal will be distorted or clipped.) A millivolt of d.c. offset becomes 20 volts after amplification of 20,000. Few electrophysiological amplifiers can produce an output as large as this, so no signal can be transmitted. To overcome this problem, most amplifiers are designed with capacitatively coupled stages to block the d.c. component of the signal. This is a.c. coupling. But suppose that the signal varies only very slowly with time; then it too will be blocked.

Single ended   Differential

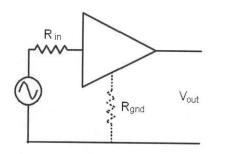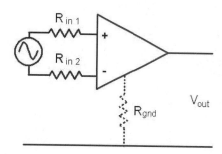

FIGURE 16.2   Single-ended and diferential amplifiers.

Thus, a.c.-coupled amplifiers filter out the lower frequencies in a signal. A good example of this is the elimination of the c-wave of the ERG in most clinical recording situations. The inclusion of multiple a.c. coupling stages in an amplifier can lead to further quite specific problems.

If the input signal multiplied by the amplifier gain exceeds the dynamic range of any stage of the amplifier, then the output of that stage will be driven to the maximum voltage that can be delivered from the power supply. This will lock up the amplifier for a time that is determined by the time constant of that stage. The recovery will not begin until the source of the overdriving is removed. If a subsequent stage of the amplifier recovers more rapidly, then the output of the amplifier will return to the normal mean level, but no signal will be able to pass. Thus, each time an artifact (such as that produced by a blink during an ERG recording) occurs, it is possible, with poor amplifier design, to add a number of blank or zero records to the stored record, thus reducing the recorded signal amplitude. Pattern electroretinogram (PERG) recordings are particularly prone to this problem because of the small signal amplitude and large amplitude that eye movement artifacts present.

FILTERS   To reduce the amount of data that must be collected and processed and the difficulties of recording, the incoming signal is usually filtered to limit the frequency range to that of specific interest. For example, to record a PERG the band-pass of the amplifiers is set to 1.0–100 Hz. The exact effect of these filters on the signal will be affected by a number of parameters associated with the filters that are used. The normally stated value of a filter is the cutoff point or shoulder frequency of the filter. It should be remembered that the filter frequency value that is normally quoted is the frequency at which the signal is reduced by 3 dB, that

is, reduced to 70% of its normal unfiltered amplitude. Therefore, a low-pass filter should be chosen that has a cutoff point sufficiently removed from the frequencies of interest. (A high-pass filter will remove frequencies below those of interest.) Another factor is the rate of attenuation with increase in frequency, or roll-off, of the filter. For an ideal filter, all frequencies above a given frequency would not be amplified, but most filters cannot achieve such a performance. For a simple resistor/capacitor (RC) network such as the decoupling capacitor used to block d.c. signals, there is an attenuation of 6 dB per octave (roll-off). Cascading multiple stages can increase this comparatively shallow roll-off, although the complexity of the required circuitry increases dramatically with increase in the number of filter stages because buffers need to be inserted between stages. However, there is an added difficulty. At or near the frequency at which the filter begins to operate, the phase of the signal alters, sometimes dramatically, depending on the filter used. To produce a filter with an improved "roll off" characteristic without the complexity of cascaded RC stages and buffers, a tuned amplifier circuit or active filter is used. There are three major categories of active filter: Bessel, Butterworth, and Chebyshev. Of these, the Chebyshev has the better amplitude versus frequency characteristic, that is, a steep roll-off and sharp shoulder (see the graph in figure 16.3). The Bessel has the better time domain characteristics, that is, minimal phase change with frequency, although this is achieved at the cost of frequency domain performance. The Butterworth is a compromise between the two; it is generally used in audio equipment. For the purposes of electrophysiology, the time domain characteristics are important because the transient responses contain numerous frequency components, which will be affected to varying degrees by these phase changes. For example, the PERG P50 peak time

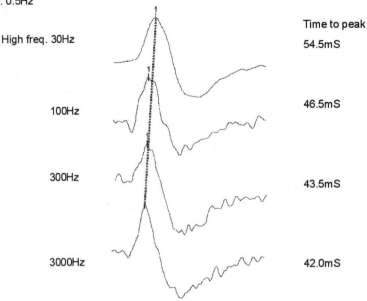

PERG

Low freq. 0.5Hz

High freq. 30Hz

100Hz

300Hz

3000Hz

Time to peak

54.5mS

46.5mS

43.5mS

42.0mS

FIGURE 16.3   The effect of low-pass filter settings on the PERG.

is of clinical significance, and this can be changed by the injudicious choice of filter (see figure 16.3). The sacrifice of frequency domain performance becomes obviously worthwhile. Thus, the filter of choice is the Bessel filter.

Another filter that is often found on modern equipment is the notch or line frequency filter. This is the inverse of a band-pass filter; that is, it attenuates only a very narrow band of frequencies, centered on-line or power supply frequency. Such a filter has a very high Q value, that is, a very steep roll-off. One problem with the use of this type of filter is that the line or mains frequency is relatively close to the frequencies that are to be recorded. This means that the phase changes that are introduced around the shoulders of this filter may well extend into the frequency band of the signal under investigation. Another problem that is encountered with notch filters but is often overlooked is the loss of an early warning of imminent electrode failure; that is, one does not pick up mains interference from an electrode in which the resistance is increasing. A preferable solution is simply to apply the electrodes correctly and set up the system properly, in which case a notch filter to remove mains frequency signals is not needed.

Real-time digital filters are becoming available, implemented using high-speed digital signal processors, a technology that was until recently very costly. While these filters are often used to mimic conventional filter designs, almost any filter configuration can be programmed. However, conventional analog filtering is still needed on the input stages.

Filters, correctly used, improve the signal-to-noise ratio. Another form of filtering, which behaves quite differently from these "real" filters, is conditioning of responses by software after they have been recorded. Various techniques are available, from three-point smoothing to Fourier decomposition of the signal, removal of power in selected frequencies, and signal reconstitution. The effect on phase information of this type of smoothing is not insignificant. It is not a substitute for predigitization filtering or good recording technique.

ANALOG-TO-DIGITAL CONVERTER (ADC)   Once amplified to manageable levels and filtered of unwanted frequency components, the signal is converted from the analog into the digital domain for processing by the computer. The two main characteristics of the analog-to-digital converter (ADC) are the voltage resolution, defined in terms of the number of discrete levels (bits) available, and the frequency at which this subsystem can make these conversions.

The minimum acceptable resolution on modern equipment is 12 bits, giving 4096 levels. It should always be remembered that this is the maximum resolution of the converter. While this degree of resolution might appear excessive, it should be considered how much of this range is actually used for the response. Thus, suppose the effective amplifier input to give full range input to the ADC is set at $\pm 0.5\,mV$ and a 2-μV PERG is to be recorded. This signal voltage is only twice the voltage separating each level of a

10-bit ADC; therefore, only 2 bits of resolution are available for the waveform to be recorded.

The temporal resolution or conversion rate of an ADC subsystem is quoted in terms of its maximum throughput. With a good-quality converter, this will represent the true speed of operation, but this is not necessarily achievable under program control. The maximum signal frequency that the unit can convert is sometimes quoted as the data throughput rate divided by 2. This is the case only for a signal that is both digital in nature and synchronous with the conversion clock. Analog signals require more than the maximum and minimum points to resolve the waveform in a satisfactory fashion.

A common source of error with converters is aliasing. This occurs when the sampling frequency is inappropriate for the signal under examination. This can result in a signal appearing to be of a totally different frequency, that is, aliasing (figure 16.4).

Because most systems use a single ADC, another device is required in multiple-channel systems; this is the sample and hold amplifier (figure 16.5). The purpose of this component is to freeze in time the input to the ADC across all channels so that, as the converter scans across the inputs, the channels are in effect, all sampled at the same time. Without the sample and hold, the output would be slewed by the channel number multiplied by the channel read time.

SIGNAL EXTRACTION   At this point, the digital signal may still be concealed within a considerable amount of noise. To extract the signal from the noise, some form of signal extraction technique is required. A number of such techniques are available. Phase-sensitive (lock-in) amplifiers extract the level of the fundamental frequency from the incoming waveform. If a stimulus is repetitive and of a frequency such that the visual system can respond to each stimulus, the incoming voltage has repetitive changes. Fourier theory states that this signal can be decomposed into a number of different sine waves (see chapter 31). In a lock-in amplifier, the input is multiplied by a sine wave of exactly the input frequency. In most equipment, there are two such amplifiers, and the internally generated sine wave in one is 90 degrees out of phase with the other. The outputs of the two amplifiers are squared and added, and this output is a measure of the amplitude of the input signal (because of the identity $\cos^2\theta + \sin^2\theta = 1$), either of its fundamental or of the second harmonic (for parts of the visual system that give ON-OFF responses). This is a powerful method and can give a rapid result, because all information about the actual waveform of the response is lost. It is an example of the general technique of cross-correlation. Full-scale Fourier analysis can now be used to similar effect by recording continuously into memory and analyzing off-line after the period of stimulation ends. The computer returns the result almost instantaneously. The power and phase that are contained at a particular frequency can be analyzed. (The fundamental here is the total duration of the record.) Such techniques have pitfalls for the inexpert user. For example, the slightest change in stimulus or internally generated sine wave frequency can have disastrous

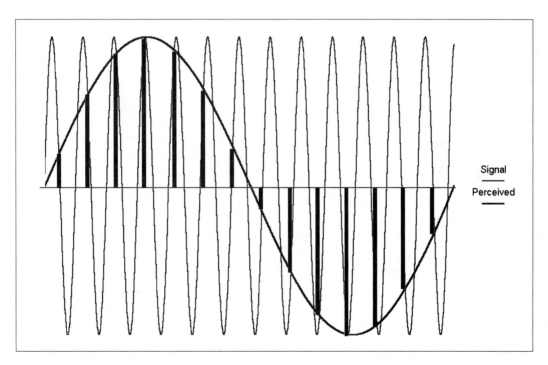

FIGURE 16.4   Aliasing. The light line represents the actual signal, a high-frequency sine wave; the vertical bars represent the sampling points; and the heavy line is the perceived signal.

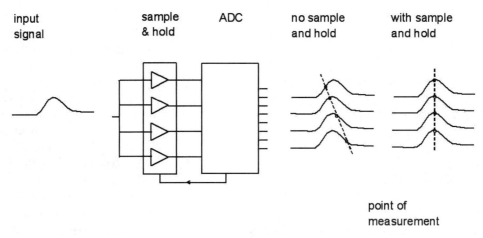

input
signal

sample
& hold

ADC

no sample
and hold

with sample
and hold

point of
measurement

FIGURE 16.5   The sample and hold amplifier.

results, and when stimuli are generated by the computer, glitches occur owing to the vagaries of operating systems. Again, if the stimulus is produced on a slow raster display and the response comes from the fovea, eye movements can alter the real frequency of the stimulus. For further analyses, see chapters 18 and 34.

The most commonly used technique is that of signal averaging. This relies on the fact that the response to be recorded is synchronous with the stimulus that is used to evoke it, whereas the background noise is random with respect to the stimulus. The technique is to record for a fixed time interval following and triggered by the stimulus, for example, a pattern reversal. When the next reversal occurs, another time interval is recorded and added to the first, and the result is divided by the number of time intervals (sweeps). The noise being a random with respect to time, the stimulus should, as the process is repeated, cancel out, leaving only the signal evoked by the stimulus. The extent to which averaging enhances the signal-to-noise ratio is given as $1/\sqrt{N}$, where N is the number of sweeps or repetitions. From this formula, it can be seen that the law of diminishing returns applies.

ARTIFACT REJECTION   One problem that can occur with signal averaging is the contamination of the "good" recording with artifacts caused, for example, by a blink or other movement. The solution to this problem is to utilize an artifact rejection system, whereby before data are passed into the signal averager, they are examined to ensure compliance with preset conditions, typically, given that the signal amplitude does not exceed preset limits at any point. If the conditions are met, then the data are passed to the averager; if not, then the entire sweep is rejected. A wide range of rejection criteria have been tried; the most successful in general

use and found on most equipment is the simplest, and is given above. The upper and lower preset limits should be variable by software. Other limits sometimes encountered include a maximum rate of change of voltage.

CONTROL SOFTWARE   Two main approaches to this vital component of the recording system exist, to allow either full control of every parameter for both stimulation and data acquisition or a series of preprogrammed tests with minimal opportunity for the operator to vary the parameters. Which option is preferred will depend on the application. An ideal solution is to have both options available so as to encompass the requirements of routine clinical examination and research.

The recording from the patient should be stored either on the local machine's fixed disk or on a network device in larger installations. Data is normally held in database form, which enables a record of all settings used during the recording to be stored attached to the traces, along with any annotation that is made during the recording. All this information should be available on printed records produced by the system, along with detailed cursor displays and measurements of timing and amplitude. An advantage of storing data in database format rather than discrete patient files is the ability to search a large number of records on specific criteria. Raw data files that can be exported for complex manipulation with third party software is a distinct advantage, although some manufacturers work with impenetrable proprietary data formats that prevent this. Adequate data backup provision on removable media is essential.

COMMERCIALLY AVAILABLE ELECTROPHYSIOLOGY SYSTEMS
Table 16.1 lists many of the currently known commercial manufacturers of visual electrophysiology systems. A

TABLE 16.1
Commercial manufacturers of visual electrophysiology systems

Commercial Visual Electrodiagnostic Systems

Caldwell Laboratories
909 N. Kellogg Street
Kennewick, WA 99336
www.caldwell.com

Diagnosys LLC
410 Great Road, Suite 6
Littleton, MA 01460-0670
www.diagnosysllc.com

Electro-diagnostic Imaging
1206 W. Hillsdale Boulevard, Suite D
San Mateo, CA 94403-3127
www.electro-diagnostic.com

Global Eye Program
Finspangsvagen 5
SE-610 14 Rejmyre, Sweden
www.globaleyeprogram.com

Jaeger-Toennies
Leibnizstrasse 7
D-97204 Hoechberg
info@jaeger-toennies.com

LKC Technologies
2 Professional Drive
Gaithersburg, MD 20879
www.lkc.com

Nicolet Biomedical, Inc.
5225-4 Verona Road
Madison, WI 53711
www.niti.com

Oxford Instruments
Manor Way
Old Woking, Surrey, GU22 9JU
United Kingdom
www.oxinst.com

Roland-Consult
J. Finger
Friedrich-Franz-Str. 19
14770 Brandenburg—Germany
www.roland-consult.de

Tomey Corporation Japan
2-11-33 Noritakeshinmachi
Nishi-ku, Nagoya 451-0051, Japan
www.tomey.de

Data Acquisition Boards and Drivers

Adept Scientific, Inc.
7909 Charleston Court

Bethesda, MD 20817
www.adeptscience.co.uk

Analog Devices
Contact: Local sales office
www.analog.com

Azectech, Inc.
123 High Street
Ashland, OR 97520
www.azeotech.com

Cambridge Research Systems Ltd.
www.crsltd.com

Data Translation, Inc.
100 Locke Drive
Marlboro, MA 01752
www.datx.com

IOTech, Inc.
25971 Cannon Road
Cleveland, OH 44146
www.iotech.com

iWorx
One Washington Street, Suite 404
Dover, NH 03820
www.iworx.com

Measurement Computing (formerly ComputerBoards)
16 Commerce Blvd
Middleton, MA 02346
www.computerboards.com

National Instruments
11500 N Mopac Expressway
Austin, TX 78759-3504
www.ni.com

NeuroScan
7850 Paseo Del Norte, Suite 101
El Paso, TX 79912
www.neuro.com

Nicolet Biomedical, Inc.
5225-4 Verona Road
Madison, WI 53711
www.niti.com

Tucker-Davis Technologies
11930 Research Circle
Alachua, FL 32615

Data Acquisition Software Packages

iWorx
One Washington Street, Suite 404
Dover, NH 03820
www.iworx.com

Neurobehavioural Systems
www.neurobehavioralsystems.com

MatLab
The MathWorks, Inc.
3 Apple Hill Drive
Natick, MA 01760-2098
www.mathworks.com

National Instruments
11500 N Mopac Expressway
Austin, TX 78759-3504
www.ni.com

Tucker-Davis Technologies
11930 Research Circle
Alachua, FL 32615

Visual Stimulators

Cambridge Research Systems Ltd.
www.crsltd.com

Grass Telefactor
Astro-Med Industrial Park
600 East Greenwich Avenue
West Warwick, RI 02893
www.grass-telefactor.com

Nicolet Instrument Technologies, Inc.
5225-4 Verona Road
Madison, WI 53711
www.niti.com

Physiological Amplifiers

A-M Systems, Inc.
PO Box 850
Carlsborg, WA 98324
www.a-msystems.com

Grass Telefactor
Astro-Med Industrial Park
600 East Greenwich Avenue
West Warwick, RI 02893
www.grass-telefactor.com

Michigan Scientific Corporation
08500 Ance Road
Charelvoix, MI 49720
www.michsci.com

Unfinished Acrylic Domes

Spherical Concepts
12 Davis Ave.
Frazer, PA
www.sphericalconcepts.com

Warner Instruments, Inc.
1141 Dixwell Avenue
Hamden, CT 06514
www.warneronline.com

number of commercial systems were originally designed for electromyographic (EMG) use and have had evoked potential capabilities added and then visual evoked potential capabilities added. A small number are designed specifically for visual electrophysiology. This situation is brought about by the very high cost of designing, manufacturing, and then marketing systems that comply with regulatory demands and the relatively small number of units carrying out visual electrophysiological examinations worldwide.

In selecting equipment, many factors need to be taken into account. High on the list of selection criteria should be the availability of technical support from the manufacturer to deal with basic system questions, setup, resolution of software bugs, and assistance with developing new protocols that are specific to the needs of the laboratory. The frequency and availability of software and equipment upgrades are important in light of the continuous evolution of testing protocols for specific disease entities. Should a system that is being considered not immediately fulfill your laboratories current and foreseeable requirements, it is advisable to treat any promise of future development with a degree of skepticism.

Systems must be user-friendly, reliable, and cost-effective, although cost is surprisingly less of a concern if it is eclipsed by the power of the system. Adherence to International Society for Clinical Electrophysiology of Vision (ISCEV) standards for all packaged testing protocols is obviously a requirement for any clinical laboratory, although the ability to exceed these standards by a significant margin is advisable.

Appropriate calibration of stimuli so that they conform to laboratory and international standards is a major concern, and some manufacturers offer calibration services and equipment for this purpose. While manufacturers are encouraged to incorporate calibration devices that automatically execute on system startup and alert users to potential calibration failures, few do, and additional independent calibration equipment is preferable and should be included in budget proposals.

Finally, data should be stored in a form that is easily exportable to other software packages. Some systems are designed with proprietary data formats, which make the raw data almost impossible to extract for further analysis.

As with any major purchase, the opinions of one's more experienced colleagues will be helpful and generally freely available.

BUILDING YOUR OWN   It is a relatively easy task to assemble a data acquisition system from individual components, provided that one possesses a moderate level of electronics and computer programming skills. The major advantage of such home-built systems is that they are relatively cheap to assemble and they can be designed to meet the specific needs of a laboratory or clinical facility. However, a major disadvantage is that the writing and debugging of the software code that makes the systems function is extremely time-consuming and laborious, frequently evolving over many years. Some device manufacturers will provide sophisticated software function calls and/or prepackaged nonspecific software code that can make the job of programming much easier. In addition, any home-built system that will be used in a clinical setting must meet all safety and locally mandated regulatory regimes.

A listing of some of the major manufacturers of specific hardware and software components needed for a typical electrodiagnostic system was given earlier in the chapter in table 16.1.

REFERENCE

1. International Society for Clinical Electrophysiology of Vision: Guidelines for calibration of stimulus and recording parameters used in clinical electrophysiology of vision. *Doc Ophthalmol* 2003; 107:185–193.

17 Electrodes for Visual Testing

STUART G. COUPLAND

Electroretinographic electrodes: general introduction

Today, many designs of electroretinographic (ERG) electrodes are available, including contact lens, gold foil, gold wire, corneal wick, wire loop, microfiber, and skin electrodes. The clinical ERG is obtained with an electrode placed at some distance from the neural elements that are producing the signals of interest. The electrical current induces an electric field within and around the eyeball and orbit, with both spatial and temporal variations.[34] The ERG signals are conducted from their retinal generator sites through various tissues to the surface electrode. Each electrode type has its own characteristic impedance, recording characteristics, and inherent artifacts. Clinical electroretinographers should be aware of electrode characteristics and should carefully choose the electrode type that is most practical for their recording situation. Typically, an ionic bridge is used to establish an electrically conductive medium between the metallic electrode and the surface of the eye or skin.

Artifacts during ERG recording can almost always be traced to the electrode system.[25,71] Characteristically, these electrode-related recording artifacts fall into one of three categories: those related to electrode polarization, those related to electrode slippage or movement, and the photovoltaic artifact. Care must be taken so that the active ERG electrode and its reference electrode are of the same metallic type. When two electrodes are made from the same metal, the potential difference between them is usually around zero, but slight impurities in the metal and possible surface contamination can cause differences in electrical potential. Potential differences between metals can be very large in comparison with the magnitude of the ERG activity measured at the cornea or surface of the skin.

Fortunately, when a.c.-coupled amplifiers are used, these steady potentials are blocked by the coupling capacitors in the input circuit, thus reducing the effect of electrode potentials. However, motion artifacts are more troublesome. But when d.c.-coupled amplification is used, the electrode potential artifacts are very important; they may cause amplifier blocking and can give rise to baseline drift that may be reduced only by using more stable electrodes. Electrode potentials can be minimized by careful preparation, by ensuring that all electrodes are of the same metal and by avoiding contamination of the electrode surfaces. Eye movement and electrode movement are two sources of potential artifact that can greatly affect the quality of ERG recordings. Electrode movement or uneven fitting of contact lens electrodes on the cornea can produce artifacts in the ERG recording. Unfortunately, ERGs recorded from any electrode can be contaminated by eye movement artifact. Techniques for the digital subtraction of eye movement artifact from flash ERGs[19] as well as pattern ERGs[20] have been described and found useful for obtaining pure ERG tracings. An additional source of artifact occurs when photic stimulation strikes the electrode surface and generates a photovoltaic signal that appears as a spike early in the ERG recordings. Fortunately, photovoltaic artifacts can be dealt with quite easily by shielding the electrode surface from the light source.

CONTACT LENS ELECTRODES   The use of contact lens electrodes for clinical ERG recording was first described by Lorrin Riggs, who developed a clear, nonirritating lens that could be fitted to the subject's eye for prolonged ERG recording sessions.[59] Several variants of contact lens electrodes have been developed over the years.[13,37,38,63,65,66] Because of their ability to give reliable and reproducible recordings,[49] contact lens electrodes are the recommended standard for clinical ERG recordings to flash stimulation. However, they are not recommended for pattern ERG recording, as they can degrade image quality on the retina.[7]

The most frequently used contact lens electrodes are the Burian-Allen (Hansen Ophthalmic Laboratories, Iowa City) and Henkes Lovac (Medical Workshop, Groningen, Holland) assemblies as illustrated in figures 17.1A and 17.1B.[13,29] Recently, the Goldlens (Diagnosys LLC, Littleton, MA) has enjoyed popularity as a well-designed low-noise contact lens electrode (see figure 17.1C). The Burian-Allen assembly makes use of a large speculum that holds the eyelids apart and contacts the scleral surface. A smaller clear corneal contact lens is held against the cornea with a spring assembly. The force exerted on the cornea by the spring mechanism of the Burian-Allen speculum contact lens has been measured at 10 g.[69]

A circular silver wire around the circumference of the contact lens makes the actual contact with the cornea and provides an active electrode. A reference electrode is formed by a coating composed of silver granules in polymerized

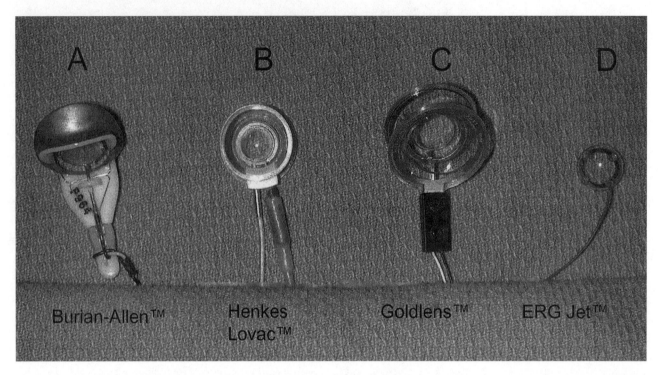

FIGURE 17.1 Contact lens electrode assemblies for clinical electroretinography. Electrodes illustrated are the Burian-Allen (A), Henkes Lovac (B), Goldlens (C), and ERG Jet (D).

plastic within the surface of the scleral speculum for bipolar ERG recordings. For monopolar ERG recordings, a forehead or indifferent ear electrode reference is used.

Although uncomfortable, the Burian-Allen electrode assembly can be used for a period of several hours, though a session of no more than 30 minutes is recommended. Disadvantages of this lens include the possibilities of corneal abrasion, conjunctival abrasion, and irritation produced by movement of the lens assembly. Although frank abrasions are uncommon, they do occur, and minor trauma can be seen in some cases if the patient's cornea is stained by fluorescein. In cooperative patients, corneal staining is often directly proportional to the skill of the examiner in inserting and removing the lenses. A 1% methylcellulose solution drop on the contact lens prior to insertion helps to protect the cornea. Naturally, contact lens electrodes are poorly tolerated by young children, who often require sedation for ERG recording.

Glass contact lens electrodes employing a dome or cup containing isotonic saline and methylcellulose have been reported.[29,33,64–66] In 1951, Henkes described an electrode that enjoys popularity today among clinical electroretinographers.[29] This corneal contact lens electrode maintains electrical contact with the surface of the cornea through a dome containing isotonic saline and methylcellulose. A low vacuum is maintained by suction, and this ensures a good electrical contact with the surface of the eye.

While the Burian-Allen and Henkes corneal contact lens electrodes have similar impedance and recording characteristics, a significant difference in the degree of susceptibility to corneal injury has been demonstrated in diabetic patients. Vey et al. investigated a series of 57 diabetic patients who underwent standard ERG recordings with subsequent slit-lamp examination utilizing fluorescein strips and cobalt blue light.[69] Twenty-eight patients were examined with the Burian-Allen speculum-type corneal electrode, and 29 patients had ERG recordings performed by using the Henkes bipolar low-vacuum corneal electrode. Subsequent biomicroscopy with fluorescein demonstrated that over 30% of the patients who were examined by using the Burian-Allen electrode demonstrated disruption of corneal epithelium, whereas corneal changes were observed in only 7% of the patients who were tested with the Henkes electrode assembly. The authors concluded that owing to the abnormal susceptibility to corneal injury displayed by diabetics, the Henkes low-vacuum electrode was their recommendation for standard ERG testing in these patients. However, it should be noted that many investigators have not found significant corneal changes from the use of Burian-Allen lenses when they are placed carefully and not left in for excessive amounts of time. Recently, there has been a reported study of the use of contact lens electrodes for recording the ERG in extremely small immature preterm infants within the nursery setting.[47] By using infant monkey size 4 bipolar contact lens electrodes (Hansen Ophthalmic Laboratories), flash ERGs were recorded in seven infants with corresponding conceptional ages of 32–34 weeks. The authors concluded that ERG recording using contact lens electrodes in preterm infants is a safe and practicable procedure.

The use of a soft contact lens under a hard lens to cushion and disperse the direct pressure on the cornea has been advocated, and comparable recording characteristics have been demonstrated.[10,23] Schoessler and Jones have described a soft hydrophilic contact lens electrode with excellent recording characteristics.[62] This electrode was formed by a fine gold or platinum wire sandwiched between two soft contact lenses. These investigators claimed that their recording electrode was more comfortable and stable than hard contact lens electrodes and provided minimum obstruction to vision. A comparison of the recording characteristics of the standard Burian-Allen speculum-type electrode assembly and a soft contact lens electrode revealed that while the amplitude of the b-wave recorded with the soft contact lens assembly was comparable, the signals were less stable over recording sessions lasting several hours.[17] This lack of recording stability was evidenced by increased high-frequency noise superimposed over the ERG waveform. Rehydration of the soft contact lens system with 0.9% saline only temporarily reduced the high-frequency noise artifact. While the soft lenses were more comfortable to wear, they required frequent rehydration, since the outer soft lens was not in contact with the moistened conjunctiva and would rapidly dehydrate. As the outer lens desiccated, it began to deform and allow air to enter the interlenticular space, thereby producing an increasingly noisy ERG recording.[17] The soft lens electrode assembly was less stable and did not remain centered on the cornea. In addition, the hydrogel lens sandwich was too delicate to be useful in clinical ERG recording situations. Other attempts at hydrogel lens construction have been more successful.[9] The ERG-Jet (Universo S.A. La Chaux-De-Fonds, Switzerland) gold foil corneal contact lens electrodes have been advocated, as they are light and relatively inexpensive and are disposable following testing. The ERG-Jet electrode is illustrated in figure 17.1D. The recording characteristics compare favorably with the Burian-Allen system.[26] However, a photoelectric artifact with longer-duration light flashes has been described.[25] As with all corneal lenses, topical anesthesia was required. While all corneal electrodes generally give excellent-quality ERG waveforms in cooperative adults, with a few exceptions,[48] they may be poorly tolerated by younger children, who may require restraint or sedation. A simple modification of the standard ERG-Jet contact lens recording electrode for use in infants and small children was developed by Brodie and Breton.[12] A small Plexiglas cylinder was fixed to the front surface of the electrode, thereby preventing lid closure and facilitating insertion and removal. The authors reported the use of this modified ERG-Jet electrode in over 400 patients and claimed that with its use, there was seldom need to use anesthesia or oral sedation in their pediatric population.

LID-HOOK ELECTRODES In addition to corneal contact lens electrodes for recording ERGs, there are circumstances in which it is preferable to use other ERG recording electrodes. An electrode that employed a polyethylene film (Mylar) strip coated on one side with aluminum and bent into a J shape was first reported to produce high-quality ERG recordings without the use of topical anesthetic.[15] Unfortunately, the aluminum coating was less than ideal because it tended to unbond from the Mylar surface at low levels of alternating current.[4,11] A gold-coated Mylar electrode was first described in which the gold surface did not unplate and with which excellent ERGs were obtained.[11] The curved tail of the J shape rode on the cornea and produced some changes in the corneal epithelium of 35% of the patients who were tested.

A low-mass, inexpensive gold foil electrode (C. H. Electrodes, Bromley, Kent) described by Arden and associates[4] was constructed from gold foil applied to Mylar (see figure 17.2A) and provided ERGs that were very similar to those obtained by more conventional contact lens electrodes. The gold foil electrode (GFE) was very flexible and, when inserted into the lower fornix and bent to lie on the cheek, barely touched the corneal margin. A junction wire was connected to the gold foil electrode and led to an insulated standard electrode wire that was also taped against the cheek. The uninsulated junction wire was not allowed to touch the skin. Although initial corneal anesthetic was recommended in the past, current practice is to use no anesthetic. In any case, once the anesthetic wears off, no additional topical anesthetic is usually required. Arden reported that the GFE produced slightly smaller responses than the Karpe lens did and had some higher-frequency components superimposed on the ERG waveform.[4] One problem with gold foil electrodes is their flexibility, in that they may shift or fall out during testing, especially in elderly patients with lid laxity, and if they are uncomfortable to the patient, tearing may effectively short the electrode and give no signal. The GFE is better tolerated by patients than standard contact lens electrode assemblies are, and this makes it possible to more easily record ERGs using the GFE on young children with congenitally malformed or narrow palpebral fissures as well as patients immediately following cataract or corneal surgery. While gold foil electrodes would appear to be less injurious to the cornea than contact lens electrodes, a small proportion of patients still suffer transient symptoms, including blurred vision, ocular discomfort, and tearing, which occasionally persists. Aylward et al. described the corneal changes in a consecutive series of 50 normal subjects undergoing electroretinography with gold foil electrodes.[6] Transient corneal changes were observed in 31 subjects (62%),

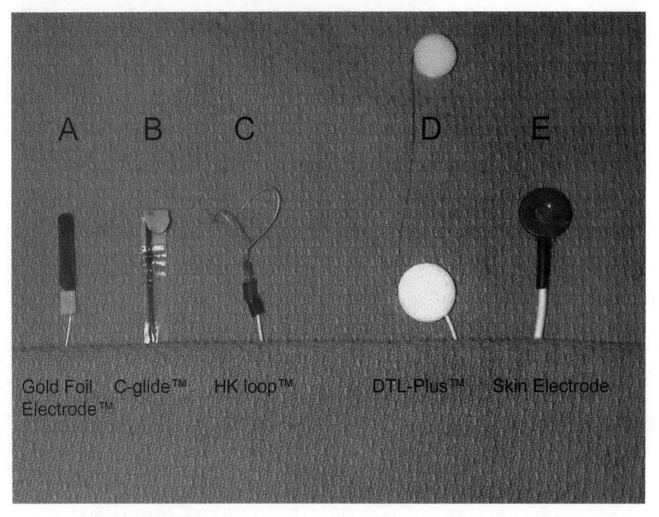

Figure 17.2   Lid-hook, microconductive fiber, and skin electrodes used in clinical electroretinography.

which included punctuate epithelial keratitis, corneal erosions, and stromal thinning. There was a significant association between the severity of corneal changes and the subject's age and the use of topical anesthetic. Because topical anesthetics typically reduce the frequency of blinking and reduce the amount of lacrimation, these may be significant factors in relation to the corneal changes.

The fact that the GFE does not interfere with the optics of the eye makes it ideal for pattern ERG recording.[7] There have been numerous reported studies in which gold foil electrodes have been compared to contact lens systems.[24,26,50,53] Gjotterberg compared several contact lens electrodes with the gold foil lid-hook assembly in 11 healthy eyes recorded on two occasions.[26] It was reported that 9 of the 11 patients preferred the GFE to the Burian-Allen or low-vacuum contact lens electrodes, although these latter electrodes produced larger-amplitude responses to scotopic flash with smaller intertest amplitude variability and therefore were deemed better for research protocols. Other disadvantages

of the GFE included the fact that it was easily blinked out, and the junction was fragile, so after several usages, the electrode became noisy. If it was placed more than 15 mm from the medial fornix, the voltage recorded declined.

Since the pattern ERG is a small evoked response, the question of an electrode's intrasessional variability and its test-retest reliability is important. Odom et al. reported a two-center study of the intrasessional variability of the pattern ERG using gold foil recording electrodes.[56] The coefficient of variation and the coefficient of repeatability were used as measures of intrasession variability or precision. They observed that for pattern ERGs recorded using gold foil electrodes, the intrasession pattern ERG reliability was 0.95 or higher, and intrasession coefficients of variability could be 0.05 or less.

Several investigators have looked at the test-retest reliability of the GFE in recording the pattern ERG.[5,57,58] Prager in two studies reported that while gold foil electrodes produced larger pattern ERG amplitudes than microconductive threads, their test-retest reliability was low.[57,58] These initial results,[57] which were repeated in a three-center study, showed that the reduction in pattern ERG amplitude and an increase in variability occurred when recordings were made with used GFEs.[58] For new gold foil electrodes, pattern ERGs were recorded with higher amplitudes than electrodes used three times in 90% of the trials. Electrodes that were used three times demonstrated an average change in the coefficient of variation of 14%. At two of these study sites, test-retest pattern ERGs on a total of 18 patients demonstrated a test-retest coefficient of variation of 30% and 47% for new and used electrodes, respectively. It was deemed that these sources of variation could have resulted from the presence of small cracks, the number and configurations varying in each electrode. Light microscopy demonstrated these small cracks, and it was proposed that constant flexion and variation would result in significantly different impedances over time. Thus, the more an electrode is used, the lower is the pattern ERG amplitude, and the resulting poorer test-retest reliability would occur. The authors recommended that gold foil electrodes be used only a single time.[58] These findings were in stark contrast to those reported in a two-center study of GFE test-retest reliability.[5] When similar gold foil electrodes were inserted in the same fashion but without using topical anesthesia, pattern ERGs were recorded after either the first or the third or fourth use in four normal subjects. The test-retest interval on the normal subjects was five to six working days, and the same electrodes were used on routine clinical patients in the interim. In these trials, the GFEs were extensively examined before and after the tenth use. The authors reported that in the results from three separate experiments, the P50 and N95 components of the transient pattern ERG do not alter significantly with electrode use. Interestingly, in some cases, the pattern ERG amplitude increased, although not significantly, with electrode use. The investigators were unable to replicate the results described by Prager et al.[57,58] In addition, they were unable to observe any cracks in the gold surface of the electrode similar to those reported by Prager et al.[57,58] Arden et al. suggested that the main source of variation was likely to be either subject related or the technical expertise of the tester rather than GFE aging.[5] Wong and Graham examined qualitative defects in gold foil electrodes and resistances in 94 used gold foil electrodes.[71] They divided the electrodes into four groups of varying resistances and gold coating defects. In addition, they measured photopic flash ERGs in a single subject with GFEs randomly selected from each group. They reported no significant difference among electrode groups for ERG peak implicit times or amplitudes, although a slightly greater amplitude variability was observed for electrode groups with more defects. Their data suggested that whether or not to use a GFE depends not on the degree of visible defects on the electrode, but rather on the overall resistance of the electrode.

Gold foil electrodes are also suitable for multifocal electroretinography. Mohidin et al. recorded multifocal electroretinograms (mERGs) from 12 subjects on three separate days to investigate the repeatability and variability of the mERG using four different electrodes.[53] They reported a coefficient of variation of 0.19 for the GFE, which was similar to the coefficient of variation of 0.21 reported by Prager et al. for the pattern ERG.[57] Prager's findings were in contrast to a two-center study reported by Odom et al.,[56] who reported a coefficient of variation as low as 0.05 for the gold foil electrode. They claimed that their low coefficient of variation was attributable to stringent technical control and use by experienced experimenters.

Other materials have been used to develop lid-hook electrodes, including carbon fiber and polyvinyl (PV) gel. Honda et al. developed a disposable electrode for ERG recording that was made from anomalous polyvinyl alcohol (PVA) gel.[32] This new PVA hydrogel electrode was made of low-cost material that could be discarded after use. The electrode was cut in the shape of a lid hook and could be inserted in the lower fornix like the gold foil lid-hook electrode. The PVA electrode was considered to be very stable without electrical polarization because it contains no metal. It was claimed that patients felt no discomfort during recordings and that the electrodes produced no corneal injury.[18,32]

The C-glide (Unimed Electrode Supplies, Farnham, Surrey, UK) is a carbon fiber lid-hook electrode that has been popular among some for ERG recording for some time (see figure 17.2B).[8] Unlike the extremely flexible gold foil lid-hook electrodes, the C-glide electrode is more rigid in construction, and it has been reported to require longer insertion time.[50] This greater rigidity may be an advantage in that the C-glide electrode may be more difficult to blink out of the eye than the highly flexible gold foil lid-hook electrode. Esakowitz et al. compared the C-glide carbon fiber electrode with other standard contact lenses, GFE, DTL, and skin electrodes for recording scotopic and photopic electroretinograms.[24] They reported that the coarse recording tip of the C-glide electrode and its preshaped plastic hook inevitably touched the eyelashes and made it the most unpopular of the eye contact electrodes tested, whereas the GFE was well tolerated and relatively simple to insert. When compared to the Burian-Allen electrode, the b-wave amplitudes produced by the C-glide were approximately 77%. The gold foil electrode produced b-wave amplitudes that were only 56% as great as those produced by the Burian-Allen contact lens electrode.[24] McCulloch et al. compared a number of electrodes including the Burian-Allen contact lens, the C-glide, and GFE in recording pattern ERGs.[50] They reported that the Burian-Allen recorded the largest amplitude pattern ERGs, whereas the C-glide and GFE gave significantly better within-session quality of recordings. From their studies, they found no compelling reason to recommend a particular type of foil or fiber electrode for pattern ERG recording, as each electrode type had advantages and disadvantages.[50] The C-glide electrode gave the largest amplitude but had the longest time for insertion and a significantly lower comfort rating than the GFE. Mohidin et al. examined the repeatability and variability of the C-glide electrode compared to several other electrode types and found that the C-glide electrode produced a significantly larger coefficient of variation of 0.31 compared to the contact lens (0.15) and GFE (0.19) when recording multifocal ERGs.[53]

A novel disposable ERG electrode was developed by Hiroi et al.[31] consisting of a thin gold filament 0.12 mm in diameter. The gold wire could be bent and placed in the lower fornix or touching the cornea. They reported electrode performance equal to that of the ERG-jet for flash and pattern ERG recording.[31] Another novel and popular noncorneal electrode for clinical ERG was developed that consists of a thin wire forming a loop modeled to fit in the lower conjunctival sac (see figure 17.2C).[27] The HK-loop electrode (HK Med, Ljubljana, Slovenia) is formed from a loop of thin stranded or monofilament silver, gold, or platinum wire that is Teflon coated over its entire length except for three small windows, which allow exposed portions of the metal. The loop is bent so that it appears U-shaped in side view, similar to a lid-hook electrode, and this portion is placed in the lower conjunctival sac, making electrical contact with the sclera, while the Teflon insulation provided shielding from unwanted extraneous potentials. The HK-loop is adaptable to unusual anatomic configurations of the patient's eye or eyelids. The ERGs that are obtained with the HK-loop electrode are similar in amplitude to those recorded with gold foil electrodes.[27,50]

DTL FIBER ELECTRODES Dawson, Trick, and Litzkow (DTL) described a very low-mass, silver-impregnated microfiber corneal electrode for clinical electroretinography.[21] This DTL electrode was based on an extremely low-mass conductive thread that makes contact with the tear film of the eye and is electrically coupled to an insulated wire. The individual fibers of the nylon thread are approximately 50 μm in diameter and are impregnated with metallic silver. The thread is usually draped in the lower fornix, although alternative methods using a holder to position the electrode across the eye have been described.[52,68] Simultaneous flash ERGs recorded from DTL fiber and Burian-Allen electrodes have been compared, and the DTL b-wave amplitudes are generally lower than the corresponding responses recorded with the Burian-Allen corneal contact lenses.[22,23,25,51]

The advantages of the DTL electrode lie in the area of subject comfort, optical quality, and reduced electrode impedance.[23] The DTL system is well tolerated by children and by adults with keratitis. Like the gold foil lid-hook elec-

trode, the DTL does not obscure the optics of the eye and therefore is superior for recording the pattern ERG. It is not blinked out of the eye like the gold foil electrode, but this may not be an advantage, for if the fiber is displaced toward the lower fornix, the signal size is reduced.[52] Hebert et al.[28] examined the reproducibility of flash ERGs recorded with DTL electrodes. Subjects were tested on two occasions separated by an interval of 7–14 days, and Naka-Rushton parameters were derived from DTL-recorded ERG responses. The Naka-Rushton parameters V_{max}, the maximum b-wave amplitude observed at the saturation point of the luminance curve, and $\log K$, the intensity necessary to produce the semisaturation of V_{max} amplitude, were examined. It was found that there was a high test-retest intraclass coefficient of $r = 0.97$ for V_{max} and $r = 0.91$ for $\log K$ in their subjects. The authors concluded that the DTL electrode yields stable and reproducible ERG recordings, provided that care is taken to ascertain proper electrode positioning.

While DTL electrodes have been found to yield highly reproducible signals for flash and pattern ERG, they were thought to represent an interesting challenge to record reproducible oscillatory potential signals.[46] Suprathreshold photopic oscillatory potentials were recorded with either a DTL electrode or a Henkes corneal contact lens electrode. While the summed oscillatory potential amplitude index recorded with the DTL electrode was one half of that obtained with the Henkes electrode, the timing and amplitude ratios were consistent for all the oscillatory potential peaks.[46] Other investigators have also found that DTL electrodes provide robust and reproducible ERG recordings compared to corneal contact lenses and gold foil electrodes for flash ERG recording,[8,24,30,45] pattern electroretinograms,[50,57,58] oscillatory potentials,[46] and multifocal electroretinograms.[51,53]

Recently, the DTL electrode has been modified, and it is now commercially available (DTL-Plus, Diagnosys LLC, Littleton, Massachusetts) and is illustrated in figure 17.2D. The DTL-Plus electrode is composed of 7-cm-long, low-mass spun nylon fibers impregnated with metallic silver. Small sponge pads at each end with adhesive backing are secured to the nasal and temporal canthi, securing the electrode and positioning the microconductive thread at the limbus.

SKIN ELECTRODES The possibility of recording ERGs in response to flash and pattern stimulation without placing electrodes in the eye has specific advantages, especially in the testing of children and infants. Although skin electrodes are in general not recommended as active recording electrodes, there are situations in which there is no other method of obtaining a reliable ERG from a patient. ERGs recorded through the periorbital skin surface have been described.[1,18,35,36,61,63,67] Tepas and Armington used skin electrodes placed on the nasal and temporal canthi and reported that averaged ERGs could be reliably recorded in a wide range of stimulus conditions.[67] Larger-amplitude ERGs have been reported with subsequent head rotation to displace the cornea toward the active electrode. The ERG signals that were produced were smaller in amplitude, noisier, less reliable, and more variable than corneal ERG recording. Signal averaging can significantly improve the signal-to-noise ratio of ERGs recorded with skin electrodes. Standardized placement of the skin electrodes is important to an individual laboratory's ability to give reliable interpretation when using this technique. The dermal electrodes (see figure 17.2E) are better tolerated, and the recording quality may be acceptable for many clinical recording situations in infants and young children, particularly if the patient will not allow testing with a corneal contact lens.[51]

While skin electrodes have been used for ERG recording for some time, there are few reports that directly compare their performance against standard contact lens assemblies.[24,44,50] The advocates of the use of skin electrodes for ERG recording have primarily been those experienced who are in pediatric electroretinography. While most, though not all, adults will accept insertion and prolonged wearing of contact lens electrodes, the majority of infants, toddlers, and young preschool children are by no means impassive and will not willingly allow insertion and wearing of contact lenses. Typically, restraint with forcible electrode placement is necessary, or electrode placement is performed while the child is sedated or anesthetized. It is in the infant population with apparently poor vision that clinical electroretinography probably plays its most crucial diagnostic role, and many pediatric electrophysiologists have turned to the skin electrode, which has allowed them to record reliable ERG recordings.[44] Kriss reported the great Ormond Street experience of over 4000 recordings using skin ERGs in a wide variety of ophthalmological and neuro-ophthalmological conditions.[44] In this study, four healthy young adults had ERG recordings from one eye using six electrode types, including skin electrodes. The researchers reported that for flash ERGs, the b-wave amplitude of skin ERGs was about 14% that recorded to a Burian-Allen electrode.[24,44] As has been previously described, several ocular and technical factors can affect skin ERGs, but the authors concluded that, provided that one recognizes these confounding factors and deals with them accordingly, skin ERGs can provide reliable and diagnostically useful information in young children.[44]

Coupland and Janaky had previously compared the performance of dermal electrodes against the popular DTL fiber and the PVA hydrogel electrode in 32 eyes,[18] where ERGs were simultaneously recorded with skin electrodes along with either DTL or PVA gel electrodes under four standardized flash conditions. The use of simultaneous skin ERG recordings ensured that any differences observed were not due to adaptation, endogenous, or environmental factors. Under all four stimulus conditions, the skin ERGs had consistently shorter a- and b-wave implicit times. This was attributed to the positioning of the skin electrode on the infraorbital ridge, the active electrode being closer to the posterior pole of the eye. Generally, the skin ERGs were about half as large in amplitude as the averaged DTL or PVA ERG recordings.

Because of the advantages of signal-averaging techniques in increasing the signal-to-noise ratio, skin electrodes have been used in detecting retinal oscillatory potentials[61] as well as in recording the pattern ERG.[1,35,36] Wali and Leguire compared skin and ERG-Jet electrodes over a wider range of luminances and compared the b-wave amplitudes for each electrode fitted by the Naka-Rushton equation.[70] As expected, V_{max} for the skin electrode was smaller than that for the corneal electrode. The value of $\log K$ differed by 0.3, with the skin electrode giving a lower value of $\log K$. There was no significant difference between the values of n for the two electrodes. A comparison of electrodes in terms of general variability as measured by the coefficients of variation showed that while the skin electrode yielded less b-wave implicit time variability, the corneal contact lens yielded less b-wave amplitude variability.[70] While skin electrodes have worked well in experienced hands, the problem of increased variability and a lower signal-to-noise ratio in ERG recording has led the ERG standardization committee of ISCEV to recommend that they should be used only in exceptional circumstances.

ERG electrode use in the world

In recent times, we have all been affected by the Internet. Instrument manufacturer Web sites for marketing and servicing have recently been implemented. A newsgroup for clinical electrophysiology of vision called CEVNet has been established by Scott Brodie. This has allowed ISCEV members to converse about challenging clinical cases, seek information about equipment and clinical practices, and communicate information of interest to the worldwide community of clinical electrophysiologists in vision. On January 6, 2003, the first international survey on ERG electrode was presented to CEVNet members, garnering over 50 individual responses from members all over the world.

Members were queried as to which electrode system they used most often and which was their second choice. Over 80% of respondents used two or more different ERG electrodes in their clinical practice. Clearly, 52% of respondents used the contact lens electrode as their first choice in clinical electroretinography. The Burian-Allen electrode was most often reported, followed by the ERG-Jet and Henkes Lovac lenses. Of interest is the fact that 36% of respondents use DTL fiber electrodes and 12% use lid-hook electrodes as their electrode of first choice. Of those using lid-hook electrodes, the majority were using gold foil electrodes, followed by C-glide carbon fiber and HK-loop configurations. There were no respondents who used skin electrodes as their electrode of first choice in all their patients. Two respondents indicated using them only in children under 5 years of age.

Of the 80% of respondents who use a second ERG electrode, lid-hook electrodes were chosen by 44%, whereas 21% of these respondents used DTL fibers or contact lens electrodes as their second choice. Interestingly, 12% of these respondents used a skin electrode as their second choice; all of these respondents were involved in testing pediatric patients.

When asked whether clinicians were using the best ERG electrode recording system, 72% of respondents expressed agreement, whereas 20% of respondents weren't sure and 8% of respondents thought that they were not using the best electrode available. The chief impediments to changing to a better ERG electrode recording system were listed as the cost and time needed to collect new normative data, the time for training staff to use the new electrode effectively, and the inability to find consistent supplies of disposable electrodes.

Respondents were also asked why they preferred the ERG electrode they were using. Those who were using contact electrodes preferred the better signal-to-noise ratio, quality, and consistency of recorded ERGs; the durability and convenience of the lid speculum were also considered important. The respondents who chose the lid-hook electrode preferred better patient acceptance, good ERG recording results, the unaltered optical quality provided by lid-hook electrodes, and their ease of use. The respondents who expressed a preference for DTL fiber electrodes were impressed with patient acceptance, the electrode's ease of use, the unaltered optical quality provided, the fact that it cannot be blinked out, the fact that the electrode is disposable, and the fact that no sterilization is needed. Skin electrodes were preferred because of ease of use, patient comfort, and the fact that no sterilization was needed.

Electrodes for d.c. electroretinography

To faithfully record the slow ocular potentials such as the c-wave and the h-wave (the "off c-wave") of the ERG, a d.c. recording system must be used. Unlike the recording of the flash and pattern ERG, for which commercial equipment is available, most laboratories that are recording the slow ocular potentials have designed apparatus specifically for this purpose. Nilsson and Andersson have described a method for d.c. recordings of slow ocular potentials.[54] Their equipment can also be used for recording the light peak and dark trough of the electro-oculogram. These investigators describe the use of a polymethylmethacrylate (PMMA)

contact lens electrode filled with a combination of methylcellulose and saline. A similar PMMA-saline-filled chamber is attached to the forehead, and the lenses are connected by means of a saline-agar bridge to matched calomel half-cells. Electrode movement was reduced by applying suction on the contact lens. This method has been used previously for studying the c-wave in both humans[41,55] and animals.[42,43] With increasing concern about HIV and hepatitis C infections, the need for disposable electrodes for d.c. recording should be considered. Carlson et al.[14] have described a d.c. ERG method that enables the recording of a-, b-, and c-waves with a disposable corneal wick electrode. Because the corneal wick electrode is disposable, easily made, and inexpensive, it was thought to be more suitable for clinical work than contact lens electrodes. While there are advantages to using the d.c. electroretinography, there are numerous technical problems related to both the electrodes and the stability of the recording system in humans limiting the value of routine clinical recording of d.c. potentials.[41,55,60]

Electro-oculogram electrodes

The electro-oculogram (EOG) was first introduced in its clinical form by Arden and colleagues to indirectly measure the standing potential of the eye.[2,3,39,40] This group pioneered the use of EOG to document retinal pigment epithelium function in normal and clinical populations. The electrodes that were used were nonpolarizable silver chloride balls sunk in plastic flanges pressed against the skin and held in place with adhesive tape. The authors claimed that bared silver wire secured by collodion gauze was equally effective but that normal electroencephalographic electrodes were not recommended; because of their large size, they could not be placed close to the canthi.[3] Since that time, subminiature Ag-AgCl skin electrodes have been developed and are most commonly used in EOG. The Arden method of using skin electrodes and a.c. recordings has become the conventional technique for recording the EOG. The standing potential of the human eye can be studied by means of d.c. recordings using a combination of suction contact lens, calomel electrodes, and d.c. amplification.[54] This procedure was described in more detail in the previous section on d.c. recording techniques.

Visual evoked potential electrodes

The visual evoked potential (VEP) is usually recorded with scalp electrodes composed of gold or silver. The best recording electrode is chlorided silver, and the worst is stainless steel.[16] Although reversible Ag-AgCl electrodes are probably better than nonreversible electrodes for a.c. recording, they are not essential unless the electrode surface area is small. Care must be taken to ensure that all electrodes are made of the same metal because potential differences between different metals can be very large when compared with the magnitude of the electrical activity of the brain.[16] Most laboratories that are recording clinical VEPs use either gold electrodes, silver disk electrodes, or chlorided silver electrodes held against the scalp with collodion-impregnated gauze or paste.[16] Isotonic electrode jelly is used to maintain the bridge between the electrode surface and the scalp. Clinical visual electrophysiologists and technicians must be aware that the electrodes are a vulnerable but vital part of the recording system and should be treated with care.

REFERENCES

1. Adachi-Usami E, Murayama K: Pattern electroretinograms recorded with a skin electrode in pigmentary retinal degeneration. *Doc Ophthalmol* 1985; 61:33–39.
2. Arden GB, Barrada A: Analysis of the electro-oculograms of a series of normal subjects: Role of the lens in the development of the standing potential. *Br J Ophthalmol* 1962; 46:468–482.
3. Arden GB, Barrada A, Kelsey J: New clinical test of retinal function based upon the standing potential. *Br J Ophthalmol* 1962; 46:449–467.
4. Arden GB, Carter RM, Hogg C, Siegel IM, Margolis S: A gold foil electrode: Extending the horizons for clinical electroretinography. *Invest Ophthalmol Vis Sci* 1979; 18:421–426.
5. Arden GB, Hogg CR, Holder GE: Gold foil electrodes: A two-center study of electrode reliability. *Doc Ophthalmol* 1994; 86:275–284.
6. Aylward GW, McClellan KA, Thomas R, Billson FA: Transient corneal changes associated with the use of gold foil electrodes. *Br J Ophthalmol* 1989; 73:980–984.
7. Bach M, Hawlina M, Holder GE, Marmor MF, Meigen T, Vaegan, Miyake Y: Standard for pattern electroretinography. International Society for Clinical Electrophysiology of Vision. *Doc Ophthalmol* 2000; 101:11–18.
8. Barber C: Electrodes and the recording of the human electroretinogram (ERG). *Int J Psychophysiol* 1994; 16:131–136.
9. Barber C, Cotterill DJ, Larke LR: A new contact lens electrode. *Doc Ophthalmol Proc Series* 1977; 13:385–392.
10. Bloom BH, Sokol S: A corneal electrode for patterned stimulus electroretinography. *Am J Ophthalmol* 1977; 83:272–275.
11. Borda RP, Gilliam RM, Coates AC: Gold-coated Mylar (GCM) electrode for electroretinography. *Doc Ophthalmol Proc Series* 1978; 15:339–343.
12. Brodie S, Breton ME: Modified ERG-jet contact lens electrodes for use in infants and toddlers. *Doc Ophthalmol* 1995; 91:141–146.
13. Burian HM, Allen L: A speculum contact lens electrode for electroretinography. *Electroencephalogr Clin Neurophysiol* 1954; 6:509–511.
14. Carlson S, Raitta C, Kommonen B, Voipio J: A DC electroretinography method for the recording of human a-, b- and c-waves. *J Neurosci Methods* 1990; 35:107–113.
15. Chase WW, Fradkin NE, Tsuda S: A new electrode for electroretinography. *Am J Optom Physiol Opt* 1976; 53:668–671.
16. Cooper R, Osselton JW, Shaw JC: *EEG Technology.* London, Butterworths, 1980.
17. Coupland SG: Time domain analysis of steady state electroretinal and visual evoked response to intermittent photic stimulation. Simon Fraser University, Burnaby, British Columbia, 1978.
18. Coupland SG, Janaky M: ERG electrode in pediatric patients: Comparison of DTL fiber, PVA-gel, and non-corneal skin electrodes. *Doc Ophthalmol* 1989; 71:427–433.
19. Coupland SG, Kirkham TH: Electroretinography and nystagmus: Subtraction of eye movement artefact. *Can J Ophthalmol* 1981; 16:192–194.
20. Coupland SG, Kirkham TH: Digital subtraction of eye movement artefact from pattern ERG recordings. *Neuro-Ophthalmology* 1983; 3:281–284.
21. Dawson WW, Trick GL, Litzkow CA: Improved electrode for electroretinography. *Invest Ophthalmol Vis Sci* 1979; 18:988–991.
22. Dawson WW, Tricke GL, Maida TM: Evaluation of the DTL corneal electrode. *Doc Ophthalmol Proc Series* 1982; 31:81–88.
23. Dawson WW, Zimmerman TJ, Houde WL: A method for more comfortable electroretinography. *Arch Ophthalmol* 1974; 91:1–2.
24. Esakowitz L, Kriss A, Shawkat F: A comparison of flash electroretinograms recorded from Burian Allen, JET, C-glide, gold foil, DTL and skin electrodes. *Eye* 1993; 7:169–171.
25. Gehlbach PL, Purple RL: An electrical artifact associated with the ERG-jet gold foil electrode. *Invest Ophthalmol Vis Sci* 1993; 34:2596–2599.
26. Gjotterberg M: Electrodes for electroretinography: A comparison of four different types. *Arch Ophthalmol* 1986; 104:569–570.
27. Hawlina M, Konec B: New noncorneal HK-loop electrode for clinical electroretinography. *Doc Ophthalmol* 1992; 81:253–259.
28. Hebert M, Lachapelle P, Dumont M: Reproducibility of electroretinograms recorded with DTL electrodes. *Doc Ophthalmol* 1995; 91:333–342.
29. Henkes HE: The use of electroretinography in measuring the effect of vasodilation. *Angiology* 1951; 2:125–131.
30. Hennessy MP, Vaegan: Amplitude scaling relationships of Burian-Allen, gold foil and Dawson, Trick and Litzkow electrodes. *Doc Ophthalmol* 1995; 89:235–248.
31. Hiroi K, Miyake M, Hashimoto T, Honda Y: Design of a new disposable ERG electrode. *Ophthalmologica* 1995; 209:299–301.
32. Honda Y, Naoi N, Kim SY, Sakaue E, Nambu M: New disposable ERG electrode made of anomalous polyvinyl alcohol gel. *Doc Ophthalmol* 1986; 63:205–207.
33. Jacobson JH: A new contact lens electrode for clinical electroretinography. *Arch Ophthalmol* 1955; 940–941.
34. Job HM, Keating D, Evans AL, Parks S: Three-dimensional electromagnetic model of the human eye: Advances towards the optimisation of electroretinographic signal detection. *Med Biol Eng Comput* 1999; 37:710–719.
35. Kakisu Y, Adachi-Usami E, Mizota A: Pattern electroretinogram and visual evoked cortical potential in ethambutol optic neuropathy. *Doc Ophthalmol* 1987; 67:327–334.
36. Kakisu Y, Mizota A, Adachi E: Clinical application of the pattern electroretinogram with lid skin electrode. *Doc Ophthalmol* 1986; 63:187–194.
37. Karpe G: The basis of clinical electroretinography. *Acta Ophthalmol Suppl* 1945; 24:1–118.
38. Karpe G: Early diagnosis of siderosis retinae by the use of the electroretinography. *Doc Ophthalmol* 1948; 2:277–299.
39. Kelsey JH: Clinical electro-oculography. *Br J Ophthalmol* 1966; 50:438–439.
40. Kelsey JH: Variations in the normal electro-oculogram. *Br J Ophthalmol* 1967; 51:44–49.
41. Knave B, Nilsson SE, Lunt T: The human electroretinogram: DC recordings at low and conventional stimulus intensities.

Description of a new method for clinical use. *Acta Ophthalmol (Copenh)* 1973; 51:716–726.

42. Knave B, Persson HE, Nilsson SE: A comparative study on the effects of barbiturate and ethyl alcohol on retinal functions with special reference to the C-wave of the electroretinogram and the standing potential of the sheep eye. *Acta Ophthalmol (Copenh)* 1974; 52:254–259.

43. Knave B, Persson HE, Nilsson SE: The effect of barbiturate on retinal functions: II. Effects on the C-wave of the electroretinogram and the standing potential of the sheep eye. *Acta Physiol Scand* 1974; 91:180–186.

44. Kriss A: Skin ERGs: Their effectiveness in paediatric visual assessment, confounding factors, and comparison with ERGs recorded using various types of corneal electrode. *Int J Psychophysiol* 1994; 16:137–146.

45. Kuze M, Uji Y: Comparison between Dawson, Trick, and Litzkow electrode and contact lens electrodes used in clinical electroretinography. *Jpn J Ophthalmol* 2000; 44:374–380.

46. Lachapelle P, Benoit J, Little JM, Lachapelle B: Recording the oscillatory potentials of the electroretinogram with the DTL electrode. *Doc Ophthalmol* 1993; 83:119–130.

47. Mactier H, Hamilton R, Bradnam MS, Turner TL, Dudgeon J: Contact lens electroretinography in preterm infants from 32 weeks after conception: A development in current methodology. *Arch Dis Child Fetal Neonatal Ed* 2000; 82:F233–F236.

48. Marmor ME: Unsedated corneal electroretinograms from children. *Doc Ophthalmol Proc Series* 1977; 13:349–355.

49. Marmor MF, Zrenner E: Standard for clinical electroretinography (1999 update). International Society for Clinical Electrophysiology of Vision. *Doc Ophthalmol* 1998; 97:143–156.

50. McCulloch DL, Van Boemel GB, Borchert MS: Comparisons of contact lens, foil, fiber and skin electrodes for patterns electroretinograms. *Doc Ophthalmol* 1998; 94:327–340.

51. Meigen T, Friedrich A: [The reproducibility of multifocal ERG recordings]. *Ophthalmology* 2002; 99:713–718.

52. Mierdel P: An improved holder for the DTL fiber electrode in electroretinography. *Doc Ophthalmol* 1995; 89:249–250.

53. Mohidin N, Yap MK, Jacobs RJ: The repeatability and variability of the multifocal electroretinogram for four different electrodes. *Ophthalmic Physiol Opt* 1997; 17:530–535.

54. Nilsson SE, Andersson BE: Corneal d.c. recordings of slow ocular potential changes such as the ERG c-wave and the light peak in clinical work: Equipment and examples of results. *Doc Ophthalmol* 1988; 68:313–325.

55. Nilsson S, Skoog K: Variations of the directly recorded standing potential of the human eye in response to changes in illumination and to ethanol. *Doc Ophthalmol Proc Series* 1977; 13:99–110.

56. Odom JV, Holder GE, Feghali JG, Cavender S: Pattern electroretinogram intrasession reliability: A two center comparison. *Clin Vis Sci* 1992; 7:263–281.

57. Prager TC, Saad N, Schweitzer FC, Garcia CA, Arden GB: Electrode comparison in pattern electroretinography. *Invest Ophthalmol Vis Sci* 1992; 33:390–394.

58. Prager TC, et al: The gold foil electrode in pattern electroretinography. *Doc Ophthalmol* 1994; 86:267–274.

59. Riggs LA: Continuous and reproducible records of the electrical activity of the human retina. *Proc Soc Exp Biol N Y* 1941; 48:204–207.

60. Rover J, Huttel M, Schaubele G: The DC-ERG: Technical problems in recording from patients. *Doc Ophthalmol Proc Series* 1982; 31:73–79.

61. Sannita WG, Maggi L, Fioretto M: Retinal oscillatory potentials recorded by dermal electrodes. *Doc Ophthalmol* 1987; 67:371–377.

62. Schoessler JP, Jones R: A new corneal electrode for electroretinography. *Vision Res* 1975; 15:299–301.

63. Stephens GM, Inomata K, Cinotti A, Kiebel G, Manev I: Canthi skin electrode method with corneal displacement. *Vision Res* 1971; 11:1213.

64. Sundmark E: Influence of the contact glass on the electroretinogram. *Doc Ophthalmol Adv Ophthalmol XVIII Concilium Belgica* 1958; 627–631.

65. Sundmark E: Recording of the electroretinogram with contact glass: Influence of the shape of the fluid layer between the glass and eye on the electroretinogram. *Acta Ophthalmol* 1958; 36:917–928.

66. Sundmark E: The electroretinogram in malignant interocular tumors. *Acta Ophthalmol* 1958; 36:57–64.

67. Tepas DI, Armington JC: Electroretinograms from noncorneal electrodes. *Invest Ophthalmol Vis Sci* 1962; 1:784–786.

68. Thompson DA, Drasdo N: An improved method for using the DTL fibre in electroretinography. *Ophthalmic Physiol Opt* 1987; 7:315–319.

69. Vey EK, Kozak WM, Danowski TS: Electroretinographic testing in diabetics: A comparison study of the Burian-Allen and the Henkes corneal electrodes. *Doc Ophthalmol* 1980; 48:337–344.

70. Wali N, Leguire LE: Dark-adapted luminance-response functions with skin and corneal electrodes. *Doc Ophthalmol* 1991; 76:367–375.

71. Wong VA, Graham SL: Effect of repeat use and coating defects of gold foil electrodes on electroretinogram recording. *Vision Res* 1995; 35:2795–2799.

18 Amplifiers and Special-Purpose Data Acquisition Systems

J. VERNON ODOM

NUMEROUS SOURCES offer practical assistance in understanding and choosing amplifiers and special-purpose systems. Some of the most practical are informational pamphlets by manufacturers. Other sources include general texts on electronics,[1] signal processing,[2,3] and electroencephalography (EEG)[3–5] and other guides.[6,7]

Amplifiers

The electrical potentials that are elicited by visual stimulation are too small to drive most recorders or to be accurately detected by the analog-to-digital converters (ADCs) that form the initial stage of most commercial systems for processing physiological signals. Therefore, a system of preamplifiers and amplifiers is required to increase the voltage of the signal. In the following sections, amplifiers and their characteristics will be described.

In discussing amplifiers, it is also necessary to consider the characteristics of the signals they will amplify and the noise that must be minimized or eliminated by them. Ideally, the signals to be amplified would only be those generated by neural activity of interest, and all other electrical features would be filtered out. To amplify the signals of interest and filter out the unwanted signals, it is helpful to consider the visual signals and the major sources of physiological and electrical noise. Table 18.1 gives the major biological signals elicited by visual stimulation, their frequency range, their amplitude range, and the gain or amplification that is required to have an output peak-to-peak voltage of 1 V. Also listed are the characteristics of other biological signals that may be noise relative to visual signals, such as the electroencephalogram and electromyogram. Naturally, these values can be only approximate. Table 18.2 presents common sources of electrical interference, their origins, and methods to minimize them.

PREAMPLIFIERS Generally, the subject's electrodes are connected to a preamplifier. The purpose of the preamplifier is to provide initial amplification (10× to 1000×) as the signal is transmitted along cables to the final amplification stage so that the effects of long cables can be minimized. Frequently, preamplifiers provide minimal filtering.

An essential concern is the patient's safety. While attached to the electrophysiological equipment, the patient is potentially part of a 110- to 220-V circuit. The several pieces of equipment in that circuit may or may not share the same ground. Many large buildings, such as hospitals, have several grounding circuits. In the unlikely event of major electrical failure of the recording equipment, the main's electricity could pass through the patient, and a ground fault could prove fatal. Consequently, the patient should be protected from the improbable event of such a major accident by electrical isolation from the equipment during the entire test.

The most frequent means of protecting the patient is to use an isolation preamplifier. Isolation amplifiers isolate the power supply of the amplifier from the power supply of the input stage or from the power supply of both the input and output stages. One must ensure that the isolation amplifier is able to isolate voltages equal to or greater than the largest voltage that is expected should an electrical accident occur. The technique that is used is to pass the input signal through a voltage-to-frequency converter. This stage uses little current, which can be provided safely. Then, by using optical means or magnetic transformers, which isolate the input from the main electronics, the frequency is transmitted to a demodulating filter, which returns the frequency to its corresponding voltage. To modulate and demodulate the input voltage, an oscillator or chopper is required. An isolation amplifier cannot handle frequencies greater than one quarter to one tenth of the oscillator frequency, depending on the quality of the amplifier. The frequency of mechanical oscillators or choppers is usually limited to the line frequency (60 Hz in the Americas, 50 Hz in Europe and Asia), but electronic choppers operate easily to several hundred kilohertz.

In addition to protecting the patient from grounding faults, isolation amplifiers can improve signal-to-noise ratios by interrupting ground loops and eliminating capacitance problems, but they may also introduce problems. At high amplifications, the carrier frequency may be seen as noise

TABLE 18.1
Visual signals and physiological noise

Signal	Frequency Range (Hz)	Amplitude range (Peak)	Amplification for 1-Volt Output
Electro-oculogram	d.c.–100	10 μV–5 mV	500
Electroretinogram			
a- and b-wave	0.2–200	0.5 μV–1 mV	1000
Oscillatory potentials	90–300	0.1 μV–100 μV	10,000
c-wave	d.c.–2	0.5 μV–1 mV	1000
Pattern ERG	0.1–200	0.1 μV–10 μV	100,000
Visually evoked potentials			
Standard	1–300	0.1 μV–20 μV	50,000
Fast wavelets	90–300	0.1 μV–5 μV	200,000
Electroencephalogram	d.c.–100	2 to 100 μV	10,000
Electromyogram	0.01–500	50 μV–5 mV	500
Electrocardiogram	0.06–1000	<5 mV	500
Galvanic skin response (electrodermal response)	d.c.–5	<1 mV	1000

TABLE 18.2
Electronic noise sources

Noise Type	Sources	Frequency Characteristics	Reduction Methods
Extrinsic noise	Electrostatic	Mains frequency	Serial grounding
	Magnetic	Mains frequency	Eliminate ground loops
	Radio frequency	>1 kHz	Shielding; low, equal electrode resistance
Thermal noise	Sensors and amplifiers	Broadband and random	Differential amplification
1/f Noise	Amplifiers	<100 Hz inversely related to frequency	Differential amplification
Blocking (saturation)	Amplifiers	All frequencies	Reduce gain or noise
Analog-to-digital converters and averaging algorithms	Quantization	<1 kHz	Choice of analog-to-digital converters
	Sampling jitter	Broadband, nonrandom	
	Aliasing		Filter high frequencies
	Round-off errors		
Trigger	Trigger jitter	>10 Hz inversely related to jitter	Stabilize trigger

added to the signal. In poor-quality filters, the higher harmonics or subharmonics of the carrier or chopper frequency may be amplified.

A second means of isolating the patient in the case of a major electrical disaster is to employ low-current, fast-acting fuses in the circuit connecting the patient to the amplifiers. The use of fuses introduces minimal alteration of the frequency or phase information of the signal. However, by increasing the number of connections or junctions through which the unamplified signal passes, the use of fuses may attenuate the signal or introduce noise. Humans can generally sense 1 mAmp at 60 Hz, and 5 mAmp is the maximum "harmless" current. Therefore, the fuses should be 1 mAmp or slightly lower and able to disconnect the circuit in no more than several milliseconds.

DIRECT CURRENT AND ALTERNATING CURRENT AMPLIFIERS
Amplifiers are characterized by a number of parameters, including bias, frequency response, input impedance, output impedance, gain (sensitivity) versus noise, slew rate versus linearity, and roll-off or attenuation versus common mode rejection ratio (CMRR).

Most amplifiers have a resistor and capacitor to separate one stage of the amplifier from the other. One consequence of the resistor-capacitor network is that direct current (d.c.) cannot be transmitted from one stage of the amplifier to the other. Very low frequencies are also attenuated.

If the stages of an amplifier are coupled directly (direct-coupled amplifiers), d.c. and higher frequencies are transmitted from one stage of the amplifier to another. Most amplifier output voltages are not zero, even when the input leads are connected together. This is called an *offset* and occurs at all stages in a d.c. amplifier; any offset voltage that is present in an earlier amplifier stage is amplified along with the signal by subsequent amplifier stages; and with high gains, the amplifier may be useless.

This problem is minimized by using a *differential amplifier*. In a differential amplifier, two inputs are provided to the amplifier, and its output is the algebraic difference of the two input signals. Practically, there is always some difference between the two circuits and their offset voltages; therefore, a bias compensation is usually provided to equalize the two halves of the amplifier.

COMMON MODE REJECTION RATIO   Whether d.c. or alternating current (a.c.), almost all contemporary physiological amplifiers are differential. In most amplifiers, the subtraction of one input from the other occurs at several of the stages of amplification. Any signal that enters both inputs is thereby drastically reduced, such as the mains or line frequency. The CMRR is determined by inputting a signal to one amplifier input and then inputting a common signal of the same amplitude to each of the two inputs. The output amplitude should be minimized when the same signal is applied to both inputs. The ratio of the input from one signal input and two signal inputs is the CMRR. With proper adjustment, a CMRR of 100,000:1 is achievable in many amplifiers. Because mains' interference (50 and 60 Hz) is a common source of artifact that may be eliminated by a high CMRR, it is often determined for these frequencies. CMRR is reduced at higher frequencies. Also, the figure given is for identical inputs. If the inputs are not identical, for example, if a corneal lens has a higher resistance than skin, the CMRR will be reduced. Hence, a major source of mains noise in modern amplifiers are differences in impedance between electrodes or other differences that lead to greater mains interference entering on one lead than another.

BIAS   The bias of an amplifier refers to the voltage output of the amplifier when the input voltage is zero. Amplifier bias should be zero. Frequently, the bias of an amplifier varies with temperature. Therefore, it is wise to measure and if necessary to adjust the bias of an amplifier only after it has been operating for several minutes (or, in extreme cases, one-half hour). A stable amplifier has a minimal variation in bias over time.

LINEARITY, GAIN, AND DYNAMIC RANGE   The output voltage of an amplifier should be a linear function of the input voltage. The slope of that linear function represents the gain of the amplifier. Real amplifiers are linear only over a range of input voltages at any one gain. The range of input voltages over which a linear function is valid is the dynamic range of the amplifier; 80–100 dB is possible.

INPUT AND OUTPUT IMPEDANCE   The input impedance of a physiological amplifier must be at least 100 times greater than that of the electrodes to avoid attenuation of the signal or the introduction of extraneous noise. If the impedance of the electrodes is 10 kΩ, the input impedance of the amplifiers must be 1–5 MΩ. For these same reasons, the output impedance of the amplifier should be low in relation to the input impedance of the averager or oscilloscope that serves as the final stage of signal processing. The characteristics of high-input impedance and low-output impedance are a common feature of all commercially available amplifiers for physiological signals.

FREQUENCY RESPONSE FUNCTION   For a specified gain and input voltage, an amplifier's frequency response function is its output voltage as a function of its input frequency. On the basis of its frequency response function, amplifiers may be classified into one of four categories based on their filter characteristics: low-pass, high-pass, band-pass, and band-reject (or notch) filters. Figure 18.1 illustrates these categories of filters. Low-pass filters pass frequencies below a certain level and reject higher frequencies. High-pass filters reject frequencies below their cutoff and pass higher frequencies. Band-pass filters pass frequencies between a low and a high frequency and reject others. A band-reject filter rejects frequencies between a high and a low cutoff frequency and pass frequencies lower than the low-frequency cutoff and higher than the high-frequency cutoff.

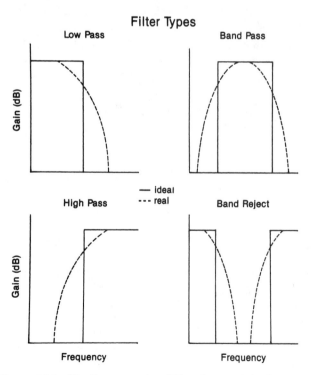

FIGURE 18.1   The four categories of filter characteristics: low pass, high pass, band pass, and band reject.

An ideal filter would have a sharp cutoff. Physically realizable filters have a range of frequencies over which the response is progressively attenuated. The characteristic frequency is where the attenuation is either 1/2 or $1/e$ (e is the base of natural logarithms). The steepness of the change or the roll-off is quantified by the rate of change of attenuation in decibels per octave or decade, outside the characteristic point at which the voltage is reduced by 50% (−6 dB) or by −3 dB (70.8%). (A decibel is 10 times the base 10 logarithm of the ratio of two powers. Alternatively, a decibel is 20 times the base 10 logarithm of the ratio of two energies or voltages. Power is energy squared—hence the difference between decibels of power and energy. An octave is the base 2 logarithm of the ratio of two numbers, that is, a halving or doubling is one octave. A decade is the base 10 logarithm of the ratio of two numbers. A 3-dB attenuation (−3 dB) of output voltage amplitude is equivalent to a voltage amplitude reduction of 29.2%. A 6-dB-per-octave roll-off indicates that the voltage amplitude decreases by 50% as the frequency doubles or halves. A 24-dB-per-octave roll-off indicates that the voltage amplitude decreases by a factor of 15.8 as the frequency increases or decreases by a factor of 2.) The roll-off of a filter consisting of a single capacitor and resistor is 3 dB per octave. To obtain steeper roll-offs, several strategies can be employed. Complex passive networks or active filters that incorporate amplifiers to "shape" the filter characteristic or that use variations on digital techniques may be employed. The penalty that is paid for roll-off includes phase changes near the characteristic frequency(s), noise, and ringing. Bessel-function filters maintain a constant phase change-versus-frequency characteristic at the expense of a shallow shoulder. The number of active stages in a filter is referred to as the number of poles. For example, a quadruple filter has four active stages.

DIGITAL AND ANALOG FILTERS   The first stage of converting the analog signals into digital voltage levels that can be inter- preted by the computer is an analog-to-digital converter (ADC). ADCs are the simplest digital filters. The characteristics of these and more complicated digital filters are important because they have become a progressively more common feature of the clinical electrophysiology laboratory. A summary of the characteristics of analog and digital filters is presented in table 18.3. Digital filters may be implemented by either hardware or software.

Any digital filter samples the incoming signal at some frequency. The accuracy of that sampling (quantization and rounding errors) and the appropriateness of the sampling frequency (aliasing and leakage errors) are important. The highest frequency in the input signal cannot be higher than half of the sampling frequency, or lower frequencies will be introduced into the signal (aliasing). Even if aliasing is avoided by appropriate low-pass filtering before the digital filter and if the sampling frequency is low relative to the frequencies of interest, voltage from some frequencies will leak or spread across several frequencies.

Despite these considerations, a well-designed digital filter has several advantages over an analog filter. Digital filters are generally more flexible. Both gain and frequency roll-offs are limited only by the digital resolution of the filter. Because the signals are digitized, noise introduced by variations in resistance, capacitance, and inductance in the various stages of the amplifier is eliminated. Finally, in most digital filters that are used for physiological applications, phase is undistorted. At high-frequency cutoffs below 60 Hz, analog filtered visual evoked potentials (VEPs) are reduced in amplitude and prolonged in latency (figures 18.2A and 18.2B). Digitally filtered signals are merely reduced in amplitude.[8]

Digital filters may be particularly useful in eliminating noise from averaged signals. For example, responses elicited by pattern reversal contain power mainly at the harmonics of the reversal rate (even harmonics of the reversal frequency). By employing digital filters, it is possible to elimi-

TABLE 18.3
Analog and digital filters

Property	Analog	Digital
Variables	Continuous in time	Discrete time (samples) discrete magnitudes
	Continuous in magnitude	
Mathematical operations	d/dt, dt, Xk +	Delay, Xk, ±
Characteristic equations	Linear differential	"Linear" difference (occasionally logical difference)
Characteristic responses	Damped sinusoids, cosinusoids	Samples of damped sinusoids, cosinusoids
Speed	To optical frequencies	To MHz
Imperfections	Initial tolerances	Coefficient rounding
"Components"	Drift	Absolutely stable
	Nonlinearity and overloading	Quantization and overflow
Noise	Thermal, shot, etc.	Quantizing, aliasing; low-level limit cycles

Effects of High Frequency
Cut-Off

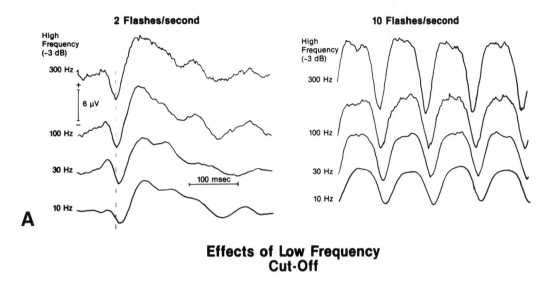

2 Flashes/second

High Frequency (−3 dB)

300 Hz

6 μV

100 Hz

30 Hz

10 Hz

100 msec

A

10 Flashes/second

High Frequency (−3 dB)

300 Hz

100 Hz

30 Hz

10 Hz

Effects of Low Frequency
Cut-Off

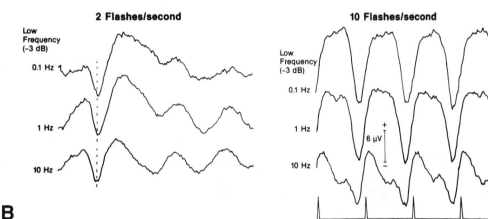

2 Flashes/second

Low Frequency (−3 dB)

0.1 Hz

1 Hz

10 Hz

B

10 Flashes/second

Low Frequency (−3 dB)

0.1 Hz

1 Hz

10 Hz

6 μV

FIGURE 18.2 A, Effects of high-frequency cut-offs on flash VEPs. All records are of 400-msec duration. The lowest trace on the right indicates the time of flashes. The figure illustrates the effects of the high-frequency cut-off on VEPs elicited by two and ten flashes per second (Grass PS-22, I-2). Notice that with increased analog filtering responses are (1) less noisy, (2) smaller in amplitude, and (3) delayed. B, Effects of low-frequency cut-offs on flash VEPs. All records are of 400-msec duration. The lowest trace on the right indicates the time of flashes. The figure illustrates the effects of low-frequency cut-offs on VEPs elicited by two and ten flashes per second. Note that higher low-frequency cut-offs (1) reduce noise, (2) reduce amplitude, (3) decrease peak latencies, and (4) alter waveforms.

nate the noise at other frequencies (Vance Zemon, personal communication, 1988).

One consideration that is frequently ignored is when an experimenter increases amplification by placing two amplifiers in cascade. (If amplifiers are cascaded, the lower-noise amplifier should be the first stage.) The roll-off of the cascaded amplifiers will be steeper, and the −3-dB points will be different from that of each device on its own. If the high-frequency cutoff f_h and the low-frequency cutoff f_l are the same for each cascaded filter, the high-frequency −3-dB point of the system will be $f_h = f'_h \times [(2^{1/n}) - 1]^{-2}$. The system's low frequency −3-dB point will be $f_l = f'_l/[(2^{1/n}) - 1]^{-2}$. The number of stages that are cascaded is represented by n.

Amplifiers that are used in clinical visual electrophysiology should amplify the entire frequency range of interest in a specific response. If recording the d.c. ERG or d.c. electrooculogram (EOG), one should use a band-pass from 0 to at least 100 Hz. For normal a.c. coupling, a band-pass of 0.3–250 Hz is adequate. However, if recording oscillatory potentials, one might choose to record from 90 to 300 Hz.

Therefore, one must alter the amplifier's[1] settings to suit the response to be recorded.

The consequences of choosing inappropriate filter settings can be dramatic alterations in response amplitude and/or waveform. Selective attenuation of the high frequencies in a response eliminates high-frequency noise. However, it may also result in a big change in waveform, latency, and amplitude of the response. A reduction of the higher frequencies will generally reduce the amplitude and prolong the latency of a response. Figure 18.2A presents the effects on averaged VEPs of variations in the high-frequency filter settings. Low-frequency attenuation will eliminate the slowly occurring changes in baseline that may be caused by eye movements or electrodermal responses. Figure 18.2B indicates the changes in VEPs that are introduced by increasing the amplifier's low-frequency filter setting. Increasing low-frequency settings will typically reduce the amplitude and latency.

AMPLIFIERS AND PHASE DISTORTIONS   Amplifiers impose a delay in the input signal. Unfortunately, the delay is not constant as a function of signal frequency. Generally, within the frequency range that is unattenuated, the phase is relatively constant across frequency. As frequencies are attenuated, large phase shifts are usually introduced. The changes in phase relationships can introduce latency changes and changes in waveform and amplitude.[3] The magnitude of phase distortion is increased as roll-off is increased. Extending the high-frequency range increases noise, and extending the low range permits slow large oscillations to be recorded, which are thought to be due to eye movements. Therefore, it is desirable to use low- and high-pass filters that have characteristic frequencies outside the region of interest.

The variations in filter settings by different laboratories and their effects on amplitude, phase, and waveform are among the major reasons explaining variation in the absolute values of amplitudes and latencies of responses obtained in different laboratories. One consequence of efforts to standardize conditions across laboratories has been the development of standards by the International Society for Clinical Electrophysiology of Vision (ISCEV) for the most common electrophysiological responses.

Special-purpose data acquisition systems

The amplifiers are usually connected to a special-purpose data acquisition system for recording a visually elicited response. The final stage may be a storage oscilloscope with camera in the case of ERGs, a chart recorder, a lock-in amplifier, or a signal-processing system such as an averager. Although the amplifiers are at the heart of the system, some means of display and storage of data must be found, and there is an increasing need for systems that analyze the visu-

ally elicited responses. This has led to the increased sophistication of the equipment that is available. In the past, much work was done with simple oscilloscopes, and data were captured on film. Chart recorders were also used, but in general, the frequency response of the pens is too low for sophisticated purposes. Now that digital computers are cheap and available, these are commonly used for display and can be used for analysis. They have generally displaced the dedicated averagers and lock-in amplifiers that were previously used.

An averager consists of a computer memory of many cells, typically 1012, that are filled sequentially at fixed intervals after a trigger; thus, the cells could be filled at 2-ms intervals, and a segment of record of just over 2 s could be obtained. When the trigger is repeated, the contents of each cell are recalled, the new voltage level is added, and the entire value is stored. At the end of N such cycles, the value in each cell is divided by N, so the contents represent the average. If the records contain both signal plus noise and the noise is random with respect to the signal, the signal-to-noise ratio is reduced by the square root of N. The limit of noise reduction is determined by the patient's endurance; for a stimulus that occurs twice a second, 100 repetitions occur in about a minute, and the noise is reduced by a factor of 10; to reduce it 20-fold would require 4 minutes, and to reduce it 100-fold would require over an hour.

However, much of what is normally considered noise may be electrical signals that are synchronized to the main's frequency, which may be phase-locked to the stimulus. Most noise is due to bad technique, and prolonged averaging is no substitute for this.

Lock-in amplifiers are averagers that basically contain two or four cells. They are used on the assumption that the stimulus is repetitive and that the response not merely is repetitive but approximates a sinusoid. If so, then one can imagine that one cell could be arranged to contain the 180 degrees of the signal that was positive and the second to contain the 180 degrees that was negative. The difference between the two would be a measure of the amplitude of the signal. However, in general, the phase relation between stimulus and response is not known. The problem is overcome by using two more cells that are filled cosinusoidally, that is, at 90 degrees of phase angle to the first pair. Now two amplitudes of signal have been determined, and by taking advantage of the relationships $\sin^2 a + \cos^2 a = I$ and $\sin a / \cos a = \tan a$, the amplitude and phase of the signal can be determined. In practical instruments, the incoming voltage from the patient is multiplied by a sine or cosine wave generated in the device, and the continuous output is summed with an integrating amplifier with a variable time constant. The amplifiers have a very high dynamic range, and their careful design ensures the success of the instrument. The assumption is that phase remains stationary; this might not be true of cortical signals, particularly when they are generated on the face of a device like a TV monitor, which is basically intermittent. The lock-in amplifier is potentially faster than an averager in reducing the signal-to-noise ratio because all waveform information is discarded, but in practice, the best results are obtained for high-frequency signals in physical systems, and the results in a slow visual system may be disappointing.

GENERAL CHARACTERISTICS OF SPECIAL-PURPOSE DATA ACQUISITION SYSTEMS   Some of the major components of a visual signal processor are presented in figure 18.3. In considering special-purpose data acquisition systems, one must consider the entire system. Even the best item is useless unless it is compatible with other parts of the system. The major considerations are how the system's components work together and whether the system satisfies the needs of the individual electrophysiological laboratory. As the ISCEV has developed standards for electrophysiology, one consideration is whether the equipment can record responses that are consistent with the standards for the responses that the laboratory will record.

To pass information from an amplifier to a computer, one requires an ADC. With the exception of some lock-in amplifiers, all contemporary data acquisition systems are based on a digital computer. The incoming amplified and filtered analog signal is converted to a digital signal by using an ADC. The digitized input may then be filtered further, be averaged, or be acted on in any fashion for which the system is programmed.

An ADC is characterized by its number of bits of resolution. The term *bit* refers to a binary exponent. For example,

an 8-bit ADC has 2^8, or 256, steps in its voltage range. If the range is programmable, the gain of the ADC may be varied. If the voltage range is ± 1 V, the ADC can resolve 0.0078125 V (1/256). Given an amplification of 10,000, this corresponds to a resolution of $0.78\,\mu$V for a single sweep. For most purposes, an 8-bit resolution for the ADC is adequate, although 10- or 12-bit resolution is desirable (a resolution of 0.2 and $0.05\,\mu$V respectively, assuming a ± 1-V range, a gain of 10,000, and a single sweep). Because the analog signal is quantized, additional noise may be introduced into the signal and may reduce the signal-to-noise ratio. In addition, the full range of the ADC cannot be employed. Thus, the amplifier gain is set so that the trace always remains on the screen. Therefore, the signal of interest will be much smaller and will extend only over, for example, one fourth of the screen, or 64 levels or fewer. This will mean that discontinuities can be seen in the waveform.

Most of the currently available commercial systems provide a software package for signal processing. The signal will be averaged or, in some older systems, summed. Signals greater than the ADC range or some predetermined smaller range may be rejected. On better systems, this artifact rejection can be turned on or off and can be adjusted within the ADC range. One or more cursors will be available, and one can determine the amplitude and latency of individual locations on the waveform. Frequently, one can transform the waveform by using a variety of mathematical functions such as adding or subtracting a constant, integrating, or differentiating the waveform, performing Fourier transforms, performing autocorrelation or cross-correlation functions, and adding or subtracting one waveform from another.

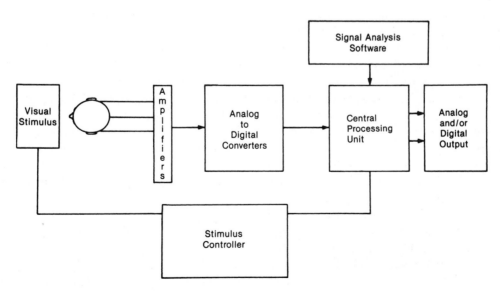

FIGURE 18.3   Major components of a typical clinical electrophysiology data acquisition system.

Artifact rejection may be accomplished in several basic ways, including filtering and subtraction of known artifacts. The most common method of artifact rejection available on commercial systems is amplitude rejection. Acquired sweeps containing voltages larger than some preset value are rejected. If the rejection level is adjustable, consideration of information in table 18.1 may be a useful guide in selecting a rejection level. The basic strategy is to choose a rejection level that rejects no real responses (or some very small percentage) and rejects any large-amplitude artifacts associated with eye movement, blinks, head movement, or muscle tension.

Particular care must be exercised in choosing and using the less common signal-processing options such as Fourier transforms. Data are not always presented in easy-to-use forms, and sometimes information is transformed. For example, the old Nicolet Med-80 failed to provide 360 degrees of phase information, and some older LKC systems report different amplitude values than those in their printouts. A useful feature of some systems is a statistical spreadsheet that allows the data to be manipulated so that one can sum the amplitudes (or powers) of various frequencies, calculate means and standard deviations, and so on.

A certain portion of the computer's memory is allocated for signal processing. The exact algorithm that is used to perform signal processing varies. Depending on the computer's speed and memory size, some unexpected effects can occur. Some computers have different data channels to divide the same region of memory. For example, if 1024 data points are allocated for data memory, one channel will have 1024 data points, two channels will have 512 data points each (1024/2), and four channels will have 256 each. Other systems have a fixed memory size per channel, so one channel occupies 1024 memory addresses, two channels occupy 2048, and so on. If a system has multiple channels, each data channel may be sampled simultaneously, or the channels may be multiplexed. If they are multiplexed, the ADC of each channel is sampled in sequence. Because the order of sampling is fixed, there may be slight but possibly significant phase or time differences between the channels.

Other portions of computer memory will be dedicated to graphics, analysis, and output of the data. Some systems provide cathode-ray tube or video displays of the incoming signal and/or averages in real time as they occur. Other systems must switch between recording data and displaying data. Therefore, one can obtain only periodic updates of the average without greatly increasing the averaging time.

Many manufacturers offer complete ERG or VEP systems. These include amplifiers, recorders, stimulators, and means of calibration and data analysis. They are often expensive and, because of the time required for development, are also often obsolete. A state-of-the art commercial system should have software control of amplifier characteristics; at least 12-bit ADCs with an upper throughput of >30,000 samples per second; 32-bit central processing units (CPUs); super video graphics array (VGA) or better with a graphics coprocessor allowing screen updates at >4/sec; a command file structure that permits the user to generate a sequence of changes in stimulus and recording parameters to be used in routine tests; a data file structure that permits the storage of multiple records from one patient in a single file; methods of analysis that permit automatic cursoring and trace measurement; recall and comparison of several records from one or more files; and deletion, addition, subtraction, and scaling of records from the same or different files. Many commercial systems do not provide these facilities, even though they may boast of features that are less important. Some obsolete systems are, however, so well engineered that they are more reliable and easy to use than their more sophisticated rivals (and they may be less expensive). The prospective purchaser should attempt to get manufacturers to loan the equipment for a real clinical trial before placing a firm order.

An alternative path is to purchase a microcomputer and special-purpose boards and connect them into a system. Several manufacturers not only provide the boards but also provide software so that data will appear in designated areas of computer memory. The code for this software is complex, for the boards must run under interrupt control, which is often very difficult to implement. The ADC boards usually contain clocks and counters and digital and analog outputs for controlling laboratory data. It is advisable to buy special graphics display boards with basic software supplied.

Some of the systems come "boxed," and the software will complete averaging routines. Then all the user has to do is to implement relatively simple routines that need not take place in real time. The advantage of this course is that the system can be combined with databases and arranged according to the user's particular requirements. However, even this software development can be time-consuming and should be attempted only by knowledgeable enthusiasts. Several centers have, however, followed this path and provide their colleagues with the programs.

The time required to perform one operation such as averaging is dependent on the speed of the computer's CPU, the design of the system, and the efficiency of the algorithms used to perform the operation. For example, after a sweep is acquired and manipulated (e.g., divided and added to the previous average), there will be some limited delay between the time the last data point of one sweep is acquired and the time the next data point can be acquired. Across averaging systems, this can vary from microseconds to milliseconds.

SOME QUESTIONS TO ASK   A sample set of questions to ask oneself when examining a system is given below. These questions are appropriate for both commercial special-purpose systems and personal computers. They are based on problems and needs that a number of users have mentioned. One's needs may be classed into several broad areas: (1) financial and physical limits, (2) equipment compatibility, (3) stimulus suitability, (4) recording suitability, and (5) analysis suitability. Each is considered briefly below. The most general and basic question is "Does the system meet your needs?" An excellent strategy is to see a system do everything one wants it to do before one purchases it. Does the system physically fit into one's laboratory? Is the system within one's financial limits?

When one buys a system, even if it seems complete apart from the cupola, one must determine whether the various components of the system are compatible, whether they can be modified, and whether they perform as desired. For example, if a xenon flash photostimulator serves as the major visual stimulus, does the central computer accept the flash trigger, or alternatively, can the computer trigger the photostimulator? Some newer systems accept only transistor-transistor logic (TTL) inputs. If one analyzes single-flash ERGs, can the signal-processing system analyze a single signal? Does the stimulator provide the types of conditions one needs? Frequently, commercial pattern stimulators provide only square-wave pattern reversal of high-contrast checkerboards. Pattern appearance, if provided, is often accompanied by a change in mean luminance. Contrast is often not variable. If one records the ERG with patients in a reclining position, can the cupola be tilted to accommodate this position?

Does the system permit averaging of enough channels to record the responses of interest? Most laboratories seldom use more than two channels, one for each eye or one for the eye and one for the cortical signals. Less frequently, one might wish to record three, four, or more channels. Does the system have a satisfactory automated EOG system? Most commercial systems either do not perform the EOG or do a poor job of EOG analysis.

Does the system provide the analysis routines that you need? Almost every system that averages will provide amplitude and latency information for at least one point. For how many points can it provide this information? Can it set up ratios or means of points or their latencies? Do you need to do spectral analysis or perform cross-correlations to calculate kernels? How does the system output the data? Are they plotted? Is a numerical output available?

Can the numbers be manipulated if needed? For example, can the values of only stimulus harmonics be presented? Last, if the system does not perform as one wishes, how difficult is it to customize the system's operation? Is the operation modifiable? If frequency information is provided, is it in useful units? One may wish to have access to the real and imaginary components in addition to amplitude (or power) and phase information.

REFERENCES

1. Brophy JJ: *Basic Electronics for Scientists*. New York, McGraw-Hill, 1966.
2. Cohen A: *Biomedical Signal Processing*, Vol 1, *Time and Frequency Domains Analysis*, and Vol 2, *Compression and Automatic Recognition*. Boca Raton, Fla, CRC Press, 1986.
3. Dawson WW, Doddington HW: Phase distortion of biological signals: Extraction of signal from noise without phase error. *Electroencephalogr Clin Neurophysiol* 1973; 34:207–211.
4. Gaumond Roger P: Round off errors in signal averaging systems. *IEEE Trans Biomed Eng* 1986; 33:365–366.
5. Glaser EM, Ruchkin DS: *Principles of Neurobiological Signal Analysis*. New York, Academic Press, 1976.
6. Kriss A: Setting up an evoked potential (EP) laboratory. In Halliday AM (ed): *Evoked Potentials in Clinical Testing*. New York, Churchill Livingstone, 1982, pp 1–44.
7. Perry NW, Childers DC: *The Human Visual Evoked Response*. Springfield, Ill, Charles C. Thomas Publishers, 1969.
8. Remond A (ed): *Handbook of Electroencephalography and Clinical Neurophysiology*. Amsterdam, Elsevier Science Publishers, 1973.
9. Walter WG, Parr G: Recording equipment and technique. In Hill D, Parr C (eds): *Electroencephalography*. New York, Mac-Millan, 1963, pp 25–64.

19 Stimulus Devices, Calibration, and Measurement of Light

CHRIS HOGG

Stimulators for visual electrophysiology

Many different light sources can be used for stimulating the visual system (with varying degrees of success). Here, we will concentrate on those in common use in visual electrophysiology at the time of writing.

Regardless of the source of stimulus energy, the peak intensity or brightness, contrast, spectral content or color, duration and enveloped shape, repetition rate, field or image size, and element size will all affect the recorded response to varying degrees and must be appropriately calibrated. The ISCEV produces guidelines for stimulus calibration, and these form a good starting point for the electrophysiologist who wishes to characterize a stimulus.[2]

Stimuli can be subdivided into two broad categories: unstructured or spatially structured. The Ganzfeld stimulator that is routinely used in the majority of laboratories for electroretinography is an example of an unstructured stimulus, to be contrasted with any device that displays a pattern. These two categories can then be further subdivided on the basis of light source or technology employed.

A Ganzfeld stimulator is simply an approximation to an integrating sphere, the object of which is to illuminate the entire retina evenly, a task that cannot be achieved by having the patient view a lamp directly. Other techniques are sometimes employed to provide an approximation to uniform retinal illumination. These include 100-diopter lenses mounted on a corneal contact lens electrode, diffusing screens or contact lenses, and half a table tennis ball held in front of the eye and back-illuminated.[4]

The Ganzfeld stimulators (figure 19.1) generally consist of a bowl of around 500-mm diameter, with ports for the injection of light from whatever source is to be utilized, commonly a xenon flash lamp for the stimulus and an incandescent bulb for background illumination. There is another, larger aperture, the exit port, for the patient's head, which is positioned in such a way that the entire visual field is occupied by the inner surface of the bowl. The bowl surface is coated with a high-reflectance white matte paint. In a true integrating sphere, light enters the bowl through one port and is subject to multiple reflections (>200) before exiting the (small) output port, thus smoothing out any irregularities in the illumination. The clinical Ganzfeld stimulator exit port must accommodate the head of a patient and is therefore as large as 300 by 250 mm for a typical adult. This significantly reduces the efficiency of a 500-mm sphere. If the sphere is made much bigger to improve the efficiency, more light is required to illuminate the interior. The dimensions given are a practical trade-off between cost and performance.

Ganzfelds for clinical use are generally equipped with filters for modifying the color and intensity of the stimuli, fixation targets and a chin rest to maintain patient position, and closed-circuit infrared video cameras to monitor the patient during the test.

The majority of Ganzfeld stimulators are powered by xenon flash lamps, such as the ubiquitous Grass PS22, although in both custom-built and commercial systems, other sources are used—mainly light-emitting diodes (LEDs) or incandescent lamps and shutter systems.

Xenon flash tubes are essentially arc lamps. They consist of a glass tube, which may be either straight, U-shaped, or coiled. An anode and a cathode (the larger electrode) are placed through the ends of the tube, and a trigger electrode is mounted on the outside of the tube between the main electrodes. The tube is filled with xenon gas at a pressure of several atmospheres.

In operation, energy is stored on a capacitor at high d.c. voltage (several hundred volts), connected in parallel with the tube. To initiate the flash, a pulse of typically 10–20 kV is applied to the trigger electrode from a step-up transformer. This causes the xenon gas to ionize and thus become electrically conductive, and the energy stored in the capacitor is rapidly discharged in the form of an arc through the gas, producing a brief, high-intensity flash of light. The wavelength composition of the light depends on the gas and on its pressure. Typically, the light is of a broad spectrum, containing significant quantities of both ultraviolet (UV) and infrared (IR) radiation in addition to the visible spectrum. (While this UV and IR radiation is beyond the human visible

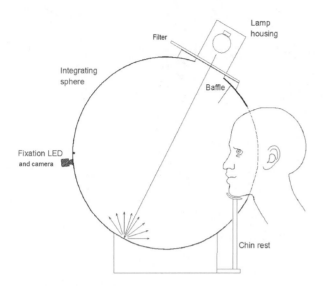

FIGURE 19.1   The Ganzfeld stimulator.

spectrum, it is capable of causing damage to the eye, so the output should be filtered accordingly.) The duration of the flash can vary from microseconds to milliseconds depending on the size of the capacitors and the impedance of the discharge circuit. This impedance consists not only of the tube, but also of the capacitors' internal resistance and that of any connecting cables.

The energy stored in the capacitors is given as

$$E = 0.5CV^2$$

where E is joules, C is capacitance (in farads), and V is voltage.

The efficiency of xenon discharge systems varies considerably, but a typical conversion rate (electrical energy to visible light) of 10–20% can be expected. The error sources associated with xenon tubes are numerous and complex. In the short term, the path of the arc through the bore of the tube may vary, resulting in a variation in the light output between flashes of apparent equal input energy. As the tube ages, the arc will erode metal from the electrodes, which will be deposited on the walls of the tube, where it will act as an optical filter. The seal around the electrode wires is subject to considerable thermal stress, which may result in the loss of gas pressure. Capacitors will age, the value of the capacitance and the internal resistance changing with time. All of these factors will affect light output to varying degrees, and several strategies have been developed to minimize these effects. The most effective methodology is to measure the light output of the tube and use this value to switch the current flowing through the tube off when the appropriate amount of light has been emitted. This may be done either by switching the power from the flash tube through a very low-impendence quench tube, thus removing power from

the light source, or by briefly switching off the power to the tube for enough time to allow the arc to collapse, thus limiting the duration of the flash and therefore its power content. Both these techniques require power in excess of that nominally required by the flash to be available.

The energy output of the flash can be controlled by three means. The method of pulse width modulation may be used, as in the Metz Mecablitz™ range of photographic flash lamps, where longer-duration (<20–1000 μs) flashes are used. The older PS22 range of Grass photic stimulators used switched capacitors to generate a range of output intensities (1.2 log units), while the more recent PS33 models use a variable voltage across fixed value capacitors to the same effect (1.0 log units).

Given periodic calibration, the author's experience is that the feedback control of flash lamps is largely unnecessary for routine ERG use. It is also the case that better alternative sources are available (see below). Assuming a stable light output, there are a number of potential problems with the use of xenon flash systems for visual electrophysiology. The first consideration must be safety; the voltage across the tube is high, typically 300–800 V, and this in itself leads to a potentially serious safety risk, as the tube can be very close to the patient. The trigger voltage is typically 10,000–20,000 V, while the peak current flow through the flash tube can be in excess of 100 amps, so all cables and connectors must be insulated and screened to an appropriate standard. Even with a well-constructed system, the potential for the generation of electrical artifacts is significant. The high-frequency and high-energy pulses in the xenon flash system are capable of radiating large amounts of electromagnetic energy both from the tube itself and transmission cables. The very fast rise and fall times of the current pulse make it difficult to filter out, a problem that is compounded by the fact that the artifact is naturally phase-locked to the trigger signal for the averager.

Because of the short duration of the flash produced by xenon flash lamps, calibration requires a photometer capable of tracking the very fast rise and fall times of the light pulse and producing an output proportional to the total emission of the source. Although a slow device that integrated light output with time could theoretically be used, the characteristics of many devices are not suitable for measurement of short, intense flashes. Lists of recommended devices are published on the ISCEV Web site.[2]

The spectral output of a typical xenon discharge system is illustrated in figure 19.2.

Incandescent lamps and shutter systems have, as was mentioned previously, been used by a number of authors[12] to illuminate Ganzfeld stimulators. Incandescent bulbs, while not having the very high output of xenon flash tubes or arc lamps, can provide a relatively high-energy output from low-voltage power supplies. Unlike the xenon flash systems, an

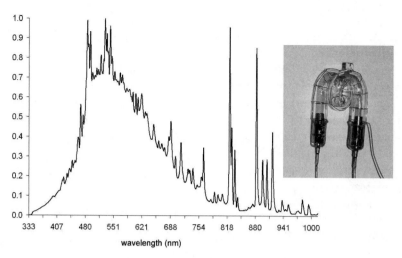

FIGURE 19.2 The spectral distribution of the light emitted by a typical xenon flash tube. The insert shows its physical appearance.

electro-optical feedback system to stabilize the light output is easily implemented, and the power supplies themselves are readily available commercially.

The drawback for routine clinical use is, however, the shutter mechanism. While large-area ferroelectric liquid crystal shutters are available, they present a number of difficulties for use in switching large amounts of light necessary for Ganzfeld illumination, such as transmission efficiency and poor contrast ratios. It should be noted that LCD switching systems are used to great effect in projection systems and may be available in suitable form in the near future. Currently, however, an electromechanical shutter is generally used to gate the light path. The disadvantages that affect electromechanical shutters are simple. Because the shutter blade has mass, it requires energy to accelerate and decelerate. With a good drive amplifier, the acceleration can be fast, but a linear shutter will still give a definite rise and fall time to the light pulse. Very fast mechanisms are available that will, with suitable maintenance, provide an effectively rectangular pulse of light from a continuous source. One major advantage of such systems is the ability to prolong the light pulse, the benefits of which are mentioned elsewhere in this book. While lamp and shutter devices have been used to good effect in several ERG research applications, they have limited application in the clinical laboratory.

Light-emiting diodes (LEDs) are also used to illuminate Ganzfeld and other stimulators. These devices are described in detail elsewhere in this chapter.

CATHODE-RAY TUBES   Cathode-ray tubes (CRTs) consist of an evacuated conical flask shaped glass vessel, the wide front surface of which is coated internally with a phosphor that is excited by an electron beam emitted from a heated cathode in the neck of the flask and accelerated toward an anode by

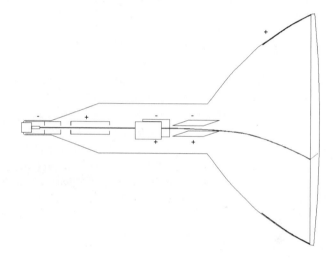

FIGURE 19.3 Schematic and cathode-ray tube showing the electron beam, lens, and deflector plates.

a high voltage (figure 19.3). When the phosphor coating is excited by this stream of electrons, light is emitted.

CRTs are driven in one of three ways. In its simplest mode, an unfocused beam of electrons excites the entire phosphor-coated area of the screen, causing this surface to be illuminated. These glow tubes can be electronically modulated relatively simply, the rise and fall times being governed by a combination of the switching speed of the electron gun and its drive circuitry and the characteristics of the phosphor used.

When used as a vector display, the electron beam is focused to a small spot, and the beam deflected in both the horizontal and vertical axis by an electrical field. In oscilloscopes, the electrodes that focus and deflect the electron beam are internal, and the field is electrostatic. Electrostatic displays are no longer in general use. In the common TV tube, the electrodes are external coils, and a magnetic field is generated by modulating the current flowing in these coils that deflects the beam. By modulating the current in the coils, the beam can be moved about the phosphor surface. All TVs and monitors develop a *raster*. The horizontal deflection is relatively fast, and repetitive while a much more slowly increasing current in the vertical coils deflects the beam downward, so a series of illuminated lines is drawn on the viewing surface from left to right across the screen. The beam is switched off while the scan returns from right to left. After each line scan the beam moves a step down the screen, progressively writing the entire visible area of the display (figure 19.4). Light emission from any point on the screen is proportional to the beam strength and lasts only for the duration of the excitation (plus the decay time of emission of the phosphor). Various phosphors are used, depending on the characteristics required from the tube. For tubes with slow refresh rates, a phosphor with a long persistence will give a high luminance output, but this would not be appropriate for high raster rate tubes, in which the long decay time would obscure subsequent scans by residual emission during the following frame.

The phosphor also determines the color of the emitted light. By utilizing three separate electron guns and three separate phosphors (red, green, and blue), a color display can be achieved. The phosphors can be placed on the surface of the tube in the form of either dots or vertical stripes arranged in triads (figure 19.5). In either case, the points on the screen (pixels) are addressed sequentially through a perforated mesh in the case of the dot phosphor or shadow mask tube, or a vertical array of fine wires in the aperture grill tube first popularized by the Trinitron tube from Sony. The shadow mask tube is generally being replaced by the aperture grill system. In the former arrangement, a significant area is inevitably covered by the masking grid arrangement; while this produces more precisely defined pixels, it

inevitably reduces the effective emitting area of the display and, with this, the luminance that is available. The striped array in the aperture grill allows for a far greater area of phosphor and thus higher luminance, while advances in control electronics largely mitigate the greater tendency to blur the pixels. A minor problem, in most applications, with the aperture grill tubes is the visibility of the grill support wires running horizontally across the display surface.

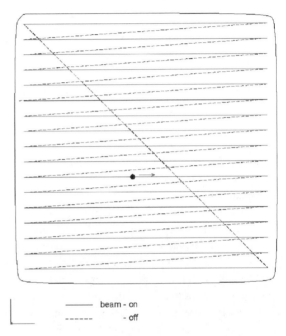

FIGURE 19.4 The raster pattern employed in all TV tubes. The external field coils move the electron beam horizontally from left to right. During the flyback (dotted lines), the electron beam is suppressed and the position deflected downwards. The number of lines in a television raster is greater than indicated. In standard 625-line TV transmission, the frames are interleaved, odd and even lines being transmitted in alternate frames. At the end of the frame, the spot returns to the upper left hand corner.

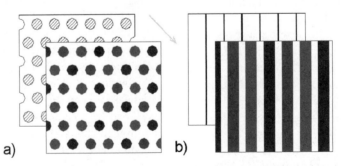

a)　　　　b)

FIGURE 19.5 A diagram showing how pixels are produced by the electron beam in color TV. A, The colored phosphor dots on the face of the tube. The red, green, and blue dots are shown as differing shades of gray. Behind them are the holes of the shadow mask. The electron beam passes through the holes and excites the dots to the required extent. The current must be changed rapidly. B, The Trinitron system. The phosphors are laid down in stripes, and the electron beam traverses a support meshwork aperture grill. The horizontal size of the spot is limited to determine the color emitted. With this arrangement a larger proportion of the screen emits light.

The way the display area of the CRT is scanned leads to a number of potential pitfalls in the use of this type of stimulus display. Although none is overly serious, they need to be considered. The time taken for the electron beam to complete a scan of the display area is given as the vertical refresh rate is normally specified in hertz. Older television displays operate at a nominal 50 or 60 Hz, depending on the region, and use an alternate-line interlaced scan, whereby the system writes half the lines of the display on alternate vertical scans or fields; thus, in a display made up of a nominal 625 lines, 262 odd-numbered lines are written in the first vertical field, and the next field writes the 263 even-numbered lines (the remaining 100 lines being used for various signaling tasks). Thus, a complete image on a 50-Hz 625-line interlaced system is written at a real rate of 25 Hz. Modern stimulus systems utilize computer displays operating in a noninterlaced mode at vertical refresh rates of typically 100 Hz, giving an image refresh rate of 10 ms.

If a stimulus is to be frame-locked, that is, the change in stimulus always occurs at a fixed point, usually the start of the sweep, to give a stable image, then the stimulus rate must be in multiples of the frame period. If the stimulus is not frame-locked, then an irregularity will be seen periodically traversing the screen. The result of using non-frame-locked stimuli affects the responses that are obtained. Assuming that the patient maintains fixation on the center of the screen but the trigger can occur at any point within the frame time, there is a jitter of plus or minus 50% of the frame period introduced. With a 100-Hz vertical refresh rate, a 10-ms period of uncertainty is introduced into the implicit time of the response. Therefore, if responses are averaged, the resultant waveform will be broadened, and the peak amplitude will be reduced. This is in some respects approximately equivalent to using a low-pass filter in the amplifier and removes the high-frequency components of the response.

A number of viewpoints exist as to the optimal trigger location and methodology with CRT displays. The ideal should be that the trigger occurs as the scan crosses the fixation point. In most cases, this will be center of the screen and can easily be achieved by adding a delay of half the frame interval to the frame initialization pulse on the monitor synchronization signal. This is readily achievable in a system in which the operator has adequate direct access to either the hardware or the software but is very difficult to do in many commercial systems. An alternative is to specify the vertical refresh rate of the stimulus display and the point at which the trigger pulse is generated with the laboratory normal values for the test in question.

Considerable effort has been applied to the development of CRT-based monitors for the television and computer displays, such that a wide range of specific characteristics are readily available, with high vertical refresh rates (>200 Hz), high luminance output, or precise color control, making these various devices readily adaptable for the display of specialized stimuli.

Liquid Crystal Displays (LCDs) LCDs are in effect variable transmission optical filters. The principle of operation is that liquid crystals rotate the plane of polarization of light to a degree that depends on the voltage across the liquid crystal layer. The two surfaces of the LCD are coated with a linear polarizer, arranged at 90 degrees to each other (extinction) (figure 19.6). This attenuates the transmission through the device. When a voltage is applied, the plane of polarization within the liquid crystal rotates, and more light is transmitted. A practical LCD device has a matrix of electrodes, in rows and columns, each of which applies charge to a very small area of the filter. Therefore, complex patterns can be displayed by altering the voltage across each pixel. In practice, color filters are incorporated into the display,

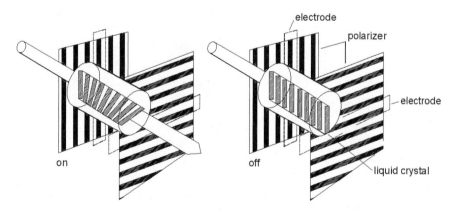

FIGURE 19.6 Principles of LCD systems. Each cell of an LCD system is coated back and front with a linearly polarizing layer, but the directions of polarization are at 90 degrees. Light transmitted through the back plane is therefore polarized, and if the LCD causes no change in the plane, transmission through the front plane is extinguished (right). However, the LCD can rotate the angle of polarization, so light passes through the front plane (left).

so each pixel consists of a triad of red-, green-, and blue-transmitting regions. The light transmission can be spatially modulated to display an image. With appropriate masking to prevent light spillage, a colored display is produced. Modern versions of these displays have individual transistors built onto the glass substrate to drive each subpixel.

LCD displays of the type commonly used as computer displays and televisions currently have two major drawbacks that limit their application as stimulus displays. The first and less problematic of these concerns color rendition. The LCD panel is normally illuminated with a cold cathode fluorescent lamp. These lamps give a very uneven spectral output, with a number of pronounced peaks. This output is then passed through RGB filters, to provide the colored display. The resultant output, while a reasonable color match, is composed of an irregular makeup of wavelengths.

Figure 19.7 shows the output spectra for a conventional CRT display and an LCD screen, both giving a white output of $x = 0.33$, $y = 0.33$ at approximately $60\,\mathrm{cd.m^{-2}}$ or $60\,\mathrm{cd/m^2}$. Although these two outputs are metameric, this means that the white is the same for both devices in humans; this is not necessarily true for other species. Furthermore, the change in the output when the color is varied will be quite different for the two displays. Therefore, the color system must be adjusted so that it is consistent with the type of display used. While this is unlikely to be problematic for black-and-white stimuli, accurate color stimulation could be difficult.

The second and more serious problem is that of response time. While high-resolution CRTs can readily sustain refresh rates in excess of 100 Hz, the refresh rate of most LCD displays is significantly slower. Most of them currently achieve a quoted rate of 40 Hz (25 ms), while the faster unit can theoretically achieve a vertical refresh rate. These figures are bound to improve with time (until recently, 34 ms was the best achievable). These low rates limit the rate of change of any stimulus. Moreover, there is a marked nonlinearity between the degree of light transmission and the rate of change to another gray level, so pixel switching times are not constant. This can, for example, result in a "fast" luminance transient on the reversal of a checkerboard display. However, an even more serious problem is the efforts of the designers of these displays to provide a smoother motion display. With a CRT display, the signal is passed directly to the screen, albeit through a significant amount of electronics. With the LCD display, the signal is held in memory until it is possible to refresh the screen, in effect a "frame grabber." The combined result of the low refresh rate and the frame delay mechanism is to introduce an unacceptable degree of uncertainty into when a transition sent from the stimulus generator will actually appear on the screen. As the display technology matures and temporal characteristics improve, such problems will become less severe, but without significant improvements in the operating characteristics, LCD displays are unsuitable for most forms of stimulus display.

Furthermore, although surmountable, problems with LCD panels relate to the comparatively narrow optimum viewing angle, which leads to both contrast and chromatic distortions experienced as the subject moves off the optical axis of the display. Contrast ratios were comparatively low with earlier displays, although this is no longer a major issue.

At the time of press, major technical advances in LCD technology are becoming available, such as 4-ms refresh rates and nonlinear pixel switching, which may make these displays suitable for use as stimulus devices.

LCD shutter devices are also commonly used in data projection systems. The color distortions that are introduced by the use of cold light fluorescent illumination in display monitors are largely overcome by the use of halogen illumination, although the temporal considerations still apply. These data projectors are capable of providing a high-luminance, large-area stimulus display and are therefore of great interest, although care should be taken with respect to the timing considerations. It should also be noted that there are wide variations between different makes and models of

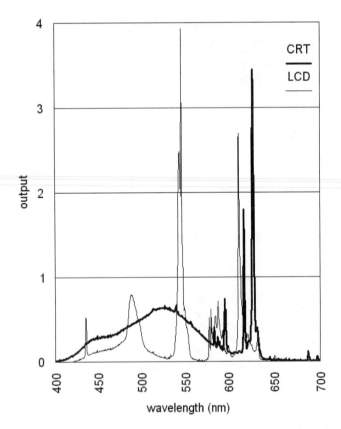

CRT / LCD

FIGURE 19.7 Comparison of the spectral variation in emission of a TV screen and an LCD screen, both of which appear "white" to the human observer.

projectors, and operating characteristics data are difficult to obtain.

Data projectors are also based around both CRTs and the Texas Instruments digital light projection system (DLP). The CRT-based projectors, while generally large and expensive, approach the conventional CRT display in temporal and chromatic performance, being based on a triplet of very high-output CRTs (one each for red, green, and blue).

Digital light projection projectors are based on a novel chip technology from Texas Instruments. The chip at the heart of these devices consists of a large number of micro-mirrors, each mounted on an individual memory cell. When the state of the cell changes, the angle of the mirror changes, thus deflecting the illumination beam through the projection lens. Intensity modulation is generated by varying the duty time each pixel is on. Almost all of the current systems based on this technology, with the exception of professional theater systems, use a single chip. The RGB separation is provided by a rapidly rotating filter wheel modulation, while the intensity variation of each color is generated, varying the duty cycle of the individual pixel mirror.

PLASMA DISPLAYS PANELS Large-area, high-resolution plasma screen video displays are available. The technology that is utilized in these displays is phosphor-based, as in a color CRT device. The display consists of an array of vertical and horizontal electrodes overlaying pixel cells containing xenon or neon gas. When the electrodes that intersect either side of a specific cell are energized, the gas fluoresces (in the same way as in a fluorescent lamp), emitting mostly UV light. This UV radiation is used to excite phosphors to produce the visible light. By arranging RGB phosphor triplets of these cells, a color display similar to that on a shadow mask color CRT is produced.

Input circuitry similar to that utilized in LCD panels is needed to control the electrodes arrays. Although the refresh rate is higher than that in LCD panels, this can lead to temporal problems. While large-area plasma displays offer some advantages for stimulus display, a cautious approach to their application is required.

ABSORPTION AND INTERFERENCE FILTERS Filters may be used to modify the characteristics of a stimulus by absorbing or blocking the passage of a portion of the light, thus reducing the energy of all or selective parts of the spectrum, thereby changing the intensity or color of the stimuli. Excluding some of the more specialized filters, such as polarizing types, two types of filters are in common use: absorption and interference filters. Neither of these is ideal. Interference filters provide very narrow pass bands but are sensitive to the direction of the incident light, the transmitted wavelengths varying with the angle of incident of the light. They are also expensive, and the largest size that is commonly available is 50 mm in diameter. There are a limited number of colored glasses that can be used as filters, but most absorption filters are made of dyes incorporated into a plastic (or gelatin) base. These absorption filters, such as those from Wratten, are relatively low in cost, are well defined, and are available in a range of sizes. However, they are subject to aging at a rate that depends on the energy they absorb. Many of the filters have quite complex absorption spectra and may pass energy at wavelengths outside the main transmission band.

For simply attenuating light intensity, without altering the wavelength composition, several alternatives to neutral density filters exist. One of the simplest and most stable alternatives is a simple aperture to reduce the area of the source that is able to transmit light into the system, a refinement being a variable aperture similar to that used in cameras. A pair of polarizing filters can be used in which the angle between the planes of polarization increases toward 90 degrees, the amount of light transmitted is reduced. This is the basis on which liquid crystal devices operate, and large-area LCD filters (as opposed to shutter mechanisms) are available as both colored and neutral electronically variable filter mechanisms, although at the time of writing, they are of limited availability, and as with other LCD mechanisms, they are subject to temperature-related variability.

As with the light source itself, calibration of filters is essential.

LIGHT-EMITTING DIODES (LEDs) Light-emitting diodes (LEDs) are nearly ideal light sources for many purposes. They are small, require low voltages and currents to drive them, and can be controlled by simple electronic means to give either continuous light outputs, extremely brief flashes, or complex waveforms (or a mixture of these) over a wide range of intensities. Their light output changes by little in intensity or relative spectral emission over extended use.[5] These properties not only simplify calibration but also reduce the frequency with which it is needed. Many different spectral outputs are available, ranging from the near ultraviolet through white to infrared in a variety of different packages with differing optical properties. The majority of the available devices are inexpensive. Until recently, the limiting factor to the use of LEDs for visual stimulation has been the relatively low outputs available; however, white LEDs are now being introduced as automobile lamps, in which a cluster of six devices gives an equivalent output of a 20-watt filament lamp. The available output energy is forecast to rise significantly over the next few years, possibly to the point at which these devices may be used as headlights. Nevertheless, even when considerable quantities of light are required (e.g., in electroretinography), LEDs can be used to advantage.

LEDs are members of the family of epitaxial semiconductor junction diodes. A junction is formed by growing a very thin crystal of a semiconductor directly onto another, slightly different, semiconductor surface. The two layers of semiconductor material (frequently gallium aluminum arsenide) contain different impurities (dopants). As a result of these impurities, one layer contains an excess of free electrons, and the other contains an excess of holes (positive charge). The energy that is required to move a charge across the junction against the concentration gradient of free electrons or holes is considerable and larger than in other types of diode (approximately 3:1). This energy band gap must be exceeded if current is to be passed through the junction. When the device is forward biased, electrons move from the negative material to the positive, and a corresponding movement of positive charge or "holes" occurs in the reverse direction. When an electron and hole pair recombine, energy is emitted as a photon. The characteristic wavelength of the photon is determined by the energy band gap. Thus, it is more difficult to produce short-wavelength LEDs, since the higher energy gap must be maintained with the controlled flow of charges. The construction of the epitaxial layer determines the direction of light that is emitted, and the absence of a resonating (reflective) cavity prevents the stimulated emission of radiation (lasing) by the photons, so the light is not coherent and contains a number of differing wavelengths. However, light is emitted over a relatively narrow bandwidth. For a typical red LED (for illustrative purposes, a Stanley HBR5566X), the peak is at 660 nm, and the half-power bandwidth is ±30 nm. This is a purer red than is readily obtainable with gelatin filters, though expensive, multilayer, complex, band-pass interference filters can produce a better approximation to a monochromatic light.

The construction of a typical LED is shown in figure 19.8. The semiconductor is mounted on a lead frame and encapsulated in a plastic (epoxy) housing with an internal spherical lens. The combination of junction structure, epoxy, and lens type determines the spatial output characteristics of the device, and for many LEDs, including all the "brightest," the light is concentrated in a cone, which can be represented in a polar diagram (figure 19.9) with a half-power spatial polar distribution of ±7.5 degrees.

A typical device requires 30 mA at around 2 V to produce its maximum output, so it is both easy to control and intrinsically safe to use in a clinical environment. The junction of most modern devices thus exhibits low electrical impedance but is nevertheless fairly robust, being able to tolerate significant overloads for short periods.

An exception and extension to this construction methodology is the white LED. In these devices, a short-wavelength-emitting junction (approximately 470 nm) is encapsulated in a phosphor material, similar to that used on the inner surface of black-and-white monochrome CRTs.

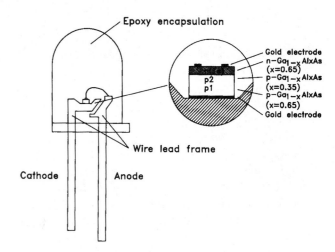

FIGURE 19.8   Construction of a typical LED.

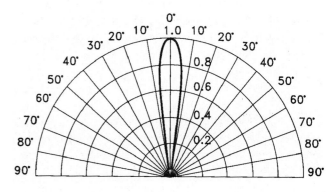

FIGURE 19.9   Polar diagram showing the spatial concentration of light from an LED.

The diode emits blue light, which excites the phosphor, which in turn emits white light. While this "white" light is a continuous broad-spectrum emission, it normally contains a major peak at the primary wavelength of the diode. The spectrum of a typical device of this type is illustrated in figure 19.10. While this continuous spectral output may offer significant advantages for ERG use when compared to white light simulated by three narrow spectral lines of red, green, and blue light, some care is required, as the phosphor, like that used in CRTs, will have a definite decay time, prolonging the trailing edge of a light pulse.

Light-emitting diode technology is advancing at a considerable pace, to the effect that devices that only a few years ago were used as indicator lamps and little else outside the laboratory are expected to be utilized as vehicle head lamps within the next two to three years. Some street lighting systems are already being installed, including an array of fewer than ten devices with suitable heat sinks potentially capable of matching the output of the current generation of xenon lamps.

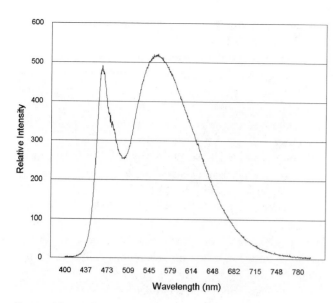

FIGURE 19.10 The emission spectrum of a typical "white" LED. Note the peak in the blue, which is the primary emission, and the second peak, due to the phosphor emission (see text).

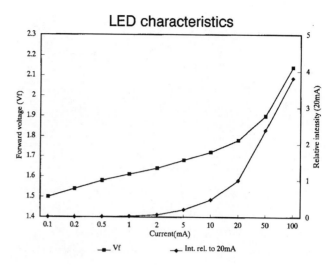

FIGURE 19.11 Relationship between applied voltage (V_f), current, and relative light output (Int) of a typical LED.

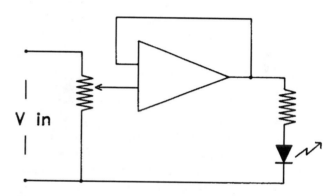

FIGURE 19.12 Voltage drive circuit of a simple flash stimulator.

Recent work suggests, however, that phosphor-enhanced white devices will age rather more rapidly than other LEDs due to a decay of the phosphor with use, similar to that which occurs in CRTs. This decay effect aside, these high output devices have the capability of producing the high luminous flux necessary for electroretinography in standard-sized Ganzfeld stimulators.

Organic LEDs (O-LEDs) are beginning to appear in numerous guises. This family of polymer-based LEDs can be printed to a plastic or glass substrate using inkjet techniques, thereby producing a low cost, high-luminance, high-resolution, RGB color display with none of the geometric limitations of LCD-based devices. It is possible that display devices based on O-LEDs will become the obvious replacement for large format CRT displays, bypassing those problems associated with the current generation of LCD-based monitors.

Various types of LEDs are available. Some are devised for special purposes—for example, alphanumeric display components or indicators. There is a great range of shape, size, and intensity. A number of devices are packaged with additional circuitry that provides a constant current flow or flashes the device on and off. Other devices contain more than one junction and can produce two or even three colors, but these are so specialized that their value for purposes other than those for which they were designed, that is, for instrument displays, is limited.

The colors that are quoted by manufacturers vary from ultraviolet to infrared, with many wavelengths being available across this range. A recent review of devices available showed that steps of 10 nm across the visible spectrum were easily achievable, although outputs varied considerably.

Until recently, the longer visible wavelengths (yellow to red) have been the brightest devices available. However, at the behest of the lighting industry, much development has been focused on the shorter (blue) end of the visible spectrum.

Certain problems and their solutions are common across the range of devices available. The relationship between applied current (or voltage) and light output of a typical device is shown in figure 19.11. For a region of about 1.5 decades, it can be seen to be approximately linear. Above or below this region, marked nonlinearities occur. Since in general, users wish to control the intensity over a much larger range, a variety of drive circuits have been devised.

For a simple flash stimulator, a voltage drive circuit may be used quite effectively (figure 19.12), and the relationship between light output and applied voltage can be determined by calibration. Better performance can be obtained by replacing the voltage drive with a current source or ideally by placing the LEDs in the feedback loop of a current drive (figure 19.13). This technique, while a significant improvement over the simple circuit in figure 19.17 still limits the

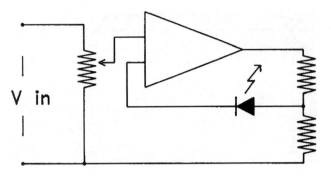

FIGURE 19.13   Feedback loop of a current drive to enhance the performance of an LED.

range of linearity available to around 2.5 decades. Thus, if a true sinusoidal output is required, the depth of modulation can never be 100%.

Two alternative techniques may be used to obtain linear control over intensity. The first consists of pulse density modulation.[7] The LEDs are driven by pulses of short duration (100-ns pulses have proved readily achievable in the author's experience), each of fixed power content. Light intensity is altered by changing the repetition rate of the pulses. An upper pulse frequency limit of 5 MHz is readily attained. For low intensities, a rate of 50 Hz is well above the critical fusion frequency of the human eye; thus, a wide range of intensity of an apparently continuous source can be achieved. If these pulses are derived from a linear voltage-controlled oscillator (VCO), a device in which the frequency of the output is related to the applied voltage, the output pulses are shaped and used to drive the LEDs through a fast switching circuit. Although good VCOs with the required range are difficult to produce, several are available as either integrated or hybrid circuits and can be driven from any waveform source so that very complex temporal changes can easily be produced. The light intensity may also be simply controlled without changing the waveform by passing the output of the VCO through frequency divider circuits. These may be readily produced by using standard logic components. Thus, a visual stimulator with a dynamic range of six orders of magnitude, consistent modulation capability, high stability, and fine control of intensity may be easily produced.

A similar effect can be achieved by using pulse width modulation, as opposed to pulse frequency modulation. This technique has gained favor recently, partially owing to the ease with which control circuits from switch mode power supplies can be utilized to control pulse width, thus eliminating the need for expensive VCOs.

One major drawback to pulse density or pulse width modulation systems derives from the high-speed switching of LEDs, especially if an array dissipating large amounts of energy is required. Each pulse contains frequency components much greater than the pulse repetition rate (5 MHz)

that are caused by damping inadequacies of the power switching circuits. Thus, the LED array acts as a very high-frequency (VHF) radio transmitter and may radiate tens of watts. (This effect can be more easily reduced in the pulse width modulation systems as the control circuits often include control of the respective rise and fall times of the pulses, thus reducing the tendency to emit the higher harmonic frequencies.)

Because the source is usually very close to both the patient and the preamplifier and because modern clinical amplifiers use high-input impedance field effect transistor input stages, which in practice make very effective FM radio receivers (the common mode rejection ratio is relatively low at very high frequencies), large stimulus artefacts are generated. Therefore, the pulse frequency modulation technique is of use primarily for psychophysical experiments.

An alternative approach is to use a low-frequency current source to drive the LEDs and continuously measure their output with a photo-sensing circuit. The output from the detector circuit is compared with the waveform input signal, and any difference is used to modify the LED drive current and thus the light output. This current modulation approach will operate effectively only over a range of three to four orders of magnitude; to go beyond this would require an unduly complex drive circuitry.

There are two significant defects affecting LEDs that the user should be aware of. The first primarily affects some older short-wavelength devices (GaN blues being a case in point), namely, a variation in emitted wavelength with current and therefore intensity. This change in wavelength can be in the region of 5–10 nm over the usable drive current range. It is, however, largely eliminated on modern devices. The shorter-wavelength blue devices also emit some energy in the ultraviolet, which can degrade the epoxy compounds that are used to encapsulate the devices, causing a loss of output through the imposition of a yellow filter. The second and potentially more serious problem affects the longer-wavelength devices. Because of the robust nature of the device junctions, it is always tempting to overdrive them for short periods and thus increase the available light intensity; indeed, most manufactures quote two maximum forward currents; one for continuous use and another significantly higher figure for reduced duty cycle operation. However, even at the maximum continuous forward current, there is a progressive fall in light output for a fixed current due to heating effects within the junction. This effect is very noticeable in the orange and red devices, becoming much less of a problem as the emitted wavelength shortens toward the green portion of the spectra.

Arrays   The low power requirements and general ease of use make LEDs an ideal choice for many types of stimulator. Because of both the size of the radiating area and the

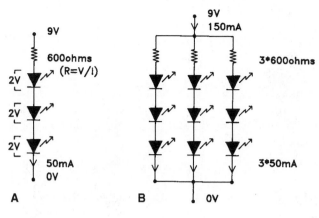

Series connection.　　Series/Parallel connection.

FIGURE 19.14　Series and parallel connections of LEDs.

relatively low radiant energy of many types of LED, it is generally necessary to use a number of devices to construct an effective stimulus. Here again, the low drive requirements make it a simple matter, provided that some care is taken in the design to interconnect a number of the diodes in an array. By using either the pulse or constant current modulation approach, an array of several hundred LEDs can be assembled to provide the required stimulus. They can be connected in series, parallel, or a combination of both. Thus, if nine devices are required for the stimulus and the power unit has an output of 9 V, three LEDs, each with a forward voltage drop of 2 V at 50 mA, could be connected in series (figure 19.14A), then three identical chains connected in parallel (figure 19.14B) will give a stimulus with maximum light output at three times the maximum continuous forward current of each device. Care should be taken to ensure that the forward voltages of the diodes are closely matched, or, preferably, select a resistor to balance the current through the three chains. This resistor will have the added benefit of protecting the drive circuits should an LED fail and short-circuit.

Applications Since Drasdo and Woodall[6] first employed LEDs for scotometry, a wide range of equipment has been described. The earlier examples are predominantly for psychophysical testing owing to the lower light intensity requirements, readily provided by the earlier generations of LEDs. Thus, LEDs have been used for determining de Lange curves in clinical circumstances, for analyzing rod-cone interactions, for measuring dark adaptation[8] and spectral sensitivity, for field screening, and for many other psychophysical and electrophysiological applications.

Commercially available stimulators include LEDs mounted in goggles similar to those used by swimmers. (A small array of LEDs is used.) They are designed for monitoring the visual evoked response (VER) in special condi-

tions, such as in operating theaters in which the small size and low voltages that are used are advantageous. Arrays of square red LEDs used to produce small high-contrast checkerboard displays suited to transportable recording systems are available from some manufacturers. In another application, LEDs were used to produce a stimulator that could be used inside an oxygen incubator for premature infants.[11]

Krakau, Nordenfelt, and Ohman[10] described the use of yellow LEDs to produce mixed rod and cone responses. Kooijman and Damhof[9] mounted red, green, and blue LEDs on a contact lens to obtain a greater range of stimulus intensity with the comparatively low light output that is available from these early devices. However, these LEDs do not generate light of intensity equivalent to that of common discharge lamps and were therefore unsuitable for illuminating Ganzfeld spheres.

Large arrays of devices were used to supply sufficient light for noncontact lens "Ganzfeld" stimulators. Arden et al.[13] used an array of 250 devices in a direct view mode to produce a 12-cm stimulator bowl capable of stimulating a full range of responses, from scotopic threshold responses to saturated b-wave ERGs, without the use of optical filters.

Other authors[1,7,12,13] have described a range of stimulus systems for the isolation of S-cones, ON–OFF bipolar cells, and retinal ganglion cells,[13] all utilizing LED-based stimulation, several of which would not be readily achievable, certainly in a clinical environment, with other light sources.

The current generation of LEDs can produce sufficient light from a moderately sized array to adequately illuminate full-size Ganzfeld spheres, with single colored or broadband white illumination, both with the considerable advantages of stability and flexibility provided by these illumination sources.

It is vital to note that several of the technologies discussed in the preceding section are advancing rapidly, to the extent that some statements may be redundant by the time of publication. Those areas most likely to be affected are the use of LEDs, which are being produced with output powers and efficiencies far in excess of those available only one year ago. Display technology is also changing rapidly: large format CRT displays are being replaced by LCD devices in consumer applications, and thus the CRT monitor is becoming a rarity. While LCD, currently the preferred format for most replacement displays, is not ideal for use as visual stimulations; new developments in LED-based technologies, however, are rapidly developing, and will offer an alternative in the future.

Amplifiers and artifacts

An amplifier is simply a device for increasing the magnitude of one or more characteristics of a signal, for example, voltage. Amplifiers that are used for routine visual electrophysiology are differential devices, sometimes referred to as *instrumentation amplifiers*. These differ from normal amplifiers in that they have two active inputs rather than one. As the name implies, they amplify the voltage difference between the two inputs, as opposed to the difference between ground and the input in the more common single-ended design. An appreciation of the operation of these devices will help the electrophysiologist to understand and ultimately remove many of the artifacts that can plague the recording of low-amplitude biological signals.

The differential input configuration does not preclude the need for a ground connection, as a current return path is still required for both inputs.

The basic design of the differential amplifier utilizes a pair of transistors arranged as a long-tailed pair (figure 19.15A). The more common three-operational-amplifier design is shown in figure 19.15B.

It is this basic amplifier design and the resultant characteristics that make routine electrophysiological recordings possible, for without the noise rejection characteristics of the differential amplifier, most signals would be irretrievably masked by noise.

Consider the operation of the circuit in figure 19.15A. With a differential input, a small signal applied on the base of Q_1 results in an identical but inverted signal being applied to Q_2. In this case, the gain is determined by the emitter resistance:

$$\text{Differential gain} = R_C/2\ (R_E + r_e)$$

However, if an identical signal is applied to both Q_1 and Q_2, that is, a common mode signal, then the gain is largely determined by the long-tailed resistor R_T:

$$\text{Common mode gain} = R_C/2\ (R_T + R_E + r_e)$$

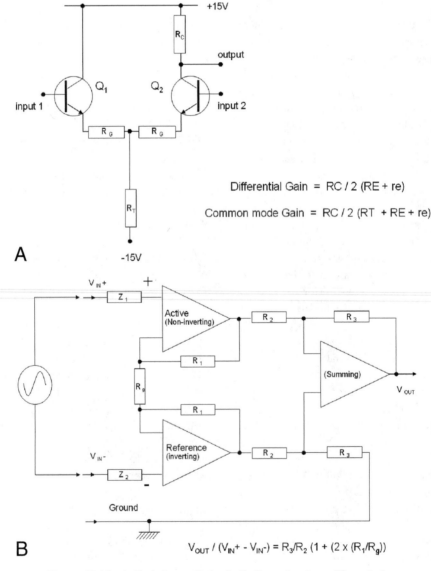

Differential Gain = RC / 2 (RE + re)

Common mode Gain = RC / 2 (RT + RE + re)

$$V_{OUT} / (V_{IN}{+} - V_{IN}{-}) = R_3/R_2\ (1 + (2 \times (R_1/R_g)))$$

FIGURE 19.15   A, Basic long-tailed pair. B, Operational amplifier solution.

Because R_T is large with respect to R_E, the differential gain is much higher than the common mode gain.

In both of these basic designs, the key factor is the amplifier's ability to selectively reject common mode signals. Thus, by placing two recording electrodes close to the source of the signal of interest, the target signal is seen as a differential mode signal by the amplifier, while other signals, by virtue of their distance from the recording site, appear as common mode sources.

CHARACTERISTICS OF AN AMPLIFIER A modern amplifier that is designed for use in a visual electrophysiology laboratory will have an input impedance of at least 100 Mohms (100,000,000 ohms). While this is very high, it is not infinite; therefore, the amplifier will draw a small current from the signal source.

The gain of the amplifier may be as high as 200,000, although much of this will be applied at later stages within the amplifier rather than at the differential front end. If the majority of the signal gain were to be applied at the differential stage of the amplifier, then the dynamic range of this stage would have to be impractically large, owing to offset voltages present on the electrodes. To avoid these large offset voltages, other features of amplifiers are needed (see below). The dynamic range of the amplifier is the peak-to-peak signal amplitude that the amplifier can handle without distortion. (This is usually around 1.5 V less than the power supply voltage at either supply rail.) So far, these considerations have applied only to the input stage, or front end, of the amplifier; if we want higher amplification (more than a few hundred times), then we have to introduce a further factor: a.c. coupling.

If a signal is applied that exceeds the dynamic range of the amplifier, then the amplifier will lock up or block. To prevent this occurring, decoupling capacitors are inserted into the circuit. The capacitor has the effect of restoring the signal mean level to zero voltage as shown in figure 19.16.

This capacitor, which forms a simple high-pass filter, removing low frequencies from the signal, exemplifies the problem of amplifier lockup. A modern amplifier will have multiple stages with decoupling capacitors separating each stage of the amplifier circuit. The problem occurs when a relatively high-amplitude artifact signal is injected into the amplifier, for example, an eye movement while recording a PERG. Because this signal exceeds the dynamic range of the amplifier, the decoupled stages are all driven to the supply rail and lock up in this position for a length of time determined by the time constant of the particular stage. (The time constant is determined by the values of the capacitor and resistor that form the basic filter [T = 0.7RC].) If a late stage of the amplifier recovers before the earlier stages, then a zero signal is passed forward into the signal averager. The decoupling capacitor or any cascaded high-pass filter stages should therefore be selected with care.

The common mode rejection ratio (CMRR) of the amplifier is the ratio differential to common mode gain and is normally expressed in decibels (dB). For a modern amplifier with balanced inputs, the CMRR should be in excess of 100 dB, or 100,000 to 1. This is with balance inputs, however. The effect of electrode impedance on the amplifier's ability to reject common mode signals is demonstrated in figure 19.17. In this figure, we have two electrodes: one good with an effective impedance of 1000 Ω and the second with failing electrode with an impedance of 50,000 Ω. If a common mode signal exists in the circuit of, say, 1 mV, then Ohm's Law dictates that a differential voltage of 0.5 μV will exist at the inputs due to the voltage drop across the electrode impedance.

The net effect of the imbalance in the electrode impedances is to significantly reduce the amplifier's effective common mode rejection ratio (CMRR). Therefore, it is important not only to reduce the impedance between any pair of electrodes to less than 5000 Ω, but also to ensure that all impedances are of approximately the same value. This effect also suggests that an amplifier's CMRR should be measured with an imbalance of 5000 Ω in the circuit, representing a more realistic scenario.

All modern amplifiers intended for clinical use should be isolated; that is, there should be no possible direct pathway

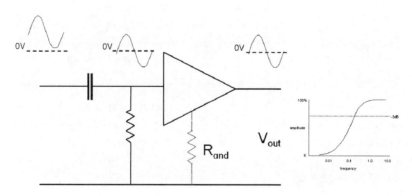

FIGURE 19.16   Simple high-pass filter.

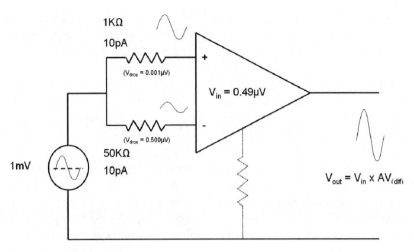

FIGURE 19.17 Effect of electrode impedance.

between the patient connections, including ground, and any other system components, including the low-voltage d.c. power supply rails. In the absence of isolation, if some component of an amplifier failed, the patient might be connected to a source of electrical current that could cause serious harm to the patient. While this galvanic barrier is primarily a safety requirement, it has additional benefits in terms of isolating the signal source, that is, the patient, from the noise with the electronic recording equipment.

This galvanic safety barrier (currently specified within the European Union and the United States, as being required to withstand 4000 V for 60 s), can be achieved by a variety of methods. The most common is the use of transformer isolation, in which a small isolating transformer is placed in the signal path and the power required for the thus isolated head stage is transferred over a separate isolation transformer, having been modulated at a high frequency and then rectified on the isolated side. Alternative isolation techniques include capacitive or optocoupled isolators to decouple the signal pathway. With optoisolation, the head stage energizes an LED source, the light output being proportional to the signal voltage, and the main amplifier contains photodiodes to convert the optical signal back to an electrical one. These LED-photodiode pairs can be obtained in a single unit, or the LEDs can be separated by several meters of fiber-optic cable. With optically coupled systems, power is usually provided by either batteries within the head stage or a separate d.c.-to-d.c. converter.

ARTIFACTS An artifact can be defined as a gardener would define a weed, that is, any signal (plant) other than the signal that we are intending to record (grow). The sources of artifactual signals are virtually limitless. First of all, there are superfluous signals of biological origin, such as electrocardiographic and muscle activity, and contamination of the target signal by components from other parts of the visual pathway; then there are the indirect biologically originating signals such as movement or perspiration effecting the electrode circuit; and finally, there are signals of a nonbiological origin. These signal sources range from the recording equipment itself to almost any device that uses electromagnetic energy.

The majority of artifactual signals not only are recorded through the electrodes, but also are generally recorded as a direct result of poor electrode technique. While improvements in amplifier design and specification, such as increasing input impedance and common mode rejection, has made electrode technique, superficially at least, less critical, the importance of electrode technique cannot to stressed too highly, both for the reduction of artifacts and for the reliability of recorded responses.

Electrodes and electrode technique are covered in detail elsewhere in this book, but a brief recap of some of the factors that will help to reduce artifacts may be helpful. Assuming that the electrode is in good condition and has been cleaned and maintained correctly and that the site of attachment has been correctly identified, then the skin should be cleaned. This is usually carried out with a proprietary cleaning compound, which both degreases the skin and gently abrades away the surface layers. Excessive abrasion leading to slight bleeding is to be avoided. The residue from the paste should then be wiped away, as the abrasive residue can prevent good adhesion. The electrode, in the case of a standard EEG disk electrode, is then filled to slightly over tilled with saline-based electrode gel and is secured to the attachment site using adhesive tape. (In the case of scalp electrodes, a combined adhesive paste and gel or colliodin adhesive and gel are used.) The electrode should be firmly in contact with the skin and secured in such a way as to prevent any movement with respect to the skin. Air bubbles in the electrode gel should be avoided. The electrode lead is then routed in such a way as to minimize movement and prevent the weight of the cable pulling on the electrode. For example, outer canthi electrode leads can be laid over the external ear. Once the surface electrodes are attached, the impedance can be measured, this should have a value of less than $5000\,\Omega$. Depending on the type of electrode that is used, a high impedance may be reduced by manipulating the electrode, abrading the skin with a blunt canula through a hole in the electrode, or removal and replacement.

The impedance of electrodes should, when measured in situ, be tested only using an a.c. impedance tester, rather than a d.c. resistance meter. The latter will polarize the electrodes, rendering them useless.

With well-positioned and securely attached electrodes, many of the sources of artifact will be significantly reduced. However, other patient-related causes of signal contamination include movement and muscle tension, the latter resulting in contamination of the recording by high-frequency electromyographic signals, observed as free-running spike activity on the real time trace. Both of these problems can be dealt with by simply positioning the subject comfortably in the correct position to observe the stimulus.

Perspiration and the presence of even very small amounts of blood have the effect of contaminating the electrochemistry of the skin-to-electrode interface. This can result in unpredictable high-amplitude, low-frequency signals being superimposed on the response under investigation. While the degree of perspiration can be reduced with a simple electric fan where air conditioning is not available, any microbleeds caused by overly aggressive skin abrasion or preexisting wounds will result in serious electrode contamination and resultant artifacts. Tears will cause significant and continuously varying changes in the effective conductance between the electrodes.

While air conditioning is an expensive option in building a laboratory, it should be remembered that for some testing, the patient and possibly an accompanying person and the operator (each equivalent to approximately 300 W) and around a kilowatt of electrical equipment, all generating a significant amount of heat, will be held within a closed box-like room, possibly for an hour or more. Apart from the comfort factor, the resultant conditions can make it very difficult to obtain satisfactory recordings.

Artifacts arising from sources other than the patient present a more diverse and interesting set of problems. While the majority of these artifacts are picked up through the patient electrode circuit, some may be transmitted directly to the recording equipment though power cabling. The sources of these signals may be within the recording equipment or room or could be some distance removed from the laboratory. Figure 19.18 illustrates four of the more commonly observed artifacts.

Figure 19.18A is by far the most commonly observed interference pattern. In this instance, 50- or 60-Hz power line noise is shown contaminating a rod ERG. While there are numerous causes for this type of interference, most of them related to poor electrodes or poor electrode technique, this is by no means the only cause of such problems. Perhaps the most difficult to trace is a ground loop. This is caused when separate components of the recording system are connected to power outlets with a difference in ground potential measured at the power sockets. For this to happen, all that is needed is a difference in the impedance of the power supply paths to ground, and this can be comparatively small. The usual causes would be having more than one power

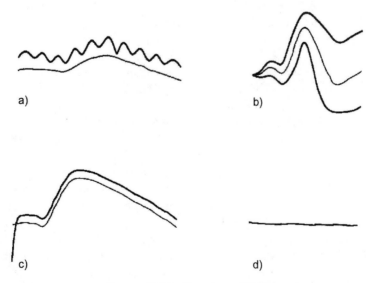

FIGURE 19.18   Common artifacts.

supply circuit in the room, fed from different sections of a building's electrical supply. The problem can then occur when equipment is moved from one power outlet to another. If the problem is not resolved by returning the power supply to its previous configuration, then the only effective method of tracing the cause of the problem is to disconnect all the supply grounds, at which point the system is not safe to use on patients, and reconnect these lines one by one until the noise returns. Then, with the cause of the problem located, appropriate remedial action can be taken.

Power supplies or power cables that are close to sensitive amplifiers or the electrodes are another source of line noise, the noise being radiated from one to the other. Power cables laid along the same cable pathway as signal cables may pick up hum by capacitive coupling. Equipment with poor or faulty earth connections can be a major source of such problems as well a significant safety risk.

This "line noise" may even be a true response, as it is possible, with older display monitors using a 50- or 60-Hz vertical refresh rate, to record both retinal and cortical signals in response to the raster pattern on a blank white screen. This type of signal is comparatively rare, as it requires very stable fixation and can easily be identified by simply placing a sheet of opaque paper between the screen and the subject. If this suppresses the signal, then it is a true evoked response. However, if it fails to do so, then it is probable that the high voltages that are used with the display are causing the transmission of electromagnetic signals to the electrodes. Where this is the case, there are several steps that can be taken. The first is obviously to ensure good closely matched electrode impedances; the second is to keep the separation between electrode leads to a minimum, reducing the volume of space enclosed by the wires and thus the magnetic flux change across the "coil" formed by the electrode circuit. Where the display is mounted on a metal table or trolley, this can act in a similar fashion to a transformer's core, especially when it is not grounded; a patient's legs under the table or trolley may then form a "secondary winding" for this effective transformer.

Line noise is not always a bad thing, however. If during a recording session a channel begins to be contaminated by line noise, this is an early warning that an electrode in that circuit is failing and requires attention. (This early warning will be lost to people who use notch filters at line frequency to conceal poor electrode technique.)

Figure 19.18B shows a PERG contaminated by "drift" or a low-frequency distortion. The more common causes for this type of distortion are blink or eye movement artifact and tears. Eye movement artifacts can be quite reproducible, in some cases mimicking a rod b-wave remarkably well during ERG recording. Tearing affecting corneal electrodes can cause this pattern of drift, as could heavy perspiration, causing a variable offset voltage on the surface electrodes.

The passage of tears from the lacrimal sac to the face may also affect the bulk tissue conductance, causing additional voltage changes.

Figure 19.18C shows an ERG contaminated by a fast negative spike. This type of current switching artifact is frequently, although not exclusively, seen on responses recorded using xenon flash lamps.

Xenon lamps are typically driven by a d.c. supply of 350–750 volts, and on discharge, pulse currents of high amperage can flow through the tube circuit, triggered by a pulse in excess of 10,000 volts. These pulses are dissipated in what is generally a poorly damped spark gap circuit, all mounted a few centimeters from the patient and electrodes. With good amplifiers and well-fitted electrodes, these spikes are rarely seen (a testimony to the design of modern equipment).

When good electrode technique fails to alleviate this problem, a common mistake is to increase the low-pass filter setting on the amplifier to remove this fast spike. However, the effect of the filter is usually to integrate the pulse, reducing the peak amplitude while prolonging the duration, in effect further distorting the important first few milliseconds of the trace. The preferred and obvious solution is to remove the source of the problem. Having eliminated the electrodes as the source of the fault, the next item to check, as with any equipment problem, is whether anything has been changed or moved. Cables from a power unit remote from the lamp head in close proximity to amplifier signal cables are a likely source, as are grounding problems within the xenon lamp system or the rest of the recording apparatus.

A further possible source of such artifacts is the photovoltaic effect. This can occur with very intense flashes, in which the light changes the energy state of the electrons in the material of the electrode, resulting in charge separation and therefore a voltage across the electrodes. If it is suspected that the origin of the discharge artifact is photovoltaic, then a simple test will isolate the problem. Interpose a sheet of opaque, although not electrically conducting material between the light source and the electrode, and record another response. If the artifact disappears, then it is likely to be photovoltaic. However, the previously mentioned causes will be found to be responsible in the vast majority of cases.

The signal in figure 19.18D might not immediately appear as one that would normally be considered an artifact as such, that is, the absence of a signal. However, in the case of an amplifier locking up and blank records being accumulated by the averager, the true nature of the signal will be distorted. Numerous potential causes other than a blocked amplifer exist for the absence of signal, ranging from power failure or other failure of a system component through an absence of stimulus or loss of connection to pathological damage of the system under investigation.

Figure 19.19 is an example of a frame pulse artifact from a CRT stimulus display. In this instance, the fast impulselike waveform of the artifact eliminates most biological signals as a possible cause, although muscle spike activity can give a similar appearance. It is, however, regular in nature (87.5 Hz—the CRT frame rate in use) and frame locked. Various solutions to this type of artifact have been tried, including grounded sheets of metalized glass between the subject and the monitor or metal cowling around the monitor, both effectively screening the patient from the source of the signal. Alternatively, adding some few milliseconds dither to trigger signal to remove the frame locking and allow the noise to average out can be beneficial in removing the noise but will have some degrading effect on the sharpness of the response. Reducing the tube current by lowering the brightness of the display will often help, especially when the display is being driven beyond the levels for which it was designed.

The recordings in figure 19.20 are presented as an interesting demonstration of several points. These are an ERG recording from an 8-year-old child. The noise on channel 2 (left eye) is measured at 400 Hz and is also present at a much lower amplitude on channel 1 (right eye). The electrodes were known not to be the cause of the problem. The second set of traces was recorded after the child's cochleal implant was switched off.

The first point is that the frequency of the artifact, measured at approximately 400 Hz, is considerably lower than the transmission frequency of a cochleal implant (>20 kHz). The second issue is that of the high-frequency transmission signal being recorded while the system has used a 3-kHz low-pass filter. Finally, why does the high frequency appear on the left channel only at a much higher amplitude?

The first issue is related to the sampling rate of 2 kHz employed for the recording. Because this is inadequate to accurately display the transmission frequency, an alias of the true signal is recorded. Second, a filter will progressively attenuate signal of increasing frequency; but with adequate amplitude in the original signal, some breakthough will occur. Finally, the implant is in the left ear and thus close enough to those electrodes to appear in part as a differential signal, while the increased distance to the right eye electrodes is sufficient that the greater part of the signal appears as a common mode signal and is therefore rejected by the amplifier's CMRR.

Sources of electromagnetic contamination of signals do not necessarily have to be in close proximity to the recording laboratory, although airborne radiation is attenuated with distance. For this reason, the proximity of high-powered electrical equipment to the laboratory should be avoided. Such equipment includes any that uses significant amounts of energy, especially electric motors (elevators, air-conditioning fans and compressors, etc.), as the motors can become very noisy as they age. One possible solution to

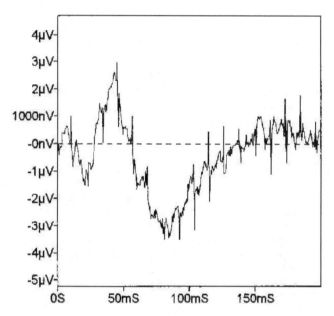

FIGURE 19.19   CRT frame breakthough.

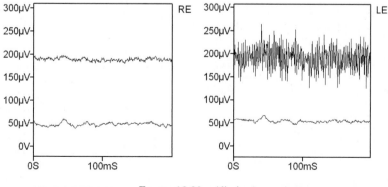

FIGURE 19.20   Aliasing.

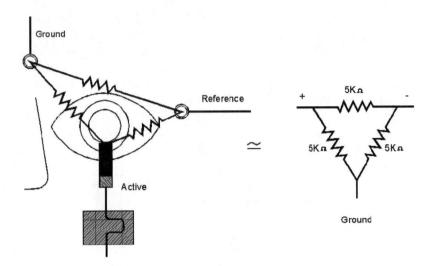

FIGURE 19.21 Dummy patient.

external electromagnetic contamination is the use of Faraday cages or fully screened rooms, although this can be costly.

If the power supply to the laboratory is shared with other sections of the hospital, then noisy equipment can transmit along the power line for considerable distances, so a faulty floor polisher several rooms or floors away, for example, can interfere with recordings. Again the solution can appear expensive, but a dedicated power supply to the laboratory back to the power inlet room will help to ensure a clean power supply. Alternatively, the power can be cleaned as it enters the laboratory with specialist equipment (uninterruptible power supplies). Do not ignore simple issues such as lighting; a.c. dimmer switches can be a serious noise source when new, degrading still further as the rheostat wears. Fluorescent lighting is employed in most large buildings, and while modern electronic units operating at high frequency (>20 kHz) have been found to cause few problems, the older 50/60-Hz units can transmit significant amounts of noise at harmonics of the base frequency and should be replaced at the earliest opportunity.

The majority of artifacts are recorded through the patient electrodes, and a significant proportion of these can be resolved by improving the electrode quality or technique. To localize the source of these problems, electophysiologists should equip themselves with a simple device known as a *dummy patient*. This simple resistive-only equivalent patient circuit is illustrated in figure 19.21. It consists of three resistors of 5000 Ω connected in a simple triangular formation, attached to three redundant electrode cables. This represents the simplest acceptable electrode circuit. (An alternative approach favored by some authors is to utilize three 2500-Ω resistors in a T configuration.) If a problem is proving intractable, then disconnect the patient electrodes and connect the dummy patient in their place. If the problem persists, then it is not electrode related but is most likely an equipment or environmental issue. In subsequently investigating the cause of the problem, due attention must be given to patient safety, as some fault-finding techniques may impair the effectiveness of in-built safety features.

REFERENCES

1. Arden GB, Wolf J, Berninger T, Hogg CR, Tzekov R, Holder GE: S-cone ERGs elicited by a simple technique in normals and in tritanopes. *Vision Res* 1999; 39:641–650.
2. Brigell M, Bach M, Barber C, Kawasaki K, Kooijman A: The International Society for Clinical Electrophysiology of Vision: Guidelines for calibration of stimulus and recording parameters used in clinical electrophysiology of vision. *Doc Ophthalmol* 1998; 95:1–14.
3. Calcagni A, Hogg CR, Spackman L, Bird AC, Holder GE: Characterisation of the normal photopic electroretinographic responses to long duration stimuli evoked by a light emitting diode stimulator. (In preparation.)
4. Cone RA: The rat electroretinogram: I. Contrasting Effects of adaptation on the amplitude and latency of the b-wave. *J Gen Physiol* 1964; 47:1089–1105.
5. Construction and performance of high efficiency red, yellow and green LED materials. Hewlett Packard application bulletin, 1975. Palo Alto, CA.
6. Drasdo N, Woodall A: Flicker fusion scotometry with solid state light sources. *Optician* 1971, pp 10–13.
7. Drasdo N, Aldebasi YH, Chiti Z, Mortlock KE, Morgan JE, North RV: The s-cone PHNR and pattern ERG in primary open angle glaucoma. *Invest Ophthalmol Vis Sci* 2001; 42:1266–1272. Erratum in: *Invest Ophthalmol Vis Sci* 2002; 43:14.
8. Ernst W, Faulkner DJ, Hogg CR, Powell DJ, Arden GB, Vaegan: An automated static perimeter/adaptometer using light emitting diodes. *Br J Ophthalmol* 1983; 67:431–442.

9. Kooijman AC, Damhof A: ERG measurements with red and yellow-green LEDs as light source for stimulation and adaptation. *Doc Ophthalmol* 1982; 31:31–38.

10. Krakau CE, Nordenfelt L, Ohman R: Routine ERG recording with LED light stimulus. *Ophthalmologica* 1977; 175:199–205.

11. Mushin J, Hogg CR, Dubowitz LMS, Skouteli H, Arden GB: Visual evoked responses to light emitting diode (LED) photostimulation in newborn infants. 1984; 58:317–320.

12. Sieving PA: Photopic ON- and OFF-pathway abnormalities in retinal dystrophies. *Trans Am Ophthalmol Soc* 1993; 91:701–773.

13. Spileers W, Falcao-Reis F, Arden GB: Evidence from human ERG a- and off-responses that colour processing occurs in the cones. *Invest Ophthalmol Vis Sci* 1993; 34:2079–2091.

V DATA ACQUISITION

20.1 Introduction to the ISCEV Standards

MICHAEL F. MARMOR AND EBERHART ZRENNER (FOR THE INTERNATIONAL SOCIETY FOR CLINICAL ELECTROPHYSIOLOGY OF VISION)

CLINICAL ELECTROPHYSIOLOGISTS should be aware that international standards or guidelines exist for the major clinical electrophysiologic responses.[1,5-7,9] These standards, established and sanctioned by the International Society for Clinical Electrophysiology of Vision (ISCEV), describe a set of basic stimuli that give rise to standard responses that should be recorded whenever electrophysiologic tests are performed clinically. Other responses or protocols may be added freely at the discretion of the examiner, but the standard responses should always be included. This ensures that electrophysiologic testing will always produce a core of data that is recognizable and comparable everywhere, whether for clinical or research purposes. This program of standardization has been highly successful. Most of the publications on clinical electrophysiology in recent years display or refer to the standard responses, and the major manufacturers of clinical electroretinographic equipment have incorporated the standards into their stimulus protocols. The standards that were current at the time of writing are reprinted in this book, but these are living documents that are revised every few years. Therefore, readers are urged to check the ISCEV Web site (www.iscev.org) to see the latest versions. There is also a useful set of ISCEV-sanctioned calibration guidelines,[2] which give advice about the evaluation and calibration of equipment for electrophysiologic testing.

Clinical electrophysiological testing became practical in the middle of the twentieth century, but a wide variety of procedures were used by different laboratories to elicit responses. Some of this variability related to changing technology, as amplifiers and recording equipment improved with the advent of transistors and later computers. By the 1970s and 1980s, the major electrophysiological tests (ERG, EOG, VEP) were established procedures, but reading the clinical electrophysiological literature was still a major challenge because the tests were performed under many different conditions. The ERG, for example, was recorded in different units after different periods of dark adaptation, with different types of lenses, with different electrical filtration settings, with different intensities and durations of light flashes, and with different colors of light. To compare data among research or clinical reports was very difficult, and this impeded both clinical care and the interpretation of clinical research.

ISCEV had recognized the need for standardization at its founding in 1961,[3,9] but serious discussions of standardization did not take place until 1987, when the National Retinitis Pigmentosa Foundation (now called Foundation Fighting Blindness) joined with ISCEV to form an international committee that collated views and practices from around the world and wrote the first standard, for clinical electrophysiology (ERG), in 1989.[4]

Once published, the ERG standard had an immediate impact. Within just a few years, most clinical electrophysiology papers incorporated the standard ERG tests or described any variations in technique relative to the ISCEV standards. Data from different patients and from procedures around the world became immediately comprehensible and comparable. This success prompted ISCEV to develop standards for the EOG and VEP and then to write guidelines for newer procedures, the pattern ERG (PERG) and multifocal ERG (mfERG). Because all of the standards rely on accurate calibration of the light stimuli and of the recording equipment, ISCEV formulated a set of calibration guidelines to summarize the best available techniques.

It is important to recognize both the power and the limitation of these ISCEV standards. The standards provide a basic core of tests that can be performed with readily available instrumentation and that are relevant to the most common clinical indications for each test. However, the standards cannot cover all possible clinical situations, all variants of testing procedure, or all of the options within the technology of testing. The introduction to each of the standards or guidelines acknowledges that there are many other test, or more specialized test, that could be performed—and indeed that should be performed in certain clinical situations. The standards responses should be obtained as a part of virtually every electrophysiological testing session but not to the exclusion of other procedures that individual clinicians or laboratories may choose to do, either routinely or as an add-on for specific patients. Furthermore, the existence of standards should not stifle innovation with respect to the development of new procedures that may eventually become standards.

The ERG standard[6] was the first to be written, and it defines five basic waveforms: dark-adapted rod response, dark-adapted maximal response, oscillatory response, light-adapted cone response, and flicker cone response. These serve to separate rod and cone function, to document inner versus outer retinal function, and to allow evaluation of waveform timing. The ERG standard uses only white-light stimuli, although some laboratories use colored stimuli as well. Additional ERG procedures, such as following responses during dark adaptation or recording responses to high-intensity flashes to show photoreceptor activity more accurately, are not included at present and remain at the discretion of individual laboratories. In clinical practice, the five standard responses will suffice to answer most diagnostic questions, but they will be amended as research shows that additional or modified responses are clinically important.

The EOG standard[7] shows the basic technique for recording the standing potential across the RPE indirectly, as the voltage changes between lid canthus electrodes when the eye looks alternately left and right. The EOG response, or light response, represents the rise in this voltage in light relative to darkness. Because there have been two established ways of setting a dark baseline, the standard allows either for the recording of a dark trough (after room illumination) or for dark-adapting over a longer time to a steady baseline level.

Establishing an effective VEP standard[8] has been a challenge because of the wide variety of clinical recording conditions that are used by different laboratories for different clinical questions. Because it is impractical for a standard to have too many variations, ISCEV settled on one basic configuration of electrodes on the scalp (central inion) and three common stimulus configurations (flash, alternating pattern, on-and-off pattern). Depending on the clinical indications, at least one of these standard responses should be included as a part of every VEP examination, even if other electrode locations or other stimuli are used as well.

As the PERG was developed and its usage increased, ISCEV elected to publish a set of guidelines that represented good practice by established laboratories. After several more years of experience, clinical expectations were codified sufficiently that standards[1] could be written. In this same spirit, guidelines have now been prepared for the mfERG,[5] which

is an even newer procedure that is gaining acceptance rapidly and is proving to have many applications in clinical ophthalmology. These guidelines provide information on how to record a basic good quality mfERG and avoid artifacts. They reflect procedures that are followed by many of the major laboratories around the world, even if it is still too early to establish binding standards.

The calibration guidelines[2] that ISCEV has prepared are intended to aid electrophysiologists in the practicalities of standardizing stimulus and recording equipment. These include recommendations on how to measure stimulus luminance, check electrodes, calibrate amplifiers, and so forth. These procedures are necessary for all types of electrophysiological recordings, since a display of standard responses has little meaning unless the stimulus and recording conditions were truly what they were intended to be.

REFERENCES

1. Bach M, Hawlina M, Holder GE, Marmor M, Meigen T, Vaegan, Miyake Y: Standard for pattern electroretinography. *Doc Ophthalmol* 2000; 101:11–18.
2. Brigell M, Bach M, Barber C, Kawasaki K, Kooijman A: Guidelines for calibration of stimulus and recording parameters used in clinical electrophysiology of vision. *Doc Ophthalmol* 1998; 95:1–14.
3. International Society for Clinical Electrophysiology (ISCERG): By-laws. *Acta Ophthalmol Suppl* 1962; 70:264–268.
4. Marmor MF, Arden GB, Nilsson SE, Zrenner E: Standard for clinical electroretinography. *Arch Ophthalmol* 1989; 107:816–819.
5. Marmor MF, Hood D, Keating D, Kondo M, Seeliger M, Miyake Y (for the International Society for Clinical Electrophysiology of Vision): Guidelines for basic multifocal electroretinography (mfERG). *Doc Ophthalmol* 2003; 106:105–115.
6. Marmor MF, Zrenner E: Standard for clinical electroretinography (1999 update). *Doc Ophthalmol* 1998; 97:143–156.
7. Marmor MF, Zrenner E: Standard for clinical electrooculography. *Doc Ophthalmol* 1993; 85:115–124.
8. Odom JV, Bach M, Barber C, Brigell M, Marmor MF, Tormene AP, Holder GE: Visual evoked potentials standard (2004). *Doc Ophthalmol* 2004; 108:115–123.
9. van der Tweel LH: Some proposals for standardization of ERG equipment. *Acta Ophthalmol Suppl* 1962; 70:87–107.

20.2 EOG Standard

MICHAEL F. MARMOR AND EBERHART ZRENNER (FOR THE INTERNATIONAL SOCIETY FOR CLINICAL ELECTROPHYSIOLOGY OF VISION)

STANDARDS OF METHODOLOGY and reporting in clinical electrophysiology are important so that clinical measures of visual function can be obtained accurately, and compared accurately, anywhere in the world. In 1989 the International Society for Clinical Electrophysiology of Vision (ISCEV) developed an International Standard for the Electroretinogram (ERG) (revised in 1994)[1] and over the ensuing decade, standards or guidelines were published for the electro-oculogram (EOG)[2], pattern electroretinogram (PERG)[3], visual evoked cortical potential (VECP)[4] and the calibration of electrophysiologic equipment[5]. These standards and guidelines show how to perform the core basic procedures for each type of electrophysiologic investigation, in a manner that will give reproducible and recognizable results anywhere. However, individual laboratories may choose to supplement the Standard responses with additional specialized procedures, or to modify a protocol to meet special needs of a particular patient.

The EOG is a widely used test which measures the light response of the retinal pigment epithelium (RPE), a slow change in the voltage of the basal RPE membrane. This signal requires light reception by the retina, and is mediated by a chemical messenger that probably comes from the photoreceptors. The EOG requires integrity of the RPE membranes, but is not a pure test of RPE function since retinal photoreception is required and since the light response is not known to be correlated with any specific RPE or retinal function (including RPE water transport, visual pigment regeneration and vision). The EOG is most specific as a marker for Best's vitelliform dystrophy, a dominantly inherited macular dystrophy in which a severely depressed light response is found more consistently with the genetic abnormality than lesions in the fundus. The measured value of the EOG (the ratio of light peak amplitude to either the dark trough or dark baseline amplitude) can vary with conditions of light- and dark-adaptation, and the EOG Standard defines a range of stimulus conditions that will make results as consistent as possible. Because the essential features of an EOG response can be elicited in several ways, the Standard allows use of either dilated or undilated pupils, and the measurement of either dark trough or dark baseline. Each laboratory should choose one of these methodologies and establish a set of normal values under their own recording conditions.

The ISCEV standards for electrophysiologic tests have been highly successful in improving the quality and comparability of data reporting in the clinical literature and the EOG is no exception. However, all of these standards are subject to quadrennial review to insure that they are up-to-date and relevant clinically. A careful review of the EOG Standard was undertaken by ISCEV in 1996–7, but no changes were recommended, and the Standard was reapproved at the Asilomar, California meeting of ISCEV, on July 24, 1997.

Thus, the ISCEV EOG Standard for Clinical Electro-oculography[2] remains active as written for another four years.

REFERENCES

1. Marmor MF, Zrenner E (for the International Society for Clinical Electrophysiology of Vision): Standard for Clinical Electroretinography (1994 Update). *Doc Ophthalmol* 1995; 89:199–210.
2. Marmor MF, Zrenner E (for the International Society for Clinical Electrophysiology of Vision): Standard for clinical electro-oculography. *Doc Ophthalmol* 1993; 85:115–124.
3. Marmor MF, Holder GE, Porciatti V, Trick GI, Zrenner E (for the International Society for Clinical Electrophysiology of Vision): Guidelines for Basic Pattern Electroretinography. *Doc Ophthalmol* 1996; 91:291–298.
4. Harding GFA, Odom JV, Spileers W, Spekreijes W: Standard for Visual Evoked Potentials 1995. *Vision Research* 1996; 36:3567–3572.
5. Brigell M, Bach M, Barber C, Kawasaki K, Kooijman A: Guidelines for calibration of stimulus and recording parameters used in visual clinical electrophysiology. *Doc Ophthalmol* 1998; 95 (1):1–14.

20.3 Standard for Clinical Electroretinography*

MICHAEL F. MARMOR, GRAHAM E. HOLDER, MATHIAS W. SEELIGER, AND SHUICHI YAMAMOTO[†] (FOR THE INTERNATIONAL SOCIETY FOR CLINICAL ELECTROPHYSIOLOGY OF VISION)

Introduction

Full-field electroretinography (ERG) is a widely used ocular electrophysiologic test. In 1989 a basic protocol was standardized so that ERGs could be recorded comparably throughout the world[1]. This standard was updated most recently in 1999[2]. Standards for five commonly obtained ERGs were presented:

1. ERG to a weak flash (arising from the rods) in the dark-adapted eye
2. ERG to a strong flash in the dark-adapted eye
3. Oscillatory potentials
4. ERG to a strong flash (arising from the cones) in the light-adapted eye
5. ERGs to a rapidly repeated stimulus (flicker)

This document is an updated version of the standard. There are no major changes in the basic ERGs, but readers should note the intensity range of the "standard flash (SF)" which had been printed differently in the 1999 version. An additional dark-adapted ERG to a higher-intensity stimulus is also suggested to users, as it is now being used widely and has diagnostic value. However, it has not yet been characterized sufficiently to be considered a required part of the standard. Because the stimulus for this additional ERG is brighter than the SF, we no longer use the term "maximal" for the dark-adapted ERG to a SF.

This standard is intended as a guide to practice and to assist in interpretation of ERGs. The five basic ERGs represent the minimum of what an ERG evaluation should include. The standard describes simple technical procedures that allow reproducible ERGs to be recorded under a few defined conditions, from patients of all ages (including infants). Different procedures can provide equivalent ERGs. It is incumbent on users of alternative techniques to demonstrate that their procedures do in fact produce signals that are equivalent in basic *waveform, amplitude, and physiologic significance* to the standard.

Our intention is that the standard method and standard ERGs be used widely, but not to the exclusion of other ERGs or additional tests that individual laboratories may choose or continue to use. There are also specialized types of ERG, which may provide additional information about retinal function (see table 20. 3.1), that are not covered by this standard. We encourage electrophysiologists to learn about and try expanded test protocols and newer tests to maximize the diagnostic value of the ERG for their patients. ISCEV guidelines for the calibration of electrophysiologic equipment[3], guidelines for recording the multifocal ERG[4], and standards for the pattern ERG[5], electro-oculogram[6] and visual evoked potentials[7] have also been published.

Because of the rapid rate of change of ERG techniques, this standard will be reviewed every four years. We have made recommendations that commercial recording equipment should have the capability to record ERGs under conditions that are outside the present standard but that are nevertheless either widely used or likely to be needed in the future. Note that this document is not a safety standard, and does not mandate particular procedures for individual patients.

The organization of this report is as follows:

Basic technology
 Light diffusion
 Electrodes
 Light sources
 Light adjustment and calibration
 Electronic recording equipment
Clinical protocol
 Preparation of the patient
Specific ERGs
 Rod ERG
 Standard combined ERG

---

*This document was approved by the International Society for Clinical Electrophysiology of Vision in Nagoya, Japan on April 4, 2003.

[†]The authors represent the ERG Standardization Committee (Dr. Marmor, Chair) of the International Society for Clinical Electrophysiology of Vision (ISCEV).

Oscillatory potential
Single-flash cone ERG
30 Hz Flicker ERG
ERG measurement and reporting
Pediatric ERG recording

Basic technology

LIGHT DIFFUSION   Full-field (Ganzfeld) stimulation should be used. With focal flashes, the area of retinal illumination is not uniform, and its extent is unknown (although focal flashes may be used for certain specialized ERG tests). Full-field dome stimulators are generally preferable to ocular diffusers (e.g., 100-diopter or opalescent contact lenses) since it is difficult with the latter to measure the extent and intensity of retinal illumination. It is incumbent on manufacturers and users of lens diffusers to verify true full-field stimulation of determinable strength.

ELECTRODES

Recording electrodes   Electrodes that contact the cornea or nearby bulbar conjunctiva are strongly recommended for basic full-field recording. These include contact lens electrodes, conductive fibers and foils, conjunctival loop electrodes and corneal wicks. For most users, contact lens electrodes will provide the highest amplitude and most stable recordings; such electrodes should be centrally transparent with an optical opening as large as possible, and incorporate a device to hold the lids apart. The corneal surface should be protected during use with a non-irritating and non-allergenic ionic conductive solution that is relatively non-viscous (e.g., no more viscous than 0.5% methyl cellulose). More viscous solutions can attenuate signal amplitude. Other types of corneal and conjunctival electrodes require more skill to use but may have certain advantages. Users should be aware that signal amplitude is reduced as the point of ocular contact moves away from the corneal apex.

Topical anesthesia is necessary for contact lens electrodes but may not be required for other types of corneal and conjunctival electrodes. It is necessary that all electrophysiologists master the technical requirements of their chosen electrode, to ensure good ocular contact, to ensure proper electrode impedance, to ensure that waveforms are comparable to standard ERGs, and to define both normal values and variability (which may be different with different electrodes) for their own laboratory. Skin electrodes are not generally recommended as active recording electrodes.

Reference electrodes   Reference electrodes may be incorporated into the contact lens-speculum assembly to make contact with the conjunctiva ("bipolar electrodes"). This is the most stable configuration electrically. Alternatively, electrodes can be placed near each orbital rim temporally as a reference for the corresponding eye. The forehead has also been used as a reference electrode site, although there is a theoretical risk of signal contamination by ocular cross-over or from cortical evoked potentials. Users are advised to avoid other positions.

Ground electrodes   A separate skin electrode should be attached to an indifferent point and connected to ground. Typical locations are on the forehead or ear.

Skin reference electrode characteristics   The skin should be prepared by cleaning, and a suitable conductive paste or gel used to insure good electrical connection. Skin electrodes used for reference or ground should have $5\,k\Omega$ or less impedance measured between 10 and $100\,Hz^{3}$. If more than one skin electrode is used (e.g., for reference and ground) they should all have similar impedance.

Electrode stability   The baseline voltage in the absence of light stimulation should be stable, whatever corneal and reference electrode system is used. Some reference electrode systems may need to be made of non-polarizable material to achieve this stability.

Electrode cleaning   Recording the ERG involves the exposure of corneal electrodes to tears and exposure of the skin electrodes to blood if there has been any abrasion of the skin surface. We advise that electrodes (if not disposable) be suitably cleaned and sterilized after each use to prevent transmission of infectious agents. The cleaning protocol should follow manufacturers' recommendations and current national standards for devices that contact skin and tears.

LIGHT SOURCES

Stimulus duration   The standard is based on stimuli of duration considerably shorter than the integration time of any photoreceptor. Thus, the light stimulus should consist of flashes having a maximum duration of about 5 ms.

Stimulus wavelength Most flash stimuli in use have a color temperature near 7000°K, and they should be used with domes or diffusers that are visibly white. Colored filters can be used to enhance the separation of rod and cone ERGs, but this is not part of the standard [Note 1].

Stimulus strength–standard flash A standard flash (SF) is defined as one of stimulus strength (in luminous energy per square meter) at the surface of the Ganzfeld bowl of 1.5–3.0 photopic $cd \cdot s \cdot m^{-2}$ (candela-seconds per meter squared) [Note 2]. This is equivalent to luminance·time, measured as $cd \cdot m^{-2} \cdot s$. Note that these are photometric units and that 3.43 $cd \cdot m^{-2} = 1\,fL$ (foot-Lambert).

Background illumination In addition to producing flashes, the stimulator must be capable of producing a steady and even background luminance of $17-34\,cd \cdot m^{-2}$ (5 to 10 fL) across the full field. A white background is used for this standard, but we recognize that colored backgrounds may also be used for special purposes.

LIGHT ADJUSTMENT AND CALIBRATION

Adjustment of stimulus and background intensity Methods of modifying both the stimulus and background intensity must be provided. We recommend that a recording system be capable of attenuating flash strength from the SF over a range of at least 3 log units, either continuously or in steps of not more than 0.3 log unit. The method of attenuation should not change the wavelength composition of either the flash or background luminance. We recognize that the stimulus and background requirements for a full range of other ERG tests will be more extensive and more stringent, and we recommend that equipment manufacturers exceed the minimum standard [Note 3].

Stimulus and background calibration The stimulus strength (in luminance·time) produced by each flash within the full-field stimulus bowl must be documented by the user or manufacturer, ideally with an integrating photometer (luminance meter) placed at the location of the eye. The light output per flash of most stroboscopes varies with the flash repetition rate; therefore, separate calibrations will need to be made for single and repetitive stimuli. The photometer should also record the background luminance of the stimulus bowl's surface, in a non-integrating mode. The photometer must meet international standards for photometric measurements based on the photopic luminous efficiency function (photopic luminosity curve), and must be capable of recording the total output of very brief flashes. Users should consult the ISCEV guidelines for calibration of electrophysiologic equipment[3] for a more detailed treatment of calibration procedures. We recommend that manufacturers of stimulators supply a suitable photometer with their equipment.

Recalibration See the ISCEV guidelines for calibration[3]. Light output from the dome varies with time from changes in the flash tube, the tube power source, line voltage, the background light bulbs, the attenuation systems, or the paint in the dome. This may be especially critical for background illumination provided by incandescent sources. Responsibility for electronic stability and warnings about sources of instability should rest with the manufacturers of the equipment; however, at present this cannot be presumed. A stabilizing transformer will minimize line voltage variations if they are a problem. The frequency with which recalibration of flashes and backgrounds is required will vary from system to system and could be as high as weekly for some units. Self-calibrating units are encouraged.

ELECTRONIC RECORDING EQUIPMENT

Amplification We recommend that the bandpass of the amplifier and preamplifiers include at least the range of 0.3 to 300 Hz and be adjustable for oscillatory potential recordings and special requirements. We advise that the input impedance of the preamplifiers be at least 10 MΩ. Amplifiers should generally be AC (alternating current) coupled (i.e., capacitively coupled) and capable of handling offset potentials that may be produced by the electrodes [Note 4].

Patient isolation We recommend that the patient be electrically isolated according to current standards for safety of clinical biologic recording systems in the user's country.

Display of data and averaging We strongly recommend that the equipment that provides the final record be able to represent, without attenuation, the full amplifier bandpass. Good resolution can be achieved with oscilloscopes or computer-aided (digitizing) systems but not with direct pen recorders. To avoid a loss of information, digitizers should sample ERGs at a rate of 1 kHz or higher per channel. With computer-aided systems, it is important that ERG waveforms be displayed promptly so that the operator can continuously monitor stability and make adjustments during the test procedure. Recording units that digitize ERG signals can usually average them as well, which may sometimes be useful.

Clinical protocol

PREPARATION OF THE PATIENT

Pupillary dilation We recommend that pupils be maximally dilated for all ERG recordings in this standard and that pupil size be noted.

Pre-adaptation to light or dark The recording conditions outlined below specify 20 min of dark adaptation before recording rod ERGs, and 10 min of light adaptation before recording cone ERGs. The choice of whether to begin with scotopic or photopic conditions is up to the user, as long as these adaptation requirements are met. If contact lens electrodes are used, the wearing time can be minimized by dark adapting first, and inserting the electrodes under dim red light at the end of the adaptation period. However, care should be used to avoid too bright a red light, and an additional 5 min of dark adaptation may be needed for recovery after lens insertion.

Pre-exposure to light   We advise that fluorescein angiography or fundus photography be avoided before ERG testing, but if these examinations have been performed, a period of dark adaptation of at least one hour is needed. It is usually preferable to record scotopic ERGs to weak flashes before the mixed and cone ERGs to more intense flashes, to minimize light adaptation, and to reduce the time that the patient wears an electrode.

Fixation   A fixation point should be incorporated into stimulus domes. A stable eye is important so that eye movements do not alter the optimal corneal electrode position, produce electrical artifacts, or allow blockage of light by the electrode or eyelid. Patients who cannot see a fixation target may be instructed to look straight ahead and keep their eyes steady. Patients should be monitored to assess compliance, and account for difficulties in eye opening or fixation.

Specific ERGs

Rod ERG   We recommend that the patient be dark-adapted for at least 20 min before recording the rod system ERG (and longer if the patient had been exposed to unusually bright light). The rod ERG should be the first signal measured after dark adaptation, since it is the most sensitive to light adaptation. The recommended stimulus is a dim white flash of strength 2.5 log units below the white SF (see above); we advise a minimum interval of 2 s between flashes. A blue stimulus is equally appropriate if equated to the white standard [Note 1].

Standard Combined ERG   The standard ERG from combined rod and cone systems is produced by the white SF in the dark-adapted eye. We recommend an interval of at least 10 s between stimuli. This ERG is normally produced by a combination of cone and rod systems.

Higher-Intensity ERG (Suggested Only)   Since publication of the last version of the ERG standard, the origins of ERG components have become better understood. It has become apparent that only the first 10–20 ms of the *a*-wave reflect photoreceptor activity. A number of laboratories have found that the dark-adapted *a*-wave is shown more clearly with the use of a brighter stimulus than the SF (approximately $10 \, cd \cdot s/m^2$). Measurement of both *a*-wave ampli-

tude and implicit time is simpler as there is generally a very well-defined single peak. There is not yet sufficient experience or universality of usage to mandate this ERG as a required part of the ERG standard, but users should be aware of its increasing acceptance and value, and consider adding it to their protocols after the standard combined ERG. An interval of 20 s is recommended between flashes of this intensity.

Oscillatory Potentials   Oscillatory potentials are generally obtained from the dark-adapted eye, using the same white SF. They may also be recorded from the light-adapted eye. The high-pass filter must be reset to 75 to 100 Hz, so that an overall bandpass of 75 to 100 Hz on the low end and 300 Hz or above at the high end is achieved. Filters should attenuate sufficiently to achieve this result. Users should be aware that there are several types of electronic and digital filters, which may have different effects upon physiologic signals (e.g., phase shifts or ringing). More information about filter selection and use is presented in the ISCEV guidelines for calibration[3].

The oscillatory potentials vary with stimulus repetition rate and change after the first stimulus. To standardize the oscillatory potentials, we recommend that white SF stimuli be given 15 s apart to the dark-adapted eyes (1.5 s apart to light-adapted eyes), and that only the second or subsequent waveforms be retained or averaged. The conditions of adaptation should be reported.

Single-Flash Cone ERG   We propose the white SF as the stimulus, and advise that to achieve stable and reproducible cone system ERGs the rods be suppressed by a background with a luminance of 17 to 34 $cd \cdot m^{-2}$ (5 to 10 fL) measured at the surface of the full-field stimulus bowl. We recommend that the higher value of the background be chosen if the stimulus flash is at the upper end of the allowable SF range and the lower background value chosen if the flash stimulus is at the lower end of the range. We recommended that patients light-adapt to the background luminance for at least 10 min before recording the cone ERG, since the cone ERGs may increase during this period. Stimuli should not be repeated at intervals less than 0.5 s. Note that the term "single-flash cone ERG" is used to distinguish this signal from flicker ERGs; it does not preclude averaging (if necessary) to improve the signal-to-noise ratio.

30-Hz Flicker ERGs   Flicker ERGs also represent the cone system, and should be obtained with SF stimuli, under the same conditions of light-adaptation as the single-flash cone ERG. Recording the flicker ERG in the light-adapted state reduces discomfort and allows the photopic adaptation to be standardized. We advise strongly that flashes be presented at a rate of approximately 30 stimuli per second, and the rate that is chosen should be constant for the laboratory. The first ERG to the flickering stimulus will be a single-flash waveform; thus, the first few waveforms should be discarded so that stable conditions are reached. Some flash tubes do not produce full output while flickering, and separate calibration or a change in neutral density filtering may be needed to keep as closely as possible to the standard.

ERG Measurements and Recording

Measurement of the ERG   In general, *b*-wave amplitude and time-to-peak (implicit time) should be measured for all ERGs (except oscillatory potentials), and the *a*-wave should also be measured when recognizable as a distinct component. According to current convention, the *a*-wave amplitude is measured from baseline to *a*-wave trough, the *b*-wave amplitude is measured from *a*-wave trough to *b*-wave peak, and the *b*-wave time-to-peak is measured from the time of the flash to the peak of the wave (see figure 20.3.1).

Oscillatory potentials   There is considerable debate in the literature about how to measure and describe oscillatory potentials [Note 5]. Their appearance is highly dependent upon stimulus conditions, adaptation and amplifier filter characteristics, but most authors describe three major peaks often followed by a fourth smaller one. Simply observing the presence of these peaks, and their normality relative to the standards of the laboratory, may be adequate for many clinical purposes at our present state of knowledge.

Averaging   Averaging is not ordinarily required to record quantifiable ERGs with the recommended types of electrodes. Averaging a limited number of ERGs may decrease variability and help to reduce background noise if present. Averaging may also be used to identify and measure very weak pathologic ERGs. Artifact rejection must be a part of any averaging system. Signal repetition rates should not exceed the recommendations in the standard for each type of ERG.

Normal values   We recommend that each laboratory establish or confirm normal values for its own equipment and patient population giving attention to an appropriate sample size. All ERG reporting (whether for local records, publication, or even for nonstandard ERGs) should include normal values and the *limits of normal*. Some manufacturers distribute norms for their standard protocols, and several large series have been published recently that give normative data. However, ERG norms for amplitude may have to be scaled up or down depending on where the user's electrode rests on cornea or conjunctiva. Note that ERG parameters change rapidly during infancy and modestly with age thereafter. Because some ERG parameters (such as *b*-wave amplitude) are not necessarily normally distributed, calculations of standard deviation may be misleading. To describe the limits of normal, we recommend listing the median value (not the mean), and the actual values on either side of the median that bracket 95% of the normal ERGs (in other words, the 95% confidence limits determined by direct tabulation of ERGs). Although circadian variations of the ERG appear to be small under ordinary recording conditions, we recommend that the time of ERG recording be noted on all records since it could become relevant for certain diseases or repeat measurements.

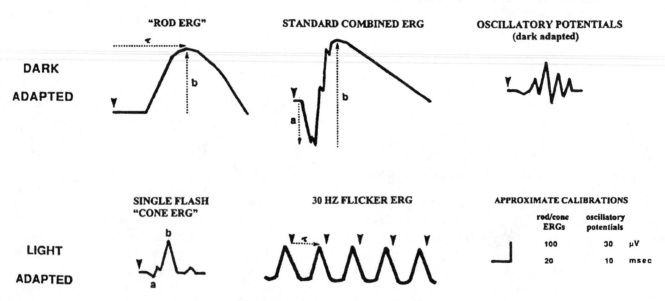

FIGURE 20.3.1   Diagram of the five basic ERGs defined by the Standard. These waveforms are exemplary only, and are not intended to indicate minimum, maximum or even average values. Large arrowheads indicate the stimulus flash. Dotted arrows exemplify how to measure time-to-peak (*t*, implicit time), *a*-wave amplitude and *b*-wave amplitude.

Reporting the ERG Standardization of ERG reporting is critical to the goal of having comparable data worldwide. We recommend that reports or communications of ERG data include representative waveforms of each of the standard ERGs displayed with amplitude and time calibrations and labeled with respect to stimulus variables and the state of light or dark adaptation. We suggest that when single flash stimuli are used without averaging, two waveforms of each ERG be displayed to demonstrate the degree of consistency or variability. The strength of stimulation (cd·s·m⁻²) and the level of light adaptation (cd·m⁻²) should be given in absolute values. *The reporting forms should indicate whether the techniques of recording meet the international standard.* We recommend that patient measurements be listed along with normal values and their variances (that must be provided on all reports). Finally, reports should note the time of testing, pupillary diameter, and any conditions that are not specified by the standard, including type and position of electrode, sedation or anesthesia, and the level of compliance.

Pediatric ERG recording

The ERG can be recorded from infants and young children but some care must be taken to account for immature eyes and limited cooperation.

Sedation or Anesthesia Most pediatric subjects can be studied without sedation or general anesthesia (topical anesthesia is necessary for contact lens electrodes). Small infants can be restrained if necessary. Uncompliant children (especially ages 2–6 for whom containment can be difficult) may become compliant with oral sedation or anxiolysis. Medical guidelines should be followed with respect to indications, risks, medical monitoring requirements and the choice of a sedative/relaxant versus general anesthesia. Considering the variability of pediatric records, there will generally be little effect on ERG amplitude or waveform with sedation or brief very light anesthesia, although full anesthesia may modify the ERG.

Electrodes Contact lens electrodes are applicable to infants and young children, but pediatric sizes will be required with speculum-containing models, and care must be used to minimize corneal and psychological trauma. Non-contact lens and skin electrodes vary in their applicability to children, and their greater comfort is often offset by greater movement or small signals that create difficulty with electrical noise or artifacts. Special care is required with children to monitor electrode position and compliance in order to avoid artifactual recordings.

Normal Values and Measurement The ERG matures during infancy, and newborn and infant signals must be interpreted with great caution. Later infantile and young childhood ERGs approach adult waveform and size. Pediatric ERGs should ideally be compared to those from normal subjects of the same age, even though there may be little normative data available. Because movement and poor fixation can make pediatric records variable in amplitude and waveform, we recommend that several repetitions of each ERG be recorded in order to recognize reproducible waveforms and choose the best examples. Standard protocols may occasionally need to be abbreviated in order to obtain the ERGs most critical to the diagnostic question under investigation. More intense stimuli may sometimes help to reveal poorly developed ERGs. Reports should note the degree of cooperation and any medications used.

Notes

1. Chromatic stimuli offer certain advantages in the separation of cone and rod ERGs, but the calibration of colored stimuli and the relation of the ERGs produced by them to the standard ERG requires special procedures. We recommend that white flashes be used for the standard ERGs, whether or not other stimuli are used in addition.

2. White stimuli produced by a combination of narrow band sources, such as red, green and blue light-emitting diodes (LEDs), may not be equivalent to broad-band white light as a stimulus for rods and cones. Manufacturers must ensure that appropriate photopic and scotopic filters are incorporated into their stimulation and calibration systems so that stimulus output is of equivalent intensity to the standard for all conditions. Separate scotopic calibration may be necessary for these LED systems, and if so the proper stimulus for eliciting rod ERGs will be 2.5 log units below a scotopically-calibrated standard flash.

3. We recommend that the flash source of commercial instruments be capable of generating strengths at least 2 log units above the SF and be attenuable through 6 log units below the SF. Regardless of whether attenuation is achieved by filters or electronic means, we also strongly recommend that commercial units incorporate a means of inserting additional colored and neutral density filters. These capabilities will allow electrophysiologists to perform a variety of useful protocols beyond the Standard, and meet possible future changes in the Standard. We also suggest that background luminance be adjustable to perform electro-oculography with the same equipment. Commercial units should also allow the insertion of colored and neutral filters into the background illumination system to meet a variety of needs.

4. DC (direct-current) amplification can produce signals identical to those from AC amplification, but it is extremely difficult to use because of drift in baseline and offset potentials; we strongly advise AC recording except for laboratories with special requirements and expertise.

5. An overall index of oscillatory potential amplitude can be obtained by adding up measurements of the three major peaks, preferably from lines spanning the bases of the adjacent troughs, but alternatively from the adjacent troughs directly (to allow use of measuring cursors with digitized systems). Some authors advise measurement of individual peaks.

REFERENCES

1. Marmor MF, Arden GB, Nilsson SE, Zrenner E: Standard for clinical electroretinography. *Arch Ophthalmol* 1989; 107:816–819.
2. Marmor MF, Zrenner E (for the International Society for Clinical Electrophysiology of Vision): Standard for Clinical Electroretinography (1999 Update). *Doc Ophthalmol* 1999; 97:143–156.
3. Brigell M, Bach M, Barber C, Moskowitz A, Robson J: Guidelines for calibration of stimulus and recording parameters used in clinical electrophysiology of vision (Revised 2002). *Doc Ophthalmol* 2003; 107:185–193.
4. Marmor MF, Hood DC, Keating D, Kondo M, Seeliger MW, Miyake Y (for the International Society for Clinical Electrophysiology of Vision): Guidelines for basic multifocal electroretinography (mfERG). *Doc Ophthalmol* 2003; 106:105–115.
5. Marmor MF, Holder GE, Porciatti V, Trick GI, Zrenner E (for the International Society for Clinical Electrophysiology of Vision): Guidelines for basic pattern electroretinography. *Doc Ophthalmol* 1996; 91:291–298.
6. Marmor MF, Zrenner E (for the International Society for Clinical Electrophysiology of Vision): Standard for clinical electro-oculography. *Arch Ophthalmol* 1993; 111:601–604.
7. Odom JV, Bach M, Barber C, Brigell M, Holder G, Marmor MF, Tormene AP, Vaegen: Visual evoked potentials standard. *Doc Ophthalmol* 2004; 108:115–123.

Note: Printed reprints of this standard are not available, but the document is available on the ISCEV website <www.iscev.org>.

20.4 Standard for Pattern Electroretinography

MICHAEL BACH, MARKO HAWLINA, GRAHAM E. HOLDER, MICHAEL F. MARMOR, THOMAS MEIGEN, VAEGAN, AND YOZO MIYAKE (FOR THE INTERNATIONAL SOCIETY FOR CLINICAL ELECTROPHYSIOLOGY OF VISION)

Introduction

The pattern electroretinogram (PERG) is a retinal biopotential that is evoked when a temporally modulated patterned stimulus of constant total luminance (checkerboard or grating) is viewed. The PERG is most often evoked by alternating reversal of a checkerboard pattern. It may be altered in dysfunction of the macula or of the inner retina selectively, which do not significantly affect the conventional full-field ERG. The PERG receives clinical and research attention in both neurological and ophthalmological practice. However, the PERG is a very small signal, typically in the region of 0.5–8 μV depending on stimulus characteristics, and PERG recording is technically more demanding than the conventional ERG. Recordings published in the literature vary considerably in technical quality as well as technique, and new users may find it difficult to choose which technique to use.

The International Society for Clinical Electrophysiology of Vision (ISCEV) feels that there is now a sufficient body of knowledge and clinical experience to propose a standard for performing a basic PERG. This document evolved from the "PERG Guidelines"[1] and is intended as a guide to practice and to assist in interpretation of PERGs. Transient PERG as described below represents the minimum of what a PERG evaluation should include. The standard describes simple technical procedures that allow reproducible PERGs to be recorded under a few defined conditions. Different procedures may provide equivalent PERG responses. It is incumbent on users of alternative techniques to demonstrate that their procedures do in fact produce signals that are equivalent in basic waveform, amplitude, and physiologic significance to the standard. Our intention is that the standard method and responses be used widely, but not to the exclusion of other paradigms that individual laboratories may use, tailored to their own requirements.

The standard is based upon equipment and analytic capabilities currently found in most neurophysiological or ophthalmological electrodiagnostic clinics. This document addresses recording conditions and technology specific to the PERG, and presumes that readers already have basic understanding and skills in clinical electrophysiology. Although much of this document will apply equally to adults and children, the standard is not necessarily appropriate to paediatric applications. The standard will be reviewed by ISCEV every four years.

Waveform nomenclature and measurement

The waveform of the PERG evoked by pattern-reversal stimuli depends on the temporal frequency of the stimulus. By convention, positivity is displayed upward.

TRANSIENT PERG At low temporal frequencies (6 reversals per second or less, equivalent to 3 Hz or less) a transient PERG is obtained (figure 20.4.1). The waveform is characterised by a small initial negative (N) component, at approximately 35 ms, which will be referred to as N35. This is followed by a later and larger positive (P) component (45–60 ms) which is typically denoted as P50. This positive portion of the waveform is followed by a large negative component at about 90–100 ms (N95).

For the transient PERG, amplitude measurements are made between peaks and troughs: The P50 amplitude is measured from the trough of N35 to the peak of P50. In some patients the N35 is poorly defined; in these cases N35 is replaced by the average between time zero and the onset of P50. The N95 amplitude is measured from the peak of P50 to the trough of N95. It should be recognised that measured in this way, N95 includes the P50 amplitude.

Latency measurements should be taken from the onset of the stimulus to the peak of the component concerned; inexperienced workers should note that the highest absolute amplitude point on a waveform will not always be appropriate for the definition of the peak if there is contamination from muscle activity or other artifacts. The peak should be designated where it would appear on a smoothed or idealised waveform.

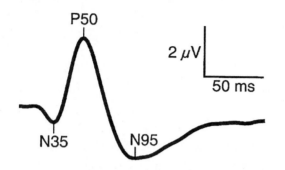

FIGURE 20.4.1 Transient PERG. Parameters: check size 0.8°, field size 15° × 15°, contrast 98%, mean luminance 45 cd/m², 4.5 reversals/s.

STEADY-STATE PERG At higher temporal frequencies, i.e. above 10 rev/s (5 Hz), the successive waveforms overlap and a "steady-state" PERG is evoked. The waveform becomes roughly sinusoidal, and Fourier analysis is required to determine the amplitude and temporal phase shift (relative to the stimulus).

Basic technology

ELECTRODES

Recording electrodes Electrodes that contact the cornea or nearby bulbar conjunctiva are recommended. This does not include contact lens electrodes or any other electrodes that degrade image quality on the retina. Thin conductive fibres, foils and loops can usually be positioned without topical anaesthesia. Those who perform the test should be aware of possible causes of artifact. Electrode integrity should be checked prior to insertion, to meet guidelines for each electrode type. Note: Some instruments can cause patient harm when impedance is measured *in situ*. Electrodes should be carefully positioned to minimise instability (a major source of artifact or interference).

• Fibre electrodes should be placed in the lower fornix. Draping the electrode across the lower eyelashes at the medial canthus, or taping it to the cheek, may help to stabilise it.

• Foil electrodes should be positioned directly under the centre of the pupil so that there is minimal or no movement of the electrode when the patient blinks. This is best achieved by having the foil curve over the lower eyelashes without contacting them, and then tethering the lead to the cheek. The junction of the electrode and lead should form as straight a line as possible and the junction should not touch the skin.

• Loop electrodes should be hooked into the lower fornix. Loops should be folded so that the contact windows on otherwise insulated wire are positioned on the bulbar conjunc-

tiva, about 5 mm under the limbus. Loop electrodes should not touch the cornea. To achieve this, the limbs of the loop should be diverged widely (15–20 mm) before entering the fornix. The lead is then taped to the cheek.

The appropriate techniques for individual electrode types are very important to achieve stable and reproducible PERG recordings. Additional sources should be consulted in relation to the specific electrode used.

Reference electrodes Surface reference electrodes should be placed at the ipsilateral outer canthi. Mastoid, earlobe or forehead locations may result in contamination of the PERG from cortical potentials or the fellow eye. If monocular PERG recording is performed, the electrode in the occluded eye may be used as a reference.

Ground electrodes A separate surface electrode should be attached and connected to the amplifier "ground input"; the forehead would be a typical location.

Surface electrode characteristics The impedance between the skin electrodes used for reference and ground, measured on the subject, should be less than 5 kΩ. The skin should be prepared with a suitable cleaning agent, and a suitable conductive paste should be used to ensure good electrical connection. Since the electrode in the eye will have a very low impedance, low impedance of the reference electrode is especially important for optimal rejection of (common-mode) electrical interference.

Electrode cleaning and sterilisation See ISCEV Standard for full-field flash ERG[2].

STIMULUS PARAMETERS This standard outlines only a basic protocol for PERG recording. Laboratories may choose to test more conditions or parameters than are described herein.

Field and check size For the "basic PERG", we recommend using a black and white reversing checkerboard with a stimulus field size between 10° and 16°, and a check size of approximately 0.8°. For some applications, such as glaucoma assessment, a larger extent such as 30° may be more appropriate.

Contrast For the "basic PERG" the contrast between black and white squares should be maximal (close to 100%) and not less than 80%.

Luminance PERGs are difficult to record with low stimulus luminance, and a photopic luminance level for the white areas of greater than 80 c.d.m⁻² is recommended. Overall screen luminance must not vary during checkerboard reversals.

Frame rate   Raster-based CRTs are typically used to present the pattern stimuli. The frame rate of the CRT is a significant stimulus parameter for PERUs, and a frequency of 75 Hz or greater is recommended.

Background illumination   The luminance of the background beyond the checkerboard field is not critical when using the suggested PERG technique as long as dim or ordinary room lighting is used; ambient lighting should be the same for all recordings. Care should be taken to keep bright lights out of the subjects' direct view.

Transient and steady-state recording   As a "basic PERG" protocol, we recommend that laboratories record the transient PERG as it allows separation of the P50 and N95 components.

There are also situations in which the steady-state PERG is useful; some laboratories favour it for glaucoma studies. Since little extra time is required, laboratories should consider recording it as well. Keep in mind, however, that the proper interpretation of steady-state PERGs requires measurement of amplitude and phase shift (relative to the stimulus) of the second harmonic by Fourier analysis. A significant first harmonic indicates technical problems. We do not recommend steady-state PERG recording without instrumentation for such analysis, and we caution that steady-state stimulation at reversal rates below our recommendation (16 rev/s) requires special equipment to modulate contrast sinusoidally.

Reversal rate   For transient PERG we recommend 2–6 reversals per second (1–3 Hz); for steady-state PERG, we recommend 16 reversals per second (8 Hz).

Recalibration   We advise regular stimulus recalibration[3].

RECORDING EQUIPMENT
Amplification systems   AC-coupled amplifiers with a minimum input impedance of 10 MΩ are recommended. Amplification systems should be electrically isolated from the patient according to the current standards for safety of biologic recording systems used clinically. We recommend that the frequency response of bandpass amplifiers should include the range from 1–100 Hz, and that notch filters (that suppress signals at the alternating current line frequency) not be used.

Some users may encounter severe electromagnetic interference that makes it difficult to obtain responses with these filter recommendations. Ideally, such interference should be eliminated by shielding or modifying equipment; rearranging the electrode leads may be of benefit.

Laboratories using stronger filtering or a notch filter must recognise that their responses may not be comparable to those from other laboratories, and should note in reports that extra filtering was applied.

Averaging and signal analysis   Because of the small amplitude of the PERG, signal averaging is always necessary. For transient PERGs the analysis period (sweep time) should be 150 ms or greater. A Fourier analysis program will be needed if steady-state PERGs are to be recorded, and the analysis period must be a multiple of the stimulus interval (e.g. 8).

Artifact rejection   Computerised artifact rejection is essential, and we recommend that this should be set at no higher than 100 μV peak-to-peak, and preferable less. The amplifiers must return to baseline rapidly following artifactual signals to avoid inadvertent storage of non-physiological data.

Data display systems   Display systems must have adequate resolution to represent accurately the characteristics of this small amplitude signal. Optimal conditions allow for simultaneous display of input signal and average. In the absence of a simultaneous display, the system should allow a rapid alternation between input signal display and average display. Thus the quality of the input signal can adequately be monitored. Even with a computerised artifact rejection system, it is important that the input signal be monitored for baseline stability and the absence of amplifier blocking.

Clinical protocol

PREPARATION OF THE PATIENT
Positioning   The patient should be positioned as comfortable as possible and leaning against a head-rest.

Pupils   The PERG should be recorded without dilatation of the pupils, to preserve accommodation and thus retinal image quality.

Fixation   A fixation spot in the centre of the screen is essential. If there are any doubts about the quality of fixation in an individual patient, an effective method is to give the patient a pointer and have them point at the middle of the screen throughout.

Excessive blinking during recording should be discouraged, pauses may be advantageous.

Refraction   Because of the nature of the stimulus, PERG examination should be performed with optimal visual acuity at the testing distance. Patients should wear the appropriate optical correction for the test distances.

Monocular and binocular recording   Proper positioning of recording and reference electrodes will permit either monocular or binocular recording of the PERG. Binocular recording of the PERG is recommended for the "basic PERG" because it is generally more stable, it reduces examination time and it allows fixation by the better eye in cases of asymmetric visual loss. Monocular stimulation is required to simultaneously record the PERG and the VEP.

Recording Typically, 150 responses should be averaged, and more may be needed with a "noisy" subject. At least two full recordings of each stimulus condition should be obtained to confirm responses (i.e. one replication).

PERG REPORTING

Reporting It is recommended that all reports contain measurements of P50 and N95 amplitude (see above), and P50 latency (the peak of N95 is often rather broad precluding accurate latency measurement of this component). If steady-state PERGs are performed, amplitude and phase shift of the second harmonic should be reported. All reports should also contain the stimulus parameters and the normal values for the laboratory concerned. Whenever practical, reporting of PERG results should include representative waveforms with appropriate amplitude and time calibrations.

Clinical norms Each laboratory should establish normal values for its own equipment and patient population. It should be noted that there are PERG changes with age.

REFERENCES

1. Marmor MF, Holder GE, Porciatti V, Trick GL, Zrenner E: Guidelines for basic pattern electroretinography. Recommendations by the International Society for Clinical Electrophysiology of Vision. *Doc Ophthalmol* 1996; 91:291–298.
2. Marmor MF, Zrenner E: Standard for clinical electroretinography (1999 update). *Doc Ophthalmol* 1999; 97:143–156.
3. Brigell M, Bach M, Barber C, Kawasaki K, Kooijman A: Guidelines for calibration of stimulus and recording parameters used in clinical electrophysiology of vision. *Doc Ophthalmol* 1998; 95:1–14.

Note: This document is available on the ISCEV website <www.iscev.org>.

20.5 Visual Evoked Potentials Standard*

J. VERNON ODOM, MICHAEL BACH, COLIN BARBER, MITCHELL BRIGELL, MICHAEL F. MARMOR, ALMA PATRIZIA TORMENE, GRAHAM E. HOLDER, AND VAEGAN (FOR THE INTERNATIONAL SOCIETY FOR THE CLINICAL ELECTROPHYSIOLOGY OF VISION)

Introduction

This document presents the current (2004) standard for the visual evoked potential (VEP). The VEP is an evoked electrophysiological potential that can be extracted, using signal averaging, from the electroencephalographic activity recorded at the scalp. The VEP can provide important diagnostic information regarding the functional integrity of the visual system.

The current standard presents basic responses elicited by three commonly used stimulus conditions using a single, midline recording channel with an occipital, active electrode. Because chiasmal and retrochiasmal diseases may be missed using a single channel, three channels using the midline and two lateral active electrodes are suggested when one goes beyond the standard and tests patients for chiasmal and retrochiasmal dysfunction.

Pattern reversal is the preferred technique for most clinical purposes. The results of pattern reversal stimuli are less variable in waveform and timing than the results elicited by other stimuli. The pattern onset/offset technique can be useful in the detection of malingering and in patients with nystagmus, and the flash VEP is particularly useful when optical factors or poor cooperation make the use of pattern stimulation inappropriate. The intent of this standard is that *at least one* of these techniques should be included in *every* clinical VEP recording session so that all laboratories will have a common core of information that can be shared or compared.

Having stated this goal, we also recognize that VEPs may be elicited by other stimuli, including moving, colored, spatially localized, or rapidly changing stimuli. These stimuli may be used to stimulate neural subsystems or to assist in localizing visual field defects. VEPs may be recorded using a full montage of electrodes covering all head regions to enable source localization. In addition to the commonly used technique of signal averaging, a variety of procedures including kernel analysis and Fourier analysis may be used to extract the VEP from background EEG activity. Some of these specialized VEPs, not covered by the standard, are listed in table 20.5.1. Equipment manufacturers are encouraged to produce equipment that can perform as many of these specialized tests as possible. We particularly encourage the ability to record a minimum of five channels.

It is clear that this standard does not incorporate the full range of possibilities of VEP recording. However, in adopting the current standard for VEPs, the society, following a principle established in earlier standards[1–5], has selected a subset of stimulus and recording conditions which provide core clinical information and which can be performed by most of the world's clinical laboratories.

By limiting the standard conditions, the intention is that the standard method and responses will be incorporated *universally* into VEP protocols *along with* more specialized techniques (table 20.5.1) that a laboratory may chose to use. The standard does not require that all stimuli should be used for every investigation on every patient. In most circumstances a single stimulus type will be appropriate. However, it is not the purpose of the standards to impede research progress, which might demonstrate that other tests are of equal or greater usefulness. This standard will be reviewed periodically and revised as needed.

The organization of this report is as follows:

Basic Technology
1. Stimulus parameters
   A. Pattern stimulus
      i. Pattern reversal stimulus
      ii. Pattern onset/offset stimulus
   B. Flash stimulus
2. Electrodes
   A. Electrode placement
3. Recording parameters
   A. Amplification and averaging systems
   B. Analysis time

*This document was approved by the International Society for Clinical Electrophysiology of Vision in Nagoya, Japan, on April 4, 2003.

TABLE 20.5.1

Some specialized types of VEP not covered by the ISCEV standard

- Steady state VEP
- Sweep VEP
- Motion VEP
- Chromatic (Color) VEP
- Binocular (dichoptic) VEP
- Stereo-elicited VEP
- Multi-channel VEP
- Hemi-field VEP
- Multifocal VEP
- Multi-frequency VEP
- LED Goggle VEP

Clinical Protocol

1. Preparation of the patient
2. Description of the three standard transient responses
   A. Pattern reversal VEP
   B. Pattern onset/offset VEP
   C. Flash VEP
3. Pediatric VEP recording
4. Multi-channel recording for assessment of the central visual pathways
5. VEP measurement and reporting
   A. Normal values
   B. VEP reporting
   C. VEP interpretation

Basic technology

STIMULUS PARAMETERS   There are two major classes of VEP stimulation, luminance and pattern. Luminance stimulation is usually delivered as a uniform flash of light and pattern stimulation may be either presented in a reversal or onset-offset fashion. The reader may refer to the ISCEV Calibration Guidelines[4] for further information regarding the measurement and definition of stimulus parameters.

Standard stimulus and recording conditions are described below and are summarized in table 20.5.2.

PATTERN STIMULUS   The recommended patterned stimulus is a black and white checkerboard. The stimulus should be defined by the visual angle subtended by the side of a single check. Visual angle is measured in degrees and minutes of arc subtended at the eye. All checks should be square and there should be an equal number of light and dark checks. Measurement of the physical check size in inches or millimeters should never be used to describe them.

Pattern stimulus luminance should be measured in candelas per meter squared ($cd \cdot m^{-2}$). The luminance of the white areas should be at least $80 \, cd \cdot m^{-2}$. The mean luminance should be uniform between the center and the periphery of the field. We recognize that some optical and electronic systems do not provide truly uniform fields and may vary by up to 30%. We encourage those following the standards to use systems that come as close to uniform as possible. The surround of the stimulus should be homogenously lit, with an average luminance equal to or below the average stimulus luminance. Practically, this can be achieved by subdued room lighting with no bright sources visible to the subject.

The Michelson contrast ($\{[L_{max} - L_{min}] / [L_{max} + L_{min}]\} \times 100$) should be at least 75%, where L = luminance, max = maximum and min = minimum. The stimulus field size should be expressed in degrees of visual angle, with an indication of field shape, i.e., rectangular field a deg × b deg or a circular field of c deg diameter or radius. The location of the fixation point should also be defined in relation to this field; i.e., in the center or d deg to the left or right of the center. The fixation point should be positioned at the corner of 4 checks when located at the center of the field.

Pattern reversal stimulus   The pattern reversal stimulus consists of black and white checks that change phase (i.e., black to white and white to black) abruptly and repeatedly at a specified number of reversals per second. There must be no overall change in the luminance of the screen. This requires equal numbers of light and dark elements in the display. Background luminance of screen and room should approximate the mean for onset/offset of each check. The stimulus should be defined in terms of the visual angle of each check, the reversal frequency, the number of reversals, the mean luminance the pattern contrast and the field size. For standard responses, at least two pattern element sizes should be used: 1 deg and 15 min per side checks. The visual field diameter should exceed 15 deg in its narrowest dimension. Reversal rates between 1 and 3 reversals per second (i.e., 0.5–1.5 Hz) should be used to elicit the standard pattern reversal response. The lower portion of this range is preferred. Stimulus rate should be reported in reversals per second to avoid the potential confusion related to the number of cycles (Hz) of a reversal stimulus being half of the number of reversals per second.

Pattern onset/offset stimulus   For pattern onset/offset a pattern is abruptly exchanged with a diffuse background. The pattern stimulus should be defined in terms of the visual angle of each check. At least two pattern element sizes should be used: checks of 1 deg and 15 min per side. The visual field stimulated should exceed 15 deg. The mean luminance of the diffuse blank screen and the patterned stimuli *must* be the same so there is no change of luminance during the transition from pattern to diffuse blank screen. This may be difficult to achieve. Background luminance should have this same value. We recommend a standard of 100 to

TABLE 20.5.2A

ISCEV standard for VEP assessment: Standard stimuli

	Field size (deg)	Stimulus type	Stimulation	Pattern element size — Checks (min)	Luminance (cd·m^{-2}) — Background	Luminance (cd·m^{-2}) — Bright element	Luminance (cd·m^{-2}) — Mean	Contrast (%)	Presentation rate
Pattern Stimulation— Pre-chiasmal	>15	Pattern reversal or onset/offset	Monocular	60, 15	Equal to mean for onset/offset	>80	>40	>75%	<1–3 reversals or ≤2 onsets per second
Flash Stimulation— Pre-chiasmal	>20	ISCEV standard luminance flash	Monocular	—	15–30	—	—	—	<1.5 flashes per second

TABLE 20.5.2B

ISCEV standard for VEP assessment: Standard recording

	Electrode montage (International 10/20 channel system) — Active	Common reference	Filters (−3 dB) — Low freq.	High freq.	Sweeps averaged
Pattern Stimulation— Pre-chiasmal	Oz	Fz	<1	>100	≥64
Flash Stimulation— Pre-chiasmal	Oz	Fz	<1	>100	≥64

200 ms pattern presentations separated by 400 ms of diffuse background. The duration of pattern presentations and diffuse background in ms should always be indicated. The data acquisition system should be set to trigger at the appearance of the stimulus.

Flash stimulus The flash VEP should be elicited by a flash that subtends a visual field of at least 20 deg. The stimulus should be presented in a dimly illuminated room. The strength (time integrated luminance) of the flash stimulus should be measured in photopic candelas seconds per meter squared ($cd \cdot s \cdot m^{-2}$). The background on which the flash is presented should be measured in candelas per meter squared ($cd \cdot m^{-2}$). The flash should have a stimulus strength of 1.5–$3\,cd \cdot s \cdot m^{-2}$ with a background of 15–$30\,cd \cdot m^{-2}$ as described in the ERG standards for the standard flash [2] and should be presented less than 1.5 times per second (<1.5 Hz).

ELECTRODES Standard silver-silver chloride or gold disc surface electrodes are recommended for recording VEPs. The electrodes should be fixed to the scalp and maintained using procedures recommended by the manufacturer. The electrode impedances should be below $5\,k\Omega$ and equal to reduce electrical interference.

Electrode placement The scalp electrodes should be placed relative to bony landmarks, in proportion to the size of the head, according to the International 10/20 system[6] (figure 20.5.1). The anterior/posterior midline measurements are based on the distance between the nasion and the inion over the vertex. The active electrode is placed on the scalp over the visual cortex at Oz with the reference electrode at Fz. Commonly used ground electrode positions include the forehead, vertex (Cz), mastoid, earlobe (A1 or A2) or linked earlobes.

Recording parameters The details of equipment calibration are given in the ISCEV Calibration Guidelines[5] and should be adhered to. The Guidelines include details on the measurement of electrode impedance as well as amplifier filtering and gain.

Amplification and averaging systems Analogue high pass and low pass filters [−3 dB points] should be set at 1 Hz or less (corresponding to a time constant 0.16 s or more) and at 100 Hz or more, respectively. Analogue filter roll-off slopes should not exceed 12 dB per octave for low frequencies and 24 dB per octave for the high frequencies. While other filter settings may be required in particular circumstances, it must be realized that all analogue filters produce an apparent change in the timing or peak latency of the components of the VEP particularly if low pass filters below 100 Hz are

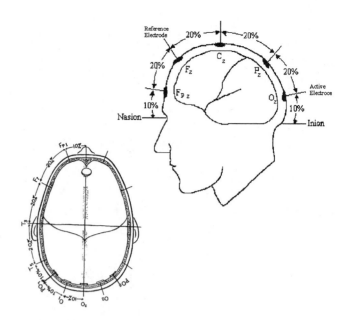

FIGURE 20.5.1 Electrode locations. Left, Location of active and reference electrodes for standard responses. The active electrode is located along the midline at Oz. The reference electrode is located at location Fz. The subscript z indicates a midline position. Right, The locations of the lateral active electrodes, O_1, O_2, PO_7, and PO_8 are indicated along with the midline active electrode location, O_z.

used. The use of notch or comb line frequency filters is not recommended.

Amplification of the input signal by 20,000–50,000 times is usually appropriate for recording the VEP. The input impedance of the pre-amplifiers must be at least $100\,M\Omega$ and the common mode rejection ratio should ideally be in excess of 120 dB. The amplifiers must be electrically isolated from the patient and international standards for safety of biological recording systems in humans should be used (IEC-601-1 type BF specification). The analogue signal should be digitized at a minimum sample rate of 500 samples per second per channel with a minimum resolution of 12 bits. Automatic artifact rejection based on signal amplitude should be used to exclude signals exceeding ±50–$100\,\mu V$ in amplitude. The amplifiers must return to baseline rapidly following artifactual signals.

The number of sweeps per average depends upon the signal to noise ratio between the VEP and the background noise. In most clinical settings, the minimum number of sweeps per average should be 64. At least two averages should be performed to verify the reproducibility of the findings. In pediatric practice, particularly with infants, a smaller number of sweeps per average may sometimes produce a clearer response. The longer recording time required to increase sample size introduces the possibility of increased variability due to loss of attention and/or increased movement.

Analysis time   The analysis time (sweep duration) for all transient flash and pattern reversal VEPs should be at least 250 ms. If one analyzes both the pattern onset and offset responses elicited by onset-offset stimuli, the analysis time (sweep duration) must be extended to at least 500 ms.

Clinical protocol

PREPARATION OF THE PATIENT   Pattern stimuli for VEPs should be presented when the pupils of the eyes are unaltered by mydriatic or miotic drugs. Pupils need not be dilated for the flash VEP.

Extreme pupil sizes and any anisocoria should be noted. For pattern stimulation, the visual acuity of the patient should be recorded and the patient should be optimally refracted for the viewing distance of the screen. Monocular stimulation should be performed. This may not be practical in infants or some other special populations, when binocular stimulation may be used to assess whether any afferent signals are reaching primary visual cortex. When a flash stimulus is used with monocular stimulation, care should be taken to ensure that no light enters the unstimulated eye. Usually this requires a light-tight opaque patch to be placed over the unstimulated eye. Care must be taken to have the patient in a comfortable, well supported position to minimize muscle and other artifacts.

The pattern onset/offset response shows a greater intersubject variability than the pattern reversal VEP but shows less sensitivity to confounding factors such as poor fixation or eye movements. It is difficult to deliberately defocus a transient pattern onset/offset stimulus. Therefore, it is an effective stimulus for detection or confirmation of malingering or evaluation of patients with nystagmus.

DESCRIPTION OF THE THREE STANDARD TRANSIENT RESPONSES The waveform of the VEP depends upon the temporal fre-

quency of the stimulus. At rapid rates of stimulation, the waveform becomes approximately sinusoidal and is termed steady-state. At low temporal frequencies, the waveform consists of a number of discrete deflections and is termed a transient VEP. Only transient VEPs form a part of this standard.

VEP peak latency, amplitude, and waveform are age-dependent. The description of standard responses below reflects the typical response of an adult aged 18–60 years of age. VEP peak latency refers to the time from stimulus onset to the maximum positive or negative deflection or excursion; thus, the term VEP peak latency corresponds to the term implicit time used to describe the time from the stimulus to the maximum deflection of electroretinograms. VEP peak latency may also be referred to as "time to peak" or peak time.

Pattern reversal VEP   The pattern reversal VEP has relatively low variability of waveform and peak latency both within a subject and over the normal population. Therefore, it is the preferred procedure in most circumstances. For pattern reversal, the VEP consists of N75, P100 and N135 peaks. The nomenclature consists of designating peaks as negative and positive followed by the typical mean peak latency (figure 20.5.2). It is recommended to measure the amplitude of P100 from the preceding N75 peak. The peak latency of P100 shows relatively little variation between subjects, minimal within-subject interocular difference, and minimal variation with repeated measurements over time. P100 peak latency is affected by non-pathophysiologic parameters such as pattern size, pattern contrast, pattern mean luminance, refractive error, poor fixation and miosis.

Pattern onset/offset VEP   The onset/offset VEP is more variable in appearance than the pattern reversal VEP. The response to pattern onset/offset stimulation typically consists

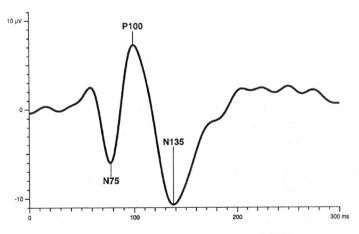

FIGURE 20.5.2   A normal pattern reversal VEP.

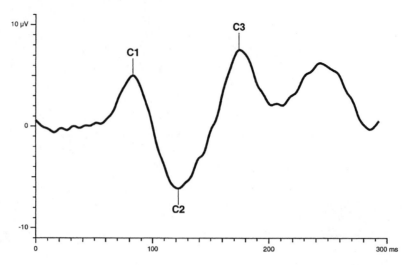

FIGURE 20.5.3   A normal pattern onset/offset VEP. Note that with a 300 ms sweep only the pattern onset response is recorded.

of three main peaks in adults; C1 (positive approximately 75 ms), C2 (negative approximately 125 ms) and C3 (positive, approximately 150 ms) (figure 20.5.3). Amplitudes are measured from the preceding negative peak.

Flash VEP   Flash VEPs are much more variable across subjects than pattern responses but show little interocular asymmetry. They may be useful in patients who are unable or unwilling to cooperate for pattern VEPs, and when optical factors such as media opacities prevent the valid use of pattern stimuli.

The visual evoked potential to flash stimulation consists of a series of negative and positive waves. The earliest detectable response has a peak latency of approximately 30 ms post-stimulus and components are recordable with peak latencies of up to 300 ms. Peaks are designated as negative and positive in a numerical sequence (figure 20.5.4). This nomenclature is recommended to automatically differentiate the flash VEP from the pattern reversal VEP. For the flash VEP, the most robust components are the N2 and P2 peaks. Measurements of P2 amplitude should be made from the positive P2 peak at around 120 ms to the preceding N2 negative peak at around 90 ms.

PEDIATRIC VEP RECORDING   Modifications to VEP recording methods and testing strategies may be required to optimize results in infants, young children or people with disabilities. In principle, the stimulation and recording methods recommended in the ISCEV standard can be applied to all populations. However, in these special populations modifications to VEP recording methods and testing strategies may be required to optimize the quality and pertinence of the result to diagnosis and visual assessment to the clinical question.

All VEPs in children should be compared with appropriate age related normal values. When recording the VEP in infants the sweep duration should be increased due to the increased peak latency in this population. By six months of age the peak latency of the main positive peak of the pattern reversal VEP for larger checks (>30') is usually within 10% of adult values.

VEPs should be recorded when the infant or child is in an attentive behavioral state. Direct interaction with the child can help maintain attention and fixation, and two testers are beneficial; one to work with the child and the other to control data acquisition. Data quality and reliability will be improved if a recording trial can be paused or interrupted when fixation wanders and then resumed as the child resumes adequate cooperation. To facilitate compliance, an infant may view the stimulus while lying across a lap, or held over the shoulder. The order of stimulus presentation also should be flexible and selected to ensure that responses most critical to the diagnostic question are obtained within an individual child's attention span. Binocular pattern stimulation, which facilitates attention and fixation, may be useful to evaluate overall visual function. Monocular testing to at least one stimulus is desirable to assess the function of each eye. It is particularly important to obtain replicate responses from children to assure that the response measured is a reliable signal and not an artifact. As for adults, additional channels of recording may be important for diagnosis of chiasmal and post-chiasmal dysfunction. When pattern VEPs cannot be reliably recorded, flash testing which is less dependent upon co-operation can usually be achieved. Pattern reversal VEPs recorded from patients with nystagmus or unstable fixation should be interpreted with caution. Pattern onset/offset stimuli can be helpful in gaining attention of children and are usually more robust in cases of nystagmus, but the waveform

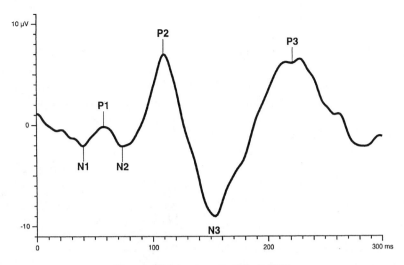

FIGURE 20.5.4   A normal flash VEP.

components change with age. Reports should note the degree of cooperation and arousal of the child.

MULTI-CHANNEL RECORDING FOR ASSESSMENT OF THE CENTRAL VISUAL PATHWAYS   Multi-channel recording is not covered by the standard. However, intracranial visual pathway dysfunction may require multi-channel recording for accurate diagnosis. With dysfunction at or posterior to the optic chiasm, or in the presence of chiasmal misrouting (as seen in ocular albinism), there is an asymmetrical distribution of the VEP over the posterior scalp. Chiasmal dysfunction gives a "crossed" asymmetry whereby the findings obtained on stimulation of one eye show an asymmetrical distribution that is reversed when the other eye is stimulated. Retrochiasmal dysfunction gives an "uncrossed" asymmetry such that the findings obtained on stimulation of each eye show an asymmetrical distribution across the hemispheres that is similar when either eye is stimulated. We suggest that for pattern reversal stimulation the stimulus should consist of high contrast black and white checks of 60' in a field of 30 deg (full-field). A minimum of two channels is needed for detection of lateral asymmetries. We suggest the use of three active electrodes, two lateral electrodes placed at O_1 and O_2, and a third midline active electrode at Oz. All three active electrodes should be referenced to Fz. This three channel montage provides the preferred montage for simultaneous detection of prechiasmal and central pathway dysfunction. Additional electrodes placed at PO_7 and PO_8, also referred to Fz, may increase sensitivity to lateral asymmetries in some cases. The position of the lateral electrodes is illustrated in figure 20.V.1B. For all stimulus conditions, normative data should include amplitude and peak latency comparisons between homologous left and right occipital channels. Particular caution is needed when interpreting the multi-channel pattern reversal VEP due to the phenomenon of paradoxical lateralization. This phenomenon, in which the response recorded at a lateral head position is generated by activity in the contralateral hemisphere of the brain, occurs with a large field, large check reversal stimulus and common reference recording to Fz.

VEP MEASUREMENT AND REPORTING   Standardization of VEP measurement and reporting is critical to the goal of having comparable data worldwide.

Normal values   Even though standardization should ensure similar responses across laboratories, each laboratory must establish its own normative values using its own stimulus and recording parameters. The construction of a normal sample for laboratory norms should include the factors of age, gender, and interocular asymmetry. Adult normative data cannot be generalized to pediatric or elderly populations. Interocular amplitude and peak latency analysis increases the sensitivity of the VEP to monocular diseases. We recommend that laboratory norms make use of descriptive statistics that do not assume a normal distribution, but are based on the calculation of the median and percentiles from the observed sample distribution. We recommend the 95% reference interval as the minimum limit of normal (i.e., the range from 2.5% to 97.5%).

VEP reporting   A minimum of two recordings of each VEP condition should be acquired, measured and displayed. Reports of the standardized conditions should specify the stimulus parameter; the field size of the stimulus, the strength (time integrated luminance) of the flash or mean luminance of the pattern, the pattern element size and contrast of pattern stimuli, the frequency of stimulation, the eye tested and the recording parameters; the filter settings and the locations of the positive (i.e., active) and negative (i.e., reference) and indifferent (i.e., ground) electrodes.

Traces should have a clear indication of polarity, time in milliseconds, and amplitude in microvolts. We recommend that VEP traces be presented as positive upwards. All VEP reports, even for non-standard responses (whether for local records or publications) should include normative values and the limits of normal.

The report should indicate whether the recordings meet this international standard. We recommend that the numerical measurements of obtained peak latency and amplitude be reported along with the normal values and the limits of normal.

VEP interpretation VEP abnormalities are not specific and can occur in a wide variety of ophthalmological and neurological problems. The interpretation should include statements about the normality and abnormality of the result in relation to normative data as well as comparison between the eyes or with previous records. The type of abnormality in the response should be described and this should be related to the clinical picture and other visual electrodiagnostic results.

Acknowledgments

ISCEV's standardization process requires the active participation of individual ISCEV members to act as consultants to the committee which writes the standard. While these contributions are too numerous to mention in detail, we wish to particularly recognize Patricia Apkarian, Jelka Brecelj, Anne Fulton, Daphne McCulloch, Dorothy Thompson, and Carol Westall for their valuable suggestions and editorial comments regarding pediatric VEPs that we have incorporated into this document.

REFERENCES

1. Marmor MF, Zrenner E: Standard for clinical electrooculography. *Doc Ophthalmol* 1993; 85:115–124.
2. Marmor MF, Holder GE, Seeliger MW, Yamamoto S: Standard for clinical electroretinography (2003 update). *Doc Ophthalmol* 2004; 108:107–114.
3. Bach M, Hawlina M, Holder GE, Marmor MF, Meigen T, Vaegan, Miyake Y: Standard for pattern electroretinography. *Doc Ophthalmol* 2000; 101:11–18.
4. Brigell M, Bach M, Barber C, Kawasaki K, Kooijman A: Guidelines for calibration of stimulus and recording parameters used in clinical electrophysiology of vision. *Doc Ophthalmol* 1998; 95:1–14.
5. Marmor MF, Hood DC, Keating D, Kondo M, Seeliger MW, Miyake Y: Guidelines for basic multifocal electroretinography (mfERG). *Doc Ophthalmol* 2003; 106:105–115.
6. American Encephalographic Society: Guideline thirteen: Guidelines for standard electrode position nomenclature. *J Clin Neurophysiol* 1994; 11:111–113.

20.6 Guidelines for Basic Multifocal Electroretinography (mfERG)

MICHAEL F. MARMOR,* DONALD C. HOOD, DAVID KEATING, MINEO KONDO, MATHIAS W. SEELIGER, AND YOZO MIYAKE* (FOR THE INTERNATIONAL SOCIETY FOR CLINICAL ELECTROPHYSIOLOGY OF VISION)

Introduction

Full-field electroretinography (ERG) is a standard clinical test for evaluating the function of the retina as a whole [1]. Multifocal electroretinography (mfERG)† is a new technique that allows analysis of local retinal function. While the technology of these recordings and the knowledge about the physiology of these responses are evolving, there is sufficient experience to propose basic guidelines for the usage of this procedure. The intention of this document, is not to mandate a "standard" of care or to fix a particular test protocol. Rather, the intention is to offer guidelines for recording the mfERG that will aid in obtaining stable and interpretable records, while minimizing artifacts. These guidelines should be especially helpful for those new to this technique, while informing the experienced user about procedures that colleagues find effective. However, we emphasize that these are guidelines and not standards. More research is needed on the applications and technology of this new technique before many aspects of these guidelines can be resolved. We anticipate that exploration of different recording protocols and their interpretation will continue, but users who are not specifically studying alternative techniques are encouraged to follow the guidelines as current "best practice". These guidelines will be re-examined in 4 years, consistent with all ISCEV practice recommendations, to make revisions as necessary and consider whether an ISCEV Standard for the mfERG should be established.

Description of multifocal electroretinography

The mfERG is a technique for assessing the local ERG from different regions of the posterior retina. Electrical responses from the eye are recorded with a corneal electrode just as in conventional ERG recording, but the special nature of the stimulus and analysis produce a topographic map of ERG responses. For the routine mfERG, the retina is stimulated with a computer monitor or other device that generates a pattern of elements (typically hexagons), each of which has a 50% chance of being illuminated every time the frame changes (figure 20.6.1). The pattern seems to flicker randomly, but each element follows a fixed, predetermined sequence (presently an "m sequence") so that the overall luminance of the screen over time is relatively stable (equiluminant). By correlating the continuous ERG signal with the on or off phases of each stimulus element, the focal ERG signal associated with each element is calculated. Data can be displayed in various ways such as a topographic array or a three-dimensional plot. Interactions between responses as a result of adaptation or non-linear response properties can also be analyzed. Different stimulus patterns and flicker sequences can be used for specialized applications.

It is important to keep in mind that the tracings of the mfERG are not "responses" in the sense of direct electrical responses from a local region of retina. The mfERG waveforms are a mathematical extraction of signals that correlate with the time that one portion of the stimulus screen is illuminated. Thus, mfERG signals may be influenced by adaptation effects (from preceding stimuli) and by the effects of scattered light on other fundus areas.

---

*Dr. Marmor was Chair of the mfERG Committee and is Director of Standards for ISCEV. Dr. Miyake is President of ISCEV.

†Multifocal electroretinography has been abbreviated in various ways in the literature, including mfERG, MERG, and MFERG. Since MERG causes confusion with other procedures in some languages, we recommend mfERG as most universally distinct and recognizable abbreviation.

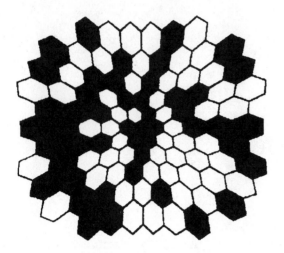

FIGURE 20.6.1 Representative hexagonal mfERG stimulus array with 103 elements, of which roughly half are illuminated at any one time.

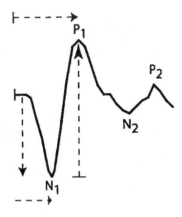

FIGURE 20.6.2 Diagram of an mfERG response to show designation of the major waveforms, and the recommended method for measuring amplitude and implicit time (time-to-peak).

WAVEFORMS

Nomenclature of peaks The typical waveform of the primary mfERG response (also called the first order response or first order kernel K_1) is a biphasic wave with an initial negative deflection followed by a positive peak (figure 20.6.2). There may be a second negative deflection after the peak. The preferred designation is to label these three peaks respectively N1, P1 and N2. There is some homology between this waveform and the conventional ERG, but they are probably not identical (see below). Thus the designations "a wave" and "b wave" are not recommended.

Cellular origin Studies in humans have shown that the N1 response includes cellular contributions from the same components as the a-wave of the full-field cone ERG, and the P1 response includes contributions from the components of the cone b-wave and oscillatory potentials. However, this body of knowledge is still incomplete, and it would be premature to assume any simple correlation between the mfERG waveform and particular classes of retinal cells.

Basic technology

ELECTRODES

Recording electrodes Electrodes that contact the cornea or nearby bulbar conjunctiva are strongly recommended for mfERG recording just as for the full-field ERG. The same recommendations as in the ERG Standard suffice, with the proviso that the optical opening or corneal lens must be clear to allow good visual acuity and refraction.

Reference and ground electrodes Proper application of suitably conductive electrodes is essential for stable mfERG recording. Follow the recommendations in the ISCEV full-field ERG and/or PERG Standards.[1,2]

Electrode characteristics, stability and cleaning Follow the recommendations in the ISCEV full-field ERG and/or pattern ERG (PERG) Standards.[1,2]

STIMULATION

Stimulus source The stimulus is generally delivered by a cathode ray tube (CRT), i.e. a monitor. Other devices are also used such as LCD projectors, LED arrays and scanning laser ophthalmoscopes. These alternative modes of stimulation may produce different waveforms and will not be discussed in these guidelines, but many of the principles of stimulation outlined below would apply to them as well.

Screen properties

Frame frequency. A CRT frame frequency of 75 Hz, has been used most widely. Users should be aware that use of a different frequency requires adjustment of the stimulus protocol and may alter the recorded signals. The frame frequency should never be line current frequency (50 or 60 Hz) which may cause interference artifacts.

Luminance. The luminance of the stimulus elements on the CRT screen should be 100–200 cd/m^2 in the lighted state and <1 cd/m^2 in the dark state. This means that the mean screen luminance during testing will be 50–100 cd/m^2.

Calibration. The luminance of dark and lighted stimulus elements should be measured with an appropriate calibrator or spot meter. Many monitor screens are not of uniform brightness over the entire screen, and variations of up to 15% are considered acceptable. If greater variation is present, stimulus size may need to be adjusted to insure equivalent effects in different regions of the retina. Techniques for calibrating stimulus and recording parameters are described in the ISCEV Guidelines for calibration.[3] We urge manufacturers of mfERG equipment to provide instruction for calibration of their devices.

Stimulus parameters

Stimulus pattern. The default hexagonal stimulus pattern was designed to compensate for local differences in signal density (and cone density) across the retina. Thus, the central hexagons are smaller than the more peripheral ones. Different patterns (e.g., equal size hexagons) can be generated and may be useful in special cases such as patients with eccentric fixation or when using specialized flicker sequences. However, these guidelines cover only the default stimulus pattern.

Flicker sequence. Commercial mfERG instruments use an m-sequence to control the order of flicker of the stimulus elements (between light and dark). This sequence is recommended for routine testing. Different sequences, or the inclusion of global light or dark frames, are possible for specialized applications, but will not be considered here.

Stimulus size. The overall stimulus pattern should subtend a visual angle of 20–30 degrees on either side of fixation. The stimulus region can be divided into different numbers of hexagons, and the choice depends on balancing the need for spatial resolution, signal-to-noise ratio, length of recording, etc. (see discussion under Clinical Protocol). The standard patterns in most frequent use at present incorporate 61, 103 or 241 stimulus elements.

Contrast and background. Contrast between the lighted and darkened stimulus elements should be 90% or greater. The background region of the CRT (beyond the area of stimulus hexagons) should have a luminance equal to the mean luminance of the stimulus array.

Fixation targets. Stable fixation is essential to obtain reliable mfERG recordings. Central fixation dots or crosses are available with most stimulus programs. They should cover as little as possible of the central stimulus element to avoid diminishing the response (but may need enlargement for low vision patients).

RECORDING EQUIPMENT

Amplifiers and filters Amplifiers should be alternating current (AC) coupled and should be capable of gain and filter adjustment. A gain of 100,000 or 200,000 is most widely used; the gain should produce recognizable signals without saturating the amplifiers. The bandpass filter removes extraneous electrical noise while preserving waveforms of interest. For general use, a filter range of 3–300 Hz or 10–300 Hz is most suitable. Users should be aware that filter settings may influence waveforms that contain components near the ends of the frequency range. The filter settings should be the same for all subjects studied by a given laboratory so that the waveforms are comparable. Line-frequency notch filters should be avoided. A masking cone (provided by some manufacturers) may reduce electrical interference.

Signal analysis

Artifact rejection. Because blinks and other movements can distort the recorded waveforms, there are "artifact rejection" programs to eliminate some of the obvious peaks or drifts from being added to the cumulative recording. Artifact rejection is often used to "clean up" a record, but should not in general be applied multiple times.

Averaging with neighbors. In order to smooth out waveforms and reduce noise, commercial programs can average the response from each stimulus element with a percentage of the signal from each of the adjacent elements. This can be useful with noisy records, but will blur the margins of small or critical regions of dysfunction. Thus, it should be used with care. With the VERIS system the percentage of neighboring responses to be averaged can be adjusted. A setting of 16% means that 50% of each trace comes from adjoining stimulus elements, and we advise using no more than 16% so that no more than 50% of each trace comes from adjoining areas. The Roland system digitally smoothes the stored data, and should be used with similar caution.

Display options

Trace arrays. All commercial programs can produce an array of the mfERG traces from different regions of the retina (figure 20.6.3). This is the basic mfERG display and should be a part of all standard display protocols. It is useful for observing areas of variation and abnormality.

Group averages. Analysis programs can average together the responses from any designated number of traces. This can be helpful for comparing quadrants, hemiretinal areas, or successive rings from center to periphery. The latter can be useful for patients who have disease that is radially symmetric or diffuse. Responses from stimulus elements relating to a local area of interest can also be averaged together for comparison with a similar area in normals.

Topographic (3-D) response density plots. These plots show the overall signal strength per unit area of retina (combining N and P components) in a 3-dimensional figure. This is sometimes useful as an overview or demonstration of certain types of pathology, but there are major dangers which need to be understood. These 3-D plots typically incorporate both negative and positive deflections, so waveform information is lost and irrelevant components (noise) can be enhanced

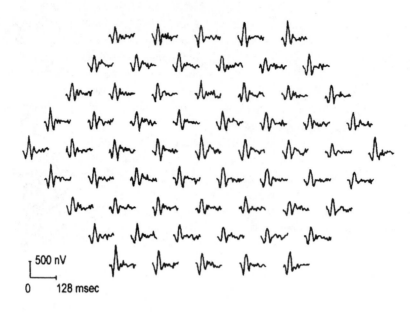

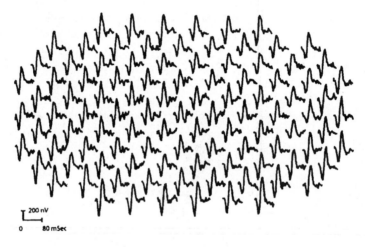

FIGURE 20.6.3   Sample mfERG trace arrays with 61 elements and 103 elements.

(see Appendix: Artifact Recognition examples for electrical noise and weak signals). The generation of 3-D plots usually involves interpolation of the responses to create the appearance of a continuous surface, and as a result spatial resolution may be modified. Finally, the appearance of the 3D plot from a given recording is dependent on whether the scaling templates were derived using averaged data from the subject or from controls, and on the duration of the displayed waveforms. A comparison of scalar plots between patients can be misleading unless the parameters and reference data are consistent for all subjects. We recommend that 3-D plots not be used by themselves to display mfERG data; they should always be accompanied by a corresponding trace array.

Kernels.   This document is aimed at the general mfERG user and only describes the measurement of the first order kernel.

Clinical protocol

PATIENT PREPARATION
Pupils   The pupils should be fully dilated.

Electrodes   These must be carefully applied according to instructions in the full-field ERG or PERG Standards.[1,2] Poor or unstable electrode contact is a major cause of poor quality records.

Patient positioning   Subjects should sit comfortably in front of the screen or instrument. The viewing distance will vary with screen size, in order to control the area (visual angle) of retina being stimulated. See the ISCEV Guidelines for calibration[3] for instructions on measuring visual angle and viewing distance.

Fixation monitoring Since good fixation is essential, fixation should be monitored in some fashion, either by direct observation of the patient or by the use of monitoring instrumentation available on some units.

Refraction Manufacturers currently recommend refraction for optimal acuity. Lenses are typically placed in a holder positioned in front of the eye. Because lenses alter the relative magnification of the stimulus, the viewing distance must be adjusted to compensate, in accordance with the scale or guidelines provided by the manufacturer. Also care must be taken to avoid inducing a ring scotoma with a plus lens. There is some controversy about whether acuity is critical to the mfERG, at least within a range of ±6D from emmetropia, so that some experts deem refraction unnecessary within these limits. It is not clear whether these data from normal eyes apply to all pathologic eyes since a small retinal lesion might be less defined in the mfERG if the stimulus cell boundaries were badly blurred.

Monocular vs. binocular recording Either monocular or binocular recording is possible, but it is incumbent on those who record binocularly to be sure that signals are not altered by decentration of either eye or by asymmetric effects from the refractive or recording lenses.

ADAPTATION

Pre-adaptation (before test) Subjects should be in ordinary room light for 15 min before testing, assuming no prior exposure to bright sun or fundus photography. Longer adaptation may be needed after such exposure. A previous full-field ERG with photopic recordings is acceptable as long as the exposure (especially flicker) was not unusually prolonged.

Room illumination Room lights should be on, and ideally produce illumination at the subject close to that of the stimulus screen. A masking cone (provided by some manufacturers) can decrease stray light.

RECORDING SEQUENCE

Stimulus

Size. 20–30 degrees of visual angle on either side of fixation.

Number of elements. Most often 61 or 103 for routine use; 241 elements for more critical localization.

Duration of recording. Total time is typically about 4 min for 61 elements, or 8 min for 103 elements (although these times might be adjusted by experienced labs according to clinical needs). The overall recording time is divided into shorter segments (e.g. 15–30 s) so that subjects can rest between runs if necessary—and also so that a poor record

(from noise, movement or other artifacts) can be discarded and run again without losing prior data. These recording times may be lengthened according to the stability of the patient and the amount of electrical interference (noise).

Choices The choice of stimulus array and recording time is a trade-off between the stability of recording and the topographic resolution of the data. Large stimulus elements (e.g. 61) give signals with less noise, but are less sensitive to small areas of retinal dysfunction. Smaller stimulus elements (e.g. 103) will show more accurately the outline of dysfunctional areas, but require longer recording time to obtain an acceptable signal to noise ratio. Large elements with a short recording time are easier for patients and suitable for a general overview of macular function. Very small elements (such as a 241 hexagon array) may sometimes be needed for disease with small or irregular effects within the macula, or for accurate tracking of functional defects. To account for trial-to-trial variability, repeat recording is recommended to confirm small or subtle abnormalities.

DATA REPORTING

Mode of display

Trace arrays. It is essential to show the trace array when reporting *on* the mfERG (see figure 20.6.3). These arrays not only show topographic variations, but also demonstrate the quality of the records, which is important in judging the validity of any suspected variations from normal.

Group averages. Arranging responses by groups can be a useful way to summarize the data. Concentric rings of traces, from the center outward, are most commonly used. Regions with fundus pathology can be averaged together if desired.

Three-dimensional scalar plots. These are optional, and should be used with caution (see discussion above). Scalar plots should never be used as the sole method of display.

Measurements

Calibration marks. Must accompany all traces or graphs. It is also important for each laboratory to establish the typical range of values for the various modes of display, so that most data from the laboratory can be plotted at the same scale to facilitate comparisons among patients.

Responses. The N1 response amplitude is measured from the starting baseline to the base of the N1 trough; the P1 response amplitude is measured from the N1 trough to the P1 peak (see figure 20.6.2). The peak latencies (implicit times) of N1 and P1 are measured from the stimulus onset. Measurements of group averages should routinely include the N1 and P1 amplitudes and peak latencies.

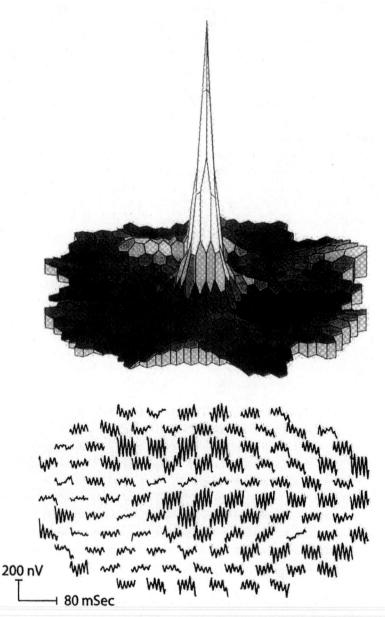

FIGURE 20.6.4 Electrical noise. The trace array shows predominately 60 Hz signals, which vary in amplitude from hexagon to hexagon because the computer correlations are randomly in or out of phase. The topographic (3-D) density plot shows a misleading tall central peak which represents noise entirely, but which might be mistaken for a foveal signal if the trace array was not also displayed.

Color scales. Optional.

Normal values Each laboratory needs to develop normative data, since variations in recording equipment and parameters makes the use of data from other sources inappropriate. Since electrophysiologic data do not necessarily follow a normal distribution about a mean, laboratories should report the median value rather than the mean, and determine 5 and 95% values as boundaries of normality. The mfERG, like the full-field ERG, diminishes somewhat with age and shows lower values in myopic eyes. While these effects are generally not large they can be relevant in some patients.

Reporting of artifacts and their resolution Reports should indicate explicitly any artifact reduction procedures or postprocessing maneuvers used to prepare the data. This should include the type and number or artifact rejection steps, the averaging of results with neighbors (noting the extent and number of iterations), and any other smoothing or averaging procedures. Any unusual causes of artifact should be noted.

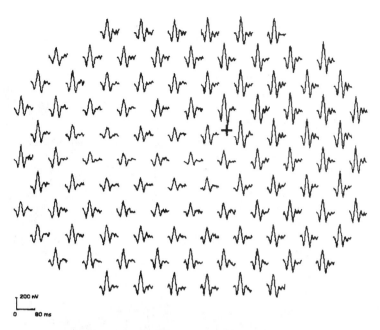

FIGURE 20.6.5 Eccentric fixation. The subject fixated at the + instead of the center. As a result, the calculated response magnitudes are altered, and there is a false appearance of central retinal dysfunction.

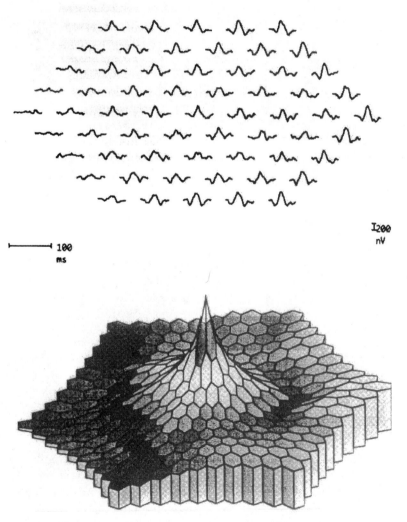

FIGURE 20.6.6 Shadowing error. The subject's view was obscured on one side by the edge of a refracting lens. As a result, both the trace array and 3-D plot show a false reduction in amplitude on one side.

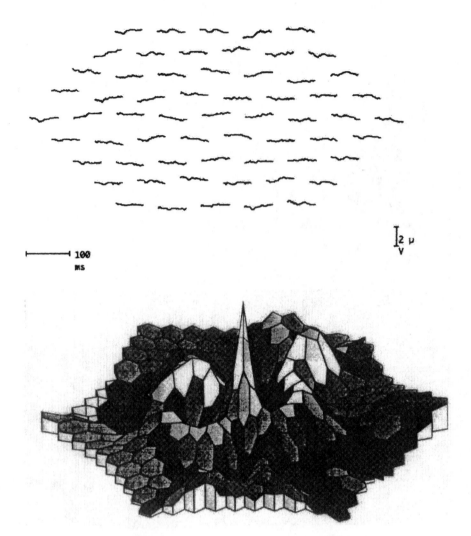

FIGURE 20.6.7 Weak signals and erroneous central peak. This patient with cone dystrophy had minimal mfERG responses, as evident from the trace array. However, the 3-D plot shows an artifactual central peak that is generated by background noise (similar to the example in figure 20.6.4) and does not represent a physiologic signal.

ACKNOWLEDGMENTS This document was approved by ISCEV in Montréal-Mont Orford, Canada, on June 21, 2001.

Appendix: Artifact recognition

There are a number of artifacts that can complicate the recording or interpretation of the mfERG. We list and illustrate some of the more common below, along with brief suggestions for avoidance or correction.

COMMON TYPES OF ARTIFACT

Electrical noise (figure 20.6.4) Poor electrode contacts, poor grounding or ambient sources can cause line current (50/60 Hz) interference that alters the physiologic patterns of responses. Noise is usually evident in trace arrays but may produce topographic (3-D) plots that appear to be physiologic even when there is no retinal response. For this reason, 3-D plots are not recommended as the sole or primary means of mfERG display. Solution: Better electrode contact, grounding or shielding.

Movement errors Inconsistent fixation and random eye movements can produce irregular signals with spikes, saturation of the amplifiers, and aberrant drifting or fluctuations in the waveforms. Milder degrees of eye movement, or unsteady fixation, cause smearing of the responses between different loci, and thus reduced resolution of small lesions. If the blind spot is not visible in a recording, this may be a clue to poor fixation. Solution: Observe the amount of noise during the recording. Contaminated runs or segments should be discarded and re-recorded. Improve fixation monitoring and fixation control.

Eccentric fixation (figure 20.6.5) This can cause trace arrays and topographic scalar plots that are depressed centrally, or show a "sloping" appearance with low signals on one side and high on the other. Solution: Check fixation, or use a special low vision target.

Orientation/shadowing errors (figure 20.6.6) These appear when a subject is poorly centered or there is shadowing from the edge of either the refraction lens or the recording contact lens. The trace arrays and topographic plots show depression in one part of the array and sometimes elevation on the opposite side. These errors must be distinguished from patterns of disease, and from the small normal nasal-temporal variation. Solution: Center the lenses and subject, and monitor eye position.

Erroneous central peak (Weak signal artifact) (figure 20.6.7) Artifactually large "responses" can appear in the center of ring averages if there is an aberrant or spurious signal that would be averaged out in more peripheral areas. Scalar topographic plots often show an artifactual central peak, even when signals are weak, because they record the strength of noise as well as physiologic signals. The effects of noise are smoothed out in peripheral areas, but become amplified in the center where the overall amplitude of noise is divided by a small area. Solution: Look at the trace array to determine whether any recognizable waveform is present in areas of interest.

Averaging and smoothing artifacts Excessive averaging or smoothing of signals can artifactually reduce spatial resolution. Severely smoothed records may not reveal small lesions, or show sharp lesion borders. Solution: Avoid unnecessary smoothing, and avoid excessive averaging with neighboring responses.

Blind spot It is not an artifact that the blind spot is less sharply defined in the mfERG than one might expect. The optic nerve may not completely cover any one stimulus patch, so that some response is always obtained. Also, it has been hypothesized that because the nerve head reflects light more than other areas of retina, there is a response to this scatter from other parts of the retina (which is attributed in mfERG plots to the blind spot).

REFERENCES

1. Marmor MF, Zrenner E (for the International Society for Clinical Electrophysiology of Vision): Standard for Clinical electroretinography (1999 update). *Doc Ophthalmol* 1999; 97:143–156.
2. Bach M, Hawlina M, Holder GE, Marmor M, Meigen T, Vaegan, Miyake Y: Standard for pattern electroretinography. *Doc Ophthalmol* 2000; 101:11–18.
3. Brigell M, Bach M, Barber C, Kawasaki K, Kooijman A: Guidelines for calibration of stimulus and recording parameters used in clinical electrophysiology of vision. *Doc Ophthalmol* 1998; 95:1–14.

21 Multifocal Techniques

DAVID KEATING AND STUART PARKS

CONVENTIONAL CLINICAL electrophysiology provides us with a range of tools to assess the visual pathway. The basic clinical test procedures are now well established, and the International Society for Clinical Electrophysiology of Vision (ISCEV) produces standards to ensure the quality control of acquisition and interpretation of the various clinical procedures. Although these base procedures are well established, they continue to contribute new information to our understanding of human visual processing and the effects of a wide range of clinical conditions on visual function.

In the last decade, multifocal electrophysiology has been a significant addition to the range of electrodiagnostic procedures. The technique adds a spatial dimension to electrophysiology and provides a new tool to investigate the nonlinear processing mechanisms of human vision. The basic details of multifocal stimulation can be found in Sutter's original papers.[57,61]

A thorough understanding of multifocal electrophysiology requires an extensive knowledge of mathematics and the engineering principles of signal detection theory. However, this detailed knowledge is not necessary for the clinical electrophysiologist who wants to use the technique for vision research or clinical investigation. The purpose of this chapter is to illustrate, for those who are familiar with conventional electrophysiology, the differences that the multifocal technique brings and provide pointers to those who may wish to explore the mathematical or engineering background in more detail. The chapter aims to give an overview of the elements of a multifocal system, describe the signal waveforms and their interpretation, explore clinical applications, and provide indications for future multifocal research.

The hardware

As with conventional electrophysiology systems, a number of commercial systems are now available for multifocal electrophysiology. In fact, there is little difference in the hardware required for multifocal electrophysiology compared to conventional systems. A multifocal system consists of the same components, and a schematic diagram is shown in figure 21.1.

The hardware must be capable of delivering the multifocal stimulus at the desired stimulus presentation time (frame rate) and to synchronize the onset of each frame with the acquisition of the analog data recovered from the subject. The most common method of delivering the multifocal stimulus is the cathode-ray tube (CRT) device, but other options such as a liquid crystal display (LCD) projection system, a scanning laser ophthalmoscope, or light-emitting diode (LED) devices are alternative methods of delivering the stimulus. The electrodes are the same as conventional electrophysiology with reports of gold foil, H-K loop, contact lens, and DTL-fiber electrodes used for multifocal electroretinograms (ERGs).[23,41] Most modern computer systems with an appropriate signal-processing card can acquire, digitize, and store in memory the raw data from a multifocal investigation. The standard method of delivering the stimulus is the CRT device, which runs at a frame rate of 75 Hz. The data acquisition card must be able to sample the data at a rate of at least 1 kHz, and a resolution of 12 bits or more is required. Advances in computer technology now allow the data to be acquired, processed, and displayed in real time.[45,47]

The software

The main difference between conventional and multifocal electrophysiology lies with the software. Standard electrophysiology usually relies on temporal serial signal averaging if transient responses are being recovered and on Fourier analysis if steady-state potentials are being recovered.

The multifocal ERG recovers transient evoked potentials but makes use of a different method of stimulation. A special group of pseudo-random binary sequences (PRBS) known as m-sequences are used. The stimuli do not have to be binary; quarternary or higher-order stimuli are possible but are less practical for multifocal ERG. Other sequences, such as random sequences generated by computerized random number generators, will have poor orthogonality properties. (Multiple sequences are termed orthogonal if they are mathematically independent of one another.) Possible sequences to consider would be Gold sequences or deBrujn sequences, which, although better than random sequences, do not have the same autocorrelation properties of m-sequences. Further details on sequence properties can be found in Klein[29] or Ireland.[22] Readers wishing to explore the mathematics of kernel analysis are directed to the work of Marmarelis and Marmarelis,[37] Volterra,[63] and Wiener.[65] Details on the

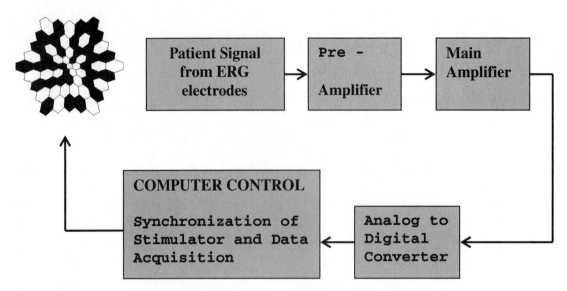

FIGURE 21.1 The hardware for a multifocal electrophysiology system. The hardware for multifocal electrophysiology can be identical to that required for standard electrophysiology. Electrodes, amplifiers, and analog-to-digital converter cards are the same. As with conventional electrophysiology, synchronization of stimulus generation and data acquisition is critical for the recovery of the response. The computer system must have adequate memory to store the data and be able to display and print the incoming and processed results.

mathematics and properties of m-sequences can be found in MacWilliams and Sloane,[36] Kruth,[33] or Davies.[4] Further details on the mathematics as applied directly to multifocal ERG are given in Sutter's original papers,[57,61] and a more intuitive approach is given in more recent publications by Sutter.[58,59]

The first application of m-sequences in electrophysiology was performed in 1975 by Fricker and Sanders,[9] who showed that the sequences could be used for global ERG measurements.

The properties of nonlinear ERG signals evoked by the sequences was further explored by Larkin in 1979[34] and described as a method of producing random VECP measurements by Collins in 1993.[3] The key breakthrough, using the sequences to stimulate many areas simultaneously by exploiting the properties of the sequences, was developed and first described by Sutter in 1992.[61] Other commercial systems have now become available. However, the power of the systems is compromised if alternative sequences to long m-sequences are used. These sequences should be carefully tested, as poorer autocorrelation properties can lead to compromises that affect the orthogonality of the sequences. Even long m-sequences themselves are prone to kernel overlap or cross-contamination. In fact, it is not possible to avoid this problem, but by careful choice of sequences, it is possible to ensure that contamination occurs outside the time windows of interest for the evoked potentials that are being investigated (ERG or VECP).

Binary m-sequences

There are different methods that are used for generation of these mathematical sequences. Mathematical methods require a knowledge of finite field theory, Euler's theorem, and Zech logarithms, and readers who wish further detail on this approach are directed to McEliece.[40] For the clinical or research electrophysiologist, the engineering method using shift register feedback generation gives an easily understandable method of sequence generation, and this is the approach that we will use here.

Shift register sequence generation

The feedback or tap positions for the shift register are taken for the terms of the defining primitive polynomial that is used for a particular m-sequence. A primitive polynomial of degree n will generate an m-sequence of length $2^n - 1$. This is best illustrated by using a short m-sequence as an example. Figure 21.2 illustrates the computation that occurs in making a short m-sequence from a root 4-bit register. This means that the highest-order term of the polynomial will be x^4, and a sequence of length $2^4 - 1$, or 15, will be generated. The example polynomial in this case is $x^4 + x + 1$. Each degree of x from this polynomial will form the tap positions of the shift register used for an exclusive OR feedback loop.

Modulo 2 arithmetic is performed or, in logic terms, an exclusive OR operation on the bits present in the tap posi-

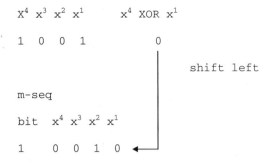

X⁴ x³ x² x¹   x⁴ XOR x¹

1 0 0 1   0

shift left

m-seq

bit x⁴ x³ x² x¹

1   0 0 1 0 ◄

Full sequence generation

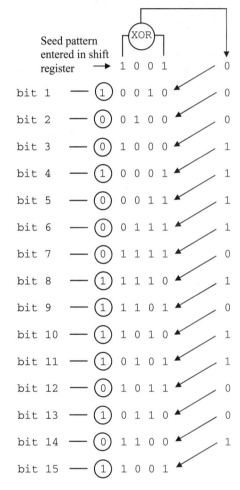

FIGURE 21.2 Generation of an m-sequence. The shift register is filled with any nonzero seed pattern. An exclusive OR operation is performed on the bits from the tap positions. The new bit is fed back into the shift register, and the first bit of the m-sequence is generated. This process is repeated until $2^n - 1$ bits are generated (in this case, 15 bits).

tions. This operation forms a new bit, which is shifted into the register from the left. The bit previously in the x^4 position is shifted out of the register, and this forms the first term or bit of the m-sequence.

For example, 1 XOR 1 gives 0. This 0 is shifted into the register from the left, and the first m-sequence bit is shifted out from the previous x^4 position. The first m-sequence bit is therefore a 1, and the shift register now contains the new bit pattern of 0 0 1 0. The procedure is then repeated until the full 15 bits have been generated as in figure 21.2. The sequence will repeat if continued in this manner.

The sequence is easily generated in software by using the code given in the appendix to this chapter. In the software segment, a slightly more efficient approach is used. In this case, the first 4 bits of the sequence are set by a seed value, and the new bit is formed by employing modulo 2 arithmetic on positions 4 back and 1 back as determined by the tap positions. This generates the same sequence as that generated in figure 21.2.

A practical m-sequence would be formed by using a higher-degree polynomial. For example, if a degree 15 primitive polynomial such as $x^{15} + x^{13} + x^{12} + x^{11} + x^6 + x^3 + x + 1$ is used, a sequence of length $2^{15} - 1$, or 32767, steps will be generated.

Sequence decimation

Decimation is the process that is used to generate a set of orthogonal sequences from an original single m-sequence. The process is illustrated for the sequence generated in figure 21.2. This sequence can be filled into a set number of columns, each column representing a stimulation area or stimulus patch. The number of columns for decimation must be a power of 2. For example, if we wish to generate a set of four orthogonal sequences from our original sequence, then we would simply fill the rows of a matrix with the bit pattern from the original sequence. This procedure should be repeated until each column is of length $2^n - 1$, or 15. The decimation process is illustrated in figure 21.3.

We now have a set of four orthogonal sequences, each of length 15. An important point to note at this stage is that all the sequences are identical but start at different positions. In this example, each sequence is shifted relative to the first sequence by four bit positions. These decimated sequences can now be used to control four stimulus areas.

Using the sequences to control a CRT stimulator

In a standard multifocal system, an m-sequence state of 1 will indicate that a stimulus element will be set to a white state, and an m-sequence step of 0 will indicate that the element is in a black state. An m-sequence base period is usually 13.33 ms for a CRT display. It is important to realize that having two consecutive m-sequence steps of 1 does not mean that an element will be in a continuous state of white for 2 × 13.33 ms; instead, each step will be a short period of white (2 ms) followed by a longer period of black (11.33 ms).

This is due to the raster nature of the CRT device. Two consecutive 1's in the sequence will therefore be two brief flashes of light separated by a black period. The visual cortex will interpret this stimulation at 75 Hz as a continuous white

Sequence 100100011110101

Decimated into 4 columns

```
1 0 0 1
0 0 0 1
1 1 1 0
1 0 1 1
0 0 1 0
0 0 1 1
1 1 0 1
0 1 1 0
0 1 0 0
0 1 1 1
1 0 1 0
1 1 0 0
1 0 0 0
1 1 1 1
0 1 0 1
```

FIGURE 21.3 Decimation of an m-sequence. The original sequence from figure 21.2 is decimated by filling the bits from the original sequence across the four columns. This process produces four sequences, which are actually shifted versions of the original sequence.

patch, but it will actually evoke two responses at the retinal level.

The cross-correlation process

We can use column 1 of our decimated m-sequence to control a stimulus element to demonstrate the cross-correlation process. To describe cross-correlation, we shall use the first-order schematic diagram illustrated in figure 21.4.

In this schematic diagram, the recovered waveform is the transition to a white stimulus minus the transition to a black stimulus. Consider the use of the m-sequence to control a single hexagonal stimulus patch (figure 21.5). The associated raw data signal from the ERG electrodes is shown above the stimulus sequence. If there is a transition to a white stimulus from a preceding black or preceding white, then a predetermined segment of data is added into a memory buffer. The data segment can be of any time period but is usually chosen to be around 300 ms or long enough to encompass the evoked potential of interest. If the transition is to a black stimulus from a preceding black or white stimulus, then the appropriate data segment is subtracted from the memory buffer. Note that the data segment can and usually is much longer than the inter-stimulus difference (typically only 13.33 ms). This is very different from conventional electrophysiology, in which the serial averaging time window is

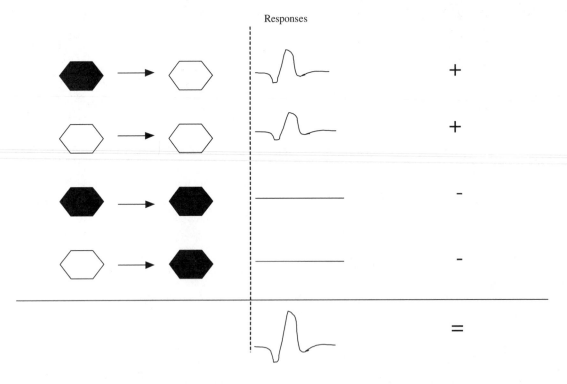

FIGURE 21.4 The first-order schematic diagram. Changes to a white stimulus are added in the cross-correlation process, and changes to black are subtracted. Note the response in row 1 (black-to-white transition) is not the same as the response in row 2 (white-to-white transition). As explained in the text, the illumination of the white hexagon lasts for a much shorter time than the base period, and the second consecutive.

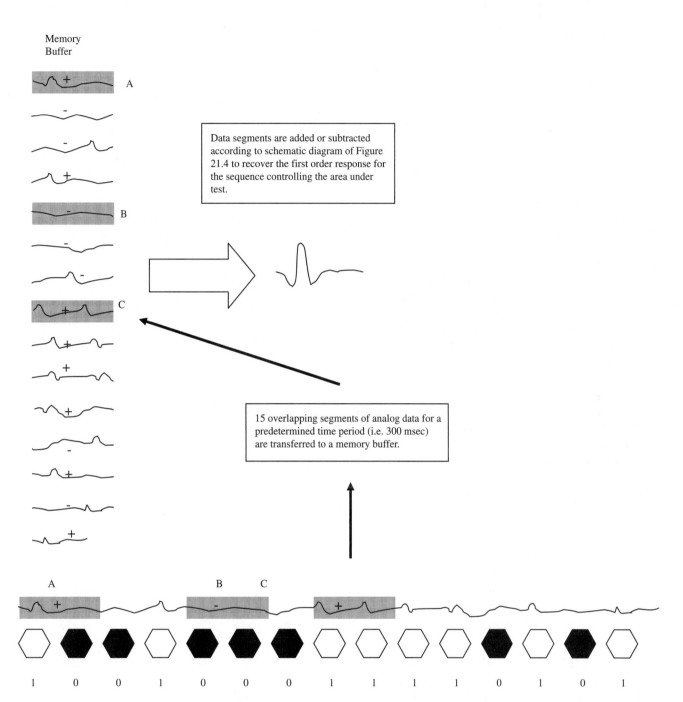

Memory
Buffer

Data segments are added or subtracted according to schematic diagram of Figure 21.4 to recover the first order response for the sequence controlling the area under test.

15 overlapping segments of analog data for a predetermined time period (i.e. 300 msec) are transferred to a memory buffer.

1 0 0 1 0 0 0 1 1 1 1 0 1 0 1

FIGURE 21.5 The cross-correlation process. The sequence generated in figure 21.2 is shown as shaded hexagons on the bottom row in the figure. A schematic version of the raw analog data from the ERG electrode is shown above the stimulus elements. If a white element is present, then a time window fol- lowing the onset of the stimulus is added to the memory buffer. Similarly, a transition to black is subtracted from the memory buffer. For the degree 4 sequence, a total of eight segments are added, and seven segments are subtracted. The resultant compos- ite response is shown.

shorter than the inter-stimulus interval. At the end of the recording period, the fully cross-correlated signal will therefore be constructed from 15 overlapping data segments, which will be the result of adding eight instances in which the stimulus was in the white state and subtracting seven segments in which the stimulus was in the black state.

Properties of m-sequences and dangers of poor sequence selection

m-Sequences have a number of properties that make them ideally suited to this type of application. The key properties are listed below.

WINDOW PROPERTY   The window property states that any bit pattern of a length n (n-tuple) for an m-sequence of degree n will occur only once in the sequence. This means that for our degree 4 m-sequence, any consecutive bit pattern that is 4 bits in length will occur only once in the sequence. This can be verified by visual examination of the sequence generated in figure 21.2.

PERIOD OR LENGTH   An m-sequence generated from a primitive polynomial of degree n will have a length of $2^n - 1$. If we continue to generate bits from the shift register, then the sequence will repeat after the $2^n - 1$ bits have been generated.

CYCLE CONTENTS   A complete m-sequence cycle has one more 1 than 0.

SHIFT AND ADD PROPERTY   The sum of any two distinct shifts of an m-sequence is a third shift of the same sequence.

We can use the shift and add property to illustrate the second-order response and to indicate the dangers of poor sequence selection.

The second-order schematic is shown in figure 21.6; it shows that instances in which there has been a change of state are added in the cross-correlation process and in instances in which there has not been a change of state, the data segments are subtracted.

Figure 21.7 shows examples of data segments added or subtracted in the cross-correlation process. If we now shift the original sequence right by 1 bit and add this new sequence to the original sequence using modulo 2 arithmetic, we form a new sequence as illustrated in row 3 of figure 21.7. This new sequence can be cross-correlated directly, as we would with the original sequence, only this time we will recover the second-order response instead of the first-order response. Figure 21.7 shows that cross-correlating the first sequence according to the rules of the schematic is the same as the standard cross-correlation using the new sequence in row 3. In effect, we can recover the second-order response direct simply by cross-correlating from row 3 of the figure. A key point to note here is that the second-order sequence is simply a shifted version of the original first-order sequence.

To illustrate the dangers of poor sequence selection, we will examine the decimated sequence of figure 21.3 in a little more detail. The first-order sequence for area B is rewritten

Flash Sequence   Responses

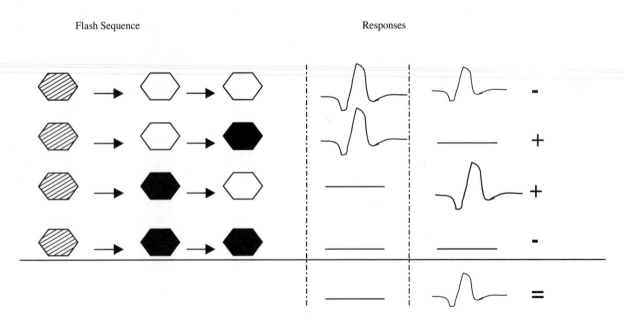

FIGURE 21.6 The second-order schematic diagram. Changes of state are added in the cross-correlation process. Two consecutive white stimuli or two consecutive black stimuli result in time windows being subtracted.

```
ABCD

1 0 0 1
0 0 0 1
1 1 1 0
1 0 1 1
0 0 1 0
0 0 1 1
1 1 0 1
0 1 1 0
0 1 0 0
0 1 1 1
1 0 1 0
1 1 0 0
1 0 0 0
1 1 1 1
0 1 0 1
```

1st order Area B	0 0 1 0 0 0 1 1 1 1 0 1 0 1 1
Shift Right	1 0 0 1 0 0 0 1 1 1 1 0 1 0 1
(Add mod 2) 2nd order Area B	1 0 1 1 0 0 1 0 0 0 1 1 1 1 0
1st order Area A	1 0 1 1 0 0 1 0 0 0 1 1 1 1 0

FIGURE 21.7   The second-order shift and add property. The decimated example in figure 21.3 is used to illustrate the second-order response. The top row shows the sequence for Area B. The next row shows the sequence shifted right by one bit. Row 3 shows the modulo 2 addition of rows 1 and 2. The bottom row shows the sequence for area A.

as the first row of figure 21.7, and if we use the shift and add technique the second row is the 1 bit shift, and row 3 is the mod 2 addition of rows 1 and 2 and represents the second-order sequence for area B. Cross-correlating the sequence from row 3 with the raw data will recover the second-order response for area B. However, examination of the decimated columns shows that this sequence is identical to the sequence that is used to control area A. This is an extreme form of kernel overlap or cross-contamination and means that cross-correlating the sequence for area A will result in a composite response that is actually the first-order response from area A combined or contaminated with the second-order response of area B. As a practical example of the use of these contaminated sequences, a photodiode placed over an area of the stimulus generates the first-order response as illustrated in figure 21.8. The photodiode is a linear device; therefore its output when a second-order cross-correlation is carried out should be zero. However, in this case, the sequences were poorly chosen, and the second-order responses from other areas are contaminated by first-order responses from the areas seen by the photodiode. Thus, signals from other hexagons that do not stimulate the photodiode produce first-order signals that appear as artefactual second-order responses to the photodiode.

There are a number of factors to consider in selecting an appropriate PRBS. When a sequence is decimated to provide a set of orthogonal sequences, we effectively have the same sequence shifted in time relative to the original sequence. To obtain clear separation of the cross-correlated responses, the shift between sequences must be larger than the time window of the evoked response. For example, if we consider using a 15-bit m-sequence, that is, a 2^{15} $(2^{15} - 1) =$ 32767 bit sequence to perform a multifocal ERG at a standard frame rate of 75 Hz and assuming an appropriate time window for the evoked response of 200 ms, then the shift between sequences must be greater than the following ratio:

$$\frac{\text{Time window}}{\text{Stimulus base period}} \text{ or } \frac{200}{13.33} = 16 \text{ sequence steps (rounded up)}$$

We must ensure that the sequences that are used to stimulate individual areas do not overlap in time. The possibility of creating flawed sequences increases as the number of stimulated areas increases, the length of the time window increases, or the length of the m-sequence is reduced. Furthermore, the primitive polynomial used will also influence the integrity of the sequences. Further details on the mathematics of sequence selection with specific reference to this cross-contamination issue can be found in a recent paper by Ireland.[22] One point to note is that *sequences of degree 12 delivered at a standard frame rate cannot be free from contamination no matter which primitive polynomial is used.* These factors are critical for the clean separation of multifocal responses, and developers must ensure that sequences fulfil these conditions. Unfortunately, manufacturers of multifocal systems do not provide the sequence information, and users must rely on the manufacturer's internal testing. The program given in the appendix to this chapter gives examples of sequences for a range of m-sequence lengths that are free from cross-contamination up to the third-order degree, assuming a standard frame rate of 75 Hz.

Software for the properties of m-sequences

Code is included in the appendix to demonstrate the generation, decimation, and empirical testing of the sequence integrity. The example code is written in an object-oriented

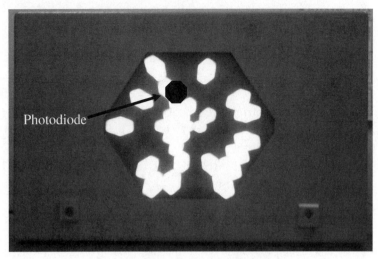

The Photodiode placed on the stimulus

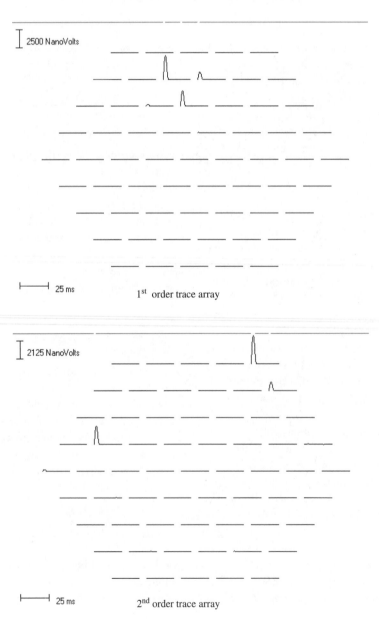

FIGURE 21.8 The photodiode experiment. The photodiode is placed on the stimulus as shown. The first trace array shows the first-order response, and the second trace array shows a contaminated second-order response.

programming language (Delphi 6) and has been simplified to enable ease of translation to other languages. The program allows the user to specify the degree of m-sequence to be generated and the number of stimulation sites required. The program will output the contamination-free time window in terms of the number of m-sequence steps or the number of milliseconds, assuming a stimulus base period of 13 ms. Specific primitive polynomials have been chosen to illustrate the influence of polynomial degree and number of stimulation sites on the duration of the contamination-free time period. Users may change the primitive polynomial simply by adjusting the appropriate tap positions in the code. The sequence testing is shown only for the first and second orders of the response; this is easily extended to further orders if desired. Copies of the program listed in the appendix are available from the authors.

Stimulus delivery

A number of options are available to deliver the multifocal stimulus. The most common method is the standard CRT monitor. The raster of a CRT device has important implications for the multifocal response. A standard CRT device will run at a frame rate of 75 Hz. A continuous white stimulus actually consists of a flickering area with each frame consisting of a period of 1–2 ms, depending on the phosphor of the device followed by a period of low luminance for the remaining time of the 13.33-ms base period. The schematic diagrams shown for the first- and second-order responses hold. There is, however, a finite time for the electron beam to traverse from the top of the screen to the bottom of the screen with lower areas typically presented 10 msec after the initial areas. This timing delay has to be corrected in the cross-correlation software. There are other methods of delivering the stimulus, such as the SLO technique described by Bultmann,[1] or Seeliger.[52] The SLO is a raster-based technique but runs at slower frame rates than the CRT device does. A further difference between SLO and CRT methods of stimulus delivery is the monochromatic light source of the SLO. The method used by our own group is that of the LCD projection system.[23,26,45] The LCD system is quite different from the CRT system in that for an m-sequence base period, the stimulus area will be in the high luminance state or the low luminance state for the full duration of the base period, that is, 13.33 ms if the frame rate is 75 Hz. The schematic diagrams for the first- and second-order responses are different from those shown in figures 21.4 and 21.6. Because a white-to-white transition is no longer two individual flashes but instead a continuous period of two base periods, that is, 26.66 ms, the schematic diagrams of figures 21.9 and 21.10 now apply. The multifocal response is therefore different from that of the CRT evoked response in that the nonlinearities of the response now include a contribution from the retina's ability to recovery from longer bleaching periods of stimulation. The LCD system does offer some attractive advantages over CRT. Wider fields of view are possible, as are higher luminance levels and improvement in signal-to-noise ratios because electromagnetic interference from the CRT scan coils is no longer present. It should be noted that the schematic diagrams are a simplification of the actual waveforms that are recovered.

LED stimulation

The use of LEDs for electrodiagnostic investigations has shown some exciting potential over the past decade or so. Several investigators[13,31,56] have used LEDs for electroretinography, and the devices are now used in several commercial electrophysiology systems. The use of solid-state devices for electrophysiology offers many advantages. Luminance does not change with time, as is the case with xenon flash tubes, and control of the stimulus pulse width is more flexible than with CRT displays.

In terms of multifocal stimulation, LEDs provide us with a versatile tool for investigation of the temporal aspects of the multifocal response but are less versatile than the high-resolution devices for examining the spatial characteristics of the response. One commercial multifocal system offers the option of LED matrix stimulation. Our own group uses a different prototype design, that consists of a fixed geometry 61-area hexagonal array.[57] From a research point of view, the LED system is versatile in that any pulse width duration can be programmed for the high luminance state. This opens up the possibility of optimizing the stimulation rate. One example of a trace array from the LED system of figure 21.8 is shown in figure 21.11. In this case, a stimulation rate of 77 Hz was used to simulate the most common method of delivering the stimulus: the CRT monitor.

Amplifier bandwidth and preservation of waveform shape

The importance of correct amplifier bandwidth needs no elaboration here (see chapters 16 and 19). Figure 21.12 shows the multifocal ERGs from a patient with an upper branch retinal vein occlusion recorded simultaneously from the same electrode with two band-pass settings. Positive P1 components are clearly seen on the 10-Hz recording, whereas the 1-Hz recording shows severe reduction of the P1 component. These results indicate that the multifocal ERG is just as susceptible to filtering artifacts as standard electrophysiology recordings are.[25] The difficulty with multifocal ERG recordings is that the signal amplitudes are

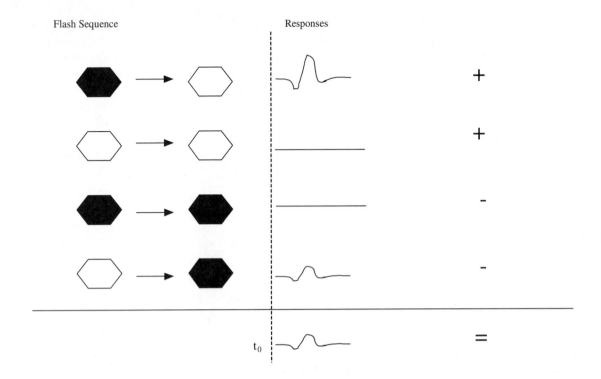

1st order LCD schematic diagram

FIGURE 21.9 First-order LCD schematic. The difference between this schematic diagram and the schematic of figure 21.4, which is for a CRT stimulus, is that no response is present for the continuous white-to-white transition.

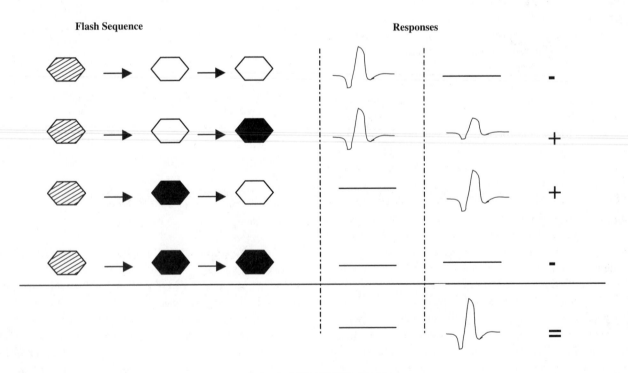

2nd order LCD schematic diagram

FIGURE 21.10 Second-order LCD response. The difference between this figure and the CRT schematic in figure 21.6 is the absence of a response for the white-to-white transition.

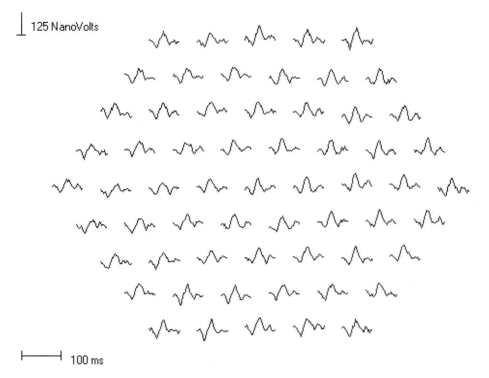

125 NanoVolts

100 ms

FIGURE 21.11 A recording using an LED stimulator. A 61-element trace array example from the LED stimulator for a control subject.

orders of magnitude smaller than ERG recordings. This means that amplifier gains are increased considerably, which in turn can lead to amplifier saturation when there are losses in fixation. In most of the early multifocal ERG recordings, a restricted filter bandwidth of 10–100 Hz was the most common. There is little doubt that wider-bandwidth recordings are more difficult to perform. Small losses of fixation can cause amplifier saturation, and the longer time constants make amplifier recovery longer. The a.c. affect of a 10-Hz filter enables the amplifier to quickly return to baseline, enabling a reduction in saturation times. However, these reductions in amplifier saturation come at a cost, as epochs of the raw data recording may be from periods when the eye is not fixating on the appropriate target, thereby causing a degradation of the cross-correlated response. The considerations of ease of recording against signal integrity has resulted in ISCEV's recommending a 3- to 300-Hz filter bandwidth in the multifocal ERG guidelines.[38] This filter bandwidth reduces the signal distortions present with the 10-Hz bandwidth and also limits the signal saturation problems associated with the 1-Hz recordings. Nevertheless, investigators should always opt for the widest bandwidth, particularly if the clinical investigation results in selective reduction of the Ganzfeld ERG b-wave or the multifocal P1 wave.

The origins of the multifocal ERG

The multifocal ERG response is a complex composite response that is a record of the various cellular retinal mechanisms response to a range of stimulation frequencies. Our knowledge of the standard full-field ERG continues to be refined. In recent years, significant evidence has pointed to OFF bipolar cells as the main contribution to the ISCEV standard photopic a-wave[2] and to the ON bipolar cells as the main contributor to the b-wave,[55] although these cells are not exclusively responsible, and it is likely that there are contributions from many sources, in particular a cone contribution to the a-wave[2] and an OFF bipolar contribution to the b-wave.[55] To understand or identify the contributing factors to the various mfERG waveform components requires analysis of data from a variety of sources. Readers should be aware that the waveforms are quite different and include contributions from nonlinear processing mechanisms such as spatial interactions, temporal processing interactions, spatiotemporal interactions, and adaptation profiles. In investigating such contributions, it is important to remember the definitions of the cross-correlated responses. The first-order response is the difference between a transition to a high-luminance state minus the transition to a low-luminance state. The second-order

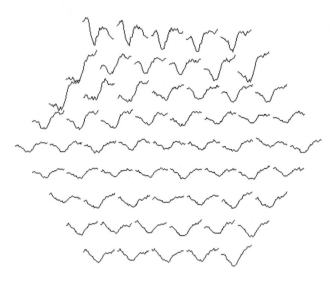

Filter bandwidth 1 – 300 Hz

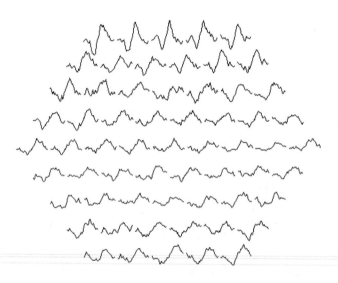

Filter bandwidth 10 – 300

FIGURE 21.12   The effect of filter bandwidth on the trace array. Corresponding trace arrays recovered simultaneously using two different filter bandwidths illustrating the waveform shape changes due to the differentiation effect of the high-pass 10-Hz filter.

response is the difference between a change of state and no change of state.

The relationship between Ganzfeld ERG and multifocal ERG

The first significant comparison of multifocal ERGs with the standard full-field ERG was performed by Hood et al. in

1996.[18] By slowing the stimulus down, Hood et al. showed that there is good correspondence between the full-field ERG a-wave and the multifocal ERG N1 component and between the full-field ERG b-wave and the multifocal ERG P1 component. Hood also showed that by increasing the stimulation rate to the standard 75-Hz frame rate, correspondence between the a-wave and the N1 waves remained intact. At the faster stimulation rates, there is less correspondence between the P1 component of the mfERG and the ERG b-wave. This is not surprising because the full-field ERG contains no information on nonlinear processing, and at fast stimulation rates, the multifocal ERG is significantly influenced by nonlinear processing. Further details on the comparison between Ganzfeld ERG and multifocal ERG are given in Chapter 14.

The previous section on amplifier bandwidth and preservation of waveform shape, in particular figure 21.12, indicates that in clinical examples in which there is a selective reduction in the b-wave, similar changes are seen in the multifocal ERG response. This means not that the waveforms are identical but that the same sources are major contributing factors to the response. The multifocal ERG response is quite different from the Ganzfeld ERG, particularly at fast frame rates. The response is not a continuous record of events with one component delayed in time relative to the other. It is not possible to meaningfully interpret the timing differences between individual components such as the N1-to-P1 times or the P2-to-N2 times. Each individual component is in itself a composite response from different pulse trains, which in turn stimulated the retina at different moments in time.

Dissecting the contributing factors to the mfERG response

Following from the previous discussion on the differences in waveform shapes between slow and fast stimulation, further light can be shed on the complexities of the multifocal response if the factors contributing to the response are examined by recovering the responses to specific pulse trains embedded in the m-sequence. A technique of selective cross-correlation to recover the response to specific pulse trains embedded in the full sequence was developed to examine the contributing components to m-sequence-controlled ERG measurements.[27] In this work, a cross-correlation is performed between the raw data signal and data segments for particular pulse trains in the m-sequence rather than using the standard first- and second-order cross-correlations previously described. Figures 21.13 and 21.14 show the contributing factors to the composite response from these different pulse trains. By dissecting the response in this way, it shows that the multifocal

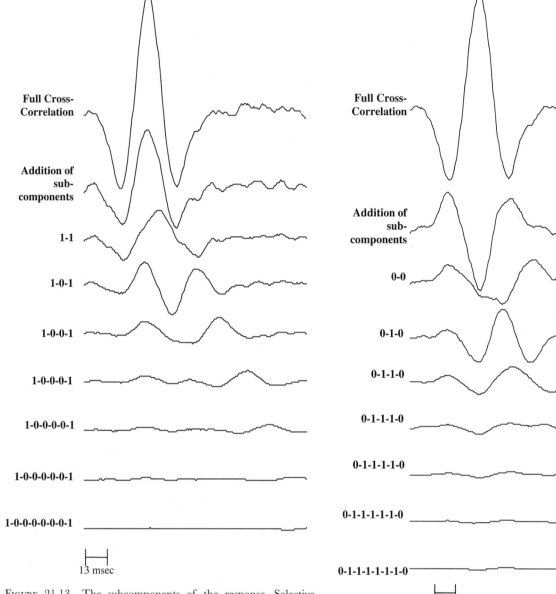

Full Cross-Correlation

Addition of sub-components

1-1

1-0-1

1-0-0-1

1-0-0-0-1

1-0-0-0-0-1

1-0-0-0-0-0-1

1-0-0-0-0-0-0-1

H 13 msec

FIGURE 21.13 The subcomponents of the response. Selective cross-correlation of the various pulse trains embedded in the m-sequence together with the addition of these components and the full cross-correlation for comparison.

Full Cross-Correlation

Addition of sub-components

0-0

0-1-0

0-1-1-0

0-1-1-1-0

0-1-1-1-1-0

0-1-1-1-1-1-0

0-1-1-1-1-1-1-0

H 13 msec

FIGURE 21.14 Further subcomponents of the response. The inverse pulse trains to those of figure 21.13. In this case, the pulse trains are differing separations of two 0's as opposed to two 1's as in fig. 21.13.

response is therefore a composite response from a number of different pulse trains that are embedded in the full m-sequence. Figure 21.15 shows that the summation of these components is identical to the full cross-correlation. In this context, it is not surprising that some of the features that are significant in the slow stimulus that is used to evoke a full-field ERG are missing from the composite multifocal response. Correspondingly, new information on the nonlinear dynamics of retinal processing is incorporated in the composite responses.

Animal studies and the use of pharmacological blocking agents

In recent years, the use of pharmacological blocking agents has played a significant role in our understanding of the origins of the conventional photopic ERG waveforms. The most notable work was performed by Sieving, who administered glutamate analogs in the monkey to study the

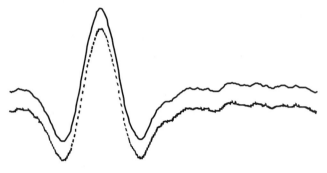

FIGURE 21.15 A comparison of subcomponent addition with the full cross-correlation. The full cross-correlation is compared with the combined subcomponents of figures 21.13 and 21.14. A vertical data shift is included here to show the two identical traces.

generation of the photopic ERG.[2,55] The effects of these blocking agents are summarized below.

APB (L-2 amino-4-phosphonobutyric acid) blocks transmission from photoreceptors to ON bipolar cells (depolarizing bipolars, or DBCs) and also blocks transmission to ON amacrine cells and ON ganglion cells.

PDA (cis-2,3 piperdine dicarboxylic acid) blocks transmission from photoreceptors to OFF bipolar cells (hyperpolarizing bipolars, or HBCs) and also to horizontal cells but does not block pathways to ON bipolar cells. It also blocks transmission from both ON and OFF bipolar cells to amacrine and ganglion cells. This implies that PDA isolates activity to photoreceptors and ON bipolar cells.

TTX (tetrdotoxin) blocks all sodium-based action potentials (generated by ganglion and amacrine cells).

In terms of the full-field photopic ERG, using intravitreal injections of APB and PDA, Bush and Sieving showed that the photopic a-wave is generated by OFF bipolar cells and cones[2] and that the b-wave is generated by a combination of OFF and ON bipolar cells.[55]

Similar studies on both the rabbit and monkey models on the multifocal ERG have now been performed and have given some insight into the possible mechanisms generating the multifocal ERG. However, one should always bear in mind that the multifocal ERG is not a single response waveform as is the case in the Ganzfeld ERG but a composite response from a number of different waveforms.[27] Nevertheless, the work of several groups detailed below does give important information on current research on the multifocal ERG origins.

In particular three separate studies by Horiguchi et al.,[19] Hare et al.,[12] and Hood et al.[15,16] have made significant advances on our knowledge of the origins of the multifocal ERG. The work of interest was conducted on the rabbit by Horiguchi et al., on monkeys (*Macaca fascicularis*) by Hare et al., and on *Macaca mulatta* by Hood et al. There are obvi-

ously species differences that make translation to the human difficult; nevertheless, Hood et al. have used this information to develop a working model of the human multifocal ERG.[15]

APB Horiguchi et al. found in the rabbit model that administering APB caused a reduction in the first-order P1 component and examination of the figures also indicates a reduction in the N2 component. In the same set of experiments for the full-field flash ERG, the b-wave of the long-duration flash was abolished by APB, and the positive peak of the short duration flash was significantly reduced by APB.

In contrast to Horiguchi et al.'s results, Hare et al. showed that APB reduces the amplitude of the b-wave but increases the amplitude of all components of the first-order mfERG. These results appear to conflict but can be partly explained by the differences in the animal models. Horiguchi et al. state that the rabbit has a significantly larger b/a ratio than the monkey does and that HBC activity makes less of a contribution to the response; this evidence is supported by absence of a cornea-positive d-wave. Hare et al. offer an explanation on the increase in N1 and P1 amplitudes, with APB as ON pathway cells driving the early phase of P1, which in turn truncates N1 and limits the later positive contribution to P1. APB is insensitive to OFF pathway contributions.

PDA In the rabbit work of Horiguchi, PDA abolished the N1 component of the mfERG first-order and had greater effect on the second-order with only a small corneo-negative component remaining. Hare et al. showed an enhancement of P1 from all eccentricities. N1 was abolished in the periphery and reduced in the center. The PDA reduction in N1 is consistent with that seen in the a-wave and indicates a contribution from activity in second and third OFF pathway cells to N1. The enhancement of P1 is also consistent with the idea of OFF pathway activity limiting the contribution of on pathway activity supported by Bush and Sieving.[2,55]

PDA shows a greater effect on the second order in both Horiguchi et al.'s and Hare et al.'s work, suggesting a greater contribution from OFF pathway activity to the second order.

TTX Hare et al. showed a slight reduction in the N1 amplitude at all eccentricities with little effect on P1 or N2 for the central responses and slight attenuation of P1 and N2 in the periphery. The second order showed a significant effect on the response from the central area with less effect on responses with increasing eccentricity. Hare et al. concluded that the effects of blocking the sodium gated channels on the first order is consistent with the full-field findings in that increasing the timing of the N1, P1, and N2 is the main effect. In the second order, a significant effect is seen on the central responses and less of an effect in the periphery, suggesting a significant contribution from amacrine and/or ganglion cells. Hare et al. also compared the effects of chronic ocular hypertension and TTX, which produced similar effects on the second order but showed significant differences in the N2 component of the first order. Important factors that may influence the results of these studies are the electrode positions and the effects of anaesthesia.[7]

A somewhat different approach was taken by Hood and coworkers. In Hood's work, TTX and N-methyl-D-aspartic acid was administered to remove all sodium-based action potentials and inner retinal potentials. At this point, the monkey multifocal ERG no longer had the fast oscillations and closely resembled the human multifocal ERG. Once these potentials were removed, then APB, PDA, and both APB and PDA were administered. This enabled the effects of OFF bipolars, ON bipolars, and photoreceptors to be estimated by careful subtraction of the various waveforms. Although some assumptions clearly have to be made, Hood et al.'s work resulted in the most comprehensive working model of the human multifocal ERG. His work supported the following chain of events for the first-order response. The leading edge of N1 is the onset of OFF bipolar cell activity with smaller receptor contribution and perhaps smaller inner retina contribution. Before the trough of N1 is reached, the shape of N1 is altered by the ON bipolar contribution. The initial portion of the leading edge of P1 is a combination of depolarization of ON bipolar and hyperpolarization of OFF bipolars. After the OFF bipolar contribution reached its trough, the leading edge of P1 is a combination of depolarization of both ON and OFF bipolars. The trailing edge of P1 is the recovery of the ON bipolars with some contribution from OFF bipolar recovery and a contribution from the inner retina.[15]

Although this work is extremely valuable in our understanding of the multifocal response, it is important to note that the multifocal ERG is not a single waveform but is a composite response from a number of interactive components. Further work on the effects of these drugs on the subcomponents that contribute to the mfERG is required. A further compounding factor is the translation of these effects from the animal to the human model.

Clinical applications

There are now several hundred publications on the multifocal technique, the majority of them on the clinical applications. In our unit, thousands of clinical investigations using the technique have been performed, and we have found the investigation to be invaluable in a wide range of conditions.[46] An overview of the clinical application was given in a recent paper by Hood.[41] To try to summarize the huge amount of published data on multifocal ERG, it is useful to try to categorize the applications into one of five areas. Throughout these publications, many authors refer to the second order

as the nonlinear or inner retinal component, but these statements are still open to debate. Evidence from our own study on the components that contribute to the multifocal ERG show that the same components exist in both first and second orders; they are simply added and subtracted in a different way. Furthermore, evidence from the animal investigations has still not clarified the contributions from the inner retina to a specific order of the response, and these investigations are further complicated in translation from the animal to the human model. It is possible that the effects of inner retinal contributions may be more evident in the second order; if so, then some effect must also be present in the first order.

Our custom-built multifocal system quantifies the quality of a recording using a reliability index. This index makes use of the fact that fixation losses cause amplifier saturation (particularly for wide filter bandwidths). The reliability index therefore measures amplifier saturation as an indicator of fixation quality.

In terms of the technical reliability of the technique on a range of conditions comprising macular disease, vascular disease, trauma, retinal dystrophies, toxicities, and inflammatory conditions, of 2151 investigations, 86 (4%) had reliability index in one or both eyes below the tolerance of 70%; 14 (0.6%) investigations were terminated before completion owing to poor patient compliance; 1694 (79%) investigations confirmed or improved localization of pathology to a retinal defect; 313 (15%) provided complementary information to discount an outer or midretinal cause for visual dysfunction; and in 44 (2%) of investigations, results remained inconclusive.

VASCULAR DISEASES OF THE RETINA
Diabetes Palmowski et al.[44] showed reduction in the first-order multifocal ERG response and also showed multifocal ERG abnormalities before clinical changes were apparent. The second-order responses in diabetic patients with or without retinopathy were also reduced, corroborating earlier work by Palmowski et al. which the authors suggest was due to inner retinal dysfunction.

Modifying the technique by using the inserted global flash also showed abnormalities in diabetic patients without retinopathy, suggesting a reduced ability of the diabetic eye to recover from a bright preceding stimulus.[53] Multifocal ERG implicit time delays could also indicate subclinical retinopathy.[8] Implicit time delays of multifocal ERG responses were also more useful indicators of diabetic macular edema than were multifocal ERG amplitude changes.[11]

Multifocal ERGs may have a role to play in assessing subclinical retinal changes in patients with diabetes. In addition, multifocal ERGs may improve objective follow-up of treatment interventions for diabetic retinopathy.

Branch retinal artery occlusion A small study on three patients with branch retinal artery occlusion showed a reduction in amplitude and a delay in implicit times of the first-order P1 and N1 mfERG responses in the affected quadrant, compared to the vertically symmetrical unaffected quadrant. The second-order responses in the affected quadrant were absent; the authors indicated that this reflected inner retinal dysfunction.[42]

Retinitis pigmentosa At advanced stages of retinitis pigmentosa (RP), the standard Ganzfeld ERG responses can be unrecordable. The spatial resolution of multifocal ERG facilitates the recording of local electrical responses from the central retina in patients with advanced RP.[17,51]

Implicit time delays of multifocal ERG responses in patients with RP could be a useful early indicator of the disease and a useful parameter for monitoring the progression of RP.[17] Multifocal ERG detects implicit time delay and amplitude reduction in a patient with early RP who was found to have normal ERG responses, indicating that in this case, multifocal ERG is a more sensitive investigative tool.[5] Furthermore, the implicit time delay of the multifocal ERG response correlated well with the reduction in visual sensitivities recorded with Humphrey visual field analysis.[17,35]

The normal multifocal ERG amplitude declines with increasing eccentricity from fixation.[61] Multifocal ERG amplitude decline is much more pronounced in patients with RP.[51] Multifocal ERG may enable the progression of RP to be followed more accurately, facilitating a better understanding of the variants of the disease.

MACULAR DISEASES

Age-related macular degeneration Multifocal ERG has been shown to be a sensitive tool in the assessment of patients with pre or early age-related macular degeneration (ARMD).[21,35] The P1 amplitude and PI latency of the central multifocal ERG responses were significantly reduced and delayed in pre-ARMD and early ARMD eyes and also in the fellow asymptomatic eyes when compared to age-matched controls.[21] Interestingly, significant delays of the peripheral retinal multifocal ERG responses were obtained from patients with ARMD, using wide-field multifocal ERG, suggesting that ARMD globally affects retinal function.[24]

Stargardt's macular dystrophy Macular multifocal ERG response amplitudes were significantly reduced in patients with Stargardt's macular dystrophy (SMD). Central multifocal ERG amplitude reductions were detected even in patients with normal visual acuity and normal visual fields.[32] These findings may have important implications in the assessment of asymptomatic relatives of affected patients with SMD.

Best macular dystrophy Central multifocal ERG amplitude reductions that correlated significantly with visual acuity loss were observed in a population of 18 patients with Best macular dystrophy. However, the multifocal ERG reductions were much more marked than those observed in eyes with ARMD or SMD.[50]

Central serous retinopathy Vajaranant et al. tested six patients diagnosed clinically and angiographically with unilateral central serous retinopathy (CSR) using multifocal electroretinography.[62] They found that multifocal ERG abnormalities of reduced amplitudes plus or minus implicit time delays were localized only to the areas that were clinically affected by the CSR, and they did not find multifocal ERG abnormalities in clinically normal areas of the affected eyes.

OTHER RETINAL DISEASES

Multiple evanescent white dot syndrome Multifocal ERG responses of a patient with multiple evanescent white dot syndrome were markedly reduced in the area corresponding to the central scotoma and moderately reduced in other parts of the central field. The reduction in amplitude of multifocal ERG responses was still apparent four months later, when visual acuity and visual fields had returned to normal.[20]

Acute idiopathic enlarged blind spot syndrome Multifocal ERG performed on seven patients diagnosed with acute idiopathic enlarged blind spot syndrome showed reduced and delayed first- and second-order multifocal ERG kernels, not only in the affected eye but also in the asymptomatic fellow eye. The retinal dysfunction that was recorded using the multifocal ERG was not confined to the optic disc area but extended into the posterior pole.[64] This small study suggests that mfERG may be a useful objective tool in the management of acquired retinal disorders.

Retinal surgery and mfERG An objective means of assessing visual function is useful for follow-up of patients after ocular surgery. Multifocal ERGs may have a key role to play in the postoperative management of patients after vitreoretinal surgery. The improvement in multifocal ERG responses after retinal detachment repair in these patients closely mirrored the subjective improvement experienced by the patients.[49] Multifocal ERG responses were markedly decreased at the fovea and, indeed, in the perifoveal areas preoperatively in patients with macular holes.[54] The loss of retinal function in the perifoveal areas was due to perifoveal retinoschisis, confirmed with optical coherence tomography. Postoperatively, multifocal ERG responses significantly improved in both the fovea and perifoveal regions. It is believed that the foveal improvement was due to closure of the hole and that the perifoveal improvement of visual function and resolution of metamorphopsia was due to the reattachment of the perifoveal retinoschsis.

Pioneering surgery has been reported in the treatment of RP involving the transplantation of intact sheets of donor foetal retina[48] into eyes with severe autosomal recessive RP. Multifocal ERG post operatively showed a small but significant negative mfERG component in the region of the transplant when the second-order response was analyzed, the significance of which has yet to be validated. These small studies indicate that mfERG potentially has an important role to play in the objective assessment of retinal function before and after retinal surgery.

Retinal toxicity and the role of mfERG Vigabatrin (VGB), an analog of gamma-aminobutyric acid, which is used in the treatment of epilepsy, has known risks of causing irreversible peripheral visual field loss.[6] Wide-field multifocal ERG (WF-mfERG) shows marked visual field constriction[39] consistent with field tests and also relatively preserved responses in the central 40 degrees in patients treated with VGB. Further work suggests a role for WF-mfERG in the assessment and early detection of retinal toxic side effects of VGB.

Multifocal ERG was found to be a sensitive indicator of retinal dysfunction in patients with chloroquine toxicity.[28] The technique was more sensitive at detecting abnormalities of retinal function than standard ERG or routine clinical tests.[28] However, only three patients were assessed in this small study.

Multifocal ERG is proving to be an easy, well-tolerated objective means of assessing retinal toxicity.

Glaucoma The role of multifocal ERG in the assessment of glaucoma patients has still not been fully explored. Current understanding suggests that multifocal ERG in its standard form is probably not as useful in the assessment of patients with inner retinal dysfunction, such as glaucoma, as it is in the assessment of patients with outer retinal or midretinal dysfunction. Some promising work on modification of the stimulation paradigms may prove useful in the isolation of inner retinal dysfunction. These techniques include the isolation of an optic nerve head component as explored by Sutter.[60] Further work is required to assess the clinical implications of such techniques. In contrast to multifocal ERG techniques, more success has been obtained with the multifocal VEP in the diagnosis of early glaucomatous changes.[10,30]

The multifocal ERG adds a new dimension to ocular electrophysiology. Significant work on the technical considerations and on the clinical application has been conducted in the past decade. The technique has been shown to be of benefit in a wide range of retinal disorders. Further work on the signal origins and on modifications of the technique for assessment of inner retinal function will take the technique further forward in the future. In parallel with the multifocal ERG work, advances on the application and understanding of multifocal VECP will eventually provide complementary information on cortical processing. The multifocal technique provides researchers with the tools to investigate visual processing and with the practical tools to assess a wide range of clinical conditions.

APPENDIX: M-SEQUENCE GENERATOR PROGRAM

```
// The program is written in Delphi 6 code with the procedures
kept to a minimum number to enable ease of translation to
other languages.

   By selecting appropriate radio buttons it is possible to gener-
ate m-sequences from degree 12 to 16 and decimate the
sequences into 64, 128, or 256 columns. The decimated arrays
are suitable for multifocal experiments. Each array is tested
empirically for cross contamination and the contamination free
period reported in the appropriate text output box.
   Authors David Keating and Stuart Parks, 2003.
   Permission is hereby given for personal use by individuals
only and not for commercial gain.


unit sequence_generator;


interface


uses
Windows, Messages, SysUtils, Variants, Classes, Graphics, Con-
trols, Forms, Dialogs, StdCtrls, Spin;

type
  TForm1 = class(TForm)
    GroupBox2: TGroupBox;
    GroupBox1: TGroupBox;
    GroupBox3: TGroupBox;
    Generate_sequence_button: TButton;
    Edit1: TEdit;
    Edit2: TEdit;
    Label1: TLabel;
    Label2: TLabel;
    Label3: TLabel;
    Label4: TLabel;
    SpinEdit1: TSpinEdit;
    RadioButton1: TRadioButton;
    RadioButton2: TRadioButton;
    RadioButton3: TRadioButton;
    procedure RadioButton1Click(Sender: TObject);
    procedure RadioButton2Click(Sender: TObject);
    procedure RadioButton3Click(Sender: TObject);
    procedure Start(Sender: TObject);
```

```
    procedure Find_Overlap_positions;
    procedure Generate_Second_order;
    procedure Decimate_sequence;
    procedure Generate_sequence;
    procedure FormCreate(Sender: TObject);
    procedure SpinEdit1Change(Sender: TObject);
  private
    { Private declarations }
  public
    { Public declarations }
    m_sequence_degree, no_of_msteps,ntaps,no_of_sites:
integer;
    window_length, site_no,step_no:integer;
    base_sequence: array[1..65535] of integer;
    m_sequence_array: array[1..65535,1..256] of integer;
    m_sequence_second_order: array[1..65535,1..256] of
integer;
    tap: array[1..16] of integer
  end;

var
  Form1: TForm1;

implementation


{$R *.dfm}

procedure TForm1.RadioButton1Click(Sender: TObject);
begin
no_of_sites:=64;
end;

procedure TForm1.RadioButton2Click(Sender: TObject);
begin
no_of_sites:=128;
end;

procedure TForm1.RadioButton3Click(Sender: TObject);
begin
no_of_sites:=256;
end;


procedure TForm1.Find_overlap_positions;
var
    site_no,step_no,l,check_step,column_shift: integer;
    first_order_runofones,second_order_runofones : integer;
    first_order_start,second_order_start, time_window:
integer;
    no_of_msecs: integer;
    seed_found: boolean;
    s: string;
begin
// find the start position of the longest run of ones in
columns 1 of first order
```

```
seed_found:=FALSE;
site_no:=1;
step_no:=0;
Repeat
        step_no:=step_no+1;
        // look for n consecutive ones
        if m_sequence_array[step_no,site_no]=1 then
                begin
                        l:=0;
                        seed_found:=TRUE;
                        Repeat
                                l:=l+1;
                                check_step:=step_no;
                                if step_no+l>no_of_msteps then
check_step:=step_no-no_of_msteps;
                                if m_sequence_array
[check_step+l,site_no]=0 then seed_found:=FALSE;
                        until l=m_sequence_degree-1;
                        if seed_found=TRUE then
first_order_runofones:=step_no;
                end;
        Until step_no=no_of_msteps;

//Where does 2nd order occur—look for n consecutive ones

seed_found:=FALSE;
step_no:=0;
site_no:=1;
Repeat
        step_no:=step_no+1;
                if m_sequence_second_order
[step_no,site_no]=1 then
                        begin
                                l:=0;
                                seed_found:=TRUE;
                                Repeat
                                        l:=l+1;
                                        check_step:=step_no;
                                        if step_no+l>no_of_
msteps then  check_step:=step_no-no_of_msteps;
                                        if m_sequence_second
_order[check_step+l,site_no]=0 then seed_found:=FALSE;
                                until l=m_sequence_degree-1;
                                if seed_found=TRUE then
second_order_runofones:=step_no;
                        end;
        Until step_no=no_of_msteps;


//Now calculate available time window—assume m-sequence
base period of 13 msec

Find lowest start position for first order
        column_shift:=(no_of_msteps+1) div no_of_sites;
        first_order_start:=first_order_runofones mod column_
shift;
```

```
        second_order_start:=second_order_runofones mod
column_shift;

        if second_order_start>first_order_start then
time_window:=second_order_start-first_order_start;
        if second_order_start<first_order_start then
time_window:=first_order_start-second_order_start;
        if (column_shift-time_window)<time_window then
time_window:=column_shift-time_window;
        if second_order_start=first_order_start then
time_window:=0;
        str(time_window,s);
        Form1.Edit1.Text:=s;
        no_of_msecs:=time_window*13;
        str(no_of_msecs,s);
        Form1.Edit2.Text:=s;
        Form1.label4.caption:='Sequence Generated';
end;


procedure TForm1.Generate_Second_order;
var site_no,step_no,next_step: integer;
begin
//generate first column of a second order array
        step_no:=0;
        site_no:=1;
        Repeat
                step_no:=step_no+1;
                next_step:=step_no+1;
                if next_step> no_of_msteps then next_step:=1;

m_sequence_second_order[step_no,site_no]:=(m_sequence_
array[step_no,site_no]+m_sequence_array[next_step,site_no])
mod 2;
        Until step_no=no_of_msteps;
end;


procedure TForm1.Decimate_sequence;
 // Now Decimate_sequence in to no of columns =
no_of_sites;
var k,step_no,site_no: integer;
begin
        step_no:=0;
        site_no:=0;
        k:=0;
        Repeat
                step_no:=step_no+1;
                site_no:=0;
                Repeat
                        site_no:=site_no+1;
                        k:=k+1;
                        If k=no_of_msteps+1 then k:=1;
                        m_sequence_array[step_no,site_no]:
=base_sequence[k];
                Until site_no=no_of_sites;
```

```
        Until step_no=no_of_msteps;
// decimation complete
end;


procedure TForm1.Generate_sequence;
var k,l,new_bit,no_of_msteps:integer;
s:string;
begin
        Form1.label4.caption:='Please Wait—Generating
Sequence';
        s:=' ';
        Form1.Edit1.Text:=s;
        Form1.Edit2.Text:=s;
        Form1.refresh;
        // first set initial seed pattern
        // equal to run of 1 bits of length n for sequence of
degree n
        For k:=1 to m_sequence_degree do
                begin
                        base_sequence[k]:=1;
                end;
        For k:=m_sequence_degree+1 to no_of_msteps do
                begin
                        new_bit:=0;
                        For l:=1 to ntaps do
                                begin
                                        // perform addition modulo 2
on bits in tap positions
                                        new_bit:=new_bit+base_
sequence[k-tap[l]];
                                end;
                        new_bit:=new_bit mod 2;
                        base_sequence[k]:=new_bit;
                end;
        Form1.refresh;
end;


procedure TForm1.FormCreate(Sender: TObject);
begin
        // set start up default values
        m_sequence_degree:=12;
        no_of_msteps:=4095;
        ntaps:=4;
        tap[1]:=12;
        tap[2]:=6;
        tap[3]:=4;
        tap[4]:=1;
        no_of_sites:=64;
end;


procedure TForm1.SpinEdit1Change(Sender: TObject);
begin
Case SpinEdit1.value of
        12:     begin
```

```
              m_sequence_degree:=12;                          tap[7]:=6;
              no_of_msteps:=4095;                             tap[8]:=5;
              ntaps:=4;                                       tap[9]:=4;
              tap[1]:=12;                                     tap[10]:=3;
              tap[2]:=6;                                 end;
              tap[3]:=4;
              tap[4]:=1;                        16:    begin
          end;                                             m_sequence_degree:=16;
                                                           no_of_msteps:=65535;
      13:    begin                                         ntaps:=4;
              m_sequence_degree:=13;                       tap[1]:=16;
              no_of_msteps:=8191;                          tap[2]:=5;
              ntaps:=4;                                    tap[3]:=3;
              tap[1]:=13;                                  tap[4]:=2;
              tap[2]:=4;                                end;
              tap[3]:=3;
              tap[4]:=1;                            end;
          end;                              end;

      14:    begin                          procedure TForm1.Start(Sender: TObject);
              m_sequence_degree:=14;         begin
              no_of_msteps:=16383;               Generate_Sequence;
              ntaps:=4;                          Decimate_Sequence;
              tap[1]:=14;                        Generate_Second_order;
              tap[2]:=5;                         Find_overlap_positions;
              tap[3]:=3;                     end;
              tap[4]:=1;
          end;                               end. {end program}

      15:    begin                           program msequence_generator;
              m_sequence_degree:=15;          uses
              no_of_msteps:=32767;              Forms,
              ntaps:=10;                        sequence_generator in 'sequence_generator.pas' {Form1};
              tap[1]:=15;
              tap[2]:=14;                      {$R *.res}
              tap[3]:=11;
              tap[4]:=10;                      begin
              tap[5]:=9;                        Application.Initialize;
              tap[6]:=8;                        Application.CreateForm(TForm1, Form1);
                                               Application.Run;
                                              end.
```

REFERENCES

1. Bultmann S, Rohrschneider K: Reproducibility of multifocal ERG using the scanning laser ophthalmoscope. *Graefes Arch Clin Exp Ophthalmol* 2002; 240(10):841–845.

2. Bush RA, Sieving PA: A proximal retinal component in the primate photopic ERG a-wave. *Invest Ophthalmol Vis Sci* 1994; 35(2):635–645.

3. Collins AD, Sawhney BB: Pseudorandom binary sequence stimulation applied to the visual evoked response: Normative data and a comparative study with pattern and flash stimulation. *Doc Ophthalmol* 1993; 83(2):163–173.

4. Davies WDT: *System Identification for Self-Adaptive Control.* New York, Wiley, 1970.

5. Dolan FM, Parks S, Hammer H, Keating D: The wide field multifocal electroretinogram reveals retinal dysfunction in early retinitis pigmentosa. *Br J Ophthalmol* 2002; 86(4):480–481.

6. Eke T, Talbot J, Lawden MC: Severe persistent visual field constriction associated with vigabatrin. *Br Med Journal* 1997; 314:180–181.

7. Fortune B, Cull G, Wang L, Van Buskirk EM, Cioffi GA: Factors affecting the use of multifocal electroretinography to monitor function in a primate model of glaucoma. *Doc Ophthalmol* 2002; 105(2):151–178.

8. Fortune B, Schneck ME, Adams AJ: Multifocal electroretinogram delays reveal local retinal dysfunction in early diabetic retinopathy. *Invest Ophthalmol Vis Sci* 1999; 40(11):2638–2651.

9. Fricker SJ, Sanders JJ: A new method of cone electroretinography: The rapid random flash response. *Invest Ophthalmol* 1975; 14(2):131–137.

10. Graham SL, Klistorner AI, Grigg JR, Billson FA: Objective VEP perimetry in glaucoma: Asymmetry analysis to identify early deficits. *J Glaucoma* 2000; 9(1):10–19.

11. Greenstein VC, Holopigian K, Hood DC, Seiple W, Carr RE: The nature and extent of retinal dysfunction associated with diabetic macular edema. *Invest Ophthalmol Vis Sci* 2000; 41(11):3643–3654.

12. Hare WA, Ton H: Effects of APB, PDA, and TTX on ERG responses recorded using both multifocal and conventional methods in monkey: Effects of APB, PDA, and TTX on monkey ERG responses. *Doc Ophthalmol* 2002; 105(2):189–222.

13. Hogg C: The use of light-emitting diodes in electrophysiology and psychophysics. In Heckenlively JR, Arden GB (eds): *Principles and Practice of Clinical Electrophysiology of Vision*. St Louis, Mosby, 1991, pp 221–227.

14. Hood DC: Assessing retinal function with the multifocal technique. *Prog Retin Eye Res* 2000; 19(5):607–646.

15. Hood DC, Frishman LJ, Saszik S, Viswanathan S: Retinal origins of the primate multifocal ERG: Implications for the human response. *Invest Ophthalmol Vis Sci* 2002; 43(5):1673–1685.

16. Hood DC, Frishman LJ, Viswanathan S, Robson JG, Ahmed J: Evidence for a ganglion cell contribution to the primate electroretinogram (ERG): Effects of TTX on the multifocal ERG in macaque. *Vis Neurosci* 1999; 16(3):411–416.

17. Hood DC, Holopigian K, Greenstein V, Seiple W, Li J, Sutter EE, et al: Assessment of local retinal function in patients with retinitis pigmentosa using multi-focal ERG technique. *Vision Res* 1997; (38):163–179.

18. Hood DC, Seiple W, Holopigian K, Greenstein V: A comparison of the components of the multifocal and full-field ERGs. *Vis Neurosci* 1997; 14(3):533–544.

19. Horiguchi M, Suzuki S, Kondo M, Tanikawa A, Miyake Y: Effect of glutamate analogues and inhibitory neurotransmitters on the electroretinograms elicited by random sequence stimuli in rabbits. *Invest Ophthalmol Vis Sci* 1998; 39(11):2171–2176.

20. Huang HJ, Yamazaki H, Kawabata H, Ninomiya T, Adachi-Usami E: Multifocal electroretinogram in multiple evanescent white dot syndrome. *Doc Ophthalmol* 1996; 92(4):301–309.

21. Huang S, Wu D, Jiang F, Ma J, Wu L, Liang J, et al: The multifocal electroretinogram in age-related maculopathies. *Doc Ophthalmol* 2000; 101(2):115–124.

22. Ireland JM, Keating D, Hoggar SG, Parks S: Identification of appropriate primitive polynomials to avoid cross-contamination in multifocal electroretinogram responses. *Med Biol Eng Comput* 2002; 40(4):471–478.

23. Keating D, Parks S, Evans A: Technical aspects of multifocal ERG recording. *Doc Ophthalmol* 2000; 100(2–3):77–98.

24. Keating D, Parks S, Evans A: Developments in ocular electrophysiology. *Curr Med Lit Ophthalmol* 2001; 11(4):85–91.

25. Keating D, Parks S, Evans AL, Williamson TH, Elliott AT, Jay JL: The effect of filter bandwidth on the multifocal electroretinogram. *Doc Ophthalmol* 1996; 92(4):291–300.

26. Keating D, Parks S, Malloch C, Evans A: A comparison of CRT and digital stimulus delivery methods in the multifocal ERG. *Doc Ophthalmol* 2001; 102(2):95–114.

27. Keating D, Parks S, Smith D, Evans A: The multifocal ERG: Unmasked by selective cross-correlation. *Vision Res* 2002; 42(27):2959–2968.

28. Kellner U, Kraus H, Foerster MH: Multifocal ERG in chloroquine retinopathy: Regional variance of retinal dysfunction. *Graefes Arch Clin Exp Ophthalmol* 2000; 238(1):94–97.

29. Klein SA: Optimizing the estimation of nonlinear kernels. In Pinter RB, Nabat EB (eds): *Non Linear Vision*. Boca Raton, Fla, CRC Press, 1992, pp 109–170.

30. Klistorner A, Graham SL: Objective perimetry in glaucoma. *Ophthalmology* 2000; 107(12):2283–2299.

31. Kondo M, Piao CH, Tanikawa A, Horiguchi M, Miyake Y: A contact lens electrode with built-in high intensity white light-emitting diodes: A contact lens electrode with built-in white LEDs. *Doc Ophthalmol* 2001; 102(1):1–9.

32. Kretschmann U, Seeliger MW, Ruether K, Usui T, Apfelstedt-Sylla E, Zrenner E: Multifocal electroretinography in patients with Stargardt's macular dystrophy. *Br J Ophthalmol* 1998; 82(3):267–275.

33. Kruth DE: *Semi-Numerical Algorithms*, ed 2. Reading, Mass, Addison-Wesley, 1981.

34. Larkin RM, Klein S, Ogden TE, Fender DH: Nonlinear kernels of the human ERG. *Biol Cybern* 1979; 35(3):145–160.

35. Li J, Tso MO, Lam TT: Reduced amplitude and delayed latency in foveal response of multifocal electroretinogram in early age related macular degeneration. *Br J Ophthalmol* 2001; 85(3):287–290.

36. MacWilliams FJ, Sloane NJA: Pseudo-random sequences and arrays. *Proc IEEE* 1977; 64:1715–1729.

37. Marmarelis PZ, Marmarelis VZ: *Analysis of Physiological Systems*. New York, Plenum Press, 1978.

38. Marmor MF, Hood DC, Keating D, Kondo M, Seeliger MW, Miyake Y: Guidelines for basic multifocal electroretinography (mfERG). *Doc Ophthalmol* 2003; 106(2):105–115.

39. McDonagh J, Stephen LJ, Dolan FM, Parks S, Dutton GN, Kelly K, Keating D, Sills GJ, Brodie MJ: Peripheral retinal dysfunction in patients taking vigabatrin. *Neurol* 2003; 61(12):1690–1694.

40. McEliece RJ: *Finite Fields for Computer Scientists and Engineers*. Dordrecht, The Netherlands, Kluwer Academic, 1987.

41. Mohidin N, Yap MK, Jacobs RJ: The repeatability and variability of the multifocal electroretinogram for four different electrodes. *Ophthalmic Physiol Opt* 1997; 17(6):530–535.

42. Ohshima A, Hasegawa S, Takada R, Takagi M, Abe H: Multifocal electroretinograms in patients with branch retinal artery occlusion [in Japanese]. *Nippon Ganka Gakkai Zasshi* 1999; 103(3):223–228.

43. Palmowski A, Bearse MA Jr, Sutter EE: Multi-focal electroretinography in diabetic retinopathy. In *Vision Science and Its Applications*. Washington, DC, OSA Technical Digest Series, 1996, pp 43–45.

44. Palmowski AM, Sutter EE, Bearse MA Jr, Fung W: Mapping of retinal function in diabetic retinopathy using the multifocal electroretinogram. *Invest Ophthalmol Vis Sci* 1997; 38(12):2586–2596.

45. Parks S, Keating D, Evans A: Wide field functional imaging of the retina. Paper presented at IEE Colloquium on Medical Applications of Signal Processing, September 1–6, 1999.

46. Parks S, Keating D, Evans A: A Review of 2151 Investigations. ARVO abstract #1794, 2002.

47. Parks S, Keating D, Hammer H, Evans A: Wide field functional imaging of the retina. *Br J Ophthalmic Phot* 1999; 2:2–5.

48. Radtke ND, Aramant RB, Seiler M, Petry HM: Preliminary report: Indications of improved visual function after retinal sheet transplantation in retinitis pigmentosa patients. *Am J Ophthalmol* 1999; 128(3):384–387.

49. Sasoh M, Yoshida S, Kuze M, Uji Y: The multifocal electroretinogram in retinal detachment. *Doc Ophthalmol* 1997; 94(3):239–252.

50. Scholl HP, Schuster AM, Vonthein R, Zrenner E: Mapping of retinal function in Best macular dystrophy using multifocal electroretinography. *Vision Res* 2002; 42(8):1053–1061.

51. Seeliger M, Kretschmann U, Apfelstedt-Sylla E, Ruther K, Zrenner E: Multifocal electroretinography in retinitis pigmentosa. *Am J Ophthalmol* 1998; 125(2):214–226.

52. Seeliger MW, Narfstrom K, Reinhard J, Zrenner E, Sutter E: Continuous monitoring of the stimulated area in multifocal ERG. *Doc Ophthalmol* 2000; 100(2–3):167–184.

53. Shimada Y, Li Y, Bearse MA Jr, Sutter EE, Fung W: Assessment of early retinal changes in diabetes using a new multifocal ERG protocol. *Br J Ophthalmol* 2001; 85(4):414–419.

54. Si YJ, Kishi S, Aoyagi K: Assessment of macular function by multifocal electroretinogram before and after macular hole surgery. *Br J Ophthalmol* 1999; 83(4):420–424.

55. Sieving PA, Murayama K, Naarendorp F: Push-pull model of the primate photopic electroretinogram: A role for hyperpolarizing neurons in shaping the b-wave. *Vis Neurosci* 1994; 11(3):519–532.

56. Smith DC, Keating D, Parks S, Evans AL: An instrument to investigate temporal processing mechanisms with the multifocal ERG. *J Med Eng Technol* 2002; 26(4):147–151.

57. Sutter EE: A deterministic approach to nonlinear systems analysis. In Pinter RB, Nabat EB (eds): *Nonlinear Vision*. Boca Raton, Fla, CRC Press, 1992, pp 171–220.

58. Sutter E: The interpretation of multifocal binary kernels. *Doc Ophthalmol* 2000; 100(2–3):49–75.

59. Sutter EE: Imaging visual function with the multifocal m-sequence technique. *Vision Res* 2001; 41(10–11):1241–1255.

60. Sutter EE, Bearse MA Jr: The optic nerve head component of the human ERG. *Vision Res* 1999; 39(3):419–436.

61. Sutter EE, Tran D: The field topography of ERG components in man: I. The photopic luminance response. *Vision Res* 1992; 32(3):433–446.

62. Vajaranant TS, Szlyk JP, Fishman GA, Gieser JP, Seiple W: Localized retinal dysfunction in central serous chorioretinopathy as measured using the multifocal electroretinogram. *Ophthalmology* 2002; 109(7):1243–1250.

63. Volterra V: *Theory of Functionals and of the Integral and Integro-Differential Equations*. New York, Dover, 1959.

64. Watzke RC, Shults WT: Clinical features and natural history of the acute idiopathic enlarged blind spot syndrome. *Ophthalmology* 2002; 109(7):1326–1335.

65. Wiener N: *Nonlinear Problems in Random Theory*. New York, Wiley, 1958.

22 The Pattern Electroretinogram

GRAHAM E. HOLDER

Introduction

The pattern electroretinogram (PERG) results from stimulation of the central retina with an isoluminant-reversing black-and-white checkerboard or grating. It arises largely in the inner retina, providing a direct assessment of retinal ganglion cell function. Furthermore, in consideration of the stimulus characteristics, the PERG enables an objective index of macular function. It can therefore play an important role in differentiation between macular and optic nerve dysfunction by facilitating improved interpretation of the cortically generated visual evoked potential (VEP) to a similar stimulus. The reader is referred to recent reviews for further details.[29,42,45]

The normal PERG: Its recording and origins

The PERG is a small signal and requires attention to technical detail perhaps even greater than that required during the recording of other visual electrophysiological tests. Particular caution has to be exercised in relation to physiological artifacts from eye movement and blink artifacts. However, given sufficient care, PERG trial-to-trial variability should be no greater than that of other electrophysiological tests.[9,62,64]

PERGs can be recorded to low temporal frequency stimuli, giving a transient waveform with separately measurable components; at higher stimulus frequencies, for example, more than 10 reversals per second, a steady-state waveform occurs, precluding individual component measurement (figure 22.1). The steady-state PERG is amenable to Fourier analysis. The separation of the PERG into individual components is probably of greater diagnostic value, and the International Society for Clinical Electrophysiology of Vision (ISCEV) standard for pattern ERG refers to the transient waveform only. This review will address the steady-state response when appropriate but will concentrate on the transient PERG.

The normal PERG, recorded in accordance with the ISCEV standard,[8] consists of three main components (figure 22.1). Many subjects have a small negative component, N35, at 30–35 ms, but this has little clinical demonstrated value and will not be considered further. The two components that are the focus for clinical diagnostic work are a prominent positive component, P50, at approximately 50 ms, and the larger negative component, N95, at 90–100 ms.[36–38] ISCEV recommends that measurement of the PERG be from peak to peak, that is, from the trough of N35 to the peak of P50 for P50 component amplitude and from the peak of P50 to the trough of N95 for N95 amplitude. P50 latency (implicit time) is measured at its peak, but N95 latency is often difficult to measure accurately due to its broader shape and is not usually considered in diagnosis.

The PERG should be recorded with electrodes that contact the cornea or nearby bulbar conjunctiva but that, unlike contact lens electrodes, do not affect the optics of the eye or degrade retinal image quality. The DTL-fiber electrode,[24] the Arden gold foil electrode,[3] and the H-K loop electrode[34] are all suitable. The gold foil electrode is that routinely used in the author's laboratories. The DTL can be draped horizontally across the cornea or placed in the lower conjunctival fornix; the latter position gives an amplitude only 80% of that obtained when the electrode is across the cornea at the level of the lower lid.[64] It is important when using the DTL that such a change in position does not inadvertently occur during recording.[85] Surface electrodes, such as silver/silver chloride EEG-type electrodes, are not recommended for routine PERG recording owing to the lower amplitude and signal-to-noise ratio than corneal electrodes but may have limited application in, for example, a pediatric population. The reference electrode for PERG recording must be at the outer canthus or ipsilateral temple to avoid contamination from the cortically generated VEP.[12] Topical anesthesia is not required for the three electrodes referred to and may be contraindicated for PERG.[5]

The properties of the recording amplifiers need careful consideration. Inappropriate amplifier design and characteristics, particularly in relation to saturation and recovery following a large artifact such as a blink, may cause PERGs of artifactually low amplitude.[31,62] On-line artifact rejection is needed during data collection to minimize intrusion from unwanted artifacts and should be set for $100\,\mu V$ or less. A satisfactory PERG usually requires the averaging of the responses to more than 150 reversals, with a minimum of two trials. The patient should refrain from facial movements and blinking during recording; suspending data acquisition every 5–10 seconds to allow the patient to blink a few times

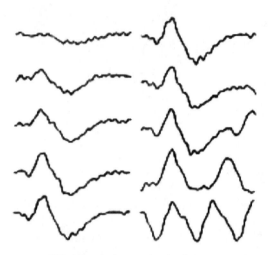

FIGURE 22.1 PERG in relation to stimulus frequency and contrast. Left, the contrast of the stimulus. Right, the rate of stimulation (reversals per second).

will reduce trial-to-trial variability. A headrest reduces head movements (and thus eye movements) and is important for artifact prevention. Binocular recording gives the lowest trial-to-trial variability[83] and is recommended, as for full-field ERG; in cases of asymmetrical visual acuity, the better eye maintains fixation. Simultaneous VEP and PERG recording may be useful, particularly in possible nonorganic visual loss, but binocular recording is preferred for routine diagnostic use. Monocular recording is necessary, however, if the patient has a squint.[43] The patient's pupils should not be dilated for PERG recording.

Stimulus parameters are important, and regular calibration is required. A linear relationship between stimulus contrast and PERG amplitude has been proposed by some authors[35,53,84,87] but is suggested by others only to apply at low stimulus temporal frequencies.[95] PERG amplitude also increases with increasing field size.[7,9,73] There are minor changes in the PERG N95 component with miosis[12] but not for P50.[44] PERG amplitude reduces with age,[19,60,67,88,89] possibly related to loss of ganglion cells,[11] and age-related normative data are required. Appropriate refraction is of crucial importance.[1,6]

Although the exact generators of the PERG have yet to be fully ascertained, the data currently suggest that the N95 component of the human PERG is a contrast-related component generated in relation to retinal ganglion cell function. P50 is partly ganglion cell derived; there is also a contribution from structures distal to the ganglion cells in the visual pathway that have not yet been ascertained.

The initial experiments on the origins of the PERG were performed on animal models and examined the effects of optic nerve section and subsequent development of retrograde degeneration to the retinal ganglion cells. Maffei and

Fiorentini[57] observed extinction of the PERG in a feline model, suggesting that the ganglion cells were responsible for the generation of the PERG. Although similar results were subsequently reported by the same group in a nonhuman primate model,[58] analogous experiments in pigeons did not produce PERG extinction but preservation of a reduced-amplitude P50 component with a shortening of P50 latency.[17] Recent pharmacological experiments in a primate model used tetrodotoxin (TTX) to block spiking cell activity.[91] These revealed severe N95 loss, and although P50 showed amplitude reduction, it was not extinguished and there was shortening of P50 latency.

Two case reports appeared of PERG change in human patients following optic nerve section (posttraumatic[78] and surgical optic nerve section[33]). Both described some PERG preservation in the affected eye despite the absence of light perception. Harrison and colleagues, recording 30 months after nerve section when retrograde ganglion cell degeneration should be complete, observed a P50 amplitude reduction of approximately 70%, accompanied by a shortening of P50 latency.[33] Similar findings have been reported in a blind eye consequent on longstanding optic nerve compression[43] and are compatible with those pharmacologically produced by Frishman's group in a macaque model.[91]

Human experimental studies utilized variations in stimulus parameters, particularly spatial tuning, a property of the retinal ganglion cells. Early studies examined only the P50 component and found no low spatial frequency attenuation.[50,90] However, N95 shows spatial tuning for a small stimulus field,[14,76] but the phenomenon is less marked with a large field.[9] Spatial tuning is also present in the N95-dominated steady-state PERG.[35] The suggestion from these data that the retinal ganglion cells are responsible for N95 generation was supported when the N95 equivalent pattern-specific response[86] correlated significantly with the volume of the ganglion cell layer.[26] The results of current source density analysis were also in keeping with a ganglion cell origin for the PERG.[10,79] The reader is referred elsewhere for a more comprehensive review of those data.[95]

Clinical data were also being amassed during the 1980s consistent with P50 and N95 having different origins.

The clinical PERG: Macular dysfunction

The PERG, in relation to the nature of the stimulus, is sensitive to macular dysfunction. The initial report of PERG abnormality in maculopathy[54] was confirmed in the early 1980s when PERG recording became more commonplace following the introduction of the gold foil and DTL electrodes. All authors reported PERG P50 component abnormalities (e.g., Groneberg,[32] Arden et al.,[6] Celesia and

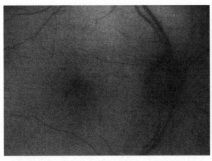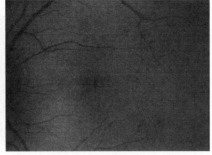

FIGURE 22.2 Fundus autofluorescence images in a 33-year-old female referred for investigation of presumed optic neuritis consequent on dengue fever. There was a two-month history of right eye visual acuity loss, but no signs other than a questionable right relative afferent pupillary defect. Right visual acuity was 6/36; left visual acuity was 6/5.

Kaufman,[20] Holder,[37,41] Clarke et al.,[22] Ryan and Arden,[72] Stavrou et al.[81]). The early studies did not separately evaluate N95, but when this component was examined,[37] it was evident that there is concomitant effect on N95 such that the N95:P50 ratio is not reduced and might even be increased.[39,42] Complete extinction of the PERG occurs in severe macular dysfunction. Although many patients with an undetectable PERG have ophthalmoscopically visible macular abnormalities, a normal-appearing macula should not be taken to imply a normally functioning macula (figures 22.2, 22.3, and 22.4).

The PERG findings in a mixed group of patients with macular dysfunction, including retinal and macular dystrophies, inflammatory retinal disease, retinal vascular disease, central serous retinopathy (CSR), and autoimmune retinopathy, are shown in figures 22.5 and 22.6. The data are displayed in relation to visual acuity. In the author's experience, all patients with visual acuity < 6/60 (20/200; 0.1) due to macular disease have an undetectable PERG, and such data are not displayed. There is a high incidence of P50 component amplitude abnormality, with a loose relationship between visual acuity and PERG P50 amplitude. P50 is subnormal in the majority of eyes with VA of 6/12 or worse. It is important to remember that appropriate refraction is needed during PERG recording so that the abnormalities reflect genuine pathology rather than suboptimal refraction.

In clinical practice, the PERG is combined with the full-field ERG. If the PERG is abnormal but the ERG is normal, then dysfunction is confined to the macula, and generalized retinal dysfunction is excluded. A pure macular dystrophy has such a pattern of dysfunction. When generalized ERG abnormalities are present, the electrophysiology defines the phenotype; if the peripheral retinal appearance is unremarkable, then an abnormal macular appearance could reflect a pure maculopathy, a generalized cone dysfunction with macular involvement, or a cone-rod dystrophy with macular involvement. This is determined by the nature of any full-field ERG abnormality.

PERG in Stargardt's disease

The most common genetically determined macular dystrophy is Stargardt-fundus flavimaculatus (S-FFM), which is usually inherited as an autosomal-recessive trait. At least some S-FFM relates to mutation in *ABCA4* (ABCR), which expresses in both rods[82] and cones,[59] but *ABCA4* has 50 exons with many polymorphisms, and it is not always evident whether the polymorphisms are disease-causing. The effect on photoreceptor function may be secondary to effect on the retinal pigment epithelium.[93] Although S-FFM can be associated with abnormalities of the full-field ERG,[55,56] such that some patients have disease confined to the macula (group 1), some have macular dysfunction plus abnormal Ganzfeld cone ERGs (group 2), and others have macular dysfunction plus abnormalities in both cone and rod full-field ERGs (group 3), a particular feature of S-FFM is that the PERG is usually undetectable, even when visual acuity may still be well preserved.[42]

It is relevant, considering the three subtypes of S-FFM, to ask whether these groups reflect different stages of the same disease or distinct diseases, perhaps in relation to different mutations in the same gene. The problems inherent in working with *ABCA4* do not easily allow this question to be answered, but there are other lines of investigation that supply suggestive results. Sibling pairs should have the same alleles, and data from a sibling pair study showed that although there could be marked intersibling differences in fundus appearance, length of history, or visual acuity, the electrophysiological grouping showed 100% sibling concordance.[56] Data from a large prospective series of patients with S-FFM were also examined to assess the relationship between the magnitude of the ERG abnormality and the duration of disease, as ascertained from direct patient questioning and hospital records. This is not as satisfactory an approach as longitudinal recordings, but they are the only available data. Groups 1 and 2 showed no significant association between the duration of the disease and the full-field

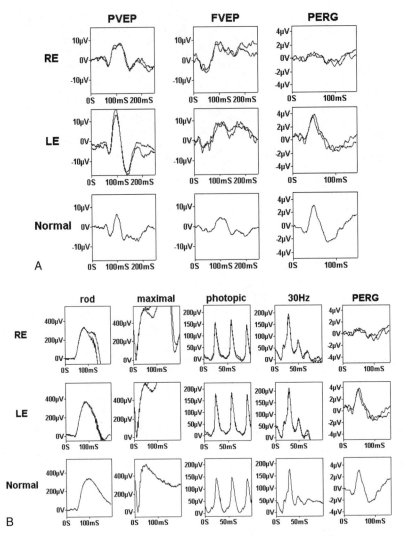

FIGURE 22.3   A, Pattern and flash VEPs and PERGs in the patient shown in figure 22.2. The right eye pattern VEP is markedly delayed, but the marked PERG P50 component amplitude reduction suggests macular rather than optic nerve dysfunction. (Source: After Holder GE: Electrophysiological assessment of optic nerve disease. *Eye* 2004; 18:1133–1143.) B, Normal full-field ERGs in the patient referred to in figure 22.2, confirming that the dysfunction is confined to the macula rather than being part of generalized retinal dysfunction. (Source: After Holder GE: Electrophysiological assessment of optic nerve disease. *Eye* 2004; 18:1133–1143.)

ERG abnormalities, but a strong association between the length of history and the severity of the electrophysiological abnormality was found for both cone and rod ERGs in group 3.[55] These data have been interpreted to suggest that only the group 3 variant of S-FFM may be progressive and, further, that a normal full-field ERG at any stage in the disorder indicates a low chance of subsequent peripheral retinal involvement, important when counseling these patients.

PERG in other maculopathies

The pattern of abnormality of a normal full-field ERG and an abnormal PERG, such that dysfunction appears confined to the macula, has also been reported in other forms of mac-ulopathy, such as CSR,[27] macular hole,[28,86] and age-related macular degeneration.[16] PERG recording was found to be more sensitive than focal ERG in the assessment of macular function in aphakic cystoid macular edema[75] and was also noted to demonstrate a degree of macular dysfunction in keeping with the reported visual acuity level even when the appearance of the macula was not thought sufficiently abnormal to explain the level of acuity. Diabetic maculopathy is also associated with abnormal PERGs.[4,23,47,61,69,72] In some instances, such as the macular dystrophy associated with the 172 mutation in *peripherin/rds*, the PERG may be abnormal before the development of acuity loss.[25] In the later stages of this disorder, the PERG becomes undetectable, but the ERG remains normal, consistent with dysfunction confined to the macula.

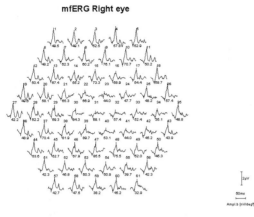

mfERG Right eye

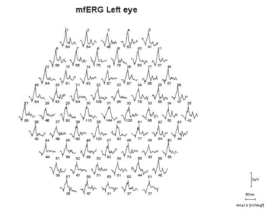

mfERG Left eye

FIGURE 22.4 mfERGs in the same patients as in figures 22.2 and 22.3 demonstrate the spatial extent of the right eye macular dysfunction. Note the preservation of the early negative component in the affected area. This may be the multifocal ERG equivalent of an electronegative ERG and thus may sug- gest sparing of the photoreceptors with the site of dysfunction being post-phototransduction. This is further supported by the normal autofluorescence. (Source: After Holder GE: Electro- physiological assessment of optic nerve disease. *Eye* 2004; 18:1133–1143.)

Usually, it is PERG amplitude that is affected in macular dysfunction. Latency changes may occur, particularly in serous detachment or macular edema.[27] It is of interest that both PERG and visual acuity may remain abnormal in CSR even when the retina has flattened.[27] A residual elevation of psychophysical threshold has also been described.[21]

The clinical PERG: Optic nerve and ganglion cell dysfunction

The pattern VEP is delayed in many disorders of optic nerve function (see chapter 25). However, because delayed VEPs are commonplace in macular dysfunction,[39,42] (see also chapter 15 of this volume), a delayed VEP should not be considered diagnostic of optic nerve disease until central retinal function has been excluded.

As retrograde degeneration to the retinal ganglion cells occurs in optic nerve disease, and the PERG has origins in relation to retinal ganglion cell function, it may be anti- cipated that the PERG would be abnormal in optic neuropathy. However, the initial expectations of PERG abnormalities in optic nerve demyelination were not met by the first studies. A variable incidence of PERG abnormality was described in the early reports, but these did not address the N95 component,[6,20,66,68,77] although it was noted in one study that the negative after potential (N95 equivalent) could be affected.[68] Some authors doubted that the PERG had any value in optic nerve demyelination.[50,63]

However, when the N95 component was also included in the analysis, it became clear that PERG abnormalities could be confined to N95, leaving P50 unaffected.[36,37] This was confirmed in later reports (e.g., Ryan and Arden,[72] Froehlich and Kaufman[31]). The incidence of PERG abnormality in optic nerve demyelination was investigated in a study of 200 eyes.[40] There was a 40% PERG abnormality, but in 85% of those abnormalities, it was the N95 component alone that was affected. A subsequent report extended those data with similar conclusions.[41] P50 component involvement occurs in a small percentage of patients, but the reduction in P50 com- ponent amplitude may be accompanied by a shortening of P50 latency (figure 22.7); P50 latency increase is not a feature of optic nerve or retinal ganglion cell disease.

The findings in acute optic neuritis, when examined within a few days of the onset of symptoms, differ from those in chronic disease;[13,40] there is marked PVEP amplitude reduction with less pronounced latency change. This may reflect edema in the optic nerve related to the acute inflam- matory lesion. At this stage, there is a reduction in the PERG P50 component that tends to resolve, and both PERG P50 and PVEP amplitude improve within a few weeks. The VEP amplitude change may reflect resolution of the initial edema. However, even though the VEP amplitude improves, greater PVEP latency delay is observed synchronous with such improvement, presumably reflecting the development of demyelination. Initially, the N95 component of the PERG is reduced parallel to the reduction in P50, with a N95:P50 ratio similar to that in the unaffected eye, but a PERG abnor- mality confined to the N95 component may be evident after the acute P50 loss has resolved with a time scale in keeping with retrograde degeneration to the retinal ganglion cells. The mechanism of the initial P50 reduction is not fully explained. It is of interest that although 8 of 17 eyes with acute optic neuritis had no detectable PVEP at presentation, this was not a predictor of final visual acuity,[42] but the only two eyes not to regain 6/12 acuity or better at follow-up had PERG P50 amplitudes of <0.5 μV at presentation (normal is >2.0 μV). Firm prognostic conclusions await a larger series.

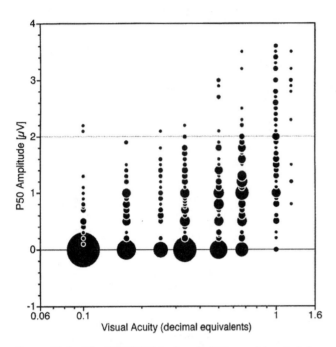

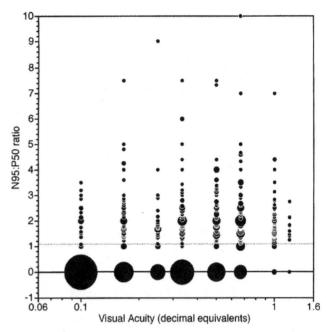

FIGURE 22.5   The PERG P50 findings in 866 eyes with retinal dysfunction. These comprise retinal dystrophies, inflammatory retinal disease, vascular disease, macular dystrophies, and so on. In no patient could a PERG be detected when visual acuity was worse than 6/60; those additional data are not shown. The format in this figure and figure 22.2 is such that the area of the circle at a given datum point reflects the number of eyes with the same value. For example, of the circles at 0.0-μV amplitude, the large circle for 6/60 (0.1) visual acuity represents 136 eyes; the medium-sized circle at 6/12 (0.5) visual acuity represents 41 eyes; and the smaller circle at 6/9 visual acuity (0.67) represents 22 eyes. The horizontal dashed line is at the lower limit of normal P50 amplitude. Note that the vast majority of eyes have abnormal PERGs, many undetectable, and that there is a clear relationship between the degree of visual acuity loss and the degree of PERG abnormality in those eyes in which a PERG was detectable. See figure 22.2 for comparison. (Source: Holder GE: The pattern electroretinogram and an integrated approach to visual pathway diagnosis. *Prog Retin Eye Res* 2001a; 20:531–561. Reproduced with permission.)

FIGURE 22.6   The PERG N95:P50 ratio findings in 866 eyes with retinal dysfunction (see the caption for figure 22.1) demonstrating that the N95 reduction is consequent upon that in P50, and is unrelated to severity of disease. See the caption for figure 22.1 for a description of the type of display used. The horizontal dashed line is at the lower limit of normal N95:P50 ratio. Note that although the vast majority of eyes have abnormal PERGs, as shown in figure 22.1, there is no relationship between the degree of visual acuity loss and the level of N95:P50 ratio in those eyes in which a PERG was detectable. This is in contrast to the data presented for P50 amplitude in figure 22.1 and demonstrates that the reduction in N95 seen in these eyes is secondary to a P50 component reduction. (Source: Holder GE: The pattern electroretinogram and an integrated approach to visual pathway diagnosis. *Prog Retin Eye Res* 2001a; 20:531–561. Reproduced with permission.)

Other disorders of optic nerve function may also be associated with PERG N95 component abnormalities. The PERG has received relatively little attention in nonarteritic anterior ischemic optic neuropathy (NAION), but N95 reduction may occur.[2,38] The P50 component is more frequently affected in NAION than demyelination, perhaps reflecting more widespread vascular-related dysfunction anterior to the retinal ganglion cells. A report has appeared showing histopathological change in both inner and outer nuclear layers of the retina in NAION.[74]

PERG abnormalities can occur in optic nerve compression[41] and may be a useful prognostic indicator for visual outcome as part of preoperative assessment.[49,71] Parmar et al.[65] found that an abnormal preoperative PERG in patients with pituitary tumor correlated with a lack of postoperative recovery.

The two most commonly occurring examples of primary ganglion cell disease are Leber hereditary optic neuropathy (LHON) and Kjer-type dominant optic atrophy (DOA).[51] LHON, related to mutation in the mitochondrial genome, usually presents with painless sequential bilateral visual loss. Most patients are between 11 and 30 years of age at presentation, but earlier and much later age of onset can occur,[18,70] with mutation-confirmed disease occurring even in patients as young as 2 years of age or as old as 80 years of age (N.J. Newman, personal communication). Females are less frequently affected than males, but the reason for this is not clear; because there is incomplete penetrance, there are probably other determining factors. There may be disk swelling at presentation, often accompanied by microangiopathic changes in the disk vessels, but there is no fluorescein leakage from the disk even in the late phase of fundus fluorescein angiography. PVEPs, when detectable, are usually markedly abnormal, with both delay and waveform distortion, but there is marked reduction in the N95 component

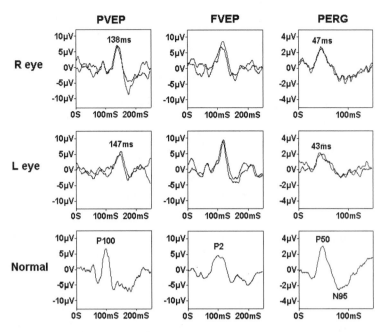

FIGURE 22.7   PERG and pattern VEP findings in a 26-year-old female who presented with blurred vision in her left eye following a hot bath. There were no physical signs, but color vision testing (Ishihara), although giving no errors, was performed very slowly. Visual acuity was 6/5 right and left. Pattern VEPs from both eyes are markedly delayed, the delay from the right eye being subclini-cal and that from the left being associated with an Uhthoff phenomenon. The patient denied ever having had any acute symptoms suggestive of retrobulbar neuritis. Note the relative reduction in PERG P50 amplitude from the left eye with a shortening of PERG P50 latency. The PERG from the right eye is normal.

of the PERG.[41] One report has suggested, in the 11778 mutation, that VEP abnormalities may precede the onset of symptoms.

DOA is related to mutation in *OPA1* on chromosome 3. There is usually progressive visual acuity loss associated with disk pallor, a centrocecal visual field defect and defective color vision.[92] Histopathological[48,52] and electrophysiological studies[15,38,46] are in keeping with degeneration of the retinal ganglion cells leading to optic atrophy. As with LHON, VEPs are often delayed, but there tends to be better preservation of the waveform in early disease. Again, in keeping with ganglion cell dysfunction, there is N95 reduction in the PERG; indeed, the PERG can occasionally be profoundly abnormal even in the absence of marked PVEP abnormality (e.g., figure 22.8). PERG abnormalities confined to N95 were reported in younger patients in a recent study of 13 patients from eight families.[46] In more advanced disease, additional P50 component involvement occurred; there was P50 amplitude reduction and shortening of P50 latency in severe end-stage disease, but the PERG P50 was always detectable even when the pattern VEP was extinguished (figure 22.8). A shortening of latency is presumed to reflect loss of the ganglion cell–derived N95 component, with additional loss of the part of P50 that arises in relation to ganglion function. The earlier, more distally generated part of P50 remains even in severe ganglion cell loss, giving apparent shortening of latency.

Patients with LHON tend to present acutely and have completely normal P50 components with very poor N95, in keeping with primary ganglion cell pathology. DOA rarely presents with an acute event, and the N95 loss in DOA is assumed to be progressive based on examination of patients in different stages of disease.[46] Diagnostically, it is often a symmetrical and marked reduction in the N95 component that suggests a primary disorder of ganglion cell function rather than dysfunction consequent on an optic nerve insult.

Concluding remarks

The PERG has an important clinical role in the evaluation of central retina, the P50 component allowing an objective assessment of macular function. In addition, the N95 component provides a direct measure of ganglion cell function. The differences between the effects of macular and optic nerve disease on the PERG enable a dramatic improvement in the accuracy of VEP interpretation, and this is perhaps the role of the PERG with the most direct clinical impact on patient management (see chapter 36). It is important always to bear in mind that clinical signs may sometimes be misleading or absent. For example, a relative afferent pupillary defect can be a feature either of optic nerve or macular dysfunction (and may not be present in bilateral disease); and the presence of a normal-appearing macula does not mean

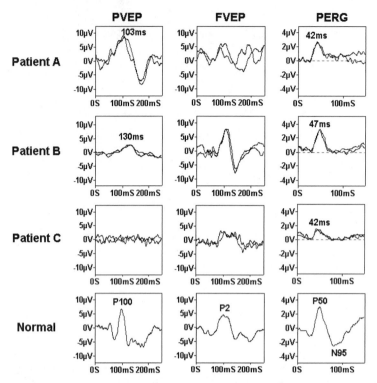

FIGURE 22.8   PERG and pattern VEP findings in three patients with dominantly inherited optic atrophy related to mutation in *OPA1*. Patient A shows N95 loss in the PERG, with shortening of P50 latency. The pattern VEP falls within the normal latency range but is of altered waveform. Patient B shows marked pattern VEP delay with N95 loss in the PERG. Patient C, with severe end-stage disease, has no detectable pattern VEP. The PERG shows amplitude loss in both N95 and P50, but the P50 amplitude reduction is associated with shortening of latency; in macular dysfunction, although P50 amplitude loss is common, a similar shortening of latency does not occur.

a normally functioning macula. Equally, a patient with disease of the ganglion cells evident on clinical examination and in the PERG can have a normal pattern VEP. The PERG, particularly as it is evoked by a stimulus similar to that used for routine clinical VEP recording, is invaluable in facilitating the distinction between optic nerve and macular disease and in the demonstration of ganglion cell dysfunction.

REFERENCES

1. Adachi-Usami E, Kuroda N, Kakisu Y: Check size and defocusing effects on equipotential maps of pattern-evoked electroretinograms. *Doc Ophthalmol* 1987; 65:367–375.

2. Almarcegui C, Dolz I, Alejos MV, Fernandez FJ, Valdizan JR, Honrubia FM: Pattern electroretinogram in anterior ischemic optic neuropathy. *Rev Neurol* 2001; 32:18–21.

3. Arden GB, Carter RM, Hogg CR, Siegel IM, Margolis S: A gold foil electrode: Extending the horizons for clinical electroretinography. *Invest Ophthalmol Vis Sci* 1979; 18:421–426.

4. Arden GB, Hamilton AMP, Wilson-Holt J, Ryan S, Yudkin JS, Kurtz A: Pattern electroretinograms become abnormal when background diabetic retinopathy deteriorates to a pre-proliferative stage: Possible use as a screening test. *Br J Ophthalmol* 1986; 70:330–335.

5. Arden GB, Hogg CR, Holder GE: Gold foil electrodes: A two centre study of electrode reliability. *Doc Ophthalmol* 1994; 86:275–284.

6. Arden GB, Vaegan, Hogg CR: Clinical and experimental evidence that the pattern electroretinogram (PERG) is generated in more proximal retinal layers than the focal electroretinogram (FERG). *Ann N Y Acad Sci* 1982; 388:214–226.

7. Aylward GW, Billson V, Billson FA: The wide-angle pattern electroretinogram: Relation between pattern electroretinogram amplitude and stimulus area using large stimuli: The wide-angle pattern electroretinogram. *Doc Ophthalmol* 1989; 73:275–283.

8. Bach M, Hawlina M, Holder GE, Marmor MF, Meigen T, Vaegan, Miyake Y: Standard for pattern electroretinography. *Doc Ophthalmol* 2000; 101:11–18.

9. Bach M, Holder GE: Check size tuning of the pattern-ERG: A reappraisal. *Doc Ophthalmol* 1996; 92:193–202.

10. Baker CL, Hess RF, Olsen BT, Zrenner E: Current source density analysis of linear and non-linear components of the primate electroretinogram. *J Physiol* 1988; 407:155–176.

11. Balaszi AG, Rootman J, Drance SM, Schulzer M, Douglas GR: The effect of age on the nerve fibre population of the human optic nerve. *Am J Ophthalmol* 1984; 97:760–766.

12. Berninger TA: The pattern electroretinogram and its contamination. *Clin Vis Sci* 1986; 1:185–190.

13. Berninger TA, Heider W: Pattern electroretinograms in optic neuritis during the acute stage and after remission. *Graefes Arch Clin Exp Ophthalmol* 1990; 228:410–414.

14. Berninger TA, Schuurmans RP: Spatial tuning of the pattern ERG across temporal frequency. *Doc Ophthalmol* 1985; 61:17–25.

15. Berninger TA, Jaeger W, Krastel H: Electrophysiology and color perimetry in dominant infantile optic atrophy. *Br J Ophthalmol* 1991; 75:49–52.

16. Birch DG, Anderson JL, Fish GE, Jost BF: Pattern-reversal electroretinographic acuity in untreated eyes with subfoveal neovascular membranes. *Invest Ophthalmol Vis Sci* 1992; 33:2097–2104.

17. Blondeau P, Lamarche J, Lafond G, Brunette JR: Pattern electroretinogram and optic nerve section in pigeons. *Curr Eye Res* 1987; 6:747–756.

18. Borruat FX, Green WT, Graham EM, Sweeney MG, Morgan-Hughes JA, Sanders MD: Late onset Leber's optic neuropathy: A case confused with ischaemic optic neuropathy. *Br J Ophthalmol* 1992; 76:571–573.

19. Celesia GG, Cone S, Kaufman D: Effects of age and sex on pattern electroretinogram and visual evoked potentials. *Electroencephalogr Clin Neurophysiol* 1986; 64:24.

20. Celesia GG, Kaufman D: Pattern ERGs and visual evoked potentials in maculopathies and optic nerve diseases. *Invest Ophthalmol Vis Sci* 1985; 26:726–735.

21. Chuang EL, Sharp DM, Fitzke FW, Kemp CM, Holden AL, Bird AC: Retinal dysfunction in central serous retinopathy. *Eye* 1987; 1:120–125.

22. Clarke MP, Mitchell KW, McDonnell S: Electroretinographic findings in macular dystrophy. *Doc Ophthalmol* 1997; 92:325–339.

23. Coupland SG: A comparison of oscillatory potential and pattern electroretinogram measures in diabetic retinopathy. *Doc Ophthalmol* 1987; 66:207–218.

24. Dawson WW, Trick GL, Litzkow CA: Improved electrode for electroretinography. *Invest Ophthalmol Vis Sci* 1979; 18:988–991.

25. Downes SM, Fitzke FW, Holder GE, Payne AM, Bessant DAR, Bhattacharya SS, Bird AC: Clinical features of codon 172 RDS macular dystrophy: Similar phenotype in 12 families. *Arch Ophthalmol* 1999; 117:1373–1383.

26. Drasdo N, Thompson DA, Arden GB: A comparison of pattern ERG amplitudes and nuclear layer thickness in different zones of the retina. *Clin Vis Sci* 1990; 5:415–420.

27. Eckstein MB, Spalton DJ, Holder GE: Visual loss from central serous retinopathy in systemic lupus erythematosus. *Br J Ophthalmol* 1993; 77:607–609.

28. Falsini B, Minnella A, Buzzonetti L, Merendino E, Porciatti V: Macular electroretinograms to flicker and pattern stimulation in lamellar macular holes. *Doc Ophthalmol* 1992; 79:99–108.

29. Fishman GA, Birch DG, Holder GE, Brigell MG (eds): *Electrophysiologic Testing in Disorders of the Retina, Optic Nerve, and Visual Pathway*, ed 2. Ophthalmology Monograph 2. San Francisco, The Foundation of the American Academy of Ophthalmology, 2001.

30. Froehlich J, Kaufman DI: Improving the reliability of pattern electroretinogram recording. *Electroencephalogr Clin Neurophysiol* 1992; 84:394–399.

31. Froehlich J, Kaufman DI: The pattern electroretinogram: N95 amplitudes in normal subjects and optic neuritis patients: *Electroencephalogr Clin Neurophysiol* 1993; 88:83–91.

32. Groneberg A: Simultaneously recorded retinal and cortical potentials elicited by checkerboard stimuli. *Doc Ophthalmol Proc Ser* 1980; 23:255–262.

33. Harrison JM, O'Connor PS, Young RSL, Kincaid M, Bentley R: The pattern ERG in man following surgical resection of the optic nerve. *Invest Ophthalmol Vis Sci* 1987; 28:492–499.

34. Hawlina M, Konec B: New noncorneal HK-loop electrode for clinical electroretinography. *Doc Ophthalmol* 1992; 81:253–259.

35. Hess RF, Baker CL: Human pattern-evoked electroretinogram. *J Neurophysiol* 1984; 51:939–951.

36. Holder GE: Pattern ERG abnormalities in anterior visual pathway disease. *Electroencephalogr Clin Neurophysiol* 1985; 61:S135.

37. Holder GE: Significance of abnormal pattern electroretinography in anterior visual pathway dysfunction. *Br J Ophthalmol* 1987; 71:166–171.

38. Holder GE: Abnormalities of the pattern ERG in optic nerve lesions: Changes specific for proximal retinal dysfunction. In Barber C, Blum T (eds): *Evoked Potentials III*. London, Butterworths, 1987, pp 221–224.

39. Holder GE: Pattern electroretinography in patients with delayed pattern visual evoked potentials due to distal anterior visual pathway dysfunction. *J Neurol Neurosurg Psychiat* 1989; 52:1364–1368.

40. Holder GE: The incidence of abnormal pattern electroretinography in optic nerve demyelination. *Electroenceph Clin Neurophysiol* 1991; 78:18–26.

41. Holder GE: The pattern electroretinogram in anterior visual pathway dysfunction and its relationship to the pattern visual evoked potential: A personal clinical review of 743 eyes. *Eye* 1997; 11:924–934.

42. Holder GE: The pattern electroretinogram and an integrated approach to visual pathway diagnosis. *Prog Retin Eye Res* 2001; 20:531–561.

43. Holder GE: The pattern electroretinogram. In Fishman GA, Birch DG, Holder GE, Brigell MG (eds): *Electrophysiologic Testing in Disorders of the Retina, Optic Nerve, and Visual Pathway*, ed 2. Ophthalmology Monograph 2. San Francisco, The Foundation of the American Academy of Ophthalmology, 2001, pp 197–235.

44. Holder GE, Huber MJE: The effects of miosis on pattern and flash ERG and pattern visual evoked potentials. *Doc Ophthalmol Proc Ser* 1984; 40:109–116.

45. Holder GE, Robson AG, Hogg CR, Kurz-Levin M, Lois N, Bird AC: Pattern ERG: Clinical overview, and some observations on associated fundus autofluorescence imaging in inherited maculopathy. *Doc Ophthalmol* 2003; 106:17–23.

46. Holder GE, Votruba M, Carter AC, Bhattacharya SS, Fitzke FW, Moore AT: Electrophysiological findings in Dominant Optic Atrophy (DOA) linking to the OPAl locus on chromosome 3q 28-qter. *Doc Ophthalmol* 1999; 95:217–228.

47. Jenkins TC, Cartwright JP: The electroretinogram in minimal diabetic retinopathy. *Br J Ophthalmol* 1990; 74:681–684.

48. Johnston PB, Gaster RN, Smith VC, Tripathi RC: A clinicopathological study of autosomal dominant optic atrophy. *Am J Ophthalmol* 1979; 88:868–875.

49. Kaufman DI, Lorance RW, Woods M, Wray SH: The pattern electroretinogram: A long-term study in acute optic neuropathy. *Neurology* 1988; 38:1767–1774.

50. Kirkham TH, Coupland SG: The pattern electroretinogram in optic nerve demyelination. *Can J Neurol Sci* 1983; 10:256–260.

51. Kjer P: Infantile optic atrophy with dominant mode of inheritance: A clinical and genetic study of 19 Danish families. *Acta Ophthalmol* 1959; 37 (suppl 54):1–146.

52. Kjer P: Histopathology of eye, optic nerve and brain in a case of dominant optic atrophy. *Acta Ophthalmol* 1982; 61:300–312.

53. Korth M, Rix R, Sembritzki O: Spatial contrast transfer functions of the pattern-evoked electroretinogram. *Invest Ophthalmol Vis Sci* 1985; 26:303–308.

54. Lawwill T: The bar-pattern electroretinogram for clinical evaluation of the central retina. *Am J Ophthalmol* 1974; 78:121–126.

55. Lois N, Holder GE, Bunce C, Fitzke FW, Bird AC: Stargardt macular dystrophy–Fundus flavimaculatus: Phenotypic subtypes. *Arch Ophthalmol* 2001; 119:359–369.

56. Lois N, Holder GE, Fitzke FW, Plant C, Bird AC: Intrafamilial variation of phenotype in Stargardt macular dystrophy–fundus flavimaculatus. *Invest Ophthalmol Vis Sci* 1999; 40:2668–2675.

57. Maffei L, Fiorentini A: Electroretinographic responses to alternating gratings before and after section of the optic nerve. *Science* 1981; 211:953–955.

58. Maffei L, Fiorentini A, Bisti S, Hollander H: Pattern ERG in the monkey after section of the optic nerve. *Exp Brain Res* 1985; 59:423–425.

59. Molday LL, Rabin AR, Molday RS: ABCR, The ABC transporter implicated in Stargardt disease, is expressed in both cone and rod photoreceptor cells. *Invest Ophthalmol Vis Sci* 2000; 41:S144.

60. Muir JA, Barlow HL, Morrison JD: Invariance of the pattern electroretinogram evoked by psychophysically equivalent stimuli in human ageing. *J Physiol (Lond)* 1996; 497:825–835.

61. Nesher R, Trick GL: The pattern electroretinogram in retinal and optic nerve disease: A quantitative comparison of the pattern of visual dysfunction. *Doc Ophthalmol* 1991; 77:225–235.

62. Odom JV, Holder GE, Fenghali JG, Cavender S: Pattern electroretinogram intrasession reliability: A two center comparison. *Clin Vis Sci* 1992; 7:263–282.

63. Ota I, Miyake Y: The pattern electroretinogram in patients with optic nerve disease. *Doc Ophthalmol* 1986; 62:53–60.

64. Otto T, Bach M: Reproducibility of the pattern electroretinogram. *Ophthalmologe* 1997; 94:217–221.

65. Parmar DN, Sofat A, Bowman R, Bartlett JR, Holder GE: Prognostic value of the pattern electroretinogram in chiasmal compression. *Br J Ophthalmol* 2000; 84:1024–1026.

66. Persson HE, Wanger P: Pattern reversal electroretinograms and visual evoked potentials in multiple sclerosis. *Br J Ophthalmol* 1984; 68:760–764.

67. Porciatti V, Burr DC, Morrone MC, Fiorentini A: The effects of aging on the pattern electroretinogram and visual evoked potential in humans. *Vision Res* 1992; 32:1199–1209.

68. Porciatti V, von Berger GP: Pattern electroretinogram and visual evoked potential in optic nerve disease: Early diagnosis and prognosis. *Doc Ophthalmol Proc Ser* 1984; 40:117–126.

69. Prager TC, Garcia CA, Mincher CA, Mishra J, Chu HH: The pattern electroretinogram in diabetes. *Am J Ophthalmol* 1990; 109:279–284.

70. Riordan-Eva P, Sanders MD, Govan GG, Sweeney MG, Da Costa J, Harding AE: The clinical features of Leber's hereditary optic neuropathy defined by the presence of a pathogenic mitochondrial DNA mutation. *Brain* 1995; 118:319–337.

71. Ruther K, Ehlich P, Philipp A, Eckstein A, Zrenner E: Prognostic value of the pattern electroretinogram in cases of tumors affecting the optic pathway. *Graefes Arch Clin Exp Ophthalmol* 1998; 236:259–263.

72. Ryan S, Arden GB: Electrophysiological discrimination between retinal and optic nerve disorders. *Doc Ophthalmol* 1988; 68:247–255.

73. Sakaue H, Katsumi O, Mehta M, Hirose T: Simultaneous pattern reversal ERG and VER recordings: Effect of stimulus field and central scotoma. *Invest Ophthalmol Vis Sci* 1990; 31:506–511.

74. Salazar JJ, Ramirez AI, De Hoz R, Triviño A, Ramirez JM: Apoptosis in optical ischaemic neuropathy. Abstracts, EVER Meeting, Palma, 1999.

75. Salzman J, Seiple W, Carr R, Yannuzzi L: Electrophysiological assessment of aphakic cystoid macular oedema. *Br J Ophthalmol* 1986; 70:819–824.

76. Schuurmans RP, Berninger TA: Luminance and contrast responses recorded in man and cat. *Doc Ophthalmol* 1985; 59:187–197.

77. Serra G, Carreras M, Tugnoli V, Manca M, Cristofori MC: Pattern electroretinogram in multiple sclerosis. *J Neurol Neurosurg Psychiat* 1984; 47:879–883.

78. Sherman J: Simultaneous pattern reversal electroretinograms and visual evoked potentials in diseases of the macula and optic nerve. *Ann N Y Acad Sci* 1982; 388:214–226.

79. Sieving PA, Steinberg RH: Proximal retinal contributions to the intraretinal 8-Hz pattern ERG of cat. *J Neurophysiol* 1987; 57:104–120.

80. Smith RG, Brimlow GM, Lea SJ, Galloway NR: Evoked responses in patients with macular holes. *Doc Ophthalmol* 1990; 75:135–144.

81. Stavrou P, Good PA, Misson GP, Kritzinger EE: Electrophysiological findings in Stargardt's–fundus flavimaculatus disease. *Eye* 1998; 12:953–958.

82. Sun H, Nathans J: Stargardt's ABCR is localised to the disc membrane of retinal outer segments. *Nature Genet* 1997; 17:15–16.

83. Tan CT, King PJ, Chiappa KH: Pattern ERG: Effects of reference electrode site, stimulus mode and check size. *Electroencephalogr Clin Neurophysiol* 1989; 74:11–18.

84. Tetsuka S, Katsumi O, Mehta M, Tetsuka H, Hirose T: Effect of stimulus contrast on simultaneous steady-state pattern reversal electroretinogram and visual evoked response. *Ophthalmic Res* 1992; 24:110–118.

85. Thompson DA, Drasdo N: An improved method for using the DTL fibre in electroretinography. *Ophthal Physiol Opt* 1987; 7:315–319.

86. Thompson DA, Drasdo N: Computation of the luminance and pattern components of the bar pattern electroretinogram. *Doc Ophthalmol* 1987; 66:233–244.

87. Thompson DA, Drasdo N: The effect of stimulus contrast on the latency and amplitude of the pattern electroretinogram. *Vision Res* 1989; 29:309–313.

88. Tomoda H, Celesia GG, Brigell MG, Toleikis S: The effects of age on steady-state pattern electroretinograms and visual evoked potentials. *Doc Ophthalmol* 1991; 77:201–211.

89. Trick LR: Age related alterations in retinal function. *Doc Ophthalmol* 1987; 65:35–43.

90. Trick GL, Wintermeyer DH: Spatial and temporal frequency tuning of pattern reversal retinal potentials. *Invest Ophthalmol Vis Sci* 1982; 23:774–779.

91. Viswanathan S, Frishman LJ, Robson JG: The uniform field and pattern ERG in macaques with experimental glaucoma: Removal of spiking activity. *Invest Ophthalmol Vis Sci* 2000; 41:2797–2810.

92. Votruba M, Fitzke FW, Holder GE, Carter A, Bhattacharya SS, Moore AT: Clinical features in affected individuals from 21 pedigrees with Dominant Optic Atrophy. *Arch Ophthalmol* 1998; 116:351–358.

93. Weng J, Mata NL, Azarian SM, Tzekov RT, Birch DG, Travis GH: Insights into the function of Rim protein in photoreceptors and etiology of Stargardt's disease from the phenotype in abcr knockout mice. *Cell* 1999; 98:13–23.

94. Zapf HR, Bach M: The contrast characteristic of the pattern electroretinogram depends on temporal frequency. *Graefes Arch Clin Exp Ophthalmol* 1999; 237:93–99.

95. Zrenner E: The physiological basis of the pattern electroretinogram. *Prog Ret Res* 1990; 9:427–464.

23 Assessing Infant Acuity, Fusion, and Stereopsis with Visual Evoked Potentials

EILEEN E. BIRCH

OVER THE PAST 25 years, there has been an explosion of new information about the maturation of vision during infancy. A growing appreciation of the role of visual experience during infancy in shaping the functional organization of the maturing visual system has driven a research effort to define the normal course of maturation and its susceptibility to disruption by early abnormal visual experience. As this research effort has bridged the transition from the laboratory to the clinical setting, the success of various treatment protocols for remediation following abnormal visual experience has come under evaluation, both in clinical trials and in clinical care of individual patients.

The study of infant visual maturation includes multiple approaches, including electrophysiology and psychophysics. Even in assessing a single visual dimension, such as visual acuity, the combination of multiple tests can provide more complete information about the infant's status than any one test alone. For example, while it is difficult to record pattern visual evoked potentials (VEPs) in patients with nystagmus or shunts, psychophysical assessment of acuity via preferential looking has a high success rate among these patients.[2,5,14] On the other hand, psychophysical testing may be insensitive to macular dysfunction and strabismic amblyopia,[9,24–26] while pattern VEPs are uniquely sensitive to these disorders because of the predominance of the central visual field in the responses.

Infant visual acuity testing is unusual in that it has bridged the gap between the laboratory and the clinic. Availability of the Teller Acuity Cards[45] has enabled psychophysical assessment of infant visual acuity during routine office examinations. While the additional expense and expertise associated with electrophysiological approaches to infant acuity assessment have limited their availability primarily to medical school hospitals and clinics, infant VEP acuity is now widely used both as an outcome measure for randomized clinical trials and for individual patient assessment. The focus of electrophysiological testing of infant visual acuity has shifted toward the use of the sweep VEP[30] in recent years. The sweep VEP is based on Fourier analysis of steady-state VEPs elicited by periodic stimulus changes, such as pattern reversal of a sine wave grating pattern. The steady-state VEP response is composed of a series of harmonically related components that are multiples of the frequency at which contrast reversal or pattern onset occurs.

To measure acuity by using the steady-state VEP, for example, the test protocol includes a series of checkerboard patterns or sine wave gratings that range from coarse to fine (low to high spatial frequency). For each pattern, 50–100 steady-state VEP responses are recorded, and the average amplitude is determined. By examining the relationship between check size (or spatial frequency) and response amplitude, the check size that corresponds to zero amplitude can be extrapolated as an acuity estimate. Ideally, many check sizes (or spatial frequencies) would be evaluated to pinpoint the exact size at which a reliable VEP could no longer be recorded. With the limited attention span of infants, this is rarely possible. In fact, in the now classic studies of the maturation of visual acuity during infancy that were conducted during the mid-1970s by Sokol[41] and by Marg et al.,[23] only four to six large-to-moderate pattern element sizes were included in each acuity test.

On the other hand, sweep VEP protocols usually present 10–20 spatial frequencies to the infant in rapid succession during a 10-second sweep. By using Fourier analytic techniques to extract the VEP responses to each of the brief stimuli (specifically, the amplitude and phase of the harmonics of the stimulation rate), sufficient information can be obtained from the VEP records to estimate visual acuity from only a few brief test trials. This technique has three significant advantages over the more classical methods. First, test time is greatly reduced. The classic steady-state VEP acuity paradigms often required an hour or more to obtain data for just a few check sizes, while data for 10–20 spatial frequencies can be collected within 15 minutes by using the sweep protocol. Second, the infant's behavioral state changes little during the recording session; since behavioral state can

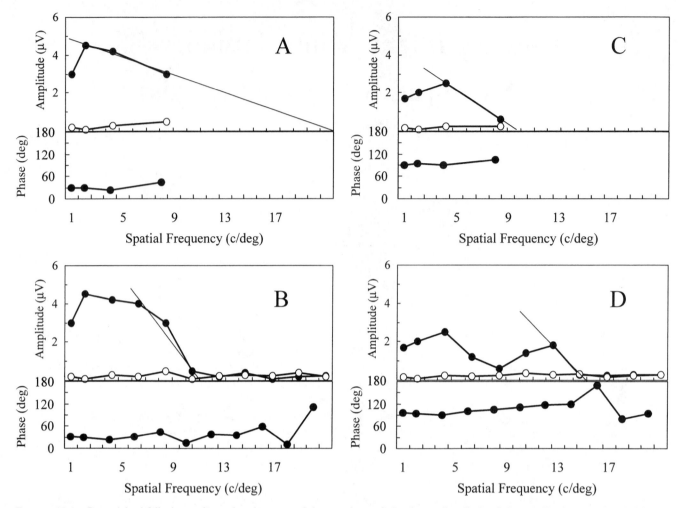

FIGURE 23.1 Potential pitfalls in acuity estimation caused by limited sampling of the amplitude versus spatial frequency function in classic VEP acuity protocols (panels A and C) that are overcome by the dense sampling and extended sampling range of the sweep VEP (panels B and D). Amplitude and phase of the VEP response (solid circles) are plotted along with amplitude at adjacent nonharmonic noise frequencies (open circles). Panel A illustrates a potential error in the acuity estimate that may occur if only low to moderate spatial frequencies are sampled (e.g., ≤8 c/deg) and the slope of the descending limb of the amplitude versus spatial frequency function is not constant. Panel B shows the more accurate acuity estimate that is derived when data are available for a larger range of spatial frequencies (1–20 c/deg). Panel C illustrates a limited sampling range (e.g., ≤8 c/deg) may also result in a poor acuity estimate because of missing a second peak in the amplitude versus spatial frequency function. Panel D shows the more accurate acuity estimate that is derived when data are available for a larger range of spatial frequencies (1–20 c/deg).

influence the quality of the data obtained, brief test protocols provide a major advantage. Third, since many more spatial frequencies can be included in the test protocol, close spacing in the series can be used, and a more accurate estimate of acuity can be obtained. Figure 23.1 illustrates two potential pitfalls in acuity estimation associated with the classic VEP acuity protocols that are overcome by the improved sampling of the amplitude versus spatial frequency function of the sweep VEP method.

Normal maturation of acuity

Over the past 10 years, we have gathered a substantial normative data set for monocular ($N = 244$) and binocular ($N =$ 347) sweep VEP acuity maturation during the first two years of life. Overall, sweep VEP acuity increases from about 0.75 logMAR (20/105 Snellen equivalent) at 6 weeks of age to about 0.37 logMAR (20/45) at 26 weeks of age and 0.25 logMAR (20/35) by 55 weeks of age (figure 23.2). This time course for acuity maturation is similar to previous reports in the literature.[16,30] The improvements in acuity parallel the considerable anatomical development that occurs postnatally. Although on fundus examination, the fovea appears mature soon after term birth,[18] the migration of cone photoreceptors toward the foveal pit is not complete during the first months of life.[47] The fine anatomical structure of the foveal cone photoreceptors is not mature until at least 4 years of age.[47] Myelination of the optic nerve and

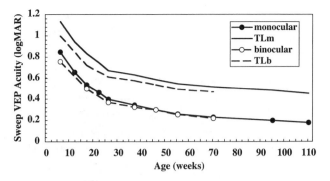

FIGURE 23.2   Mean monocular (solid circles; $N = 244$) and binocular (open circles; $N = 347$) sweep VEP acuity as a function of age in weeks (E. Birch, unpublished data). Also shown are the lower 95% tolerance limits for the normative range of individual monocular and binocular scores. Note that binocular sweep VEP acuity is consistently slightly better than monocular sweep VEP acuity and that the tolerance limits are narrower during the first year of life.

tract continues to increase for 2 years postnatally.[22] While the number of cells in the primary visual cortex appears to be complete at birth, there are considerable increases in cell size, synaptic structure, and dendritic density during the first six to eight months of life,[11,17] and elimination of supernumerary synapses in visual cortex continues until about 11 years of age.[17]

Mean binocular sweep VEP acuity is better than mean monocular sweep VEP acuity by about 0.03 logMAR. The variability of binocular sweep VEP acuity within an age group (e.g., 17-week-old infants), defined as 95% of the normal distribution, is about ±0.23 logMAR around the mean. Variability is slightly greater for monocular sweep VEP acuity: ±0.29 logMAR. These values are roughly comparable to the 0.6 logMAR range of sweep VEP acuities reported by Norcia and Tyler[31] for normal infants in a single age group.

Within the normative sample, mean interocular acuity differences are small in each age group, averaging less than 0.1 logMAR. However, the range of interocular differences comprising 95% of the normal distribution varies with age. At 6 weeks, 95% of interocular differences fall within ±0.29 logMAR while, by 46 weeks, 95% of interocular differences fall within ±0.18 logMAR. The latter value is consistent with previous reports of the range of normal interocular differences in sweep VEP acuity during infancy.[16]

Normative longitudinal measurements of sweep VEP acuity over the first 18 months of life have also been reported.[37,38] These data have direct clinical utility in that they provide a method for determining whether a change in an individual's acuity over time represents a significant change. In other words, such data provide a baseline for the evaluation of progression, recovery, and/or response to treatment in individual patients. The rate of sweep VEP

acuity development (slope) ranged from −0.34 to −0.89 logMAR/log weeks in a normative sample of 53 healthy term infants tested on five occasions during the first 18 months of life. Preliminary studies have suggested that rate of acuity development during infancy may be more predictive of long-term visual acuity outcome than the infant's acuity determined from a single acuity test.[19]

Preterm birth

Preterm birth potentially plays an important role in visual development; premature exteriorization removes the visual system from the nurturing intrauterine environment during its period of rapid maturation. The immature visual system is unnaturally subjected to external visual stimulation, and its tissues can no longer depend on placental maternal-to-fetal transfer of essential nutrients. While the basic organization of the structures of the visual system appear to be specified innately, it is clear that postnatal visual experience and nutrition can modify the fine structure and function of the visual system.

Both stimulating and harmful effects of early precocious exposure to light or patterned visual stimulation are possible. Damage could be inflicted, for example, by changing the rate of synaptic production, interfering with the normal process of elimination of supernumerary synapses, or by disrupting the normal sequential differentiation of neurons or their connections. Stimulating effects could result from early activation of visual experience-dependent neuronal pathways, enhancing their rate of maturation. In general, VEP acuity studies have found slight or no accelerating effect on the rate of acuity development (figure 23.3). In fact, while there appears to be little difference in acuity between healthy preterm and term infants during the first 57 weeks postconception, preterm infants may have an overall slower rate of acuity development so that by 66 weeks postconception, acuity is significantly poorer in the preterm group.[37]

Just as it is clear that there are critical periods during which abnormal visual experience may result in permanent adverse changes in the way that the visual system matures, it has become clear recently that some dietary deficiencies during infancy may have adverse effects on the maturation of visual function. Recently, there has been a focus on the differences in omega-3 long-chain polyunsaturated fatty acid levels in human milk versus infant formula. Over 60% of the structural material in the brain is lipids, including cholesterol and phosphoglycerides of neural membranes, which are rich in docosahexaenoic acid (DHA) and arachidonic acid (AA). As a component of the central nervous system with a common embryonic origin, the retina contains similarly high levels of DHA and AA to structural lipids, particularly in the metabolically active photoreceptor outer segments. Changes in the relative proportions of different brain and retinal

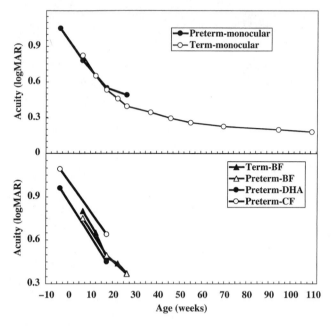

FIGURE 23.3 Top, Monocular sweep VEP acuity of healthy preterm and term infants.[31,37] (E. Birch, unpublished data). Bottom, VEP acuity of healthy breast-fed (BF) preterm[3] (E. Birch, unpublished data) and term infants along with VEP acuity data from preterm infants who were fed control formula (CF)[3] or experimental formula supplemented with docosahexaenoic acid (DHA).[3]

phospholipids, especially the large changes in DHA levels and the DHA/AA ratio, during late fetal development and infancy may be reflected in cellular and neural maturation. Evidence from randomized clinical trials suggests that formula-fed preterm infants are at particular risk from DHA deficiency because they are deprived of the last trimester of placental maternal-to-fetal transfer of DHA because they have limited capacity to endogenously synthesize DHA from the precursor fatty acids that are provided by most infant formulas, and because they are the least likely to be breast-fed. Preterm infants who are fed formulas without DHA show lower DHA levels in red blood cell membranes and cerebral cortex and poorer VEP acuity than are infants who receive DHA in their diet (figure 23.3).

Reliability and validity of sweep VEP acuity

The reliability of infant sweep VEP acuities has been evaluated in both normal and clinical cohorts. In normal infants, Norcia and Tyler[31] reported that 65–75% of individual sweep responses reach criterion to provide an acuity score and that 95% of individual sweep acuity scores were within ±0.16 logMAR. This is similar to the 22% (±0.17 logMAR) test-retest variability reported by Prager et al.[35] Norcia and Tyler[31] also report that the best acuity from a single sweep differed from the vector average of multiple sweeps by less than 0.11 logMAR. Within a single age group of normal

infants (e.g., 17-week-olds), the cross-sectional variability of sweep VEP acuity is about 0.6 logMAR. Since this intersubject variability far exceeds intrasubject variability, it appears that most of the cross-sectional variability is due to true individual differences and not to measurement error. Test-retest reliability data from pediatric patients are almost nonexistent, but reliability may be poorer than in normative cohorts. In patients with cortical visual impairment, retest varied by ±0.3 logMAR from the original acuity score.[12] This is likely the worst-case scenario for assessing reliability, since VEP recording in this cohort of patients is often complicated by the presence of seizure activity, nystagmus, and visual inattention. Nonetheless, these data demonstrate that caution must be exercised in extending normative reliability data to patient groups.

The validity of sweep VEP acuity estimates has been evaluated through concordance across centers, through concordance with other acuity estimates in both normative and clinical cohorts, and by evaluating the predictive value of early sweep VEP acuity estimates for long-term optotype acuity outcomes. As was discussed in more detail in the section entitled "Normal maturation of acuity," there is excellent concordance between the normative sweep VEP acuity data obtained in our laboratory and in Norcia's laboratory for mean acuity development, variability around the mean within age groups, monocular-binocular acuity differences, and interocular differences. In addition, three separate sites in two independent studies[36–38] that tested normal infants with both sweep VEP and Teller Acuity Cards found the same trends in acuity development. Sweep VEP acuity was generally higher than Teller Acuity Card acuity during the first few months of life, but the rate of development was steeper for Teller Acuity Card acuity. Thus, the ratio of sweep VEP to Teller Acuity Card acuity decreased with age.

The concordance between sweep VEP acuity and optotype acuity has been evaluated for defocus due to refractive error. Sweep VEP acuity and optotype acuity are correlated, but the predictive power of sweep VEP acuity for an individual's optotype acuity in the presence of refractive error is limited. Optotype acuity can be predicted only within two lines for 95% of individuals.[46] In general, for no defocus to modest defocus, sweep VEP acuity tends to be equal to or poorer than optotype acuity, while for moderate to severe defocus, sweep VEP acuity tends to be better than optotype acuity.[20] Sweep VEP is unlikely to be recordable at all if optotype acuity is poorer than 20/200.[42]

The concordance between sweep VEP acuity and optotype or grating acuity has been evaluated for various ophthalmopediatric disorders. Gottlob et al.[13] initially reported a good correlation between best single sweep acuity and optotype acuity in 135 children with diverse visual disorders, but in a follow-up study of patients with organic diseases, nystagmus, strabismus, or ptosis, Gottlob et al.[14] reported that the accuracy of sweep VEP acuity depended on the particular disease. Overall, the correlation between sweep VEP acuity and optotype acuity was high ($r = 0.84$), but the slope of the regression line was significantly less than 1.0 because acuities worse than 0.33 logMAR had better sweep VEP than optotype acuity, while for better optotype acuities, sweep VEP acuity underestimated optotype acuity. The best correlation and the slope closest to 1.0 was found for the subset of patients with organic diseases (e.g., retinopathy of prematurity, persistent hyperplastic primary vitreous, optic nerve glioma, Leber's amaurosis), and the poorest correlation was found for patients with nystagmus. In the largest study to date, Arai et al.[1] reported that 77% of eyes in 100 patients with various ocular pathologies and optotype acuities, ranging from 20/15 to 20/400, had sweep VEP acuity agreement within one octave and that the poorest concordance was found for patients with optic nerve disease.

Concordance between sweep VEP acuity and preferential-looking grating acuity, either by forced-choice preferential looking or by the Teller Acuity Card Procedure, shows a similar pattern of results. Namely, overall there is a good correlation but sweep VEP acuity tends to be better than grating acuity when acuity is poor and grating acuity tends to be better than sweep VEP acuity when acuity is normal or only mildly impaired.[12,20,31,33]

The predictive value of infant sweep VEP acuity for long-term optotype acuity outcome also has been evaluated. Jeffrey et al.[19] evaluated a cohort of patients with cortical visual impairment. They reported that both the initial sweep VEP acuity, obtained at a mean of 8 months of age, and the rate of sweep VEP acuity development over the first 18 months of life were correlated with the acuity outcome at ≥5 years of age ($r = 0.45$ and $r = 0.57$, respectively). However, the rate of acuity development was a more sensitive predictor of visual impairment (75%) than was the initial acuity (50%), and rate also was a more specific predictor (86%) than initial acuity (46%). In a recent study of 47 low-birth-weight children,[32] sweep VEP grating acuity was not predictive of optotype acuity outcome at ≥4 years of age when the VEP was assessed before 6 months adjusted age but was predictive when acuity was assessed at 7–12 months. In addition, the rate of sweep VEP acuity maturation during the first 2 years of life was predictive of optotype acuity outcome.

Fusion and stereopsis

Particularly for the evaluation of fusion and stereopsis, the cortical magnification of the foveal area and visual cortical topography favor VEP protocols, since responses reflect macular function regardless of stimulus size. Two steady-state VEP protocols have been employed to assess sensory fusion. In the correlogram protocol, originally developed by Petrig,[34] the stimulus is an anaglyphic dynamic random dot

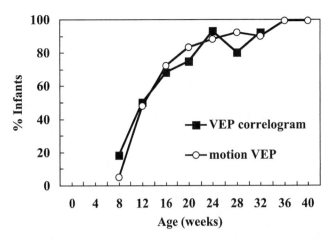

FIGURE 23.4 The percentage of infants who have a reliable VEP in the correlogram or motion VEP protocols as a function of age in weeks. Note that few infants have fusion before 4 weeks of age, while most infants have fusion by 26 weeks[6] (E. Birch, unpublished data).

pattern that alternates in time between correlated ($r = 1.0$, bright dots fall on corresponding points in the two eyes, fusion stimulus) and anticorrelated ($r = -1.0$, bright dot in one eye and dark dot in the other eye fall on corresponding points, rivalry stimulus). VEPs in response to changes from the correlated state to the anticorrelated state assess the infant's ability to appreciate fusion and rivalry. As is shown in figure 23.4, few infants under 4 weeks of age demonstrate fusion, while by 12–16 weeks, virtually all infants demonstrate sensory fusion.[6]

In the motion VEP protocol, originally developed by Norcia et al.,[27,28] a sine wave grating is jittered back and forth; whether the motion VEP is symmetric for nasalward and temporalward motion is assessed. Healthy children older than 1 year of age and adults have symmetric responses to both directions of motion (approximately equal in amplitude); therefore, a steady-state VEP at twice the jitter rate (F_2 harmonic) can be recorded. Nasal-temporal asymmetry of the motion VEP is a routine finding in healthy infants aged 2–6 months[4,27] (figure 23.5). Symmetry of the motion VEP has been shown to be highly correlated with foveal fusion; asymmetry has been shown to be highly correlated with monofixation.[4,10] The maturation of sensory fusion from both protocols is shown in figure 23.4. In each protocol, few infants under 4 weeks of age demonstrate fusion, while by 26 weeks (6 months), virtually all infants demonstrate sensory fusion.[4,6]

The maturation of stereopsis has been determined by using dynamic random dot stereograms. The onset of stereopsis occurs at about 15 weeks of age (figure 23.6).[6] After onset, the rate of stereoacuity maturation is rapid, with the infant achieving stereoacuity of 50 arc sec by 35 weeks (figure 23.6).[6] The relationship between VEP amplitude and

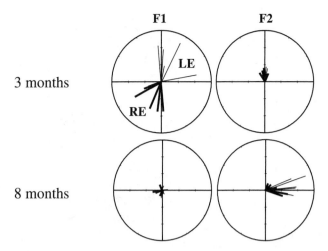

F1   **F2**

3 months

8 months

FIGURE 23.5   Polar plots of infant motion VEP fundamental and second harmonic response amplitude and phase. Five responses were obtained for the right eye (RE; thick lines) and left eye (LE; thin lines) at each test age. At 3 months of age, the infant shows a nasal-temporal asymmetry in the motion VEP, that is, a motion response primarily at the fundamental frequency, with an approximate 180-degree interocular phase difference. At 8 months of age, the infant shows symmetry of the motion VEP, that is, a motion response primarily at the second harmonic, with no interocular phase difference.

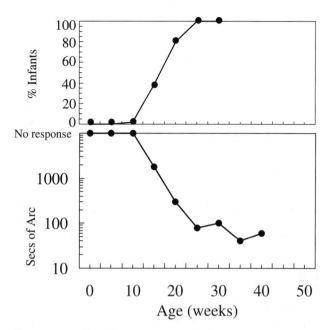

FIGURE 23.6   Top, The percentage of infants who have a reliable VEP in the dynamic random dot stereogram protocol as a function of age in weeks.[6] Note that few infants have random dot stereopsis before 10 weeks of age, while most infants have random dot stereopsis by 26 weeks. Bottom, VEP random dot stereoacuity as a function of age in weeks.[6] Stereoacuity improves rapidly from about 2000 arc sec at 15 weeks of age to about 100 arc sec by 24 weeks and 60 arc sec by 40 weeks of age.

binocular disparity is complex, with a linear relationship from threshold to about 15 min arc, a dip in amplitude and loss of phase coherence at intermediate disparities, and large amplitude response with a different phase for coarse disparities (figure 23.7).[6] The two distinct ranges of VEP response to disparity may represent independent coarse and fine disparity-sensitive mechanisms.[29]

Multiple stimulus sweep VEP paradigms

A useful twist on standard sweep VEP test protocols is to present two or more stimuli simultaneously. As long as each stimulus is presented at a different, nonharmonic temporal rate, it will have an independent temporal signature associated with it. Clearly, it has an advantage in speed of data acquisition and in controlling for differences in arousal, optical focus, and fixation (which might be more variable if testing was conducted sequentially for each location).

The multiple stimulus approach becomes even more useful when it is joined to a test-probe paradigm. In such a paradigm, a constant test stimulus is presented simultaneously with a swept probe stimulus. For example, while the subject fixates a 10% contrast 3 c/deg grating phase alternating at 6 Hz, a second grating that is phase alternating at 7 Hz can be presented simultaneously at the same retinal location to examine contrast masking (by sweeping contrast) or spatial frequency masking (by sweeping spatial frequency).[43] Alternatively, dichoptic masking can be examined

if the test stimulus is presented to one eye and the swept probe stimulus is presented to the other eye.[43] Recently, this approach has been used to assess rivalry (alternate suppression) in both adults and infants. Adults show clear VEP amplitude waxing and waning for each eye that correlates with the perceptual dominance of that eye.[8] On the other hand, in 35 normal infants age 5–15 months, rivalry could not be detected with this approach.[7] This finding contrasts with those of psychophysical studies, which suggest that rivalry develops along a similar time course to stereopsis, at about 3–6 months of age.[15,39]

Special considerations for recording VEPs from infant patients

In the topographic projection from the retina to the occipital cortex, the central 6–8 degrees of the visual field is predominant, with the peripheral visual field more sparsely represented. The VEP recorded from the scalp over the occipital lobe even more strongly reflects the macular area because its projection is on the exposed surface of the occipital cortex, while the peripheral projection lies deep within the calcarine fissure. This certainly enhances the sensitivity of the VEP to disruption of central vision, which subserves acuity and fine stereoacuity. On the other hand, a child with

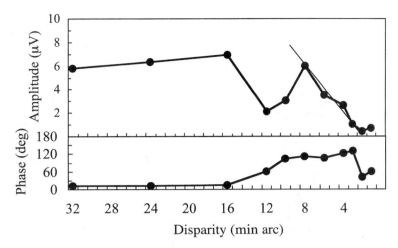

FIGURE 23.7 VEP amplitude and phase as a function of disparity. The amplitude versus disparity function is nonmonotonic, with two amplitude peaks. A dip in amplitude occurs at about 15 min arc. Response phase at disparities coarser than 15 min arc differs from response phase for disparities finer than 15 min arc by about 90 degrees. The straight line indicates the best fit by linear regression over the fine disparity range that was used to estimate stereoacuity.

poor macular function and/or eccentric fixation may fail to produce a reliable VEP response despite substantial residual visual function.

Two other factors that can limit the ability to obtain VEPs in infant patients include state and visual attention. Sleepy infants, sedated infants, and anesthetized infants all produce poor or variable VEP results. Head and body movements, including yawning, crying, or sucking, can lead to muscle artifacts in the VEP records. Infants who are unable to maintain gaze near the center of the stimulus may produce variable or absent VEP responses even when significant visual function is present; nystagmus is a particular problem, since the eye movements also may generate artifacts in the VEP records. Failure to accommodate appropriately and/or uncorrected refractive errors substantially reduces the amplitude of responses and may lead to nondetectable VEPs in infants who see quite well when the stimuli are in proper focus.

Infants with neurological diseases present additional challenges because gross disorganization of the electroencephalogram (EEG) usually precludes successful VEP testing.[2,40,44] While medications can reduce disorganization of the EEG, they often result in an infant who is not sufficiently alert or visually attentive to produce reliable VEP responses. Accurate electrode placement, which is accomplished via careful measurement relative to skull landmarks, may not be possible in patients with abnormal brain anatomy. Surgical alterations in brain anatomy, such as the placement of shunts, also may interfere with the ability to record a signal at some sites on the scalp.

As a final note, it is worth stating that with few exceptions, the clinical value of sweep VEP testing does not lie in the detection or differential diagnosis of ophthamopediatric diseases. Instead, the strength of VEP assessment lies in quantitative measurement of the degree of visual impairment. In addition to its utility for determining the natural history of ophthalmopediatric disorders and their response to treatment, determination of sweep VEP acuity can be of great value in establishing eligibility for educational and social services and for providing parents with a clear picture of their child's abilities. Sweep VEP acuity in conjunction with preferential looking acuity using Teller Acuity Cards can provide a more complete picture. While each test has its strengths and weaknesses in terms of sensitivity, accuracy, and physical demands of the patient, the two tests together can provide immensely useful information about visual impairment and its response to treatment.

ACKNOWLEDGMENTS   This research was supported in part by NIH grants EY05236 and HD22380.

REFERENCES

1. Arai M, Katsumi O, Paranhos F, Lopes De Faria J, Hirose T: Comparison of Snellen acuity and objective assessment using the spatial frequency sweep PVER. *Graefes Arch Clin Exp Ophthalmol* 1997; 235:442–447.
2. Bane M, Birch E: VEP acuity, FPL acuity, and visual behavior of visually impaired children. *J Pediatr Ophthalmol Strabismus* 1992; 29:202–209.
3. Birch EE, Birch DG, Hoffman DR, Uauy R: Dietary essential fatty acid supply and visual acuity development. *Invest Ophthalmol Vis Sci* 1992; 33:3242–3253.
4. Birch E, Fawcett S, Stager D: Co-development of VEP motion response and binocular vision in normal infants and infantile esotropes. *Invest Ophthalmol Vis Sci* 2000; 41:1719–1723.
5. Birch E, Hale L, Stager D, Fuller D, Birch D: Operant acuity of toddlers and developmentally delayed children with low vision. *J Pediatr Ophthalmol Strabismus* 1987; 24:64–69.

6. Birch E, Petrig B: FPL and VEP measures of fusion, stereopsis and stereoacuity in normal infants. *Vision Res* 1996; 36:1321–1327.

7. Brown R, Candy T, Norcia A: Development of rivalry and dichoptic masking in human infants. *Invest Ophthalmol Vis Sci* 1999; 40:3324–3332.

8. Brown R, Norcia A: A method for investigating binocular rivalry in real-time with the steady-state VEP. *Vision Res* 1997; 37:2401–2408.

9. Ellis G, Hartmann E, Love A, May J, Morgan K: Teller acuity cards versus clinical judgment in the diagnosis of amblyopia with strabismus. *Ophthalmology* 1988; 95:788–791.

10. Fawcett S, Birch E: Motion VEPs, stereopsis, and bifoveal fusion in children with strabismus. *Invest Ophthalmol Vis Sci* 2000; 41:411–416.

11. Garey L: Structural development of the visual system of man. *Hum Neurobiol* 1984; 3:75–80.

12. Good W: Development of a quantitative method to measure vision in children with chronic cortical visual impairment. *Trans Am Ophthalmol Soc* 2001; 99:253–269.

13. Gottlob I, Fendick M, Guo S, Zubcov A, Odom J, Reinecke R: Visual acuity measurements by swept spatial frequency VECPs: Clinical application in children with various visual disorders. *J Pediatr Ophthalmol Strabismus* 1990; 27:40–47.

14. Gottlob I, Wizov S, Odom J, Reinecke R: Predicting optotype visual acuity by swept spatial visual-evoked potentials. *Clin Vision Sci* 1993; 8:417–423.

15. Gwiazda J, Bauer J, Held R: Binocular function in human infants: Correlation of stereoptic and fusion-rivalry discriminations. *J Pediatr Ophthalmol Strabismus* 1989; 26:128–132.

16. Hamer R, Norcia A, Tyler C, Hsu-Winges C: The development of monocular and binocular VEP acuity. *Vision Res* 1989; 29:397–408.

17. Huttenlocher P, De Courten C: The development of synapses in striate cortex of man. *Hum Neurobiol* 1987; 6:1–9.

18. Isenberg S: Macular development in the premature infant. *Am J Ophthalmol* 1986; 101:74–80.

19. Jeffrey B, Weems J, Salomão S, Birch E: Prediction of visual acuity outcome following perinatal cortical insult. Paper presented at American Association for Pediatric Ophthalmology and Strabismus, San Diego, CA, 2001.

20. Katsumi O, Arai M, Wajima R, Denno S, Hirose T: Spatial frequency sweep pattern reversal VER acuity vs. Snellen visual acuity: Effect of optical defocus. *Vision Res* 1996; 36:903–909.

21. Katsumi O, Denno S, Arai M, De Lopes Faria J, Hirose T: Comparison of preferential looking acuity and pattern reversal visual evoked response acuity in pediatric patients. *Graefes Arch Clin Exp Ophthalmol* 1997; 235:684–690.

22. Magoon E, Robb R: Development of myelin in human optic nerve and tract: A light and electron microscope study. *Arch Ophthalmol* 1981; 99:655–659.

23. Marg E, Freeman D, Peltzman P, Goldstein P: Visual acuity development in human infants: Evoked potential measurements. *Invest Ophthalmol Vis Sci* 1976; 15:150–152.

24. Mayer D, Fulton A, Hansen R: Visual acuity of infants and children with retinal degenerations. *Ophthalmol Paediatr Gen* 1985; 5:51–56.

25. Mayer D, Fulton A, Rodier D: Grating and recognition acuities of pediatric patients. *Ophthalmology* 1984; 91:947–953.

26. Mayer D, Fulton A, Rodier D: Grating acuity of esotropic infants does not always agree with fixation. *Invest Ophthalmol Vis Sci* 1984; 25 (suppl):218.

27. Norcia A, Garcia H, Humphry R, Holmes A, Hamer R, Orel-Bixler D: Anomalous motion VEPs in infants and in infantile esotropia. *Invest Ophthalmol Vis Sci* 1991; 32:436–439.

28. Norcia A, Hamer R, Jampolsky A, Orel-Bixler D: Plasticity of human motion processing mechanisms following surgery for infantile esotropia. *Vision Res* 1995; 35:3279–3296.

29. Norcia A, Sutter E, Tyler C: Electrophysiological evidence for the existence of coarse and fine disparity mechanisms in human. *Vision Res* 1985; 25:395–401.

30. Norcia A, Tyler C: Spatial frequency sweep VEP: Visual acuity during the first year of life. *Vision Res* 1985; 25:1399–1408.

31. Norcia A, Tyler C: Infant VEP acuity measurements: Analysis of individual differences and measurement error. *Electroencephalogr Clin Neurophysiol* 1985; 61:359–369.

32. O'Connor A, Birch E, Leffler J, Salomão S: Visual Evoked Potential (VEP) and Preferential-looking (PL) grating acuity as predictors of long-term visual impairment in low birth weight children. *Invest Ophthalmol Vis Sci* 2003; 44:E-abstract 2712.

33. Orel-Bixler D, Haegerstrom-Portnoy G, Hall A: Visual assessment of the multiply handicapped patient. *Optom Vis Sci* 1989; 66:530–536.

34. Petrig B, Julesz B, Kropfl W, Baumgartner G, Anliker M: Development of stereopsis and cortical binocularity in human infants: Electro-physiological evidence. *Science* 1981; 213:1402–1404.

35. Prager T, Zou YL, Jensen C, Fraley J, Anderson R, Heird W: Evaluation of methods for assessing visual function of infants. *J AAPOS* 1999; 3:275–282.

36. Riddell P, Ladenheim B, Mast J, Catalano T, Nobile R, Hainline L: Comparison of measures of visual acuity in infants: Teller acuity cards and sweep visual evoked potentials. *Optom Vis Sci* 1997; 74:702–707.

37. Salomão S, Berezovsky A, de Haro F, Cinoto R, Ventura D, Birch E: Longitudinal visual acuity development in healthy preterm infants. *Invest Ophthalmol Vis Sci* 2000; 41:S728.

38. Salomão S, Birch E: Individual growth curves for infant visual acuity measured by sweep VEP and FPL in the first 18 months of life. *Vision Res*, in press.

39. Shimojo S, Bauer J, O'Connell K, Held R: Pre-stereoptic binocular vision in infants. *Vision Res* 1986; 26:501–510.

40. Smith D: The clinical usefulness of the visual evoked response. *J Pediatr Ophthalmol Strabismus* 1984; 21:235–236.

41. Sokol S: Measurement of infant visual acuity from pattern reversal evoked potentials. *Vision Res* 1978; 18:33–39.

42. Steele M, Seiple W, Carr R, Klug R: The clinical utility of visual-evoked potential acuity testing. *Am J Ophthalmol* 1989; 108:572–577.

43. Suter S, Suter P, Perrier D, Parker K, Fox J, Rossler J: Differentiation of VEP intermodulation and second harmonic compinents by dichoptic, monocular, and binocular stimulation. *Vis Neurosci* 1996; 13:1157–1166.

44. Taddeucci G, Fiorentini A, Pirchio M, Spinelli D: Pattern reversal evoked potentials in infantile spasms. *Hum Neurobiol* 1984; 3:153–155.

45. Teller D, McDonald M, Preston K, Sebris S, Dobson V: Assessment of visual acuity in infants and children: The acuity card procedure. *Dev Med Child Neurol* 1986; 28:779–789.

46. Wiener D, Wellish K, Nelson J, Kuppersmith M: Comparisons among, Snellen, psychophysical, and evoked potential visual acuity determinations. *Am J Optom Physiol Opt* 1985; 62:669–679.

47. Youdelis C, Hendrickson A: A qualitative and quantitative analysis of the human fovea during development. *Vision Res* 1986; 26:847–855.

24 Aging and Pattern Visual Evoked Cortical Potential

EMIKO ADACHI-USAMI

THE DECREASE IN visual acuity and other visual functions with aging has been reported extensively. This decline of visual function has been attributed to anatomical aging changes in the eye and the visual pathway. Opacities of the crystalline lens and vitreous body, miosis, and a loss of neurons at both the retina and the visual cortex have been considered to be the factors responsible for the loss of function.

With the development of surgical techniques for cataracts and the prolongation of life, patients older than 90 years often have a visual acuity over 20/20. Are their cells and neurons in the visual pathway still functioning as in youth?

Visually evoked cortical potentials (VECPs) to pattern stimulation have been known to reflect several visual functions related to neuronal function, and the effect of age on pattern VECP has been studied by a number of authors. There is general agreement that the P100 peak latency increases and amplitude decreases in the elderly. However, the ophthalmological findings described in the literature are not sufficiently clear. The present chapter deals with the aging effects on pattern VECPs mainly in elderly subjects.

General changes in visual evoked cortical potentials with age

WAVEFORM There have been a few reports that described the development of VECP waveforms.[3,18,24] Generally, the waveforms change from a single positive peak to a negative-positive complex with age. The pattern-onset response consists mainly of a single positive peak with a latency of about 150 ms until about 10 months, a negative component becomes recognizable at the age of 20 months, and the initial positive component splits into two positive waves at puberty.

Figure 24.1 shows the pattern-reversal VECP responses to three check sizes from one infant that were recorded at three different ages. At the age of 10 weeks, simple, large, slow positive peaks with a peak latency at about 150 ms are observed. At 15 weeks the peak latencies of positive waves become shorter—about 120 ms. At 19 weeks the positive peak and the negative troughs become sharp and clear. The check size that elicits the largest responses in amplitude is

80 min at 10 weeks but becomes smaller—40 min at 15 weeks and 20 min at 19 weeks. No obvious alternation of VECP waveforms was observed after that. This development of waveforms is concurrent with the anatomical development of the macula and myelin sheath as well as with synaptic development.

Amplitude changes with aging There has been a variant of opinion regarding the aging effects on VECP amplitude. Halliday et al.[10] reported that there was no significant effect of age on amplitude. Celesia and Daly[6] also found no correlation between age and the amplitude of P100.

In contrast, Shaw and Cant[15] reported that the P100 amplitude was greatest in childhood, declined until the fourth decade, increased again, and then decreased after the sixth decade. Wright et al.[21] found that the amplitude of the component of the pattern-reversal VECPs was very high in the teenage group but, once reduced, became constant from the twenties onward and showed no further consistent age changes.

We found that the P100 amplitude decreased with aging as shown in figure 24.2. A progressive reduction in the amplitude of the P100 component with age for lower temporal frequency ranges was observed up to the ages of 30 to 39 years; however, the temporal tuning curve tended to shift toward lower frequencies with age after 30 years.

PEAK LATENCY CHANGES WITH AGING Most of the related literature refers to the increase in P100 latency in the elderly. However, a delay of the P100 is also known as an important criterion for diagnosing optic neuritis caused by multiple sclerosis. We have to be very careful when judging abnormal delay of the P100 because it can be found not only in the elderly but also in normal controls by changing the stimulus conditions such as lower vs. upper visual field, monocular vs. binocular viewing, luminance, defocusing, and spatial frequency of stimuli.

In 1975 Asselman and others[5] reported that the latency of the P100 was unaffected by aging until about 60 years but that thereafter there was a tendency for it to increase. In subjects under the age of 60 years the mean latency was

Check size, minutes

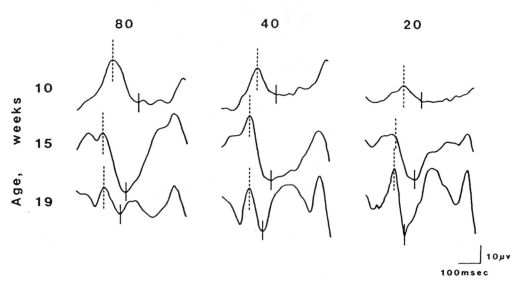

FIGURE 24.1   Pattern-reversal VECP responses to three check sizes from one infant that were recorded at the ages of 10, 15, and 19 weeks after her birth.

90.5 ms, but over the age of 60 years it was significantly longer at 97.2 ms.

Still later, in 1977, Celesia and Daly[6] reported a linear increase in mean latency with age. They showed an annual increase of 0.18 ms in the delay of the P100 during the age range from 15 to 70 years; it increased from 93 to 103 ms over that period. More precisely, Shearer and Dustman[17] stated that the rate of the P100 delay accelerates from young adulthood through the sixth decade. The rate of increase has been demonstrated to be greater for smaller than for larger check sizes.[7,19,22] Shaw and Cant[16] showed that the relationship between age and latency is influenced by pattern luminance and that at lower levels of luminance there is an increase in latency after the fourth decade.

In order to exclude the effect of senile opacity of the crystalline lens, we compared the P100 latency between phakic eyes and aphakic eyes with an intraocular lens (figure 24.3). Peak latency changes by aging were similar in the two groups showing a significant delay in the age group beyond 70 years, suggesting that reduced transparency of the medium in the elderly was not the reason for the delay of the P100, but rather it was possibly due to senile changes in the neural pathway.

Some authors suggested a gender effect for the P100 increase in the elderly. Halliday et al.[10] found that the increase in mean latency from the age of 50 years was seen only for the female group. We also found shorter latencies in elderly females, although such a tendency has been observed throughout their life spans (figure 24.4). On the contrary, Mitchell et al.[14] reported that a significant age effect (increasing values with age) was demonstrated, but

none in relation to gender. Further studies on gender and age relationships are necessary.

In summary, it might be true that the increase in P100 latency with age begins rather late in life, over 60 years, and is uncertain at ages below 50 years.

Temporal frequency characteristics

Few VECP studies have been performed on age-related changes in temporal frequency characteristics. Wright and Drasdo[21] found by psychophysical measurements that contrast sensitivity was significantly lowered with age, especially for high temporal frequency stimulation.

Adachi-Usami et al.[1a] recorded pattern VECPs from 70 normal volunteers aged 4 to 70 years. Eleven reversal frequencies between 1 and 20 reversals per second (rps) were presented. A progressive reduction in the amplitude of the P100 component with age for lower frequency ranges of less than 10 rps was shown up to the ages of 30 to 39 years, and the temporal tuning curve followed a constant pattern after 40 years. However, there was a tendency for the maxima of the tuning curve to shift toward lower frequencies with age after 30 years. The youngest group, 0 to 9 years, had two peaks at 3 and 10 rps, contrary to the single peak found in older groups (see figure 24.2).

Contrast thresholds

An increase in contrast threshold in spatial vision with age is well known.[4,8,12,20,21] Most of the studies were based on psychophysical measurements.

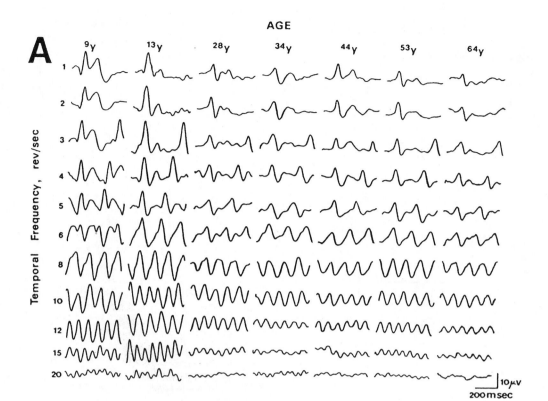

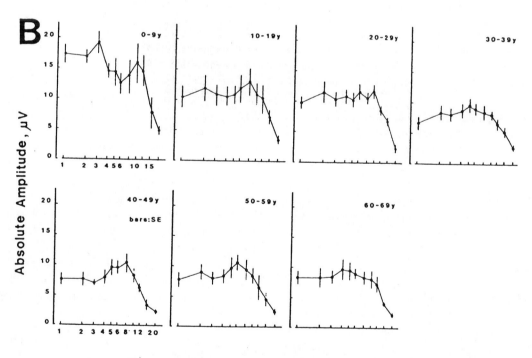

FIGURE 24.2   A, Pattern-reversal VECPs to 11 different reversal frequencies for seven age groups. B, P100 amplitude of the pattern-reversal VECPs vs. temporal frequency curves measured in seven age groups. Each age group contains ten subjects. Each point represents the mean ±1 SE. (From Adachi-Usami E, Hosoda L, Toyonaga N: *Doc Ophthalmol* 1988; 69:139–144. Used by permission.)

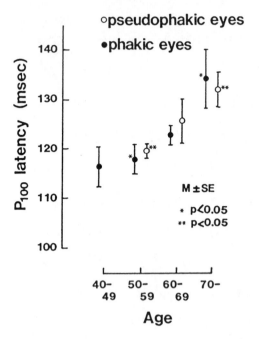

FIGURE 24.3 Effect of age on P100 peak latency of pattern-reversal VECPs obtained from phakic and pseudophakic eyes.

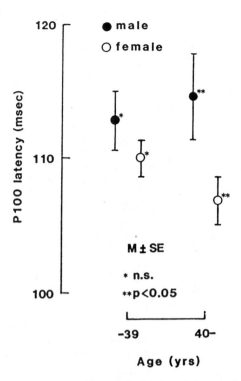

FIGURE 24.4 Gender difference in P100 peak latency for young and elderly groups.

Our study[25] could verify this by means of pattern VECPs (figure 24.5). The subjects, 38 normal volunteers ranging from 20 to 79 years old, were divided into three age groups. An artificial pupil of 3 mm was used to eliminate senile miosis effects. All patients' visual acuities were more than 1.0. With decreasing pattern contrast, the P100 peak latency decreased linearly as log contrast rose. The contrast threshold was determined by extrapolating the regression line of the line of the latency vs. log contrast to 140 ms for each check size. Contrast thresholds in elderly subjects were significantly higher than those of middle-aged or younger subjects at higher spatial frequency stimuli.

Luminance thresholds

The threshold levels for both rods and cones are significantly affected by age. However, the form of the psychophysically measured dark adaptation curve is the same for all age groups, although there is evidence that the amount of light reaching the retina is interfered with by the crystalline lens, which loses its transmittance with age, as well as by senile miosis. On the other hand, it is known that the decrease in pattern luminance increases the P100 latency of VECPs.[2,11]

In order to determine the luminance threshold increase in the elderly by means of VECPs, the factors that interfere with the optical transmittance need to be excluded. We therefore studied the luminance threshold in 39 normal phakic eyes and 25 pseudophakic eyes after posterior-chamber lens implantation.[26] The regression line was obtained from the VECP P100 amplitude vs. luminance data. Then, VECP luminance threshold was estimated by extrapolating to the light which produced a zero response. The threshold was seen to increase with age. The difference in thresholds between young subjects (aged 30 to 39 years) and elderly subjects (aged 60 to 79 years) was approximately 0.8 log units in neutral-density filter value (figure 24.6A). VECP luminance thresholds in pseudophakic eyes were a bit higher than those of the normal controls (figure 24.6B).

These results suggested that the increase in the luminance threshold in the elderly was not due to a lesser transparency of the crystalline lens but rather to aging changes of the neural pathway.

Pupillary size

The pupil becomes smaller with age, which means that retinal luminance will be reduced to a certain extent. So the delay and reduction of the P100 in the elderly could be partly caused by miosis, not only by the senescence of the neural pathway.

According to Wright et al.[22] the mean pupil diameter decreased from 4.9 mm in the 10- to 19-year-old age group

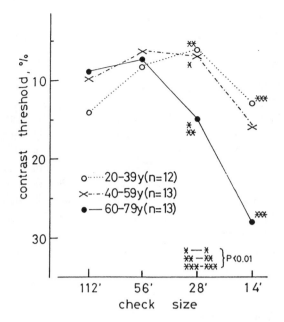

FIGURE 24.5 Mean contrast thresholds for each check size in three age groups. The spatial frequency characteristics of the contrast thresholds are observed to be equally shaped in all groups. The contrast thresholds are significantly increased in the elder group with small check size stimuli (P < .01). (From Yamazaki H, Adachi-Usami E: *Acta Soc Ophthalmol Jpn* 1988; 92:1662–1665. Used by permission.)

to 3.15 mm in the 70- to 79-year-old age group, with a difference in retinal luminance of 0.38 log units. Halliday et al.[11] and Adachi-Usami and Lehmann[2] found that a 1-log unit decrease in pattern luminance resulted in a 15- to 18-ms increase in P100 latency. According to our data,[25] a 0.38-log luminance decrease evoked an increase of 7 ms, whereas Wright et al.[22] calculated this increase to be 5.7 ms.

In an earlier section, the increase in luminance threshold in the elderly was described as being 0.8 log units, which could not be caused by the reduction in pupil size alone.

Therefore, we studied the effect of the pupillary area on contrast threshold based on the P100 latency in normal and young subjects (figure 24.7).[9] The pupil was dilated with cyclopentolate, and VECP contrast thresholds were measured at pupil sizes of 2, 3, 4, 5, and 6 mm with the use of an artificial pupil. The VECP latency contrast threshold (T) was defined as the contrast necessary for obtaining a criterion latency of P100 from the upper limit of age-matched normal subjects with 4-mm artificial pupil size. The pupillary area was represented by A, and a relation of $\log T = -k \log A + C$ was found, where C is a constant. The contrast threshold obtained was higher in the elderly group than in the young group, but the differences were small with small pupil size. There were fewer differences in contrast threshold between the young and elderly groups with small pupils.

It was thus again proved that the increase in contrast thresholds in the elderly was not influenced by miosis.

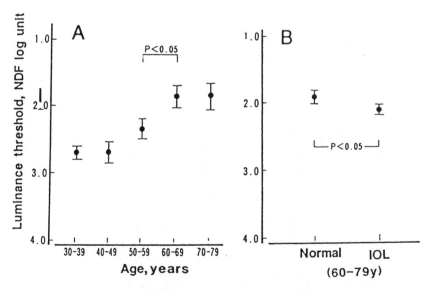

FIGURE 24.6 A, Aging effects on VECP luminance thresholds. Luminance thresholds increase with age. B, VECP luminance threshold in normal phakic subjects and pseudophakic eyes. (From Adachi-Usami E: *Jpn J Ophthalmol* 1990; 34:81–94. Used by permission.)

Accommodation

The amplitude of accommodation decreases with age from about 20 D at 5 years to 0.5 D at 60 years.

Millodott et al.[13] applied steady-state pattern VECPs for objective measurements of accommodation and demonstrated its attenuation with advancing age. We[23] employed

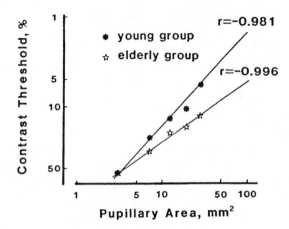

FIGURE 24.7 Contrast threshold vs. pupillary area in a young group (aged 20 to 30 years) and an elderly group (55 to 70 years). (From Fujimoto N, Adachi-Usami E, Ito Y: *Acta Soc Ophthalmol Jpn* 1988; 92:1185–1189. Used by permission.)

transient VECPs instead (figure 24.8) and recorded them by increasing minus-power lenses in 1-D steps in front of the eye up to the range where no response was recordable. It was found that the amplitude of the P100 component was attenuated linearly with increased accommodation stimulus. The regression line was calculated from the pattern VECP amplitude vs. accommodation stimulus (in diopters) plots, and the accommodation power was determined by extrapolating the line to the 0-μV amplitude. The gradient of the regression line increased with age. The accommodation obtained when measured with pattern VECPs was attenuated significantly in the groups over 40 years of age (figure 24.9), and there was also a remarkable delay in P100 peak latencies (see figure 24.8).

The accommodation determined subjectively was found to be smaller at approximately 3 D than that obtained by the pattern VECP measurements.

Conclusion

As mentioned above, there is no doubt that aging increases the latency of VECPs, and the effect is also clear in regard to amplitude. A more precise description is available in our latest work.[1a]

Accordingly, we should evaluate the delay in latency with care and precision when diagnosing diseases. It is recom-

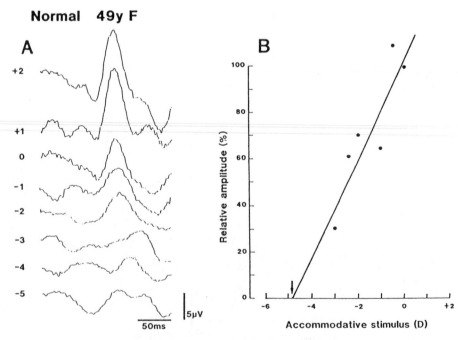

FIGURE 24.8 A, Pattern VECPs of a 49-year-old normal female. A minus-power lens was placed in front of the eye, and the power was increased in 1-D steps. B, The relative amplitude of P100 to the one for 0 D was plotted against lens power. The diopters of difference between −2 D and the lens power of the zero-amplitude point, defined by extrapolating the regression line (dotted line), were determined as the objective amplitude of accommodation. (From Yamamoto S, Adachi-Usami E, Kuroda N: *Doc Ophthalmol* 1989; 72:31–37. Used by permission.)

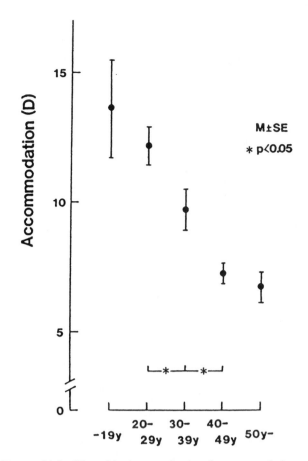

FIGURE 24.9 The objective amplitude of accommodation as measured by patterns VECPs were averaged for each decade. Accommodation power was reduced significantly over 30 ($P < .05$) and over 40 years of age ($P < .05$). (From Yamamoto S, Adachi-Usami E, Kuroda N: *Doc Ophthalmol* 1989; 72:31–37. Used by permission.)

mended that normative data for every age group be readily available in all clinical facilities.

REFERENCES

1a. Adachi-Usami E: Senescence of visual function as studied by visually evoked cortical potentials. *Jpn J Ophthalmol* 1990; 34:81–94.

1. Adachi-Usami E, Hosoda L, Toyonaga N: Effects of aging on the temporal frequency characteristics determined by pattern visually evoked cortical potentials. *Doc Ophthalmol* 1988; 69:139–144.

2. Adachi-Usami E, Lehmann D: Luminance effects on latency and topography of average pattern-evoked potentials. *Doc Ophthalmol Proc Ser* 1983; 37:353–360.

3. Apkarian A, Reits D, Spekreijse H: Component specificity in albino VEP asymmetry: Maturation of the visual pathway anomaly. *Exp Brain Res* 1984; 53:285–294.

4. Arundale K: An investigation into the variation of human contrast sensitivity with age and ocular pathology. *Br J Ophthalmol* 1978; 62:213–215.

5. Asselman P, Chadwick DW, Marsden CD: Visual evoked responses in the diagnosis and management of patients suspected of multiple sclerosis. *Brain* 1975; 98:261–282.

6. Celesia GG, Daly RF: Effects of aging on visual evoked responses. *Arch Neurol* 1977; 34:403–407.

7. Celesia GG, Kaufman D, Cone S: Effects of age and sex on pattern electroretinograms and visual evoked potentials. *Electroencephalogr Clin Neurophysiol* 1987; 68:161–171.

8. Derefeldt G, Lennenstrand G, Lundh B: Age variations in normal human contrast sensitivity. *Acta Ophthalmol* 1979; 57:679–690.

9. Fujimoto N, Adachi-Usami E, Ito Y: The effect of pupillary area on senescence on contrast threshold as determined by human PVECP latency. *Acta Soc Ophthalmol Jpn* 1988; 92:1185–1189.

10. Halliday AM, Barrett G, Carroll WM, Kriss A: Problems in defining the normal limits of the VEP. In Courjon J, Mauguire F, Revol M (eds): *Clinical Application of Evoked Potentials in Neurology*. New York, Raven Press, 1982, pp 1–9.

11. Halliday AM, McDonald WI, Mushin J: Delayed pattern-evoked responses in optic neuritis in relation to visual acuity. *Trans Ophthalmol Soc U K* 1973; 93:315–324.

12. Kline DW, Schieber F, Andrew CC: Age, the eye, and the visual channels: Contrast sensitivity and response speed. *J Gerontol* 1983; 38:211–216.

13. Millodott M, Newton I: VEP measurement of the amplitude of accommodation. *Br J Ophthalmol* 1981; 65:294–298.

14. Mitchell KW, Howe JW, Spencer SR: Visual evoked potentials in the older population: Age and gender effects. *Clin Phys Physiol Meas* 1981; 8:317–324.

15. Shaw NA, Cant BR: Age-dependent changes in the amplitude of the pattern visual evoked potential. *Electroencephalogr Clin Neurophysiol* 1981; 51:671–673.

16. Shaw NA, Cant BR: Age-dependent changes in the latency of the pattern visual evoked potential. *Electroencephalogr Clin Neurophysiol* 1980; 48:237–241.

17. Shearer DE, Dustman RE: The pattern reversal evoked potential: The need for laboratory norms. *Am J Electroencephalogr Technol* 1980; 20:185–200.

18. Sokol S, Jones K: Implicit time of pattern evoked potentials in infants: An index of maturation of spatial vision. *Vision Res* 1978; 19:745–755.

19. Sokol S, Moskowitz A, Towle VL: Age-related changes in the latency of the visual evoked potential: Influence of check size. *Electroencephalogr Clin Neurophysiol* 1981; 51:559–562.

20. Weale RA: Senile changes in visual acuity. *Trans Ophthalmol Soc U K* 1975; 95:36–38.

21. Wright CE, Drasdo N: The influence of age on the spatial and temporal sensitivity function. *Doc Ophthalmol* 1985; 59:385–395.

22. Wright CE, Williams DE, Drasdo N, Harding GFA: The influence of age on the electroretinogram and visual evoked potential. *Doc Ophthalmol* 1985; 59:365–384.

23. Yamamoto S, Adachi-Usami E, Kuroda N: Accommodation power determined with transient pattern VECPs in diabetes. *Doc Ophthalmol* 1989; 72:31–37.

24. Yamazaki H: Pattern visual evoked cortical potential waveforms and spatial frequency characteristics in children. *Doc Ophthalmol* 1988; 70:59–65.

25. Yamazaki H, Adachi-Usami E: Aging effects on spatial frequency characteristics measured by VECPs. *Acta Soc Ophthalmol Jpn* 1988; 92:1662–1665.

26. Yamazaki H, Adachi-Usami E: VECP luminance threshold in pseudophakic eyes. *Acta Soc Ophthalmol Jpn* 1988; 92:767–772.

25 Aberrant Albino and Achiasmat Visual Pathways: Noninvasive Electrophysiological Assessment

P. APKARIAN AND L. J. BOUR

Introduction

Classic and enduring percepts of albinism include pale-skinned, white-haired, dancing pink-eyed individuals. It is now well established, however, that the albino phenotype per se ranges from extreme hypopigmentation of the hair, skin, and ocular fundi, oculomotor instabilities (e.g., idiopathic congenital nystagmus), and interocular misalignments to the albino phenotype of dark skin pigmentation (including black skin or ready ability to tan), dark brown or black hair, ocular pigmentation, and absence of ocular motor instabilities and/or misalignments (figure 25.1). Basically, and despite the wide range of albino genetic features within and between phenotypes, inherited albino abnormalities of melanin metabolism and synthesis result in two major visual pathway anomalies: foveal hypoplasia (figure 25.2) and misrouted optic nerve fibers (figures 25.3 and 25.4).[44,45] While foveal hypoplasia is a consistent and obligate albino feature, as reflected by the absence of a foveal reflex, albinos may present, albeit rarely, with normal fundus pigmentation, normal iris pigmentation, and/or ocular stability. Diagnostic ambiguity arises under these conditions and is further exacerbated in the normal infant or young child whose visual systems, including foveal hypoplasia, reflect normal fundus immaturity. In general, full foveal development, under normal conditions, is not reached before 45 months of age.[50] Therefore, a poorly defined or absent foveal reflex may simply reflect normal visual system immaturity rather than foveal hypoplasia. Diagnostic ambiguity can be resolved by noninvasive electrophysiological assessment of the visual pathways. That is, pathognomonic to albinism per se is primary optic pathway misprojection with a preponderance of misrouted temporal retinal fiber projections that erroneously cross at the optic chiasm. Thus, in albinism, regardless of genotype or phenotype, a dominant portion of temporal retinal fibers erroneously decussate at the chiasm rather than maintaining appropriate ipsilateral projections and organization (figures 25.3 and 25.4). Of interest is that

albino mammals of all species have this remarkable anomalous optic pathway feature.[74,79]

Regarding ipsilateral projections, it is also of interest to note that most recently, an inborn, isolated achiasmatic syndrome (figures 25.2B, 25.3, 25.4) also was identified in humans via the albino visual evoked potential (VEP) misrouting test,[11,13,14] albeit in this instance, following monocular, full-field stimulation, the achiasmatic evoked potential responses reflect significant ipsilateral asymmetry rather than the classic albino contralateral asymmetry (e.g., figure 25.3). Such unusual ipsilateral VEP distributions following full-field stimulation reflect a unique achiasmatic condition; VEP ipsilateral misrouting results indicating an isolated achiasmatic condition were confirmed and defined via magnetic resonance imaging.[11–13] Within the same time period, the isolated achiasmatic condition with an autosomal-recessive genotype[73] also was reported in a breed of achiasmatic Belgian sheepdogs.[78]

Returning to the albino mammalian primary visual pathways per se, the anomalous albino optic pathway condition was initially described in rats.[62] Thereafter, the aberrant albino visual pathways were confirmed across several albino mammalian species, including mice, mink, monkeys, and humans.[43,67] Within this period, studies of melanin metabolism during embryogenesis also began to demonstrate the prominent role of melanin in normal retinal neurogenesis and axonal trajectory along the immature optic cup and stalk.[71,72] Preclusion of normal melanogenesis of neural ectoderm derivatives, as in albinism, was found to result in abnormal histogenesis of retinal pigment, abnormal retinal ganglion cell metabolism, and differentiation and the consequent inappropriate guidance, projection, and organization of retinal-fugal fibers. The deleterious effects of abnormal melanin metabolism that disturb the delicate embryological processes that are involved in retinal differentiation and patterning of chiasmal decussation are evident at birth and predetermine the final course of visual pathway maturation.[49,70] Recent magnetic resonance imaging (MRI)

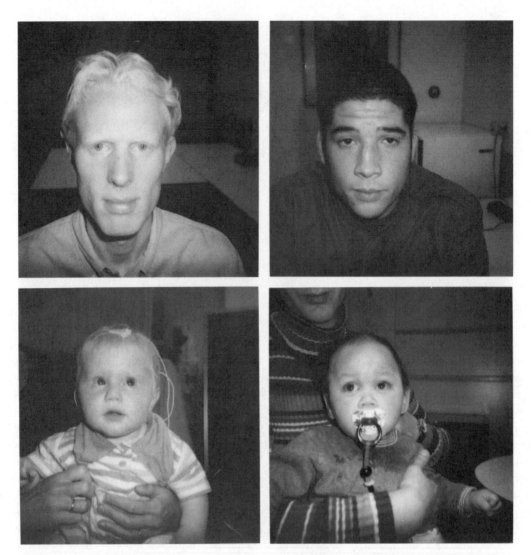

FIGURE 25.1 Variable genotype and phenotype in a representative sample of albinos including autosomal-recessive oculocutaneous, tyrosinase-negative albinism (left column), X-chromosomal ocular albinism, and autosomal-recessive oculocutaneous, tyrosinase-positive albinism (right column). Foveal hypoplasia, reduced visual acuity, and VEP optic pathway misrouting are common features regardless of inheritance mode or phenotypic expression. (See also color plate 17.)

assessment of the albino visual pathways also has demonstrated that the size and configuration of the optic chiasm, reflecting aberrant optic fiber decussation, differs significantly in albinos compared to normal age-matched controls. Compared to normal controls, the albinos showed significantly smaller chiasmal widths, smaller optic nerves and tracts, wider angles between nerves and tracts, and a distinctly different size and configuration of the optic chiasm.[68] In addition, ascending further along the primary visual pathway, anatomical studies have shown via the lateral geniculate nuclei (LGN) of albinos that near the vertical meridian, a central segment of temporal retinal fibers erroneously terminates within contralateral rather than ipsilateral projection sites. As a result of the misrouting, the medial portion of LGN layers A1, representing a portion of the ipsilateral visual field, is misaligned. The albino LGN receives

aberrant crossed input from temporal fibers, thus displacing portions of the normal ipsilateral temporal projections. Each albino hemiretina maps to the appropriate LGN layer: however, the abnormal segment represents the mirror symmetric portion of the visual field, disrupting normal alignment from layer to layer (see figure 25.4).

Adaptation to these and various other LGN layer incongruencies demonstrates remarkable plasticity of the albino visual system. For example, given the albino mismapping of retinal projections, albino visual field loss also is expected. However, if visual field testing in a given albino is performed accurately (i.e., account is taken of accompanying albino ocular motor instabilities, misalignments, and reduced acuities), the albino visual fields prove perfectly normal.

While optic pathway misrouting including an abnormal preponderance of contralateral retinal fiber projections

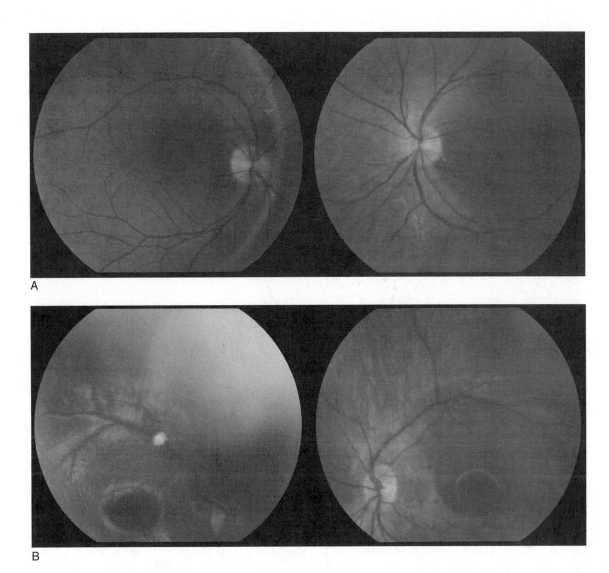

A

B

FIGURE 25.2   Fundi of left and right eye (A) of an 18-year-old albino and (B) of a 16-year-old achiasmat. For comparison, note the presence of foveal hypoplasia only in the albino fundi; foveal hypoplasia, pathog- nomonic to albinism, is absent in the achiasmat. (See also color plate 18.)

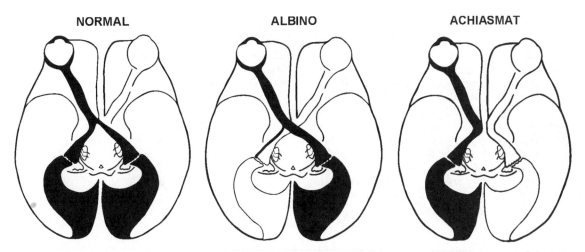

FIGURE 25.3   Simplified schematic of the primary visual pathways emphasizing normal organization of retinal-fugal projections within the chiasmatic region compared to abnormal projections characteristic of albinos and achiasmats.

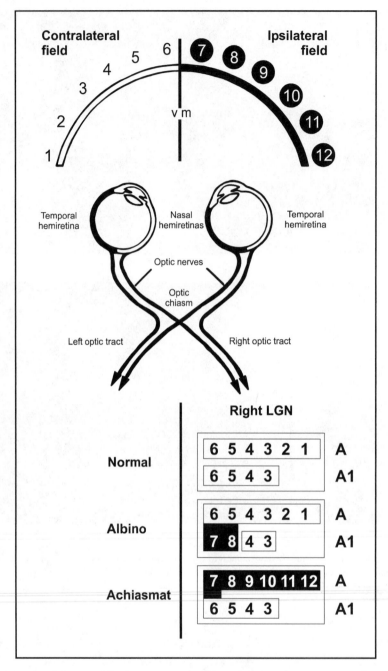

FIGURE 25.4 Simplified schematic of the visual field representation onto two adjacent right dorsal LGN layers. Normally, LGN layers receive, in strict alignment of visual space coordinates, nasal retinal projections from the contralateral eye (LGN layer A) and temporal retinal projections from the ipsilateral eye (LGN layer A1). Note also that the representation in laminae A and A1 are in register. For the albino, a central segment of temporal retinal fibers erroneously decussate. As a result, the medial portion of layer A1 representing a part of the ipsilateral visual field is misaligned with the corresponding projections of layer A and is also represented in mirror reversal. The order of the abnormal projections is reversed as indicated by the descending numbers (dark sections reflect abnormal ipsilateral field representation). In comparison, for the isolated achiasmat, all nasal fibers fail to decussate, and the entire ipsilateral hemifield is represented in LGN layer A; temporal retinal projections from the same eye project, as under normal conditions, to ipsilateral LGN layer A1. However, with both nasal and temporal retinal projections from a single retina projecting ipsilaterally, the entire visual field now is represented in layers A and A1 in complete mirror reversal; congruency is present only at the vertical midline (VM). (Source: Adapted from Williams et al., 1994, figure 4, page 639.)

defines the albino condition via molecular, biological, and genetic assessment, two primary genetic forms of albinism have been defined: autosomal-recessive albinism and X-linked albinism. Autosomal-recessive albinism, is further subdivided into tyrosinase-positive albinism with melanin pigment present in hair, skin, and ocular structures; tyrosinase-negative albinism with melanin pigment sparse or absent; and brown oculocutaneous albinism. Brown oculocutaneous albinism is phenotypically distinct from tyrosinase-related oculocutaneous albinism (OCA1) and genetically distinct from protein P-gene-related oculocutaneous albinism (OCA2). The occurrence of OCA1 and OCA2 in the general Western population is approximately one in 40,000 individuals. The majority of affected individuals are compound heterozygotes with distinct maternal and paternal mutations. Of clinical relevance, however, is that regardless of albino genotype or phenotype, albinism, as was stated above, fosters two primary pathognomonic albino features: foveal hypoplasia with corresponding visual acuity reduction and misrouted temporal retinal projections with corresponding high incidence of ocular motor misalignments and instabilities. In addition to reduced visual acuity due to albino fovea hypoplasia and misrouted primary optic pathway projections, auxiliary albino ophthalmic features include photophobia, iris transillumination, and refractive errors.

For clinical albino diagnosis, regardless of genotype or phenotype and across the age range from neonate to the elderly, the obligate albino optic pathway misrouting of retinal fugal fibers can be readily recorded from the surface of the scalp via appropriate VEP testing (figure 25.5). Protocol details of the VEP misrouting test protocol are described in more detail below in the section on optic pathway misrouting detection. In general, however, the albino VEP response demonstrates contralateral hemispheric response lateralization following full-field monocular stimulation. That is, with right eye viewing, albino VEP topography across the electrode array shows a relatively early latency window of left hemispheric response dominance; with left eye viewing, an early latency window of right hemispheric response dominance is effected. Thus, via appropriate and age-dependent stimulus profiles, monocular albino VEPs measured across the electrode array demonstrate contralateral interocular asymmetry. This pattern of lateralization is specific to albinism and should not be confused with VEP asymmetries resulting from optic pathway lesions, malformations, or tumors. Nor should this form of interhemispheric and/or interocular asymmetry be confused with normally occurring hemispheric response dominance, which, in normal controls, can reflect remarkable intersubject variability. That is, VEP topography across the occiput, in any given test group and regardless of age, can alter from midline dominance, midline attenuation, left hemispheric response dominance, or right hemispheric response dominance. However, of direct relevance to VEP albino misrouting detection is that in nonalbinos, the recorded interhemispheric asymmetry remains constant with either left or right eye viewing. In addition to the relevance of interhemispheric response profiles, it is of considerable significance to note that the VEP misrouting test protocol is age dependent. The age variable has proven critical in optimizing the VEP misrouting test across the age span.

With positive results from VEP detection of albino pathognomonic contralateral VEP response dominance, initial queries during establishment of the albino VEP misrouting test protocol concerned the optimum surface electrode loci as well as the minimum number of electrode derivations. To address these issues, principal component analysis was applied to the monocular VEP profiles of several normal controls as well as albino patients; VEP recordings were performed with 24 electrode derivations (figure 25.6). Basically, the multielectrode dipole studies revealed that a primary, five-channel, albino optic pathway misrouting response with pattern onset stimuli reflected both striate and extrastriate VEP components. With aberrant retinogeniculate projections and abnormal visual field representation identified within cortical areas 17 and 18,[61] it is of interest to note that in clinical practice, the albino VEP "signature" is found consistently for the VEP component from cortical area 18. The latter is due to the fact that cortical area 18 is more accessible than cortical area 17 to scalp electrodes;[60] area 17's contribution to the albino VEPs is generally reduced. As a result, responses generated from cortical area 18 constitute (at least in adults) the most likely indicator for albino VEP asymmetry. Of practical relevance in the multielectrode tests was that the results accurately defined the optimum electrode montage, including number

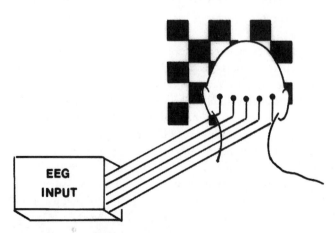

FIGURE 25.5 Schematic of an optimum electrode montage for VEP assessment in albinos. Ag/AgCl electrodes are positioned with an equal spacing of 3 cm in a horizontal row 1 cm above the inion. Reference is either linked ears or Fz.

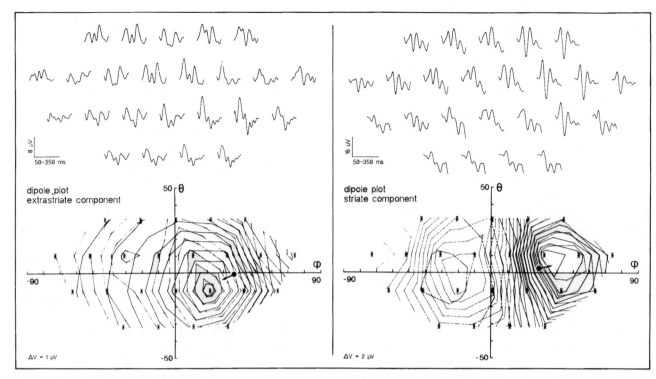

FIGURE 25.6   Principal component analysis (PCA) applied to the VEP response with monocular (OS) stimulation. Left and right panels show the VEP pattern-onset response of an oculocutaneous and an ocular albino, respectively. PCA with a time interval of 71–179 ms was used to identify cortical sites of albino asymmetry with a 24-electrode derivation. Contralateral VEP asymmetry within this early time window clearly is demonstrated by the equipotential lines (faded contours) and the fitted equivalent dipole potential distributions (darker contours). Location and orientation of the equivalent dipoles are indicated by the dots with arrow. In albinism, the strongest contralateral asymmetry generally is obtained from the extrastriate component (as shown in the left panel). The albino VEP response at the right panel also demonstrates contralateral asymmetry for the striate component. Horizontal and vertical axes are at 0° azimuth and elevation angles. Electrodes, in both horizontal and vertical planes are spaced 3 cm apart. The lowest row of electrodes is positioned 1 cm below the inion; the second row of electrodes is positioned 2 cm above the inion. (See also chapter 15.)

and loci of recording channels, for application of the albino VEP misrouting test across the age range.

While the precise electrical sources and loci of the recorded VEPs remain under investigation, it is understood that, in general, the VEPs are derived from extracellular field potentials of the apical dendrites of pyramidal cells. The dendridic trees that generate the evoked potentials that are recorded at the scalp surface are parallel to each other and are also oriented perpendicularly to the cortical surface. Therefore, electrical activity in the neurons causes current to flow in the extracellular medium over considerable distances. VEPs that are recorded at the scalp therefore reflect the summed ion current that is generated from a plethora of synchronously activated neuronal assemblies, including retinogeniculocortical, intracranial, and corticocortical processing. Although VEP measures are generated within different brain regions, it is also of interest to note that VEPs reflect not only retinogeniculate cortical processing (figure 25.6), but also intracranial and corticocortical processing. As such, if the anatomic structures and underlying extracellular electrical field potentials are defined, VEP evaluation serves as a non-invasive probe for characterizing and localizing maturational and/or anomalous developmental processes throughout the primary visual pathways. As a caveat, however, it is of clinical relevance to acknowledge that the albino VEP misrouting test protocol per se is both age dependent and stimulus specific.

Via indexes of interhemispheric asymmetry derived from interocular comparisons of VEP profiles across the electrode array, the presence or absence of albino misrouting can be reliably determined. Note, however, that until proven otherwise, the degree of asymmetry does not reflect or demonstrate any relationship with the percentage of erroneously crossed chiasmal fibers and/or various phenotypic characteristics such as cutaneous pigmentation.

While the present study promotes albino assessment via VEP testing, most recently, the abnormal visual pathway projections associated with albinism also have been investigated via nonfunctional[68] as well as functional magnetic resonance imaging.[49,64] The latter has revealed that the albino visual cortex is activated by both the contralateral visual field and by abnormal input representing the ipsilateral visual field.

Methodology for primary optic pathway misrouting detection

ELECTROPHYSIOLOGICAL METHODS Monocular and binocular transient and steady-state luminance and checkerboard pattern VEPs are recorded from five tinned, copper-cup electrodes positioned (with collodion) in a horizontal row across the occiput, 1 cm above the inion (figure 25.5). One electrode is placed on the midline; left and right occipital electrode sites are equally spaced about 3 cm apart. In infants and children, the reference electrode preferentially is placed at the midline, frontal cortex about 1 cm above the hairline; common ground is located near the vertex (see, e.g., Apkarian,[7,8] Apkarian et al.[20]). For more mature patients, the reference electrodes are linked earlobes. Bandwidth of the EEG preamplifiers is set either at 0.5–70 Hz or, for higher stimulus frequencies, at 0.5–120 Hz (12 dB/oct). The sample frequency is greater than 250 Hz. For all averaged VEP data depicted, response positivity is plotted upward. The choice of using the number of five active electrodes and of using the above-mentioned electrode locations for misrouting detection with pattern onset/offset was derived from principal component analysis of the VEP potential distributions across the occipital lobe as depicted in figure 25.6. The figure illustrates that albino optic pathway misrouting is reflected primarily within VEP components demonstrated to originate from both cortical areas 17 and 18. In clinical practice, the albino "signature" is found consistently for the components from cortical area 18. This particular response selectivity is due to the fact that cortical area 18 activity is more accessible to occipital scalp electrodes[60] and because of the generally reduced contribution of area 17 to albino VEPs. To ensure inclusion of cortical areas of maximum positivity and negativity in the VEP potential distribution of particularly the extrastriate components and to optimally detect contralateral VEP asymmetry in albinism with luminance flash and pattern-onset/offset stimulus protocols, five electrodes are necessary and also sufficient. However, for testing albino neonates, the active electrode number, if necessary, can be reduced to three. The optimum position of the electrode array across the occiput can be derived from the dipole plot of figure 25.6, which shows that the extrastriate components optimally are detected about 1 cm above the inion.

STIMULUS For transient evoked potentials, the stimuli include checkerboard pattern-onset/offset (40 ms/460 ms and 300 ms/500 ms) and/or luminance flash (1 Hz, 0.6 and 2J). Viewing distance for luminance flash is set at 30 cm. Checkerboard patterns are generated on a high-resolution CRT monitor with 90% contrast or more and a mean luminance of approximately 90 cd/m². Full-field and partial-field (left half-field or right half-field) pattern stimulation sub-tending 15° at a distance of 114 cm is typically employed. The viewing distance for pattern stimuli is set at 114 cm and extended to 228 cm or reduced to 57 cm depending on the patient's pattern VEP responses.

VEP DATA ANALYSIS The distribution of recorded signals across the occiput is evaluated by visual inspection of VEP response lateralization.[7–9,20,24] A difference potential, in which a right occiput response is subtracted from that of a left, facilitates misrouting detection. Misrouting asymmetry is revealed in the form of polarity reversals of the difference potential from left to right eye stimulation. A schematic display of how VEP responses lateralize and the corresponding difference potential is depicted in figure 25.7.

INTERHEMISPHERIC ASYMMETRY INDEX A quantitative estimate of hemispheric lateralization for each eye and stimulus condition is derived from interhemispheric surface area calculations across the five-electrode array (figure 25.7). That is, the amplitude versus electrode function was subdivided into left and right occiput derivations. The area under the respective half-curves (L_s and R_s) was then calculated with baselines (zero-offset) determined by the lowest VEP amplitude measured across the five electrodes (figure 25.8).

A lateralization ratio for both left (OD) and right (OS) stimulation is obtained by dividing the lower area for each homologous pair by the higher area.[76] If the left-half area amplitude is greater than the right half ($L_s > R_s$), lateralization is defined as the right-half pair divided by the left (R_s/L_s), irrespective of which eye has been stimulated. For all remaining conditions, lateralization is defined as 2 minus the left-half pair divided by the right-half ($2 - (L_s/R_s)$). For instance, when there is contralateral asymmetry (as in albinism) with OD stimulation, L_s (OD) > R_s (OD); thus, the lateralization for OD stimulation is Lat (OD) = R_s(OD)/L_s(OD). With OS stimulation, L_s(OS) < R_s(OS); thus, the lateralization is Lat (OS) = $(2 - L_s(OS)/R_s(OS))$. If the lateralization equals 0, this indicates left-hemispheric lateralization; a value of 1 indicates interhemispheric symmetry; and a value of 2 indicates right-hemispheric lateralization. Finally, it is important to compare the lateralization for OD stimulation, Lat (OD), with the lateralization for OS stimulation, Lat (OS). Thus, an interocular asymmetry index I_{asym} is defined that equals lateralization OS minus lateralization OD. Consequently, if both OD and OS stimulation VEP responses laiteralize to the left or right, the asymmetry index varies around 0. If the peak of the potential distribution lateralizes across the left occiput following right eye stimulation and the response lateralizes to the contralateral or right occiput following left eye stimulation, the asymmetry index will be positive, and when it approaches 2, it reflects maximum contralateral asymmetry. An asymmetry index of −2 reflects maximum ipsilateral asymmetry; that is, the right eye response peaks across the

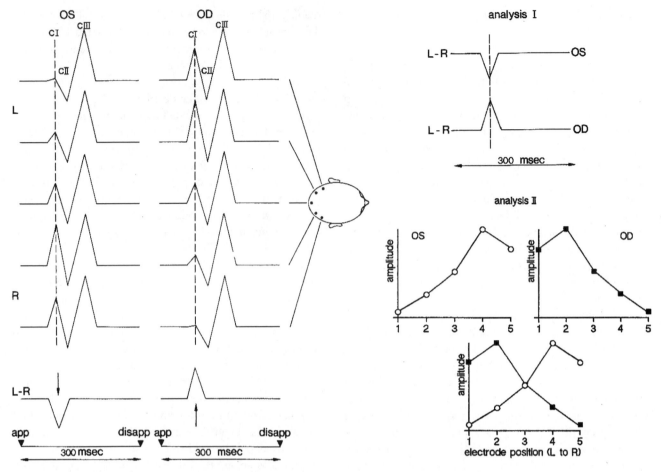

FIGURE 25.7 Schematic of analysis procedures for determining left (OS) and right (OD) eye VEP response asymmetry with pattern-onset stimulation (300/500 ms). The dashed line is drawn 90 ms after pattern onset. Visual inspection within an early latency window reveals contralateral hemispheric asymmetry, that is, left eye VEPs following full-field stimulation lateralize to the right hemisphere; right eye VEPs lateralize to the left hemisphere. Hemispheric laterality can also be observed from a bipolar derivation in which trace 2, immediate left of midline, is subtracted from trace 4, immediate right of the midline. Polarity reversal is indicated by arrows and by a dashed line. VEP amplitude distribution as a function of electrode position from left (electrode positions 1 and 2) to right (electrode positions 4 and 5) occiput at a latency of 90 ms for OS and OD stimulation and their combined distribution is depicted below the label "analysis II").

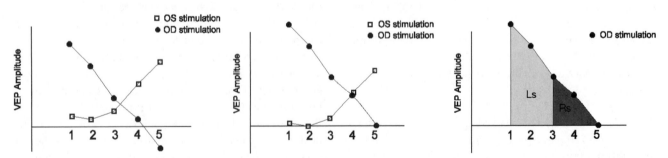

FIGURE 25.8 The leftmost schematic shows the VEP amplitude distributions for right eye (solid dots) and left eye stimulation (open squares) at the optimum latency for VEP asymmetry detection. The schematic at the middle displays the same data points except that the baseline for both distributions is shifted such that the minimal VEP amplitude is set to zero. The schematic at the right shows how the surface beneath the VEP amplitude distribution with OD stimulation is subdivided into left of the midline, labeled L_s(OD), and right of the midline, labeled R_s(OD). A similar surface subdivision for OS stimulation yields L_s(OS) and R_s(OS).

right occiput, and the left eye response peaks across the left occiput. Significant negative interocular asymmetry indices have been found in the achiasmatic condition with ipsilateral projections of the optic fibers.

Normative laboratory standards for normal and albino subjects tested under the same conditions indicate significant (Kolmogorov-Smirnov, $P > .001$) contralateral or ipsilateral asymmetry for an index value of $+0.7$ or -0.7, respectively (see e.g., Apkarian,[7,8] Apkarian and Shallo-Hoffmann[21]). With age-appropriate application,[7,8,24] the VEP misrouting test has proven highly sensitive and specific.[26,36,46,58,66,81]

Ocular motor disorders and concomitant VEP assessment in albinism

OCULAR MOTOR ASSESSMENT   Albino ocular motor profiles in two dimensions were assessed in mature as well as pediatric patients by using the double magnetic induction (DMI) method[14,30,31] and the scleral search coil method.[35,40,65] The scleral search coil methodology provides the option of either two-dimensional[12] or three-dimensional ocular motor recording;[10,15,17,28] the DMI methodology provides two-dimensional recording. However, for pediatric application, despite custom-designed scleral search coils, the DMI method proved more patient-friendly and thus more practical.[14,29,57]

With the DMI method, gold metallic scleral rings are placed on each eye following application of topical anesthesia. For implementation in pediatric patients, the recording rings were custom-designed for the immature eye, including immature corneal size, scleral curvature, and palpebral fissure length.[16] The three DMI ring parameters of particular importance were the inner and outer diameters and the coil top angle. DMI recording resolution is 5–10 minutes per arc with a sample frequency greater than 250 Hz.

Following application of either the scleral search coils or DMI rings, the patient is positioned within a coil system in a homogeneous alternating primary magnetic field (30 kHz horizontal, 40 kHz vertical) with constant amplitude. For pediatric testing, the patient is seated upright in the tester's lap. The actual coil/ring pickup system is centered and aligned at a distance of about 1 cm from the patient's nasion. Accurate and stable alignment of the patient within the eye movement recording system is facilitated by on-line video feedback together with markers.

Via the DMI method, two-dimensional recording was implemented. Horizontal as well as vertical eye positions were derived from a secondary magnetic field picked up by a detection coil placed in front of the eye. The custom-designed golden rings attached to the infant's left and right eyes generate this secondary field, the strength of which is related to the rotation of the rings. To calibrate the positions of both the left and right eyes, at the beginning of each experimental session, the infants were reinforced to track laser spots that jumped either horizontally or vertically -10 to $+10$ degrees from straight ahead, that is, the zero degree position.[57]

Measurement of ocular rotation in three dimensions (3D) was implemented via the dual scleral induction coil technique.[28,40] To account for the various offsets, corrective alterations were added to the calibration procedures.[52] Calibration consisted of an in vitro and an in vivo protocol. Via a rotation matrix,[65] sine and cosine components of direction and torsion coils were converted to 3D Fick coordinates. After Haustein,[48] Fick coordinates were converted to rotation vectors. Zero-fixations were also parsed into foveation periods.[1,6,27,33,38,80] Criteria for foveation periods included target fixation accuracy to within ±30 minutes in both vertical and horizontal planes and eye velocity of less than 7.5 deg/s in both vertical and horizontal planes. Mean velocities and standard deviations (derived from all trials) were calculated for foveation periods across the duration of the fixating epoch.

In contrast to two-dimensional eye movement recording with the DMI method, recording with either two- or three-dimensional search-coil methodology proved nonviable in infants and young children. Application of soft silicone search coils onto the ocular sclera requires cooperative subjects/patients and was not feasible for the younger patients because the scleral search coils per se irritated the patients, rendering them uncooperative. In addition, the delicate wiring of the search coils was readily impaired either during attempted application or soon thereafter. However, while three-dimensional scleral search coil ocular motor recording in pediatric patients proved inappropriate, two-dimensional DMI recording proved highly feasible.

MISALIGNMENTS AND OCULAR MOTOR INSTABILITY   Although about 30% of albinos present with anisotropia including hypodeviation,[41,59] the VEP misrouting test is dependent on interocular comparisons rather than impaired interocular alignment and/or binocular function. Because monocular VEP testing is required for the detection of possible contralateral hemispheric asymmetry, interocular misalignments as such also do not create conflicting interocular images. With binocular VEP testing, interocular misalignments also do not affect the albino VEP misrouting test results, as the latter test is based on interocular/monocular comparisons rather than on binocularity. However, of significant relevance for VEP evaluation is that almost all albinos present with ocular motor instabilities[2,34,39,47,51,53,63] in the form of classic congenital nystagmus (CN). Previous studies have shown that for patients with congenital nystagmus, visual acuity is optimal during so-called foveation periods.[1,6,27,33,38,42] Concerning ocular motor activitiy, note that the term *foveation period* refers to temporary (i.e., with a duration of approximately 50–300 ms) low or zero (i.e., less than 5–10 degrees/s) retinal velocity. During visual pathway maturation, patients with CN learn to make so-called snapshots of the visual world during the foveation periods; gaze strategies are also implemented to increase both the duration and the amount of foveation periods.[4,75] The latter is achieved, for example, by interocular convergence and/or by tilting the head such that eye position with respect to head tilt corresponds with a so-called null point or null zone.[3,5] Within the null point or null zone, the amplitude and frequency of the nystagmus are at minimum intensity. Image stabilization during these foveation periods has a particularly favorable effect on spatial vision, such as visual acuity. As an aside, it is of interest to note that while albino congenital nystagmus profiles readily present with so-called foveation periods, albinism visual acuity per se is limited by the degree of foveal hypoplasia, the latter being pathognomonic to the albino condition. Nonetheless, the term *foveation periods* with respect to ocular motor profiles in albinism is implemented with the understanding that in albinos, this conditions refers to cyclic but brief millisecond periods when the ocular orbit is still.

Figure 25.9 portrays a three-dimensional ocular motor profile recorded from a mature albino. The profile and position of the right and left eyes in the horizontal planes are

depicted in the upper traces, middle traces depict vertical plane ocular motor profiles, and lower traces depict torsional plane ocular motor profiles. Classic CN waveforms in the horizontal planes together with well-defined foveation periods are presented. In this particular albino, the congenital nystagmus profile demonstrates a unidirectional jerk right with extended foveation. Note also the "micro seesaw" nystagmus in the vertical and torsional planes; that is, with upward movement, the right eye rotates counterclockwise, while with simultaneous downward movement, the left eye rotates clockwise. With downward movement of the right eye, the opposite occurs with primarily the right eye rotating clockwise.[18] However, most common in albinism is that ocular motor instabilities are predominantly present in the horizontal planes in the form of classic congential nystagmus. Concomitant instabilities in vertical and torsional planes, if at all present, are generally of significantly smaller amplitude.

Another important feature of CN is that the amplitude and frequency of the ocular motor instabilities may depend on viewing conditions, including direction of gaze, monocular versus binocular viewing, convergence, room lighting, stimulus level of brightness, visual attention, and/or stress.[2,4,56] Figure 25.10, for example, clearly depicts significant differences between the ocular motor profile recorded during OU viewing compared to OD viewing. During monocular viewing, the intensity of the congenital nystagmus, as depicted, tends to increase. Also during monocular viewing, vertical instabilities, particularly of the eye under cover, generally are of larger amplitude than ocular motor instabilities of the viewing eye. In figure 25.11, the effect of increased visual attention on the CN profile also is demonstrated. Increased visual attention presents with the occurrence of significantly more frequent foveating saccades and foveation periods, resulting in improved spatial vision.

CHECKERBOARD STIMULUS AND FOVEATION PERIODS The results of VEP testing in albinism particularly with pattern stimuli (e.g., checkerboard patterns of varying check size) are influenced by the amplitude and frequency of the congenital nystagmus and consequently by the number and duration of so-called ocular motor foveation periods. As such, image stability during visual stimulation with checkerboard configurations is essential, particularly in the majority of albinos with CN. Concerning temporal parameters of the stimulus profile, it is important to note that transient pattern reversal and/or steady-state sweep techniques are particularly unfavorable with respect to fixation stability.[23] Even in normal subjects with stable fixation, both pattern reversal and pattern sweep stimuli invoke motion perception artifacts, which, in turn, induce ocular tracking movements. For example, figure 25.12A depicts, in a normal control subject, traces of a three-channel EEG recording concomitant with

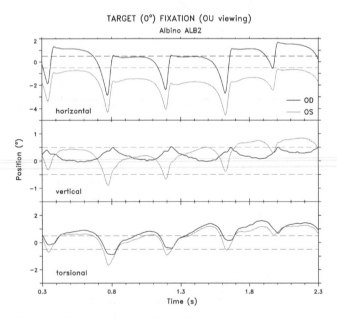

TARGET (0°) FIXATION (OU viewing)
Albino ALB2

FIGURE 25.9 A 2-s-duration binocular eye movement recording of a mature albino. Ocular motor instabilities follow the waveform profile of idiopathic congenital nystagmus (CN) in the horizontal planes (upper traces) and a "micro seesaw" nystagmus (SSN) in the vertical (middle traces) and torsional planes (bottom traces). Positive deflections represent rightward, upward, and clockwise rotation, respectively. Upward movement of OD is associated with intorsion; simultaneous downward movement of OS is associated with extorsion. Fast phases of nystagmus in the horizontal planes are phase-locked to the seesaw nystagmus.

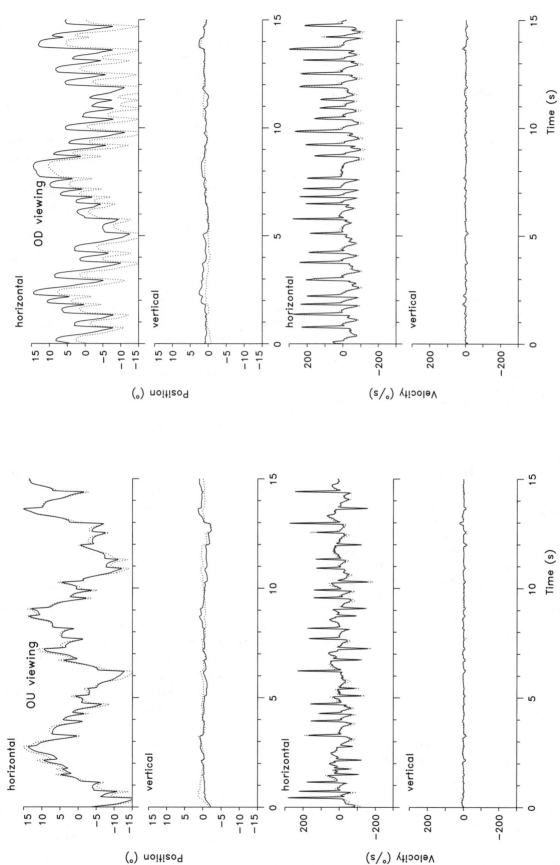

FIGURE 25.10 Smooth tracking of an albino to a triangular waveform stimulus is depicted. With binocular (OU) viewing (left column), CN with a profile of bidirectional jerk is recorded, whereas with monocular (OD) viewing (right column), the CN presents with a profile of unidirectional jerk right. Amplitude of the fast phases of nystagmus is greater during OD viewing; the latter is readily observed from the ocular velocity traces (lower traces).

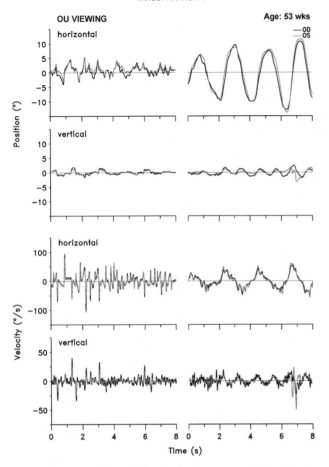

EFFECT OF VISUAL ATTENTION
TARGET FIXATION: 0°

FIGURE 25.11 Effects of visual attention on the CN profile of a 53-week-old albino are depicted. Traces at the left column depict recorded eye movements when the infant is attentive; traces at the right column depict eye movements during an absence of visual attention. During epochs of visual attention, frequently occurring foveating saccades in the horizontal planes are observed. The latter ensure that the fixation target is positioned onto the central retinal region. During epochs of visual inattention, large-amplitude, pendular eye movements are recorded; with the latter, there is no attempt to bring the eye position onto target. Note also that vertical eye position is significantly more stable when the albino infant is attending to the target.

simultaneous horizontal and vertical eye movement recordings. The stimulus profile (middle) indicates brief periods of pattern onset (check size of 55′) stability. Except for a few insignificant fixation saccades, eye position also is stable within ±15 degrees. In contrast, figure 25.12B demonstrates that in the same normal healthy control, pattern reversal stimulus (reversal rate = 5 Hz, check size = 55′) induces tracking in the form of optokinetic nystagmus with fast phases to the left and with an amplitude of about 1 degree. The slow phase of nystagmus in horizontal directions varies between 1 and 2 degrees per second.

In general, with the vast majority of albinos who present with ocular motor instabilities, it is of significance to note that the nystagmus per se actually creates additional motion artifacts within the VEP response profiles. Therefore, implementation of pattern reversal stimulus protocols in patients with ocular motor instabilities and/or reduced acuity renders the VEP response profiles invalid. Pattern reversal also should not be implemented in the assessment of spatial vision (e.g., VEP acuity estimates), nor should pattern reversal be implemented in the assessment of VEP albino asymmetry test. In addition, half-field stimulation is not recommended. The use of half-fields requires stable fixation within 1 degree, which for the majority of albinos with CN is possible only during a short period of time, that is, during their foveation periods. Particularly in albino infants and children with varying visual attention, half-field stimulation definitely is not recommended.[23]

The use of pattern-onset stimulus considerably reduces the problem of image instability due to CN. Contrary to the pattern-reversal stimulus, during which a checkerboard always is visible, the sudden onset of a checkerboard pattern on a gray background does not induce motion artifacts in patients with ocular motor instabilities and/or in patients with poor fixation. Thus, an optimum pattern stimulus presentation profile includes pattern onset of 40-ms duration and pattern offset of 460-ms duration, particularly when the duration of the pattern-onset stimulus is brief (40/460 ms). Furthermore, with the use of monocular full-field pattern-onset stimulation, the presence of CN and the concomitant difficulties with image stability will have minimal contaminating effects on the VEP acuity and VEP asymmetry test results.

To demonstrate contamination of ocular movement artifacts on VEP recordings, averages of VEPs recorded during foveation periods were compared to averages of VEPs recorded during nonfoveation periods.[12,29] Figure 25.13 shows simultaneous EEG and eye movement recording during pattern onset stimulation in an albino adult. Vertical dashed bars indicate time periods when pattern onset stimulation coincides with foveation periods. About 100 ms after the majority of these periods, a VEP response with a clear positive peak is observed in the raw EEG recording obtained from three occipital electrodes.

Figure 25.14 shows schematically how two sets of VEP averages are obtained from simultaneous EEG and eye movement recordings shown in figure 25.13. One set of VEP averages is calculated from responses following a low eye velocity period during visual stimulation, and the other set of VEP averages is obtained from responses following a period with higher retinal velocity during pattern-onset stimulation. The averages of these two sets of VEP responses are displayed in Figure 25.15. The finer lines are VEPs from an adult albino when mean retinal image velocity during time

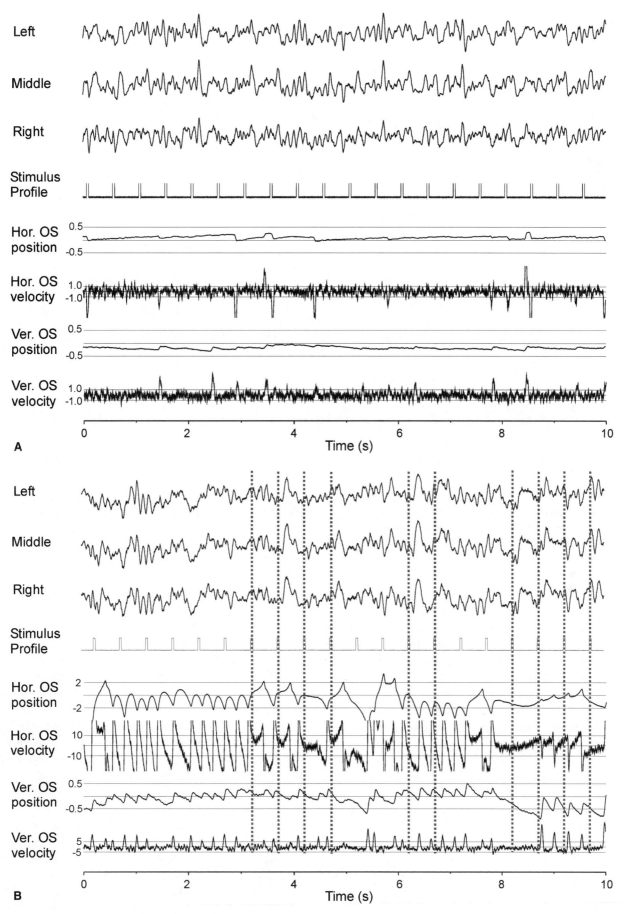

FIGURE 25.12 Simultaneous EEG and eye movement recordings (10 seconds) in a normal control during (A) pattern onset/offset stimulation and (B) pattern-reversal (steady-state) stimulation. The upper three traces show the raw EEG as recorded from three occipital loci. The fourth trace illustrates the stimulus profile. OS horizontal eye position, horizontal eye velocity, vertical eye position, and vertical eye velocity also are depicted (lower four traces). Note that with pattern-reversal stimuli, there is significant rightward artifact drift in the horizontal plane.

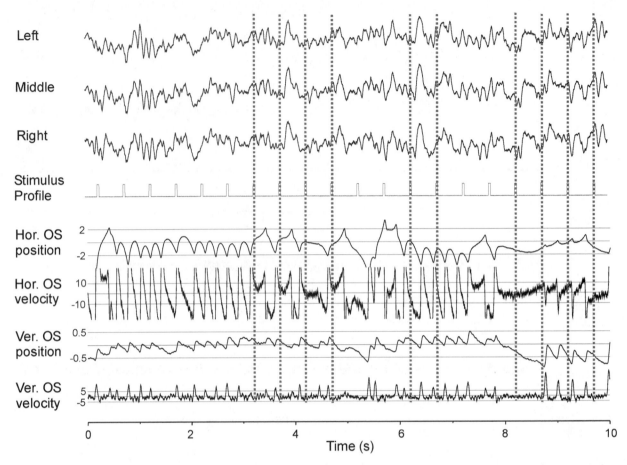

FIGURE 25.13 Comparable to Figures 25.12A and 25.12B but now measured in an albino adult during pattern-onset/offset stimulation (check size = 110′). Note that the CN profile intermittently reflects ocular motor profiles of unidirectional jerk right and also bidirectional jerks with slow eye movement foveation. The dashed vertical lines indicate when a pattern-onset stimulus of 40 ms coincides with reduced eye velocity (i.e., less than 10 degrees/s).

of stimulation was, on average, 36 degrees/second. The heavier lines are VEPs from VEP averages recorded from pattern-onset responses within foveation periods when mean retinal image velocity was, on average, less than 4 degrees/second. The VEP averages locked to foveation periods are significantly more robust; these foveation-linked VEP averages during OD and OS stimulation also more clearly demonstrate the albino asymmetry.

In conclusion, with oculomotor instabilities in albinism, retinal motion of VEP stimuli may significantly reduce the VEP response to retinal contrast per se. Moreover, VEP responses will reflect both an image contrast component and an image motion component. Therefore, to assess VEP acuity (equivalent to Snellen acuity) and also VEP asymmetry in albinism, the use of pattern-onset (40/460 ms) stimuli is strongly recommended. In addition, the VEP responses can be improved by creating stimulus conditions for albino patients, including visual attention, zero-position, and reduced stress, that increase the number of foveation periods and prolong their duration.

VEP topography in normal controls and albinism

The electrophysiological correlate of albino optic pathway misrouting is apparent from visual inspection of the raw traces with a difference in hemispheric response amplitude from OD to OS viewing. Because the VEP misrouting signature is age dependent, the latency window of asymmetry becomes more restricted as VEP responses, in general, become more mature. Regardless of age, however, the VEP latency window of asymmetry occurs primarily within initial, earlier latency VEP components. Thus, one need only attend to an early time window of the response (figure 25.16); the latency window of asymmetry is earlier in more mature patients. In albinos older than 3–5 years of age, contralateral asymmetry via the pattern-onset response typically is most pronounced at a latency from about 80 to 110 ms. In the mature pattern-onset response, this latency window corresponds to the first major positive waveform deflection, classically labeled C_1.[54,55] Principal component analysis (figure 25.6) has confirmed that in more mature albinos (older than

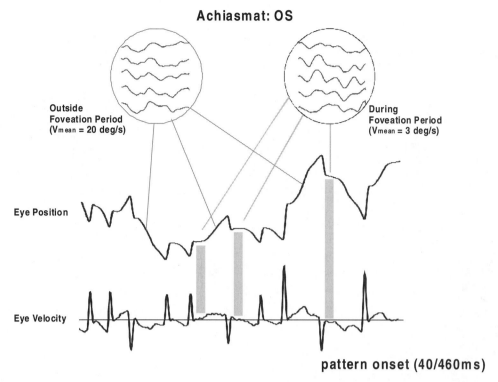

Achiasmat: OS

Outside
Foveation Period
(Vmean = 20 deg/s)

During
Foveation Period
(Vmean = 3 deg/s)

Eye Position

Eye Velocity

pattern onset (40/460ms)

FIGURE 25.14 Schematic of an eye movement recording of a patient with CN. Vertical yellow bars indicate foveation periods when retinal velocity approaches zero. This can readily be observed from the lower velocity trace. Two sets of VEP averages are depicted: one obtained from VEP responses following visual stimulation outside foveation periods and another obtained from VEP responses following visual stimulation during foveation periods. The latter are significantly more robust. (See also color plate 19.)

Albino

OU   OD   OS

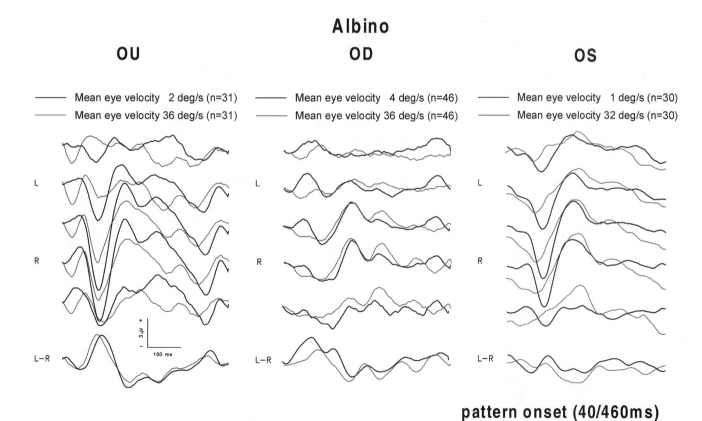

——— Mean eye velocity 2 deg/s (n=31)
········· Mean eye velocity 36 deg/s (n=31)

——— Mean eye velocity 4 deg/s (n=46)
········· Mean eye velocity 36 deg/s (n=46)

——— Mean eye velocity 1 deg/s (n=30)
········· Mean eye velocity 32 deg/s (n=30)

L

R

L−R

pattern onset (40/460ms)

FIGURE 25.15 Depicted are VEP averages (black traces) in an albino during OU, OD, and OS viewing extracted from periods with low mean ocular velocity (less than 5 degrees/second). Also depicted are VEP averages (red traces) extracted from responses to pattern-onset stimulation during high mean ocular velocity. Five channels positioned across the occiput and one difference channel (i.e., VEP channel 4 positioned at left occiput subtracted from VEP channel 2 positioned at right occiput) also are presented. (See also color plate 20.)

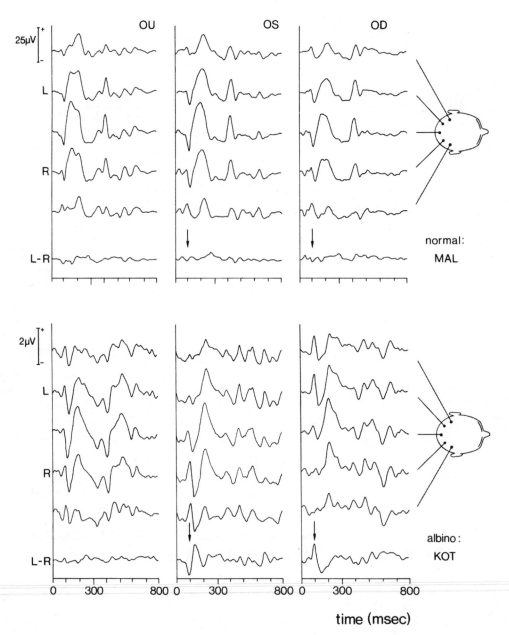

FIGURE 25.16 Binocular (OU), left eye (OS), and right eye (OD) pattern onset/offset (300ms/500ms) VEP responses (check size = 55′) from a normal control (upper panel) and an albino (lower panel). Reference electrode was linked ears. For derivations, see figure 25.7, wherein the sixth (bottommost) trace is a bipolar derivation representing the difference between the second L trace (left hemispheric derivation) and the fourth R trace (right hemispheric derivation).

3–5 years), reliable VEP albino asymmetry is determined via the C_1 component. Thus, stimulus and recording procedures that optimize the C_1 component should be employed. The C_1 component in the pattern-onset VEP is typically considered to reflect primarily local luminance variation in the response. The second negative component, C_2, which is absent in the VEP profiles of infants and children owing to visual pathway immaturity, reflects contrast mechanisms and, as such, is particularly sensitive to pattern size and defocus. Because of the foveal hypoplasia and reduced acuity in albinos, it is common to find an absent or relatively weak C_2 component concomitant with a robust, readily identifiable C_1 component, at least in more mature albino VEP profiles. While the pattern of interhemispheric asymmetry as described is specific to albinism, VEP topographical asymmetries per se should not be confused with normally occurring hemispheric response dominance owing primarily to individual variation in cortical neuroanatomy. The latter, which is of standard normal occurrence, will reflect the same hemispheric response dominance regardless of left or right

eye viewing. An example of hemispheric response dominance in normal controls is depicted in the four panels on the left in figure 25.17. Herein, VEPs were evoked binocularly and monocularly in normal controls; amplitude of the pattern-onset C_1 component is plotted as a function of electrode position from left to right occiput (see the schematic in figure 25.7). Figure 25.17 shows that cortical topography of VEP responses in normal controls can present with midline dominance, midline attenuation, and/or varying degrees of hemispheric lateralization. For the latter, the peak of the potential distribution is located either to the left (lower left) or to the right (lower right) occiput region. These normal but varying profiles of asymmetric VEP topography are unrelated to any significant interocular asymmetry indexes (see the black bars in figure 25.17). Similar variation in hemispheric response dominance can also be observed in albinos, but it is the interocular asymmetry per se that defines the pathognomonic albino optic pathway misrouting condition. For example, the four panels at the right of figure 25.17 show varying profiles of VEP topography obtained from

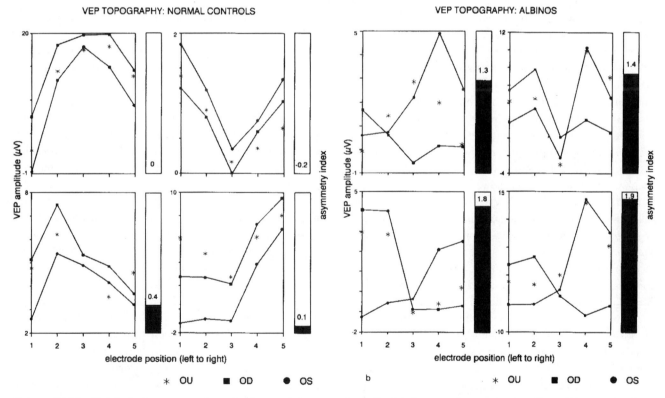

FIGURE 25.17 Hemispheric response lateralization and intersubject lateralization variability in a sample of normal controls (left four panels) and a sample of albinos (right four panels). Unconnected star symbols denote binocular VEP amplitude of the pattern onset (300/500 ms; check size = 55′) C1 component across the electrode array. Results from right eye (OD) and left eye (OS) stimulation are indicated by solid squares and solid circles, respectively. Asymmetry index values for each monocular data set are represented by vertical bars. Response

lateralization in normal controls as well as albinos varies from midline dominance (upper left) to midline attenuation (upper right) to left (lower left) or right (lower right) hemispheric response lateralization. Profiles of monocular topography plots for the normal observers are comparable and, in all four controls, result in nonsignificant asymmetry indexes. In contrast, for the albinos, left and right eye potential distributions across the occiput show significant contralateral asymmetry (asymmetry indexes are indicated by vertical black bars).

monocular and binocular stimulation. In contrast to the four normal control topography plots shown at the left, all four albinos present with significant interocular asymmetry indexes as indicated by the vertical bars.

The pattern of hemispheric asymmetry, characteristic to albinism, also should not be confused with VEP asymmetry resulting from optic pathway lesions, malformations, tumors, and/or other non-albino-related visual pathway anomalies. In this respect, it is interesting to note that, opposite to the contralateral asymmetry observed in albinism, a VEP topography distribution is found in nondecussating retinal-fugal fiber syndrome[13,14] that reflects ipsilateral asymmetry (figure 25.18). In general, the VEP misrouting test is particularly sensitive to aberrant chiasmal conditions, including the condition of achiasma, in which there is an absence of crossing optic fibers. Note that in the latter condition, ipsilateral asymmetry is associated with a *negative* interocular asymmetry index.

While all albinos demonstrate VEP misrouting, heterozygote carriers characteristically do not, although some carriers show iris diaphany and retinal hypopigmentation. In figure 25.19, the VEP response profile from an X-chromosomal ocular albino carrier is presented along with the response from her albino son. A partial family pedigree across four generations is depicted. The 39-year-old carrier presented with reduced acuity, significant iris diaphany, and patchy retinal pigmentation. However, there was no nystagmus, foveal and macular reflexes were normal, and the VEP misrouting test was negative, as seen by inspection of the monocular responses following full-field pattern-onset stimulation. As was expected, the albino son (proband) who presented with nystagmus, fundus hypopigmentation, foveal hypoplasia, iris diaphany, and photophobia showed clear evidence of optic pathway misrouting both for pattern-onset and luminance flash. Furthermore, the albino misrouting test is positive regardless of genotype. Two albinos, one classified as autosomal-recessive oculocutaneous and the other as having X-chromosomal ocular albinism, show clear evidence of VEP misrouting as depicted in figure 25.20A. Finally, as is shown in figure 25.20B, obligate heterozygotes for autosomal-recessive forms of albinism do not show the misrouting trait. In this case, the VEP profile of the proband's father (upper traces) and paternal aunt (lower traces) of the upper albino shown in figure 25.20A show no evidence of aberrant retinofugal projections. These negative misrouting findings in the human albino carrier are of interest in light of reports of abnormal retinogeniculocortical pathways in normally pigmented cats that carry a recessive albino allele.[8] However, to date, there is no clear evidence indicating aberrant visual pathways in the human albino carrier; therefore, albino carrier detection with the VEP is not feasible.

The pattern of hemispheric asymmetry described is specific to albinism also is not observed in patients with con-

genital nystagmus (CN) who manifest one or more albinotic symptoms (figure 25.14). In such cases, differential diagnosis based on clinical evaluation may remain equivocal. Particularly in young patients with oculomotor instabilities, foveal and/or macular hypoplasia is difficult for the physician to judge. It has been demonstrated[69] that family members with inherited CN did not show evidence of VEP contralateral asymmetry, indicating that the CN that was manifested was unrelated to optic pathway misprojections indicative of albinism. However, the classic albino misrouting profile was revealed only in the albino proband patient of this family. Figure 25.21 shows the VEP pattern-onset responses, together with the topography plots in three age-matched children. Contralateral asymmetry and a significant interocular asymmetry index are obtained only in the albino child (upper traces) and not in the CN control (middle traces) and albino control (lower traces).

An important caveat in albino misrouting test with luminance flash and pattern onset concerns component specificity and visual pathway maturation.[19,24] The consequence is that while a pattern-onset paradigm yields high test sensitivity selectively in the older albinos, for the albino infant, test performance with a similar paradigm has a much lower reliability. Compared to the adult pattern-onset waveform, which is triphasic (positive C1, negative C2, and positive C3; see also figures 25.16 to 25.21), the immature pattern-onset response consists of a primarily single positive peak. Despite the presence of recordable pattern-onset responses, for the albino infant, the VEP potential distributions and corresponding topography plots quite frequently do not show evidence of misrouting. Therefore, in childhood, the misrouting detection can be demonstrated primarily with luminance flash. Figure 25.22 shows a VEP luminance flash response in an autosomal-recessive oculocutaneous albino at the age of 21.4 weeks (lower traces) and an age-matched normal control (upper traces). Interocular amplitudes between both subjects are comparable; however, the albino clearly shows contralateral asymmetry with a significant asymmetry index value of 1.79.

Although VEP misrouting correlates in the adult human albino were first demonstrated with a luminance flash paradigm, the original experimental tests yielded rather poor detection rates and were therefore limited usefulness for clinical application.[37] The inferior performance rates of the luminance flash in older albinos is due, at least in part, to the fact that the luminance flash response undergoes a dramatic maturational course, showing increasing complexity in waveform with age.[22,24,25,32] As a consequence, hit rates and test reliability also diminish significantly when a luminance flash misrouting test is attempted in older albinos. Figure 25.23A shows the monocular VEP luminance flash response in four albinos younger than 1 year of age. It is interesting to observe for these four albino infants in figure 25.23B the

VEP MISROUTING TEST

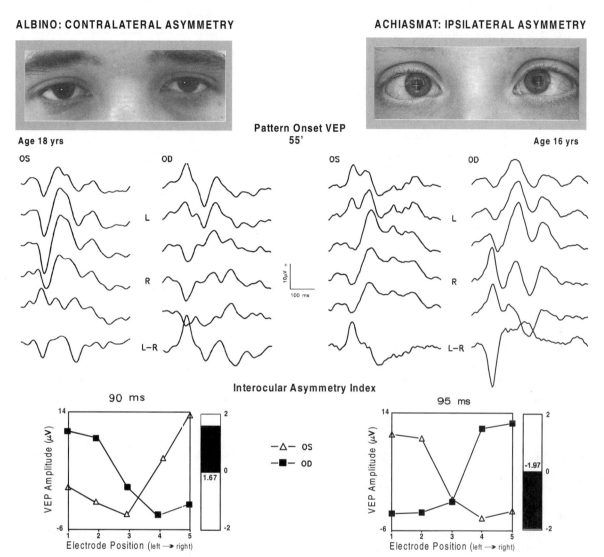

Pattern Onset VEP
55'

ALBINO: CONTRALATERAL ASYMMETRY

Age 18 yrs

ACHIASMAT: IPSILATERAL ASYMMETRY

Age 16 yrs

Interocular Asymmetry Index

FIGURE 25.18 Left eye (OS), and right eye (OD) pattern onset/offset (40 ms/460 ms) VEP responses (check size = 55′) from an X-chromosomal ocular albino (left panel) and a patient with nondecussating retinal-fugal fiber syndrome (right panel). Fundi of both patients are shown in figures 25.2A and 25.2B, respectively. VEP amplitude distribution across the electrode array for OD and OS stimulation is depicted below the VEP traces. In the case of contralateral asymmetry (left) in the albino, following left eye stimulation (OS), a major positive peak of the pattern onset response lateralizes to the right occiput, and with right eye stimulation, a major positive peak lateralizes to the left occiput. This interocular occipital lateralization yields a highly significant interocular asymmetry index of 1.67 at 90 ms. For comparison, occipital lateralization in an achiasmat is also presented. In the case of ipsilateral asymmetry (right) in an achiasmat, following left eye stimulation (OS), a major positive peak of the pattern onset response lateralizes to the left occiput, and with right eye stimulation, a major positive peak lateralizes to the right occiput. This rare interocular ipsilateral VEP response lateralization results in a highly significant interocular asymmetry index of −1.97 at 90 ms. (See also color plate 21.)

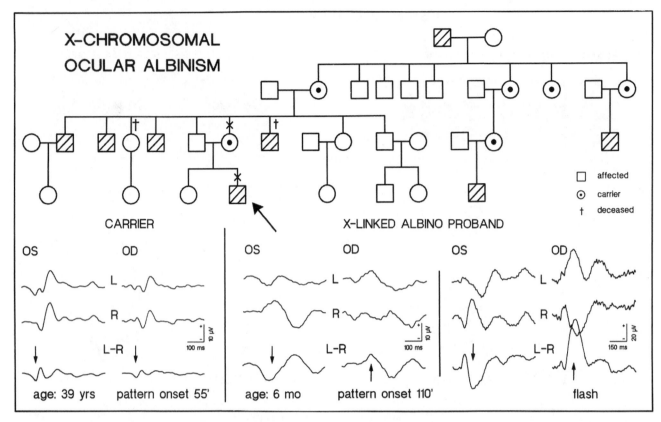

FIGURE 25.19 Family pedigree of the X-chromosomal mode of albino inheritance across four generations. VEP misrouting detection is negative for the 39-year-old obligate heterozygote albino carrier (lower left). In contrast, the carrier's 6-month-old son, the proband (see arrow on the pedigree profile), clearly demonstrates the albino misrouting profile for both flash and pattern-onset stimulus conditions. Starred symbols indicate the two family members who underwent VEP testing. Note also that the immature responses do not show component-specific asymmetry; rather, the whole positive peak appears to shift from the right to the left hemisphere following left and right eye stimulation, respectively.

contralateral asymmetry index as a function of VEP latency. Solid symbols indicate an asymmetry index higher than 0.7, which demonstrates that there are time windows of significant asymmetry for luminance flash that also depend on age.

Figure 25.24 illustrates the sensitivity and selectivity of the interocular asymmetry index for pattern onset as well as luminance flash as a function of age. For a group of 47 normal controls older than 6 years of age, no hemispheric asymmetry is found higher than 0.5, whereas for a group of 61 albinos, no hemispheric asymmetry is found lower than 0.9 (two upper panels). If a value of 0.7 is chosen for the hemispheric asymmetry index, the sensitivity of the misrouting test for albinism in this case is 100%: None of the 61 albinos has an asymmetry index lower than 0.7. In addition, an asymmetry index greater than 0.7 clearly is pathognomonic for aberrant chiasmal crossing associated with albinism; also, specificity is 100%. It is important to note that 100% sensitivity as well as 100% selectively can be obtained only when the correct misrouting protocol is followed, that is, full-field monocular stimulation, test during wakefulness, and stimulation of the central visual field. Furthermore,

figure 25.24 illustrates that there is an age recipe for albino misrouting detection.[24] Comparison of the upper right panel with the lower left panel shows that the pattern-onset VEP misrouting test has a considerable amount of false negatives when the albino is younger than 6 years of age. However, comparison of the lower left panel with the lower right panel of figure 25.24 shows that below the age of 6 years, the luminance flash can be used for misrouting detection instead of pattern onset. With a cutoff value of 0.7, no false negatives are found for a group of 73 albinos; sensitivity again reaches 100%. Finally, figures 25.25, 25.26, and 25.27 show an extensive overview of a large albino patient population. The three contour plots show the hemispheric asymmetry index as a function of age and a function of VEP response latency. Figure 25.25 represents only the results for luminance flash. Note that for the luminance flash VEP, the age axis has a logarithmic scale. This shows more clearly the windows of significant asymmetry at the younger ages. Figures 25.26 and 25.27 show on a linear scale for age similar results as shown in figure 25.25 for pattern onset with check sizes of 55′ and 110′, respectively. Across subjects, the average of the

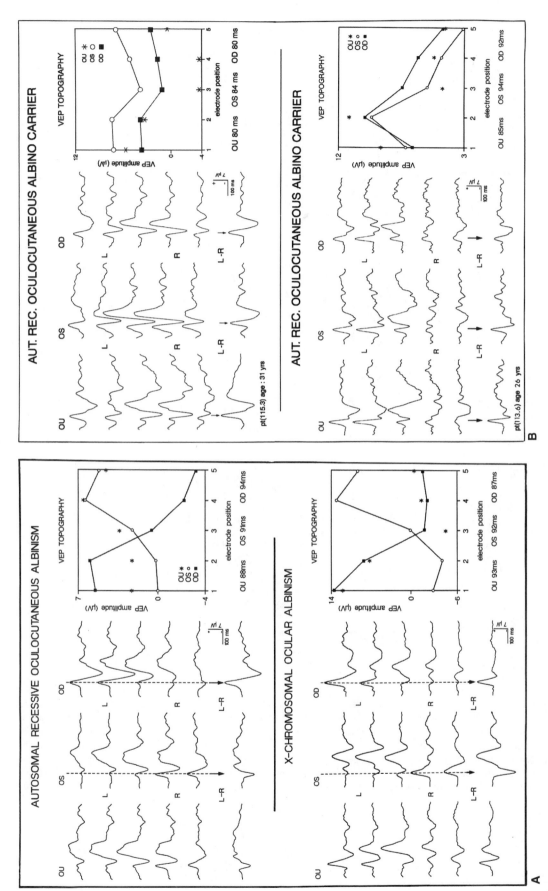

FIGURE 25.20   A, Binocular (OU), left eye (OS), and right eye (OD) pattern-onset/offset (40/460 ms; check size = 55′) VEP responses of an oculocutaneous albino (upper traces) and an X-linked ocular albino (lower traces). VEP responses follow the interocular interhemispheric asymmetry profiles depicted in figure 25.7. Vertical dashed lines indicate the latency window of maximum asymmetry; arrows denote the polarity reversal of the difference potential at a latency of about 90 ms. Both interocular VEP potential distributions (rightward panels) show a crossed pattern of interocular asymmetry. In addition, binocular (OU) stimulation (asterisks) shows a right hemisphere dominance for the oculocutaneous albino and a left hemisphere dominance for the ocular albino. B, Binocular (OU), left eye (OS), and right eye (OD) pattern-onset/offset (40/460 ms; 55′ check size) VEP responses recorded from two adult albino carriers. The VEP topography profiles are definitely negative for a crossed pattern of interocular asymmetry via monocular (OD, OS) full field stimulation. Note that OD, OS, and OU topography profiles follow comparable VEP topography distributions across the electrode array, reflecting primarily left hemispheric response dominance across viewing conditions at a latency of the first major positive peak; see also difference potentials (sixth trace).

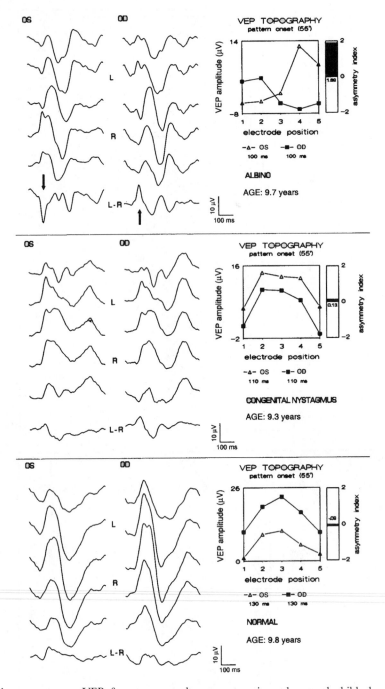

FIGURE 25.21 Monocular pattern-onset VEPs from two controls, age-matched to an albino child (uppermost traces) tested at the age of 9.7 years. The format is comparable to the schematic, figure 25.7. The age-matched 9- to 10-year old controls include a child with hereditary (X-chromosomal) congenital nystagmus (middle traces) and a normal child (lowermost traces). The albino shows interocular contralateral asymmetry; the congenital nystagmic and normal child show interocular symmetry. Note the polarity reversal of the difference potentials (see arrows), the crossover of the monocular response amplitudes plotted across the electrode array, and the high asymmetry index (1.89) of the albino child. Topography plots at the right are derived from amplitude values across the electrode array at the latencies denoted.

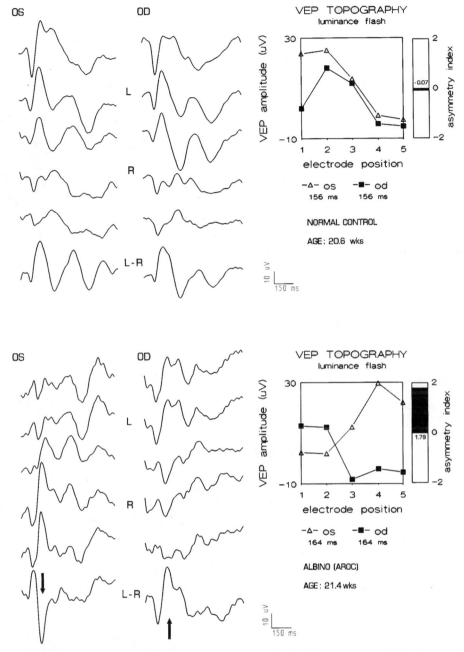

FIGURE 25.22   Monocular luminance flash VEPs from a normal control (upper) and an albino (lower) tested at approximately age 20–21 weeks. The format is similar to that of figure 25.7. Topography plots at the right show left hemispheric response dominance for the normal control but no significant interocular asymmetry. In contrast, the albino topography plot shows contralateral asymmetry with a highly significant asymmetry index value of 1.79.

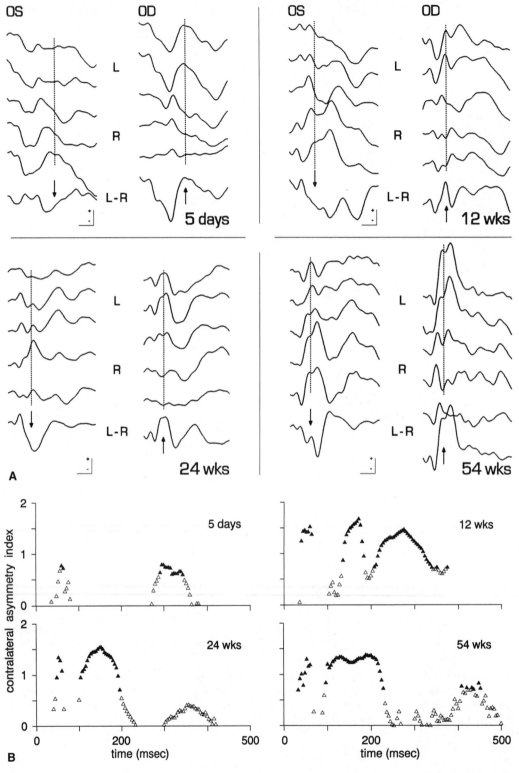

FIGURE 25.23   A, Left (OS) and right (OD) eye luminance flash responses from the left (L) to right (R) occiput from an albino infant at 5 days (upper left), 12 weeks (upper right), 24 weeks (lower left), and 54 weeks (lower right) of age. VEP response traces also follow the format of figure 25.7 schematic. The vertical dashed line is positioned at the latency reflecting the optimum contralateral asymmetry index. The polarity reversal (see arrows) of the difference potentials from left to right eye stimulation also is indicative of albino VEP asymmetry. Calibration angle equals 10 μV in the vertical plane and 100 ms in the horizontal plane. B, Contralateral asymmetry index values (positive values depicted) as a function of VEP response latency derived from the four albino monocular VEPs shown in part A. Two time windows of significant (>0.7) contralateral asymmetry are observed (solid triangles). An early asymmetry region occurring around 60 ms, appears within an age-stationary, narrow window; a more robust and longer-latency cluster of asymmetry shifting toward shorter latencies across the age range reflects maturation of the visual response.

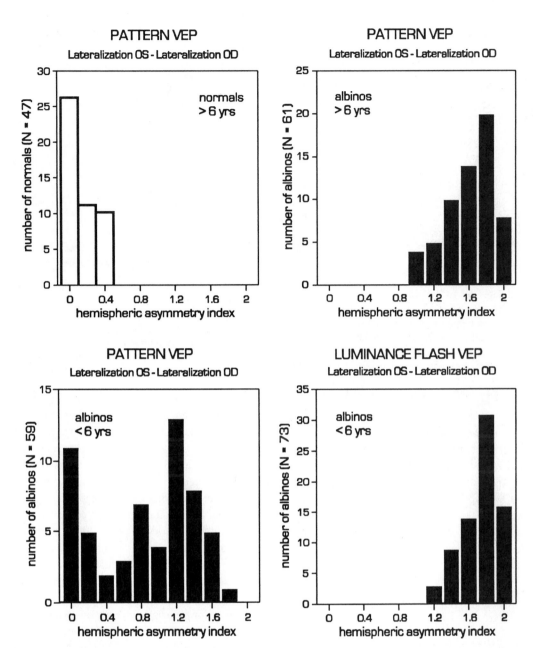

FIGURE 25.24 Upper histograms, Asymmetry index distributions with the pattern-onset paradigm (55′ and 110′ check size) for normal controls and albinos older than 6 years of age. The two groups show no overlap. Normal controls present with asymmetry index values below 0.7; albinos present with asymmetry index values above 0.7. Lower histograms, Asymmetry index distributions with pattern-onset paradigm (left) and luminance flash (right) for albinos younger than 6 years of age. Reliable and significant albino contralateral asymmetry within this younger age group is detected with the luminance flash paradigm. For the younger age group, pattern onset is neither selective nor sensitive.

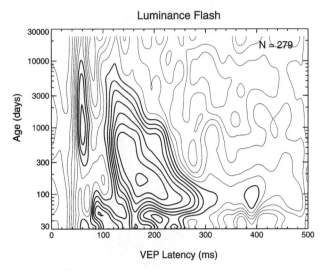

Luminance Flash

FIGURE 25.25 Contour plot of interocular asymmetry indexes across the age span as a function of latency of the luminance flash VEP response is depicted (upper asymmetry contour plot). VEP latency is presented in milliseconds; age is presented in days. The contour plot is an average of 279 independent recordings. The sample rate is 500 ms along the horizontal axis and 100 ms along the vertical axis. Contour lines representing asymmetry index values equal to or greater than 0.7 (value of significant asymmetry) are plotted in bold.

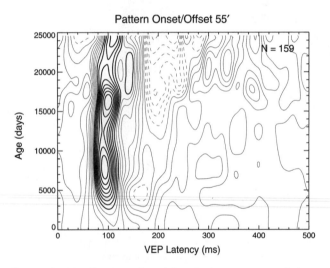

Pattern Onset/Offset 55′

FIGURE 25.26 Contour plot of interocular asymmetry indexes across the age span as a function of latency of the pattern-onset (55′ check size) VEP response is depicted. The contour plot is an average of 159 independent recordings. Contour lines that represent asymmetry index values equal to or greater than 0.7 (value of significant asymmetry) are plotted in bold.

hemispheric asymmetry, determined from monocular full-field stimulation (see methodology), is calculated. When this average is equal or greater than 0.7, isocontour lines are plotted in bold. Figure 25.25 clearly shows for the luminance flash VEP an early window of significant contrateral asymmetry between 50 ms and 70 ms, which latency is independent of age. However, the optimal significance of this early

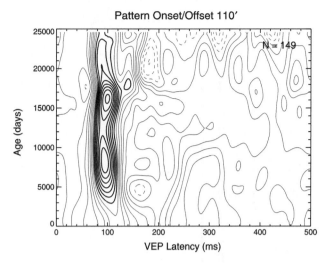

Pattern Onset/Offset 110′

FIGURE 25.27 Comparable to figures 25.24 and 25.25, but now the contour plot of interocular asymmetry index across the age span as a function of latency of the pattern-onset (110′ check size) VEP response is depicted. The contour plot is an average of 149 independent recordings. Contour lines that represent asymmetry index values equal to or greater than 0.7 (value of significant asymmetry) are plotted in bold.

window is at the age of 3 years and gradually loses significance at older ages. In addition, a later and more important window of greater significance is present between 100 ms and 300 ms. Figure 25.25 demonstrates that the optimal latency of significant contralateral asymmetry for this window decreases with age from 250 ms to 120 ms. At birth, the optimal latency for significant contralateral asymmetry in albino infants varies between 200 and 300 ms. Between the age of 2 and 6 years, the maximum contralateral symmetry for luminance flash gradually decreases, and at 6 years of age, the optimum latency of significant asymmetry for detection of albinism is about 140 ms. Figures 25.26 and 25.27 show for pattern onset only one window of significant contralateral asymmetry that varies between 80 and 120 ms. Optimal latency decreases slightly with age from 110 ms at 3 years of age to 90 ms in adulthood. Contralateral asymmetry for pattern onset already can be found at a very early age (a couple of months). However, more reliable and significant results for misrouting detection with pattern onset start at the age of 3 years. The maximum of the average of contralateral asymmetry increases considerably from the age of 3 years to the age of 18–20 years. Through adulthood, the average of optimal latency and the average of maximum asymmetry remain constant. A slight increase in latency and a decrease of maximum asymmetry may be present at ages older than 50–60 years. A check size of 55′ gives some better results than 110′ because response to the latter contains more VEP components of local luminance. However, when the albino patient has a low visual acuity, stimulation with 110′ check size has an advantage over 55′ check size.

From figures 25.24 through 25.27, the following age recipe may be derived for routine clinical application. For practical purposes, use the luminance flash paradigm for albinos under 3 years of age, use both the luminance flash and pattern-onset paradigm for albinos between 3 and 10 years of age, and for albinos older than 10 years, the pattern onset paradigm is sufficient. For a more accurate misrouting detection, it is better to use both paradigms across all ages. Moreover, for albino infants, the pattern-onset response also can be used to assess the VEP visual acuity.

Conclusions

Interocular VEP asymmetry in albinism reflects misrouted optic pathway projections in which a preponderance of temporal retinal fibers erroneously decussate at the optic chiasm. The latter, pathognomonic to albinism, disrupts functional and anatomical organization throughout the optic pathways. VEP misrouting results comparable to those depicted are present in all albinos regardless of phenotype, genotype, or age.[24] Interocular VEP hemispheric asymmetry reflecting albino misrouting was first demonstrated in adult albinos via a luminance flash paradigm.[37] Because the latter yielded rather poor detection rates, clinical application was limited. However, subsequent studies emerged[9,23] in which various transient stimulus profiles, such as luminance flash, pattern reversal, and pattern onset/offset, were evaluated in albinos across the age span. The former led to a "practical" albino VEP test protocol that included employment of (1) the luminance flash paradigm for patients younger than 3 years of age, (2) both the luminance flash and pattern onset paradigms for patients between about 3 and 6 years of age, and (3) the pattern-onset paradigm for patients older than 6 years of age. During actual VEP testing, luminance flash is presented to all patients across the age range for comparison with international standards; pattern onset also is presented across the age range to assess spatial maturation and VEP acuity. As a caveat, it is important to take into consideration the fact that luminance flash and pattern-onset results from the VEP misrouting test in particularly young patients are considered valid only when the results recorded during wakefulness and full attention.

In general, the 100% detection rate of VEP asymmetry in albinos across the age range concomitant with zero false positives in normal age-matched controls, heterozygote family members, and nonalbino patients with comparable albino symptoms (e.g., nystagmus, reduced acuity, retinal hypopigmentation) indicates and confirms that the VEP misrouting test follows a decisive protocol for albino detection and differential diagnosis. The fact that all albinos have neural ectoderm anomalies that preclude normal visual pathway development ensures detection by appropriate VEP assessment regardless of albino age, genotype, or phenotype.

Furthermore, since the albino VEP signature is age specific, corresponding electrophysiological response profiles also contribute to the objective assessment of visual pathway maturation and function.

In conclusion, it is of interest to note that several centuries ago, an excerpt from Vesalius was published[77] in which normal mammalian optic pathways were erroneously described as having an absence of mammalian optic pathway decussation. While we now certainly have a correct overview of mammalian visual pathway structure and function, primary visual pathways, particularly concerning the topic of visual pathway decussation, have for millennia, as can be seen from the Vesalius reference, attracted the interest and passions of philosophers, anatomists, and artists in the vigorous quest to understand the sensory appreciation of visual space, ocular motor control, and single binocular vision. The present overview attempts to gain more insight into these issues by outlining and describing objective VEP and ocular motor assessments of visual function across the age range.

REFERENCES

1. Abadi RV, Dickinson CM: Waveform characteristics in congenital nystagmus. *Doc Ophthalmol* 1986; 64:153–167.
2. Abadi RV, Bjerre A: Motor and sensory characteristics of infantile nystagmus. *Brit J Ophthalmol* 2002; 86:1152–1160.
3. Abadi RV, Pascal E: Periodic alternating nystagmus in humans with albinism. *Invest Ophthalmol Vis Sci* 1994; 35:4080–4086.
4. Abadi RV, Scallan C: Manifest latent nystagmus and congenital nystagmus waveforms in the same subject. *Neuro-ophthalmology* 1999; 21:211–221.
5. Abadi RV, Whittle JP, Worfolk R: Oscillopsia and tolerance to retinal image movement in congenital nystagmus. *Invest Ophthalmol Vision Sci* 1999; 40:339–345.
6. Abadi RV, Worfolk R: Retinal slip velocities in congenital nystagmus. *Vision Res* 1989; 29:195–205.
7. Apkarian P: Methodology of testing for albinism with visual evoked cortical potentials. In Heckenlively JR, Arden GB (eds): *Handbook of Clinical Electrophysiology of Vision Testing*. St Louis, Year Book Medical Publishers, 1991, pp 425–434.
8. Apkarian P: Albinism. In Heckenlively JR, Arden GB (eds): *Handbook of Clincial Electrophysiology of Vision Testing*. St Louis, Year Book Medical Publishers, 1991, pp 773–782.
9. Apkarian P: A practical approach to albino diagnosis: VEP misrouting across the age span. *Ophthalmic Paediatr Genet* 1992; 13:77–88.
10. Apkarian P: Chiasmal crossing defects in disorders of binocular vision. *Eye* 1996; 10:222–232.
11. Apkarian P, Barth PG, Wenniger-Prick L, Bour L: Non-decussating retinal fugal fibre syndrome: VEP detection of a visual system anomaly associated with visual loss, nystagmus and aberrant optic chiasm. *Invest Ophthalmol Vis Sci* 1993; 34 (suppl.):711.
12. Apkarian P, Bour L: Concurrent DMI ocular motor and pattern onset VEP measures in patients with metabolic and/or chiasmal midline disorders. *Invest Ophthalmol Vis Sci* 2001; 42 (suppl):844.

13. Apkarian P, Bour L, Barth PG: A unique achiasmatic anomaly detected in non-albinos with misrouted retinal-fugal projections. *Eur J Neurosci* 1994; 6:501–507.
14. Apkarian P, Bour LJ, Barth PG, Wenniger-Prick L, Verbeeten B Jr: Non-decussating retinal-fugal fibre syndrome: An inborn achiasmatic malformation associated with visuotopic misrouting, visual evoked potential ipsilateral asymmetry and nystagmus. *Brain* 1995; 118:1195–1216.
15. Apkarian P, Bour L, Bruno P, Berg vd AV: Three dimensional eye movement recordings in non-decussating retinal fugal fibre syndrome: An inborn achiasmatic malformation identified with congenital and see saw nystagmus. *Invest Ophthalmol Vis Sci* 1995; 36 (suppl):175.
16. Apkarian P, Bour LJ, de Faber JTHN: Developmental aspects of inborn ocular motor instabilities and misalignments: Double magnetic induction method (DMI) eye movement recordings in paediatric patients. *Invest Ophthalmol Vis Sci* 1999; 40 (suppl):962.
17. Apkarian P, Bour L, van der Steen J, Collewijn H: Ocular motor disorders associated with inborn chiasmal crossing defects: Multi-planar eye movement recordings in see-saw and congenital nystagmus. In Becker W, Deubel H, Mergner T (eds): *Current Oculomotor Research: Physiological and Psychological Aspects.* New York, Plenum, 1999, pp 403–413.
18. Apkarian P, Bour LJ, van der Steen J, De Faber JTHN: Chiasmal crossing defects in disorders of ocular motor function: Three dimensional eye movement recordings in albinism and non-decussating retinal fugal fibre syndrome. *Invest Ophthalmol Vis Sci* 1996; 37 (suppl):228.
19. Apkarian P, Reits D, Spekreijse H: Component specificity in albino VEP asymmetry: Maturation of the visual pathway anomaly. *Exp Brain Res* 1984; 53:285–294.
20. Apkarian P, Reits D, Spekreijse H, van Dorp D: A decisive electrophysiological test for human albinism. *Electroencephalogr Clin Neurophysiol* 1983; 55:513–531.
21. Apkarian P, Shallo-Hoffmann J: VEP projections in congenital nystagmus: VEP asymmetry in albinism: A comparison study. [Published erratum appears in *Invest Ophthalmol Vis Sci* 1992; 33:691–692.] *Invest Ophthalmol Vis Sci* 1991; 32:2653–2661.
22. Apkarian P, Spekreijse H: The VEP and misrouted pathways in human albinism. In Cracco RQ, Bodis-Wollner I (eds): *Evoked Potentials.* New York, Alan R. Liss, 1986.
23. Apkarian P, Spekreijse H: The VEP and misrouted pathways in human albinism. In Cracco RQ, Bodis-Wollner I (eds): *Evoked Potentials.* New York, Alan R. Liss, 1986, pp 211–226.
24. Apkarian P, Thijssen R: Detection and maturation of VEP albino asymmetry: An overview and a longitudinal study from birth to 54 weeks. *Behav Brain Res* 1992; 49:57–67.
25. Apkarian P, Van Veenendall W, Spekreijse H: Albinism: An anomaly of maturation of the visual pathways. *Doc Ophthalmol Proc Ser* 1986; 45:271–284.
26. Bach M, Kommerell G: Albino-type misrouting of the optic nerve fibers no found in dissociated vertical deviation. *Graefes Arch Clin Exp Ophthalmol* 1992; 230:158–161.
27. Bedell HE, White JM, Abplanalp PL: Variability of foveations in congenital nystagmus. *Clin Vis Sci* 1989; 4:247–252.
28. Bour LJ, Apkarian P: Three-dimensional eye movement calibration using search coils in patients. *Proceedings of the First Ophthalmology Society Congress,* September 1996, pp 59–61.
29. Bour LJ, Apkarian P: A novel approach for objective visual function assessment: Simultaneous EEG/VEP and DMI Rings/search coils recordings. *Invest Ophthalmol Vis Sci* 2001; 42 (Suppl):624.
30. Bour LJ, Aramideh M, Ongerboer de Visser BW: Neurophysiological aspects of eye and eyelid movements during blinking in humans. *Neurophysiol* 2000; 83(1):166–176.
31. Bour LJ, Van Gisbergen JAM, Bruijns J, Ottes FP: The double magnetic induction method for measuring eye movement: Results in monkey and man. *IEEE* 1984; 419–427.
32. Boylan C, Clement RA, Harding GFA: Lateralization of the flash visual-evoked cortical potential in human albinos. *Invest Ophthalmol* 1984; 25:1448–1450.
33. Chung STL, Bedell HE: Velocity criteria for "foveation periods" determined from image motions simulating congenital nystagmus. *Optom Vis Sci* 1996; 73:92–103.
34. Cogan DG: Congenital nystagmus. *Can J Ophthalmol* 1967; 2:4–11.
35. Collewijn H, Van der Mark F, Jansen TC: Precise recording of human eye movements. *Vision Res* 1975; 15:447–450.
36. Creel DJ, Summers CG, King RA: Visual anomalies associated with albinism. *Ophthalmic Paediatr Genet* 1990; 11:193–200.
37. Creel D, Witkop CJ, King RA: Asymmetric visually evoked potentials in human albinos: Evidence for visual system anomalies. *Invest Ophthalmol* 1974; 13:430–440.
38. Dell'Osso LE, Daroff RB: Congenital nystagmus waveforms and foveation strategy. *Doc Ophthalmol* 1975; 39:155–182.
39. Farmer J, Hoyt CS: Monocular nystagmus in infancy and early childhood. *Am J Ophthalmol* 1984; 98:504–509.
40. Ferman L, Collewijn H, Jansen TC, van den Berg AV: Human gaze stability in the horizontal, vertical and torsional direction during voluntary head movements, evaluated with a three-dimensional scleral induction coil technique. *Vision Res* 1987; 13:811–828.
41. Glaser JS: *Neuro-ophthalmology,* ed 3. Philadelphia, Lippincott Williams & Wilkins, 1999.
42. Goldstein HP, Gottlob I, Fendick MG: Visual remapping in infantile nystagmus. *Vision Res* 1992; 32:1115–1124.
43. Gross KJ, Hickey TL: Abnormal laminar patterns in the lateral geniculate nucleus of an albino monkey. *Brain Res* 1980; 190:231–237.
44. Guillery RW: Why do albinos and other hypopigmented mutants lack normal binocular vision, and what else is abnormal in their central visual pathways? *Eye* 1996; 10:217–221.
45. Guillery RW, Ookoro AN, Witkop CJ: Abnormal visual pathways in the brain of a human albino. *Brain Res* 1973; 96:373–377.
46. Guo SQ, Reinecke RD, Fendick M, Calhoun JH: Visual pathway abnormalities in albinism and infantile nystagmus: VECPs and stereoacuity measurements. *J Pediatr Ophthalmol Strabismus* 1989; 26:97–104.
47. Harcourt B: Hereditary nystagmus in early childhood. *J Med Genet* 1970; 7:250–257.
48. Haustein W: Considerations on Listing's law and the primary position by means of a matrix description of eye position control. *Biol Cybern* 1989; 60:411–420.
49. Hedera P, Lai S, Haacke EM, Lerner AJ, Hopkins AL, Lewin JS, Friedland RP: Abnormal connectivity of the visual pathways in human albinos demonstrated by susceptibility-sensitized MRI. *Neurology* 1994; 44:1921–1926.
50. Hendrickson AE, Yuodelis C: The morphological development of the human fovea. *Ophthalmology* 1984; 91:603–612.
51. Hertle RW, Tabuchi A, Dell'Osso LF, Abel LA, Weismann BM: Saccadic oscillations and intrusions preceding the postnatal

appearance of congenital nystagmus. *Neuroophthalmol* 1988; 8:37–42.

52. Hess BJM, van Opstal AJ, Straumann D, Hepp K: Calibration of three-dimensional eye position by using search coil signals in rhesus monkey. *Vision Res* 1992; 32:1647–1654.

53. Hoyt CS: Nystagmus and other abnormal ocular movements in children. *Pediatr Ophthalmol* 1989; 34:1415–1423.

54. Jeffreys DA, Axford JG: Source locations of pattern specific components of human visual evoked potentials: I. Component of striate cortical origin. *Exp Brain Res* 1972; 16:1–21.

55. Jeffreys DA, Axford JG: Source locations of pattern specific components of human visual evoked potentials: II. Components of extrastriate cortical origin. *Exp Brain Res* 1972; 16:22–40.

56. Kommerell G, Zee DS: Latent nystagmus: Release and suppression at will. *Invest Ophthalmol Vis Sci* 1993; 34:1785–1792.

57. Korff CM, Apkarian P, Bour LJ, Meuli R, Verrey JD, Roulet Perez E: Isolated absence of optic chiasm revealed by congenital nystagmus, MRI and VEPs. *Neuropediatrics* 2003; 34:219–223.

58. Kriss A, Timms C, Elston J, Taylor D, Gresty M: Visual evoked potentials in dissociated vertical deviation: A reappraisal. *Br J Ophthalmol* 1989; 73:265–270.

59. Leigh RJ, Zee DS: *The Neurology of Eye Movements*, ed 3. New York, Oxford University Press, 1999.

60. Lesèvre N, Joseph JP: Modifications of the pattern evoked potential in relation to the stimulated part of the visual field. *Electroencephalogr Clin Neurophysiol* 1979; 47:183–203.

61. Leventhal AG, Creel DJ: Retinal projections and functional architecture of cortical areas 17 and 18 in the tyrosinase-negative albino cat. *J Neurosci* 1985; 5:795–807.

62. Lund RD: Uncrossed visual pathways of hooded and albino rats. *Science* 1965; 149:1506–1507.

63. McCarty JW, Demer JL, Hovis LA, Nuwer MR: Ocular motility anomalies in developmental misdirection of the optic chiasm. *Am J Ophthalmol* 1992; 113:86–95.

64. Morland AB, Hoffmann MB, Neveu M, Holder GE: Abnormal visual projection in a human albino studied with functional magnetic resonance imaging and visual evoked potentials. *J Neurol Neruosurg Psychiatry* 2002; 72:523–526.

65. Robinson DA: A method of measuring eye movement using a scleral search coil in a magnetic field. *IEEE Trans Biomed Electronics* 1963; 10:137–145.

66. Roy MS, Milot JA, Polomeno RC, Barsoum-Homsy M: Ocular findings and visual evoked potential response in the Prader-Willi syndrome. *Can J Ophthalmol* 1992; 27:307–312.

67. Sanderson KJ, Guillery RW, Shackelford RM: Congenitally abnormal visual pathways in mink (Mustela vision) with reduced retinal pigment. *J Comp Neurol* 1974; 154:225–248.

68. Schmitz B, Schaefer T, Krick CM, Reith W, Backens M, Käsmann-Keller B: Configuration of the optic chiasm in humans with albinism as revealed by magnetic resonance imaging. *Invest Ophthalmol Vis Sci* 2003; 44:16–21.

69. Shallo-Hoffmann J, Apkarian P: Visual evoked response asymmetry only in the albino member of a family with congenital nystagmus. *Invest Ophthalmol Vis Sci* 1993; 34:682–689.

70. Shatz CJ, Kliot M: Prenatal misrouting of the retinogeniculate pathway in Siamese cats. *Nature* 1982; 300:525–529.

71. Silver J, Sapiro J: Axonal guidance during development of the optic nerve: The role of pigmented epithelia and other extrinsic factors. *J Comp Neurol* 1981; 202:521–538.

72. Strongin AC, Guillery RW: The distribution of melanin in the developing optic cup and stalk and its relation to cellular degeneration. *J Neurosci* 1981; 1:1193–1204.

73. Tang O, Williams RW, Goldowitz D: Mapping the achiasmatic mutation in the dog: A progress report [abstract]. *Soc Neurosci Abstr* 1994; 20:1504.

74. Taylor WOG: Visual disabilities of oculocutaneous albinism and their alleviation. *Trans Ophthalmol Soc UK* 1978; 98:423–445.

75. Tusa RJ, Zee DS, Hain TC, Simonsz HJ: Voluntary control of congenital nystagmus. *Clin Vis Sci* 1992; 7:195–210.

76. Varner JL, Peters JF, Ellingson RJ: Interhemispheric synchrony in the EEGs of full-term newborns. *Electroencephalogr Clin Neurophysiol* 1978; 45:641–647.

77. Versalius A: De humani corporis fabrica: Caput IIII. De primo nervorum a cerebro originem. In *Basileae*. Ioannis Oporini, 1543, pp 324–325.

78. Williams RW, Hogan D, Garraghty PE: Target recognition and visual maps in the thalamus of achiasmatic dogs [see comments]. *Nature* 1994; 367:637–639.

79. Witkop CJ Jr, Jay B, Creel D, Guillery RW: Optic and otic neurologic abnormalities in oculocutaneous and ocular albinism. *Birth Defects Orig Art Ser* 1982; 18:299–318.

80. Yee RD, Wong EK, Baloh RW, Honrubia V: A study of congential nystagmus: Waveforms. *Neurology* 1976; 26:326–333.

81. Zubcov AA, Fendick MG, Gottlob I, Wizov SS, Reinecke RD: Visual-evoked cortical potentials in dissociated vertical deviation. *Am J Ophthalmol* 1991; 112:714–722.

26 Clinical Psychophysical Techniques

KENNETH R. ALEXANDER

Visual psychophysics

INTRODUCTION: COMPARISON OF PSYCHOPHYSICAL AND ELECTROPHYSIOLOGICAL APPROACHES Electrophysiological procedures have proven to be of considerable value in assessing the functional properties of classes of neurons within the visual pathway in both normal visual systems and those with pathology. For example, the a-wave of the ERG has provided important information about the integrity of the rod and cone photoreceptors in retinal degenerations such as retinitis pigmentosa (RP).[46]

In many applications, the electrophysiological response represents the summed activity of neurons that are responding to stimuli covering a broad region of visual space. However, with the advent of focal and multifocal ERG and multifocal VEP techniques (reviewed by Hood[45]; see also chapter 14), it has become possible to record the electrical activity of neurons responding to stimuli that are presented within spatially delimited regions. Nevertheless, the ability to record specifically from spatially localized generators of electrophysiological responses remains somewhat limited, owing in part to the need to achieve adequate signal-to-noise ratios.

By comparison, psychophysical procedures can provide a measure of visual function within a quite small region of the visual field, with stimuli sometimes subtending less than 1 minute of visual angle. However, unlike electrophysiological responses, psychophysical responses represent the properties of the entire visual pathway, from photoreceptors to cortex. Furthermore, psychophysical measurements are subject to the potential influence of cognitive factors such as attention, and they are also dependent on the motor skills that are involved in producing a response.

Nevertheless, psychophysical procedures, particularly in combination with electrophysiological techniques, can provide important insights into the site and nature of defects within the visual pathway in disorders of the visual system. For example, Seiple and colleagues[92] investigated the retinal site of adaptation defects in patients with RP by comparing increment thresholds that were derived from psychophysics with those that were derived from the focal ERG. On the basis of similarities in the results obtained with the two approaches, they concluded that the adaptation defects shown by the patients with RP had an outer retinal locus.

As was discussed by Seiple et al.,[91] however, any direct comparison between psychophysical and electrophysiological procedures should consider a number of factors before firm conclusions can be drawn about the relationship with the disease process. These factors include the size and duration of the stimulus, the mechanism of response generation (whether the response is generated by the most sensitive unit or is the summed response of a number of units), the gain of the response, and the adaptation level. Additional discussions of the linking hypotheses or propositions that should be considered in specifying the relationship between psychophysical results and physiological states can be found in the work of Brindley,[16] Teller,[100] and Lee.[58]

FUNDAMENTAL CONCEPTS OF PSYCHOPHYSICS In current usage, the term *psychophysics* refers both to a set of methods and to a body of knowledge about the visual system that has been gathered with these methods. The general aim of psychophysical methods is to relate sensory states to the physical properties of visual stimuli in a quantitative manner. The physical properties of visual stimuli can be easily obtained through the appropriate instrumentation, such as photometers. Information about sensory states is less readily available. Observers typically communicate information about sensory states through a verbal response, such as "yes, those two lights look the same," or by a motor response, such as the press of a particular button or the reaction time to stimulus presentation.

It is important to note that sensory states can vary in either quantity or quality. Sensations that vary in quantity, such as brightness, are termed *prothetic*, and can be plotted on a scale of magnitude. For example, a light of $100\,cd/m^2$ presented in darkness appears to have a greater brightness than does a light of $10\,cd/m^2$ under the same conditions, and so brightness is considered to be a prothetic sensation. Sensations that vary in quality but not quantity, such as hue, are termed *metathetic* and cannot be plotted on a magnitude scale. For example, the hue "green" is neither more nor less in quantity than the hue "red," so no magnitude scale of hue is justified. However, both prothetic and metathetic sensations are amenable to psychophysical measurements.

The usual goal of a psychophysical experiment is to determine a person's threshold. The term *threshold* refers to the stimulus magnitude that provides a transition between two sensory states, either between "no sensation" and "sensation" or between two different sensations. In some applications, the outcome measure is termed *sensitivity*, which is the reciprocal of threshold.

In current usage, the threshold is not a fixed stimulus value but varies stochastically. That is, owing to various sources of variability, such as quantal fluctuations in the light output or intrinsic noise within the visual system, there is no one stimulus magnitude that forms the absolute boundary between two sensory states. Instead, stimuli that are near a certain value may be reported as "seen" on some occasions and not others. As a consequence, when one plots the percent of trials on which a stimulus is reported "seen" versus the values of the stimulus, the data typically form an S-shaped function rather than a function with an abrupt step at some particular stimulus value.

There are two general classes of thresholds: detection thresholds and difference thresholds. The detection or absolute threshold represents the minimum stimulation necessary to detect the presence of a stimulus. The difference or increment threshold refers to the change in visual stimulation that is necessary for the observer to discriminate between a test stimulus and a reference stimulus. Detection can be considered to be a special case of discrimination in which the reference stimulus has a value of zero.

A clinical example of a detection threshold is the quantal flux necessary for detecting a flash of light that is presented to the visual field periphery in dark-adapted perimetry. An example of a difference threshold can be found in the anomaloscope test of color vision defects. In this test, the observer's task is to determine whether a mixture of middle- and long-wavelength lights is different from a reference light of intermediate wavelength. Static perimetry is an additional example of the clinical application of the difference or increment threshold. In static perimetry, the observer's task is to discriminate a small flash of light (an increment) from the adapting field of the perimeter bowl.

CLASSICAL PSYCHOPHYSICAL TECHNIQUES   Three basic psychophysical methods for measuring thresholds were introduced by Gustav Fechner in the 1800s. Perhaps the most straightforward of these classical psychophysical techniques is the method of adjustment, in which the observer manipulates the test stimulus until it is just detectable or is just noticeably different from a reference stimulus. Typically, the threshold is defined as the mean of a series of such measurements. A variation of the method of adjustment is the tracking procedure, in which the observer continuously adjusts the stimulus to maintain it at a threshold level. Tracking has proven useful in measuring sensory events that change over time, such as the recovery of sensitivity following exposure to a bleaching light. Because the observer has direct control over the stimulus, however, the method of adjustment is open to potential artifacts. For example, the observer may adjust the stimulus by some fixed, arbitrary amount on each trial without regard to sensory events. Furthermore, the tracking method can be influenced by any changes that may occur in the observer's response criterion over time.

A second classical psychophysical procedure is the method of limits. In this procedure, the experimenter initially sets the stimulus to a value that is either below or above the estimated threshold and then alters the stimulus value in small steps until the observer signals that the stimulus has just been detected (ascending method) or that it has just disappeared (descending method). The threshold is defined as the mean of a series of such measurements. The method of limits has proven valuable in the clinical setting but is also vulnerable to artifacts. These include errors of habituation, in which the observer maintains the same response ("seen" or "not seen") from trial to trial without regard to sensory events, and errors of anticipation, in which the observer reports prematurely that the stimulus has become visible or has disappeared.

The third classical approach is the method of constant stimuli. In this technique, a fixed number of different test stimuli are presented whose values span the region of the estimated threshold in discrete steps. Each stimulus is presented the same number of times in a random order. The observer responds "seen" or "not seen" on each trial. The percentage "seen" is plotted for each stimulus value, resulting in a psychometric function, as illustrated in figure 26.1. The data are typically fit with an ogival function such as a cumulative normal distribution, or with a sigmoidal function, such as a logistic function or a Weibull function. The threshold is defined typically as the value that is reported "seen" on 50% of the trials. In the method of constant stimuli, catch trials are often used, in which no test stimulus is presented. If the observer responds that a stimulus was seen on such a trial, he or she is informed of the mistake and is urged to try harder.

SIGNAL DETECTION THEORY   Although the classical psychophysical techniques have proven useful in a clinical setting, it is apparent that they do not take into account the observer's response bias or criterion, which can have a substantial effect on the threshold estimate. An alternative approach is the set of methods derived from signal detection theory (SDT), in which there is no assumption of a sensory threshold. Instead, an emphasis is placed on the decision strategies that are employed by the observer, who is required

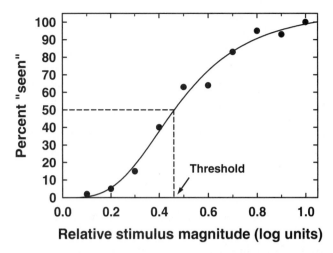

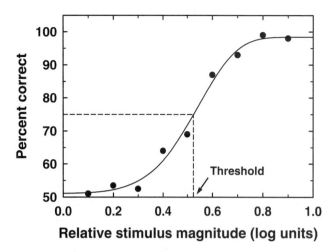

FIGURE 26.1 An example of a psychometric function derived from the method of constant stimuli, in which the percent of trials on which a stimulus was reported "seen" is plotted against the stimulus magnitude. The curve fit to the data points represents a logistic function. The threshold refers to the stimulus value that was reported "seen" on 50% of the trials, as derived from the fitted curve.

FIGURE 26.2 An example of a psychometric function derived from a two-alternative forced-choice procedure, in which the percent correct value is plotted for each stimulus value. The curve fit to the data points represents a Weibull function. The threshold refers to the stimulus value at which the observer was correct on 75% of the trials, as derived from the fitted curve.

to detect a signal in the presence of noise. The noise is usually considered to consist of some combination of external noise (outside the observer) and internal noise (within the observer). The SDT approach provides a way to separate an observer's actual sensitivity from his or her response criterion. It should be noted that the term *sensitivity* in this context refers to an observer's ability to discriminate a signal from noise, not to the reciprocal of threshold.

A standard SDT method is the "yes-no" procedure, in which there is a single observation period that contains either noise alone or a signal embedded in noise. An example of this approach is the detection of a grating patch (signal) that has been added to external white noise.[74] The observer responds either "yes," a signal was present, or "no," a signal was not present. Various values of the signal are presented across trials. For simplicity of analysis, it is often assumed that the probability density distributions of both the noise and the signal-plus-noise are Gaussian. In an analysis of the results, the two most important events are hits, in which the observer correctly responds that a signal was present, and false alarms, in which the observer reports that a signal was present when it was not.

For a given signal strength, a plot of hit rate versus false alarm rate yields a point on a function termed a *receiver operating characteristic (ROC) curve*. To generate an ROC curve with multiple points, the observer's criterion is usually manipulated by varying the payoffs associated with hits and false alarms and/or by varying the probability of signal presentation. The distance of the ROC curve from chance performance provides an index of the observer's sensitivity. Although it is an excellent method for distin-

guishing between an observer's sensitivity and his or her response criterion, the yes-no procedure is generally a time-consuming technique that has seen limited clinical application.

A related SDT procedure that has been widely used in the clinical setting is the forced-choice procedure. In this technique, the observer is presented with two or more observation intervals. These may be separated spatially (i.e., the test stimulus is presented at one of several possible test locations within the visual field) or temporally (i.e., the test stimulus is always presented at the same location but in one of two or more well-defined time periods). Only one of the observation intervals contains a signal, and the observer's task is to report the interval in which the signal occurred.

In the forced-choice procedure, a fixed set of stimulus values is presented multiple times across a series of trials, and the percentage correct value is derived for each stimulus magnitude. The percentage correct value is then plotted as a function of stimulus magnitude to derive a psychometric function, from which the observer's sensitivity can be derived. An example of a psychometric function derived from a two-alternative forced-choice (2AFC) procedure is given in figure 26.2.

A typical (although arbitrary) measure of sensitivity is the stimulus that results in a percentage correct value that lies halfway between chance performance and perfect performance. Chance performance, or the "guessing rate," is equal to $1/n$, where n is the number of alternatives (e.g., chance performance in a 2AFC procedure is 50%). The results of a 2AFC procedure are related quantitatively to those of a comparable yes-no procedure in that, for a given signal strength, the percentage correct value is equal to the area under the ROC curve.[31]

The forced-choice procedure is often termed *criterion free*, because it provides a way to measure an observer's sensitivity independent of the response criterion. The forced-choice method is not without potential drawbacks, however. First, it depends on an observer's cooperation. As an extreme example, a malingering observer might decide to respond incorrectly on some trials, thereby affecting the estimate of sensitivity. Frequently, an observer may be inattentive on a certain percentage of trials, which leads to a *lapsing rate*, or less-than-perfect performance at high stimulus values. Another potential drawback to the forced-choice procedure is that it is based on the idea of an unbiased observer, and this is not likely to be the case. Observers tend to exhibit nonrandom behavior, such as an avoidance of long strings of identical responses, even though these can occur statistically. Observers may also have a position bias in a spatial forced-choice procedure or an interval bias in a temporal forced-choice procedure such that they tend to prefer one response interval over another. In addition, observers may become confused by the number of possible choices if there are more than two alternatives.

In the forced-choice approach, certain observers, especially patients, may be unwilling to give a response when they are certain that they see nothing or when they feel that they cannot discriminate between alternatives. Consequently, an "unforced-choice" method has been proposed, in which the response "I don't know" is allowed. The properties of the unforced-choice procedure have been analyzed statistically,[50,53] and it has been shown that under certain conditions, this technique can have advantages over the standard forced-choice approach.

One of the useful concepts derived from SDT is that of the "ideal observer." An ideal observer is one who has access to all the information that is present in the stimulus. The stimulus can be defined either as a distal stimulus (before it has entered the eye) or, more commonly, as a proximal stimulus (one that has been subjected to some degree of optical and/or neural processing). The efficiency of human performance can then be derived from a comparison of the results of an actual human observer with that of the ideal observer. This approach has been applied to a wide variety of visual tasks, ranging from simple two-point discrimination,[36] in which the optical and photoreceptoral properties of the eye are taken into account, to complex tasks such as reading,[60] in which visual, lexical, and oculomotor sources of information are included.

ADAPTIVE PSYCHOPHYSICAL TECHNIQUES The classical psychophysical methods and those of SDT tend to be time-consuming and inefficient, because they typically present a set of stimuli that span a range of values, from those that are

non-detectable to those that are detected with a high degree of probability. A more efficient strategy is to concentrate on stimulus values that lie near the presumed threshold. This is the approach taken by adaptive psychophysical procedures. In adaptive psychophysics, the stimulus to be presented on a given trial depends on the observer's prior responses. An example of a simple adaptive technique is the tracking method, described earlier. A number of different adaptive psychophysical procedures have been devised that use various decision rules to guide the stimulus choice on any given trial. An excellent historical overview of these adaptive procedures has been given by Leek.[59]

Adaptive procedures can be divided into two general categories: those that are parametric, in which there is an explicit assumption about the nature of the underlying psychometric function, and those that are non-parametric, in which there is no particular assumption about the psychometric function except that it is monotonic with stimulus magnitude. Non-parametric techniques are generally variations of the staircase method, which is related in turn to the tracking method. In the simplest staircase procedure, a response of "seen" (or a correct response in a forced-choice procedure) results in a decrease in stimulus magnitude on the subsequent trial. A response of "not seen" (or an incorrect response in a forced-choice procedure) results in an increase in the stimulus magnitude.

This conceptually simple "up-down" staircase approach has not proven effective, however. For example, a "seen/not seen" staircase is subject to changes in an observer's response criterion over time, just as is the tracking procedure. Furthermore, in a 2AFC staircase, the observer will be correct on 50% of the trials by chance alone, independent of the detectability of the stimulus. Therefore, chance plays too large a role in governing the decision as to whether to increase or decrease the step in the simple up-down forced-choice staircase.

As a result of these inadequacies, the simple up-down staircase was replaced by the transformed up-down staircase.[63] In the transformed staircase, the stimulus value to be presented on a given trial depends on the outcome of more trials than just the preceding one. In deciding which stimulus value to use on each trial, a number of different decision rules can be applied. A common rule is the "two-down, one-up" decision rule. According to this rule, two consecutive correct responses are required before the stimulus magnitude can be decreased, whereas only one incorrect response is sufficient to increase the stimulus magnitude. An illustration of a forced-choice staircase using a "three-down, one-up" decision rule is given in figure 26.3. Different staircase decision rules can be used to estimate specific points on a psychometric function.[63] For example, the "two-down, one-up" rule provides an estimate of the 70.7% correct point. Staircase procedures often use step sizes that are equivalent for the

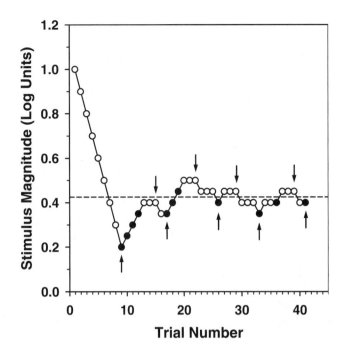

FIGURE 26.3 An illustration of an up-down transformed staircase based on a two-alternative forced-choice procedure, with the stimulus magnitude plotted for each trial. The staircase used a "one-down, one-up" decision rule until the first reversal was reached. Subsequently, a "three-down, one-up" decision rule was used, in which three consecutive correct responses were required to decrease the stimulus value by one step, whereas a single incorrect response was sufficient to increase the stimulus value by one step. The open circles represent correct responses; the solid circles represent incorrect responses. The arrows indicate the staircase reversal points. The dashed line represents the threshold, which was defined as the mean of the last six reversal points.

upward and downward directions, but some advantages of using asymmetrical steps (larger up than down) have been discussed by Garcia-Perez.[34]

In the staircase approach, sensitivity is often defined as the mean of a number of staircase reversal points, as illustrated in figure 26.3. Sensitivity can also be derived by fitting a psychometric function to the complete data set by using a maximum likelihood procedure and then obtaining the stimulus magnitude that corresponds to a particular percentage correct value. A discussion of the relative merits of these two approaches has been provided by Klein.[53]

In addition to the transformed staircase, non-parametric staircase approaches include parameter estimation by sequential testing (PEST),[99] which uses a heuristic set of rules to define the step size, with the staircase terminating when the step size reaches a predefined value, and the modified binary search (MOBS),[102] which uses a bisection method to define the step size. The parametric approach is typified by QUEST,[104] in which the stimulus value on a given trial is based on the most probable estimate of sensitivity as derived

from a Bayesian statistical analysis of the results of previous trials. In QUEST, the underlying psychometric function is assumed to correspond to a Weibull function. A comprehensive, quantitative analysis of the various parametric and non-parametric adaptive techniques and their advantages and disadvantages has been provided by Treutwein.[101]

Because of their relative efficiency, adaptive psychophysical techniques have seen widespread use in the clinical setting. One common application is in static perimetry, in which the goal is the rapid, accurate assessment of increment thresholds at multiple locations throughout the visual field. Some of the adaptive algorithms that are commonly used in commercial static perimeters have been discussed by Johnson.[49]

Interactive examples of some of the psychophysical methods described in the preceding sections can be found on the CD-ROM that accompanies the textbook on sensation and perception by Levine.[62]

SUPRATHRESHOLD PSYCHOPHYSICAL TECHNIQUES Although psychophysical procedures are used primarily to derive thresholds, much of sensory experience results from suprathreshold stimulation. The assessment of visual responses to suprathreshold stimulation is readily performed using electrophysiological procedures, such as the measurement of an ERG luminance-response function. However, the assessment of visual responses to suprathreshold stimuli is problematic for psychophysical techniques. Nevertheless, sensory scaling procedures have been developed, in large part by S. S. Stevens, that can potentially assess the suprathreshold properties of the human visual system (reviewed by Marks and Gescheider[70]).

One approach to sensory scaling is the method of magnitude estimation, in which an observer is asked to assign a number to the magnitude of the sensory experience that is elicited by a stimulus presentation. The technique of magnitude production has also been used, in which the observer manipulates the stimulus value in order to generate sensory events of particular magnitudes. The stipulation in both magnitude estimation and magnitude production is that the assigned numbers or stimulus settings reflect the magnitude of sensory experience on a ratio scale (i.e., this light is twice as bright as that one). From such techniques, it is possible to derive a scale of the relationship between stimulus magnitude (S) and sensation magnitude (R). Experiments of this nature have typically reported a power law relationship between these two variables:

$$R = kS^n \qquad (1)$$

in which k is a constant of proportionality and n is an exponent that varies with the sensory modality. Psychophysical methods for sensory scaling have found limited application in the clinical setting but have proven useful in specialized circumstances, such as in characterizing the nature of suprathreshold contrast perception in amblyopia.[65]

CLINICAL APPLICATIONS OF PSYCHOPHYSICAL METHODOLOGY
Psychophysical methods are of considerable interest in their own right, but they are also of immense practical value in the clinical setting by virtue of their ability to provide important information about disease processes that is not readily available by other means. For this reason, psychophysical techniques have long played a key role in the clinical evaluation of various forms of visual deficits, whether applied informally, as in the measurement of Snellen visual acuity or, more formally, as in the sophisticated adaptive algorithms used in commercial static perimetry. The aim has generally been to provide information about the characteristics, time course, and underlying pathophysiology of visual system disorders, which is useful in patient management and in determining whether visual disorders are amenable to therapeutic intervention.

It has become increasingly apparent, however, that the traditional clinical psychophysical tests such as those of visual acuity and perimetry might not reveal the full extent of damage in disorders of the visual system.[83] As an example, people with melanoma-associated retinopathy, a form of night blindness associated with a malignant skin cancer, have normal visual acuity but a substantial reduction in their sensitivity to motion that is not apparent on standard clinical vision tests.[106] Therefore, new clinical psychophysical approaches are being developed that take into account the fact that the visual system consists of parallel pathways that may be differentially vulnerable to ocular disease processes.

A number of different parallel pathways have been identified in electrophysiological recordings from the primate visual system, and it is generally assumed that these pathways are applicable to human vision as well. Examples include the red-green and blue-yellow chromatic pathways for spectral coding;[25] the ON and OFF pathways, which code information about light increments and decrements, respectively;[89] the magnocellular and parvocellular pathways, which have different contrast coding properties as well as other distinctive features;[51] and dorsal and ventral streams, which are thought to process information about "where" an object is in space and "what" it is, respectively.[71]

These multiple processing streams can be viewed as consisting of sets of filters or analyzers that extract specific types of information from the visual environment.[38,83] Traditionally, standard clinical psychophysical procedures have tended to emphasize only first-order analyzers, which encode luminance variations, while neglecting other types of analyzers, such as the second-order system that responds to local variations in contrast or texture.[66]

By choosing the appropriate stimuli and visual tasks, it is possible to emphasize specific visual subsystems to test for "hidden" losses that are not readily apparent by standard clinical psychophysical procedures. As an example of this approach, patients with glaucoma were tested with specialized perimetric procedures that consisted of red-on-white increments, blue-on-white increments, and critical flicker frequency.[73] The goal was to evaluate relative sensitivity losses within a red-green chromatic mechanism, a "blue-on" chromatic mechanism, and an achromatic temporal mechanism, respectively. Chromatic defects were more apparent than achromatic defects in the glaucoma patients, emphasizing the need to test for specific pathway deficits in patients with ocular disease.

In summary, a wide variety of psychophysical procedures have been developed by which to evaluate and understand visual function, of both visually normal individuals and those with visual system disorders. The psychophysical method of choice in any given situation depends ultimately on trade-offs among a number of different factors, including the necessity for the control of the observer's criterion, the efficiency of the threshold estimation procedure, the cost in terms of the observer's and experimenter's time, and the nature of the visual task. Applied optimally, clinical psychophysical techniques provide a powerful noninvasive means for defining the pathophysiology of visual system disorders and for assessing the impact of potential treatment methods.

Duplicity theory

It has been well established that human vision is mediated by two classes of photoreceptor systems: rods and cones.[28] This has been termed the *duplicity theory*, although it is more an experimentally validated fact than a theory. The rod system functions optimally under conditions of dim (scotopic) illumination but provides no way to discriminate among wavelengths of light and has relatively poor spatial and temporal resolution. The cone system is optimized for relatively high (photopic) light levels, is less sensitive to light than the rod system, but provides good spatial and temporal resolution and mediates color vision. It should be noted that the terms *scotopic* and *photopic* are used in reference both to the receptor system that mediates vision and to the level of illumination, regardless of receptor type. This potential ambiguity of usage is further complicated by the term *mesopic*, which refers to intermediate light levels. Under mesopic conditions, it is possible that both rod and cone systems can mediate vision, depending on such factors as stimulus wavelength and size.

The human retina contains a single type of rod photoreceptor, with rhodopsin as its visual pigment (other vertebrates may have more than one type of rod photoreceptor[28]).

There are three types of cone photoreceptors in the human visual system, which differ in the spectral absorption characteristics of their photopigments.[90] The spatial density of rods and cones varies with eccentricity and meridian.[24] The peak spatial density for rods occurs at approximately 15 degrees of eccentricity. The peak spatial density for middle- (M) and long-wavelength-sensitive (L) cones occurs in the foveal center. The peak spatial density for short-wavelength-sensitive (S) cones occurs at approximately 1 degree of eccentricity, with an absence in the foveal center.[26] The luminosity functions for rod and cone systems differ considerably, which results in a noticeable change in the apparent brightness of spectral lights ("Purkinje shift") as the visual system shifts from rod-dominant vision to cone-dominant vision or vice versa.

An important consideration in assessing the response properties of rod and cone systems, both in visually normal individuals and in those with visual disorders, is that information transfer within the visual pathway is limited both by the properties of the photoreceptors and by those of the postreceptoral network into which the photoreceptor signals feed. Suction electrode recordings from individual primate photoreceptors have shown that the cone photoreceptor response to a light flash is faster than that of rod photoreceptors, while the rods are somewhat more sensitive to light,[11] so some of the functional differences between rod and cone systems appear to be related to the properties of the photoreceptors themselves. However, the great differences between rod- and cone-mediated vision are due to a considerable extent to synaptic and postsynaptic influences on the visual signals. These postreceptoral processes play a large role in limiting the response properties of the rod and cone systems. As an example, there is now substantial evidence from anatomy, physiology, psychophysics, and electroretinography that there are two primary rod pathways.[93] A sensitive "slow" rod pathway involves signal transmission from rod photoreceptors to ganglion cells via the rod bipolar cells, AII amacrine cells, and ON and OFF cone bipolar cells. An insensitive "fast" rod pathway involves signal transmission from rod photoreceptors to the cone pathway via gap junctions between rods and cones. These two rod pathways are likely responsible for the duplex critical flicker frequency (CFF) function of the rod system that is found not only in visually normal individuals,[20,21] but also in rod monochromats.[43] Thus, the evidence indicates that the limited temporal resolution that is often thought to characterize the rod system results in large part from postreceptoral limitations on signal processing. Similarly, the relatively poor temporal resolution of the S cone system[105] also appears to result from postreceptoral constraints, because the temporal response properties of the S cone photoreceptors do not differ from those of the M and L cone photoreceptors.[11]

It has sometimes been assumed that rod and cone systems function independently. However, there is a large body of evidence that the sensitivity of one system can be modified significantly by the other.[12,56] Interactions between rod and cone systems are often most apparent when stimuli are small and/or temporally modulated. Rod-cone interactions can be observed in ERG recordings[5,88] as well as psychophysically. There appear to be several fundamentally different types of rod-cone interactions with different underlying mechanisms.[27,56]

Dark adaptometry

It is well known that following the eye's exposure to a bright light, visual sensitivity requires a substantial period of time to recover. If the light exposure is sufficiently intense, complete recovery can take as long as 45–50 minutes.[79] The typical time course of dark adaptation is illustrated in figure 26.4. This bleaching recovery curve was measured in the peripheral retina of a normal individual by using a test flash of 500 nm, a wavelength to which both rod and cone systems are sensitive. Thresholds are plotted relative to those measured in the completely dark-adapted state before exposure to a bleaching light.

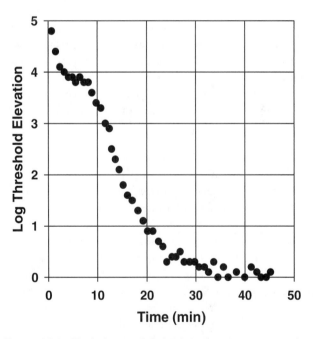

FIGURE 26.4 Typical normal dark adaptation curve measured at 20 degrees in the nasal visual field using a 500-nm, 1.7-degree, 500-ms test flash following a 2-minute exposure to a full-field bleaching light of 3.6 log cd·m^{-2}. Thresholds are plotted relative to their dark-adapted (prebleach) value. A transition between cone-mediated and rod-mediated detection (rod-cone break) occurs at about 10 minutes. Complete recovery of the rod system typically requires approximately 45 minutes.

The dark adaptation curve in figure 26.4 follows a characteristic two-branched course, with an inflection occurring at approximately 10 minutes. In accordance with duplicity theory, the early branch represents the recovery of cone system sensitivity. Thresholds measured during the later branch are mediated by the rod system, and the inflection point is termed the rod-cone break (*Kohlrausch knick*). Consequently, as dark adaptation proceeds, a chromatic test flash initially appears colored and later appears colorless as detection shifts to the rod system.

The difference between the absolute (colorless) threshold and the threshold for color has been termed the *photochromatic interval*. The threshold for color does not correspond exactly with the cone detection threshold, because the rod system can influence the threshold for color.[2,64,96] This type of rod-cone interaction has been attributed variously to a desaturation of the chromatic cone signal by an achromatic rod signal[64] and to a rod-induced shift in the balance of color-opponent cells,[97] most likely involving nonlinear processes.[18]

To a first approximation, the dark adaptation curves of the rod and cone systems may be quantified according to the following exponential equation:

$$\log I_t = A + B \exp[-(t - t_r)/\tau] \qquad (2)$$

in which I_t is the threshold at any given time t during dark adaptation; t_r is either 0 (for the cone portion) or the time of the rod-cone break (for the rod portion); and A, B, and τ are free parameters.[79] This equation provides a quantitative description of dark adaptation that can be helpful in the clinical assessment of abnormalities in the time course of bleaching recovery. However, significant departures from this relationship have been noted for both the rod[54,72] and cone[7,17,32] systems.

MECHANISMS OF DARK ADAPTATION   The recovery of sensitivity following light exposure depends ultimately on the regeneration of bleached photopigment.[75] For example, if the concentration of photopigment within the photoreceptors is reduced through vitamin A deprivation, then the time course of psychophysical dark adaptation is prolonged, and thresholds may never reach normal levels.[52,76] In addition, there is a general correspondence between the time course of rhodopsin regeneration and the rate of return of rod system sensitivity.[85] Yet psychophysical dark adaptation is not due simply to the recovery of a light absorber. That is, when 90% of rhodopsin has regenerated following an intense bleach, the rod threshold remains elevated by about 2 log units,[54,72] although the threshold elevation due to a reduced quantal catch would be only approximately 0.1 log unit.

Despite decades of study, uncertainty still remains about the exact biochemical events that are responsible for the desensitization of the rod system following a bleach and for the subsequent recovery of rod sensitivity (for an extensive review, see Lamb and Pugh[55]). It is likely that various bleaching intermediates, such as metarhodopsin products and "free" opsin, activate the visual cascade that leads to the loss of visual sensitivity. The recovery of sensitivity then depends on the removal or inactivation of these bleaching intermediates, as well as the return of 11-*cis* retinal from the retinal pigment epithelium to the rod photoreceptor outer segments.[33,55,61]

To complicate matters, there is considerable evidence that postreceptoral as well as photoreceptoral processes are involved in the recovery of sensitivity during dark adaptation. First, changes in test flash size can influence the shape of the dark adaptation curve,[6,14,85] although test size should have no influence on the rate of photopigment regeneration. The concept of an "adaptation pool" was introduced by Rushton[86] to account for the observations that changes in sensitivity appear to result from the pooling of signals from many photoreceptors. Second, dim lights that bleach a trivial amount of photopigment and that have no effect on the receptor potential or on horizontal cell responses in the skate retina nevertheless result in an elevation of b-wave and ganglion cell thresholds that requires several minutes to recover.[39] It has been proposed that threshold elevations observed following weak bleaches and/or early in the course of dark adaptation result from non-photoreceptoral or "network" mechanisms, whereas threshold elevations observed later in the course of dark adaptation result from "photochemical" processes occurring within the photoreceptors (reviewed by Dowling[28]).

Although the recovery of sensitivity during dark adaptation is thought to depend primarily on events that occur within the retina of the bleached eye, binocular interactions during dark adaptation have been reported. For example, the time course of dark adaptation for a test flash that is presented to one eye is affected by the presence of a small, dim light presented to the nontested eye during bleaching recovery.[57,68] Furthermore, rod thresholds during bleaching recovery can be lowered by pressure-blinding the dark-adapted, nontested eye.[68] In addition, the rod absolute threshold for a test flash that is presented to one eye can be reduced by intense long-wavelength adaptation of the contralateral eye.[82] To account for these findings, it has been proposed that the dark-adapted, nontested eye generates noise that interferes with detection.[68,82]

In addition to a recovery of sensitivity, other phenomena accompany the dark adaptation process. After the offset of a bleaching light, the pupil is initially constricted, and then, following a transient series of oscillations, it dilates with a time course similar to that of the recovery of rod sensitivity.[4] Following the offset of a bleaching light, an afterimage may be apparent, which then fades over time. The initial afterimage, which typically appears colored, originates from the cone system. If the bleaching exposure is of high intensity, particularly in aphakic individuals, erythropsia may result, in which the visual environment appears to be tinged with red. A prolonged, colorless afterimage that originates from the rod system[67] is also often visible. It has been suggested that the rod afterimage is related to the noisy residual excitation of photoreceptors that has been observed following the cessation of an adapting light.[11]

The apparent correlation between the disappearance of the rod afterimage and the recovery of rod sensitivity gave rise to the concept of the *equivalent background*,[10,98] according to which bleached photoreceptors produce a continuing signal in darkness that reduces the detectability of a test flash. The basis for this equivalent background of "dark light" may be the presence of bleaching intermediates such as metarhodopsin products and opsin that act like real light in activating the G-protein cascade. Although real light and dark light have many similar properties, they are not always identical, however.[35,61]

FACTORS AFFECTING DARK ADAPTATION In the measurement of dark adaptation, the parameters of the test flash have a marked effect on the nature of the recovery curve. One of the primary factors is the test stimulus wavelength, as illustrated in figure 26.5. This figure presents dark adaptation curves obtained from a visually normal subject using

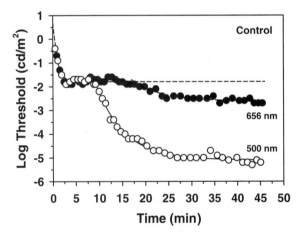

FIGURE 26.5 Dark adaptation curves for a visually normal observer using 500-nm (open circles) and 656-nm (solid circles) test flashes, with bleaching and test conditions equivalent to those of figure 26.4. The solid line through the open circles represents the best fit of Equation (2) to the rod-mediated portion. This curve has been shifted vertically to fit the filled circles. The dashed curve represents the fit of Equation (2) to the thresholds during the cone plateau. Because the data are plotted in photopic units, thresholds for the two chromatic stimuli are identical during the cone plateau. The curves subsequently diverge, and the magnitude of the threshold difference between the curves indicates that both curves represent rod-mediated thresholds. The rod-cone break occurs later in time for the 656-nm test flash than for the 500-nm test flash.

a middle-wavelength (open circles) and a long-wavelength (solid circles) test flash. It is apparent that the test flash wavelength influences the time of the transition from cone-mediated to rod-mediated detection (rod-cone break). With a middle-wavelength test flash, the transition occurs at approximately 10 minutes under these conditions. For a long-wavelength test flash, there is an extended cone plateau, and the rod-cone break occurs considerably later in the course of bleaching recovery.

The change in the time course of the rod-cone break is predictable from the relative sensitivity of the rod system to the two wavelengths of test flash. This is illustrated by the solid line through the filled circles in figure 26.5. This is the same curve that was fit to the open circles, but it was shifted vertically in proportion to the differential sensitivity of the rod system to the long-wavelength versus the middle-wavelength test flash. Although it is often assumed that the threshold for a long-wavelength test flash is cone-mediated in the retinal periphery, this is not necessarily the case. Large, long-wavelength test stimuli can be detected by the rod system in the periphery following complete dark adaptation, as shown in figure 26.5.

Although not illustrated in figure 26.5, the characteristics of cone-system dark adaptation are also influenced by the wavelength of the test flash. If a short-wavelength test flash is used to measure dark adaptation following a long-wavelength bleaching light, the cone-mediated portion of the recovery curve typically has two branches. The first branch represents detection by the short-wavelength cone system; the second branch is mediated by the middle-wavelength cone system.[7] Even when dark adaptation is measured with a test stimulus that is detected solely by the long-wavelength cone system, recovery does not necessarily proceed along a single exponential time course. Temporary plateaus and losses of cone system sensitivity are observed that have been attributed to the influence of postreceptoral mechanisms.[17,32]

The retinal locus of the test flash also has an important influence on the nature of the dark adaptation curve.[42] A small test flash that is presented to the fovea typically results in a dark adaptation curve that is cone-mediated throughout bleaching recovery. As illustrated in figure 26.5, a test flash that is presented to the parafovea can be detected by either the cone system or the rod system, depending on test flash and bleaching parameters and the time during recovery at which the threshold is measured.

Although it is often assumed that detection is mediated either by the rod system or the cone system independently, evidence for rod-cone interactions during dark adaptation has been presented. For example, the foveal cone threshold has been observed to fall slightly during the later part of dark adaptation, an effect that has been attributed to the influence of the rod system.[29] Furthermore, during the later part of the cone plateau in the peripheral retina, threshold variability may increase, and the cone-mediated threshold may rise slightly, effects that have been attributed to the influence of the rod system.[107]

Bleaching parameters can also have a marked effect on the time course of dark adaptation. One important consideration is the wavelength of the bleaching light. Short wavelengths are more effective than long wavelengths in desensitizing the rod system. Therefore, short-wavelength bleaches result in a longer cone plateau with a more distinct rod-cone break. Long-wavelength bleaches affect primarily the cone system, so the rod-cone break occurs relatively early in bleaching recovery or may be absent altogether, with thresholds being rod-mediated throughout dark adaptation.

The duration and intensity of the bleaching light also have an important effect on dark adaptation. The relationship between p, the fraction of unbleached pigment, and t, the bleaching time measured in seconds, has been described by the following relationship:

$$-\frac{dp}{dt} = \frac{pI}{Q} - \frac{(1-p)}{t_0} \tag{3}$$

where I is the retinal illuminance in trolands (either photopic or scotopic, as appropriate), Q is the energy of the pulsed stimulus (in td·s) required to bleach p from 1 to $1/e$ (photosensitivity), and t_0 is the time constant of regeneration in seconds.[3,44] For the rod system, $Q = 1.57 \cdot 10^7$ scotopic td·s and $t_0 = 519\,s$; for the cone system, $Q = 5.0 \cdot 10^6$ photopic td·s and $t_0 = 130\,s$.[108] However, significant departures from this first-order kinetic equation have been observed.[15,22,84,95]

For relatively brief bleaching lights (e.g., less than 45 s for the rod system), there is a reciprocal relationship between light energy and duration,[87] such that p depends on It_0 in td·s:

$$\log(\log 1/p) = \log(It_0) - \log Q \tag{4}$$

For longer bleaching lights, for which significant photopigment regeneration has occurred, the relationship can be described as

$$p = I_0/(I + I_0), \tag{5}$$

where $I_0 = Q/t_0$.[3] An extremely brief (microsecond to millisecond range), high-intensity flash does not have the same bleaching effect as does a longer-duration light that delivers an identical total number of quanta. This phenomenon, which has been termed *Rushton's paradox*,[79] results from photoreversal, in which the absorption of some of the incident quanta by bleaching intermediates reisomerizes the photopigment.[40] Photoreversal occurs primarily with short-wavelength bleaching lights, and it increases the quantal catching capacity of the photoreceptors, thereby potentially contributing to retinal light damage.[41]

If the bleaching light is relatively weak, there is a rapid recovery of sensitivity following light offset that has been termed *early dark adaptation*,[9] or *Crawford masking*.[23] Depending on the adapting level and the photoreceptor system that is involved, the recovery of sensitivity can require only a few milliseconds or as much as a few minutes. Under certain conditions, the threshold elevation at the offset of the adapting field is substantially greater than would be expected from the extent of photopigment bleaching.[87] It is likely that the temporal dynamics of sensitivity changes during early light and dark adaptation depend in large part on the contrast-response properties of postreceptoral pathways.[78]

It is typically the case that sensitivity begins to recover immediately following the offset of an adapting light. However, under certain conditions, thresholds may become transiently elevated rather than reduced during the initial period of dark adaptation. An example is transient tritanopia, in which the cone system threshold for a short-wavelength test flash is elevated transiently following the offset of a yellow adapting field.[8,80] Similar results can be observed under other conditions of chromatic adaptation.[81] Transient tritanopia is thought to represent the action of a "restoring force" that temporarily elevates the threshold by driving a postreceptoral opponent mechanism to a polarized state.[80] Because transient tritanopia can be observed in the b-wave of the primate ERG,[103] the site of the chromatic interaction appears to be at or distal to the generators of the photopic b-wave, which are thought to be the retinal bipolar cells.[94]

CLINICAL EVALUATION OF DARK ADAPTATION   For the clinical measurement of dark adaptation, the most widely used instrument has been the Goldmann-Weekers Dark Adaptometer, but this device currently has limited availability. An alternative, commercially available instrument is the SST-1 Scotopic Sensitivity Tester (LKC Technologies). A comparison of these two instruments has been provided by Peters et al.[77] In addition, perimeters such as the Humphrey Field Analyzer (Carl Zeiss Meditech) can be modified to evaluate dark adaptation,[19] but an appropriate bleaching source is also necessary.

An informal test of dark adaptation is the macular photostress recovery test.[69] In this procedure, visual acuity is first measured by conventional procedures, and then the macula is exposed to a bright light, such as that from a direct ophthalmoscope. The patient is then asked to read the acuity chart again, and the time that is required to return to within one line of the prebleach visual acuity is measured. It has been suggested that this technique can differentiate between macular disease and disorders of the optic nerve,[37] but the interpretation of results is complicated by the wide range of normal findings.[69]

In the clinical evaluation of dark adaptation abnormalities, it is important to distinguish between threshold elevations per se and delays in the time course of bleaching recovery. Some diseases that affect the photoreceptors

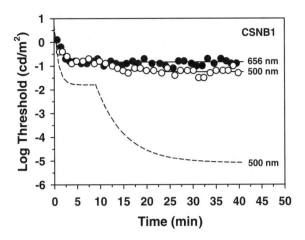

FIGURE 26.6 Dark adaptation curves for an individual with the complete form of congenital stationary night blindness, measured under conditions similar to those described in figure 26.5. The use of chromatic test flashes distinguishes between rod- and cone-mediated thresholds. Thresholds for the 656-nm test flash are cone-mediated throughout dark adaptation. Thresholds for the 500-nm test flash are rod-mediated after approximately 10 minutes, but are elevated substantially above normal (dashed line, replotted from figure 26.5). Despite the extreme elevation of the rod-mediated thresholds, the rod-cone break occurs at about the normal time.

and/or retinal pigment epithelium can result in threshold elevations without an accompanying abnormality in the time course of dark adaptation, whereas other disorders of the outer retina may be accompanied by delayed bleaching recovery. Without a measurement of prebleach thresholds, it may be difficult to distinguish between these two alternatives.[1] Furthermore, it is important to compare dark adaptation results obtained from patients with the results from control subjects of equivalent ages, because aging can result in a delay of the recovery of rod sensitivity.[47]

In assessing the time course of dark adaptation, it is of value to identify the photoreceptor system that mediates detection thresholds in order to determine whether a dark adaptation abnormality is specific to the rod or cone system. For this purpose, dark adaptation should be measured with at least two wavelengths of test flash to which the rod and cone systems have markedly different sensitivities. For example, figure 26.6 shows dark adaptation curves measured at 20 degrees in the nasal visual field of an individual with the "complete" form of congenital stationary night blindness (CSNB1) (see Alexander et al.[2] for patient characteristics). During the first few minutes of dark adaptation, the superimposition of the data points for the two wavelengths of test flash indicates that thresholds are cone-mediated for this patient during this period. Thresholds for the long-wavelength test flash (solid circles) then remain constant throughout the remainder of bleaching recovery. However, at the normal time of the rod-cone break (approximately 10 minutes, as shown by the dashed line), thresholds for the

middle-wavelength test flash (open circles) show a slight decline for this patient.

The small but consistent difference between the thresholds for the two wavelengths of the test flash during the later portion of dark adaptation indicates that thresholds for the middle-wavelength test flash are rod-mediated at the end of bleaching recovery, although the threshold is elevated by approximately 4 log units above normal. Without such a comparison, it might have been concluded erroneously that thresholds obtained with the middle-wavelength test flash represented a delayed recovery of cone sensitivity. Furthermore, anomalous plateaux that have the action spectrum of rods can occur during the course of dark adaptation following small bleaches.[19] Without an evaluation of spectral sensitivity, it might be thought that these plateaux represented delayed rod-cone breaks.

TREATMENT FOR DEFECTS IN DARK ADAPTATION The administration of vitamin A can be effective in treating abnormalities of dark adaptation in people with vitamin A deficiency due to systemic conditions, such as Crohn's disease.[52] Nutritional approaches have also been successful in treating some forms of retinal degeneration that are accompanied by disturbances in dark adaptation, such as Sorsby's fundus dystrophy.[13,48] The development of other potential approaches to treating dark adaptation abnormalities is being facilitated by the rapid advances in identifying the molecular genetic basis of such night blinding disorders as fundus albipunctatus and Oguchi disease.[30,55] Nevertheless, complete success in treating the various disturbances in bleaching recovery that can occur in patients with retinal diseases will require a more comprehensive understanding of the complex photochemical and neural events that govern the dark adaptation process, not only in the rod system, but in the cone system as well.

REFERENCES

1. Alexander KR, Fishman GA: Prolonged rod dark adaptation in retinitis pigmentosa. *Br J Ophthalmol* 1984; 68:561–569.
2. Alexander KR, Fishman GA, Derlacki DJ: Mechanisms of rod-cone interaction: Evidence from congenital stationary nightblindness. *Vision Res* 1988; 28:575–583.
3. Alpern M: Rhodopsin kinetics in the human eye. *J Physiol* 1971; 217:447–471.
4. Alpern M, Ohba N: The effect of bleaching and background on pupil size. *Vision Res* 1972; 12:943–951.
5. Arden GB, Frumkes TE: Stimulation of rods can increase cone flicker ERGs in man. *Vision Res* 1986; 26:711–721.
6. Arden GB, Weale RA: Nervous mechanisms and dark adaptation. *J Physiol* 1954; 125:417–426.
7. Auerbach E, Wald G: The participation of different types of cones in human light and dark adaptation. *Am J Ophthalmol* 1955; 39:24–40.
8. Augenstein E, Pugh EN Jr: The dynamics of the pi-1 colour mechanism: Further evidence for two sites of adaptation. *J Physiol* 1977; 176:56–72.

9. Baker HD: Initial stages of light and dark adaptation. *J Opt Soc Am* 1963; 53:98–103.

10. Barlow HB, Sparrock JMB: The role of afterimages in dark adaptation. *Science* 1964; 144:1309–1314.

11. Baylor DA: Photoreceptor signals and vision. *Invest Ophthalmol Vis Sci* 1987; 28:34–49.

12. Benimoff NI, Schneider S, Hood DC: Interactions between rod and cone channels above threshold: A test of various models. *Vision Res* 1982; 22:1133–1140.

13. Berson EL: Nutrition and retinal degenerations. *Int Ophthalmol Clin* 2000; 40:93–111.

14. Blakemore CB, Rushton WAH: The rod increment threshold during dark adaptation in normal and rod monochromat. *J Physiol* 1965; 181:629–640.

15. Bonds AB, MacLeod DIA: The bleaching and regeneration of rhodopsin in the cat. *J Physiol* 1974; 242:237–253.

16. Brindley G: *Physiology of the Retina and Visual Pathways*, ed 2. Baltimore, Williams and Wilkins, 1970.

17. Brown AM: Dark adaptation of the long-wavelength sensitive cones. *Vision Res* 1983; 23:837–843.

18. Buck SL, Knight RF, Bechtold J: Opponent-color models and the influence of rod signals on the loci of unique hues. *Vision Res* 2000; 40:3333–3344.

19. Cideciyan AV, Pugh EN Jr, Lamb TD, Huang Y, Jacobson SG: Plateaux during dark adaptation in Sorsby's fundus dystrophy and vitamin A deficiency. *Invest Ophthalmol Vis Sci* 1997; 38:1786–1794.

20. Conner JD: The temporal properties of rod vision. *J Physiol* 1982; 332:139–155.

21. Conner JD, MacLeod DIA: Rod photoreceptors detect rapid flicker. *Science* 1977; 195:698–699.

22. Coolen ACC, van Norren D: Kinetics of human cone photopigments explained with a Rushton-Henry model. *Biol Cybern* 1988; 58:123–128.

23. Crawford BH: Visual adaptation in relation to brief conditioning stimuli. *Proc R Soc (Lond) B* 1947; 134:283–302.

24. Curcio CA, Sloan KR Jr, Packer O, Hendricksen AE, Kalina RE: Distribution of cones in human and monkey retina: Individual variability and radial asymmetry. *Science* 1987; 236:579–582.

25. Dacey DM: Parallel pathways for spectral coding in primate retina. *Ann Rev Neurosci* 2000; 23:743–775.

26. de Monasterio FM, McCrane EP, Newlander JK, Schein SJ: Density profile of blue-sensitive cones along the horizontal meridian of macaque retina. *Invest Ophthalmol Vis Sci* 1985; 26:289–302.

27. Denny N, Frumkes TE, Goldberg SH: Differences between summatory and suppressive rod-cone interaction. *Clin Vis Sci* 1990; 5:27–36.

28. Dowling JE: *The Retina: An Approachable Part of the Brain.* Cambridge, Mass, Belknap Press, 1987.

29. Drum B: Rod-cone interaction in the dark-adapted fovea. *J Opt Soc Am* 1981; 71:71–74.

30. Dryja TP: Molecular genetics of Oguchi disease, fundus albipunctatus, and other forms of stationary night blindness: LVII Edward Jackson Memorial Lecture. *Am J Ophthalmol* 2000; 130:547–563.

31. Egan JP: *Signal Detection Theory and ROC Analysis.* New York, Academic Press, 1975.

32. Eisner A: Multiple components in photopic dark adaptation. *J Opt Soc Am A* 1986; 3:655–666.

33. Fain GL, Matthews HR, Cornwall MC, Koutalos Y: Adaptation in vertebrate photoreceptors. *Physiol Rev* 2001; 81:117–151.

34. Garcia-Perez MA: Forced-choice staircases with fixed step sizes: Asymptotic and small-sample properties. *Vision Res* 1998; 38:1861–1881.

35. Geisler WS: Comments on the testing of two prominent dark-adaptation hypotheses. *Vision Res* 1980; 20:807–811.

36. Geisler WS: Sequential ideal-observer analysis of visual discriminations. *Psychol Rev* 1989; 96:267–314.

37. Glaser JS, Savino PJ, Sumers KD, McDonald SA, Knighton RW: The photostress recovery test in the clinical assessment of visual function. *Am J Ophthalmol* 1977; 83:225–260.

38. Graham NVS: *Visual Pattern Analyzers.* New York, Oxford University Press, 1989.

39. Green DG, Dowling JE, Siegel IM, Ripps H: Retinal mechanisms of visual adaptation in the skate. *J Gen Physiol* 1975; 65:483–502.

40. Grimm C, Reme CE, Rol PO, Williams TP: Blue light's effects on rhodopsin: Photoreversal of bleaching in living rat eyes. *Invest Ophthalmol Vis Sci* 2000; 41:3984–3990.

41. Grimm C, Wenzel A, Williams T, Rol P, Hafezi F, Reme C: Rhodopsin-mediated blue-light damage to the rat retina: Effect of photoreversal of bleaching. *Invest Ophthalmol Vis Sci* 2001; 42:497–505.

42. Hecht S, Haig C, Wald G: Dark adaptation of retinal fields of different size and location. *J Gen Physiol* 1935; 19:321–339.

43. Hess RF, Nordby K: Spatial and temporal limits of vision in the achromat. *J Physiol* 1986; 371:365–385.

44. Hollins M, Alpern M: Dark adaptation and visual pigment regeneration in human cones. *J Gen Physiol* 1973; 62:430–447.

45. Hood DC: Assessing retinal function with the multifocal technique. *Prog Retin Eye Res* 2000; 19:607–646.

46. Hood DC, Birch DG: Abnormalities of the retinal cone system in retinitis pigmentosa. *Vision Res* 1996; 36:1699–1709.

47. Jackson GR, Owsley C, McGwin G Jr: Aging and dark adaptation. *Vision Res* 1999; 39:3975–3982.

48. Jacobson SG, Cideciyan AV, Regunath G, Rodriguez FJ, Vandenburgh K, Sheffield VC, Stone EM: Night blindness in Sorsby's fundus dystrophy reversed by vitamin A. *Nat Genet* 1995; 11:27–32.

49. Johnson CA: Recent developments in automated perimetry in glaucoma diagnosis and management. *Curr Opin Ophthalmol* 2002; 13:77–84.

50. Kaernbach C: Adaptive threshold estimation with unforced-choice tasks. *Percept Psychophys* 2001; 63:1377–1388.

51. Kaplan E, Lee BB, Shapley RM: New views of primate retinal function. *Prog Retin Res* 1990; 9:273–336.

52. Kemp CM, Jacobson SG, Faulkner DJ, Walt RW: Visual function and rhodopsin levels in humans with vitamin A deficiency. *Exp Eye Res* 1988; 46:185–197.

53. Klein SA: Measuring, estimating, and understanding the psychometric function: A commentary. *Percept Psychophys* 2001; 63:1421–1455.

54. Lamb TD: The involvement of rod photoreceptors in dark adaptation. *Vision Res* 1981; 21:1773–1782.

55. Lamb TD, Pugh EN Jr: Dark adaptation and the retinoid cycle of vision. *Prog Retin Eye Res* 2004; 23:307–380.

56. Lange G, Denny N, Frumkes TE: Suppressive rod-cone interactions: Evidence for separate retinal (temporal) and extraretinal (spatial) mechanisms in achromatic vision. *J Opt Soc Am* 1997; 14:2487–2498.

57. Lansford TG, Baker HD: Dark adaptation: An interocular light adaptation effect. *Science* 1969; 164:1307–1309.

58. Lee BB: Single units and sensation: A retrospect. *Perception* 1999; 28:1493–1508.

59. Leek MR: Adaptive procedures in psychophysical research. *Percept Psychophys* 2001; 63:1279–1292.

60. Legge G, Hooven T, Klitz T, Stephen Mansfield J, Tjan B: Mr. Chips 2002: New insights from an ideal-observer model of reading. *Vision Res* 2002; 42:2219–2234.

61. Leibrock CS, Reuter T, Lamb TD: Molecular basis of dark adaptation in rod photoreceptors. *Eye* 1998; 12:511–520.

62. Levine MW: *Levine and Shefner's Fundamentals of Sensation and Perception*, ed 3. New York, Oxford University Press, 2000.

63. Levitt H: Transformed up-down methods in psychoacoustics. *J Acoust Soc Am* 1970; 33:467–476.

64. Lie I: Dark adaptation and the photochromatic interval. *Doc Ophthalmol* 1963; 17:411–510.

65. Loshin DS, Levi DM: Suprathreshold contrast perception in functional amblyopia. *Doc Ophthalmol* 1983; 55:213–236.

66. Lu ZL, Sperling G: Three-systems theory of human visual motion perception: Review and update. *J Opt Soc Am A* 2001; 18:2331–2370.

67. MacLeod DIA, Hayhoe M: Rod origin of prolonged afterimages. *Science* 1974; 185:1171–1172.

68. Makous W, Teller DY, Boothe R: Binocular interaction in the dark. *Vision Res* 1976; 16:473–476.

69. Margrain TH, Thomson D: Sources of variability in the clinical photostress test. *Ophthalmic Physiol Opt* 2002; 22:61–67.

70. Marks LE, Gescheider GA: Psychophysical scaling. In Wixted, J (ed): *Steven's Handbook of Experimental Psychology*, ed 3, Vol 4: *Methodology*. New York, John Wiley, 2002, pp 91–138.

71. Mishkin M, Ungerleider LG: Contribution of striate inputs to the visuospatial functions of parieto-preoccipital cortex in monkeys. *Behav Brain Res* 1982; 6:57–77.

72. Nordby K, Stabell B, Stabell U: Dark-adaptation of the human rod system. *Vision Res* 1984; 24:841–849.

73. Pearson P, Swanson WH, Fellman RL: Chromatic and achromatic defects in patients with progressing glaucoma. *Vision Res* 2001; 41:1215–1227.

74. Pelli DG, Farell B: Why use noise? *J Opt Soc Am A* 1999; 16:647–653.

75. Pepperberg DR, Brown PK, Lurie M, Dowling JE: Visual pigment and photoreceptor sensitivity in the isolated skate retina. *J Gen Physiol* 1978; 71:369–396.

76. Perlman I, Barzilai D, Haim T, Schramek A: Night vision in a case of vitamin A deficiency due to malabsorption. *Br J Ophthalmol* 1983; 67:37–42.

77. Peters AY, Locke KG, Birch DG: Comparison of the Goldmann-Weekers dark adaptometer and LKC Technologies Scotopic Sensitivity Tester-1. *Doc Ophthalmol* 2000; 101:1–9.

78. Pokorny J, Sun VCW, Smith VC: Temporal dynamics of early light adaptation. *J Vision* 2003; 3:423–431.

79. Pugh EN Jr: Rushton's paradox: Rod dark adaptation after flash photolysis. *J Physiol* 1975; 248:413–441.

80. Pugh EN Jr, Mollen JD: A theory of the pi-1 and pi-3 color mechanisms of Stiles. *Vision Res* 1979; 19:293–312.

81. Reeves A: Transient desensitization of a red-green opponent site. *Vision Res* 1981; 21:1267–1277.

82. Reeves A, Peachey NS, Auerbach E: Interocular sensitization to a rod-detected test. *Vision Res* 1986; 26:1119–1127.

83. Regan D: A hypothesis-based approach to clinical psychophysics and to the design of visual tests: The Proctor Lecture. *Invest Ophthalmol Vis Sci* 2002; 43:1311–1323.

84. Ripps H, Mahaffey IM III, Siegel IM, Ernst W, Kemp CM: Flash photolysis of rhodopsin in the cat retina. *J Gen Physiol* 1981; 77:295–315.

85. Rushton WAH: Rhodopsin measurement and the regeneration of rhodopsin. *J Physiol* 1961; 156:166–178.

86. Rushton WAH: Visual adaptation (the Ferrier lecture). *Proc R Soc Lond [Biol]* 1965; 162:20–46.

87. Rushton WAH, Powell DS: The rhodopsin content and the visual threshold of human rods. *Vision Res* 1972; 12:1073–1082.

88. Sandberg MA, Berson EL, Effron MH: Rod-cone interaction in the distal human retina. *Science* 1981; 212:829–831.

89. Schiller PH: The ON and OFF channels of the visual system. *Trends Neurosci* 1992; 15:86–92.

90. Schnapf JL, Kraft TW, Nunn BJ, Baylor DA: Spectral sensitivity of primate photoreceptors. *Vis Neurosci* 1988; 1:255–261.

91. Seiple W, Greenstein VC, Holopigian K, Carr RE, Hood DC: A method for comparing psychophysical and multifocal electroretinographic increment thresholds. *Vision Res* 2002; 42:257–269.

92. Seiple WH, Holopigian K, Greenstein VC, Hood DC: Sites of cone system sensitivity loss in retinitis pigmentosa. *Invest Ophthalmol Vis Sci* 1993; 34:2638–2645.

93. Sharpe LT, Stockman A: Rod pathways: The importance of seeing nothing. *Trends Neurosci* 1999; 22:497–504.

94. Sieving PA, Murayama K, Naarendorp F: Push-pull model of the primate photopic electroretinogram: A role for hyperpolarizing neurons in shaping the b-wave. *Vis Neurosci* 1994; 11:519–532.

95. Smith VC, Pokorny J, van Norren D: Densitometric measurements of human cone photopigment kinetics. *Vision Res* 1983; 23:517–525.

96. Spillmann L, Conlon JE: Photochromatic interval during dark adaptation and as a function of background luminance. *J Opt Soc Am* 1972; 62:182–185.

97. Stabell B, Stabell U: Effects of rod activity on colour threshold. *Vision Res* 1976; 16:1105–1110.

98. Stiles WS, Crawford BH: Equivalent adaptational levels in localized retinal areas. In *Report of a Joint Discussion on Vision*, Physical Society of London. Cambridge, England, Cambridge University Press, 1932, 194–211. (Reprinted in Stiles WS: *Mechanisms of colour vision*. London, Academic Press, 1978.)

99. Taylor MM, Creelman CD: PEST: Efficient estimates on probability functions. *J Acoust Soc Am* 1967; 41:782–787.

100. Teller DY: Linking propositions. *Vision Res* 1984; 24:1233–1246.

101. Treutwein B: Adaptive psychophysical procedures. *Vision Res* 1995; 35:2503–2522.

102. Tyrrell RA, Owens DA: A rapid technique to assess the resting states of eyes and other threshold phenomena: The modified binary search (MOBS). *Behav Res Meth Instr Comp* 1988; 20:137–141.

103. Valeton JM, van Norren D: Transient tritanopia at the level of the ERG b-wave. *Vision Res* 1979; 15:689–693.

104. Watson AB, Pelli DG: QUEST: A Bayesian adaptive psychometric method. *Percept Psychophys* 1983; 33:113–120.

105. Wisowaty J, Boynton RM: Temporal modulation sensitivity of the blue mechanism: Measurements made without chromatic adaptation. *Vision Res* 1980; 20:895–909.

106. Wolf JE, Arden GB: Selective magnocellular damage in melanoma-associated retinopathy: Comparison with congenital stationary nightblindness. *Vision Res* 1996; 36:2369–2379.

107. Wooten BR, Butler TW: Possible rod-cone interaction in dark adaptation. *J Opt Soc Am* 1976; 66:1429–1430.

108. Wyszecki G, Stiles WS: *Color Science: Concepts and Methods*, ed 2. New York, John Wiley, 1982.

27 Measurement of Contrast Sensitivity

GEOFFREY B. ARDEN

Definition of contrast

If a visual stimulus varies in intensity, either in space or in time, it is possible to define a maximum and minimum intensity. The ratio between these intensities is known as contrast. If the output of a source changes from I_1 at t_1 to I_2 at t_2, the contrast is

$$\frac{(I_1 - I_2)}{(I_1 + I_2)}$$

This measure of contrast is often termed *modulation*. It is evident that the maximum value for contrast is 1.0 when $I_2 = 0$. A similar definition can be used when contrast is measured in a complex spatial scene. Sometimes, however, if the image consists of a single edge, the contrast is taken as $\Delta I / I_{avg}$, where averaging over the entire image occurs.

Flicker and gratings

In visual science, it is often desirable to use stimuli that are repetitive in space or time: a simple example is the repetition of a flashing light. If one views a homogeneous field that alters in this way, it appears to flicker, and this is an example of temporal luminance contrast; if a repetitive pattern of varying luminance is seen (for example, a series of stripes), then the pattern can be described in terms of spatial luminance contrast. A stimulus can have both temporal and spatial contrast, for example, a pattern of vertical stripes can drift horizontally, the darker and lighter portions can be rhythmically interchanged (pattern reversal), or the pattern can be made to appear and disappear from a uniform background. Temporal and spatial color contrasts—without luminance changes—can also be produced. Analysis of visual performance is then reduced to determining the minimum contrast or contrast sensitivity associated with a stimulus that has given spatiotemporal (or color) properties. Chapters 31 and 34 in this book deal with the mathematical specification of stimuli in time and space, and chapter 19 describes methods whereby such stimuli may conveniently be produced. The theory of threshold determination is discussed in chapter 26. This introduction assumes that the changes are simple, repetitive, and sinusoidal.

Temporal contrast

It is evident that temporal contrast sensitivity varies with the temporal frequency changes of the object. Detection of objects is usually best at intermediate frequencies and reduced at higher and lower frequencies. The "low-frequency falloff" can only be seen with sinusoidal temporal changes. Likewise, if temporal frequency change is too fast, the object appears not to change at all. The frequency at which this occurs is the flicker fusion frequency. Familiar examples of objects that change so rapidly in time that they appear continuous are the images on TV or cinema screens. All parts of our retinas do not have similar capabilities: the flicker from a TV, which is invisible or nearly invisible with foveal viewing, can be readily seen with the peripheral retina. Also, the ability to see flicker depends upon a number of other parameters. The cinema image is renewed less frequently than that of a TV, but the flicker is less obvious because the screen luminance is lower.

The exact form of temporal contrast sensitivity was first investigated by DeLange,[6] and the set of curves describing the behavior of the visual system (figure 27.1) are often called DeLange curves. Note that the dependent variable is retinal illumination.[10] At low illuminations where rods subserve vision, only low temporal frequencies can be seen. The performance of the photopic system improves up to high retinal illuminations. There are irregularities at intermediate frequencies due to rod-cone interactions (see chapter 28). The frequency at which 100% modulated stimuli cannot be distinguished from constant illumination is the flicker fusion frequency.

Temporal contrast sensitivity (like any form of contrast) is determined by how far the modulation of the stimulus can be reproduced by the photoreceptors and the intermediate neurons. The membrane potential of photoreceptors increases in illumination and decreases in darkness. The modulation of the potential depends not only upon the rate of change of potential at the onset of a flash but also upon the rate of recovery. Thus, for weak flashes, rods are "slower" than cones. For intense flashes, rods can respond very quickly to increases of illumination, but the recovery is very slow, and this is the reason why flicker becomes invisible in

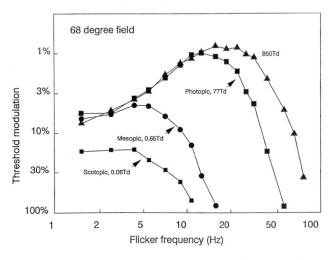

FIGURE 27.1 Threshold modulation of a sinusoidally modulated light, as a function of temporal frequency. Note the logarithmic scales. The "low frequency fall off" is exaggerated, and the frequency of maximum sensitivity is elevated, due to the very large field size. (After Kelly.[10])

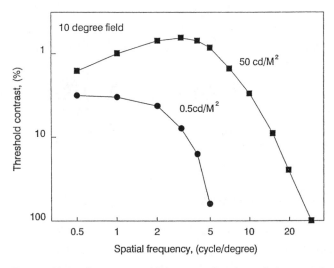

FIGURE 27.2 Contrast sensitivity as a function of the spatial frequency of the sinusoidal grating. Scotopic contrast sensitivity is considerably worse than at 0.5 cd/M². (After Arden.[2])

photopic conditions at low temporal frequencies. In cones, the recovery is much faster, so higher flicker rates can be transmitted. The highest frequency of stimulation that can be detected without attenuation of the signal (the characteristic frequency) is a convenient measure of the temporal response characteristics. In bipolar and ganglion cells, the characteristic frequency is higher than for cones. Thus diminution in flicker fusion frequency can be due to postsynaptic mechanisms as well as photoreceptor disturbance. An important instance is the recent finding that primate blue cones respond with the same dynamics as do red and green cones. The fact that the blue "channel" can only respond slowly has been well documented by psychophysicists, but this must be a function of postsynaptic mechanisms. The fusion frequency of retinal mechanisms is higher than that of higher cortical mechanisms. Thus, electroretinograms (ERGs) may follow flicker rates above psychophysical fusion frequency.

Spatial contrast

Spatial contrast has attracted more interest than has temporal because the ability to resolve a pattern of high spatial frequency, i.e., a grating consisting of a series of fine lines, bears an obvious relationship to the common clinical test of visual acuity. In practice, no one would replace optotypes with fine gratings, and it is worthwhile discussing why. Optotypes are of course familiar. More importantly, differentiation of letters is a very powerful psychophysical tool: a "26-way forced-choice test." If the patient is asked to discriminate a grating from a uniform field, either we have to accept his estimate or else ask if the grating is vertical,

horizontal, or oblique; this is a far less discriminative test. A "bell-shaped curve" relates spatial frequency to contrast threshold (figure 27.2). For 2 to 4 cycles per degree, a contrast of 0.5% or even less may be detected; at the upper frequency limit (approximately 30 cycles per degree), a contrast of 100%—black on white—is required. Only this one point is determined in conventional measurement of visual acuity, and therefore nearly the whole spectrum of spatial vision is not detected by routine clinical examination. Figure 27.3 shows various types of contrast sensitivity functions that occur in association with a loss of the ability to see high spatial frequencies. Panel A shows the effect of minimal ametropia: only high-frequency vision is affected. However, a loss of contrast sensitivity may occur for every spatial frequency (panel B), and then visual discrimination is more severely impaired. In some form of cataract, only low-spatial-frequency vision may be affected: then the patient will complain of impairment in his vision although visual acuity is normal. Therefore it is well worthwhile testing contrast sensitivity, providing this can be done quickly and simply. At low spatial frequencies, the contrast on the retina is not reduced by optical blur; therefore, if contrast sensitivity is reduced for such targets, either complex abnormalities (such as cataracts) are present, or there must be neurophysiological damage to the visual pathway. Another virtue of determining contrast sensitivity is that at low spatial frequencies the image covers a portion of the retina that is much larger than the fovea and, especially if a grating is used, detection depends upon the operation of the extramacular retina.

It is easy to become too enthusiastic about the need for measuring contrast sensitivity, and it must always be remembered that defects in acuity are related to foveal damage and

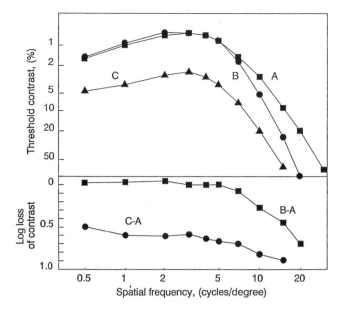

FIGURE 27.3 Pattern of loss of spatial contrast. Upper panel, Normal result, B, contrast loss at higher spatial frequencies such as occurs in minimal ammetropia. C, loss at all spatial frequencies, such as occurs in cataract. Lower panel, Although visual acuity, the cut-off spatial frequency at 100% contrast or a higher contrast (e.g., 10%) is not greatly different between B and C, the subjective visual disturbance is quite different, as shown by the visuograms, B–A and C–A. (After Arden.[2])

that, in practice, this is usually much more important to the patient than anything else. So great is the foveation of the visual system that a loss of low–spatial frequency sensitivity in practice indicates foveal damage, unless specific measures are taken to test the peripheral retina. Thus (see below), contrast sensitivity may appear to be normal in patients with defects in the peripheral field unless peripheral retinal contrast sensitivity is measured. Also, measurement of the cutoff spatial frequency with gratings of relatively high contrast, for example, 10% (see chapter 26), is unlikely (except in special cases) to provide useful clinical information. Testing in this manner is sometimes described as measuring "grating acuity." In this author's view, it should be abandoned, especially since there are now adequate means of rapidly assessing contrast thresholds. Furthermore, not all visual defects lead to a loss of contrast sensitivity. In amblyopia contrast sensitivity is often quite good, even though the ability to read and recognize letters is poor: contrast sensitivity is determined by the retinal mechanisms, while the cortical analyzers of more complex functions suffer from an added disability.

Means of producing stimuli for testing contrast sensitivity

Temporal contrast sensitivity is best measured by equipment with electronic control of light intensity, and for most

instances, the light-emitting diode is adequate since it is simple to control and provides a high source brightness. In applications where high spectral purity is required, light from a conventional optical system can be passed through filters or a spectrometer and then gated by a flicker wheel, with profiles cut to ensure sinusoidal output, or by using variable filters. Rotating Polaroids can also be employed, although a "cosine-squared" relationship results; electronic means of obtaining intensity variation can also be obtained with CROs, liquid crystals, or composites such as PZLT.

Spatial contrast sensitivity is often tested with gratings, which should be of sinusoidal profile. These may be produced electronically, and various systems are commercially available. They produce the best results but are in general not mobile and are expensive. Alternatively, such gratings may be photographed and printed. Various versions of such tests exist: the best is backlighted, so contrast can be determined accurately and does not vary with ambient illumination. Near-vision and remote versions of such tests are available. Various low-contrast optotypes have also been described. These have certain advantages (see above), but the number of contrast levels are usually limited, and the letters are not filtered. While such tests may be adequate for spatial frequencies higher than that for maximum sensitivity, they will not do for lower frequencies. This can be checked by any myopic user: the visibility of the optotype should be unaffected by a spectacle correction.

Methods of testing

Electronic test methods, often computer driven, can incorporate sophisticated psychophysical paradigms. "Forced-choice" techniques are preferable. When a number of spatial frequencies are to be tested, they should not be measured in order of ascending or descending frequency to avoid fatigue or learning effects. The speed of making measurements is often of practical importance in the clinic. For this reason, techniques used in laboratories—ascending ramps, receiving operator curves, random blocks—are rarely employed. Modified binary search routines (MOBS) with "quick and dirty" algorithms for threshold determination are widely employed.

Clinical results

TEMPORAL FREQUENCIES There are not many references to disease states in the literature. Responses are abnormal in retinitis pigmentosa and hypertension,[3,16,18,19] optic nerve disease,[8] and cerebrovascular insufficiency. A recent review article by Tyler summarizes the results.[15]

SPATIAL CONTRAST SENSITIVITY In many conditions, the patient's capability may be reduced below what is expected from visual acuity as a result of additional low-spatial-frequency loss, and this has been described by numerous authors.[7,9,11-14,17] Contrast sensitivity has also been used to diagnose eye diseases ranging from the corneal edema resulting from contact lens wear to glaucoma. References are to be found in recent reviews.[1,2,4]

REFERENCES

1. Arden GB: Advances in diagnostic visual optics. In Breinin GM, Siegel IM (eds): *Proceedings of the 2nd International Symposium. 1982*. Berlin, Springer-Verlag, 1983, pp 198–206.

2. Arden GB: Testing contrast sensitivity in clinical practice. *Clin Vis Sci* 1988; 2:213–224.

3. Attwell D, Wilson M, Wu SXM: A quantitative analysis of interactions between photoreceptors in the salamander (*Ambystoma*) retina. *J Physiol (Lond)* 1984; 352:703–737.

4. Bodis-Wollner I, Storch RL: Overview of contrast sensitivity and neuro-ophthalmic disease. In Nadler M, Miller D, Nadler DJ (eds): *Glare and Contrast Sensitivity for Clinicians*. Princeton, NJ, Princeton University Press, 1990, pp 85–112.

5. Buncic JR, Tytla ME, Trope GE: Flicker sensitivity in ocular hypertension before and during hypotensive treatment. *Invest Ophthalmol Vis Sci* 1986; 27 (suppl):158.

6. DeLange H: Research in the dynamic nature of the human fovea-cortex systems with intermittent and modulated light: I. Attenuation characteristics with white and colored light. *J Opt Soc Am* 1958; 48:777–784.

7. Fleishman JA, Beck RW, Linares OA, et al: Deficits in visual function after recovery from optic neuritis. *Ophthalmology* 1987; 94:1029–1035.

8. Hess RF, Plant GT: The psychophysical loss in optic neuritis: Spatial and temporal aspects. In Hess RF, Plant GT (eds): *Optic Neuritis*. Cambridge, England, University of Cambridge Press, 1986.

9. Hess R, Woo G: Vision through cataracts. *Invest Ophthalmol Vis Sci* 1978; 17:428–435.

10. Kelly DH: Visual responses to time-dependent stimuli: I. Amplitude sensitivity measurements. *J Opt Soc Am* 1961; 51:422–429.

11. Kupersmith MJ, Siegel IM, Carr RE: Reduced contrast sensitivity in compressive lesions of the anterior visual pathway. *Neurology* 1981; 31:550–554.

12. Kupersmith MJ, Siegel IM, Carr RE: Subtle disturbances of vision with compressive lesions of the anterior visual pathway measured by contrast sensitivity. *Ophthalmology* 1982; 89:68–72.

13. Loshin DS, White J: Contrast sensitivity: The visual rehabilitation of the patient with macular degeneration. *Arch Ophthalmol* 1984; 102:1303–1306.

14. Ross JE: Clinical detection of abnormalities in central vision in chronic simple glaucoma using contrast sensitivity. *Int Ophthalmol* 1985; 8:167–177.

15. Tyler CW: Two processes control variations in flicker sensitivity over the life span. *J Opt Soc Am [A]* 1989; 4:481–490.

16. Tyler CW, Ernst WJK, Lyness AL: Photopic flicker sensitivity losses in simplex and multiplex retinitis pigmentosa. *Invest Ophthalmol Vis Sci* 1986; 25:1035–1042.

17. Watson AB, Robson JG: Discrimination at threshold: Labelled detectors in human vision. *Vision Res* 1981; 21:1115–1122.

18. Wolf E, Gaeta AM, Geer SE: Critical flicker frequencies in flicker perimetry. *Arch Ophthalmol* 1968; 80:347–351.

19. Wright CE, Drasdo N: The influence of age on the spatial and temporal contrast sensitivity function. *Doc Ophthalmol* 1985; 59:385–395.

28 Suppressive Rod-Cone Interaction

THOMAS E. FRUMKES

ROD- AND CONE-VISION do not operate independently: cone-mediated pathways are tonically inhibited by dark-adapted rods. This latter phenomenon is referred to throughout this article as *suppressive rod-cone interaction (SRCI)*, although other names have been used in the literature.

Background

SRCI was discovered by four independent psychophysical investigations of flicker.[2,14,27,34] Sensitivity to cone-mediated flicker *decreases* during the rod-recovery phase of dark adaptation (e.g., see figure 28.1); similarly, cone-mediated flicker sensitivity *increases* as the illuminance of rod-stimulating backgrounds increases (e.g., see figure 28.2). Action spectra showed SRCI to reflect an influence of the dark-adapted state of rods upon cone-mediated vision.[2,26] Furthermore, this effect clearly reflects a tonic inhibitory influence of dark-adapted rods, not a facilitatory effect produced by light-adapted rods (see below).

SRCI has been documented by electroretinographic (ERG) procedures in normal humans.[6] The technique is quite difficult, and psychophysical procedures are much more fruitful for clinical investigation. However, our knowledge of this effect is considerably enhanced by intracellular recordings in subhuman species. SRCI has been clearly documented in cat horizontal cells and has been observed in all types of neurons in the amphibian retina except rods and color-opponent cells.[21,29,40] In the mud puppy, SRCI is blocked in *all* retinal neurons by divalent ions such as lead, which selectively block the rod input to second-order neurons, or by excitatory amino acid analogues such as D-O-phosphoserine, which selectively block the light response of horizontal cells; in the presence of such agents, cone-mediated flicker responses are considerably *enhanced*.[18,22] This strongly suggests that SRCI reflects a tonic *inhibitory* influence of dark-adapted rods upon cone pathways that is synaptically mediated by horizontal cells.

In the mud puppy, SRCI is seen in the cones themselves and is again blocked when horizontal cell responses are prevented pharmacologically, thus suggesting that SRCI must partially reflect a direct inhibitory influence upon cones. In amphibians, SRCI can be modified by the application of either agonists or antagonists of the putative neurotransmitter substances γ-aminobutyric acid (GABA), glycine, or dopamine[19,20,44]; however, these substances do not really mimic or totally block SRCI. In summary, the neurotransmitter(s) as well as the specifics of the neural pathway underlying this horizontal cell–mediated influence are at present unclear. It is clear that SRCI reflects one or several different rod-modulatory influences upon cone pathways within the retinal outer plexiform layer.

When using either psychophysical or neurophysiological procedures, SRCI has been shown to be limited by three parameters.[10,21,27,40] First, SRCI is very small with low-frequency flicker, but increases to a $>1 \log_{10}$ effect with flicker frequencies $>15\,Hz$. Second, background enhancement of flicker increases with illuminance of the background field up to a limiting value. In the cat, human, and mud puppy, the limiting irradiance for a 500-nm background is about $1\,nW/cm^2$, which corresponds to a retinal illuminance of about 1 troland (or under free viewing conditions with an unrestricted pupil, a luminance of about $1\,cd/m^2$).

Third, the magnitude of SRCI decreases as the size of the flicker probe increases and generally cannot be observed with Ganzfeld stimuli.[4,6,22,40] Pflug and Nelson[40] and Frumkes and Eysteinsson[22] have interpreted this to indicate that SRCI is limited by well-known electrical coupling properties of horizontal cells (e.g., see Lamb[31] and Nelson[38]). SRCI is also largely attributed to the adapted state of rods in retinal areas *adjacent to* rather than *within* the area stimulated by the cone probe.[26,27] This suggests that SRCI serves as the means for rods to modulate lateral inhibitory influences within the distal retina. As would be expected therefore, rod adaptation exerts as great an influence upon cone-mediated spatial (grating) acuity as on flicker.[15,37] Flicker is preferred in most studies for its ease in experimentation.

Many other forms of rod-cone interaction are known in addition to SRCI, three of which are noteworthy. First, cone adaptation exerts an influence upon rod-mediated flicker.[25] This phenomenon has not been studied by other psychophysicists, but a very similar effect has been described in the cat retina by electrophysiological procedures.[39,41] When using ERG procedures, this "reverse effect" may have considerable clinical utility. Second, rod and cone signals summate together: depending upon their relative phase, the signals will either add together to produce a larger sensation or cancel one another out.[16,35,46] Third, dark-adapted rods also exert an inhibitory effect upon a specific (correct color detection) threshold.[32] Although much less is known about these other three types of rod-cone interaction, it is quite

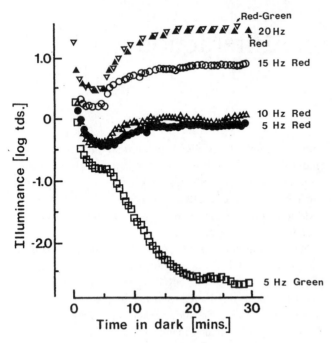

FIGURE 28.1 Illuminance of a 2-degree, 20-minute sinusoidally flickered test stimulus presented 7 degrees parafoveally that produces just perceptible flicker as a function of time in the dark. Stimuli were presented in maxwellian view, and flicker was generated by either a red or green light-emitting diode and was either 5, 10, 15, or 20 Hz. Data represented by inverted open triangles were obtained with red and green flicker presented in counterphase and matched in scotopic illuminance. (From Goldberg SH, Frumkes TE, Nygaard RW: *Science* 1983; 221:180–182. Used by permission.)

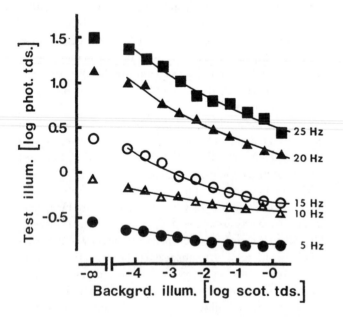

FIGURE 28.2 Illuminance of a 2-degree, 20-minute-diameter red flickering test stimulus that produces just perceptible flicker as a function of the illuminance of a 28-degree continuously exposed adapting field of 512-nm wavelength. For the test stimulus, 1 photopic troland is equal to −1.3 log scotopic trolands. Other parameters are as listed in figure 28.1. (From Goldberg SH, Frumkes TE, Nygaard RW: *Science* 1983; 221:180–182. Used by permission.)

clear that they are all distinct from each other and from SRCI.[5,16,25]

Clinical perspective

In most psychophysical and clinical studies of SRCI, the observer adjusts the intensity of a cone-stimulating probe until flicker is just perceived. The probe is flickered at a fixed frequency (usually between 15 and 25 Hz) and size (between 1 and 2.5 degrees). The magnitude of SRCI is assessed by determining the amount that cone flicker sensitivity is influenced by selective rod adaptation. Although SRCI can be seen with flicker probes placed at virtually any retinal position including the fovea,[4,14,16] most investigators prefer to systematically vary rod adaptation and study at most a few retinal positions (e.g., figures 28.1 and 28.2). In contrast, Alexander and Fishman[1–3] prefer to study only two levels of adaptation but to systematically vary retinal position, as shown in figure 28.3. I stress this methodological difference at the outset because their conclusions often differ strikingly from those reported by other groups, thus suggesting that sweeping generalizations may be unwarranted.

Night blindness

SRCI has been studied in a variety of night blindness conditions. Arden and his colleagues have reported three types of abnormalities in SRCI that are associated with retinitis pigmentosa (RP). First, SRCI is sometimes lacking or considerably reduced in retinal areas in which rod vision is absent[10]; this was confirmed by Alexander and Fishman.[3] Second, in some patients with dominantly inherited RP, the amount of SRCI was carefully probed on both sides of the "cliff" separating areas of the retina where rods were clearly affected from areas where they were functioning more normally. Obviously, SRCI is missing in the affected retinal areas, but this deficit extended several degrees into "unaffected" areas.[11] Such a finding would be anticipated from a horizontal cell lateral inhibitory model. Third, in some patients in which rod dark adaptation measured by usual psychophysical threshold or fundus reflectometry procedures is slower than normal, the growth of rod inhibition upon cones nevertheless proceeds at a normal rate.[10] A similar dissociation between the time course of rod threshold changes and the growth of inhibition of cones during dark adaptation has been seen also in patients with fundus flavimaculatus.[42,45] In normals, the antiphosphodiesterase theophylline specifically influences the time course of inhibition upon cones during rod adaptation while having little influence upon rod threshold per se.[30] Since cyclic nucleotides play so critical a role in rod phototransduction, this suggests that in patients with slowed dark adaptation there is some dissocia-

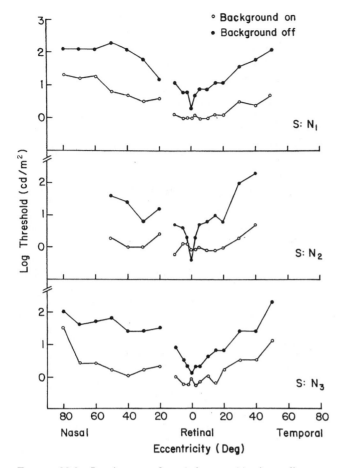

○ Background on
● Background off

S: N₁

S: N₂

S: N₃

80 60 40 20 0 20 40 60 80
Nasal   Retinal   Temporal
Eccentricity (Deg)

FIGURE 28.3 Luminance of a 1-degree, 44-minute-diameter square-wave flickering test probe of 25 Hz that was just perceived as flickering as a function of position on the retina. The stimuli were presented by means of a modified Tübinger perimeter and were presented in the dark (closed circles) or against a Ganzfeld background of 0.5 log cd/m². Results are from three observers. (From Alexander KR, Fishman GA: *Br J Ophthalmol* 1984; 60:303–309. Used by permission.)

tion between photopigment bleaching and the release of neurotransmitter in the dark.

A number of studies have investigated patients with stationary night blindness. This condition is characterized by normal rod rhodopsin content and absent or considerably reduced rod sensitivity; sometimes the ERG has a fairly normal rod a-wave but a considerably reduced or absent rod b-wave. Two groups of investigators have found SRCI to be absent in the six patients they examined.[8,10,28,43] On the other hand, Alexander and Fishman[3,5] (also personal communication) have found normal SRCI in the three patients they examined. Although there remains the possibility that different groups are describing different diseases with similar symptoms, it is probable that these conflicting findings may reflect some unresolved methodological difficulty. Indeed, a third possible change in SRCI that is associated with this condition has recently been suggested by ERG procedures.[36]

In a much different vein, Arden and Hogg[9] studied three individuals who appeared absolutely normal after even the most intense traditional clinical testing but who all complained of night vision difficulties: all refused to drive an automobile at night. In all three, the change in cone-mediated flicker sensitivity occurring during rod-dark adaptation was >2.5 log₁₀ units as opposed to about 1 log unit in normals. Recall that SRCI exerts as big an influence upon cone-mediated *spatial* acuity as upon flicker.[37] Apparently, too much rod inhibition upon cone pathways is a "new" cause for night blindness.

Disorders of color vision

SRCI has been studied in males with common X-linked forms of dichromacy, namely, deuteranopes and protanopes (respectively lacking normal green and red cones). SRCI is apparently normal in the two deuteranopes carefully investigated but is totally lacking in the four protanopes carefully investigated.[13,22,26] Although these results have yet to be fully published, several results from the two protanopes investigated by the author prove particularly intriguing. Because inhibition upon cones is lacking, the flicker sensitivity of these individuals in the dark was considerably superior to normal (i.e., the sensitivity level of normals in the presence of an optimal rod-adapting field). One of these men was additionally studied using grating acuity procedures: rod suppression of cone grating acuity is lacking, and hence, his spatial vision is similarly supernormal in the dark. The other protanope studied by the author showed another form of rod-cone interaction involving the use of Stiles' two-color increment threshold procedure.[12,23] But Alexander and Fishman question the generality of these findings. That is, although they failed to find SRCI in two "extremely protanomalous" individuals,[1] they have since found a normal pattern for SRCI in two protanopes (personal communication). More recently, they suggest that SRCI has little to do with the rod influence upon color perception.[5]

X-linked inherited conditions

SRCI is lacking in males with a number of X-linked conditions including protanopia and RP (see above). Although SRCI reflects distal retinal function, Arden and Hogg[8,10] also find it to be missing in individuals with X-linked retinoschisis, a result again disputed by Alexander and Fishman[3] (also personal communication). More recently, there have been several studies in female obligatory carriers who lack the phenotypical expression of this disease. Arden et al.[7] fail to find SRCI in such women. Arden (personal communication) now has some evidence that SRCI might be similarly absent in carriers of X-linked RP. SRCI is also lacking in individuals with choroideremia and reduced in others who are carriers for this condition.[48]

Newer developments

It is probable that SRCI has value for assessing visual functioning for a wide variety of other disease conditions. Lorenz and Zrenner[33] have associated a number of the complaints of myopes to a reduction in rod inhibition upon cones! The use of SRCI for assessing function in more general conditions such as diabetic retinopathy is still unexplored.

The value of SRCI as a test of visual functioning can be vastly improved. Zrenner and his associates[42,45,48] have found alterations in SRCI to be associated with alterations in color vision and particularly the phenomenon of transient tritanopia; Arden also has associated changes in SRCI with changes in color vision. This author can foresee several developments in the near future that will greatly expand the clinical usefulness of SRCI. First, SRCI should be more clearly related to horizontal cell functioning and lateral inhibition. Other than the *Werblin-Westheimer* procedure developed by Enoch,[17] SRCI is probably the only known measure of lateral inhibitory effects in humans that is specifically attributable to the distal retina. Second, SRCI testing should be specifically associated with other types of rod-cone interaction. For example, Denny et al.[16] have developed procedures for testing both a summation of rods and cones as well as SRCI in a single-sitting time period and show that the underlying mechanism must differ considerably. Their procedure should be of great value for studying individuals (RP or fundus flavimaculatus patients) in which the time course of rod threshold recovery and the growth of rod inhibition during dark adaptation are dissociated. If the claim by Alexander et al.[5] for dissociation between SRCI and rod inhibition of color perception is replicated, this too should be of clinical value. Finally, it now seems probable, based upon neurophysiological findings in lower species,[22,44,47] that SRCI possibly reflects a number of distinct mechanisms. If these can be teased apart by simple stimulus manipulation, their value for clinical investigation will be greatly enhanced.

ACKNOWLEDGMENTS Supported in part by National Eye Institute Grant EY05984 and grants from the National Science Foundation.

REFERENCES

1. Alexander KR, Fishman GA: Rod-cone interaction: Evidence for a distal retinal locus. *J Opt Soc Am* 1983; 73:1915.
2. Alexander KR, Fishman GA: Rod-cone interaction in flicker perimetry. *Br J Ophthalmol* 1984; 68:303–309.
3. Alexander KR, Fishman GA: Rod-cone interaction in flicker perimetry: Evidence for a distal retinal locus. *Doc Ophthalmol* 1985; 60:3–36.
4. Alexander KR, Fishman GA: Rod influence on cone flicker detection: Variation with retinal eccentricity. *Vision Res* 1986; 26:827–834.
5. Alexander KR, Fishman GA, Derlacki DJ: Mechanisms of rod-cone interaction: Evidence from congenital stationary nightblindness. *Vision Res* 1988; 28:575–583.
6. Arden GB, Frumkes TE: Stimulation of rods can increase cone flicker ERGs in man. *Vision Res* 1986; 26:711–721.
7. Arden GB, Gorin MB, Polkinghorne PJ, Jay M, Bird AC: Detection of the carrier state in X-linked retinoschisis. *Am J Ophthalmol* 1988; 105:590–596.
8. Arden GB, Hogg CR: Absence of rod-cone interaction in nyctalopia and retinoschisis. *J Physiol* 1984; 353:19.
9. Arden GB, Hogg CR: A new cause for difficulty in seeing at night. *Doc Ophthalmol* 1985; 60:121–125.
10. Arden GB, Hogg CR: Rod-cone interactions and analysis of retinal disease. *Br J Ophthalmol* 1984; 69:405–415.
11. Arden GB, Hogg CR, Moore AT, Ernst WJK, Kemp CM, Bird AC: Abnormal rod-cone interaction in dominant retinitis pigmentosa. *Invest Ophthalmol Vis Sci* 1987; 28 (suppl):235.
12. Bauer GM, Frumkes TE, Nygaard RW: The signal-to-noise characteristics of rod-cone interaction. *J Physiol* 1983; 337:121–135.
13. Coletta NJ, Adams AJ: Loss of flicker sensitivity on dim backgrounds in normal and dichromatic observers. *Invest Ophthalmol Vis Sci* 1985; 26 (suppl):187.
14. Coletta NJ, Adams AJ: Rod-cone interactions in flicker detection. *Vision Res* 1984; 24:1333–1340.
15. Coletta NJ, Schefrin BE, Adams AJ: Rod adaptation influences cone spatial resolution. *Invest Ophthalmol Vis Sci* 1986; 27 (suppl):71.
16. Denny N, Frumkes TE, Goldberg SH: Differences between summatory and suppressive rod-cone interaction. *Clin Vis Sci* 1990; 5:27–36.
17. Enoch JM: Quantitative layer-by-layer perimetry. *Invest Ophthalmol Vis Sci* 1978; 17:208–257.
18. Eysteinsson T, Frumkes TE: Physiology and pharmacological analysis of suppressive rod-cone interaction in *Necturus* retina. *J Neurophysiol* 1989; 61:866–877.
19. Eysteinsson T, Frumkes TE, Denny N: The importance of horizontal cell coupling for rod-cone interaction. *Invest Ophthalmol Vis Sci* 1987; 28 (suppl):403.
20. Frumkes TE, Denny N, Sliwinski M, Eysteinsson T: The role of horizontal cell coupling for suppressive rod-cone interaction (abstract). *Neuroscience* 1987; 13:26.
21. Frumkes TE, Eysteinsson T: Suppressive rod-cone interaction in distal vertebrate retina: Intracellular records from *Xenopus* and *Necturus*. *J Neurophysiol* 1987; 57:1361–1382.
22. Frumkes TE, Eysteinsson T: The cellular basis for suppressive rod-cone interaction. *Vis Neurosci* 1988; 1:263–273.
23. Frumkes TE, Goldberg SH: Rod-cone interaction in dichromats and abnormal trichromats. *J Opt Soc Am* 1982; 72:1741–1742.
24. Frumkes TE, Naarendorp F, Goldberg SH: Abnormalities in retinal neurocircuitry in protanopes: Evidence provided by psychophysical investigation of temporal-spatial interactions (abstract). *Invest Ophthalmol Vis Sci* 1988; 29 (suppl):163.
25. Frumkes TE, Naarendorp F, Goldberg SH: The influence of cone stimulation upon flicker sensitivity mediated by adjacent rods. *Vision Res* 1986; 26:1167–1176.
26. Goldberg SH: Tonic suppression of cone flicker by dark-adapted rods. Unpublished portions of a doctoral dissertation, City University of New York, 1983.

27. Goldberg SH, Frumkes TE, Nygaard RW: Inhibitory influence of unstimulated rods in human retina: Evidence provided by examining cone flicker. *Science* 1983; 221:180–182.

28. Greenstein VC, Hood DC, Siegel IM, Carr RE: A possible use of rod-cone interaction in congenital stationary nightblindness. *Clin Vis Sci* 1988; 3:69–74.

29. Hassin G, Witkovsky P: Intracellular recording from identified photoreceptors and horizontal cells of the *Xenopus* retina. *Vision Res* 1983; 23:921–932.

30. Kohen L, Zrenner E, Schneider T: Der Einfluss von Theophyllin und Coffein auf die sensorische Netzhautfunktion des Menschen. *Fortschr Ophthalmol* 1986; 83:338–344.

31. Lamb TD: Spatial properties of horizontal cell responses in the turtle retina. *J Physiol* 1976; 363:239–255.

32. Lie I: Dark adaptation and the photochromatic interval. *Doc Ophthalmol* 1963; 17:411–510.

33. Lorenz B, Zrenner E: Warum sind Myope mit chorioidaler Degeneration blendungsempfindlich? *Forschr Ophthalmol* 1987; 84:468–473.

34. Lythgoe RJ, Tansley K: The relation of the critical frequency of flicker to the adaptation of the eye. *Proc R Soc Lond [Biol]* 1929; 105:60–92.

35. MacLeod DIA: Rods cancel cones in flicker. *Nature* 1972; 235:173–174.

36. Miyake Y, Horiguchi M, Ota I, Shiroyama N: Characteristic ERG flicker anomaly in incomplete congenital stationary night blindness. *Invest Ophthalmol Vis Sci* 1987; 28:1816–1823.

37. Naarendorp F, Denny N, Frumkes TE: Rod light and dark adaptation influence cone-mediated spatial acuity. *Vision Res* 1988; 28:67–74.

38. Nelson R: Cat cones have rod input: A comparison of the response properties of cones and horizontal cell bodies in the retina of the cat. *J Comp Neurol* 1977; 172:109–135.

39. Olsen BT, Schneider T, Zrenner E: Characteristics of rod driven off-responses in cat ganglion cells. *Vision Res* 1986; 26:835–845.

40. Pflug R, Nelson R: Enhancement of red cone flicker by rod selective background in cat horizontal cells (abstract). *Neuroscience* 1986; 16:406.

41. Schneider T, Olsen BT, Zrenner E: Characteristics of the rod-cone transition in electroretinogram and optic nerve response. *Clin Vis Sci* 1986; 1:81–91.

42. Schneider T, Zrenner E: Rod-cone interaction in patients with fundus flavimaculatus. *Br J Ophthalmol* 1987; 71:762–765.

43. Siegel IM, Greenstein VC, Seiple WH, Carr RE: Cone function in congenital nyctalopia. *Doc Ophthalmol* 1987; 65:307–318.

44. Stone S, Witkovsky P: Center-surround organization of *Xenopus* horizontal cells and its modification by GABA and strontium. *Exp Biol* 1987; 47:1–12.

45. Ulbig M, Zrenner E, Schneider T: Funktionelle und morphologische Variationen bei Fundus flavimaculatus. *Fortschr Ophthalmol* 1988; 85:312–316.

46. van den Berg TJTP, Spekreijse H: Interaction between rod and cone signals studied with temporal sine wave stimulation. *J Opt Soc Am* 1977; 67:1210–1217.

47. Yang X, Wu S: Effects of background illumination on the horizontal cell responses in the tiger salamander retina. *J Neurosci* 1989; 9:815–827.

48. Zrenner E, Kohen L, Krastel H: Einschraenkungen der Netzhautfunktion bei Konduktorinnen der Chorioideremie. *Fortschr Ophthalmol* 1986; 83:602–608.

29 The Use of Fluorescein Angiography as an Adjunct to Electrophysiological Testing

JOHN R. HECKENLIVELY

WHILE THERE ARE A number of retinal diseases where the electrophysiological test results are distinctive and often highly characteristic, the usual case undergoing evaluation needs to have other parameters assessed in order for a diagnosis to be reached. Typically, the diagnostic information considered includes the age of onset, inheritance pattern, symptoms, and morphological changes as seen on examination or in photographs; these are correlated with the results of electrophysiological and psychophysical testing.

One test that normally might not be thought to be of much value in electrodiagnosis is fluorescein angiography (FA) and fundus photography (FP). However, there are a number of situations where the FA and FP can strongly support or give the correct diagnosis. On occasion, additional information is learned about the disease process that may have clinical importance.

Basic principles of fluorescein angiography

Briefly, FA testing is based on the fact that blue light stimulates or excites fluorescein molecules to emit bright green light, which can be recorded selectively by the use of transmission filters on film or by video camera.[2,18,19] The fluorescein is normally injected as a bolus in an antecubital vein and reaches the eye through the circulatory system in about 10 seconds. Since the fluorescein dye is blood borne and is a moderately large molecule, it normally does not leave retinal blood vessels because of the endothelial cells' tight junctions. If the vessels are involved in an active inflammatory process, or have lost their tight junctions due to scarring, dye leaks or stains the tissue.

Since choroidal vessels do not have tight junctions, free passage of fluorescein takes place in the choroid, which contributes to the "choroidal flush" seen in the early transit phase of the FA. The confluent nature of the retinal pigment epithelial (RPE) monolayer, which also has tight junctions, prevents leakage of the fluorescein into the subretinal space.

If the RPE is damaged, it may diffusely or focally leak in recognizable patterns, or if the cells are filled with pigmented material, the choroidal flush is blocked and gives what has been termed the "dark choroid effect."[1,5] Changes in the status of the retinal and choroidal vasculature systems are easily seen with FA. How quickly the fluorescein appears, what layer is affected, whether it is a diffuse slow active early leak or stain or late stain all give important diagnostic information.

Hereditary retinal diseases with distinctive fluorescein angiograms

CHOROIDEREMIA The choroideremia pattern is not always obvious on fundus examination, particularly in children or in patients who have more choroidal pigmentation. Visual physiological studies usually demonstrate a rod-cone loss pattern on the electroretinogram (ERG), elevation of the rod thresholds, and often ring scotomas or constricted fields.[13,17] Usually an X-linked recessive inheritance pattern can be established.

The FA in choroideremia shows a distinctive scalloped loss of the choriocapillaris, which is hypofluorescent next to brightly hyperfluorescent patent choriocapillaris (figures 29.1A and 29.1B). With only the clinical history and ERG results, the diagnosis of X-linked retinitis pigmentosa (RP) might be made, yet this conclusion would miss the more precise diagnosis of choroideremia, which can be made by the examination of the fundus directly and confirmed by FA in cases where choroidal pigmentation masks the choriocapillaris/RPE dropout.

The appearance of lobular loss of RPE and choriocapillaris on FA that is confined primarily to the posterior pole can also be seen in Bietti's crystalline retinal dystrophy (figures 29.2A and 29.2B). Pericentral RP will have selective loss of RPE and choriocapillaris at the edge of the posterior pole to the midequator, but there is also an associated pigmentary retinopathy.

CONFIRMING MACULAR SCHISIS VS. EDEMA Cystoid macular edema is a known complication that may occur in a number of panretinal degenerations including RP. Occasionally a patient with the appearance of cystoid edema on direct

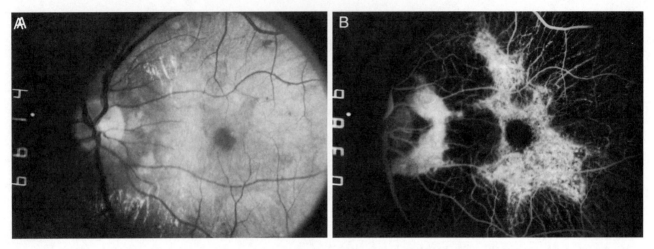

FIGURE 29.1 Choroideremia in a 22-year-old Japanese man from an X-linked recessive family pedigree. A, A red-free photograph, left eye, demonstrates choroidal pigmentation that almost masks an island of intact RPE in the macula. B, FA of the same area demon-strates two islands of patent choriocapillaris in the macula and parapapillary area, with loss of choriocapillaris and small choroidal vessels outside the patent areas. The fovea is hypofluorescent, prob-ably from thickened RPE.

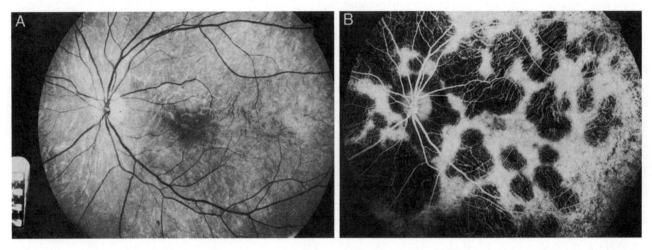

FIGURE 29.2 Bietti's crystalline retinal dystrophy in a 45-year-old man with no family history; his visual acuity was OD 20/20, OS 20/25; the ERG was abnormal in a rod-cone pattern; and the light peak–dark trough ratio on the electro-oculogram (EOG) was 1.2. A, Wide-angle red-free photography shows cyrstalline dots throughout the posterior pole and more apparent choroidal circu-lation than usual. B, FA of the same area reveals lobule loss of choriocapillaris with retention of larger choroidal vessels. In Bietti's dystrophy, the choriocapillaris loss is usually confined to the poste-rior pole.

ophthalmoscopy will be found to have no accumulation of dye in the foveal area on late frames of the FA. Stereo observation will usually demonstrate a schisis-like breakdown of the retinal tissue that may look cystic. The most common conditions where this may occur are Goldmann-Favre disease, juvenile retinoschisis, and Usher's syndrome. The lack of late macular staining in these cases can be most helpful in arriving at a better understanding of the patient's visual acuity problems.

X-linked retinoschisis has a distinctive ERG, although severe cases can be confused with RP, particularly if older members in the family develop a pigmentary retinopathy.[12,20] The negative waveform in the dark-adapted bright-flash

ERG may be ignored in the face of concurrent poor pho-topic and scotopic rod tracings. However, the macular and, if present, the peripheral schisis changes can be distinctive although at times subtle. Red-free photography, which is part of the usual FA protocol, often gives the clearest demon-stration of macular schisis, which is reinforced by no stain-ing or leakage in the area, so that the changes are not mistaken for cystoid macular edema (figure 29.3). The pres-ence of macular schisis on red-free photos in face of a neg-ative wave would eliminate the diagnosis of congenital stationary night blindness, which also has a negative wave-form (see table 49.3 and chapter 72).

The other common retinal dystrophy that occasionally has foveal schisis-like degeneration, i.e., a cystoid macular change without leakage, is Usher's syndrome[6] (figure 29.4). Many of these patients demonstrate cystic-like changes that look like cystoid edema but do not show leakage on FA.[11] In these cases the macular cysts eventually degenerate and leave an atrophic macula.

Deutman reported five pedigrees with dominant cystoid macular edema in which the older individuals had atrophic macular degeneration while younger members had cystoid edema.[3] Moderate to high hyperopia, astigmatism, strabismus, and punctate opacities in the vitreous were common. Capillaries of the posterior pole and disc were dilated; the ERG was normal, and the EOG was subnormal.

PATTERN DYSTROPHIES/RPE DISEASE FA is particularly useful in bringing out subtle lesions of the RPE and therefore can be quite useful in evaluating patients with hereditary macular dystrophies such as cone-rod, cone, or the pattern dystrophies.[3] Similarly, more subtle cases of sector RP can be diagnosed because there is often a clear demarcation line between apparently unaffected (or functioning) retina and areas of nonfunctioning retina (figure 29.5). Wide-angle FA may be helpful in this documentation. While the FA would not be used alone in making the diagnosis, some carrier states might be identified such as choroideremia, X-linked ocular albinism, or RP. Early dominant type II RP will often show heavy granularity and focal dropout of the RPE and telangiectasia of the posterior pole and disc vessels before there are significant ERG changes.

PRESERVED PARA-ARTERIOLAR RETINAL PIGMENT EPITHELIAL RETINITIS PIGMENTOSA In 1981, Heckenlively described an autosomal recessive form of RP that, in more advanced states, is characterized by preserved para-arteriolar RPE (PPRPE) adjacent and under retinal arterioles; diffuse atrophy of surrounding RPE is necessary in order to observe the PPRPE pattern.[8] Patients have been uniformly hypermetropic when typical RP patients are myopic, and the age of onset has usually been childhood to adolescent years. Many of the cases have had disc drusen. The ERG, when present, is in a rod-cone pattern, and the rod threshold on dark adaptometry is elevated. These patients tend to be severely affected by the time the PPRPE pattern is apparent.

FA is very effective in bringing out subtle cases of the PPRPE pattern (figure 29.6A), which may be difficult to distinguish on fundus examination alone. It should be noted that cases of diffuse retinal edema in advanced RP may occasionally show hypofluorescence next to arterioles, which could be confused with PPRPE (figure 29.6B).

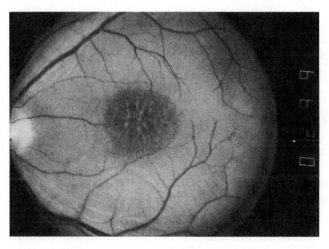

FIGURE 29.3 Juvenile retinoschisis. A red-free fundus photograph of a 38-year-old man demonstrates a stellate pattern in the macula. Red-free photography most clearly demonstrates the macular schisis pattern characteristic of this disorder.

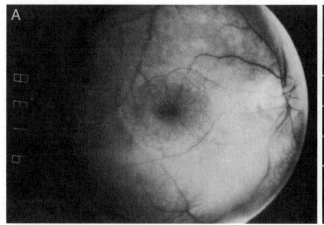
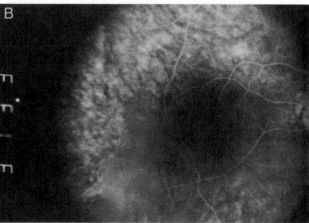

FIGURE 29.4 Twenty-five-year-old man with Usher syndrome, type 1. A, A red-free photograph demonstrates cysticlike macular changes.

B, FA shows no late leakage in the macular area. Careful inspection of the fovea with the 90-D lens showed irregular cystic disintegration.

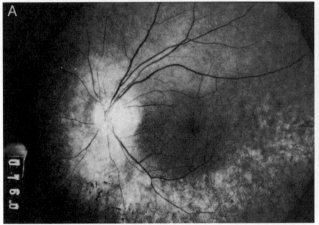 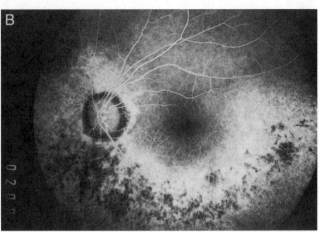

FIGURE 29.5 Red-free photograph (A) and FA (B) of a 63-year-old woman with sector RP. The patient reported a 4-year history of visual symptoms and superior field loss. The RPE loss is evident inferior to the vascular arcade on FA.

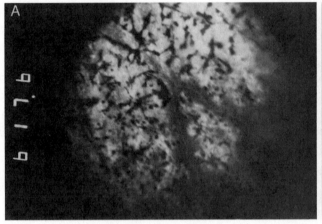 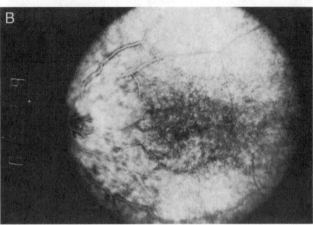

FIGURE 29.6 A, FA in PPRPE in a 33-year-old lady with advanced RP from a family with consanguineous parents and presumed autosomal recessive inheritance. B, Autosomal dominant RP patient who does not have PPRPE but has severe posterior pole edema where perivascular hypofluorescent changes which mimic fluorescein changes seen in PPRPE RP.

DARK CHOROID EFFECT Bonnin et al. described a "silent choroid sign" in tapetoretinal degenerations that since has been termed the *dark choroid effect* or *sign*.[1] Histopathological correlation by Eagle and associates in a case of fundus flavimaculatus with dark choroid demonstrated lipofuscin-like deposits filling the RPE, thereby blocking the choroidal fluorescence.[4] The importance of this diagnostic sign was clarified by Fish et al. in 1981, who examined 91 patients with various types of hereditary macular disease with FA.[5] Forty-seven patients in the study had retinal flecks, 34 of whom had a dark choroid effect. An additional 3 retinal dystrophy patients had the effect.

As suggested by the study of Fish et al., the most common retinal condition with dark choroid is fundus flavimaculatus (figures 29.7A and 29.7B), but occasionally recessive cone dystrophies or cases with inverse RP starting with posterior pole flecks will show the dark choroid effect, particularly in areas surrounding the macular area, and the dark choroid helps to identify this group of diseases. Some patients with RP have hypofluorescent fovea centralis areas on FA that likely represent the same process as dark choroid, that is, blockage of choroidal flush by thickened or less transmissive RPE.

While patients with fundus flavimaculatus typically have only mild or subnormal ERG and EOG values, some more advanced cases may have macular atrophy with minimal flecks and cone-rod ERG patterns, and the FA finding of dark choroid and full peripheral visual fields helps to establish the correct diagnosis. Some of these latter patients may be diagnosed as having central areolar choroidal sclerosis, but if a dark choroid effect is present, then the diagnosis of fundus flavimaculatus is more likely.

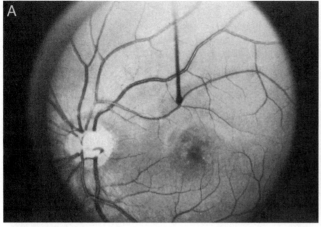 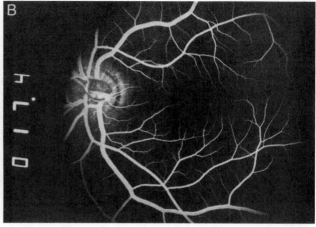

FIGURE 29.7 Dark choroid effect in Stargardt's disease. A, Red-free photography of a 22-year-old woman with 20/200 vision since 11 years of age demonstrates subtle macular atrophy and a few foveal flecks. B, FA shows profound hypofluorescence with only faint window defects in the macular area.

OTHER FINDINGS ON THE FLUORESCEIN ANGIOGRAM FA may assist in better understanding the ocular status of patients with a number of retinal degenerations since in advanced stages many will have diffuse retinal or macular edema. In other cases window defects may be seen that may not be obvious on clinical examination and indicate areas of atrophy or scarring. A nonspecific finding in a number of retinal dystrophies in early stages is telangiectasia of the optic nerve head and sometimes the macular area. This appears to occur more frequently in the cone-rod degeneration[1] or cone degenerations. Some patients with retinal dystrophy will also have marked hyperfluorescent disc staining on late phases, which on an otherwise normal examination may be an indication to pursue a diagnosis with electrophysiological testing. Optic nerve temporal atrophy has been reported in a number of diseases and may be more easily seen in some patients by FA[10,14,15] (figure 29.8).

Rarely patients with retinal dystrophy will have subretinal or retinal neovascularization, leaking or telangiectatic vessels giving retinal edema or even a Coats' exudative reaction, all of which can be better understood with FA.[9,21] Of particular importance to find are patients with RP and the Coats' reaction, who should be treated with photocoagulation, since if present the retinal or subretinal neovascularization may hemorrhage and lead to severe scarring and even phthisis bulbi (figure 29.9).

Peripheral retinal telangiectasia is a prominent feature of facioscapulohumeral muscular dystrophy with deafness, an autosomal dominant disorder with variable expressivity.[7] Likewise, dominant exudative vitreoretinopathy is a hereditary dystrophy that has prominent vascular changes.[16] Retinal electrophysiological studies have not been reported in this disease.

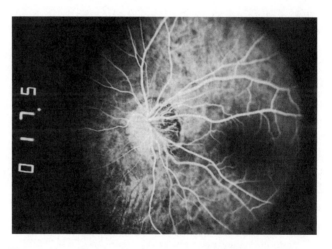

FIGURE 29.8 Temporal optic atrophy and disc telangiectasia in a 33-year-old woman with RP cone-rod degeneration. Temporal optic atrophy may be seen in cone dystrophy, cone-rod degenerations, and congenital stationary night blindness; it is a strong indication to do an ERG if other symptoms are present. Temporal atrophy may be difficult to distinguish from tilted discs of high myopia, but FA often shows papillary vessels in the area where disc tissue should be present.[15]

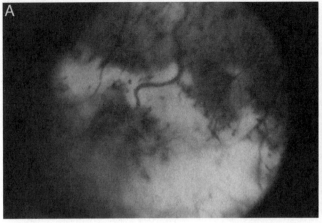

FIGURE 29.9 Coats's reaction in a 32-year-old woman with advanced simplex RP. A, Red-free photography shows pigmentation, subretinal exudates, and dilated retinal vessels. B, FA demonstrates telangiectasia and neovascularization. Initially, she responded to xenon photocoagulation with regression for 2 years, after which despite several photocoagulation treatments, the neovascularization progressed with vitreal hemorrhage and phthisis bulbi. Early subretinal neovascularization was found in her other eye, which regressed with panretinal photocoagulation.

REFERENCES

1. Bonnin P, Passot M, Triolaire MTh: Le signe due silence choroidien dans les degenerescences tapetoretiennes posterieures. *Doc Ophthalmol Proc Ser* 9:461–463, 1976; 9:461–463.
2. Bursell SE, Mainster MA: Methods of vitreoretinal evaluation. In Newsome DA (ed): *Retinal Dystrophies and Degenerations.* New York, Raven Press, 1988, pp 5–10.
3. Deutman AF: Dominant macular dystrophies: Cystoid macular edema and butterfly dystrophy. *Doc Ophthalmol Proc Ser* 1976; 9:415–431.
4. Eagle LRC, Lucier AC, Bernardino VB, et al: Retinal pigment epithelial abnormalities in fundus flavimaculatus. *Ophthalmology* 1980; 87:1189–1200.
5. Fish G, Grey R, Sehmi KS, Bird AC: The dark choroid in posterior retinal dystrophies. *Br J Ophthalmol* 1981; 65:359–363.
6. Fishman GA, Vasquez V, Fishman M, Berger D: Visual loss and foveal lesions in Usher's syndrome. *Br J Ophthalmol* 1979; 63:484–488.
7. Gurwin EB, Fitzsimons RB, Sehmi KS, Bird AC: Retinal telangiectasis in facioscapulohumeral muscular dystrophy with deafness. *Arch Ophthalmol* 1985; 103:1695–1700.
8. Heckenlively JR: Preserved para-arteriolar retinal pigment epithelium (PPRPE) in retinitis pigmentosa. *Br J Ophthalmol* 1982; 66:26–30.
9. Heckenlively JR: Retinitis pigmentosa, unilateral Coats's disease and thalassemia minor: A case report. *Metab Pediatr Syst Ophthalmol* 1981; 5:67–72.
10. Heckenlively JR: RP cone-rod degeneration. Thesis for membership in the American Ophthalmological Society. *Trans Am Ophthalmol Soc* 1987; 85:438–470.
11. Heckenlively JR: RP syndromes. In Heckenlively JR (ed): *Retinitis Pigmentosa.* Philadelphia, JB Lippincott, 1988, pp 226–227.
12. Heckenlively JR: Simplex retinitis pigmentosa. In Heckenlively JR (ed): *Retinitis Pigmentosa.* Philadelphia, JB Lippincott, 1988, p 194.
13. Heckenlively JR, Bird AC: Choroideremia. In Heckenlively JR (ed): *Retinitis Pigmentosa.* Philadelphia, JB Lippincott, 1988, pp 176–187.
14. Heckenlively JR, Martin DA, Rosales TR: Telangiectasia and optic atrophy in cone-rod degenerations. *Arch Ophthalmol* 1981; 99:1983–1991.
15. Heckenlively JR, Martin DA, Rosenbaum A: Loss of electroretinographic oscillatory potentials, optic atrophy and dysplasia in congenital stationary night blindness. *Am J Ophthalmol* 1983; 96:526–534.
16. Kaufman SJ, Goldberg MF, Orth Dh, Fishman GA, Tessler H, Mizuno K: Autosomal dominant vitreoretinochoroidopathy. *Arch Ophthalmol* 1982; 100:272–278.
17. McCulloch C, McCulloch RJP: A hereditary and clinical study of choroideremia. *Trans Am Acad Ophthalmol Otolaryngol* 1948; 542:160–190.
18. Schatz H: *Essential Fluorescein Angiography: A compendium of 100 Classic Cases.* San Anselmo, Calif, Pacific Medical Press, 1983.
19. Schatz H: Fluorescein angiography: Basic principles and interpretation. In Schachat AP, Murphy RP, Patz A (eds): *Retina,* vol 2. St. Louis, CV Mosby Co, 1989, pp 1–77.
20. Tanino T, Katsumi O, Hirose T: Electrophysiological similarities between the eyes with X-linked recessive retinoschisis. *Doc Ophthalmol* 1985; 60:149–161.
21. Uliss AE, Gregor Z, Bird AC: Retinitis pigmentosa and retinal neovascularization. *Ophthalmology* 1986; 93:1599–1603.

VI DATA ANALYSIS

30 Experimental Design and Data Analyses in Vision Function Testing

STEVEN NUSINOWITZ

WHEN IS A PARAMETER that reflects visual function abnormal? When is a change in some aspect of visual function meaningful, and when is it just a random chance variation? When is a therapeutic intervention helpful in slowing the progression of disease? When might an intervention be harmful? These are just some of the areas in which statistical analyses can be extremely helpful and informative. In this chapter, basic issues of experimental design and statistical analysis are discussed. Detailed discussion of a variety of statistical issues is beyond the scope of this chapter. Whenever possible, the reader will be referred to primary sources for expanded discussion.

Summarizing the characteristics of a sample using descriptive statistics

The most basic way of summarizing functional data is by using descriptive statistics. Three pieces of information are usually provided in summarizing the characteristic of a randomly drawn sample of data. First, the number of separate and independent observations made regarding any one variable or the number of individual subjects is denoted by N. In eye research, for example, observations made by two individuals by the right eye are independent (or uncorrelated) for statistical purposes, and $N = 2$, but observations made by the left and right eyes of the same individual are *not* independent. This is a fact that is frequently overlooked in many experimental designs. Most parametric statistical tests (see below) require that the assumption of independence be met. If the assumption of independence is ignored, an increase in the Type I error rate is likely to occur (see below).[1]

The second piece of information used in describing sample data is the average, or center, of the distribution of scores. The three measures of a distribution's center are the *mean, median,* and *mode.* The mean is the most widely used measure of the center and is defined as the sum of all scores divided by the number of scores. The median is the score at the fiftieth percentile, that is, the score that exactly divides the upper half of the scores from the lower half of the scores. Finally, the mode is defined as the most popular scores in the distribution. The mode is the crudest of averages, since it is not necessarily unique; a distribution of scores might have two or three popular scores, or modes.

The estimates of the mean, median, and mode are influenced by the nature of the underlying distribution. If a sample of data is *normally* distributed, the mean, median, and mode will be very close. However, there are other types of sample distributions, called *skewed* distributions, in which the mean, median, and mode can be very different.

The third descriptive statistic is a measure of how the scores vary around the center of the distribution. Commonly used measures of variability are the *range, standard deviation,* and *variance.* (There are several other measures of variability, such as the average deviation and the quartile deviation, that will not be described here.) The range is the difference between the highest score and the lowest score in the distribution. The standard deviation is the most common measure of the variability of a sample. In statistics, it is usually denoted S, although in nonstatistical applications *sd* or *st dev* is commonly used. It is defined as the square root of the sum of the squared deviations from the mean divided by N. The variance, which is computed as the square of the standard deviation, also indicates how representative of the individual scores the mean is.

The specific applications and methods of computation of the measures of the average and variability of test scores can be found in most elementary statistics textbooks.

A common application of descriptive statistics is in establishing *normative* data for some specific testing protocol. Normative data are defined by the nonpathological visual system and provide a guideline for deciding whether a particular electrophysiological or psychophysical parameter lies within normal limits or is outside the normal range and perhaps indicative of underlying pathology. Normal limits are usually defined arbitrarily as, for example, ±2.0 standard deviations (S) from the mean. For example, if the mean of a sample of electroretinogram (ERG) b-waves is $300\,\mu V$ and the standard deviations of the distribution of b-waves is $50\,\mu V$, then the scores from 200 to $400\,\mu V$ represent the mean $\pm 2.0\,S$. If the distribution of scores is normally distributed, $\pm 2.0\,S$ will capture approximately 98% of the distribution of normal scores. Of course, the caveat here is that roughly 2.0% of the normal population of scores would be considered abnormal by chance alone.

Estimating population parameters

It is of course not practical to measure an entire population, say, those with normal vision, to estimate the mean and variability of a specific functional parameter, such as the amplitude of the b-wave of the ERG. Instead, if an investigator wants to learn about the mean and standard deviation of the population, called μ and σ, respectively, a representative sample of individuals is drawn from the population of interest, and then this sample is studied. (Greek letters designate population parameters.)

There are two ways to estimate μ, the population mean. One is called a *point estimate*. For this method, a random sample of individuals is drawn from the population of interest, and the mean of this sample is taken as the best estimate of μ. A second way of estimating μ is called an *interval estimate*. Instead of computing a single estimate of μ, a range of likely values is computed so that there is a high probability that this range contains the population μ. The range is called a *confidence interval*, and its boundaries are called *confidence limits*. The confidence interval can be set at different levels. For example, the 95% confidence limits means that the mean drawn from a sample falls with the specified range. If the mean of the sample falls outside this range, and with a 95% confidence interval there is a 5% chance that this will occur, then the sample must have been drawn from a different population from that defining the confidence interval. To set broader limits, an investigator might establish the 99% confidence limits, that is, that 99% of the sample means would fall within the specified range and 1% would fall outside the range. It should be apparent that setting confidence limits allows testing of specific hypotheses about a sample data, as, for example, when one asks whether one group of patients generates b-wave amplitudes that are different from those of a normal population of b-waves.

Investigators frequently report the *standard error of the mean* in studies testing whether one sample is significantly different from another sample. If one were to draw 100 random samples from a population, then the standard deviation of the 100 sample means is called the *standard error of the mean*, denoted σ_x. The term is related to the standard deviation of the scores in the entire population of interest (σ) and is defined as $\sigma/\sqrt{N}$. The σ_x has a huge advantage in testing the difference between sample means: that even in cases of extreme skewness and kurtosis, σ_x has a Gaussian distribution. However, in the clinic in which the issue is to determine whether a particular individual's score is abnormal, the σ_x is not particularly useful.

When does a parameter estimate indicate pathology?

Of importance to the clinician is whether a particular set of responses lie within or outside normal limits. For example, if an ERG is performed, a clinician would be interested in knowing whether a rod- or cone-mediated response lies within normal limits or whether it falls outside normal limits. Scores that fall outside normal limits are suggestive of underlying pathology.

To answer these questions, statistical methods are employed. Most established clinical laboratories will have normative data derived from a normal population for the parameters of interest. A mean and the boundaries of normal function, or the confidence limits, will be established. Some laboratories set 95% or 99% confidence limits, and if a particular parameter estimate falls outside this range, it is considered abnormal. Other laboratories arbitrarily set these limits at 2.0 or even 3.0 standard deviations from the mean.

While normative data can be found in the literature for some electrophysiological tests (see, e.g., Birch and Anderson[2] and Birch, Anderson, and Fish[3] for the ERG), it is commonly recommended that laboratories collect their own normative data. The rationale for this point of view is that performance on a particular test depends not only on the characteristic of the observer, but also on how the data were collected. An important point to remember is that the normative data should be representative of the population of interest. Normative data collected in Australia, for example, might not be representative of individuals in North America, so the concept of global norms seems foolish. Variations in stimuli, equipment, and data analysis can affect not only the average performance on a test, but also the variability associated with the test scores. What might be considered within normal limits in one laboratory might be outside in another. However, if a laboratory can ensure that the populations, stimulus conditions, and data collection are consistent with the normative data reported in the literature, it is probably safe to use those data as a guideline.

Basic elements of experimental design and hypothesis testing

There is considerable interest in evaluating the effectiveness of therapeutic interventions for the prevention or even reversal of a progressive eye disease. The intervention might involve administering a drug or some sort of genetic therapy. In the simplest experimental design to evaluate the effectiveness of a treatment, the drug or gene therapy would be administered in a *treatment condition* and a placebo in a *control condition*, and the effectiveness of the treatment would be evaluated with some outcome measure such as a change in the amplitude of an ERG signal. In this example, the placebo is assumed to be a sham condition in which no treatment is delivered. However, the control condition need not be the absence of a treatment. In a drug trial, for example, an available alternative drug that has already been accepted as the current standard of care might be used as the control condition. The main point is that one needs an appropriate control group against which the treatment effect is evaluated.

One type of possible experimental design to evaluate a treatment is called the *independent groups design*. In this instance, a group of subjects are selected at random from the population of interest and then split, with random assignment to either the treatment or control condition. In every respect, the treatment and control groups are treated alike. Ideally, the experiment should be run *double-blind*: Neither the experimenter nor the subject knows who is receiving the drug.

In the above example, the subjects are randomly assigned to one or the other condition, but it is conceivable that by chance alone, the groups might differ in some irrelevant way. For example, by chance, one group might be older or might be disproportionately higher in males than females. This factor alone and not the particular treatment could be responsible for any observed differences.

To avoid the influence of irrelevant factors, experimenters will make their groups as comparable as possible. Suppose age is a relevant factor; the experimenter will then equate the two groups for age. If gender were a relevant factor, then the experimenter would balance the groups to avoid gender differences, either using only males or only females or using equal numbers of each gender in each group. One possible experimental design is to select pairs of subjects from the population of interest who have been equated on as many relevant variables as possible and then assigning one of each pair to either the treatment or the control condition. This design is called a *groups with matched-subjects design*.

Ideally, the matched subjects should be identical in every important way. If an experiment could be administered to identical twins, then the match would be very good, but this is often impractical. A more feasible approach would be to test the same individual under both conditions. For example, a patient might be tested before and after administration of a drug or gene therapy. This is the ultimate in matching and is generally considered to be the most powerful experimental design if it can be run. This particular design is called a *repeated measurements design*.

The experimental designs just described are the most basic of designs. More frequently than not, however, exper-imental designs are significantly more complicated. For example, an investigator might be interested in examining the effects of different doses of a drug treatment on more than one disease entity (a two-factor design). The experimental design might have X number of dose levels and Y number of disease entities. If $X = 4$ and $Y = 5$, then this experimental design would require 20 groups of subjects (4 doses × 5 diseases) if an independent groups design were used. In another experimental design, an experimenter might be interested in the before and after effects of administration of a drug on each subject within each disease entity. This is called a *mixed design* because each subject acts as its own control (repeated measures on the same subject) and they are nested within disease group (independent groups). The particular experimental design that is developed depends in large part on the questions that are being asked. The main goal of any experimental design is to have the most powerful possible design to answer relevant questions and control for irrelevant variables. Of course, the more complicated the design, the more difficult are the computational analysis and interpretation of the statistical findings. It is good practice to design an experiment and simulate potential outcomes to ensure that the design unambiguously answers the questions of interest.

Type I and II errors

When tests of significance evaluating the differences between conditions or subjects are made, two types of errors can occur. These errors are referred to as *Type I* and *Type II* errors. For demonstration, assume that there are two groups of subjects, say, patients with X-linked retinitis pigmentosa (*xlrp*) and patients with autosomal-dominant retinitis pigmentosa (*adrp*) and the performance measure to be compared is the amplitude of the cone b-wave. If an investigator rejects the hypothesis of no difference in the cone b-wave amplitude between *xlrp* and *adrp* (referred to as the null hypothesis, or H_0) when in fact H_0 is true, an error is made, and this type of error is called a Type I error. Alternatively, an investigator might fail to reject H_0, when in reality, the hypothesis of no difference is false—in reality, there is a real difference in b-wave amplitudes between *xlrp* and *adrp*. This is also an error and is called a Type II error. The main goal of any statistical hypothesis testing is to make correct decisions, that is, to reject H_0 when it is false and to not reject H_0 when it is true.

The probability of making a Type I error is called by a number of different names, including *alpha* (α), *significance level*, or *p-value*. For example, when testing the difference in the cone b-wave amplitude between *xlrp* and *adrp*, an investigator might find that the significance, or *p-value*, of the test is 0.05. This means that the difference that is observed in the performance of the two groups has a 5% likelihood of occurring by chance alone. In rejecting the hypothesis of no difference between the groups (H_0), therefore, the investigator will have a 5% chance of making a Type I error—rejecting H_0 when it is in fact true. Frequently, an investigator will set α at a higher level, say, 0.01. This means that an investigator will have only a 1% chance of making a Type I error. However, in setting a more stringent α or *p-value* for the test, the investigator is making the test less sensitive to real differences that might exist between the groups, and this can lead to a Type II error. The probability of making a Type II error is referred to as *beta* (β). The probability of making a Type II error and the probability of making a correct rejection of H_0 are determined by a number of variables discussed in the section below on the power of a statistical test.

Power

The *power* of a statistical test is the ability of the test to correctly reject the hypothesis of no difference between samples (the null hypothesis) when in fact there are real differences. The power of a test is determined by a number of variables, including the level of significance that is set for the test, the size of the sample, the magnitude of the population variability, the magnitude of the difference between population means, and whether a one- or two-tailed test is used.

In some experimental designs in vision research, calculation or consideration of statistical *power* is not an important consideration. An example of such a situation would be when there are large differences between groups on some performance measure such as the amplitude of the b-wave of the ERG, as in the case of normal subjects and patients with X-linked retinitis pigmentosa. Another example would be when the populations of interest are so unique and rare that sufficient numbers of subjects cannot be obtained to meet the requirements of power.

However, in some experimental designs, a researcher might decide that it is important to reject the hypothesis of no difference, H_0, if the difference between two groups of patients is greater than some predetermined value. For example, a researcher might decide that a difference of 100 μV on an ERG response is a meaningful difference betweeen a treatment and a control group; smaller differences might be rejected as being of little practical or clinical importance. Thus, the researcher would test the hypothesis of no difference, H_0, that μ, the difference in population means of the two groups, is $\leq 100 \mu$V against the alternative hypothesis that $\mu \geq 100 \mu$V. The question then is what power does the test of H_0 have when the alternative hypothesis is true.

As was stated above, the power of the test would depend on several factors. First, power increases as α increases; α is an arbitrary value that defines the likelihood of a particular event or occurrence and is traditionally set at 0.05. Power increases as α increases because a larger range of values is included in the rejection region. Second, power will be affected by whether H_0 and the alternative hypothesis, H_1, are one- or two-tailed tests. In two-tailed tests, there are two critical regions that scores must exceed in order for H_0 to be rejected, whereas in a on-tailed test, there is only one critical region, making the one-tailed test a more powerful test to reject H_0 in some specific experimental situations.

Finally, the population variance (a measure of variability) and sample size are two additional factors affecting power. In general, a smaller population variance and a larger sample size will yield lower estimates of the standard error of the mean (S.E.). If H_0 is true, a smaller S.E. increases the probability of rejecting the H_0 in favor of the alternative hypothesis; power is increased.

Traditionally, sample size will depend on what specific power is desired as well as the smallest difference between two groups that must be exceeded with that level of power in order to reject H_0. Procedures for calculating sample size can be found in a number of standard statistical design references, including Cohen[6] and Kirk.[9] The reader is referred to Brewer,[5] Cohen,[7] and Meyer[11] for a helpful and in-depth discussion of the practical considerations of power calculations.

Assessing physiological change in the clinic

Frequently, clinicians are asked to evaluate patients who are undergoing a treatment for a systemic disease where the treatment may adversely affect vision. Treatment of systemic lupus erthymatosis with Plaquenil (hydroxychloriquine) is such an example. The clinician's task is to select a test or a battery of tests that reliably detect the onset of drug toxicity. Finding the appropriate test(s) that can discriminate normal patients from those with a potentially toxic response is typically accomplished by deriving receiver operating characteristic (ROC) curves. A ROC curve is a graphical representation of the trade-off between false-positive and false-negative rates for selected values obtained from a test. Conventionally, the plot shows the false-positive rate on the X-axis and the false-negative rate on the Y-axis. Equivalently, the ROC curve is the representation of the trade-off between sensitivity and specificity. Accuracy, which refers to the test's ability to discriminate normal from abnormal, is measured by the area under the ROC curve. A zero-effect ROC curve, which would be consistent with a test that is a poor discriminator, would have an area of 0.0, and a perfect discriminator would have an area of 1.0, when sensitivity and specificity are expressed as fractions of unity. In a plot of the true positive rate against the false-positive rate, a zero-effect test would be indicated by a diagonal line with a slope of 1.0 and an origin at 0.0. From the ROC curves, one can select any pass/fail measure and then compare the performance of the test with a gold standard that is known to discriminate between groups of patients.

ROC curves can also be constructed from clinical prediction rules. For example, one might find that changes in the electro-oculogram, an abnormal color vision test, depressed macular function on the multifocal ERG, and changes in the retinal pigment epithelium are predictive of Plaquenil toxicity. ROC curves can be constructed by computing the sensitivity and specificity of increasing numbers of these clinical findings (0–5). The ROC curves would indicate whether this set of clinical findings adequately discriminates normal from toxic responses and what minimum number of clinical findings would have the most predictive power. A more detailed discussion of ROC analysis can be found in Metz[10] and Zweig and Campbell.[15]

Here the issue is that of change. How much change in some physiological parameter would need to occur for the researcher to conclude that a treatment has positive or negative consequences? Clearly, a one-time evaluation of visual function is inadequate. Serial testing is required, which usually involves obtaining pretreatment baseline measures and then repetitive testing at appropriate time intervals during treatment. Electrophysiological and psychophysical test results are notoriously variable and are influenced by many factors. Variability can originate from factors inherent in the subject or patient, such as diurnal rhythms and attention, or from factors external to the patient, such as stimulus variations and the quality of the tester.

Waiting for the test scores to fall outside normal limits is not acceptable if termination of treatment and drug washout will reverse the negative consequences for visual function. Such dramatic change in an individual might suggest that irreparable damage has resulted. Instead, the question becomes: How much change is acceptable? How much change is attributable to the treatment and how much is random variation in the parameter estimate?

One strategy is to obtain test-retest reliability measurements for the specific test for normal observers. Published databases of this sort are becoming available (see, e.g., Birch, Hood, Locke, Hoffman, and Tzekov[4]). Then one can say that 15%, 20%, or 50% variation in a particular physiological or psychophysical parameter is random variation. If the change is greater than the prescribed amount, then the treatment can be assumed to have some effect. An alternative strategy would be to obtain test-retest reliability measurement on the particular patient before treatment and then use this estimate of variability to evaluate treatment for this individual. A within-subject design is generally accepted as being a more powerful experimental design but would require more extensive testing that might be beyond the scope of most clinical laboratories.

An additional question would be whether a single negative finding would be sufficient to conclude a treatment effect. In patients with glaucoma or a progressive retinal disease, it is common to observe visual function over many test sessions before concluding that progressive change has occurred and determining the amount of that change. In drug therapies, this kind of luxury is not afforded to the clinician who must decide whether a drug treatment should be discontinued. Correlation with other clinical findings is very important in this context. Finally, the trend in visual function must be reversible when drug washout has occurred to conclude definitively that the drug caused the progressive change in visual function.

Parametric and nonparametric statistical testing

There are two broad classes of statistical tests: *parametric* and *nonparametric* tests. Each of these classes of tests relies on certain assumptions. Parametric tests, for example, rely on the assumption (among other assumptions) that test scores obtained from a population are normally distributed. That is, in a distribution of test scores, the assumption is made that there are just as many high and above-average scores as there are low and below-average scores. In comparing two groups of scores using a parametric test, it is assumed that the two groups of scores are normally distributed around a mean and have more or less equal variability. A parametric test, such as an analysis of variance (ANOVA) or a *t*-test, is inappropriate when this assumption is not met.

Sometimes, however, data sets and experimental designs do not allow this assumption of normality to be made. For example, distributions of test scores may have unequal variability; one set might be normally distributed, but a second set of test scores might have substantially greater numbers of higher than lower scores. In such cases, it is sometimes possible and legitimate to transform the raw test scores into another numeric form, as in the conversion to logarithms, to normalize and equate the distributions and then to continue with an appropriate parametric test.

In other situations, the nature of the test scores themselves prevents the use of a parametric test. For example, in a drug toxicity study, an investigator might simply ask whether there is a positive or negative change in a visual field rather than actually quantifying, for example, the percent change in area of the visual field. Or the outcome measure might require a two-alternative forced choice, such as "Yes, I see it" or "No, I don't see it." Or the test scores might be in the form of a rating scale, say, from 1 to 5, as in the scale for rating the density of cataracts. These types of experimental test results would be better suited to nonparametric than to parametric statistical analyses.

In general, nonparametric tests are less powerful than parametric tests. If the assumptions for the use of a parametric test can be met, then a parametric test will be a more sensitive test to detect small differences. Nonparametric tests tend to overlook or miss small differences and produce a Type II error: accepting the hypothesis of no difference between groups when in reality it should not have been accepted. (A broad discussion of the use of nonparametric tests can be found in Seigel.[13])

Regression analyses

In some research questions, an investigator might be interested in understanding how a particular physiological or psychophysical parameter changes with time. For example, an issue that has been investigated extensively in the literature is whether the mode of inheritance affects disease progression associated with retinitis pigmentosa. Alternatively, an investigator might be interested in knowing whether the presence or absence of a particular antigen affects disease progression as measured by the changes in visual field area or a physiological parameter, such as the amplitude of the b-wave.

This class of question is best addressed with a regression analysis. The simplest form of a regression analysis is called a *linear regression analysis*. In this type of regression, it is assumed that a straight line defines the relationship between two variables, such as ERG amplitude and age. By using a least-squares minimization procedure, the best fit straight line is found that describes the relationship between the two variables, and the relationship is defined by an equation of the form

$$Y = b_0 + b_1 X$$

where b_0 and b_1 are constants and X and Y are the variables that are to be related, such as ERG amplitude and age, respectively, in the above example. The constant b_1 is called the slope of the line and indicates the rate of change of Y with X. This constant can be used to indicate how much in the way of amplitude loss occurs on average with each year of change. The constant b_0 is the Y-intercept, that is, the value of Y when X is equal to zero.

In the discussion thus far, the relationship between two variables is assumed to be linear; that is, a straight line is assumed to describe the relationship between two variables. It is conceivable, however, that for some physiological and psychophysical variables, a straight line is not the best way of describing the relationship. For example, a curved line might describe the relationship better. In this instance, the regression equation is best fit by a polynomial equation of the form

$$Y = b_0 + b_1 X + b_2 X^2 + \cdots + b_p X^p + \cdots + B_{a-1} X^{a-1}$$

where X and Y are described as above and $b_{0-(a-1)}$ are the slope coefficients. As can be see, in a nonlinear relationship between two variables, it is impossible to state a single value to define the rate of change of one variable with the other. One possible remedy to this is to transform scores into some form that will better define a linear relationship.

Defining and modeling the relationship between two variables can be complicated, filled with assumptions and fraught with difficulties. The reader is referred to Myers and Well[12] and Darlington[8] for discussions of computational and practical issues in linear and nonlinear regression analysis.

Univariate and multivariate statistical analyses

Univariate statistical analyses refers to the situation in which there is only one outcome measure, called a *dependent variable*. There can be one or more *independent variables*, which is either a variable that is manipulated by an experimenter or some naturally occurring category. For example, in a drug intervention study, the empirical question might involve testing the effects on the b-wave of the ERG (the dependent variable) for different doses of a particular drug (the independent variable). Or the study might be expanded to study the interaction effects of gender (a second independent variable) and drug dose on ERG amplitudes. Analysis of variance (ANOVA) and *t*-tests are examples of univariate statistical analyses.

In some experimental designs, however, there may be more than one outcome measure or dependent variable. For example, if an experimental design called for performing an entire ERG protocol that conforms to the International Society for Clinical Electrophysiology standards, there could be as many as five or six dependent variables. Or one might have an ERG measure and a psychophysical measure, such as the area of a visual field, as outcome measures. In these situations, the empirical question might be which ERG measure is a better indicator of drug toxicity or whether an ERG measure does better than a psychophysical measure.

In vision research, data are typically analyzed with multiple univariate analyses. For example, one might use a *t*-test to test the significance of gender differences on the amplitude of an ERG response. A second *t*-test might be used to test the significance of gender differences on the area of the visual field. An experimenter might continue with multiple *t*-tests to examine differences in outcome measures for each independent variable separately.

In general, this analytical approach is acceptable provided that the number of comparisons is small. When the number of comparisons is relatively large, the results of multiple *t*-tests may be misleading and statistically suspect. Each *t*-test is accompanied by a margin of error that is dictated by the *p*-value or α. If $\alpha = 0.05$, then there is a 5% chance of a difference being observed in sample means based on chance alone. If several independent univariate tests are performed on the same sample of subjects, the error rate increases with the number of univariate tests. In addition, when numerous outcome measures are obtained from the same sample, these outcome measures are also interrelated in complex ways, and the probability of error increases even further.

These increases in error rates are frequently overlooked in clinical vision studies or, alternatively, are dealt with by asserting a more stringent criterion level for significance. For example, one might set $\alpha = 0.01$ or 0.001, which would reduce the rejection level of the hypothesis of no difference to 1% and 0.1%, respectively. However, such approaches would reduce the power of the test to detect real differences that might exist between the samples (see the section on power), thereby increasing the probability of a Type II error. With the use of multivariate statistics, complex interactions between multiple independent (outcome) measures and independent (experimental) variables can be assessed while keeping the overall error rate at some stated level, say, 5%, independent of the number of comparisons that are made. Experimental designs in clinical and experimental vision science are becoming increasingly complex, particularly in studies in which one is trying to find the most sensitive measure of change. These experimental designs call for multivariate analyses, and there are numerous statistical analysis packages, such as SPSS, SYSTAT, and SAS, that can make the job of computation less painful. However, while the computational part of multivariate statistics can be made relatively easy, the interpretation of the statistics in terms of understanding relationships between many variables can be very difficult. The reader is referred to Tabachnick and Fidell[14] for a comprehensive discussion of multivariate statistical designs and interpretation issues.

Summary

Exploring experimental questions involves complicated experimental designs and statistical analyses. Experimental design addresses the issue of how an experiment is to be constructed so that it best answers the questions of interest. Statistical analyses allow one to quantify and summarize the data obtained from an experiment and allow tests of the significance of experimental findings. The major goal of any experimental design and statistical analysis is to provide the most powerful possible mechanism to answer experimental questions and to test specific hypotheses. It is recommended that an experiment be simulated with generated data to ensure not only that the data can be analyzed appropriately, but also that the interpretation of the analysis will be unambiguous.

REFERENCES

1. Anderson LR, Ager JW: Analysis of variance in small group research. *Personality Social Psychol Bull* 1978; 4:341–345.
2. Birch DG, Anderson JL: Standardized full-field electroretinography: Normal values and their variation with age. *Arch Ophthalmol* 1992; 110:1571–1576.
3. Birch DG, Anderson JL, Fish GE: Yearly rates of rod and cone functional loss in retinitis pigmentosa and cone-rod dystrophy. *Ophthalmology* 1999; 106:258–268.
4. Birch DG, Hood DC, Locke KG, Hoffman DR, Tzekov RT: Quantitative electroretinogram measures of phototransduction in cone and rod photoreceptors: Normal aging, progression with disease, and test-retest variability. *Arch Ophthalmol* 2002; 120:1045–1051.
5. Brewer JK: Issues of power: Clarification. *Am Educ Res J* 1974; 11:189–192.
6. Cohen J: *Statistical Power Analysis for the Behavioural Sciences*. New York, Academic Press, 1969.
7. Cohen J: Statistical power analysis and research results. *Am Educ Res J* 1973; 10:225–230.
8. Darlington RB: *Regression and Linear Models*. New York, McGraw-Hill, 1990.
9. Kirk R: *Experimental Design: Procedures for the Behavioural Sciences*. Pacific Grove, CA, Brooks/Cole, 1982.
10. Metz CE: Basic principles of ROC analysis. *Sem Nucl Med* 1978; 8:283–289.
11. Meyer DL: Statistical tests and surveys of power: A critique. *Am Educ Res J* 1974; 11:179–188.
12. Myers JL, Well AD: *Research Design and Statistical Analysis*. New York, HarperCollins, 1991.
13. Siegel S: *Nonparametric Statistics for the Behavioural Sciences*. New York, McGraw-Hill, 1956.
14. Tabachnick BG, Fidell LS: *Using Multivariate Statistics*. New York, Harper and Row, 1989.
15. Zweig MH, Campbell G: Receiver-operating characteristic (ROC) plots: A fundemental evaluation tool in clinical medicine. *Clin Chem* 1993; 39(4):561–577.

31 Analytical Techniques

L. HENK VAN DER TWEEL AND OSCAR ESTÉVEZ

VISUAL ELECTROPHYSIOLOGISTS have at present a wide choice of instruments at their disposal, from direct recorders to sophisticated computers. This enables them to record ever smaller responses and to improve their quality. "Thresholds," defined as the weakest stimuli evoking recognizable responses, are continuously dropping, and the range and type of electroretinogram (ERG) and visual evoked potential (VEP) stimuli have been regularly extended. In addition, computer-based analytical methods are increasingly being used for the characterization of responses.

A proper selection from these modern methods requires knowledge about the principles of signal analysis on which they are based. These same principles apply to many quantitative aspects of visual function. The present chapter is meant to help the researcher and the clinician to find their way among the multitude of published methods. Emphasis will be laid less on mathematical rigor than on the understanding of fundamental concepts. The topics to be covered are (1) the recording and processing of electrical responses and (2) analytical questions concerning the stimulus and response characterization.

The unavoidable presence of noise (e.g., the background electroencephalogram [EEG]) demands procedures for noise reduction, especially if weak stimuli are presented. This can be done in a variety of ways, but in clinical practice it is often most important to reduce the recording time, which has encouraged the use of more "efficient" methods such as, for instance, the so-called steady-state stimulation. It is intended that the present chapter will enable the evaluation of such techniques.

For a long time nearly all ERGs and VEPs were recorded with flashes. The responses obtained in this way are often complex and more prone to the effects of strong nonlinearities (for a definition of this term, see below). However, by employing stimuli with other waveforms, among which sinusoidal modulation is the most frequent, it is easier to recognize deviations from linearity and to identify significant nonlinear properties of the system under study. An added advantage of sinusoidal stimuli is that linearity can often be approximated to a satisfactory degree, which facilitates analysis and description.

More recently homogeneous field stimulation has been superseded by the use of spatially structured fields such as checkerboards and sine wave gratings. This type of research has developed in two main directions:

1. Characteristics such as amplitude, wave shape, and latency are used to discriminate between normal and pathological responses. In this case only rather elementary methods of signal improvement need be employed.

2. The responses are used as a criterion for the "effectiveness" of a changing stimulus, e.g., when the size of checks in a checkerboard or the periodicity and the contrast of a grating are manipulated to obtain a constant response. The results of such studies are often expressed as a contrast sensitivity function (transfer function). The theoretical background, however, is complicated and requires among other things an analytical characterization of the stimulus, e.g., that of a checkerboard.

Basic concepts of signal analysis

LINEARITY One approach to analyzing the results of clinical electrophysiology is to treat all stimuli as if they were transduced and processed by a "black box" between the stimulus and recorded response. The simplest assumption that can be made about the black box is that of linearity, even though no biological system strictly fulfills such a condition.

The definition of a linear system is that it obeys the "superposition principle." Assume that A and B are (quantifiable) input signals (e.g., stimuli) that result respectively in outputs C and D of the system under study. Let us use $\rightarrow$ to signify "produces the response" so that we have $A \rightarrow C$ and $B \rightarrow D$. In this case we say that a system is linear if $A + B \rightarrow C + D$. A consequence of linearity is that the amplitude of the response is strictly proportional to that of the input. Input and output do not need to belong to the same physical category; they may, for instance, represent light values and voltage respectively as in figure 31.1, where the upper traces represent the voltage of the ERG of an anesthesized cat and the lower ones the modulation of the intense light source that was employed.[17]

A cardinal property of linear systems concerns the harmonic function $A \sin 2\pi ft$ (figure 31.2). It is the only function that retains its identity (its sinusoidal shape and its

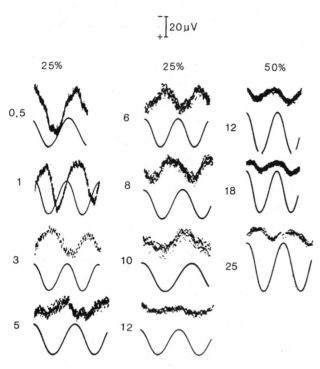

FIGURE 31.1 An early example of the responses of a reasonably linear "black box" in which light is translated into voltage. The ERG of an anesthetized cat is recorded with sinusoidally modulated light (retinal illumination, 50,000 trolands; field, 56 degrees; 25% respectively; 50% modulation depth; range, 0.5 to 25 Hz; upper traces, ERG; lower traces, photocell signal of illumination). Responses approach the sinusoidal shape, a property of linear systems. (From van der Tweel LH, Visser P: Electrical responses of the retina to sinusoidally modulated light. In *Electroretinographia*. Acta Facultatis Medicae Universitatis Brunensis, 1959, pp 185–196, Lekarska Fakulta University Brne. Used by permission.)

period) when submitted to a linear transformation; a light input $A \sin 2\pi ft$ will, for instance, evoke a response $B \sin(2\pi ft + \Phi)$ with, in general, B different from A and Φ an added phase shift. A direct consequence of this property is that, at the output of a linear system, no new frequencies are generated from any input, no matter how complex that input is.

In physics, basic (passive) elements like capacities, inductances, resistances, and their combinations are the simplest linear elements; however, complex (active) devices like electronic amplifiers can also approach linearity to a large degree.

FREQUENCY DEPENDENCE The ratio of output to input amplitudes of harmonic functions will in general depend on frequency; this is expressed in the "amplitude characteristic," i.e., the normalized ratio of output to input amplitude as a function of frequency. Similarly the "phase characteristic" is defined as the function representing the phase shift between the output and the input for all frequencies. Together they fully define the input-output relation of any linear "black box" for arbitrary signals. In filter theory often the two characteristics are combined into the "transfer function."

As an example of the usefulness of this representation, we show in figure 31.3 the amplitude and phase characteristics of the occipital VEPs of two subjects to sinusoidally modulated light.[16] The responses of both subjects A and B are approximately sinusoidal and show preference for frequencies around 10 Hz. The sharpness (selectivity) of the amplitude plot, however, is much more prominent in B than in A, which is also reflected (as should be expected in a quasilinear system) in the steep course of the phase characteristics around 10 Hz of subject B. At the same time, B exhibits a strong monorhythmic persistent alpha rhythm. The responses have been proved to add to the spontaneous activity without any indication of entrainment phenomena.

Note that there is no sense in talking about phase relations between sinusoidal signals with different frequencies. If a signal contains more than one frequency, the phase relationship between any two frequencies will vary according to the moment of observation. This applies even to the harmonically related frequencies of a periodic wave shape. For example, figure 31.4 shows a sine wave and its second harmonic. The phase relationship during one period is different for each point along the x-axis. For certain purposes a characteristic point may be chosen as a reference, for instance, when the voltage changes its sign from negative to positive (positive zero-crossing).

MINIMUM-PHASE RULE, DELAY, AND LATENCY In every physically realizable system a nonconstant amplitude/frequency response is necessarily accompanied by phase shifts that are a function of frequency. In systems without active components (i.e., if only capacities, inductances, and resistances are present) the phase characteristic can be fully calculated from the amplitude characteristic. This is a consequence of what is known as the "minimum-phase rule." If active components are included, phase shifts will often be larger but can never be smaller than the calculated minimum phase for a passive system. The attenuated high-frequency signal at the output of a single low-pass filter, for instance, must be accompanied by a phase shift up to 90 degrees for frequencies approaching infinity. Different amplitude characteristics are necessarily accompanied by different phase characteristics. However, the reverse is *not* true: different phase characteristics can be associated with the same amplitude plot.

An important example of phase shifting without amplitude changes is when a pure delay or latency is involved. In that case the phase changes proportionally to the frequency. The relation is as follows:

$$\tau = (\Phi_2 - \Phi_1)/2\pi(f_2 - f_1) \qquad (1)$$

with τ the delay and Φ the phase shift in radians. In figure 31.5, the "responses" are subject to a delay of 25 ms. For sinusoidal stimulus "A" at 30 Hz the phase delay is 450

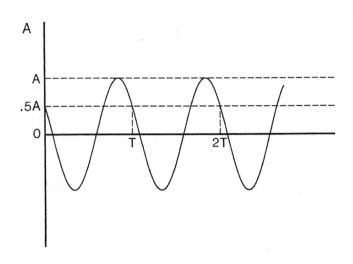

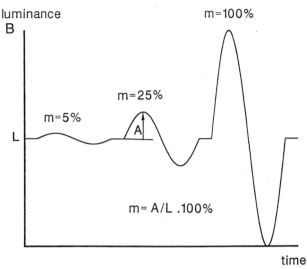

FIGURE 31.2 A, An elementary sine wave: $A \sin(2\pi ft + \Phi)$ with the period $T = 1/f$. In the example $\Phi = 5\pi/6$ (150 degrees). An equivalent mathematical representation of the same curve is A $\cos(2\pi ft - \Phi)$ with $\Phi = \pi/3$ (60 degrees). B, In case light is modulated, amplitude is given in percent modulation depth (percentage of the average light level).

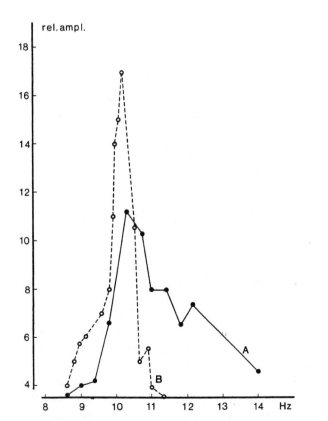

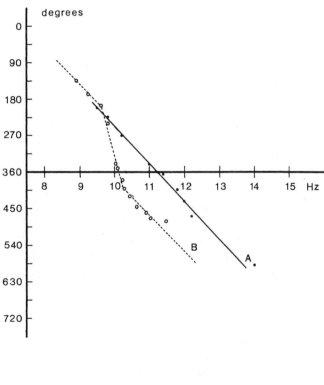

FIGURE 31.3 Amplitude and phase characteristics of human occipital VEPs to sinusoidally modulated light. The subjects A (solid lines) and B (dashed lines) show large differences in the selectivity of the response. This is reflected in the amplitude as well as in the phase plot; the high selectivity in subject B is clearly expressed in an extra phase jump of approximately 180 degrees, while in subject A such a jump was not found. Note that the frequency axis is on a linear scale and not on the conventional logarithmic one. The linear phase shift with frequency is equivalent to a delay of approximately 250 ms. (From van der Tweel LH, Verduyn Lunel HFE: Human visual responses to sinusoidally modulated light. *Electroencephalogr Clin Neurophysiol* 1965; 18:587–598. Used by permission.)

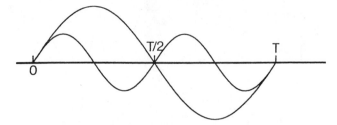

FIGURE 31.4 Two harmonically related frequencies. Both phases were chosen to be zero at $t = 0$. At point $T/2$, the phase at frequency $f_1 = 1/T$ is π; at frequency $f_2 = 2/T$ the phase is zero again, i.e., 2π (shifted a whole period).

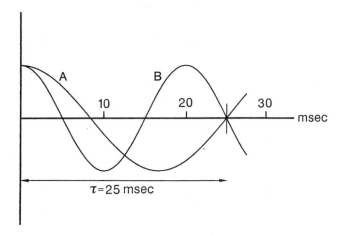

FIGURE 31.5 Phase shifts ($5\pi/2$ and $3\pi/2$) at frequencies of 50 Hz (B) and 30 Hz (A) due to a delay of 25 ms. This delay obeys the formula: $\tau = (\Phi_2 - \Phi_1)/2\pi(f_2 - f_1)$.

degrees, more than one full cycle; B exhibits a phase shift of 270 degrees at 50 Hz. The difference is 180 degrees (π). The formula then reads $\tau = \pi/(2\pi \cdot 20)$, which yields a delay of 25 ms, as expected. Note that, if the delay were to be much longer, the phase angles at both frequencies would include more periods, and these extra periods should also be taken into account. If one wishes to avoid ambiguities, a series of closely spaced frequencies should be used. The ensuing phase-frequency regression line should (minimum-phase corrections applied) within experimental accuracy pass either through the origin ($f = 0$, $\Phi = 0$) or through $\Phi = \pm\pi$.

With due caution, therefore, the formula allows for an efficient way to estimate VEP or ERG latencies: by using a frequency band where the response is reasonably sinusoidal and its amplitude does not change too much with frequency. If the amplitude dependency is strong, there will be extra phase shifts that can be estimated from the minimum-phase rule and used for correction.

From the above, it follows that in principle one should not use the phase shift (or, for instance, the peak of the sinusoidal response) at a given frequency as a criterion for delay. Not only are there extra phase shifts possible due to the minimum-phase rule, but there is still another source of error that can trap even the most eminent: due to the periodic character of the stimulus, as was explained above, one or more periods may be missed. This mistake will be mostly evident when unrealistic delays are obtained, but also ambiguities of only half a period may occur. The point to keep in mind is that an increase in light, for instance, has no obligatory relation to the polarity of an electrical response. This is self-evident when recording VEPs because their polarity will also depend on electrode placement. Even when different frequencies are employed, the results must be interpreted with care. For example, figure 31.1 shows the cat ERG in response to bright, flickering, sinusoidally modulated light of various frequencies. Since the responses are reasonably sinusoidal, linearity is approached. At 0.5 Hz, the phase angle is about 90 degrees and at 3 Hz about 180 degrees. Applying our equation for delay suggests that the latency would be about 100 ms. Now this is quite unlikely, and the probable explanation is that the ERG to this bright modulated light is generated by more than one process, one cornea-positive and the other cornea-negative, and the amplitude characteristics of the two are very different.

There is a special problem with regard to latency determination of (steady-state) VEPs with pattern reversal. Whereas for homogeneous fields sinusoidal modulation is to be preferred, the same is not the case for patterns because abrupt reversal gives a much better defined moment of activation than sinusoidal modulation does. In the latter case the actual moment of excitation will be dependent on the contrast. On the other hand, because abrupt transitions will dominate observation, sine wave modulation is better suited for psychophysical experiments.

DISTORTION We have already mentioned that every linear system made of real physical components will exhibit frequency-dependent characteristics. This means that the relation between the original input amplitudes and phases at different frequencies will be subject to alteration, i.e., the output wave shape will not in general resemble the input: it will be distorted. This is called *linear* distortion because the superposition principle applies all the same to the output components. According to Fourier theory, as will be explained below, the shape of an arbitrary input signal is determined by the amplitudes and phases of the frequencies of which it is composed. Since in any real system the relation between input and output amplitudes and phases will depend on frequency, the output shape must differ from that of the input. Shape distortion is only absent in cases where the input is a pure harmonic function, when a sinusoidal input results in a sinusoidal output.

A type of linear distortion that will nearly always be present is attenuation of high frequencies. In mechanics this attenuation is due to inertia, in electricity to (stray) capacitances, and in electrophysiology, diffusion processes (among others) play a similar role. Flicker fusion is an example of high-frequency attenuation, but the ERG and the VEP are also subject to this form of attenuation.

Nonlinear distortion, on the other hand, differs fundamentally from linear distortion. Nonlinearity means that proportionality between input and output does not hold for all signal amplitudes, for instance, often for a large input signal the responses do not grow any more (saturation). Therefore, in the presence of nonlinearities, the superposition principle is *not* obeyed. In principle, all real systems are subject to nonlinear distortion, saturation and thresholds being the most frequent ones (although modern electronic devices can approximate linearity to a large degree). Nonlinearity is an inherent and common property of biological systems. Although the division is not absolute, for our purpose it is useful to distinguish "essential" from "nonessential" nonlinearities. For instance, logarithmic and exponential functions as well as saturation are nonessential: the distortion is strongly dependent on the strength (amplitude) of the phenomenon. If an incremental or decremental signal δ is made small enough, the system may approach linear behavior (because, e.g., $\log(1 + \delta) \approx \delta$). When the input signal is enlarged, quadratic and higher-order terms are playing a role. Rectification, however, belongs to the class of essential nonlinearities; in the ideal case—no matter how small the input signal—the system transmits only one polarity. This means the introduction of significant quadratic and higher-order terms. In reality, rectification will not always be abrupt, i.e., it will not occur at a given break point, but it will be a smooth transition over some small interval and will—for certain small inputs—obey linearity. Nevertheless, in VEP studies rectification can exhibit astonishingly sharp discontinuities, as is shown in figure 31.6.[12] In this figure it is demonstrated that even for modulations as small as 1.25% of the average light intensity one still obtains a second harmonic response (although with decreasing relative amplitude). Because of the selectivity of the responses to sinusoidally modulated light, as shown in figure 31.3, rectification expresses itself especially at 5-Hz stimulation; the second harmonic is then 10 Hz, just at the maximum of the response characteristic. In fact, at stimulation with 10 Hz the response itself is to a high degree sinusoidal. With respect to rectification, this has been demonstrated in the ganglion cells of the goldfish.[10] It must be noted that distortions caused by rectifiers and by saturation are usually frequency independent. This type of distortion is called static, and such nonlinear elements are called *static* nonlinearities, in contrast to elements whose parameters would change with frequency, which exhibit *dynamic* nonlinearities. Adaptation belongs to the last category.

A consequence of nonlinearity in general is that the response to a combination of harmonic functions will

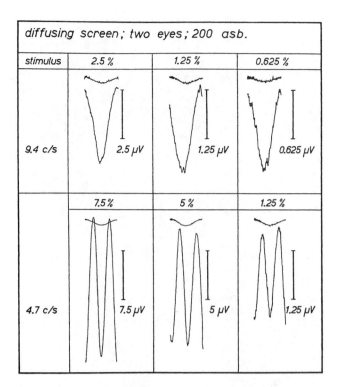

FIGURE 31.6 Occipital VEPs to sinusoidally modulated light at 4.7 and 9.4 Hz. The sinusoidal responses at 9.4 Hz are strictly proportional to modulation depth (note the changing amplification factor). At 4.7 Hz sinusoidal second-harmonic responses can be recorded down to 1.25%, although less than proportionally. (From Spekreijse H, Van der Tweel LH: *Proc Kon Ned Akad van Wetensch* 1972; 75:77–105. Used by permission.)

contain new nonharmonic frequencies. For example, if two frequencies f_1 and f_2 are presented and there is a quadratic term in the nonlinearity, the frequencies $2f_1$, $2f_2$, $f_1 + f_2$, and $f_1 - f_2$ will also appear in the output. In fact such a property has been used in visual studies to analyze the system, especially if rectification could be expected.

It is interesting to realize, with regard to the above considerations, that we do not appear to be aware of the inherent logarithmicity of the intensity transformation within our own visual system. Neither do we notice the distortions of considerable intensity that usually occur in black-and-white photographs. In hearing, however, even small nonlinearities in the chain of sound transformations may be intolerable. They can add "extraneous" and disturbing frequencies: hi-fi was not invented for nothing! On the other hand, the visual system is very sensitive to *linear* distortion that introduces phase shifts in an image. Figure 31.7A shows two of the bars of a medium-contrast square wave grating on an oscillograph screen.[13] The white lines at the bottom represent the screen luminance. As will be described in the following chapter, the generating signal of the grating can be resolved into or synthesized from a number of sinusoids, each representing a certain (harmonic) spatial frequency with specific

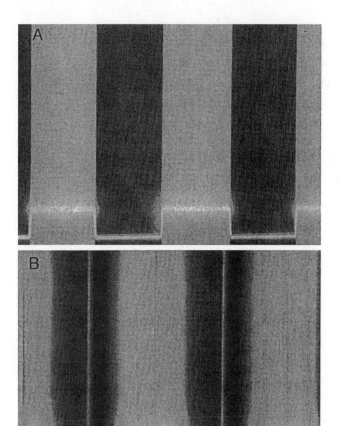

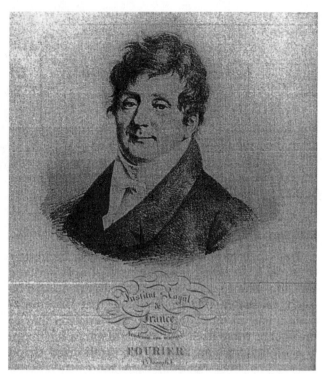

FIGURE 31.8 Portrait of Joseph Fourier, lithograph. (Courtesy of the Museum Boerhaave, Leyden, The Netherlands.) The text below reads: "Membre de la Légion d'honneur, etc. Né à Auxerre, le 21 Mars 1768, élu en 1817 et Sécretaire perpétuel pour les sciences mathématiques en 1822." Translated: "Member Legion of Honor, born Auxerre, France, March 21, 1768, elected in 1817 and Permanent Secretary for Mathematical Sciences in 1822."

FIGURE 31.7 Two cycles of a square wave pattern (*A*) generated on a cathode ray tube. *B*, Drastic phase shifting has been performed without affecting the amplitudes of the Fourier components. The generating signals are displayed at the bottom of the patterns. (From van der Tweel LH: In Spekreijse H, van der Tweel TH (eds). *Spatial Contrast*. Amsterdam, Elsevier Science Publishers, 1977, pp 9–12. Used by permission.)

amplitude and phase. The phase relationship of the composing frequencies determines the exact shape of the grating. By electronic means it is possible to shift the relative phases without affecting the amplitudes. As can be seen, the appearance of the grid changes dramatically by such a procedure (figure 31.7B).

Again in contrast to the behavior of the visual system, hearing is very tolerant of phase distortion, in any case for periodic signals (Helmholtz's rule). If the two generating wave forms of figure 31.7 are played into a loudspeaker at, e.g., 300 Hz, A and B sound identical because the same harmonics are present in the same relative amplitudes.

Fourier analysis

In 1807 Fourier (whose portrait is shown in figure 31.8) submitted his epoch-making manuscript on heat conduction to the Institut de France for publication, but it was not until 1822 that his book *Théorie Analytique de la Chaleur* appeared.[9]

In this book one of the most fundamental theorems of physics was developed. According to Fourier's theory, every *periodic* function can be decomposed into or synthesized from an (in principle) infinite number of harmonic functions. The lowest frequency is the inverse of the fundamental period, and all other frequencies are multiples thereof. In addition, there is a term representing the average level of the function. The lowest frequency is also called the *fundamental* or *first harmonic*, and all others form the *higher harmonics*. Their various amplitudes and phases are such that, when added together, they reproduce the shape of the original function.

Fourier's formula for periodic time functions reads as follows:

$$F(t) = a_0/2 + \sum_{n=1}^{\infty} (a_n \cos 2\pi nft + b_n \sin 2\pi nft) \qquad (2)$$

where $F(t)$ is a *periodic* function with the period T and a_0 is a constant that represents twice the mean of the function, also conventionally (and sloppily) called the DC-term or, when light is considered, the average illumination.

The frequency f (in hertz) is the inverse of T in seconds. If $n = 2, 3, 4$, etc., one speaks of the second, third, fourth, etc., harmonic. Often the sine and cosine terms are taken together:

$$F(t) = A_0/2 + \sum_{n=1}^{\infty} A_n \cos(2\pi n f t + \Phi_n) \qquad (3)$$

where $A_0 = a_0$, $A_n^2 = a_n^2 + b_n^2$, and $\tan \Phi = b_n/a_n$.

If distance (x) is the variable, then we use P instead of T: $f = 1/P$. For spatial periodic phenomena in vision, spatial frequency is given in cycles per degree and period in visual angle (degree). The terms a_n and b_n can be respectively computed from the equations

$$a_n = 2/T \cdot \int_{-T/2}^{+T/2} F(t) \cos 2\pi n f t \, dt \qquad (4)$$

and

$$b_n = 2/T \cdot \int_{-T/2}^{+T/2} F(t) \sin 2\pi n f t \, dt \qquad (5)$$

For computational reasons harmonic functions are often displayed in complex notation as $C_n \exp(jn\Omega t)$, with j being the square root of -1 and Ω, $2\pi f$. This is identical with the sin-cos treatment because $\exp(jn\Omega t) = \cos n\Omega t + j \sin n\Omega t$.

STANDARD PERIODIC SIGNALS   The scope of Fourier analysis can best be understood by considering the analysis of simple periodic functions like a square wave. Its components can be easily calculated (figure 31.9). Note that the fundamental has an amplitude $(4/\pi)$ that exceeds that of the square wave itself. As the third and a few more of the harmonics are added, the synthesized shape approaches the square pattern more and more. There remains, however, a narrowing overshoot of about 18% that shifts toward the steep flanks of the square wave as more and more harmonics are included; this is called Gibbs' phenomenon.

Another important standard signal is that formed by periodic impulses. Theoretically the impulse (or $\delta-$) function is by no means simple, but for the present purpose, the following explanation will suffice. It is supposed that each impulse is infinitely short and infinitely high. For instance, electrical current impulses can be given with diminishing duration δt and increasing strength i in order to keep the total charge per impulse constant. This total is normalized to *unity*, and the mean charge (dc or zero-frequency component) becomes then $1/T$; light flashes can be treated in a similar way. The Fourier spectrum of these repetitive impulses consists of equally spaced spectral lines of constant amplitude at frequencies f, $2f$, $3f$, etc. These are again impulse functions, but on a frequency axis (figure 31.10A), the amplitudes are $2/T$. Since the average of periodic unit impulses is by definition $1/T$, all sinusoidal components extend into the negative part of the amplitude axis (figure 31.10B). At present, comparatively simple computer programs are available that easily perform on-line Fourier analysis of any signal, periodic or not, so quickly that the calculations seem instantaneous. Note that the Fourier analysis of a nonperiodic signal is technically performed as if the analyzed interval is part of one period of a repetitive signal! This period should be chosen with due care.

THE FOURIER INTEGRAL   Theoretically, the Fourier series represents of reproduces a *periodic* function that continues *forever*. In practice this can never be achieved, although a sufficiently long interval may be considered to approach the ideal situation. For single events or transients, i.e., signals of the "one-in-a-lifetime" sort, the discrete sum Σ is substituted by an integral. Figure 31.11 gives an example to better understand the meaning of this extrapolation. In figure 31.11, we start with the presentation of a square wave with

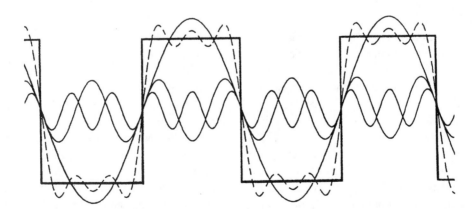

FIGURE 31.9   The first three harmonics of a square wave and their sum (dashed line). The amplitude of the fundamental exceeds that of the square wave. The overshoot does not disappear but becomes narrower when more frequencies are included.

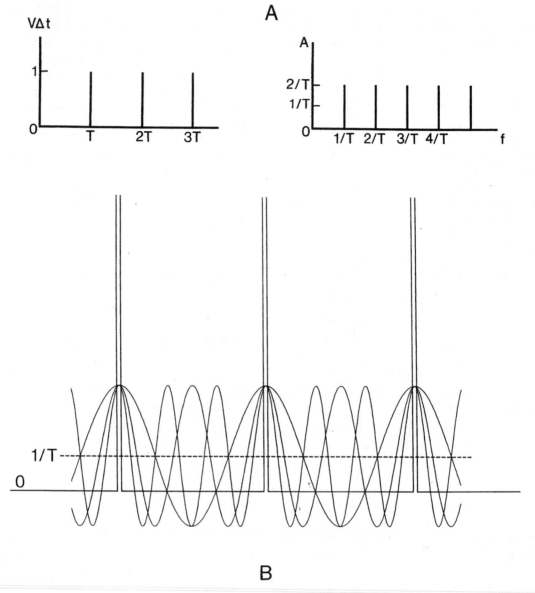

A

B

FIGURE 31.10 *A*, Fourier spectrum of periodic impulses normalized to $V \cdot \delta t = 1$. All amplitudes are $2/T$; "DC" level, $1/T$. Note that the impulses in the time domain have the dimension volt·seconds and *not* volt. *B*, Periodic impulse functions (period T) as they are built up from cosine waves of frequencies n/T ("DC" level, $1/T$). The virtual modulation depth of all components is 200%.

its Fourier line spectrum as was treated before in figure 31.9. Subsequently, one period of this square wave is isolated and repeated with progressively longer periods. The spectral representation for the signals with lengthened periods is indicated in figure 31.11. In accordance with the increase in period T, the fundamental frequency $1/T$ decreases, which results in more closely spaced spectral lines.

If this procedure were to be continued (i.e., is extrapolated to an infinitely long interval), the spectral lines would become infinite in number and therefore approach a continuum, at which moment they represent the Fourier transform of a single event; the Fourier *series* (the line spectrum of equation 3) has become the Fourier *integral*:

$$F(t) = 1/2\pi \cdot \int_{-\infty}^{+\infty} A(\Omega) \exp j\Omega t d\Omega \qquad (6)$$

with $\Omega = 2\pi f$ and f the frequency. At the same time this forms the (nonnormalized) envelope of the former line spectra.

Especially revealing is the case of a single impulse. If the procedure just described is applied to the case of figure 31.10A, extrapolating to a single impulse, the continuous spectrum that results exhibits a constant amplitude at all frequencies. All composing harmonic functions reach maximal amplitudes at the moment of the occurrence of the impulse (see also figure 31.10B). Therefore they are represented by

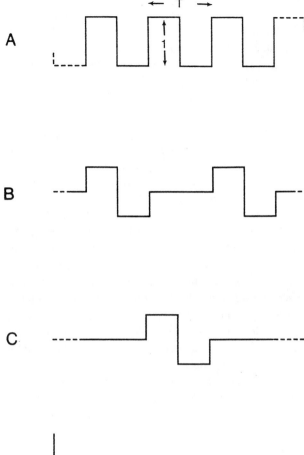

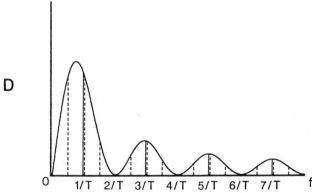

FIGURE 31.11 A square wave (A) of period T is dissected and presented with increasing intervals: 2T (B), . . . , infinity (C). D, The original line spectrum at $f = 1/T$, $1/3T$, . . . etc., is filled up at increasing periods until the Fourier integral is approached (continuous curve). All spectra are normalized.

by Fourier analysis of the input and output signals. In practice, impulses and step functions are usually preferred as test signals. The impulse function is a natural choice because of its constant amplitude spectrum and well-defined phase spectrum. All constituting frequencies have an equally large, although vanishing, small maximum at $t = 0$ ($A \cos 2\pi f t$). Because of this equal amplitude spectrum the Fourier coefficients of the response directly yield the transfer function.

The response to a *unit step* function, i.e., the integral of the impulse function, can also fully define a system. Step functions are typically useful in slow systems because their low-frequency content is high. Another technique is to directly determine the frequency response with a close enough series of sine waves of different frequencies. In vision research nonlinearities of the saturation type should also be considered; when one wants to avoid them, either weak incremental or decremental flashes (sudden decreases of a certain luminance) with long enough pauses may be employed, or sinusoidal modulation with restricted modulation depth can be used to probe the frequency range of interest. In principle, the two methods will be just as time-consuming to arrive at equally reliable results. If one wants to study nonlinearities, sinusoidal modulation will often be preferable above strong flashes because distortions of the sinusoidal shape are easily detected. Moreover, the adaptation state of the eye is well defined. Which of these techniques is to be preferred depends upon the question at hand and the system to be analyzed.

DOMAINS Notwithstanding the fact that Fourier analysis is mathematically a straightforward procedure, conceptually it is by no means simple. As previously mentioned, a variable quantity (e.g., luminance) that is a function of time or space can equally well be represented by means of its Fourier transform as a function of frequency. Although probably superfluous, it must be stressed that in the frequency domain "time" or "space" have themselves disappeared as a dimension.

An example from acoustics is probably the most revealing: if we were to perform Fourier analysis on a symphony of Mozart of, say, 30 minutes, we would obtain a fundamental frequency of $1/1800$ Hz. If the frequencies present in the music extend to 20 kHz, there will be no less than 3.6 $\times 10^7$ lines in the amplitude spectrum and as many points in the phase spectrum. *The original representation of the physical phenomenon is replaced by a set of numbers, and time itself is lost.* These numbers, if used to code corresponding physical generators (including phase information), would allow one to reproduce the original phenomenon. (Note: In a recent lecture, Stan Klein has advanced the idea that a musical score can be considered a Fourier representation *avant la lettre*.)

Our auditory system indeed allows a musical person to extract separate pitches from a complex sound, apparently

cosine functions at $t = 0$. Even though their relative amplitudes will be (infinitely) small, they will add significantly at time zero and nowhere else.

TEST SIGNALS In theory, the characteristics of a linear system can be determined from its response to nearly any transient signal; the transfer function follows from the ratios of the amplitudes of each component, which are obtained performing some kind of Fourier analysis (Ohm's acoustical law). In agreement with this, a sound wave is in general perceived as an entity, and no individual pressure vibrations are heard. Of course, if a really simple form of Fourier analysis were being performed by the ear, we could only "hear" the symphony after it has been played, and it would be just the same whether played forward or backward. In reality, the ear performs a sort of running frequency analysis with a sliding time window of approximately 50 ms, and in this way there is both frequency analysis *and* flow of time.

Theoretically the duality of the frequency and space domains applies in a similar way to the visual scene as to sound waves. However, in contrast to the perceived uniqueness of a sound wave as described above, each and every element of a grating is always perceived as a distinct entity, even at levels approaching threshold. Therefore the number of periods of a grating plays a much less important role in perception than do the number of oscillations in audition.[5]

There have been suggestions that for certain visual tasks such as recognition of blurred faces the visual system would employ a kind of piecemeal Fourier analysis because this would be technically advantageous. From the above exposition it should be evident that the representations in time or space carry the same information as those in the frequency domain. Both representations will therefore need the same amount of computation, although of course the physical or/and anatomical properties of the brain may confer practical advantages to one or the other modes.

PRACTICAL CONSIDERATIONS ON USING FOURIER ANALYSIS
In practice, a recorded response will always be restricted to a certain duration T or, in space, to a certain restricted region S. In the execution of a Fourier transform, however, the phenomenon is usually interpreted as periodic in T or S, as was mentioned before. Therefore the Fourier transform will not be continuous but display a discrete although dense spectrum with line distances of $1/T$ or $1/S$. In case of repetitive stimulation this is evident: if an ERG or a VEP is presented for 0.5 seconds, the lowest meaningful frequency will be 2 Hz, and harmonics will also occur in multiples of 2 Hz. Although there are programs that will enable a higher resolution by artificially extending the time interval being analyzed, no information is gained by this. If a frequency spectrum is to be computed from an *averaged* signal, it makes no sense to extend the analyzed interval beyond that section of the recording that can be considered to exceed the noise. In practice, such a section will be extended to a longer analysis period to obtain a dense enough spectrum.

An important consideration is that periodicity can only be an idealization in practice. One must realize that in reality a finite number of periods is always present; time or space will be the restricting factor. This means in Fourier terms that the theoretical discrete lines of exact periodicity will

broaden: the spectrum is continuous. In figure 31.12 the effect on the Fourier spectrum of restricting the number of periods of a square wave is demonstrated. An important rule of thumb is that the width of the spectrum δf around the center frequency f multiplied by the number of periods N is approximately constant, thus

$$\delta f \cdot N = K. \qquad (7)$$

The spectral lines of higher harmonics are subject to the same *absolute* widening, i.e., δf. This is of special concern for gratings because even if the number of periods in the optical stimulus is large, the effective number of periods on the retina will be different for various spatial frequencies. As a consequence, the effective bandwidth will be also different for different frequencies. Another complicating factor is due to eccentricity effects: along the bars of a centrally presented grating the effective length will be less for fine gratings than for coarse ones. The implications of all this are difficult to oversee and will certainly affect the experiments in different ways. For a system performing Fourier analysis, discrimination of periodicity or frequency will be impaired if only one or a few periods are present due to the broad maxima in the Fourier transform. This is easily demonstrated in hearing: if one or a few cycles of a sine wave are presented to the ear, a transient is heard with very little pitch. However, the fact that this effect has no equivalent in spatial vision suggests that vision does not primarily rely on harmonic analysis. We discuss this question in the next section.

Real signals also deviate from ideal ones in other ways. For instance, neither strict periodicity nor constant amplitude are really achieved in practice, although in our case deviations will be mostly negligible. More important is that in recording VEPs and ERGs people blink, move their eyes, and shift their attention; therefore even for an ideal stimulus, VEPs will exhibit latency jitter and fluctuations of amplitude. Attention to this will be paid when discussing averaging, but here it can be said that in principle fluctuations will also influence the initial Fourier line spectrum of signals that are in origin periodic.

Although the concept of noise will be treated extensively later, one aspect deserves attention within this framework: white noise is defined by its Fourier spectrum as consisting of a continuum of frequencies with constant amplitude. The only difference between this noise spectrum and that of the impulse function is found in their phase spectra. For noise, phases are distributed at random, instead of being equal (cosine functions) at a prescribed time, as in the case for an impulse function. This again demonstrates the importance of phase, which is of such special significance in the visual world.

Just as in the real world the width of an impulse function cannot be reduced infinitely, similarly the frequency spectrum of noise will be restricted at the high-frequency end.

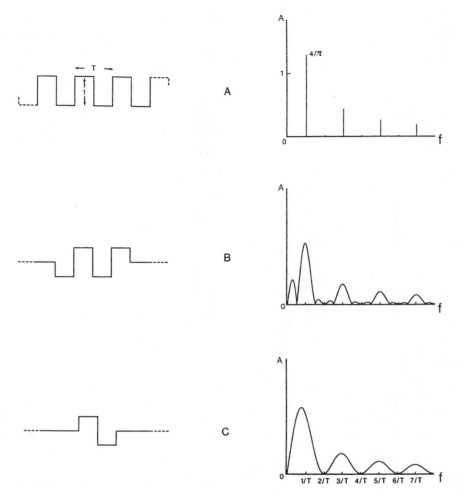

FIGURE 31.12 A, The line spectrum of an infinite square wave. B, Spectrum of two periods of the same. C, Spectrum of one period, equal to 11 D (Spectra normalized).

Some aspects of spatial Fourier analysis

LINEARITY   All optical systems, contrary to physiological ones, are linear in so far as the relative light distribution of an optical image is independent of intensity. However, it is a misunderstanding to think that optical systems are linear in their *reproduction* of images. For example, if a sinusoidal grid is imaged through a simple lens, the image may expand toward the edges and introduce new frequencies in the Fourier spectrum. Only in well-corrected optical systems do harmonic functions retain their harmonic character.

TIME VS. SPACE   There is an essential difference between space and time phenomena: time has an inherent direction, whereas space does not. Therefore, smoothing in time is always accompanied by phase shifts, whereas smoothing in space will generally be performed without phase distortion. Actually the minimum-phase rule is a consequence of causality. So-called phase-free filtering has recently been developed, but it can only be performed by computer or by

reversing the playback of a tape.[19] Because the signal is processed artificially, the result is not anymore restricted to the past; it may be looking into the "future," i.e., causality can be violated: the "response" can precede the stimulus. Figure 31.13 gives a schematic explanation of elementary phase-free low-pass filtering.[15] In modern practice filtering is mostly performed digitally but digitally does not necessarily imply "phase-free." In principle time reversal is then an essential condition and therefore physical laws are no longer valid. In the figure the signal is filtered twice, once in the normal direction and once backward. The reversed result of the latter is then added to the first. One can see that the result spreads from $+\infty$ to $-\infty$, which makes estimation of latencies dubious. This in contrast to real-time low-pass filtering when, in principle, the start of a transient can always be found (in the noiseless case), even if more filtering stages are present. On the other hand, peak latencies will generally be much more reliable with phase-free filtering, which is especially advantageous for high-pass filtering of repetitive signals.

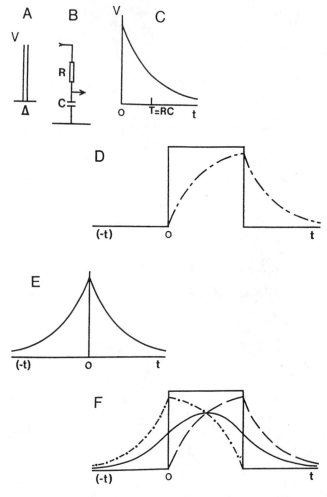

FIGURE 31.13 Principle of phase-free filtering. A, A (voltage) impulse function (Δ-function). B, The circuit—a simple RC network through which it is passed. C, The resulting output. D shows a square pulse (full line), and dashed lines indicate the output after filtering. In a computer or tape the memory can contain all values from −t to +t, where t is a large number, so the filter can be made to act upon the signal not only in "real time" but also in the future! The mathematical effect of this is shown in E for an impulse response and in F for a square pulse. The dashed lines in F show the operation in the "forward" mode, and the dash-and-dotted lines indicate the reverse operation. The resulting (normalized) output is shown by the full line. The result may be pretty, and the peaks may not be "displaced," but the time of origin of the response is lost. (From van der Tweel LH, Estévez O, Strackee J: Measurement of evoked potentials. In Barber C (ed): *Evoked Potentials.* Lancaster, England, MTP Press, Ltd, 1980, pp 19–41. Used by permission.)

In space the situation is different. Often blurring will be more or less circular symmetrical; with modern compound lenses, more complicated defocused patterns may be produced. Most optical systems can be adequately characterized by either their point or their line spread function. The line spread function has much in common with the impulse function in time. Just as the impulse response of a filter gives the frequency response, the Fourier transform of the line spread function directly gives the optical transfer function. The line spread function is very often symmetrical due to the already mentioned equivalency of right and left in space. In optical systems that are not well corrected and also in vision, both point and line spread functions will depend on eccentricity. Moreover, in general, line spread functions should be determined with line elements that are not too long.

A fact that deserves special attention in applying spatial Fourier techniques is that of the axial alignment of object and image. This alignment has to be accurate; if not, linear phase shifts will occur. For instance, a misalignment of 1 degree will give a phase shift of 4 × 360 degrees for spatial frequencies of 4 cycles per degree (period of 15 minutes) etc., because distance is translated in phase, *including whole periods*.

SPATIAL FREQUENCY Fourier theory is obviously also valid in space: any distribution of light can theoretically be obtained by a composition of spatial harmonic functions. However, whereas Fourier analysis in time is straightforward, the two dimensionality of space requires more complicated techniques and raises its own questions when applied to the study of the visual system. The most fundamental problem arises when light distributions are to be expressed in terms of their Fourier spatial harmonic content; it is due to the nonexistence of negative light. Consider the case of a 100% contrast bar pattern (black and white): according to our discussion in the section "Standard Periodic Signals," the fundamental exceeds in amplitude that of the original light distribution, which means that this "component" would go negative!

For an electrical signal there are no such problems because negative and positive are symmetrical. Neural processes also permit encoding of negativity, and therefore in principle Fourier processing of neural signals would be feasible— assuming that the average can also be properly encoded. On the other hand, there being no negative light, a given light distribution cannot in general be synthesized from physical harmonic gratings.

Fourier analysis of one-dimensional patterns, for instance, square or triangular grids, is straightforward; the extension along the elements is in principle infinite, but the resultant normalized Fourier spectrum will not change if shorter elements are employed. In experiments with grids, the length of the grid elements may influence the amplitude of VEPs or as such the threshold. If we take as an example a square grid with a contrast of A% and a period (twice the bar width) of X degrees, this will be represented by the average level (luminance) and frequencies of $(2n + 1) \cdot 1/X$ c/degree with respective amplitudes of $4A/\pi$, $4A/3\pi$, etc. It is interesting to note that the eccentricity effect will influence the harmonics differently. As far as the authors know, no systematic research has been performed on this matter.

Note that, depending on the sharpness of the bars, many "frequencies" are present in this representation. In this respect, "bar width" is a simpler characterization of a square grid than is spatial frequency. "Frequency" can better be reserved for sinusoidal gratings.

CHECKERBOARDS AND FOURIER ANALYSIS   To understand the meaning of Fourier analysis of two-dimensional figures, namely, that of the checkerboards that are so often used in VEP research, consider in Figure 31.14A, the heavy arrowed lines.[14] The mean luminance along these lines is then half that of the white squares. Therefore there is no periodicity perpendicular to these lines in the sense of Fourier analysis, i.e., no spatial frequency of $1/2a$ (Figure 31.14A). For the tilted rays of Figure 31.14B, alternate diagonals fall in the black or in the white fields, and thus the first true Fourier components are at 45 and 135 degrees. The profile is perpendicular to the diagonals and is triangular with identical maximum contrast as that of the checkerboard elements. The period P in this direction is equal to $a\sqrt{2}$; the spatial frequencies belonging to this triangular profile are therefore the inverse of this and are subsequently $P/3$, $P/5$, etc. The amplitudes will be $8/\pi^2$, and respectively $1/9$, $1/25$, etc., times this. All the above applies for both diagonal directions. At the position of Figure 31.14C the integrated contrast will be zero again. The orientation *selectivity* will depend on the number of checks included; for large numbers orientation selectivity will be very sharp. For the orientation in figure 31.14D, by the same reasoning a triangular grid will be produced with a contrast of $^1/_3$ and a spatial frequency $1/2a \cdot \sqrt{10}$. Due to the symmetry of the checkerboard there are now four identical orientations. *Note that there is no harmonic relation anymore between the main components.* Therefore one can never speak of the *fundamental* of a checkerboard, and analysis and synthesis is by no means as simple as for a bar pattern. As in the case of bars, the only unambiguous definition of a checkerboard, and also the simplest, is by the size of its elements.

RECEPTIVE FIELDS   There is a considerable amount of literature about receptive fields and their representation in the frequency domain.[4] As long as one accepts linearity, the two representations are perfectly equivalent. For not too complicated receptive fields, the representation in the frequency domain is necessarily broad because the lowest frequency has to fit more or less the field size and, as we have seen, the Fourier transform of one single period has a very broad representation. For receptive fields with straight edges the transform remains rather elementary with equidistant zeros. Circular fields are much more complicated in this context, however. For instance, no harmonic relations exist anymore between zeros or maxima.

It is of course possible to imagine receptive field structures, including inhibitory zones, that would provide sharper frequency selectivity. A discussion of these problems is beyond the scope of this chapter, but it should be understood that the mathematical background necessary to treat the "receptive field" concept in Fourier terms is much more complicated than is often appreciated.

Correlation techniques, noise, and power spectrum

AUTOCORRELATION   Autocorrelation and cross-correlation functions are of great help in defining and understanding linear (and also certain classes of nonlinear) systems, as well as in performing system analysis. We shall treat functions of time as an example, but our discussion is equally valid for functions of variables with other dimensions.

The definition of the autocorrelation function $R(\tau)$ of $f(t)$ is as follows:

$$R(\tau) = 1/2T \cdot \int_{-T}^{+T} f(t)f(t-\tau)dt \tag{8}$$

with T going to infinity (figure 31.15).

If $f(t) = A\cos(2\pi ft + \Phi)$, it is easily calculated that

$$R(\tau) = A^2/2 \cdot \cos 2\pi f\tau \tag{9}$$

(see figure 31.16).

Note that τ is a time lag or time difference and must not be confused with time itself: the autocorrelation function is *not* a process in time but a purely mathematical construct. For $\tau = 0$ the autocorrelation function is always maximal because it is then exactly the integrated square of $f(t)$. $R(0)$ is conventionally normalized to 1. Another property of this function is that $R(\tau) = R(-\tau)$, that is so say, $R(\tau)$ is symmetrical around the origin. This symmetry corresponds with the loss of phase information for harmonic functions. In figure 31.16 some examples are given of autocorrelation functions of common signals.

GAUSSIAN NOISE   The concept of autocorrelation is especially useful to define noise. An important case is that of white noise; this is a signal whose autocorrelation function is an impulse. Only for the delay $\tau = 0$ is there a net value, normalized to 1; everywhere else it approaches 0. This definition in fact formalizes the inherent unpredictability that characterizes noise. In practice, the frequency band of the noise will be always restricted; therefore the autocorrelation function will be a broadened impulse function, as is exemplified in figure 31.16C, where the autocorrelation function of noise filtered by a one–RC stage, low-pass filter is shown. The result is a symmetrical exponential.

We shall consider here only the most elementary form of noise, i.e., noise with an amplitude distribution:

$$P(x) = 1/s\sqrt{2} \cdot \exp\left(-x^2/2s^2\right) \tag{10}$$

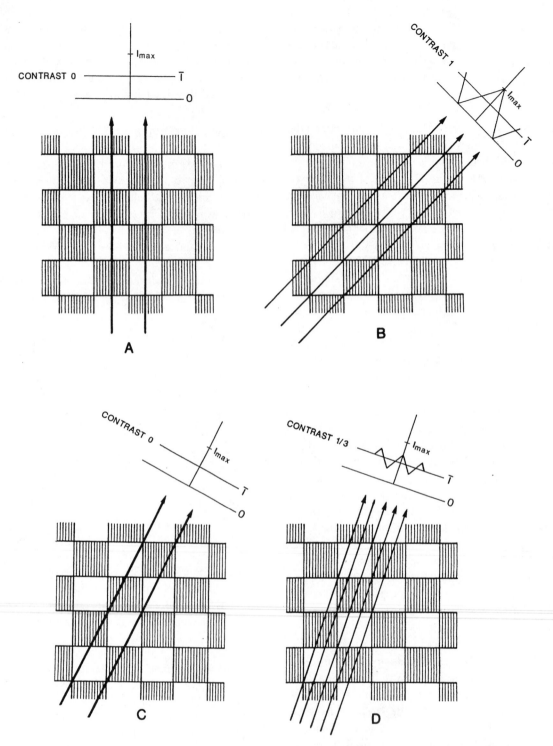

FIGURE 31.14 The integrated luminance along the elements of a checkerboard (of 100% contrast, i.e., black and white) in some main directions. A, In the horizontal and vertical directions there is no variation. Therefore there is no component with a spatial frequency of $1/2a$. B, Diagonally, a triangular distribution with the original contrast is obtained. This forms the first spatial frequency present: $1/2a \cdot \sqrt{2}$. C, In this direction and in its counterpart, again, no net result is obtained. D, Two of three checks cancel, and the contrast is reduced to $1/3$. Four equivalent directions exist. (From van der Tweel LH, Estévez O, Pijn JPM: *Doc Ophthalmol Proc Ser* 1983; 37:439–452. Used by permission.)

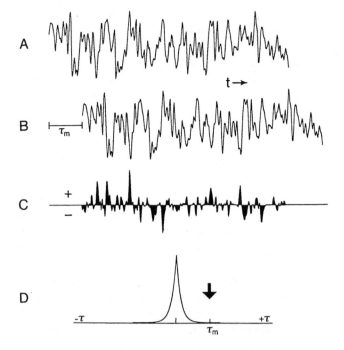

FIGURE 31.15 Principle of calculating the autocorrelation function. The signal (A), filtered Gaussian noise, is multiplied with a copy of itself (B), but shifted with a (discrete) lag τ_m. C shows the outcome of the multiplication. The values at all sampling points are added. The result is point τ_m of D, where the total function with m ranging from $-\infty$ to $+\infty$ is presented.

with $P(x)$, the probability that amplitude x occurs, obeying a Gaussian distribution function with standard deviation s.

If Gaussian "white" noise (i.e., noise with a flat spectrum) is passed through a linear filter, we obtain "colored" noise. An important property of Gaussian noise is that its amplitude distribution remains Gaussian after linear filtering, independent of the filter characteristics.

With correlation techniques it could be proved that often the alpha rhythm has the characteristics of selectively filtered Gaussian noise. This is not only of interest theoretically but also for techniques of signal extraction. Moreover, the amplitude histograms of samples of alpha rhythm often show close resemblance to a Gaussian distribution.

POWER The power of an electrical signal is given by the average of V^2/R. In ERG and VEP, however, the resistances R are undefined and thus the powers are also unknown. It is common practice in electrophysiology to ignore R and to express "power" as amplitude squared of the Fourier components (in either μV^2 or V^2).

An important theorem in this respect is that of Parseval, which states that the time average of the square of a function $F(t)$ with period T equals half the sum of the squared amplitudes of its Fourier components:

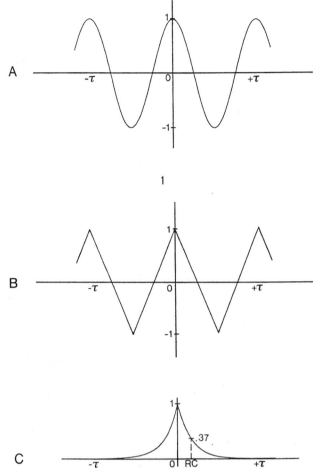

FIGURE 31.16 A, Autocorrelation functions of $A\cos(2\pi ft + \Phi)$. B, A square wave. C, One-stage low-pass filtered noise with the time constant $t_c = RC$.

$$1/T \cdot \int_{-T/2}^{+T/2} F^2(t)dt = 1/4 \cdot a_0^2 + 1/2 \cdot \sum_{n=1}^{\infty} A_n^2 \qquad (11)$$

This result is obtained when we consider the Fourier series representation of the function $F(t)$ and the *orthogonality* property of harmonic functions, i.e., that only integrals of the form

$$A_n A_m \int \cos 2\pi f_n t \cdot \cos 2\pi f_m t dt \qquad (12)$$

with $m = n$ will contribute to the time average. In this context orthogonality means that the normalized integrated product of any two harmonic functions with different frequencies, if sufficiently long, will equal zero. The only terms that contribute to the autocorrelation are then the squares of the amplitudes at each frequency (see the previous section).

In the case of *nonperiodic* signals, e.g., noise or any transient, the discrete sum at the right side of equation 11 becomes also an integral (similar to what was described in the section on the Fourier integral). ΣA_n^2 will change into a continuous function of frequency, i.e., $A^2(f)$. This is known as the "power spectrum" of $F(t)$.

Although we shall not go into detail considering the physical and mathematical problems regarding the representation of the (power) spectrum, some remarks may be made: as was discussed before, the natural restrictions to true periodicity mean that in practice no Fourier spectrum will exhibit pure spectral lines; therefore the energy or power will always be distributed over a finite frequency band. As a consequence, the power at an *exact* frequency will be zero. The problem is circumvented by taking not power but the power per infinitesimal frequency range *df*, "power density." Therefore instead of "power spectrum," the term *power density spectrum* is also often used. Since power is additive, the total power in the frequency domain is obtained by integration over the frequency range.

The advantage of power density (dimension V^2/Hz) as a measure in the frequency domain, especially if noise is involved, is found in the well-defined properties of power such as additivity. However, it must be realized that power seems to have no specific meaning as a measure of properties of electrophysiological phenomena; in any case, ERGs and VEPs are conventionally recorded as an amplitude function of time. This is one of the reasons why, if their frequency spectrum is wanted, often it is not the power spectrum that is given but the amplitude spectrum. In recent publications the term "amplitude density" is used analogously to power density with the "dimension" $V/\sqrt{Hz}$. This may be confusing, however, because "amplitude" is not additive along the frequency axis. Only Gaussian noise obeys strict rules; in other cases there will be ambiguity.

CROSS-CORRELATION AND SYSTEM ANALYSIS   An important step in the analysis of systems can be made by using the cross-correlation function R (note we use the same symbol R as above) between the output g and the input f. This function is defined by the formula

$$R(\tau) = 1/2T \cdot \int_{-T}^{+T} f(t)g(t-\tau)dt \qquad (14)$$

for T going to infinity. It expresses the relation between two (time) functions f and g in the same way that the autocorrelation function expresses the relation of a function to itself. If the two functions f and g have nothing in common, the result will be zero. If they are identical, the cross-correlation function becomes the autocorrelation function defined before. A common (hidden) signal embedded in two independent sources of noise will emerge in the cross-correlation function if a long enough sample can be processed.

Cross-correlation is especially effective in identifying transport delays between two signals: the cross-correlation

will exhibit a maximum at τ = transport delay. If both signals are subject to noise of different origin, this influences only the normalized value of the maximum and its statistical significance, but not its delay. If, for instance, the EEGs from the two hemispheres have a cross-correlation function differing from zero, it can be concluded that either one hemisphere influences the other or both are acting under a common influence. In the latter case there may be zero delay (i.e., the cross-correlation function will show a maximum at $\tau = 0$). However, such a maximum should in general be interpreted with due caution because in all recordings electrical cross talk can be expected. Even if the common (parasitic) signal is at a very low level, a long enough recording period may eventually produce a significant result at $\tau = 0$. Results with zero delay will have to be specially examined and the power spectra of the initial signals taken into account. Cross-correlation functions with a maximum different from $\tau = 0$ can in general be considered trustworthy. Note that, as observed before, the cross-correlation functions of any two harmonic functions of different frequencies will be zero due to the orthogonality principle.

An important application of the cross-correlation function arises when white noise is used as an input. When the input noise is correlated with the output of the system, the result is identical to the impulse response, and its Fourier transform directly yields the transfer function of the system. The reason is that both the impulse and white noise have the same flat spectrum. The difference between the impulse function and white noise is only found in their respective phase spectra. However, the phase *shifts* after transmission through the system are the same for *each* separate frequency, whether the input is noise or an impulse, and therefore, the results will indeed be identical. Usually band-limited noise is employed with a flat spectrum simulating white noise in the region of interest. In case of noise-modulated light, the effective modulation depth (determined by the standard deviation of the noise signal) is necessarily restricted to about 30%; otherwise noise peaks will (too) often produce prolonged black periods (virtual negativity of light).

The transfer function determined by this method is equal to the product of all transfer functions of the series of linear processes involved. It is fundamentally impossible to separate or to identify, for instance, low-pass and high-pass stages. This means that, for example, in visual physiology distal and proximal frequency-dependent processes (filters) as identified by linear analysis cannot be separated—neither can their sequence be determined.

The equality of the noise and impulse response functions is only generally valid in linear systems. Nonetheless, there is one important class of nonlinearities in which cross-correlation can be usefully applied: cross-correlating white noise input with the output of a system with one static nonlinearity (i.e., a nonlinearity that is frequency independent like a rectifier) yields the shape of the impulse response of the totality of the linear processes involved. This is due to the fundamental property of Gaussian noise, described above, that its Gaussian character is retained after linear filtering. Therefore, the input to the nonlinearity is also Gaussian independent of the linear distal filters mostly present. The only difference with the result in the absence of static nonlinearity is found in the absolute value of the cross-correlation function, which depends on the characteristics of the nonlinearity (Bussgang's theorem[1]). Together with other advanced techniques, this property of Gaussian noise has been successfully employed in VEP studies to determine the transfer functions of various stages in the system.[11]

In contrast, however, to the equivalent use of noise and impulse functions in linear system analysis, in *nonlinear* systems the response to an impulse input, e.g., a flash, will in general *not* represent the impulse response of the linear elements. Already the reversing of the polarity of the impulse will give rise to different results, which makes interpretation difficult if not impossible. For instance, if there is an early nonlinearity like strong saturation, a "positive" unit impulse will yield a different result from a "negative" one; these differences may become crucial when the nonlinearity is interleaved with linear elements.

Averaging

Although Fourier analysis has become very popular in visual electrophysiology due to the wide availability of simple programs and personal computers, averaging can still be considered the method of choice in recording weak responses. Averaging is conceptually much simpler than Fourier analysis and is, in principle, maximally effective in noise reduction.

THE STIMULUS FOR AVERAGING   Classic averaging is performed by synchronizing the start of data collection with the stimulus and measuring (digitally) the response at a number of consecutive intervals that are then saved into a buffer in the computer's memory. The process is repeated, and in consecutive stimulus periods the amplitudes of corresponding samples are added by a computer. The stimulus can be periodic or not, as long as the period of interest is kept in synchrony with the stimulus and does not exceed the shortest stimulus interval. Averaging is in fact identical to cross-correlating a signal (ERG or VEP) with a chosen number of impulses of unit size. It is a linear method and as such also subject to treatment by using Fourier theory. (Actually, periodic averaging is equivalent to a filtering procedure that only allows frequencies belonging to the fundamental period and its harmonics to pass through while rejecting all other frequencies; furthermore, the "filter sharpness" of this process increases with the number of responses recorded.)

The stimulus in the case of averaging should have a stable amplitude and, in principle, should also be periodic. Otherwise, dynamic interactions may be a confounding factor. Strong adaptation effects have been described by Jeffreys,[6] from which it also follows that for transient stimulation there is a lower limit to the stimulation period.

IMPROVING THE SIGNAL-NOISE RATIO WITH AVERAGING Averaging originally was based on the assumption that responses are stable and noise reasonably Gaussian. From this it follows that the signal-to-noise improvement (expressed in power) is proportional to the number of periods added. Because VEPs are characterized by amplitude and shape rather than by power, the rule of thumb is that noise amplitude is reduced relative to the response by the square root of n (the number of intervals added).

In relation to the above, there rises an important question: *What is the signal-to-noise ratio?* In a strict sense the signal-to-noise concept makes only sense for two Gaussian processes, one of which is considered to be the "signal" and the other the "noise" and the other being the superposition of harmonic signals and noise. A requirement is then that figures of signal-to-noise ratio be expressed per frequency band because at some frequencies the signal may be larger than the noise and at other frequencies this may be the other way around. Especially in the case of transient responses, the signal-to-noise concept can be difficult to apply and can easily give rise to ambiguities, for instance, when the frequency spectrum of the transient is very different from that of the noise. Suitable filtering may reduce such problems.

When averaging, both the frequency spectrum of the noise and the stimulus repetition rate may play an important role. Often there is a strong alpha rhythm of, say, 10 Hz with a high selectivity. If the stimulus rate were to be 1, 2, 5, or 10 Hz, the effective noise would be relatively amplified depending on the selectivity of the alpha process and the sweep period chosen: the lower the rate, the lesser the enhancing. A signal-to-noise ratio calculated on the basis of total power would then be highly overestimated, although the improvement will still go with $\sqrt{n}$. When the stimulus period is chosen such that it just fits an odd multiple of half a period of the alpha frequency, the recording interval will fall between alternating polarities of the alpha rhythm. Because of this, the result will be much improved: the effective signal-to-noise ratio is increased because the alpha rhythm will tend to cancel in successive sweeps.[11]

RESPONSE FLUCTUATIONS   VEPs and ERGs are subject not only to noise contamination but also to inherent fluctuations. There is a fundamental difference between the disruptive effects of additive noise and those due to variability of the response itself. If, as sometimes has been described, response and noise interact, then simple rules cannot be given.

Theoretically there are two main types of response irregularities: latency jitter and amplitude fluctuations. Because their effects are comparatively small in routine measurements, they will only be treated briefly.

Latency jitter of the response or of parts of it will lead to smoothing during averaging. Actually, time jitter is the most effective low-pass filter that can be physically realized. Techniques have been described to implement adaptive filtering that counteracts these smoothing effects.[19] If the responses occur in clusters with different latencies, interesting methods exist to separate these clusters.[8] Analysis of conventional pattern VEPs in our laboratory by using sophisticated filtering has shown, however, that even near threshold the latency spread was not more than a few milliseconds. Concerning amplitude fluctuations, Dagnelie et al.[3] have found fluctuations on the order of 25% for a 50% modulated, 20 Hz luminous stimulus. In our own experience with recordings between 100 and 200 sweeps, reproducibility of pattern responses is generally very good.

An instrumental artifact is caused by the property that in certain TV stimulators the stimulus is not synchronized with the TV frame rate in order to prevent pickup from the mains or VEPs to TV flicker.[18] Since mostly only the central part of the TV screen is fixated (or as such has a dominant position), this will cause jitter of the stimulus on the order of 20 ms, equivalent to low-pass filtering using a "square" unit impulse response of 20-ms duration (in case of 50 Hz mains). Although this is not unequivocally translatable in a frequency cutoff, it means approximately an attenuation of 3 dB at a frequency of 22 Hz.

In some cases, one might wish to extract individual responses. Those interested in suitable techniques, like *a posteriori* filtering, are referred to the extensive literature covered and discussed by Lopes da Silva.[7]

PRACTICAL CONSIDERATIONS ON AVERAGING   In our type of experiments time is often at a premium. Therefore stimulus period and sweep time should be strictly coupled so that there are no loose periods in between. This self-evident facility is often lacking in simple averagers, or no attention has been paid to it in computer programs. In the case of pattern reversal responses, it is advisable to record two responses per sweep. This allows one to check the symmetry of the stimulus while, at the same time, it gives an impression of the stability of the experimental situation. Early artifact rejection can also be strongly recommended.

Synchronous amplification

Related to cross-correlation and to Fourier analysis is the technique of synchronous detection. (Lock-in amplifiers are a technically different realization of synchronous detection with the same advantages and disadvantages.) This technique is especially useful when repetitive stimulation at higher frequencies is employed: so-called steady-state experiments. The principle of the method is multiplication of the signal that contains the expected periodic response, with two harmonic functions of the same frequency and 90 degrees phase shift, i.e., a sine and a cosine. The outcome is smoothed (integrated) over a chosen time, e.g., by a resistor-capacitor (RC) filter, but separately for the sine and cosine. After this, the square root of the sum of squares is taken and recorded. For long RC times this approximates performing Fourier analysis on *one* frequency only: that of the fundamental of the stimulus. In other words, one is computing the Fourier series' coefficients a_1 and b_1, and from these the amplitude A is computed in real time. Note that any smoothing should be done before squaring a and b. This optimizes noise reduction. One can also obtain the (tangent of the) phase by using $tg\Phi = b/a$, although this is not common practice.

In most commercial synchronous amplifiers the multiplication is in fact replaced by synchronous rectification (figure 31.17). In this figure it is supposed that the stimulus evokes a sinusoidal response that is passed through a synchronized full-wave rectifier. This is equivalent to alternately multiplying the signal by +1 and −1 during each half-period. In the top half of the figure, the sign of the multiplier changes when the sine wave crosses zero, and the sum of the shaded areas is maximal. When the sign change is delayed by 90 degrees (lower part), the net result is zero. Other phases are usually encountered in practice since there is no telling, a priori, the phase angle (or delay) between stimulus and response. Then the two channels will both record a response of which the sizes will depend on that angle. An estimate of the response amplitude, however, is independent of the phase. The further procedure is the same as described above for true multiplication.

An important consequence of using this technique is that not only will the fundamental component of the response determine the result, but also odd harmonics will because the multiplying function itself contains these harmonics. Therefore, the results of synchronous amplification are only unambiguous when the response itself is nearly a sine wave, as is generally the case at high stimulation frequencies. It should be realized that this type of simple quantification is at the cost of losing all information about possible components in the VEP.

Synchronous techniques are also treacherous at low frequencies when the fundamental is not the main contributor anymore (see the response at four reversals per second in figure 31.18); low-frequency cutoff may even be suggested simply because the period extends beyond the most prominent part of the response; in other words, the contribution of the fundamental becomes smaller when the frequency is lowered.

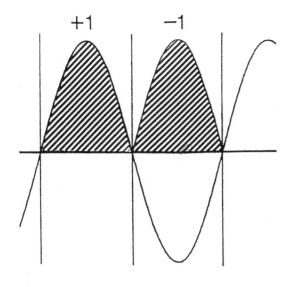

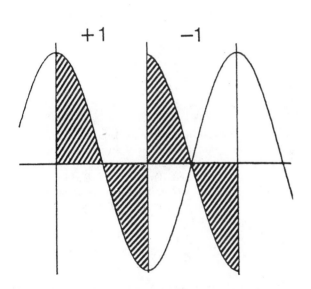

FIGURE 31.17   Scheme of synchronous detection.

Note that synchronous detection is governed by the stimulus interval and that with pattern reversal the reversal rate is twice that of the luminance modulation of the elements. Therefore, the detection procedure or the multiplication must be governed by the second harmonic of the modulation frequency of the two sets of elements. This is the reason why in the literature the response is often characterized as "second harmonic." The term is not only confusing but even wrong in the case of pure contrast responses because the response has evidently the same frequency as the true stimulus, i.e., that of the reversal itself. There is only sense in talking about second harmonics of the modulation frequency if the responses are governed mainly by luminance, as is the case with large elements or probably in part of the pattern ERGs.

The advantages of synchronous detection are those of simplicity and the possibility of continuous recording that they allow. The signal-to-noise improvement is dependent on the smoothing time constant and can be arbitrarily large at the cost of time resolution. This is sometimes expressed as equivalent bandwidth. For a similar noise reduction the consumption of time for averaging and synchronous amplification is comparable. For automatic tracking procedures, however, synchronous amplification is indeed a very appropriate technique.

Conclusion

We remarked in the introduction about the need to reconsider concepts such as "threshold." The point is that, even if signal-to-noise improvement may proceed comparatively slowly, the only restriction in improving the sensitivity of a recording is that imposed by the endurance of the subject. In practice, it has proved to be possible under favorable conditions to measure VEPs to modulated light at less than 5% of the psychophysical threshold.[12] The reason is that the computer memory by far exceeds the integration time of flicker perception and also the electrodes cover a much larger visual area than contributes to sensation. In such situations, it will depend on the patience of experimenter and subject what can be considered a nonrecordable response. It is clear that an unambiguous statement will be that at a noise level of x μV no response could be recorded, but this does not give an indication whether recording for a longer period would have yielded a VEP or that a "hard" threshold has indeed been passed, as is common with pattern evoked potentials. Probably the earliest example demonstrating a true electrophysiological threshold is the work of Campbell and Maffei,[2] where the objective threshold and the extrapolated electrophysiological one were shown to coincide very well. It is therefore recommended that the experimental technique used be stated exactly in order to enable judgment by the reader.

Whatever techniques are employed, Fourier theory is as important for the quantification of the responses themselves as it is for the signal analytical description of the stimulus-response relation. As was already stated, linear system analysis is exhaustive, and there remains only the question of choosing the most practical solution. Nonlinear system analysis has no general recipes, but there are groups of systems, e.g., those with one static nonlinearity that are accessible to systematic analysis. But also in those cases Fourier stands central!

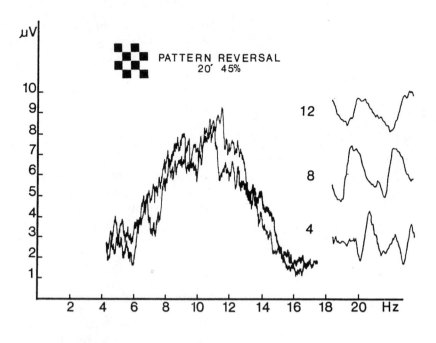

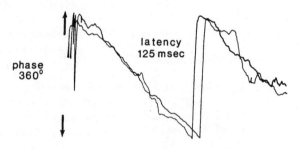

FIGURE 31.18 Continuous recording with synchronous detection of the amplitude (upper trace) and phase (lower trace) of the response to a reversing checkerboard at various frequencies. Two successive averaged evoked potentials at three frequencies are inserted. From approximately 8 reversals per second on, the fundamental dominates. At 4 Hz the higher harmonics become stronger but do not contribute to the synchronously detected response, which contains mainly the fundamental. Therefore, the smaller response at low frequencies is an instrumental artifact. However, latency determination by means of phase shift as a function of frequency is still valid. (From van der Tweel LH, Estévez O, Strackee J: Measurement of evoked potentials. In Barber C (ed): *Evoked Potentials.* Lancaster, England, MTP Press, Ltd, 1980, pp 19–41. Used by permission.)

REFERENCES

1. Bussgang JJ: Crosscorrelation functions of amplitude distorted Gaussian signals. *MIT Research Laboratory Electronics* Technical Report 216. Cambridge, Mass, MIT Press, 1952.
2. Campbell FW, Maffei L: Evidence for the existence of orientation and size detectors in the human visual system. *J Physiol* 1970; 207:635–652.
3. Dagnelie G, van den Berg TJTP, Reits D: Unfamiliar effects of flicker on the human EEG. *Doc Ophthalmol Proc Ser* 1977; 15:173–178.
4. Enroth-Kugel C, Robson JG: Functional characteristics and diversity of cat retinal ganglion cells. *Invest Ophthalmol Vis Sci* 1984; 25:250–267.
5. Estévez O, Cavonius CR: Low frequency attenuation in the detection of gratings: Sorting out the artifacts. *Vision Res* 1976; 16:497–500.
6. Jeffreys DA: The physiological significance of pattern visual evoked potentials. In Desmedt JE (ed): *Visual Evoked Potentials: New Developments.* Oxford, England, Clarendon Press, 1977, pp 134–167.
7. Lopes da Silva FH: Event related potentials: Methodology and quantification. In Niedermeyer E, Lopes da Silva FH (eds): *Electro-Encephalography.* Baltimore, Urban & Schwarzenberg, 1982, pp 655–664.
8. Pfurtscheller G, Cooper R: Selective averaging of the intercerebral click evoked responses in man: An improved method of measuring latencies and amplitudes. *Electroencephalogr Clin Neurophysiol* 1975; 38:187–190.
9. Regan D: *Human Brain Electrophysiology.* New York, Elsevier Science Publishing Co, Inc, 1989.
10. Spekreijse H: Rectification in the goldfish retina: Analysis by sinusoidal and auxiliary stimulation. *Vision Res* 1969; 9:1461–1472.

11. Spekreijse H, Estévez O, Reits D: The physiological analysis of visual processes in man. In Desmedt JE (ed): *Visual Evoked Potentials: New Developments*. Oxford, England, Clarendon Press, 1977, pp 16–89.

12. Spekreijse H, van der Tweel LH: System analysis of linear and nonlinear processes in electrophysiology of the visual system. *Proc Kon Ned Akad van Wetensch* 1972; 75:77–105.

13. van der Tweel LH: In Spekreijse H, van der Tweel LH (eds): *Spatial Contrast*. Amsterdam, Elsevier Science Publishers, 1977, pp 9–12.

14. van der Tweel LH, Estévez O, Pijn JPM: Notes on Fourier methods in vision research. *Doc Ophthalmol Proc Ser* 1985; 37:439–452.

15. van der Tweel LH, Estévez O, Strackee J: Measurement of evoked potentials. In Barber C (ed): *Evoked Potentials*. Lancaster, England, MTP Press, Ltd, 1980, pp 19–41.

16. van der Tweel LH, Verduyn Lunel HFE: Human visual responses to sinusoidally modulated light. *Electroencephalogr Clin Neurophysiol* 1965; 18:587–598.

17. van der Tweel LH, Visser P: Electrical responses of the retina to sinusoidally modulated light. In *Electroretinographia*. Acta Facultatis Medicae Universitatis Brunensis, Lekarska Fakulta University Brne, 1959, pp 185–196.

18. Van Lith GHM, van Marle GW, van Dok-Mak GTM: Variation in latency times of visually evoked cortical potentials. *Br J Ophthalmol* 1978; 62:220–222.

19. Verburg J, Strackee J: Phaseless recursive filtering applied to chestwall displacements and velocities, using accelerometers. *Med Biol Eng* 1974; 12:483–488.

20. Woody CD: Characterization of an adaptive filter for the analysis of variable latency neuroelectric signals. *Med Biol Eng* 1967; 5:539–553.

32 Reverse Correlation Methods

BEVIL R. CONWAY AND MARGARET S. LIVINGSTONE

Introduction

Reverse correlation is a method that is often used to characterize the response properties of neurons and to answer the simple question "What is the correlation between the response of a neuron and the stimulus used to elicit a response?" In any given sensory area within the brain, say, primary visual cortex, a given neuron will respond only to a restricted portion of that sensory domain, say, the upper left quadrant of the visual field. This phenomenon is captured by the notion of the receptive field, and our example neuron would be said to have a receptive field in the upper left quadrant of the visual field. In addition to spatial localization, receptive fields also describe the particular stimulus configuration to which the neuron is most responsive. Importantly, different neurons respond specifically to some stimuli and are indifferent or respond poorly to other stimuli. A visual neuron might be responsive to a small black spot on a white background, a line of a particular orientation, or a specific color, for example. Moreover, a given neuron may respond in opposite ways to two different stimuli, with different time courses. For example, a given cortical color cell might respond with excitation at a short latency and suppression at a long latency to one color and suppression at a short latency and excitation at a long latency to the opponent color. Thus, receptive fields have spatial and temporal structure. And a complete description of a receptive field includes both *where* in a sensory field a neuron is responsive to stimuli and *to what* stimuli the cell responds best. Although we will focus on visual neurons for this chapter, the concept of receptive field is useful in all sensory systems; for example, one can investigate the response properties of a neuron in somatosensory cortex to different kinds of stimuli applied to a specific region on the skin, the response properties of a neuron in auditory cortex to different frequencies, and the response properties of a neuron in olfactory cortex to different odors. In fact, reverse correlation techniques were originally developed for characterizing cells in the auditory cortex.[1,8]

The problem of how to characterize a given neuron's receptive field is not trivial; in fact, it took several decades before neuroscientists appreciated that single retinal ganglion cells in the cat's eye respond only to small spots of light in a specific location of the retina.[19] Previously, scientists had attempted without much success to elicit responses using full-field illumination, which they naively considered to be the "best" visual stimulus. We can sympathize. After all, what good would a visual neuron be if it could not report the difference between the room lights "on" and the room lights "off"? We now appreciate the sophistication of center-surround receptive fields and that these are a rather elegant way to encode the maximum amount of information (contrast borders) about the visual world with the smallest number of neurons—even if center-surround neurons do not respond very well to global illumination changes. In the primary visual cortex, the characterization of receptive fields was an even greater challenge. Having just established that retinal ganglion cells and cells in the lateral geniculate nucleus prefer small spots of light, scientists were rather discouraged to find that these stimuli were largely ineffective at driving cells in the next stage of visual processing, the primary visual cortex (V-1). It took an accident of experimental design to discover that most cells in V-1 actually respond best to oriented lines.[15,16] As David Hubel describes it in his Nobel lecture:[13]

For 3 or 4 hours [of recording from a single V-1 cell] we got absolutely nowhere. Then gradually we began to elicit some vague and inconsistent responses by stimulating somewhere in the mid-periphery of the retina. We were inserting the glass slide with its black spot into the slot of the ophthalmoscope [used to stimulate the retina by projecting the spot onto a screen in front of the animal's eyes] when suddenly over the audiomointor the cell went off like a machine gun. After some fussing and fiddling we found out what was happening. The response had nothing to do with the black dot. As the glass slide was inserted its edge was casting onto the retina a faint but sharp shadow, a straight dark line on a light background. That was what the cell wanted, and it wanted it, moreover, in just one narrow range of orientations.

The experimental procedure employed by Kuffler and Hubel and Wiesel in their pioneering studies of the visual system can be characterized as follows:

Place an electrode into an area of the visual system and isolate a single cell → *Flash a stimulus on the retina* → *Measure the neuron's response and decide what stimulus to try next*

As more and more different stimuli were tested, it became clear that cells are rather specialized, responding really well to some stimulus features (e.g., lines and edges) and not very well at all to others (e.g., different colors). Moreover, a given cell might respond best not just to lines and edges, but to lines and edges of a specific orientation. In fact, one might have one's electrode immediately adjacent to a cortical cell and not be able to elicit any response at all from the cell with a 45° line if the cell's preferred stimulus is an 80° line. Thus, in trying to fully characterize both the spatial and temporal response properties of a given neuron, one is faced with two problems: First, the particular stimuli that you choose to use will influence your decisions about what stimuli the cell is responsive to (you might mischaracterize an orientation-selective cell if you test it only with small spots), and second, it takes quite a long time to test a cell's response to every stimulus you can think of (as you would like to, so as not to miss the cell's actual stimulus preferences).

Reverse correlation methods overcome both of these problems, though they have limitations, which should be appreciated so as not to misinterpret the results. (We will discuss these at the end of the chapter.) Moreover, in addi-

tion to providing a full characterization of the spatial and temporal response properties of single neurons, reverse correlation methods have also proved useful in characterizing the receptive fields of multiple neurons simultaneously.[9] We will first describe this powerful technique in general terms, as it is used to study the visual system, and will then use some specific examples to outline the limitations.

Reverse-correlation methods: The generic case

The stimulus for a reverse correlation sequence is usually presented on a computer monitor and consists of a random sequence of images. In figure 32.1, each letter represents a unique stimulus. The neuron's action potentials are recorded continuously during stimulus presentation. These spikes are shown as tick marks beneath the stimulus sequences (figure

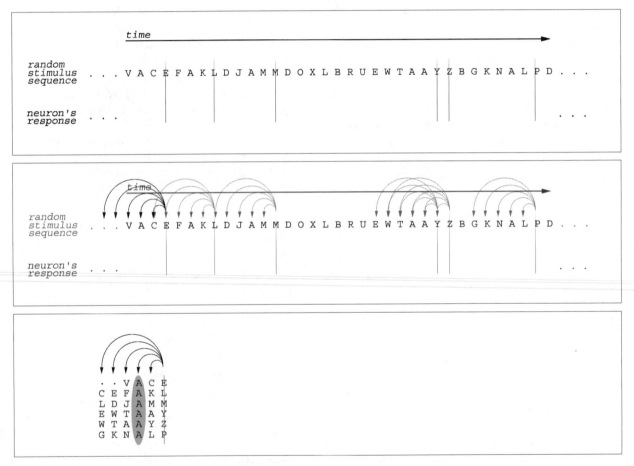

FIGURE 32.1 The basic idea of reverse correlation. Top, A random sequence of stimuli (represented by letters) is used to elicit a neuron's response while the neuron's activity (vertical lines) is continuously recorded. Middle, Following thousands of stimuli presentations, one correlates the stimuli that occurred before each action potential, keeping track of the stimuli that occurred one, two, three, four, and so on frames before each action potential. Bottom, One then aligns all of the stimuli sequences that preceded action potentials to reveal correlations between the stimuli and the neuron's response. In this case, the stimulus represented by the letter "A" occurred with a high probability two stimuli before each action potential. We could conclude that this neuron responds well to the stimulus represented by "A," with a physiological latency of two stimulus frames.

32.1, top panel). As with real neurons, there is no correlation between the neuron's spikes and the stimuli that occurred at exactly the same time; the spikes coincide with the letters E, L, M, Y, Z, and P in this example. In real neurons, this is because there is a visual latency—a finite amount of time that it takes for the visual stimulus to be encoded into neural activity and transmitted to the cell from which you are recording. But after running an extended sequence of stimuli and collecting the neural activity concurrently, one can determine the prior probability that a given stimulus occurred at a given length of time before a spike. We can look at the stimuli that occurred immediately before each spike (CKMAYL), the stimuli that occurred two stimuli before each spike (AAAAAA), and so on (figure 32.1, middle panel). If one then aligns all the letters that occurred before a spike, one can begin to see patterns emerge. In our example case, it is clear that the stimulus "A" occurs with a very high probability two stimuli before each spike (figure 32.1, bottom panel). Therefore, we would conclude that this neuron has a visual latency of two stimulus frames and responds best to the stimulus represented by the letter "A." Note that this way of correlating a neuron's activity with a stimulus is different from forward correlation in several ways. First, stimuli are constantly being presented. This means that the number of stimuli that can be presented in a given amount of time is much greater with reverse correlation than with forward correlation. Second, the stimuli are presented randomly, which eliminates scientist-introduced biases. Third, the result is an average *stimulus* preceding a spike by a given amount of time as opposed to an average *response* following a spike by a given amount of time (although these are mathematically equivalent because the response is a discrete element: a spike).

The stimuli, represented in figure 32.1 by letters, can be anything you like. They can, for example, be used to map the spatial structure of receptive fields. In this case, each letter might represent a single frame of a computer monitor that has been divided (invisibly) into a grid. Each frame would then have just a few squares in the grid illuminated and would look like a disorganized checkerboard (e.g., figure 32.2A); different frames would have different randomly assigned squares illuminated. An important feature of reverse-correlation mapping is that the configuration of each frame is random with respect to those preceding and following it; that is, there is no temporal structure. After presenting many of these stimuli (a sequence that looks like coarse television "snow"), one can then determine which frames precede action potentials, from which we can determine which are more likely to have caused excitation. We can then generate an "average" frame for a given delay by averaging all the frames that preceded an action potential by that delay. We can do this for several "reverse-correlation" delays to generate a "movie" of average stimuli. (An example

is discussed in the next section; see figure 32.2.) This is useful because with one major assumption, the resulting maps can be used to infer the receptive field and to predict the "optimal" stimulus. These maps are often referred to as *first-order receptive fields* or *first-order kernels*.

The assumption that enables us to use these first-order kernels to predict the optimal stimulus is that the underlying neural response is linear. A cell is considered linear if it responds to two spots presented simultaneously in a way that is matched by the sum of the cell's response to the two spots presented separately. Because the stimuli are presented in quick succession, it is implied either that the response to a given stimulus ends before the following stimulus is presented or that the response to a previous stimulus does not affect the cell's response to the subsequent stimulus. As it turns out, most real neurons are not linear. For most orientation-selective cells, for example, the sum of the responses to a series of stimuli, each a single spot that would make up a line if presented simultaneously, is generally much weaker than the cell's response to an actual line. But the response of the cell to a spot is not negligible, so if the cell is presented with many such stimuli, the average response can be a fair approximation of the response to a complete stimulus and can be used, with caution, to infer the cell's receptive field. Because the stimuli that are used in a reverse-correlation experiment are random with respect to each other, all the nonlinear interactions average out when an adequately long stimulus sequence is used. As we will discuss in the section entitled "Reverse-Correlation Methods: Determining Second-Order Kernels," some cells appear to perform a function that is decidedly nonlinear. For these cells, the assumption of linearity, along with the first-order kernels that are extracted from a reverse-correlation experiment, are poor, even misleading, characterizations of the cells' receptive fields.

Mapping the spatial structure of simple cell receptive fields

Simple cells, first described in primary visual cortex of the cat by Hubel and Wiesel, respond best to a light bar next to a dark bar in just one particular location of the visual field and at only one orientation of bar. Hubel and Wiesel[15] discovered this by astute observation of an accident (see quote above). When cat simple cells were subsequently mapped with reverse correlation, using single spot stimuli or checkerboards in which the black or white value at any given position is randomly determined, they show an average stimulus that matches the optimal stimulus;[3,18,25,28] the average stimulus appears as oriented white region(s) next to oriented dark region(s) (figure 32.2A). In figure 32.2A, the first panel in the top row (beside the example stimulus frame) represents the average stimulus that coincided, at exactly the same time,

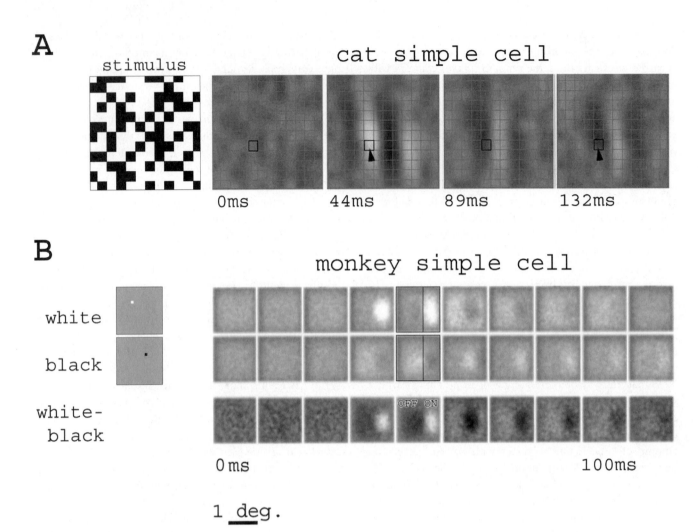

A

stimulus

cat simple cell

0ms 44ms 89ms 132ms

B

monkey simple cell

white

black

white-
black

0 ms 100ms

OFF ON

1 deg.

FIGURE 32.2 Spatial first-order response maps of simple cells in primary visual cortex revealed by reverse-correlation techniques. A, left panel, A single frame of a checkerboard stimulus used to stimulate the anesthetized cat simple cell whose response maps are shown to the right. Right panels, The average blurred stimulus that preceded an action potential by 0, 44, 89, and 132 ms (adapted from Reid et al., 1987, with generous permission from R. Clay Reid). Whiter regions in each response map represent a higher probability that the preceding stimulus had a white square at that location; blacker regions represent a higher probability that the preceding stimulus had a black square at that location. From this first-order response map, we can infer that this cell responded best to an almost vertically oriented white next to black next to white bar, with a visual latency of 44 ms. Note that regions that are white at one delay are black at a later delay (arrowhead). See text for discussion. B, left panels, Single frames from single contrast stimuli, used to stimulate the alert monkey simple cell whose response maps are shown to the right. Right panels, The average blurred stimulus that preceded an action potential by 0, 13, 25, 38, 50, 63, 75, 88, 100, and 113 ms for the white stimulus (top panels) and black stimulus (bottom panels). Whiter regions represent a higher probability that the given white or black stimulus preceded an action potential at the given delay. The response to white is subtracted from the response to black (bottom panels) to show the spatial antagonism of the white "ON" subregion and the black "OFF" subregion. (Adapted from Livingstone MS, Conway BR: Substructure of direction-selective cell receptive fields in macaque V1. *J Neurophysiol* 2003; 89:2743–2759.)

with the cell's action potentials. As you can see, there is not much structure in this panel, which makes sense; the cell's activity can correlate with the stimulus only after some visual latency. This is because the stimulus has to be detected by the photoreceptors, converted into action potentials by the retinal ganglion cells, and transmitted through the lateral geniculate nucleus to the neuron from which we are recording in primary visual cortex (layer 4). All this takes some

time, which we call the *visual latency*. We can gauge how long the visual latency is by how far before an action potential the average stimulus starts to show structure.

The second panel in figure 32.2A shows the average stimulus at a reverse-correlation delay of 44 ms. This was the average preceding stimulus at the optimal delay and can be interpreted as a probability map. Whiter regions indicate regions of the stimulus that were more likely to have been white at a delay of 44 ms before a spike; conversely, blacker regions represent regions of the stimulus that were more likely to have been black at a delay of 44 ms before a spike. These average stimuli are often referred to as *response maps* or *stimulus-response functions*. Note that the gray value (i.e., probability) averaged over an entire response map at any given delay is the same for each average response map at any delay, but in the response maps that correspond to the visual latency of the cell, the probability is distributed nonrandomly. We can follow the structure of the probability at different reverse-correlation delays, shown in the remaining panels of figure 32.2A. So we can ask, "How does the average optimal stimulus compare at different reverse-correlation delays?" If we take our simple cell as an example (figure 32.2A), it turns out that regions that are excited at short delays are suppressed at long delays and regions that are suppressed at short delays are excited at long delays (see the arrowhead in figure 32.2A). For some cells, the relationship at different delays is not so simple. This is in fact the case with the cat cell in figure 32.2A. By inspection, you can see that white regions are subtly shifted from one reverse-correlation delay to another: at 44 ms, the dominant white region is centered on the blackened reference square; at 89 ms, it is to the right; and at 132 ms, it is farther to the right. Therefore, we would predict that the optimal stimulus for this cell is not only an oriented white bar next to a black bar, but also one that moves location from right to left across the receptive field. Importantly, the first-order kernels that are produced for this cell, typical of simple cells, correspond well with the receptive field properties of the cell; the cell does in fact respond best to a white bar next to a black bar and, moreover, one that moves. But many, if not most, visual cells are not adequately described by first-order kernels alone (see the section below entitled "Reverse-correlation methods: Determining second-order kernels").

Early technical limitations

Reverse-correlation mapping is an elegant way to describe the spatial and temporal response properties of visual neurons. But it requires a relatively large amount of data storage because one needs to have a continuous record of the stimulus configuration and spike activity. Early attempts at reverse correlation were hampered by the storage limitation of computers. In a creative solution to this problem, Sutter[30] used photographic film to capture the stimuli that preceded action potentials. He would expose the same piece of photographic film to all the stimuli that preceded action potentials. The experimental details are not available (he published this as an abstract to the Society for Neuroscience) but presumably were not optimal because he subsequently developed m-sequences.[31] An m-sequence is a sequence of numbers derived from a simple formula that is used to define the luminance value of each square in a checkerboard. The sequence of stimuli characterized by an m-sequence has no temporal structure, yet each stimulus can be derived from a mathematical formula. Although the whole ensemble of stimulus frames appears as coarse TV snow, a given stimulus frame at a particular time in the sequence can be reconstructed with the m-sequence formula. Thus, one needn't record the stimuli, only the spike history. The cat simple cell shown in figure 32.2A was mapped with m-sequences.[28] Today, computers are powerful enough that storage capacity is no longer a limitation, and most reverse-correlation studies use randomly generated stimuli, not m-sequences. It should be reiterated, however, that the stimulus sequences that are used will affect how well the stimulus response functions characterize the cell's physiological properties. A tremendous amount of mathematics is involved in determining what sort of stimuli should be used so as to avoid acquiring spurious response functions. M-sequences remain a nice way of doing this. The interested reader is directed elsewhere for details of this mathematics,[24] but it should suffice to say here that the variables for spatial mapping include the number of squares illuminated in any given frame (sparse versus dense) and the way in which each frame relates to the next. Most important, each frame should be random compared to the next so that with very long stimulus sequences, there is no pattern relating the stimuli.

Reverse-correlation methods in the alert animal

The earliest studies of the primary visual cortex were done in alert cats.[14] But as you can imagine, it was not easy to determine where the cat was looking, so it was even harder to determine the correlation between stimulus and neural response. This led to the development of recordings in paralyzed and anesthetized animals, in which eye position can be accurately determined. Although these studies provided valuable insights, one could not rule out the effect of anesthetic on the recordings. But with the development of eye-movement-monitoring systems, one could once again record in alert animals and determine, after the fact, where the stimuli were in retinal coordinates, by maintaining a continuous record of eye position and stimulus position.[21] This could then be coupled with reverse-correlation to enable high-resolution receptive field maps in the alert animal. In these experiments, monkeys are trained to fixate on a small dot presented on a computer monitor. Having the monkeys perform this task eliminates large saccadic eye movements but does not reduce constantly occurring smaller eye movements. The monkeys' eyes are monitored by using an eye coil placed inside a magnetic field coil: An insulated wire loop is sutured to the sclera around the eye, and the ends of the loop are mounted to a connector attached to the monkeys' skull, which allows one to monitor the current through the wire. The monkey's head is placed inside a magnetic field coil so that a current is induced in the monkey's eye coil every time the monkey moves its eyes. The magnetic flux through the eye coil, and the induced current, changes proportionally with the monkey's eye movements; the system can be calibrated so that by monitoring the current through the coil, one has a remarkably precise measure of eye position.

The details of reverse-correlation mapping using this alert animal preparation are similar to those used in the anesthetized cat except that one accounts for eye position by subtracting it from the stimulus position for any given frame. The resulting maps for a simple cell recorded in monkey primary visual cortex are shown in figure 32.2B.[20] For this particular case, only a single square was illuminated in any given frame, and this square was not constrained to a stimulus grid, as in the m-sequence mapping. The stimuli were either white on a gray background (figure 32.2B, top panel) or black on a gray background (figure 32.2B, middle panel). Thus, unlike m-sequence maps, which use a checkerboard, responses to white and black spots are mapped with separate stimulus runs. The response maps for both black and white spots are shown according to the same grayscale, where whiter regions indicate a higher probability. So white in the black maps shows the part of the receptive field that was excited by black at that delay. Note that at the optimal reverse-correlation delay (the fifth panel from the left), the probability that a white stimulus preceded an action potential is roughly the inverse of the probability that a black stimulus preceded an action potential (compare the boxed regions in figure 32.2B). Thus, the cell was "push-pull"[11]: It was excited by white and suppressed by black in one part of the receptive field and was suppressed by black and excited by white in an adjacent part of the receptive field. This can be summarized by subtracting the black response functions from the white response functions (figure 32.2B, bottom row). The size of the stimulus frame was much smaller in the maps of the monkey cell because the monkey cell receptive fields are considerably smaller than those of cells in the cat. The scale bar is the same for both cells, and both cells were recorded at roughly the same eccentricity (within 5 degrees of the fovea/area centralis). Despite the difference in scale, however, the monkey simple cell shows many of the same features of the cat simple cell: White regions at early reverse-correlation delays are replaced by dark regions at late reverse-correlation delays, and this transition is gradual—the black region of the monkey cell gradually shifts to positions more rightward at longer reverse-correlation delays, so one would predict that the cell would respond best to a black bar moving right to left.

Because for some cells, the peak response in the response maps shifts over different reverse-correlation delays (e.g., figures 32.2A and 32.2B), it is sometimes useful to generate

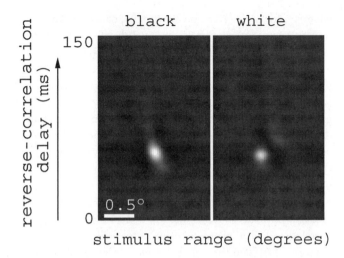

FIGURE 32.3   First-order space-time maps for a direction-selective simple cell in monkey primary visual cortex. The probability that an optimally oriented black bar (left map) or a white bar (right map) preceded an action potential is given according to a grayscale map on which whiter regions indicate a higher probability. This cell showed a complementary pattern of probabilities for white and black maps, indicating that the cell is "simple"; however, the response probabilities shift over time. Maps like these are often called "slanted" space-time maps and reflect the direction preference of the cell. The slant in this map is from upper left to lower right. (In the black map, it is evident as a diagonal white blob of increased probability, and in the white map, it is evident as a black region that moves diagonally between two temporally offset white blobs.) The horizontal striations throughout the maps reflect the cell's average, uncorrelated response to the continuously presented stimuli. (Adapted from Livingstone MS, Conway BR: Substructure of direction-selective cell receptive fields in macaque V1. *J Neurophysiol* 2003; 89:2743–2759.)

space-time maps that display the spatial shift over time in one figure (figure 32.3). To generate the space-time maps shown in figure 32.3, a monkey simple cell was stimulated with optimally oriented black and white bars, presented on a gray background; the bars were moved along a stimulus range, along one spatial dimension (x-axis), through the center of the receptive field. The probability that a given stimulus preceded a spike at a given delay (y-axis) is shown according to a grayscale: Whiter regions indicate a higher probability. You can see that this cell had not only spatial structure (the probabilities for the white and black maps are complementary), but also temporal structure (the spatial distribution of the probabilities for each map shift as reverse-correlation delay is changed), suggesting this cell's optimal stimulus was not just a bar but one that moved over time. This cell and the ones shown in figure 32.2 were in fact directionally selective, though as we will see in the next section, first-order maps give only a weak account of directionally-selective cells' receptive fields, especially those of complex direction-selective cells (see figure 32.4).

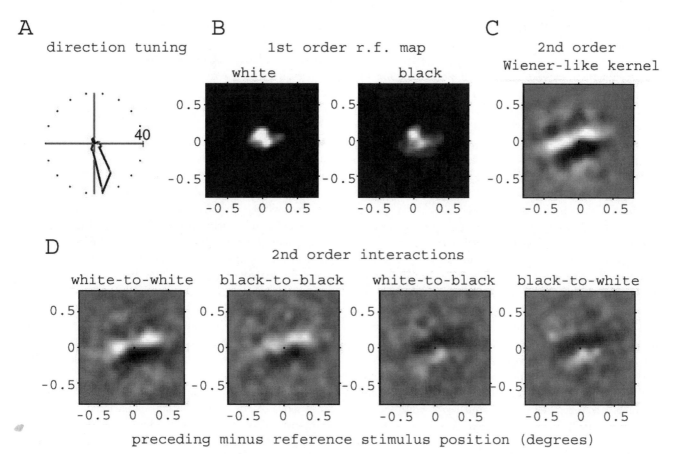

A direction tuning

B 1st order r.f. map

white   black

C 2nd order Wiener-like kernel

D 2nd order interactions

white-to-white   black-to-black   white-to-black   black-to-white

preceding minus reference stimulus position (degrees)

FIGURE 32.4   Spatial second-order response maps for a complex, direction-selective cell in monkey visual cortex. A, Direction tuning curve. This cell preferred bars of almost horizontal orientation moving down and slightly to the right. B, First-order response maps to white spots (left) and black spots (right) at the optimal reverse-correlation delay, reflecting the cell's receptive field (r.f.). The horizontal and vertical axes are in degrees of visual angle, centered on the stimulus range, which was centered on the receptive field. Note that these maps show very little spatial structure and reveal little about the receptive field of the neuron, unlike the first-order maps of the simple cells shown in figure 36.2. C, Second-order response map (Wiener-like kernel). This is derived from the individual maps shown in (D). D, Responses to pairs of spots were extracted from the same spike train used to generate the first-order receptive field maps (A); this involved a long reverse-correlation experiment in which a single white and a single black spot were presented in every stimulus frame, with a random spatial relationship to each other. From this stimulus, four sequences of spots could be extracted: white preceding white, black preceding black, black preceding white, and white preceding black. The maps show the responses to such sequential pairs of spots presented anywhere in the receptive field; one spot was defined as the reference spot, and the other spot as the preceding spot. The reference spot's position, though it could

have been anywhere in the receptive field, is normalized to the center. The gray values throughout the map indicate the response of the cell when the preceding spot occupied that location. These maps reflect the direction preference of the cell. For example, this cell was suppressed by preceding white spots located below and to the right of reference white spots (black region in the leftmost panel) and excited by preceding white spots located above and to the left of reference white spot (white region in the leftmost panel). Sequential black spots show a similar pattern of second-order interactions (second panel from the left). Interestingly, sequential spots that invert contrast (last two panels) show an inverted pattern of second-order interactions. This pattern of interactions shows that the cell prefers inverting-contrast sequences if the sequences progress in the direction opposite to the cell's actual direction preference. This is the neural correlate of the visual illusion called reverse-phi motion: a stimulus that is made to change contrast in mid movement appears to move in the opposite direction to the physical progression of the stimulus. This shows that the fundamental stage of motion processing is contrast-sign specific. Note that these second-order maps are much more informative than the first-order maps. (Adapted from Livingstone MS, Conway BR: Substructure of direction-selective cell receptive fields in macaque V1. *J Neurophysiol* 2003; 89:2743–2759.)

Reverse-correlation methods: Determining second-order kernels

The technique discussed so far is used to describe the average optimal *single* frame at any given reverse-correlation delay preceding an action potential. The average optimal stimuli are sometimes referred to as *first-order kernels*. These first-order kernels show the amount of the cell's response that is linear and are useful in characterizing the receptive fields of simple cells whose responses are largely linear. But as we discussed in a previous section ("Reverse-correlation methods: The generic case"), most visual cells are not linear; that is, their responses to two spots presented simultaneously or in sequence cannot be adequately predicted by summing the responses to the two stimuli presented independently.[2,26] This is epitomized by the so-called complex cells in the cat's primary visual cortex. A complex cell responds preferentially to a bar of a given orientation, but unlike simple cells, for which the bar needs to be situated in a specific portion of the receptive field, a complex cell will respond to the bar if it is placed anywhere within the receptive field.[15] Moreover, complex cells do not respond well to spots; they require a bar to give a good response. Thus, mapping a complex cell with a sequence of spots will not provide an enlightening first-order map (see figure 32.4B). In fact, for most visual neurons, some fraction of the neurons' response depends on the particular sequence or configuration of frames.[27] We can ignore this when we generate a first-order kernel because the sequence of stimulus frames is random—it has no temporal structure. But how then do we adequately study cells that fire well only when a black spot is preceded by a white spot, cells that fire only to a sequence of spots moving through visual space (directionally selective cells), or cells that fire only to two adjacent spots presented simultaneously (complex cells)? Such nonlinear cells exist, and the nonlinearities that they encode are certainly important for processing visual information. We would not want to prevent ourselves from studying such cells by looking only at linear properties.

Fortunately, one can use reverse correlation to examine both first-order interactions and second-order interactions. In the schematic shown in figure 32.1, the letters would then represent sequences of frames, not just single frames (if one were interested in mapping sequential interactions), or each letter would represent a pair of spots (if one were interested in mapping simultaneous interactions). Of course, to use the same stimulus run to map the first-order interactions, one still has to make sure that there is no overall temporal structure to the stimulus and that the spatial location of each spot in any given frame is random and independent of the other spot in that frame if pairs of spots are used.

How then, you might ask, can we examine second-order interactions using a stimulus sequence that has no overall tem-poral or spatial structure? The answer is that the sequence of stimuli used is enormous: it contains every possible combination of spatial and temporal structures, many times over, but no overall spatial or temporal structure. Using our analogy of the letters of the alphabet to represent the stimulus sequence, it is as if all 26 letters are presented, in a random sequence, so many times over that every letter is, at some point in the sequence, preceded and followed by every other letter but no subsequence of letters predominates. The challenge, then, is to extract from the responses to this huge stimulus sequence those responses to all spatial and temporal combinations.

Theoretically, this has been solved by Wiener[34] and Marmarelis and Marmarelis,[24] who stipulated not only the appropriate stimulus sequence that should be used (Gaussian white noise, much like television "snow"), but also a very powerful analysis that extracts the first-order and second-order kernels. (It actually can extract the third-order, fourth-order, fifth-order, and so on kernels too.) Wiener's method is analogous to the cross-correlation method shown in figure 32.1. Wiener's analysis also tells you how much of the cell's response is accounted for by each kernel. Simple cells, for example, would have a lot of their response accounted for by first-order kernels (figure 32.2), while complex cells would have more of their response accounted for by second- or third-order kernels (figure 32.4). The method described by Wiener and Marmarelis and Marmarelis is potentially extremely powerful because it allows one to fully characterize the receptive field of a neuron without prior hand mapping. (Hand mapping is the crude form of forward correlation that Kuffler and Hubel and Wiesel used to determine receptive field location, orientation and/or direction-preference.) One needn't, for example, just acquire the first-order kernel as a means of quantifying a simple cell; rather, one can use the technique to demonstrate that a given cell is in fact simple by showing that the majority of the variance of its response is accounted for by the first-order map. Unfortunately, the white noise stimuli prescribed by this rigorous approach would require an almost infinite amount of time to execute, which is practically not feasible and further confounded by the fact that visual cells adapt rather quickly to white noise. Simpler stimuli, such as the checkerboards or spots that were used to map the cells in figure 32.4, have proven more useful. Such stimuli yield "Wiener-like" kernels,[10] which have proven enlightening in understanding the mechanism underlying direction selectivity, in which the neuron's job is to compute the spatial configuration of the stimulus across time (figure 32.4).[6,20] One can see just on cursory inspection that the second-order Wiener-like kernels for a complex direction-selective cell have much more structure than the first-order kernels (compare figures 32.4B and 32.4C). Modifications of the technique have also been very useful in determining the substructure of complex cell receptive fields.[26,32]

Mapping multiple stimulus dimensions: Orientation and color

Reverse-correlation techniques have also been used to investigate the mechanisms of orientation selectivity[29] (figure 32.5), color selectivity (figure 32.6),[4,5,7] and depth selectivity.[12,23,33] In these cases, the letters in the schematic in figure 32.1 represent bars or sine-wave grating stimuli of different orientations; different colors, either equiluminant (i.e., roughly the same value if reproduced in grayscale) or cone isolating (i.e., selectively changing the activity of a single cone while maintaining constant activity of the remaining two cone classes); or bars presented independently to the two eyes.

When orientation is tested with reverse correlation, the response maps show that cells in layer 4B have an orientation preference,[29] a nice confirmation of the results obtained with forward correlation.[16] The peak response of these first-order kernels occurs around a reverse-correlation delay of 53 ms (figure 32.5). Conversely, when the cone inputs to color cells are examined with reverse-correlation, the spatial first-order response maps at the optimal reverse-correlation delay show that the cells are both spatially and chromatically, or "double," opponent.[4] In these maps, high probability of cell firing is represented by whiter regions. For each cone class, the response profile shows that the cell is suppressed by stimuli in one location and excited by the same stimuli in a different location, while a comparison of the cone maps shows that in any given location the cell is excited by one cone class (L) and suppressed by the opponent cone classes

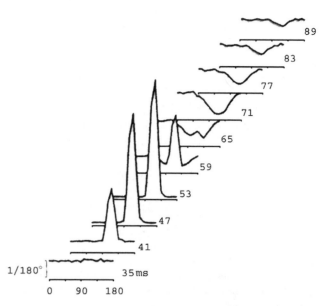

FIGURE 32.5 Dynamics of orientation tuning in monkey primary visual cortex using a reverse-correlation technique in which the stimuli are gratings of different orientations. Responses to each orientation (horizontal axis, 0°, 90°, 180°) are shown at various reverse-correlation delays. The cell's optimal orientation is ~135° at an optimal reverse-correlation delay of 47 ms. Note the rebound suppression to this optimal orientation at longer reverse-correlation delays. (Adapted from Ringach DL, Hawken MJ, Shapley RM: Dynamics of orientation tuning in macaque primary visual cortex. *Nature* 1997; 387:281–284.)

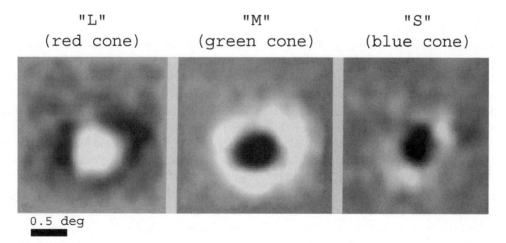

FIGURE 32.6 Spatial structure of the first-order response maps, at the optimal reverse-correlation delay, of a cone-opponent cell in monkey visual cortex using reverse-correlation and cone-isolating stimuli. These maps show that the cell's receptive field is both spatially and chromatically opponent. Whiter regions indicate a higher probability that the given stimulus preceded an action potential; blacker regions indicate a lower probability. The maps predict that the optimal stimulus for this cell is a red spot surrounded by a green annulus. Such cells likely underlie spatial color contrast. (Adapted from Conway BR: Spatial structure of cone inputs to color cells in alert macaque primary visual cortex [V-1]. *J Neurosci* 2001; 21:2768–2783.)

(M + S). Such "double-opponent cells" are found in the cytochrome oxidase blobs[22] in layers both above and below layer 4 in the monkey. As with the simple cell receptive fields that showed opposite responses to opposite contrast spots at different reverse-correlation delays, oriented cells and color cells are suppressed at long reverse-correlation delays by stimuli that cause excitation at optimal reverse-correlation delays. This phenomenon is loosely described as *rebound*.

Potential pitfalls of reverse correlation

One must be careful in interpreting the results of a reverse-correlation experiment. One potential pitfall of spatial maps involves the interpretation of regions in a stimulus-response function that correspond to the absence of a spot—the dark regions in the response function for the monkey color cell, for example. These regions show that the average optimal stimulus X ms before the cell's spikes did not contain a spot at that location. This is often interpreted as "spots at these locations cause suppression of cell firing," which is sometimes misstated as "spots at these locations cause inhibition of cell firing." The potential difficulty in interpretation arises because the dark regions might simply represent the cell's complete disinterest in the stimulus—neither excitation nor suppression. If one stimulated a cell in the visual system with auditory stimuli, it would be unlikely to show any correlated response or any response at all. This does not mean that the auditory stimuli cause suppression. So how does one determine whether a region is actually suppressed by a given stimulus, on the basis of the reverse-correlation response profile? For the maps shown in figure 32.6, one can compare the response probability in a region under question to the response probability that one knows is well outside the receptive field, where stimuli do not correlate with the cell's activity. Thus, we can see that the dark regions in figure 32.6 that form an annulus in the "L" map and the center of the annulus in the "M" and "S" map do correlate with a much lower probability of firing than the average probability outside the receptive field. Therefore, we can safely conclude that these stimuli, when located in particular configurations corresponding to the black regions, cause suppression of firing. But we have to be even more careful. We still do not know whether the suppression is attributed to an inhibition of the cell from which we are recording. It may be inhibition of a cell in the retina or lateral geniculate nucleus. Therefore, even though these regions represent significant suppression of firing, because we cannot record a firing rate of less than zero spikes per second, we cannot attribute this suppression to the mechanism "inhibition." To establish this, we would have to record from the cell intracellularly.[11]

Similarly, what does one make of the reduced firing of a cell to nonoptimal orientated stimuli at the optimal reverse-correlation delay (compare the response to 180° at the reverse-correlation delay of 35 ms with response at 53 ms; see figure 32.5)? Can we conclude that these nonoptimal stimuli inhibit the cell because the response probability is lower at the optimal reverse-correlation delay? Just as in the spatial maps in which the probability averaged across a given response map at any given delay is the same regardless of the delay (i.e., the average grayscale is the same for all panels in figure 32.6), the average response for all orientations at any given delay will be the same. Thus, at reverse-correlation delays that are shorter than the visual latency, the response for any given orientation will be roughly equal to the response for any other orientation; any orientation could have coincided with an action potential because there is no correlation between the action potential and the randomly presented stimulus. But as one approaches the cell's visual latency, the probability distribution shifts, revealing the cell's optimal orientation. This necessarily means that the probability at nonoptimal orientations will go down and does not mean that the cell is inhibited, or even suppressed, by these nonoptimal orientations. But the temporal evolution of the response profile shows not only that the cell is suppressed by optimal stimuli at long reverse-correlation delays (a rebound at 71 ms; see figure 32.5), but also that it is suppressed by nonoptimal stimuli at long delays. This is shown as the so-called Mexican hat response profile at a reverse-correlation delay of 59 ms. This might be evidence that inhibition of a cortical origin, which has a longer visual latency than the feedforward excitation that establishes orientation selectivity, sharpens orientation selectivity.

Finally, one must be careful not to use reverse correlation to blindly assign function to neurons in the visual system. One could imagine, for example, measuring the orientation-tuning response of a strongly cone-opponent cell and achieving some weak orientation bias. This need not mean that the cell is using the orientation bias to encode information about the visual scene. Thus, one is left with a compromise between two experimental approaches. On the one hand, there are advantages and disadvantages to studies that examine all neurons with the same battery of stimuli (e.g., cone-isolating, orientation, spatial luminance, moving). These studies can produce nice population results that can be used to categorize cells.[17] But these sorts of studies are cumbersome because one usually is not able to maintain recording from a single cell long enough to allow one to measure the responses to all the stimuli. Moreover, for any given stimulus parameter (say, orientation), one usually has to use a less than optimal stimulus for any given cell (say, nonoptimal spatial frequency) to allow one to use the same stimulus (differently oriented bars of a fixed spatial frequency) to test every cell. On the other hand, there are advantages and disadvantages to screening cells with hand-mapping before testing with reverse correlation. The major disadvantage is that one cannot make very secure conclusions about how a given aspect of the visual world (say, color) is processed by a population of cells. But screening does permit one to reach more accurate and in-depth conclusions about how a given visual attribute is processed.[4] Fortunately, different investigators have their biases, so both kinds of studies continue to be done.

Conclusion

In summary, reverse correlation is a powerful tool that has provided insight into the mechanisms of visual processing by permitting a thorough characterization of the spatial and temporal properties of the receptive fields of cells in the early visual system along multiple stimulus dimensions, including spatial structure, luminance, orientation, direction, and color. Undoubtedly, reverse correlation will assist us as we begin to study more closely the transformations of this information in higher visual areas.

ACKNOWLEDGMENTS *We gratefully acknowledge Chris Pack and Tom Davidson for useful comments on the manuscript.*

REFERENCES

1. Aertsen AMHJ, Johannesma PIM: A comparison of the spectro-temporal sensitivity of auditory neurons to tonal and natural stimuli. *Biol Cybern* 1981; 42:145–156.
2. Barlow HB, Levick WR: The mechanism of directionally selective units in rabbit's retina. *J Physiol* 1965; 178:477–504.
3. Citron MC, Emerson RC: White noise analysis of cortical direction selectivity in cat. *Brain Res* 1983; 279:271–277.
4. Conway BR: Spatial structure of cone inputs to color cells in alert macaque primary visual cortex (V1). *J Neurosci* 2001; 21:2768–2783.
5. Conway BR, Hubel DH, Livingstone MS: Color contrast in macaque V1. *Cereb Cortex* 2002; 12:915–925.
6. Conway BR, Livingstone MS: Space-time maps and two-bar interactions of direction-selective cells in macaque V1. *J Neurophysiol* 2003; 89:2726–2742.
7. Cottaris NP, De Valois RL: Temporal dynamics of chromatic tuning in macaque primary visual cortex. *Nature* 1998; 395:896–900.
8. DeBoer E, Kuper P: Triggered correlation. *IEEE Biomed Eng* 1968; 15:169–179.
9. Eckhorn R, Krause F, Nelson JI: A cross-correlation technique for mapping several visual neurons at once. *Biol Cybern* 1993; 69:37–55.
10. Emerson RC, Citron MC, Vaughn WJ, Klein SA: Nonlinear directionally selective subunits in complex cells of cat straite cortex. *J Neurophysiol* 1987; 58:33–65.
11. Ferster D: Linearity of synaptic interactions in the assembly of receptive fields in cat visual cortex. *Curr Opin Neurobiol* 1994; 4:563–568.
12. Freeman RD, Ohzawa I: On the neurophysiological organization of binocular vision. *Vision Res* 1990; 30:1661–1676.
13. Hubel DH: Exploration of the primary visual cortex, 1955–78. *Nature* 1982; 299:515–524.
14. Hubel DH, Wiesel TN: Receptive fields of single neurones in the cat's striate cortex. *J Physiol* 1959; 148:574–591.
15. Hubel DH, Wiesel TN: Receptive fields, binocular interaction and functional architecture in the cat's visual cortex. *J Physiol* 1962; 160:106–154.
16. Hubel DH, Wiesel TN: Receptive fields and functional architecture of monkey striate cortex. *J Physiol* 1968; 195:215–243.
17. Johnson EN, Hawken MJ, Shapley RM: The spatial transformation of color in the primary visual cortex of the macaque monkey. *Nature Neurosci* 2001; 4:409–416.
18. Jones JP, Palmer LA: The two-dimensional spatial structure of simple receptive fields in cat striate cortex. *J Neurophysiol* 1987; 58:1187–1211.
19. Kuffler SW: Discharge patterns and functional organization of mammalian retina. *J Neurophysiol* 1953; 16:36–68.
20. Livingstone MS, Conway BR: Substructure of direction-selective cell receptive fields in macaque V1. *J Neurophysiol* 2003; 89:2743–2759.
21. Livingstone MS, Freeman DC, Hubel DH: Visual responses in V1 of freely viewing monkeys. *Cold Spring Harbor Symp Quant Biol* 1996; 61:27–37.
22. Livingstone MS, Hubel DH: Anatomy and physiology of a color system in the primate visual cortex. *J Neurosci* 1984; 4:309–356.
23. Livingstone MS, Tsao DY: Receptive fields of disparity-selective neurons in macaque striate cortex. *Nat Neurosci* 1999; 2:825–832.
24. Marmarelis PZ, Marmarelis VZ: *Analysis of Physiological Systems.* New York, Plenum Press, 1978.
25. McLean J, Palmer LA: Contribution of linear spatiotemporal receptive field structure to velocity selectivity of simple cells in area 17 of cat. *Vision Res* 1989; 29:675–679.
26. Movshon JA, Thompson ID, Tolhurst DJ: Receptive field organization of complex cells in the cat's striate cortex. *J Physiol* 1978; 283:79–99.
27. Reid RC, Soodak RE, Shapley RM: Linear mechanisms of directional selectivity in simple cells of cat striate cortex. *Proc Natl Acad Sci U S A* 1987; 84:8740–8744.
28. Reid RC, Victor JD, Shapley RM: The use of m-sequences in the analysis of visual neurons: Linear receptive field properties. *Vis Neurosci* 1997; 14:1015–1027.
29. Ringach DL, Hawken MJ, Shapley RM: Dynamics of orientation tuning in macaque primary visual cortex. *Nature* 1997; 387:281–284.
30. Sutter EE: Electrophysiological investigation of visual units in the cat: A revised conception of receptive fields. *Soc Neurosci Abstr* 1974; 4:444.
31. Sutter EE: The fast m-transform: A fast computation of cross-correlations with binary m-sequences. *SIAM J Computing* 1992; 20:686–694.
32. Szulborski RG, Palmer LA: The two-dimensional spatial structure of nonlinear subunits in the receptive fields of complex cells. *Vision Res* 1990; 30:249–254.
33. Tsao DT, Conway BR, Livingstone MS: Receptive fields of disparity-selective neurons in macaque V1. *Neuron* 2003; 38:103–114.
34. Wiener N: *Nonlinear Problems in Random Theory.* New York, Wiley, 1958.

33 Stimulus-Response Functions for the Scotopic b-Wave

ANNE B. FULTON AND RONALD M. HANSEN

THE RELATIONSHIP OF stimulus intensity to ERG response has been widely studied in healthy and diseased retinas.[9–11,13–15,23,24,34,61,66,67] The ERG stimulus-response functions summarize the graded responses of the distal retinal cells to a range of flash intensities. Stimulus-response (S-R) functions for the amplitudes and implicit times of the several components of the intact ERG waveform in human and animal subjects have been described and provide a foundation on which the interpretation of cellular processes is built. This chapter will focus on scotopic b-wave functions. Other chapters are devoted to derivation of the photoreceptor response from the a-wave (chapter 35) and postreceptoral components such as the oscillatory potentials (chapter 43).

The hyperbolic function

$$V/V_{max} = I^n/(I^n + \sigma^n) \tag{1}$$

reasonably well describes[2,3,23,44,61] the relationship of the scotopic b-wave potential, V, to stimulus intensity, I. The value of I that produces a half-maximum (semisaturated) response is σ. Thus, $1/\sigma$ is an index of sensitivity. The exponent in equation (1) indicates the slope of the function at σ.

As is shown in figure 33.1, the two parameters $\log\sigma$ and V_{max} provide a compact representation of a large number of b-wave responses (figure 33.1A). On a log-log plot of the S-R function, response voltage increases linearly as low-intensity lights are incremented and then, as I is increased further, approaches a maximum (figure 33.1B). The implicit time of the response decreases with increasing intensity (figure 33.1C). If n is 1, as usually is the case,[3,5,6,18,19,25,26,38,44,46,69] the linear range covers about 1.8 decadic log units of stimulus intensity.[59] With progression to higher flash intensities at which the a-wave is present, a second limb of the S-R function becomes apparent.[51] The complete b-wave function (figure 33.1B) is not monotonic. The fit of equation (1) does not include the second limb.[16,23,51,61] For normal adults, the reported values[3,4,6,16,23,44,52,58] of $\log\sigma$ range from 0 to −0.5 log scotopic troland seconds with standard deviations less than 0.2 log unit. Normal adult values of V_{max} range from 281 μV to 521 μV with a standard deviations of less than 100 μV.[3,4,6,16,23,44,52,58]

In the first reports that equation (1) summarizes the voltage of the response of distal retinal cells to a range of stimulus light intensities, Naka and Rushton[47,48] noted that the mathematical function also represents a logistic growth curve[64] such as describes the growth of the U.S. population between 1790 and 1940. Perhaps more relevant to changes in potential across the membranes of retinal cells are models of enzyme[45] or adsorption[42] kinetics that may be cast as a hyperbolic function and summarized by equation (1). Examples of physical events fulfilling the prediction of this mathematical model are enzyme and adsorption kinetics.[42,45] As substrate is added, enzyme velocities increase linearly until enzyme sites approach saturation and velocities approach a maximum.[42] Adsorption of particles on a surface proceeds linearly until sites become occupied, and then, no matter how many more particles are made available, the rate of adsorption reaches a never-to-be-exceeded rate.[42]

Since the first mathematical summary of ERG S-R functions,[26] a good deal more has been learned about the S-R functions of the photoreceptors and the postreceptoral cells and the origins of the components of the ERG (chapter 12). No single class of cells accounts entirely for the behavior of b-wave S-R functions.[53,57] The current understanding is that the scotopic b-wave S-R function represents the observed relationship of the mass activity of ON-bipolar cells with lesser contributions from other second- and third-order neurons.[1,29,30,49,50,65,68,70]

To obtain S-R curves such as those shown in figure 33.1, stimulus intensities sufficiently low to establish the linear portion of the curve and sufficiently high to establish saturation are needed. In practice, a several log unit range of stimuli, incremented in 0.2–0.5 log unit steps, are used to obtain data sets from which the parameters of equation (1) can be determined. Curve-fitting programs minimize the root mean square deviation of the observed responses from equation (1). Larger step sizes and fewer experimental points may reduce the precision with which the parameters of equation (1) can be determined.

Procedural and technical explanations are usually offered for the scotopic b-wave S-R functions that are not well described by equation (1). The most straightforward and common explanations are that the stimuli are not well

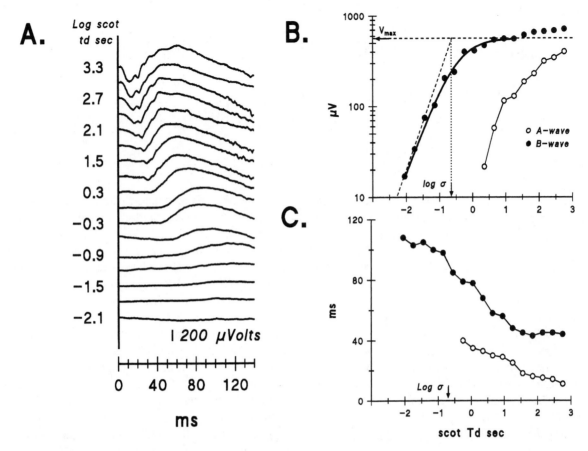

FIGURE 33.1 The scotopic stimulus-response (S-R) functions. A, Sample ERG records from a normal subject. The amplitude of the b-wave response increases with increasing stimulus intensity. At the higher intensities, a-waves are also seen. The troland values of the stimuli are indicated to the left of every other trace. B, The amplitudes of the a- and b-wave responses in panel A are shown as a function of stimulus intensity on a log-log plot. The arrow indi- cates $\log \sigma$, the flash intensity that elicits a half-maximum b-wave amplitude. The smooth curve represents equation (1) (see the text) with $n = 1$ fit to the monotonic portion of the S-R function. The upper limb is ignored in the curve fit. The dashed lines are an oblique with a slope of 1.0 and a horizontal at V_{max}. The dashed lines intersect at $\log s$. C, The implicit times of the a- and b-waves are plotted as a function of log stimulus intensity.

placed. For instance, definition of the lower end of the func- tion depends on sufficient stimulation with low intensities. In the normal adult eye, stimuli producing approximately −1 to −2 log scotopic troland seconds retinal illuminance evoke small b-waves. At very low intensities, producing approximately −3 log scotopic troland seconds retinal illu- minance, the small (≤20 μV) scotopic threshold response (STR) is evoked from the thoroughly dark-adapted eye.[17,57,63] Besides being evoked by lower-intensity stimuli, the STR is a corneal-negative potential and has longer implicit times, typically in the range of 100–180 ms. Insufficient intensity and large step size would leave the upper portion of the curve, including the second limb (figure 33.1B), incompletely defined. The lack of demonstrable saturation at higher intensities may be due to several factors that are not neces- sarily mutually exclusive. These include the failure to limit responses to those mediated by one class of photoreceptors and, especially at higher stimulus intensities, repetition rates that suppress amplitudes of subsequent responses. The sco-

topic b-wave S-R functions in normal subjects are similar, whether the cone contribution is subtracted or not. However, the cone contribution may have a significant effect on the b- wave S-R functions recorded from dark-adapted patients with retinal disease.[52,60]

Responses to test lights that uniformly stimulate as much of the retina as possible[39,40] are more readily interpreted than those elicited by smaller, nonuniform fields. International Society for Clinical Electrophysiology of Vision (ISCEV) standards recommend full-field stimulation.[43] An integrating sphere or a flash lamp and diffuser at close range are used. It is recognized that the integrating sphere does not provide perfectly uniform intensity of stimulation over the entire retinal surface.[39,40] Full-field and less than full-field stimuli yield nearly identical S-R functions in normal subjects.[21] However, valid comparisons of responses from normal and diseased retina are best based on responses to full-field stim- ulation. Disease may reduce the area of functional retina and alter the parameters of the S-R function.[12,37,62]

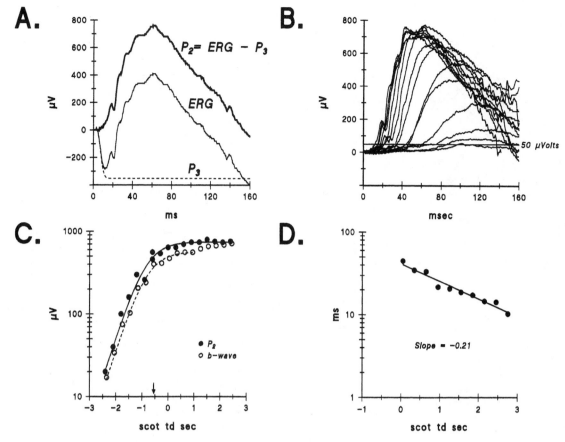

FIGURE 33.2 Derivation of the postreceptoral response, P_2. A, P_2 is derived by subtraction of the rod photoresponse (labeled P_3) from the intact ERG waveform. B, The family of P_2 waves in a normal subject is shown. A horizontal line marks the 50-mV level. C, The points show the amplitude of P_2 (waves displayed in B) as a function of stimulus intensity on a log-log plot. The smooth curve is the equation $P_2/P_{2max} = I/(I + K_{P2})$ fit to the points. The dashed curve

shows the S-R function for the b-wave from which the P_2 records were derived. The arrow indicates the semisaturating stimulus ($\log s$ or $\log K_{p2}$), which, for the normal retina, is the same for the b-wave and P_2. The saturated amplitude of P_2 (P_{2max}) exceeds that of the b-wave (V_{max}). D, For the records shown in B, the latency of P_2 at 50 mV is shown as a function of stimulus intensity of a log-log plot.

In retinal degenerative disorders or in early infancy, the range of response amplitudes between the noise level and saturation is attenuated. To improve signal-to-noise ratio, signal averaging becomes necessary if interpretable S-R data are to be obtained. Maintenance of a constant state of retinal adaptation is critical. Care must be taken that repeated stimulations do not themselves attenuate the response. The on-line observation of the trough-to-peak amplitudes of successive b-waves is often used to make this determination. At high stimulus intensities, 60-s or longer intervals may be necessary.

In an analysis reminiscent of that of Granit,[27,28] the ERG waveform is considered to be the sum of the photoreceptor and postreceptoral retinal responses.[33,35] Contemporary analyses digitally subtract the rod photoreceptor response, which is derived mathematically from the a-wave and called P_3,[34,41,54] from the intact ERG waveform to obtain P_2

(figure 33.2A). P_2 is thought to represent mainly the ON-bipolar cell response but also activity in other second- and third-order retinal neurons.[1,29,30,33,35,50,55,56,65,68] The isolated P_2 component (figure 33.2B) may be a clearer representation of the postreceptoral activity than is the b-wave.[15] In a mathematical analysis similar to that using equation (1) for the b-wave, the P_2 S-R function (figure 33.2C) is fit with

$$P_2/P_{2max} = I/(I + K_{P2})$$

where P_{2max} is the saturated amplitude and K_{P2} is the semi-saturation constant. The ON-bipolar cells have their own G-protein cascade. To evaluate the kinetics of the G-protein cascade,[55] the latency at which P_2 reaches 50 μV is noted (figure 33.2D). In the normal retina, this latency, plotted as a function of stimulus intensity on log-log coordinates, is a linear function with slope approximately −0.2. Departures

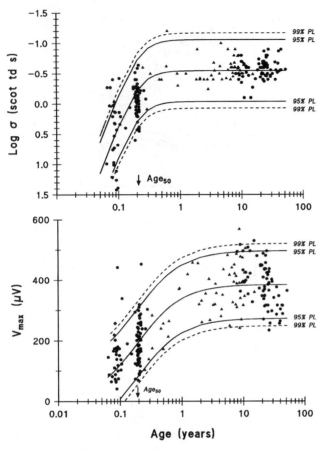

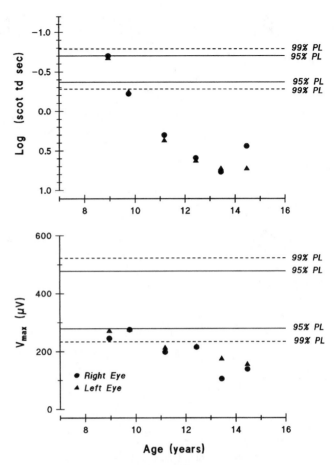

FIGURE 33.3 Normal development of the parameters of the b-wave S-R function, log s (upper panel) and V_{max} (lower panel) are shown. The solid line is a logistic growth curve fit to these data,[23] and the upper and lower 95% and 99% prediction limits of normal are shown. The data are log σ and V_{max} values of 166 subjects with normal eyes (circles) recruited for studies of visual development[23] and 54 patients (triangles) referred for ERG testing who were found to have normal eyes.[22,23]

FIGURE 33.4 The course of the scotopic b-wave parameters, log s (upper panel) and V_{max} (lower panel), in a patient with cone-rod degeneration. The b-wave sensitivity (log σ) decreased approximately 1.5 log units, and V_{max} declined by about 0.25 log unit. Responses to the ISCEV cone stimulus averaged less than 15% of normal during this interval.

from this relationship are taken as evidence of dysfunction of the ON-bipolar cells' G-protein cascade.[55]

Theoretical and experimental studies of P_2 have led to more complete specification of factors that control the parameters of the S-R function.[14,15,33,35] For instance, low photoreceptor sensitivity[33,35] alone shifts log σ and log K_{P2}. Also, low saturated amplitude[33,35] of the rod photoresponse alone shifts log σ and log K_{P2}. Furthermore, there is evidence that if rod outer segment function is intact (that is, rod photoreceptor sensitivity and amplitude the saturated response are normal), rod inner segment dysfunction is transmitted to the bipolar cell so as to shift log σ and log K_{P2}.[15]

Analyses of S-R functions have found applications in studies of development,[19–23,31] aging,[4,7,67] photoreceptor degenerations,[3,6,18,19,25,44,46] and retinal vascular diseases.[8,38,66] The two parameters of the b-wave S-R function, log σ and V_{max}, can be examined separately as shown for studies of normal development (figure 33.3). In normal human devel-

opment, log σ and V_{max} follow indistinguishable courses of maturation.[23] The age at which log σ and V_{max} are half the adult value is approximately 10 weeks (figure 33.3). In some retinal diseases, log σ and V_{max} follow disparate courses (figure 33.4). Study of the behavior of the parameters of the S-R functions, log σ and V_{max}, offers an opportunity to consider cellular mechanisms such as variation in number of retinal cells and photopigment or simple response compression.[32,36]

ACKNOWLEDGMENTS Supported by National Eye Institute Grant EY 10597.

REFERENCES

1. Aleman T, LaVail MM, Montemayor R, Ying G-S, Maguire MM, Laties AM, Jacobson SG, Cideciyan AV: Augmented rod bipolar cell function in partial receptor loss: An ERG study in P23H rhodopsin transgenic and aging normal rats. *Vision Res* 2001; 41:2779–2797.

2. Arden G: The retina. In Davson H (ed): *Neurophysiology in the Eye*, vol 2A, ed 2. New York, Academic Press, 1976.

3. Arden G, Carter R, Hogg C, Powell D, Ernst W, Clover G, Lyness A, Quinlan M: A modified ERG technique and the results obtained in X-linked retinitis pigmentosa. *Br J Ophthalmol* 1983; 67:419–430.

4. Birch DG, Anderson JL: Standardized full-field electroretinography: Normal values and their variation with age. *Arch Ophthalmol* 1992; 110:1571–1576.

5. Birch DG, Fish G: Rod ERGs in children with hereditary retinal degeneration. *J Pediatr Ophthalmol Strabismus* 1986; 23:227–232.

6. Birch DG, Fish GE: Rod ERGs in retinitis pigmentosa and cone-rod degeneration. *Invest Ophthalmol Vis Sci* 1987; 28:140–150.

7. Birch DG, Hood D, Locke K, Hoffman D, Tzekov RT: Quantitative electroretinogram measures of phototransduction in cone and rod photoreceptors. *Arch Ophthalmol* 2002; 120(8):1017–1124.

8. Breton ME, Montzka DP, Brucker AJ, Quinn GE: Electroretinogram interpretation in central retinal vein occlusion. *Ophthalmology* 1991; 98(12):1837–1844.

9. Burian H, Burns C: Electroretinography and dark adaptation in patients with myotonic dystrophy. *Am J Ophthalmol* 1966; 61:1044–1054.

10. Burian H, Pearlman J: Evaluation of the amplitude of the b-wave of the human electroretinogram: Its intensity dependence and relation to the a-wave. *Am J Ophthalmol* 1964; 58:210–216.

11. Bush RA, Sieving PA: A proximal retinal component in the primate photopic ERG a-wave. *Invest Ophthalmol Vis Sci* 1994; 35:635–645.

12. Cideciyan AV, Hood DC, Huang Y, Banin E, Li ZY, Stone EM, Milam AH, Jacobson SG: Disease sequence from mutant rhodopsin allele to rod and cone photoreceptor degeneration in man. *Proc Nat Acad Sci U S A* 1998; 95(12):7103–7108.

13. Cideciyan AV, Jacobson SG: An alternative phototransduction model for human rod and cone ERG a-waves: Normal parameters and variation with age. *Vision Res* 1996; 36:2609–2621.

14. Cooper LL, Hansen RM, Darras BT, Korson M, Dougherty FE, Shoffner JM, Fulton AB: Rod photoreceptor function in children with mitochondrial disorders. *Arch Ophthalmol* 2002; 120:1055–1062.

15. Cox G, Hansen R, Quinn N, Fulton AB: Retinal function in carriers of Bardet Biedl syndrome. *Arch Ophthalmol* 2003; 121:804–811.

16. Evans LS, Peachey NS, Marchese AL: Comparison of three methods of estimating the parameters of the Naka-Rushton equation. *Doc Ophthalmol* 1993; 84(1):19–30.

17. Frishman LJ, Reddy MG, Robson JG: Effect of background light on the human dark adapted electroretinogram and psychophysical threshold. *J Opt Soc Am A Opt Image Sci Vis* 1996; 13:601–612.

18. Fulton A: Background adaptation in RCS rats: *Invest Ophthalmol Vis Sci* 1983; 24:72–76.

19. Fulton AB, Hansen RM: Electroretinography: Application to clinical studies of infants. *J Pediatr Ophthalmol Strabismus* 1985; 22:251.

20. Fulton AB, Hansen RM: The relation of retinal sensitivity and rhodopsin in human infants. *Vision Res* 1987; 27:697.

21. Fulton AB, Hansen RM: Scotopic stimulus response relations of the b-wave of the electroretinogram. *Doc Ophthalmol* 1988; 68:293–304.

22. Fulton AB, Hansen RM: Workup of the possibly blind child. In Isenberg SJ (ed): *The Eye in Infancy*, 2 ed. St: Louis, Mosby, 1994, ch 38.

23. Fulton AB, Hansen RM: The development of scotopic sensitivity. *Invest Ophthalmol Vis Sci* 2000; 41:1588–1596.

24. Fulton A, Hansen R, Petersen R, Vanderveen D: The rod photoreceptors in retinopathy of prematurity: An electroretinographic study. *Arch Ophthalmol* 2001; 119:499–505.

25. Fulton A, Manning K, Baker B, Schukar S, Bailey C: Dark-adapted sensitivity, rhodopsin content and backgound adaptation in pcd/pcd mice. *Invest Ophthalmol Vis Sci* 1982; 22:386–393.

26. Fulton AB, Rushton WA: The human rod erg: Correlation with psychophysical responses in light and dark adaptation. *Vision Res* 1978; 18:793–800.

27. Granit R: The components of the retinal action potential in mammals and their relation to the discharge in the optic nerve. *J Physiol* 1933; 77:207–239.

28. Granit R: The components of the vertebrate electroretinogram. In *Sensory Mechanisms of the Retina*. London, Hafner, 1963, ch 3.

29. Gurevitch L, Slaughter MM: Comparison of the waveforms of the ON bipolar neuron and the b-wave of the electroretinogram. *Vision Res* 1993; 33:2431–2435.

30. Hanitzsch R, Lichtenberger T, Mattig W-U: The influence of MgCl2 and APB on the light induced potassium changes and the ERG b-wave of the isolated superfused retina. *Vision Res* 1996; 36:499–507.

31. Hansen R, Fulton AB: Electroretinographic assessment of background adaptation in 10 week old human infants. *Vision Res* 1991; 31:1501–1507.

32. Hood DC: Testing hypotheses about development with electroretinographic and increment threshold data. *J Opt Soc Am A Opt Image Vis Sci* 1988; 5:2159–2165.

33. Hood DC, Birch DG: A computational model of the amplitude and implicit time of the b-wave of the human ERG. *Vis Neurosci* 1992; 8:107–126.

34. Hood DC, Birch DG: Rod phototransduction in retinitis pigmentosa: Estimation and interpretation of parameters derived from the rod a-wave. *Invest Ophthalmol Vis Sci* 1994; 35:2948–2961.

35. Hood D, Birch D: Beta wave of the scotopic (rod) electroretinogram as a measure of the activity of human on-bipolar cells. *J Opt Soc Am A Opt Image Vis Sci* 1996; 13(3):623–633.

36. Hood DC, Birch DG, Birch EE: Use of models to improve hypothesis delineation: A study of infant electroretinography. In Simons K (ed): *Early Visual Development, Normal and Abnormal*. New York, Oxford University Press, 1993.

37. Hood DC, Shady S, Birch DG: Heterogeneity in retinal disease and the computational model of the human rod photoresponse. *J Opt Soc Am A Opt Image Vis Sci* 1993; 10:1624–1630.

38. Johnson M, Marcus S, Elman M, McPhee T: Neovascularization in central retinal vein occlusion: Electroretinographic findings. *Arch Ophthalmol* 1988; 106:348–352.

39. Kooijman A: Ganzfeld light distribution on the retina of human and rabbit eyes: Calculations and in vitro measurements. *J Opt Soc Am A Opt Image Sci Vis* 1986; 3:2116–2120.

40. Kooijman AC: The homogeneity of the retinal illumination is restricted by some ERG lenses. *Invest Ophthalmol Vis Sci* 1986; 27(3):372–377.

41. Lamb TD, Pugh EN Jr: A quantitative account of the activation steps involved in phototransduction in amphibian photoreceptors. *J Physiol* 1992; 449:719–758.

42. Langmuir I: The constitution and fundamental properties of solids and liquids: I. Solids. *J Am Chem Soc* 1916; 38:2221–2295.

43. Marmor MF, Zrenner E: Standard for clinical electroretinography. *Doc Ophthalmol* 1995; 89:199–210.

44. Massof R, Wu L, Finkelstein D, Perry C, Starr S, Johnson MA: Properties of electroretinographic intensity response functions in retinitis pigmentosa. *Doc Ophthalmol* 1984; 57:279–296.

45. Michaelis L, Menten M: Die kinetik der invertinwirkung. *Biochem Z* 1913; 49:333–369.

46. Moloney J, Mooney D, O'Conner M: Retinal function in Stargardt's disease and fundus flavimaculatus. *Am J Ophthalmol* 1983; 96:57–65.

47. Naka K, Rushton W: S-potentials from colour units in the retina of fish (cyprinidae). *J Physiol* 1966; 185:536–555.

48. Naka K, Rushton W: The generation and spread of S-potentials in fish (Cyprinidae). *J Physiol* 1967; 192:437–461.

49. Newman EA: Current source-density analysis of the b-wave of frog retina. *J Neurophysiol* 1980; 43(5):1355–1366.

50. Newman EA, Odette LL: Model of electroretinogram b-wave generation: A test of the K+ hypothesis. *J Neurophysiol* 1984; 51(1):164–182.

51. Peachey NS, Alexander KR, Fishman GA: The luminance-response function of the dark-adapted human electroretinogram. *Vision Res* 1989; 29:263–270.

52. Peachey NS, Charles HC, Lee CM, Fishman GA, Cunha-Vas JG, Smith RT: Electroretinographic findings in sickle cell retinopathy. *Arch Ophthalmol* 1987; 105:934–938.

53. Pugh EN Jr, Falsini B, Lyubarsky AL: The origin of the major rod and cone driven components of the rodent electroretinogram and the effect of age and light rearing history on the magnitude of these components. In Williams TP, Thistle AB (eds): *Photostasis and Related Phenomena.* New York, Plenum Press, 1998.

54. Pugh EN Jr, Lamb TD: Amplification and kinetics of the activation steps in phototransduction. *Biochem Biophys Acta* 1993; 1141:111–149.

55. Robson J, Frishman L: Response linearity and kinetics of the cat retina: The bipolar cell component of the dark-adapted electroretinogram. *Vis Neurosci* 1995; 12(5):837–850.

56. Robson JG, Frishman LJ: Photoreceptor and bipolar cell contributions to the cat electroretinogram: A kinetic model for the early part of the flash response. *J Opt Soc Am A Opt Image Vis Sci* 1996; 13:613–622.

57. Robson JG, Frishman LJ: Dissecting the dark adapted electroretinogram. *Doc Ophthalmol* 1999; 95:187–215.

58. Roecker EB, Pulos E, Bresnick GH, Severns M: Characterization of the electroretinographic scotopic B-wave amplitude in diabetic and normal subjects. *Invest Ophthalmol Vis Sci* 1992; 33(5):1575–1583.

59. Rushton W: S-potentials. Estratto da Rendiconti della scuola Internazionale di Fisica. *Enrico Fermi* 1973; 63:256–269.

60. Sandberg MA, Miller S, Berson EL: Rod electroretinograms in an elevated cyclic guanosine monophosphate-type human retinal degeneration. *Invest Ophthalmol Vis Sci* 1990; 31:2283–2287.

61. Severns ML, Johnson M: The care and fitting of Naka-Rushton functions to electroretinographic intensity response data. *Doc Ophthalmol* 1993; 85(2):135–150.

62. Shady S, Hood DC, Birch DG: Rod phototransduction in retinitis pigmentosa: Distinguishing alternative mechanisms of degeneration. *Invest Ophthalmol Vis Sci* 1995; 36:1027–1037.

63. Sieving PA, Nino C: Human scotopic threshold response. *Invest Ophthalmol Vis Sci* 1986; 29:1608–1614.

64. Snedecor GW, Cochran WG: *Statistical Methods*, ed 7. Ames, Iowa State University Press, 1980.

65. Stockton R, Slaughter RM: B-wave of the electroretinogram: A reflection of ON-bipolar cell activity. *J Gen Physiol* 1989; 93:101–121.

66. Sverak J, Peregrin J: Electroretinographic intensity response curves in central retinal artery occlusion. *Arch Ophthalmol* 1968; 79:526–530.

67. Sverak J, Peregrin J: The age-dependent changes of the electroretinographic (ERG) intensity-reaction curves. *Sb Ved Pr Lek Fak Karlovy University Hradci Karlov* 1972; 15:473–483.

68. Tian N, Slaughter MM: Correlation of dynamic responses in the ON bipolar neuron and the b-wave of the electroretinogram. *Vision Res* 1995; 35(10):1359–1364.

69. van Norren D, Valeton M: The human rod ERG: The dark-adapted a-wave response function. *Vision Res* 1979; 19:1433–1434.

70. Wurziger K, Lichtenberger T, Hanitzsch R: On-bipolar cells and depolarising third order neurons as the origin of the ERG b-wave in the RCS rat. *Vision Res* 2001; 41:1091–1101.

34 Kernel Analysis

J. VERNON ODOM

CHAPTER 33 DEALT with linear systems and stated that there is no general method of describing nonlinearities. Nevertheless, these are so common and important in the visual system that methods of description are important, none more so than *kernel analysis*. The aims of this chapter are, first, to give a nonrigorous account of this method that will enable the clinical electrophysiologist to use the method and interpret the results and, second, to briefly indicate the rationale for using kernel analysis and the choice of strategy to fit particular situations. Finally, some clinical and experimental results of this method will be given. For a more mathematically rigorous treatment of many of these same points, the reader is referred to other sources.[15,18,21–23,25,26,32,35,37]

The definitions of a linear system are given in the previous chapter. It will be recalled that if the response to a brief impulse is known, the response of a linear system to any other stimulus can be predicted. This is not true of a nonlinear system. Figure 34.1 provides an example of a nonlinear system. Figure 34.1A is a diagram of two stimulus pulses—the stimulus that is readily obtained from Grass stroboscopes, for example; figure 34.1B shows the response. The early part of the response is shown as a solid line. In the absence of a stimulus, the record would continue according to the dotted line, but in the presence of a second flash, the record corresponding to the lower full line is obtained. If the responses to the first and second of the paired flashes were equal (a linear system), the upper of the two lines would be followed. Figure 34.1C shows the difference between the actual response and the larger response that is expected from a linear system. The waveform (for ease, look at the peak times) of the residual "real" second response and also the waveform of the difference bear a complex relationship to the impulse response. Many systems that are nearly linear have thresholds and saturation points, and stimuli of appropriate intensity can evoke nonlinear behavior. Such nonlinearities are typically referred to as nonessential nonlinearities. An example of a nonessential nonlinearity is the clipping observed from the output of a linear filter when the input is too large. Other systems exhibit nonlinearities throughout the full range of their operations. These are referred to as essential nonlinearities. A rectifier is a typical example of a physical system that demonstrates essential nonlinearities. As was indicated with the previous examples, nonlinearities can be modeled by electronic components (e.g., rectifiers, amplifiers, filters). In the case of figure 34.1,

which behaves in a way very similar to the electroretinogram (ERG), the nonlinearity occurs at various voltage levels and is time dependent, that is, it demonstrates an essential nonlinearity.

Several strategies exist to characterize a system so that its response to an arbitrary stimulus can be predicted. In the time domain, these strategies are based on computing cross-correlations between the stimulus and the response.[15,18,20,22,23,25,26,32,37] Stimuli that are used to determine kernels are presented in figure 34.2. Typical stimuli are white noise or pseudorandom sequences (PRS), such as M-sequences. In the frequency domain, the system's responses to a set of sine waves are described by Fourier analysis, and the responses of appropriate order (second order, etc.) are summed.[20,21,26,35]

In using these input signals, it is possible to calculate a series of integrals that fully characterize the system's response to any arbitrary stimulus. Kernels are the weights of these integrals; as such, they are analogous to the coefficients of a polynomial. The zero-order kernel represents the bias or mean response of a system. The first-order kernel, analogous to the polynomial's first-order coefficient, represents the best linear approximation (in a least mean square error sense) of the response elicited by the stimulus and estimates the impulse response. The second-order kernel is analogous to the second-order coefficient in a polynomial equation; it represents the interactions of two stimulus pulses or variations in stimulus pulse amplitude on the response. It is difficult to record enough response samples to characterize higher-order kernels accurately. Consequently, it is uncommon to calculate kernels beyond the second order. Figure 34.3 illustrates some of the difficulties of linear approximations of nonlinear systems. A linear approximation of a nonlinear system varies with the range of stimulus conditions over which the estimate is made.

First-order kernels and systems

If a system were linear, the first-order kernel would completely characterize the system and would be exactly equivalent to the normalized impulse response. In a nonlinear system, the first-order kernel represents a linear approximation to the system's impulse response. Because higher-order odd nonlinearities (third, fifth, etc.) can influence the estimate of the first-order kernel, it does not represent or

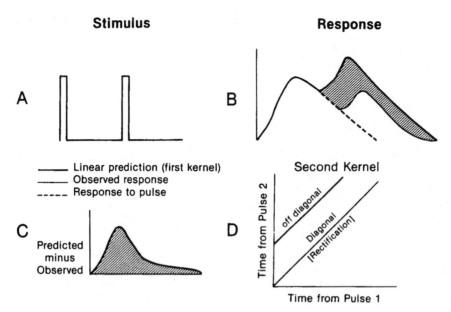

Stimulus　　　　　　　　　　**Response**

A

B

　　── Linear prediction (first kernel)
　　── Observed response
　　---- Response to pulse

C　Predicted
　　minus
　　Observed

D　**Second Kernel**

Time from Pulse 2 / off diagonal / Diagonal [Rectification]

Time from Pulse 1

FIGURE 34.1　First- and second-order kernels. The four panels illustrate several of the major points of first- and second-order kernels. A, Two impulses with a fixed separation. B, (1) The response to a single pulse, (2) the linear prediction of the response to two pulses with the delay illustrated in A (the response of two single flashes added together with the appropriate delay), and (3) the obtained response. C, The difference between the predicted response and the response obtained in B. D, One way of presenting the second-order kernel. The second-order kernel has three dimensions. Time from pulse 1 is on the abscissa, and time from pulse 2 is on the ordinate. The difference between linear predic-

tions and obtained results (e.g., C) could be plotted either on the *z*-axis (not displayed) or as contour lines on the *xy*-coordinates. The main diagonal represents the response when the two pulses were at the same time and reflects second-order nonlinear ties related to amplitude differences in the pulses. One physical system with second-order amplitude dependent nonlinearities is a rectifier. Off diagonals represent the differences between predicted and obtained responses for a specific difference in time between the two pulses. C would represent an off diagonal, with the time between pulses illustrated in A.

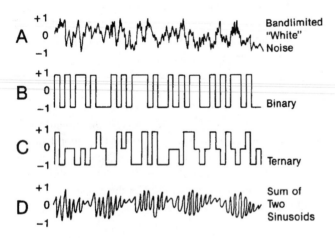

Stimuli for Kernel Analysis

A　Bandlimited "White" Noise

B　Binary

C　Ternary

D　Sum of Two Sinusoids

FIGURE 34.2　Stimuli for kernel analysis. The values of +1, 0, and −1 represent arbitrary dimensions. They may be thought of as input voltages, logic levels, or intensity levels. A, An effort to represent band-limited white noise. It should have a flat frequency spectrum and a Gaussian amplitude distribution. White noise may be approximated by using a sum of sinusoids (usually eight or more different frequencies). Binary pseudorandom sequences (B), ternary sequences (C), and sums of two sinusoids (D) have useful properties. Deterministic signals such as B, C, and D may have greater contrast, are computationally easier to analyze, and may be averaged.

estimate the system's linear elements or processes directly. However, given a model of the visual system, such as a sandwich model, one can evaluate the appropriateness of the models.[15,23,25,26,35]

The visual system is highly nonlinear. The visual system's nonlinearity is indicated by its response to pattern stimulation, especially as recorded by visual evoked potentials (VEPs). Figure 34.4 illustrates that a linear system's response to either pattern appearance or reversal as recorded by scalp electrodes cannot be observed if (1) there is no change in the mean luminance with pattern appearance or change and (2) the receptor elements are homogeneously spaced and one assumes that the elements respond symmetrically to light increase and decrease.[25,40] Despite the visual system's essential nonlinearity, it is possible to calculate a first-order kernel.

Second-order kernels

In the time domain, the second-order kernel is a three-dimensional construct that represents the response as a function of time from a first impulse and a second impulse. It indicates the nonlinear effect of the time between two pulses on the response.[15,18,23,36] Usually, the second-order kernel is plotted as a two-dimensional contour map (see figure 34.1D)

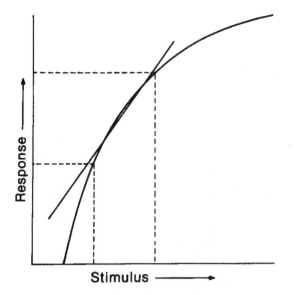
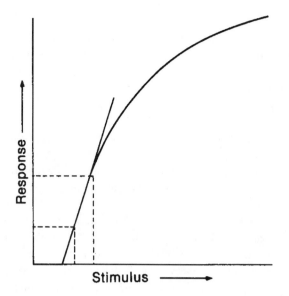

FIGURE 34.3 Linear approximations of the response of a non-linear system. The dashed lines extending to the abscissa indicate the limits of the stimulus conditions; those extending to the ordinate indicate the limits of the observed responses. The straight lines were best fit through the indicated regions. Linear estimates of a nonlinear process will be different depending on the input condi-

tions, such as mean luminance or contrast, and are highly dependent on the stimulus values used. Consequently, different experiments can yield very different estimates of the first-order kernel. The presence of a strong, reliable first-order kernel for a particular stimulus range does not mean that the system or the response is linear.

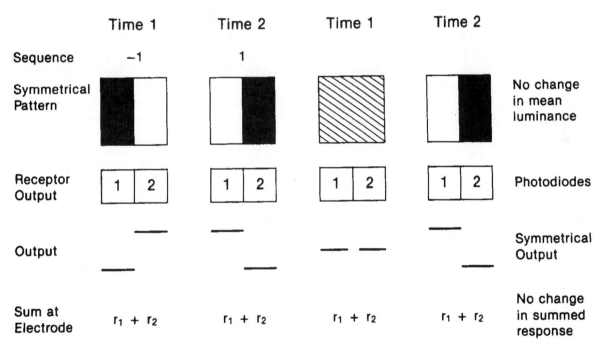

FIGURE 34.4 If the visual system were composed of linear elements, the response recorded by ERG and VEP electrodes to pattern reversal and to pattern appearance would be zero. Top row, The stimuli observed at two time periods: time 1 and time 2. Second row, The two sensors that detect the light level in the two regions of

the figure. Third row, The voltage outputs of the sensors at the two times, low output for dark and higher outputs for light. Fourth row, Any ERG or VEP electrode sums the output of the two sensors. In each case, the sums are the same in time 1 and time 2, and there would be no change in response recorded by the electrode.

with the x- and y-axes representing time from the first and second pulses, respectively. In the frequency domain, the second-order kernel is the sum of all of the second-order frequencies present in the response.[20,21,35]

Stimuli

Theoretically, Gaussian white noise is the most appealing stimulus with which to characterize a system. It has equal power at all frequencies and a Gaussian amplitude distribution and is equivalent to all frequencies of sine waves, with their phases random with respect to one another. If white noise has a Gaussian amplitude distribution, most of the changes in stimulus values are small, and if the stimulus is light, the nonnegative nature of light requires a truncation of range about the mean value. Therefore, the signal-to-noise ratio of responses elicited by white noise stimuli is often small and requires longer recording periods to acquire reliable kernel estimates. The same considerations apply to sums of sinusoids. The larger the number of frequencies that are used, the lower is the maximum contrast of individual sine waves because the total contrast of the sum of sinusoids must be 100% or less. For example, if one employed a sum of eight sine waves, the maximum contrast of any one frequency would be about 12%.

If a PRS of two or three stimulus levels or a sum of sinusoids with two or three sine waves is selected as the stimulus, the system characterization will be less complete, but there will be an improved response signal-to-noise ratio because the stimuli can be presented at higher contrasts. Therefore, shorter recording periods may be used to acquire the response. Because the stimulus is deterministic, more efficient analysis procedures may be used to calculate the kernels, and the responses may be signal averaged.

In determining kernels from PRS, several constraints are important. First, if a binary PRS controls stimulus polarity, it is impossible to establish the main diagonal of the second-order kernel (table 34.1). Second, in using PRS, general principles of digital sampling must be observed. The accuracy of the kernels is primarily determined by the total duration of the experiment,[13,37] and the highest-order kernel that can be calculated is limited by the recording period.

To avoid what are termed deconvolution errors in kernel estimation, the stimulation frequency should be high relative to the high-frequency limit of the visual system (e.g., the ERG or VEP critical flicker fusion frequency) at the particular mean luminance and contrast that are selected. To avoid transduction errors, the stimulus must be accurately presented, that is, the stimulus-generating interface must be able to follow a stimulus of at least twice the maximum stimulus frequency. For example, a video display cannot follow stimuli of greater than 30 Hz in the Americas or 25 Hz or so

TABLE 34.1
Effect of binary sequence control sequence

Sequence Value	Polarity		Change/Reversal	
	Light	Pattern	Light	Pattern
−1	Off	1	Off	1
+1	On	2	On	2
+1	On	2	Off	1
−1	Off	1	Off	1
+1	On	2	On	2
−1	Off	1	On	2
+1	Off	1	Off	1
−1	Off	1	Off	1
+1	On	2	On	2
−1	On	2	On	2
−1	Off	1	On	2
+1	On	2	Off	1

in Europe and Asia. The luminance of xenon flash units often varies with the frequency or interstimulus interval. If a xenon flash is used, it must be stable in these characteristics. A cathode-ray tube (CRT) display, a light-emitting diode display, or a bright light with a shutter or chopper as the stimulus should work well.

To understand the meaning of a kernel, one must know which stimulus events were controlled by the PRS (see table 34.1). If the stimulus is light and a PRS controls stimulus polarity (light on or light off), the impulse is a rapid change from the minimum light level to the maximum light level employed in the PRS and has a duration of one time period in the PRS. If the stimulus is pattern, the PRS may control stimulus polarity (e.g., pattern phase 1 or 2) or the presence or absence of a reversal. The impulse is a pattern reversal in the second case. In the first case, it is the rapid change from pattern phase 1 to phase 2 and back to phase 1. Until recently, only a few VEP or ERG experiments have employed kernel analysis.[1,3–5,13,14,17,22,24,26–40] Determinations of the first- and second-order kernels permit the detection of different frequency regions of VEP activity[22,23,26] and isolation of the characteristics of different stages of monocular[13,20,40] and binocular[1,19,39] visual processing and demonstrate the feasibility of using kernel analysis in clinical situations.[4,5,24] The isolation of particular pathways or stages of visual processing opens exciting possibilities for clarifying the nature of disease processes or detecting and diagnosing different diseases.

VEP[4] and cone ERG[5,13,17] first-order kernels elicited by luminance are reported to be acquired more rapidly and/or to be more reliable than their averaged equivalents. Cone ERG first-order kernels are abnormal in some amblyopes.[14] Rod ERG first-order kernels are considerably smaller than the clinical dark-adapted flash ERG[13] because (1) it is difficult to achieve the same level of dark-adaptation in the PRS conditions as in the clinical situation, (2) the flash intensity is usually lower, and (3) the clinical ERG reflects linear and nonlinear processes.

Pattern-reversal stimulation has been employed successfully to determine first-order kernels of VEPs[14,24] and ERGs[14] (see table 34.1). Patients with multiple sclerosis generally have altered VEP pattern-reversal kernels,[24] and amblyopes have smaller VEP and pattern ERG responses in the amblyopic eye.[14]

Recently, arrays of as many as 200 light sources have been employed to estimate ERG and VEP first- and second-order kernels. From these kernels, it is possible to compute ERG[34]

or VEP[33] visual fields with finer spatial resolution than automated perimetry in a recording session of less than 30 minutes for both eyes. ERG fields were initially reported to be abnormal in blind spot syndrome and age-related maculopathy patients.[34] These multiple input stimuli have come to be termed *multifocal stimuli*. One may record a multifocal ERG (mfERG) or multifocal VEP (mfVEP), depending on the choice and placement of electrodes and recording obtained. These multi-input stimuli may be patterns, but more commonly, one uses lights or regions of a CRT that are turned on and off (figure 34.5). The mfERG has been

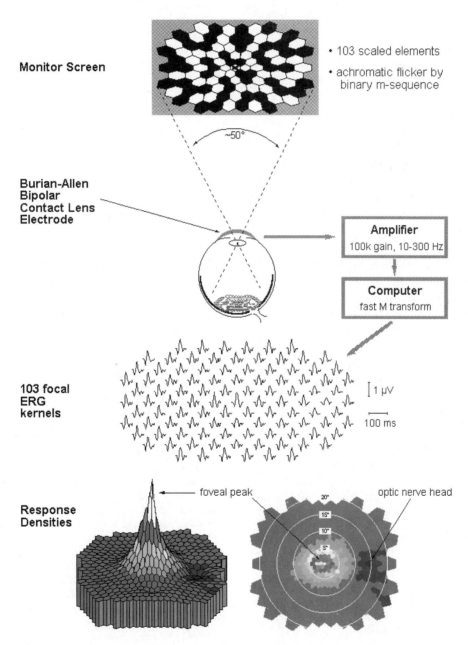

FIGURE 34.5 Schematic representation of a typical multifocal ERG setup using the VERIS system. (Illustration used with the permission of Interzeag Corporation at: http://www.octopus.ch/products/fr3_veris_description.htm.)

useful in detecting a number of central retinal dystrophies.[7,8] The mfERG is already sufficiently widely used that the International Society for Clinical Electrophysiology of Vision has established a standard for clinical mfERG.[16]

The reasons for desiring an objective map of visual function are numerous. A map of visual function should correlate better with localized lesions than does the standard ERG and should provide information about central retinal function, which the standard ERG does not. In addition, there is an issue of familiarity; ophthalmologists are familiar with looking at visual fields and thinking of retinotopic variations in function as correlating with specific diseases.

The fact that the mean luminance of the stimulus is in the photopic range and the frequency of stimulation is quite high suggests that the origins of the standard mfERG are more like those of photopic fast flicker; that is, the first order kernel involves little or no photoreceptor activity and is predominantly determined by postreceptoral cells with some ganglion cell layer involvement in its generation while the second order kernel has some postreceptoral level activity and considerable inner retinal (amacrine and ganglion cell) input.[2,6,9–12,36]

The uses of multifocal techniques are a trade-off between spatial resolution, recording time, and size of the signal. The finer the spatial resolution, the smaller is the signal and the more recording time is required. Using relatively fine resolution, one records signals that are typically in the nanovolt range using a recording time of at least 8 minutes per eye, divided into several shorter intervals. Therefore, careful attention to recording details is essential. Otherwise, signals are overwhelmed by environmental and physiological noise sources. Similarly, stable fixation is essential to obtain reliable mfERG recordings with relatively fine spatial resolution. These issues of stable fixation and small signal size may limit the utility of multifocal techniques in those whom one cannot trust to maintain stable fixation, such as children, patients with nystagmus, and malingerers. In patients with small central lesions, one can usually obtain satisfactory recordings with instructions to fixate the center of the screen. In a few cases, it may be advisable to reduce the spatial resolution to decrease the recording time and the need for precise fixation.

ACKNOWLEDGMENTS   Although the author takes full responsibility for the section, he wishes to acknowledge the helpful comments, suggestions, and ideas of many people and to acknowledge the inspiration of Henk Spekreijse and Dik Reits in the year of their retirement, 2003.

REFERENCES

1. Baitch LW, Levi DM: Evidence for nonlinear binocular interactions in human visual cortex. *Vision Res* 1988; 28:1139–1143.

2. Fortune B, Cull G, Wang L, VanBuskirk EM, Cioffi GA: Factors affecting the use of multifocal electroretinography to monitor function in primate model of glaucoma. *Doc Ophthalmol* 2002; 105:151–178.

3. Fricker SJ, Kuperwaser MC: Is linear analysis sufficient to reveal abnormalities of the visual system under dichoptic viewing conditions? *Ann N Y Acad Sci* 1982; 388:622–627.

4. Fricker SJ, Sanders JJ III: Clinical studies of the evoked response to rapid random flash. *Electroencephalogr Clin Electrophysiol* 1974; 36:525–532.

5. Fricker SJ, Sanders JJ: A new method of cone electroretinography: The rapid random flash response. *Invest Ophthalmol* 1975; 14:131–137.

6. Hare WA, Ton H: Effects of APB, PDA, and TTX on ERG responses recorded using both multifocal and conventional methods in monkey. *Doc Ophthalmol* 2002; 105:189–222.

7. Hood DC: Assessing retinal function with the multifocal technique. *Prog Retin Eye Res* 2000; 19(5):607–646.

8. Hood, DC (ed): The multifocal technique: Topographical ERG and VEP responses. *Doc Ophthalmol* 2000; 100:49–251.

9. Hood DC, Bearse MA Jr, Sutter EE, Viswanathan S, Frishman LJ: The optic nerve head component of the monkey's (Macaca mulatta) multifocal electroretinogram (mERG). *Vision Res* 2001; 41:2029–2041.

10. Hood DC, Frishman LJ, Saszik S, Viswanathan S: Retinal origins of the primate multifocal ERG: Implications for the human response. *Invest Ophthalmol Vis Sci* 2002; 43:1673–1685.

11. Hood DC, Frishman LJ, Viswanathan S, Robson JG, Ahmed J: Evidence for a ganglion cell contribution to the primate electroretinogram (ERG): Effects of TTX on the multifocal ERG in macaque. *Vis Neurosci* 1999; 16:411–416.

12. Hood DC, Greenstein V, Frishman L, Holopigian K, Viswanathan S, Seiple W, Ahmed J, Robson JG: Identifying inner retinal contributions to the human multifocal ERG. *Vision Res* 1999; 39:2285–2291.

13. Larkin RM, Klein S, Ogden TE, et al: Nonlinear kernels of the human ERG. *Biol Cybern* 1979; 35:145–160.

14. Levi DM, Manny RE: The pathophysiology of amblyopia: Electrophysiological studies. *Ann N Y Acad Sci* 1982; 388:98–112.

15. Marmarelis PZ, Marmarelis VZ: *Analysis of Physiological Systems: The White-Noise Approach*. New York, Plenum, 1978.

16. Marmor MF, Hood D, Keating D, Kondo M, Seeliger M, Miyake Y: Guidelines for basic multifocal electroretinography (mfERG). *Doc Ophthalmol* 2003; 106:105–115.

17. Ogden TE, Larkin RM, Fender DF, et al: The use of nonlinear analysis of the primate ERG to detect retinal dysfunction. *Exp Eye Res* 1980; 31:381–388.

18. O'Leary DP, Honrubia V: On-line identification of sensory systems using pseudorandom binary noise perturbations. *Biophys J* 1975; 15:505–532.

19. Pinkhasov E, Zemon V, Gordon J: Models of binocular interaction tested with VEP's. *Invest Ophthalmol Vis Sci* 1987; 28 (suppl):127.

20. Ratliff F: Form and function: Linear and nonlinear analyses of neural networks in the visual system. In McFadden D (ed): *Neural Mechanisms in Behavior*. New York, Springer-Verlag, 1988.

21. Regan MP, Regan D: A frequency domain technique for characterizing nonlinearities in biological systems. *J Theor Biol* 1988; 133:293–317.

22. Reits D: *Cortical Potentials in Man Evoked by Noise Modulated Light* (unpublished dissertation). University of Utrecht, Netherlands, 1975.

23. Reits D, Spekreijse H: Sequential analysis of a lumped non-linear system; a model for visual evoked brain potentials. In Kunt M, de Coulon F (eds): *Signal Processing: Theories and Applications*. New York, Elsevier Science, 1980.

24. Schoon DV, Wong EK: First-order Wiener kernel visually evoked potentials obtained from multiple sclerosis patients. *Doc Ophthalmol* 1987; 65:125–134.

25. Spekreijse H, Estevez O, Reits D: Visual evoked potentials and the physiological analysis of visual processes in man. In Desmedt JE (ed): *Visual Evoked Potentials in Man: New Developments*. Oxford, England, Clarendon Press, 1977.

26. Spekreijse H, Reits D: Sequential analysis of the visual evoked potential system in man: Nonlinear analysis or a sandwich model. *Ann N Y Acad Sci* 1982; 388:72–97.

27. Srebro R: Would an evaluation of binocularity using algebraic interaction between the two eyes be modified using the pseudorandom binary sequence method? *Ann N Y Acad Sci* 1982; 388:628–630.

28. Srebro R: An analysis of the VEP to luminance modulation and of its nonlinearity. *Vision Res* 1992; 32:1395–1404.

29. Srebro R, Sokol B, Wright WW: The power spectra of visually evoked potentials to pseudorandom contrast reversal of gratings. *Electroencephalogr Clin Neurophysiol* 1981; 51:63–68.

30. Srebro R, Wright WW: Visually evoked potentials to pseudorandom binary sequence stimulation. *Arch Ophthalmol* 1980; 98:296–298.

31. Srebro R, Wright WW: Pseudorandom sequences in the study of evoked potentials. *Ann N Y Acad Sci* 1982; 388:98–112.

32. Sutter EE: A practical nonstochastic approach to nonlinear time-domain analysis. In Marmarelis VZ (ed): *Advanced Methods of Physiological System Modeling, vol. 1*. Los Angeles, Biomedical Simulations Resource, 1987.

33. Sutter EE: Field topography of the visual evoked response. *Invest Ophthalmol Vis Sci* 1988; 29 (suppl):432.

34. Sutter EE, Dodsworth-Feldman B, Haegerstrom-Portnoy G: Simultaneous multifocal ERGs in diseased retinas. *Invest Ophthalmol Vis Sci* 1986; 27 (suppl):300.

35. Victor JD, Knight B: Nonlinear analysis with an arbitrary stimulus ensemble. *Q Appl Math* 1979; 37:113–136.

36. Viswanathan S, Frishman LJ, Robson JG: Inner-retinal contributions to the photopic sinusoidal flicker electroretinogram of macaques. *Doc Ophthalmol* 2002; 105:223–242.

37. Wickesberg RE, Geisler CD: Artifacts in Wiener kernels estimated using Gaussian white noise. *IEEE Trans Biomed Eng* 1984; 31:454–461.

38. Zemon V, Conte M, Jindra L, et al: *Evoked potential estimates of temporal filters in the human visual system*. Paper presented at the Seventh Annual Conference of the IEEE Engineering in Medicine and Biology Society, 1985, pp 431–436.

39. Zemon V, Pinkhasov E: Dichoptic visual-evoked potentials and nonlinear mechanisms in human vision. *J Opt Soc Am* 1983; 73:1923–1924.

40. Zemon V, Ratliff F: Intermodulation components of the visual evoked potential. *Biol Cybern* 1984; 50:401–408.

35 Measuring the Health of the Human Photoreceptors with the Leading Edge of the a-Wave

DONALD C. HOOD AND DAVID G. BIRCH

DURING THE 1980s, there was an explosion of information about the physiology of single retinal cells. Although electroretinogram (ERG) research became more sophisticated with modern recording and computer technology, the analysis of the human ERG did not keep pace with the new information that was gained from retinal physiologists. In 1989, we started our study of the cellular bases of the human ERG with a simple strategy. We asked, "Would a quantitative comparison between single-cell physiology and aspects of the ERG help to reveal the cellular bases of the human ERG?" In particular, the analyses of the human ERG at that time did not make use of the new information about primate receptors. In fact, the prevailing analysis of the ERG was actually inconsistent with the single-cell results.[19]

Our starting point was the model of the ERG proposed by Granit in the 1930s.[15,16] The vertebrate ERG potential shows two prominent peaks: the a- and b-waves (see chapters 15 and 26). These waves result from the algebraic sum of a number of components with different cellular bases (see chapter 15). Figure 35.1A (from Hood and Birch[22]) presents a simplified version of the ERG based on Granit's classic analysis.[15,16] According to this view, the ERG is the result of the algebraic summation of the negative potential P3 produced by the receptors with the positive potential P2 produced by the cells of the inner nuclear layer.

We asked, "Is the leading edge of the a-wave the sum of rod receptor activity?" While it was clear that the a-wave largely reflected photoreceptor activity,[7,42] other evidence suggested that postreceptoral contributions could influence the a-wave.[6,40] We argued that if the leading edge of the a-wave is the sum of rod receptor activity, then it should be possible to fit the leading edge of the human rod a-wave with the quantitative model that Baylor et al.[2] fitted to the responses of single primate rod photoreceptors. In 1990, we showed that the same model, fitted to recordings from single rods, fit the leading edge of the human a-wave.[20,21] The solid curves in figure 35.1B are human rod ERGs to a series of high-intensity flashes presented to the dark-adapted eye. The dashed curves are the predictions from a version of the

Baylor et al.[2] model. These results provided strong support for Granit's view that the leading edge of the a-wave was the response of the receptors.

In this chapter, we review how models of phototransduction have been fitted to the leading edge of the human a-wave and illustrate how the parameters of these models provide a way to evaluate the effects of retinal disease on the human photoreceptors.

The need for high-intensity flashes

Figure 35.2A shows the ERG response to a brief (<1 ms) flash of white light of moderate intensity (2 log sc td s) presented to the dark-adapted eye. This flash is the highest intensity that is currently recommended by the International Society for Clinical Electrophysiology of Vision (ISCEV) standards (see chapter 26). The dashed curve shows the receptor contribution to this response. At this intensity, only a small portion of the rod photoreceptors' response is seen. (In fact, the rods are still in their linear range.[21]) Notice that the amplitude of the peak of the a-wave (small arrow) does not represent the peak of the receptor's response. A mix of photoreceptor and postreceptor activity determines the peak of the a-wave at this intensity (see chapter 15; see also Bush and Sieving,[8] Jamison et al.,[36] and Robson et al.[47]). In fact, the negative a-wave, elicited by moderately intense flashes (e.g., figure 35.2A), has a negative postreceptoral contribution.[8] (See figure 10 in Robson et al.[47] for an illustration.) On the other hand, the leading edge of the response to a flash that is about a hundred times more intense (e.g., 4.0 log sc td s) provides a good estimate of the receptors' responses, as shown in figure 35.2B.

High-intensity ERG protocols

To study receptor activity, protocols have been designed to isolate rod and cone a-waves at relatively high flash intensities. (Technically, the flashes are expressed in energy units, but we will use the common convention and refer to flash

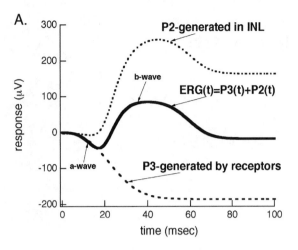

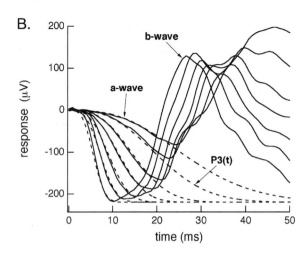

FIGURE 35.1 A, A simplified version of Granit's model[15,16] of the vertebrate rod ERG. (From Hood DC, Birch DG: Human cone receptor activity: the leading edge of the a-wave and models of receptor activity. *Vis Neurosci* 1993; 10:857–871.) B, The ERGs elicited by flashes of intensities higher than are typically used in the clinic. (Modified from Hood DC, Birch DG: The relationship between models of receptor activity and the a-wave of the human ERG. *Cl Vis Sci* 1990; 5:293–297.)

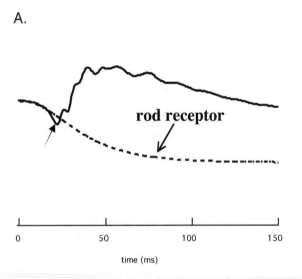

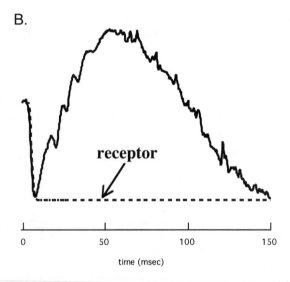

FIGURE 35.2 A, The ERG elicited by a brief flash of moderate intensity (about $2 \log \text{sc td s}$) presented to the dark-adapted eye. B, The ERG elicited by a brief flash 100 times more intense (about $4 \log \text{sc td s}$) presented to the dark-adapted eye.

intensity rather than flash energy.) The protocols must meet three criteria:

1. The flashes must be intense enough to allow for a good estimate of the maximum receptor response.

2. The contributions of the rods and cones must be isolated. In particular, the a-wave response to an intense flash in the dark is a mixed rod and cone response. Although the cone contribution is relatively small in normal control subjects, the cone contribution can be a significant part of the dark-adapted a-wave from patients with diseases of the rod receptors.[25]

3. The yellowing of the lens or cornea can affect the estimate of receptor sensitivity, especially if blue flashes are used and older populations are studied.

These problems have been addressed in different ways by the protocols described in the literature.[5,10,11,20,25,37]

In the protocol that we prefer,[29] both rod and cone a-waves are obtained by using a single series of white flashes. The flashes are first presented to the dark-adapted eye. Typically, we use four flashes ranging in intensity from 3.2 to 4.4 $\log \text{sc td s}$. (Higher intensities can be used as well.) To obtain an estimate of the cone contribution to these responses, the same flashes ($2.8–4.0 \log \text{phot td s}$) are then presented on a steady field of about 30cd/m^2 (ISCEV standard white background). Assuming an 8-mm pupil, this background is about $3.2 \log \text{td}$. The choice of the background intensity is critical. If it is too dim, a rod contribution will be present in the ERG. If the background is too intense, the cone response will be reduced in amplitude. While no background intensity can

A.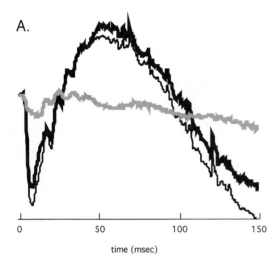

B.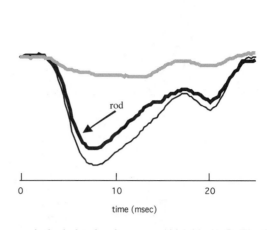

FIGURE 35.3   A, The ERG responses elicited by a 4.0 log sc td s flash presented in the dark (thin black) and on a rod-saturating background (thick gray). The difference between these two responses is the isolated-rod response (thick black). B, The first 25 ms of the records in panel A.

strictly satisfy these criteria, in our experience the 3.3 log sc td background reduces the rod a-wave to close to zero and has a very small effect on the cone a-wave amplitude.[23,24,26,29] A two-flash technique can also be employed to obtain isolated cone responses.[4,12,41,43,47] The two-flash technique has the advantage that it does require a background, and thus, with the appropriate time interval between flashes, one can obtain a truer measure of the "dark-adapted" cone response. On the other hand, it is harder to incorporate into a clinical protocol.

Figure 35.3A contains the responses to a 4.0 log sc td s flash presented in the dark (thin black trace) and on the rod-saturating background (thick gray trace). The difference between these two responses is the isolated rod response (thick black trace). Figure 35.3B shows the first 25 ms of these records. The thick black curve is the rod-isolated a-wave for this flash intensity. The response on the background, shown as a thick gray curve, is the cone response.

Figure 35.4 shows the rod-isolated (panel A) and cone (panel B) ERGs for a control subject. The solid curves correspond to the leading edges of the four flash intensities that make up our white flash protocol. The dashed curves are a fit of the model described below.

To summarize the white flash protocol, there are four flash intensities extending up to about 4.4 log sc td s. (Assuming an 8-mm pupil, 4.4 log sc td s corresponds to 500 sc cd s/m² or 210 cd s/m².) The same flashes are presented in the dark and on a white background of about 30 cd/m². We typically average three dark-adapted responses and ten light-adapted responses; more might be needed in studying patients with retinal diseases that reduce a-wave amplitudes. The rod-only response is obtained by subtracting the light-adapted responses from the dark-adapted responses. The responses on the background are the cone-only responses. As we will see below, this protocol could be reduced to two flash intensities. (For more details about the white flash protocol, see Hood and Birch.[29])

Fitting a model to the leading edge of the a-wave

FITTING A MODEL OF THE ROD PHOTORECEPTORS   In our initial work, we fitted the Baylor et al.[2] model to the leading edge of the rod-isolated a-wave. In 1992, Lamb and Pugh[39] suggested an equation based on the kinetics of the activation phase of rod phototransduction. For the leading edge of the a-wave, their formulation is computationally similar to that of Baylor et al.[2] (see the discussion in Hood and Brich[23]). The parameters of the Lamb and Pugh model, however, can be more easily interpreted in terms of parameters of transduction. In our expression of this model,[23,25] the leading edges of the rod a-waves are fitted with the following equation:

$$R(I,t) = \left\{ 1 - \exp\left[-I \cdot S \cdot (t - t_d)^2 \right] \right\} \cdot R_{\max} \qquad \text{for } t > t_d \quad (1)$$

where the amplitude R is a function of flash energy I and time t after the occurrence of a brief, essentially instantaneous, flash. S is a sensitivity parameter that scales I (flash energy); $R_{\max}$ is the maximum amplitude; and t_d is a brief delay. Values of t_d from about 2.5 to 4 ms have been reported from different laboratories.[5,10,23,25] Part of the parameter t_d is a constant that depends on the duration of the test flash and the properties of the recording equipment, and part depends on the properties of the receptors and the transduction process. (See Breton et al.,[5] Cideciyan and Jacobson,[11] Hamer and Tyler,[17] Lamb and Push,[39] and Robson et al.[47] for a discussion.) We find that for practical purposes, t_d can

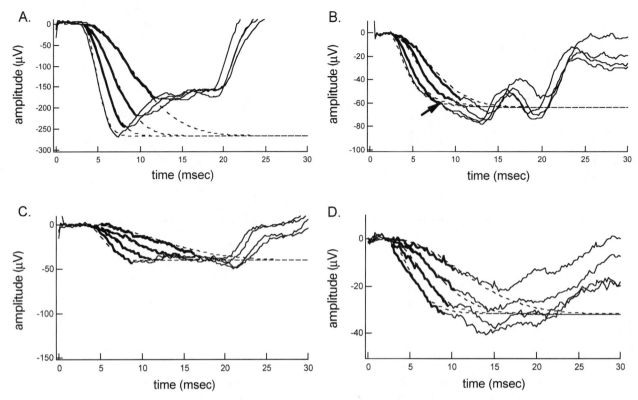

FIGURE 35.4   A, The rod-isolated responses to flashes ranging in intensity from 3.2 to 4.4 log sc td s. The portion of the leading edge of the a-wave shown in bold black was fitted with equation (1). The dashed curves are the results from the model for the best fitting parameters (R_{max} of 251.2 mV and log S of 0.84). B, The cone responses to flashes ranging in intensity from 2.8 to 4.0 log phot td s. The portion of the leading edge of the a-wave shown in bold black was fitted to the cone version[26,33] of the Lamb and Pugh model.[39] The dashed curves are the results from the model for the best fitting parameters (R_{max} of −63.1 mV and log S of 1.57). C,

Same as in panel A for the rod-isolated responses from a patient with retinitis pigmentosa. The best fitting parameters were −40.1 mV (R_{max}) and 0.64 (log S). D, Same as in panel B for the cone responses from a patient with retinitis pigmentosa. The best-fitting parameters were −32.0 mV (R_{max}) and 1.14 (log S). The vertical scale for the patient in panels B and D are twice those for the control subject in panels A and C. (Modified from Tzekov RT, Locke KG, Hood D, Birch DG: Cone and rod ERG phototransduction in retinitis pigmentosa. *Invest Ophthal Vis Sci* 2003; 44:3993–4000.)

be considered a constant for any given recording system. The value of t_d is determined by fitting equation (1) to the records from normal control subjects with t_d, S, and R_{max} that are allowed to vary for the best fits. The value of t_d is then fixed at this averaged control value, and the data from normal controls and patients are then refitted, allowing S and R_{max} to vary. This leaves only two parameters, S and R_{max}, that need to be estimated. (For our system, the value of t_d is 3.2 ms.) Note that in equation (1), flash intensity is expressed in scotopic troland seconds. The flash intensities given in scotopic troland seconds in this chapter assume a pupil diameter of 8 mm. The diameter of the dilated pupil can vary from 7 mm to 9 mm depending on the individual and may be much smaller in subjects with glaucoma and other conditions that affect pupil size. Therefore, we measure each individual's dilated pupil diameter and use the actual flash intensities expressed in scotopic troland seconds when fitting equation (1). Thus, individual differences in pupil diameter will not affect the results.

The dashed curves in figure 35.4 show the fit of the model to the leading edge of the rod a-wave of a control subject (panel A) and of a patient with dominant retinitis pigmentosa (RP) (panel C). The bold parts of the records are the portions of the wave that are fitted. For normal control subjects and patients with near normal values of S, the model is fitted to the three lowest flash intensities, that is, up to 4.0 log sc td s. If S is substantially elevated, then the response to the highest flash intensity is also used in the fitting procedure. (Technical note: The range of flash intensities that we use can be expressed in values of log ($I \times S$) from about 4.6 to 6.0. Equation (1) provides a good fit up to a value of log ($I \times S$) of about 5.3. As we discuss below, there are alternative models that can be used to fit responses to higher flash energies.)

The fit of the model yields estimates of S and R_{max}. For the patient's records in figure 35.4C, R_{max} is substantially reduced to about 15% of the normal value. (Note the change in the vertical scale between panels A and C.) The value of

normal   Patient with delayed b-wave

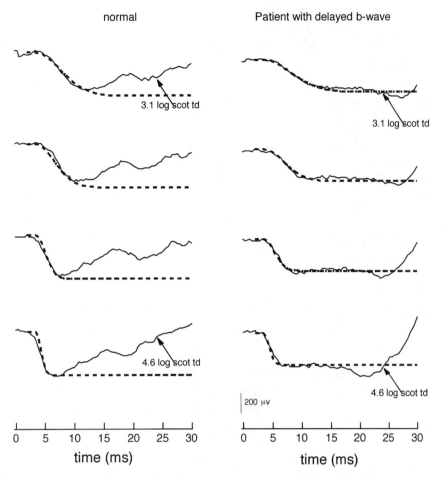

FIGURE 35.5 The rod-isolated responses from a normal control subject (A) and a patient with abnormally delayed postreceptoral responses (B). The fit of equation (1) is shown as the dashed curves.

(From Hood DC, Cideciyan AV, Halevy DA, Jacobson SG: Sites of disease action in a retinal dystrophy with supernormal and delayed rod electroretinogram b-waves. *Vision Res* 1996; 36:889–901.)

$\log S$ is slightly lower, by 0.2 log unit, than the value of $\log S$ for controls of a similar age.

Postreceptoral contributions can intrude on the leading edge of the a-wave (e.g., see chapter 15). Although the manner in which these contributions affect the peak of the a-wave is not completely understood, they do not appear to affect the fit of equation (1).[13,14] Two lines of evidence suggest that the influence of postreceptoral contributions are relatively minor in our recordings. First, the postreceptor responses in many of the patients with RP are delayed, providing a better picture of the photoreceptor response. Notice in figure 35.4C, for example, that the model fits the rod a-wave well beyond 12 ms. Figure 35.5 (right panel) provides another example from Hood, Cideciyan, Roman, and Jacobson.[30] This patient has a disorder that is known to delay the postreceptoral responses. The left panel shows the records from a control subject from the same experiment. In both cases, the model was fitted in the same way and for the same range of times. The model fits the leading edge of the a-wave well in both cases. For the patient, however, the model fit the rod a-wave out to 20 ms and beyond.

The second line of evidence suggesting that the influence of postreceptoral contribution is relatively minor comes from a study of adaptation. These results are shown in figure 35.6 (from Pepperberg, Birch, and Hood[44]). The 4.4 log sc td s flash was presented on a series of backgrounds from 0 (dark) to 2.8 sc td s. Notice that weak backgrounds reduce the peak of the a-wave by about 5%. The peak of the a-wave is not reduced further until the background reaches levels that are known to affect the rod photoreceptors.[2] Taken together, the results in figures 35.4 through 35.6 suggest that the peak a-wave in our fully dark-adapted recordings is only slightly influenced by a small negative contribution from postreceptoral cell(s). (Interestingly, the published fits of equation (1) often fall below the peak of the a-wave, suggesting an early, postreceptoral contribution that is positive. It is not clear to what extent these small differences are due to different states of adaptation or the way the model is fitted.)

THE IMPORTANCE OF A GOODNESS-OF-FIT MEASURE   The a-waves from patients with disease of the receptors can be

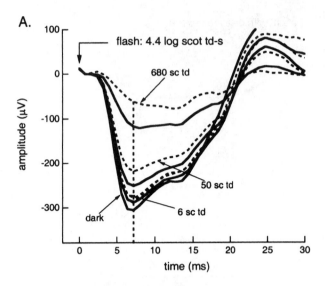

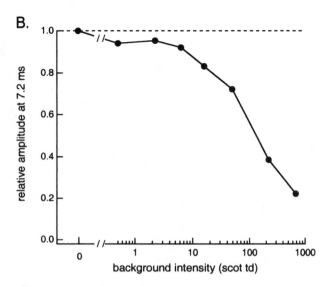

FIGURE 35.6 A, Responses to a 4.4 log sc td s flash presented on a series of steady background fields ranging from darkness to 680 sc td s. B, The relative amplitude of the response at 7.2 ms (see dashed line in panel A) is shown as a function of the intensity of the background. (Modified from Pepperberg DR, Birch DG, Hood DC: Electroretinographic determination of human rod flash response in vivo. *Methods Enzymol* 2000; 316:202–223.)

small, and the model can therefore be difficult to fit. A goodness-of-fit measure provides an objective way to eliminate poor fits. In particular, we calculate a least-squares, goodness-of-fit measure defined as follows:

$$\text{statfit} = \frac{\sqrt{\sum (x_i - m_i)^2}}{\sqrt{\sum (x_i - \mu)^2}} \qquad (2)$$

where x_i is the value of the response at point i in time, m_i is the value of the model fitted at the same point in time, and μ is the mean of the response for the time period evaluated. A perfect fit to the data would produce a statfit of 0.0, whereas a value of 1.0 indicates that the model does no better than using the mean of the data.[32] In general, statfit values less than 0.15 represent good fits, and we reject fits if the statfit is greater than 0.5. (Note that the statfit statistic can be related both to signal-to-noise ratios and to false-positive rates.[32])

FITTING A MODEL OF THE CONE PHOTORECEPTORS The a-wave of the cone-driven response, obtained on the rod-suppressing background, can be fitted with a modification of equation (1). To fit the cone a-wave, Hood and Birch[24,26] added a stage of low-pass filtering with a time constant of 1.8 ms. They showed that the cone a-waves from control subjects and patients with RP were well described by setting t_d to 1.7 ms and letting S and $R_{\max}$ vary. The dashed curves in figure 35.4 show the fit to a normal control (panel B) and a patient with RP (panel D). As the postreceptor contributions to the photopic ERG intrude on the leading edge of the a-wave at these intensities (see Bush and Sieving[8] and Robson et al.[47] and chapter 15), the model is fitted to the first 8–

10 ms of the response. Notice that the responses from the control subject deviate from the model as early as 8 ms at the higher intensities that are used (arrow in figure 35.4B). Robson et al.[47] found that the intrusion of a postreceptoral component can occur even earlier at the highest intensities. As in the case of the rods, this does not mean, however, that we cannot get a good estimate of the cone photoreceptors' response. In fact, the results from patients with RP confirm that we are, in fact, obtaining a good estimate. The postreceptoral portions of the responses are delayed in many of these patients, providing a better picture of the photoreceptor response. Notice in figure 35.4D, for example, that the model (dashed curves) fits the a-wave well beyond 10 ms. Figure 35.7 (right panel) provides another example. This patient with a dominant form of RP had reasonably large cone a-waves with a clearly delayed postreceptoral contribution. The model fitted the a-wave out to nearly 20 ms. (See also figure 4A in Hood and Birch.[26])

A SIMPLER EQUATION FOR THE CONE A-WAVE Fitting the cone model requires convolving equation (1) with the equation for an exponential filter. However, there is a simpler approach that does not require a convolution operation and therefore can be more easily implemented. In particular, Hood and Birch[26] adapted the Lamb and Pugh expression in equation (1) so that the saturating nonlinearity had the form of a Michaelis-Menton equation and the exponent had a value of 3. In particular, they showed that the leading edge of the cone a-waves was equally well fitted by

$$R(I,t) = \left\{ \frac{I \cdot S_c \cdot (t - t_d)^3}{I \cdot S_c \cdot (t - t_d)^3 + 1} \right\} \cdot Rm_{p3} \quad \text{for } t > t_d \qquad (3)$$

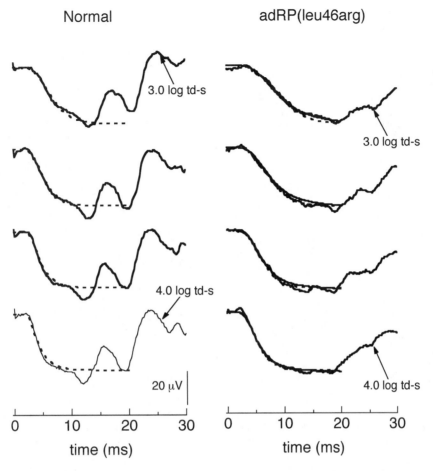

FIGURE 35.7   The cone responses from a normal control subject (A) and a patient with retinitis pigmentosa (B). The fit of a cone version[26] of the Lamb and Pugh model[39] is shown as the dashed curves and the fit of equation (3) as the smooth bold curve.

(Modified from Hood DC, Birch DG: Phototransduction in human cones measured using the alpha-wave of the ERG. *Vision Res* 1995; 35:2801–2810.)

where the terms have similar meaning as the terms in equation (1). S_c is a sensitivity (gain) parameter that scales flash energy I and has as its units $(td\,s)^{-1}(s)^{-3}$; R_{max} is the maximum amplitude; and t_d is a brief delay. The solid, bold curves in figure 35.7 (right panel) are the fit of equation (2). These curves are nearly indistinguishable from the fit of equation (1) followed by low-pass filtering.

NORMATIVE VALUES AND REPEAT RELIABILITY   Figure 35.8 shows the parameters for 100 control subjects reported by Birch et al.[3] The rod and cone values of $\log S$ significantly decrease with age, but the values of $\log R_{max}$ do not.[11] In particular, on average, the values of $\log S$ for the rods and cones decreased by 0.06 (rod) and 0.04 (cones) log unit per decade. In other words, on average, the value of rod S for someone 70 years old would be one half (0.3 log unit) the value for someone who is 20 years old.[3] As with all electrophysiological testing, each clinic needs to establish its own normative values. For example, R_{max} will vary with electrode composi-

tion and configuration (e.g., bipolar versus monopolar electrode configurations).

The repeat reliability of the a-wave measures is good. In fact, the results of Birch et al.[3] strongly suggest that R_{max} is a better outcome measure for prospective studies than are the more traditional measures of the ISCEV standard ERGs. In addition to being stable with age, the repeat reliability of R_{max} is better than that of the traditional measures (e.g., b-wave amplitude) of the ISCEV standard flashes.

ALTERNATIVE MODELS   The original Lamb and Pugh[39] model has a major weakness: Equation (1) does not fit the first few milliseconds of the response to high flash intensities. Figure 35.9 shows the first 20 ms of the isolated rod responses to five flash intensities. The model was fitted to the lower three intensities (bold records), but the theoretical curves (dashed curve) are shown for all responses. The theoretical curves become increasingly poor at fitting early times as flash intensity is increased.[5,11] While these deviations

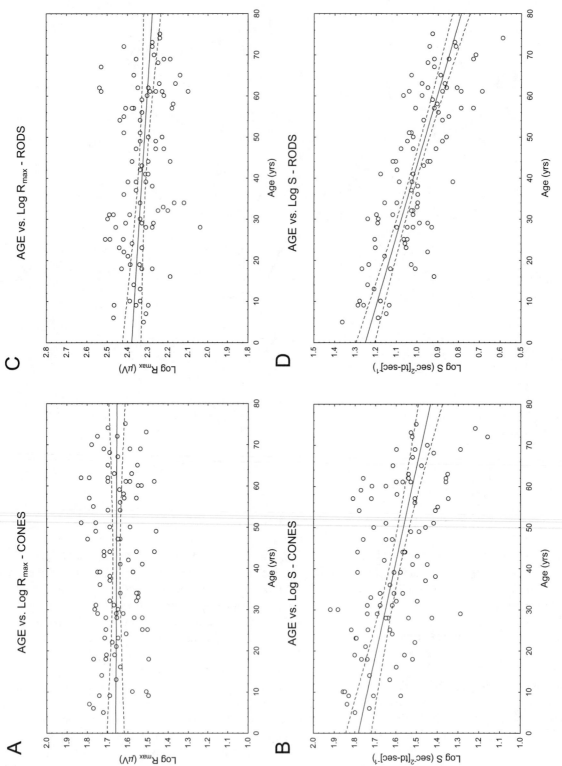

FIGURE 35.8   A, Log R_{max} values for the fit of a cone version[26] of the Lamb and Pugh model[39] to the cone a-waves of control subjects are shown as a function of the age of the subject. B, Log S values for the fit of the cone model as a function of the age of the subject. C, Log R_{max} values for the fit of equation (1) to the rod-isolated a-waves of control subjects are shown as a function of the age of the subject. B, Log S values for the fit of equation (3) as a function of the age of the subject. (From Birch DG, Hood DC, Locke KG, Hoffman DR, Tzekov RT: Quantitative electroretinogram measures of phototransduction in cone and rod photoreceptors: normal aging, progression with disease, and test-retest variability. *Arch Ophthalmol* 2002; 120:1045–1051.)

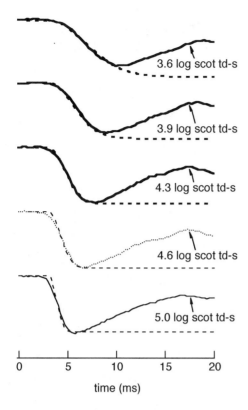

FIGURE 35.9 The rod-isolated responses from a control subject to flashes ranging in intensity from 3.6 to 5.0 log sc td s. The dashed curves are the results from the fit of equation (1) to the leading edge of the a-waves for the three lowest flash intensities.

were originally thought to be due to a breakdown in the assumptions underlying the biochemical model,[5,39] it is now clear that the problem is a result of lumping a number of factors into the single delay parameter, t_d.[11,17,52] Three groups have produce alternatives to equation (1) for the human rod a-wave.[11,47,52] The alternative models differ in detail, but they share the following characteristics: First, they all improve the fit to responses at early times after intense flashes. Second, these models are more difficult to implement than equation (1) because more parameters need to be estimated or calculated. Furthermore, a convolution operation is required, meaning that the model cannot be implemented in most spreadsheet programs. Third, the models all have two parameters that are essentially the same as S (a gain parameter) and R_{max} (the maximum response). Fourth, it is likely that if all other parameters except these two are fixed for a group of normal controls, then reasonably comparable estimates of the effects on S and R_{max} should result. From the viewpoint of basic science, none of these models is based entirely on parameters that can be independently estimated from the steps of phototransduction, although the Robson et al. model[47] has the most biochemical detail. From a clinical point of view, it remains to be seen whether the resulting parameters will be sufficiently different from those estimated from equation (1) to justify the added difficulty in

fitting these models. However, if flash intensities greater than about 4.4 log sc td s are used, then one of these alternative models should be employed.

Diseases of the photoreceptors and the leading edge of the a-wave

UNDERSTANDING THE MEANING OF THE S AND R_{max} PARAMETERS   Figure 35.10 provides a simple way to understand the parameters S and R_{max}. This figure illustrates two hypothetical, and very different, effects that a disease process might have on the rod a-waves. The dashed curves in both panels are the first 60 ms of the rod ERG to a brief (1 ms) flash of light of about 4.0 log sc td s. Suppose that a disease process decreased the sensitivity parameter, S, of the rods without changing their maximum response. A change in S is like a change in flash intensity. (Note in equation (1) the term $(I \times S)$.) The solid curve in figure 35.10 (left panel) is the response of a control subject to a flash of light that is one fourth (0.6 log unit) less intense than the flash that produces the dashed curve. This change in flash intensity mimics a change in S by a factor of one fourth (a change in log S of 0.6 log unit). The right panel of figure 35.10 illustrates a change in the maximum response R_{max}. A change in R_{max} is defined as one that decreases the a-wave by a multiplicative factor. The solid curve is the normal curve divided by 4.

The dotted curves in figure 35.10 show the fit of equation (1) to the hypothetical responses. The model is fitted only to the leading edge of the a-wave (bold part). From the fit of the model, changes in S and R_{max} can be obtained. As indicated in the figure, a change in the parameter S by a factor of one fourth is equivalent to a change in flash intensity by the same factor. Similarly, a change in R_{max} by a factor of one fourth is equivalent to scaling the entire receptor response by a factor of one fourth.

DISEASES OF THE RETINA AND CHANGES IN ROD PHOTORECEPTOR PARAMETERS   Diseases of the retina can affect S and/or R_{max}. In figure 35.11A, the change in log S is plotted against the change in log R_{max}. The mean normal values are shown as the solid lines at zero, and the dashed lines show the 95% limits. Thus, the points that fall to the left of the vertical dashed line have abnormal R_{max} values, and the points that fall below the horizontal dashed lines have abnormal S values. Johnson and Hood[37] found that patients with CRVO who develop neovascularizaton had decreased values of S but relatively normal values of R_{max} (solid circles in figure 35.11A). The change in S in these patients is probably due to a slowing of one or more of the steps of phototransduction, which results in a decrease in the amplification or sensitivity of transduction. The authors speculated that these changes are secondary to hypoxia. Other conditions that are thought to produce hypoxia of the receptors have

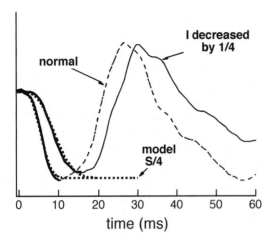

decreased S
(sensitivity 1/4 normal)

decreased R_{max}
(maximum amplitude 1/4 normal)

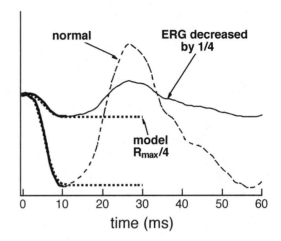

FIGURE 35.10 Two effects that a disease process could have on the rod receptor and thus on the leading edge of the rod a-wave (shown as bold). The dashed curve is the dark-adapted rod response to a flash of 4.0 log sc td s. A, A change in sensitivity, *S*, is defined as a change that acts as if the flash intensity were decreased. The solid curve shows the ERG response to a flash that is one fourth as intense as the flash producing the dashed curve. The bold dotted curve labeled "model" is the fit of equation (1) assuming that the flash intensity has not changed. B, A decrease in the maximum response (R_{max}) is defined as a change that scales the entire leading edge (bold) by the same factor. The solid curve shows a hypothetical ERG response created by dividing the dashed curve by 4. The bold dotted curve labeled "model" is the fit of equation (1).

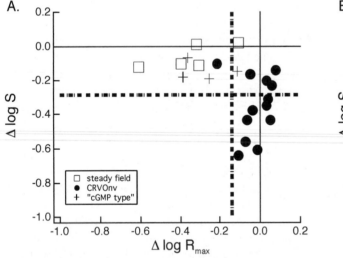

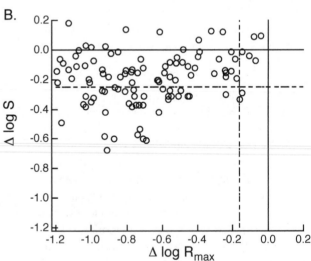

FIGURE 35.11 A, The change in log rod *S* versus the change in log rod R_{max} for individual subjects with central retinal vein occlusion (solid circles) and "cGMP-type" enhanced b-wave (plus signs). The open squares show the effects of steady backgrounds on the rod parameters of a control subject. B, The change in log rod *S* versus the change in log rod R_{max} for individual subjects with RP. In both panels, the mean normal values are shown as the solid lines at zero, and the dashed lines show the 95% limits. (Data from Tzekov RT, Locke KG, Hood D, Birch DG: Cone and rod ERG phototransduction in retinitis pigmentosa. *Invest Ophthal Vis Sci* 2003; 44:3993–4000.)

been shown to produce changes in S.[13,18,45,46] Reynaud, Hansen, and Fulton[46] speculated that metabolic acidosis may be the cause.

Figure 35.11A shows two conditions that can affect R_{max} while leaving S relatively unchanged. The open squares show the effects of a steady background on the leading edge of the rod a-wave of control subjects. Increasing the background intensity (the square symbols) decreases R_{max} owing to response compression while producing relatively small changes in S.[26,29,53] The second example of a decrease in R_{max} with a relatively normal S value comes from a study of patients with delayed, and supernormal, rod b-waves.[31] This is an unusual retinal dystrophy that has been described by a number of groups.[1,14,38,48,49,55] The results from fitting the rod a-waves from four of these patients are shown in figure 35.11A (plus signs). The value of S was normal, while R_{max} was reduced in three subjects.

Some diseases, such as RP and the cone dystrophies, have been found to produce changes in both S and R_{max}. While some patients show only changes in R_{max},[9,35] others show changes in both S and R_{max}.[4,25,51,54] Figure 35.11B contains the results for 157 patients with RP.[54] RP clearly decreases R_{max} as expected. In some cases, there is also a change in S, while in others, the S value is within normal limits (dashed horizontal line in figure 35.11B). Diseases that affect the phototransduction cascade directly are most likely to affect S, although other factors may be involved as well.[54] It is likely that the R_{max} changes are due to missing and/or shortened rod receptors, while the S changes imply that transduction is abnormal in at least some of the remaining rod photoreceptors.[25,33]

RP and Changes in Cone Photoreceptor Parameters

Because the cone signals are smaller, there are fewer studies that have reported cone parameters. However, the cone parameters have been studied for RP. Interestingly, RP, a primary disease of the rod photoreceptors, decreases the sensitivity S of the cones.[26–28,54] Figure 35.12 shows the results from 157 patients with RP plotted as in figure 35.11B.[54] On average, the loss in cone R_{max} is less severe than the loss in rod R_{max} (figure 35.11B), while the loss in cone S values is more severe than in the case of the rods. While the decrease in cone R_{max} is easy to understand, the decreases in S values are more interesting, especially considering that they can be larger than the change in the rod S values. Tzekov et al.[54] note that choroidal and retinal blood flow are reduced in many patients with RP and suggest that this may be the underlying cause of the depressed S values. (Remember that decreases in S have been associated with conditions that produce hypoxia.) In any case, there are other pathologic changes in the outer retina that could be causing the decrease in S; a discussion of these can be found in Tzekov et al.[54]

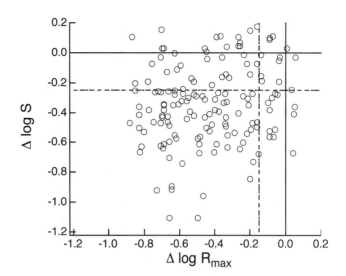

FIGURE 35.12   The change in log cone S values versus the change in log cone R_{max} values for individual patients with retinitis pigmentosa. (Data from Tzekov RT, Locke KG, Hood D, Birch DG: Cone and rod ERG phototransduction in retinitis pigmentosa. *Invest Ophthal Vis Sci* 2003; 44:3993–4000.) In both panels, the mean normal values are shown as the solid lines at zero, and the dashed lines show the 95% limits.

Distinguishing Among Alternative Explanations of Receptor Damage

With careful assumptions, the parameters S and R_{max} can be related to parameters of the initial phases (activation) of phototransduction.[25,29] However, there are only two parameters, and each can be affected by a number of possible disease mechanisms. Therefore, by themselves, these parameters cannot necessarily distinguish among alternative hypotheses. For example, a change in S has been attributed to changes in the amplification or speed of transduction, to preretinal absorption, and to a decrease in the density of rhodopsin in individual disks. Likewise, a change in R_{max} has been attributed to response compression (light adaptation), the loss of large sections of the retina, and shortened outer segments. Presumably, most patients with RP show decreased R_{max} due to a combination of a loss of regions of receptors and local losses of rod outer segment membrane. To distinguish among alternative hypotheses, other measures can be used, including measures of preretinal absorption, b-wave (or derived P2) implicit times and amplitudes,[22,33,51] densitometry, phototransduction deactivation[4,12,41,43,47] (see chapter 39), visual fields,[51] focal ERGs, and computer simulations.[33,34]

Assessing human receptor activity in the clinic

Traditionally, human rod receptor activity has been evaluated by measuring the slope and/or the peak amplitude of the a-wave to flashes of moderate intensity (see figure 35.2A). The peak a-wave amplitude does not represent the peak receptor response, and the slope is affected similarly by changes in R_{max} or S. Adding high-intensity flashes to the standard clinical protocol would allow the clinician to directly evaluate receptor function. In addition, there are diseases that are better identified with high-intensity flashes, such as enhanced S-cone syndrome and X-linked juvenile retinoschisis. In this section, we consider how the high-intensity techniques can be modified for the clinic.

CLINICAL PROTOCOLS   The ISCEV-recommended "high-intensity" flash is about 100 times too dim for an adequate measure of receptor activity. This standard intensity was set at a time when commercially available equipment could not produce flashes of higher intensities. Newer systems are capable of flash intensities 1000 or more times higher. Thus, there appears to be little reason not to modify the clinical standards. The four flash protocol[29] described above adds about 10 minutes to a testing session.[3] However, the additional testing time could be reduced to between 2 and 5

minutes, as excellent results can be obtained with one or two flash intensities.[11,29] In fact, Cideciyan and Jacobson[11] showed that two flash intensities (4.6 and 2.3 log sc td s) were sufficient to obtain reliable estimates of S and R_{max}. If the current "high-intensity" flash in the ISCEV protocol were dropped, the time that is added to the test would be negligible.

NO NEED FOR A FITTING PROGRAM   In principle, it should be possible to incorporate the software needed to fit equation (1) into commercial equipment, and at least one manufacturer has expressed plans to do so. Until this feature is generally available, a fear of curve fitting should not dissuade someone from using the a-wave to estimate receptor parameters. Hood and Birch[29] suggest a procedure that could be easily implemented by anyone who is capable of using a spreadsheet program. Here, we demonstrate an even easier, although slightly less precise, technique.

Figure 35.13 illustrates a procedure that requires only a pencil and a ruler. Figure 35.13 shows the rod-isolated

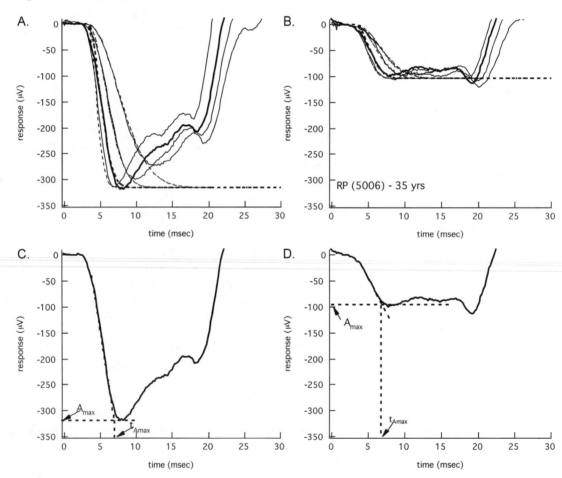

FIGURE 35.13   A, The first 30 ms of the rod-isolated ERG responses from a normal control subject. The dashed curves are the fit of equation (1) to the leading edge of the responses to the lowest three flash intensities. B, As in panel A for a patient with retinitis pigmentosa. C, Illustration of the simple method for obtaining estimates of A_{max} and t_{Amax} for the records in panel A. The values of A_{max} and t_{Amax} are proxies for the model parameters S and R_{max}. D, As in panel C for a patient with retinitis pigmentosa whose records are shown in panel B.

A.

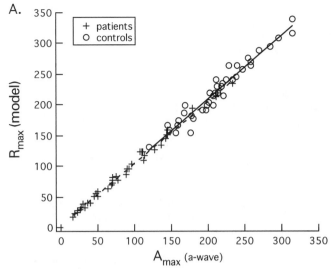
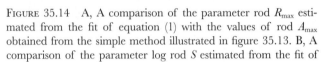

B.

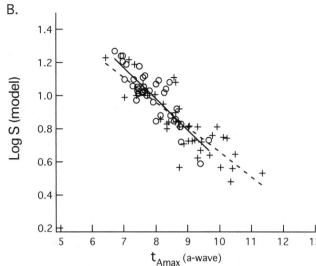

FIGURE 35.14   A, A comparison of the parameter rod R_{max} estimated from the fit of equation (1) with the values of rod A_{max} obtained from the simple method illustrated in figure 35.13. B, A comparison of the parameter log rod S estimated from the fit of equation (1) with the values of rod t_{Amax} obtained from the simple method illustrated in figure 35.13. In both panels, the straight lines are the best-fitting linear regression line for the patients (dashed) and normal controls (solid).

responses from a normal control (panel A) and a patient with RP (panel B) for the four-flash protocol. In the lower panels, the response to 4.0 log sc td s is shown. The simple method involves first drawing two lines: A horizontal line at the point of the maximum a-wave and a diagonal line along the leading edge of the a-wave. Next, two measures are obtained: A_{max}, which is the y-axis value of the horizontal line, and t_{Amax}, which is the x-axis value of the point at which the two lines intersect. These measures, A_{max} and t_{Amax}, are the proxies for R_{max} and S. Figure 35.14 compares the parameter values that are obtained by the simple method with those estimated from the fit to the full protocol. Each point represents a pair of values for one of 40 control subjects (open circles) or for one of the 40 patients with RP (plus signs). The value of A_{max} is an excellent measure of R_{max}, with r^2 of 0.95 for the controls and 0.99 for the patients (figure 35.14A). The t_{Amax} values provide a reasonably good measure of S, with r^2 of 0.71 for the controls and 0.76 for the patients (figure 35.14B). There are two possible reasons why the correlation between S and t_{Amax} is lower than that between A_{max} and R_{max}. First, unlike S, the t_{Amax} measure does not take pupil diameter into consideration. This factor can affect log S by about 0.1 log unit (i.e., in our experience, the pupil diameters ranged from 7 to 9 mm for the 80 subjects). A correction factor could be incorporated into this method.[50] Second, at the 4.0 log sc td s intensity, t_{Amax} changes relatively little with changes in intensity (see figure 35.13A) and thus relatively little with S. The fit to the model may provide a better measure of S because it makes use of the responses

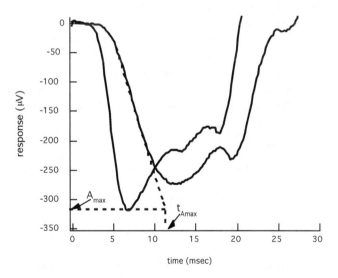

FIGURE 35.15   A version of the simple method that uses two flash intensities. A_{max} is estimated from the response to the more intense flash (4.4 log sc td s), and t_{Amax} is estimated from the response to the less intense flash (3.1 log sc td s).

to lower flash intensities, at which the curves change more with flash intensity or S changes.

Figure 35.15 shows a second version of a simple method; in this case, two flash intensities are employed. The higher flash intensity (4.4 log sc td s) provides the measure of A_{max}, and the lower flash intensity (3.1 log sc td s) provides the measure of t_{Amax}. Compared to the simple method based on one flash, the values of t_{Amax} obtained with the two-flash method should correlate better with S, while the values of A_{max} should correlate as well.

This analysis suggests that the ISCEV ERG protocol should be modified to include two flashes of higher intensity presented in the dark and on a $30\,cd/m^2$ background. The lower intensity of two flashes should be about $3\log sc\,td\,s$, and the higher should be about $4.4\log sc\,td\,s$. The rod-isolated and cone responses can be analyzed by fitting one of the models, although for most purposes, a pencil and ruler technique will do.

Summary

The analysis of the leading edge of the a-wave offers a way to answer the question "How does a particular disease or treatment affect the phototransduction process of the human rod and cone receptors?" Furthermore, when combined with information from other techniques, an alternative hypothesis about the effects of a disease process can be distinguished. Although alternative equations have been suggested and more work is needed to distinguish among them, any of these equations can be used to improve our understanding of receptor function. In fact, as we have shown, it is even possible to estimate the parameters of phototransduction without fitting an equation. While an a-wave analysis has been used in the laboratory study of animal models and in the clinical study of patients with retinal diseases, it has not made its way into the standard (ISCEV) ERG protocol (see chapter 26). To be of use in the clinic, flashes of higher intensity need to be added to this protocol.

ACKNOWLEDGMENTS   This work was supported in part by Grants EY-05235 and EY-09706 from the National Eye Institute and support from the Foundation Fighting Blindness. We thank Dr. Karen Holopigian for comments on the manuscript.

REFERENCES

1. Alexander KR, Fishman GA: Supernormal scotopic ERG in cone dystrophy. *Br J Ophthalmol* 1984; 68:69–78.
2. Baylor DA, Nunn BJ, Schnapf JL: The photocurrent, noise and spectral sensitivity of rods of the monkey Macaca fascicularis. *J Physiol* 1984; 357:575–607.
3. Birch DG, Hood DC, Locke KG, Hoffman DR, Tzekov RT: Quantitative electroretinogram measures of phototransduction in cone and rod photoreceptors: Normal aging, progression with disease, and test-retest variability. *Arch Ophthalmol* 2002; 120:1045–1051.
4. Birch DG, Hood DC, Nusinowitz S, Pepperberg DR: Abnormal activation and inactivation mechanisms of rod transduction in patients with autosomal dominant retinitis pigmentosa and the pro-23-his mutation. *Invest Ophthalmol Vis Sci* 1995; 36:1603–1614.
5. Breton ME, Schueller AW, Lamb TD, Pugh EN Jr: Analysis of ERG a-wave amplification and kinetics in terms of the G-protein cascade of phototransduction. *Invest Ophthalmol Vis Sci* 1994; 35:295–309.
6. Brown KT: The electroretinogram: Its components and their origins. *Vision Res* 1968; 8:633–677.
7. Brown KT, Watanabe K, Murakami M: The early and late receptor potentials of monkey cones and rods. *Cold Spring Harb Symp Quant Biol* 1965; 30:457–482.
8. Bush RA, Sieving PA: A proximal retinal component in the primate photopic ERG a-wave. *Invest Ophthalmol Vis Sci* 1994; 35:635–645.
9. Cideciyan AV, Hood DC, Huang Y, et al.: Disease sequence from mutant rhodopsin allele to rod and cone photoreceptor degeneration in man. *Proc Natl Acad Sci U S A* 1998; 95:7103–7108.
10. Cideciyan AV, Jacobson SG: Negative electroretinograms in retinitis pigmentosa. *Invest Ophthalmol Vis Sci* 1993; 34:3253–3263.
11. Cideciyan AV, Jacobson SG: An alternative phototransduction model for human rod and cone ERG a-waves: Normal parameters and variation with age. *Vision Res* 1996; 36:2609–2621.
12. Friedburg C, Thomas MM, Lamb TD: Time course of the flash response of dark- and light-adapted human rod photoreceptors derived from the electroretinogram. *J Physiol* 2001; 534:217–242.
13. Fulton AB, Hansen RM: Photoreceptor function in infants and children with a history of mild retinopathy of prematurity. *J Opt Soc Am A Opt Image Sci Vis* 1996; 13:566–571.
14. Gouras P, Eggers HM, MacKay CJ: Cone dystrophy, nyctalopia, and supernormal rod responses: A new retinal degeneration. *Arch Ophthalmol* 1983; 101:718–724.
15. Granit R: *Sensory Mechanism of the Retina.* London, Oxford University Press, 1947.
16. Granit R: The components of the retinal action potential in mammals and their relation to the discharge in the optic nerve. *J Physiol* 1933; 77:207–239.
17. Hamer RD, Tyler CW: Phototransduction: Modeling the primate cone flash response. *Vis Neurosci* 1995; 12:1063–1082.
18. Holopigian K, Greenstein VC, Seiple W, Hood DC, Carr RE: Evidence for photoreceptor changes in patients with diabetic retinopathy. *Invest Ophthalmol Vis Sci* 1997; 38:2355–2365.
19. Hood DC, Birch DG: The relationship between models of receptor activity and the a-wave of the human ERG. *Clin Vis Sci* 1990; 5:293–297.
20. Hood DC, Birch DG: A quantitative measure of the electrical activity of human rod photoreceptors using electroretinography. *Vis Neurosci* 1990; 5:379–387.
21. Hood DC, Birch DG: The A-wave of the human electroretinogram and rod receptor function. *Invest Ophthalmol Vis Sci* 1990; 31:2070–2081.
22. Hood DC, Birch DG: A computational model of the amplitude and implicit time of the b-wave of the human ERG. *Vis Neurosci* 1992; 8:107–126.
23. Hood DC, Birch DG: Light adaptation of human rod receptors: The leading edge of the human a-wave and models of rod receptor activity. *Vision Res* 1993; 33:1605–1618.
24. Hood DC, Birch DG: Human cone receptor activity: The leading edge of the a-wave and models of receptor activity. *Vis Neurosci* 1993; 10:857–871.
25. Hood DC, Birch DG: Rod phototransduction in retinitis pigmentosa: Estimation and interpretation of parameters derived from the rod a-wave. *Invest Ophthalmol Vis Sci* 1994; 35:2948–2961.

26. Hood DC, Birch DG: Phototransduction in human cones measured using the alpha-wave of the ERG. *Vision Res* 1995; 35:2801–2810.

27. Hood D, Birch DG: Abnormal cone receptor activity in patients with hereditary degeneration. In Anderson RE (ed.): *Degenerative Diseases of the Retina*. New York, Plenum, 1995, pp 349–358.

28. Hood DC, Birch DG: Abnormalities of the retinal cone system in retinitis pigmentosa. *Vision Res* 1996; 36:1699–1709.

29. Hood DC, Birch DG: Assessing abnormal rod photoreceptor activity with the a-wave of the ERG: Applications and methods. *Doc Ophthalmol* 1997; 92:253–267.

30. Hood DC, Cideciyan AV, Halevy DA, Jacobson SG: Sites of disease action in a retinal dystrophy with supernormal and delayed rod electroretinogram b-waves. *Vision Res* 1996; 36:889–901.

31. Hood DC, Cideciyan AV, Roman AJ, Jacobson SG: Enhanced S cone syndrome: Evidence for an abnormally large number of S cones. *Vision Res* 1995; 35:1473–1481.

32. Hood D, Li J: A technique for measuring individual multifocal ERG records. In *Non-invasive Assessment of the Visual System: Trends in Optics and Photonics, vol. 11*. Washington, D.C., Optical Society of America, 1997, pp 33–41.

33. Hood DC, Shady S, Birch DG: Heterogeneity in retinal disease and the computational model of the human-rod response. *J Opt Soc Am A* 1993; 10:1624–1630.

34. Hood DC, Shady S, Birch DG: Understanding changes in the b-wave of the ERG caused by heterogeneous receptor damage. *Invest Ophthalmol Vis Sci* 1994; 35:2477–2488.

35. Jacobson SG, Kemp CM, Cideciyan AV, Macke JP, Sung CH, Nathans J: Phenotypes of stop codon and splice site rhodopsin mutations causing retinitis pigmentosa. *Invest Ophthalmol Vis Sci* 1994; 35:2521–2534.

36. Jamison JA, Bush RA, Lei B, Sieving PA: Characterization of the rod photoresponse isolated from the dark-adapted primate ERG. *Vis Neurosci* 2001; 18:445–455.

37. Johnson MA, Hood DC: Rod photoreceptor transduction is affected in central retinal vein occlusion associated with iris neovascularization. *J Opt Soc Am A* 1996; 13:572–576.

38. Kato M, Kobayashi R, Watanabe I: Cone dysfunction and supernormal scotopic electroretinogram with a high-intensity stimulus: A report of three cases. *Doc Ophthalmol* 1993; 84:71–81.

39. Lamb TD, Pugh EN Jr: A quantitative account of the activation steps involved in phototransduction in amphibian photoreceptors. *J Physiol* 1992; 449:719–758.

40. Murakami M, Kaneko A: Differentiation of P3 subcomponents in cold-blooded vertebrate retinas. *Vision Res* 1966; 6:627–636.

41. Nusinowitz S, Hood DC, Birch DG: Rod transduction parameters from the a-wave of local receptor populations. *J Opt Soc Am A* 1995; 12:2259–2266.

42. Penn RD, Hagins WA: Kinetics of the photocurrent of retinal rods. *Biophys J* 1972; 12:1073–1094.

43. Pepperberg DR, Birch DG, Hood DC: Photoresponses of human rods in vivo derived from paired-flash electroretinograms. *Vis Neurosci* 1997; 14:73–82.

44. Pepperberg DR, Birch DG, Hood DC: Electroretinographic determination of human rod flash response in vivo. *Methods Enzymol* 2000; 316:202–223.

45. Reynaud X, Chunguang RM, Hansen RM, Fulton AB, Aouididi S, Dorey CK: Morphological and ERG evidence of retinal hypoxia in interrupted oxygen induced retinopathy in the neonatal rat. *Invest Ophthalmol Vis Sci* 1994; 35:1378.

46. Reynaud X, Hansen RM, Fulton AB: Effect of prior oxygen exposure on the electroretinographic responses of infant rats. *Invest Ophthalmol Vis Sci* 1995; 36:2071–2079.

47. Robson JG, Saszik SM, Ahmed J, Frishman LJ: Rod and cone contributions to the a-wave of the electroretinogram of the macaque. *J Physiol* 2003; 547:509–530.

48. Rosenberg T, Simonsen SE: Retinal cone dysfunction of supernormal rod ERG type: Five new cases. *Acta Ophthalmol (Copenh)* 1993; 71:246–255.

49. Sandberg MA, Miller S, Berson EL: Rod electroretinograms in an elevated cyclic guanosine monophosphate-type human retinal degeneration: Comparison with retinitis pigmentosa. *Invest Ophthalmol Vis Sci* 1990; 31:2283–2287.

50. Seaman CR, Locke KG, Hood D, Birch DG: Rapid clinical assessment of a-wave photoreceptor function. *ARVO Abstract* 2003; 1884.

51. Shady S, Hood DC, Birch DG: Rod phototransduction in retinitis pigmentosa: Distinguishing alternative mechanisms of degeneration. *Invest Ophthalmol Vis Sci* 1995; 36:1027–1037.

52. Smith NP, Lamb TD: The a-wave of the human electroretinogram recorded with a minimally invasive technique. *Vision Res* 1997; 37:2943–2952.

53. Thomas MM, Lamb TD: Light adaptation and dark adaptation of human rod photoreceptors measured from the a-wave of the electroretinogram. *J Physiol* 1999; 518(2):479–496.

54. Tzekov RT, Locke KG, Hood D, Birch DG: Cone and rod ERG phototransduction in retinitis pigmentosa. *Invest Ophthalmol Vis Sci* 2003; in press.

55. Yagasaki K, Miyake Y, Litao RE, Ichikawa K: Two cases of retinal degeneration with an unusual form of electroretinogram. *Doc Ophthalmol* 1986; 63:73–82.

VII PRINCIPLES OF CLINICAL TESTING

36 Localizing Lesions in the Visual System

GRAHAM E. HOLDER

THE ABILITY OF electrophysiological testing to provide objective evidence of function at different levels of the visual system enables accurate localization of dysfunction in the vast majority of patients. This chapter provides an overview of lesion localization in clinical practice; it does not set out to address specific diseases in detail; those are covered elsewhere in this volume. The patients and disorders chosen to illustrate diagnostic points have been selected merely to be representative for the nature of the associated electrophysiological findings. Referencing has also been restricted, and the reader is referred to the relevant chapters of this volume or to another standard text (e.g., Fishman et al.[4]) for more information, particularly clinical details, on specific diseases.

Conventional clinical diagnosis relates the symptoms, history, and family history reported by the patient to the signs found on examination. The difficulties in accurate lesion localization based purely on this approach are clearly manifest in the visual system. For example, night blindness can arise from disorders of the photoreceptors, such as retinitis pigmentosa (RP) or enhanced S-cone syndrome, or may arise post-phototransduction, as in X-linked congenital stationary night blindness or melanoma-associated retinopathy. Fundus examination might not be helpful; a retina may look grossly normal on ophthalmoscopic examination but not function normally, as in Leber congenital amaurosis or vitamin A deficiency. Also, the degree of intraretinal pigment deposition in a patient with RP may be a poor indicator of the extent of retinal degeneration; there may be only mild pigmentary changes but profound loss of function. Equally, an abnormal retinal appearance may be associated with normal function, such as in a choroideremia carrier. Further, blurring of vision, central field loss, color vision disturbance, and a relative afferent pupillary defect can occur in macular dysfunction but are more commonly associated with optic nerve disease. Many diagnostic dilemmas can be resolved by appropriate electrophysiological testing.

The approach adopted relates to the nature of the electrophysiological findings. In summary, the electro-oculogram (EOG) will give information regarding the function of the retinal pigment epithelium (RPE) and its interaction with the photoreceptors. Electroretinography (ERG) assesses the photoreceptor and inner nuclear layers of the retina, with additional diagnostic dissection enabled in the cone system by the use of short-wavelength stimulation to assess the function of the S-cone pathway and long-duration stimulation to separate the function of the ON (depolarizing) and OFF (hyperpolarizing) pathways associated with L- and M-cones. If disease is confined to the macula, the full-field ERG will be unaffected, and pattern electroretinography (PERG) or multifocal electroretinography (mfERG) is needed. The reader is reminded that these tests of central retinal function are technically demanding; both are small signals, and the latter is particularly dependent on the ability of the patient to maintain accurate fixation. The PERG consists of two main components: P50 and N95. Although much of P50 arises in relation to spiking cell function, it is driven by the macular photoreceptors, and P50 component amplitude may be used to assess macular function quantitatively. The function of the retinal ganglion cells, which do not significantly contribute to the routine clinical full-field ERG, is objectively measured using the PERG N95 component. The cortical visual evoked potential (VEP) enables conclusions to be drawn regarding the intracranial visual pathways, including the optic nerves, the optic chiasm, and the visual cortex. However, it should always be borne in mind that the VEP is a "downstream" response that arises largely in the visual cortex and, as such, can be affected by disease anywhere "upstream" in the visual system, exemplified by the delayed pattern VEP common in macular disease. Thus, a combined approach, incorporating and integrating information from different tests, might be needed for accurate disease characterization and lesion localization.[7]

Abnormal EOG light rise: RPE dysfunction

The majority of patients with an abnormal light rise in the EOG have disturbance of function at the level of the photoreceptors, and reduction in EOG light rise is consequent upon photoreceptor dysfunction. The main exception to this is Best vitelliform macular dystrophy, a dominantly inherited

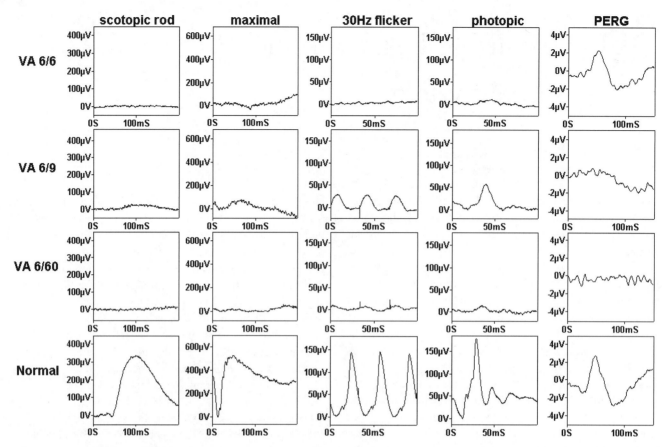

FIGURE 36.1 Data from three patients with rod-cone dystrophy (RP). The findings illustrate the complimentary nature of full-field ERG, reflecting the mass responses of the retina, and pattern ERG, reflecting macular function. See text for further details. (After Holder GE: The pattern electroretinogram. In Fishman GA, Birch DG, Holder GE, Brigell MG: *Electrophysiologic Testing in Disorders of the Retina, Optic Nerve, and Visual Pathway,* 2 ed. Ophthalmology Monograph 2. San Francisco: The Foundation of the American Academy of Ophthalmology; 2001. Reproduced with permission.)

disorder related to mutation in *VMD2*. In Best disease, a profoundly reduced, often abolished, EOG light rise is associated with normal ERGs. The diagnosis is usually first suggested by the appearance of characteristic vitelliform foveal lesions, but once these have progressed to the vitelliruptive stage, there may occasionally be difficulties in making the distinction between Best disease and adult vitelliform macular dystrophy or pattern dystrophy. In the latter case, although there may be mild EOG light rise reduction, the profound loss of EOG light rise characteristically present in Best disease does not occur.

Abnormal rod-specific b-wave, abnormal maximal ERG response a-wave: rod photoreceptor dysfunction

Although the rod-specific response of the International Society for Clinical Electrophysiology of Vision standard ERGs is the most sensitive measure of rod system dysfunction, an abnormality of this response, which consists of a rod-specific b-wave but no a-wave, does not allow accurate lesion localization. The b-wave arises in the inner nuclear layer of the retina in relation to rod ON-bipolar cell function (see chapter 12), and an abnormality of the rod-specific b-wave may reflect either photoreceptor disease or dysfunction arising post-phototransduction. The first 10–12 ms of the maximal response a-wave relate to photoreceptor hyperpolarization; thus, it is an a-wave abnormality that accurately localizes dysfunction to the rod photoreceptors. RP (rod-cone dystrophy) is the most frequently occurring example of this, and the findings from three patients are illustrated in figure 36.1. In rod-cone dystrophy, the rod ERG, by definition, is more affected than the cone ERG; the opposite applies in cone-rod dystrophy; most genetically determined generalized photoreceptor degenerations fall into these two categories. Note the complementary infor-

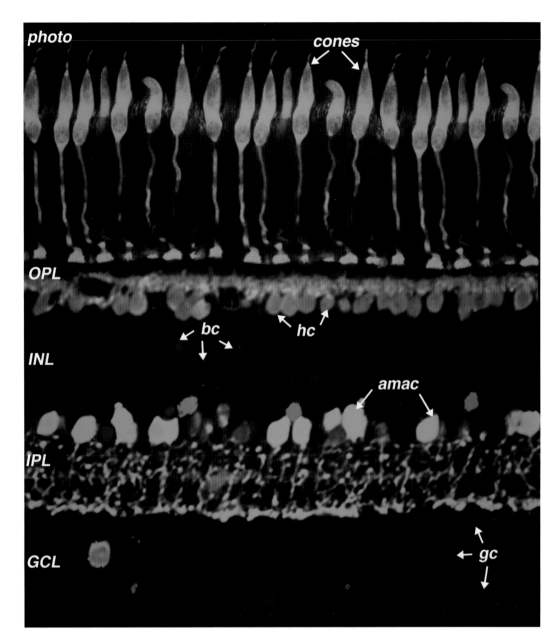

PLATE 1   Immunostained monkey retina close to the fovea. Some neurons of each of the layers are immunolabeled with antibodies against GCAP (photoreceptors), calbindin (horizontal cells and some bipolar cells), calretinin (AII amacrine cells and two other varieties of amacrine cells), and parvalbumin (ganglion cells). Photo, photoreceptor layer—rods and cones; OPL, outer plexiform layer; bc, bipolar cells; hc, horizontal cells; INL, inner nuclear layer; amac, amacrine cells; IPL, inner plexiform layer; GCL, ganglion cell layer; gc, ganglion cells. (See figure 6.4.)

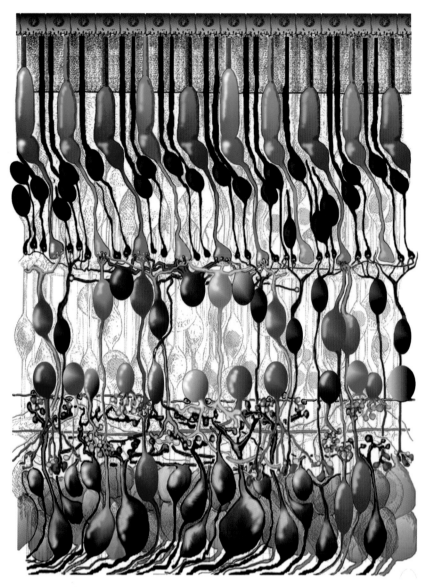

PLATE 2   A drawing of a slice of the human retina showing all the nerve cells we currently understand on the basis of their shape, function, and neurocircuitry. The photoreceptors lie deep at the back of the retina against the pigment epithelial cells (top of drawing), and the ganglion cells lie at the superficial surface of the retina (bottom of drawing). Bipolar cells and horizontal and amacrine cells pack the middle of the retina with two plexiform layers dividing them, where synaptic interactions take place. (See figure 6.5.)

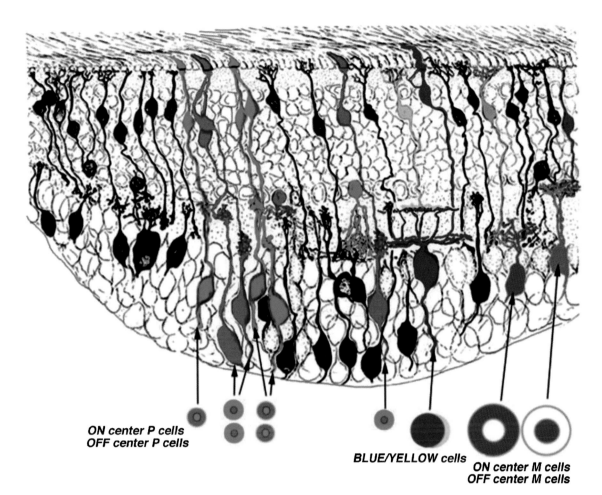

ON center P cells
OFF center P cells

BLUE/YELLOW cells

ON center M cells
OFF center M cells

PLATE 3 A drawing, based on an original from Polyak (1941), showing the neurocircuitry of the fovea in the primate retina. Midget or P cell pathways consist of a single cone, two midget bipolar cells, and two midget ganglion cells. Because P cells carry information from only one cone, it will also be spectrally tuned. Red and green cones pass either ON center/OFF surround information or OFF center/ON surround information concerning which are both spectrally and spatially opponent (small red and green circles and rings). Blue cones have their own pathway through a dedicated blue ON center bipolar cell feeding to the lower dendrites of a bistratified blue/yellow ganglion cell type. The yellow message carried to the top tier of the bistratified ganglion cells dendrites comes from a diffuse bipolar cell (yellow) that contacts green and red cones. M ganglion cells of the fovea carry a message from diffuse ON center or OFF center bipolar cells (orange and brown bipolar cells) and form the parallel OFF and ON center, achromatic channels (gray and white circles and rings) concerned with movement and contrast to the brain. (See figure 6.11.)

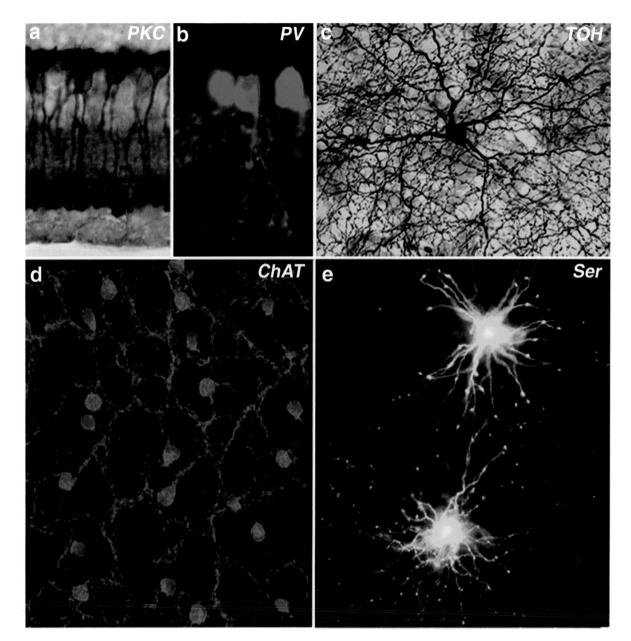

PLATE 4 A, An immunostained image of rod bipolar cells immunostained with antibodies against protein kinase c (PKC). B, Small-field bistratified AII amacrine cells are immunostained with antibodies to parvalbumin (PV). C, Dopamine-containing cells are immunostained with antibodies to tyrosine hydroxylase (TOH) as seen in a flat mount of the retina. Thousands of dopamine cell processes cross each other and make a dense network of processes in the top part of the inner plexiform layer, to synapse on various cell types, among them the AII amacrine cell. D, Two mirror symmetric amacrine cell populations, known as starburst cells, are immunostained for their acetylcholine neurotransmitter (ChAT) and seen in flat mount of retina. One set of starburst cells sits in the ganglion cell layer, and the other sits in the amacrine cell layer. Their respective dendritic plexi run and synapse in sublamina b and sublamina a. Starburst amacrine cells are thought to influence ganglion cells to be able to transmit messages concerning direction of movement in the visual field. These cells are particularly well developed in animals with visual streaks in their retinas. E, A17 amacrine cells immunolabeled with antibodies to serotonin (Ser) and also to GABA. A17 cells connect rod bipolar axon terminals in reciprocal GABAc receptor–activated circuits across the entire retina. (E from Vaney DI: Many diverse types of retinal neurons show tracer coupling when injected with biocytin or Neurobiotin. *Vision Res* 1998; 38:1359–1369.) (See figure 6.14.)

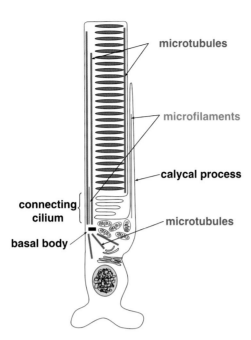

PLATE 5   The cytoskeleton of photoreceptors is composed principally of microtubules and microfilaments. The axoneme in the connecting cilium is composed of nine microtubule doublets, typical of nonmotile sensory cilia, and project to nearly the distal end of the outer segment. Microfilaments are found in the connecting cilia as well. In the inner segment, microtubules form the molecular train tracks between the Golgi complex and the connecting cilium. (See figure 7.2.)

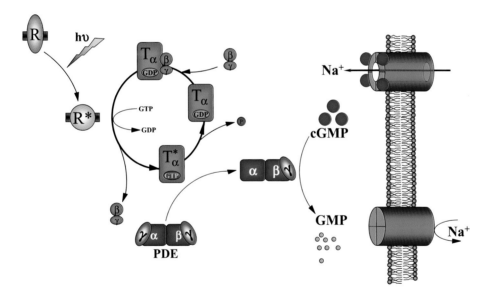

PLATE 6   The activation cascade of the phototransduction pathway. Light is absorbed by rhodopsin (R). Photoactivated rhodopsin (R*) binds heterotrimeric transducin (T), catalyzing the exchange of GTP for GDP on the α-subunit. Activated transducin removes an inhibitory subunit from the cGMP phosphodiesterase (PDE), which hydrolyzes cGMP to GMP. Reduction of cGMP causes the cyclic nucleotide-gated channels to close. (See figure 7.3.)

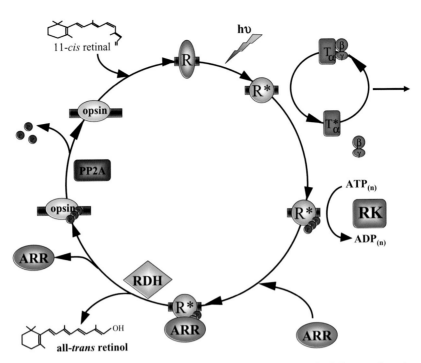

PLATE 7   The rhodopsin cycle. Light is absorbed by rhodopsin (R), becoming photoactivated (R*). R* is phosphorylated on C-terminal serine and threonine residues by rhodopsin kinase (RK). Phosphorylated, photoactivated rhodopsin is bound by arrestin, blocking the ability of R*P to bind to transducin (T). Arrestin remains bound until the all-*trans* retinal chromophore is reduced by a retinal dehydrogenase (RDH) to all-*trans* retinol and released from the phospho-opsin. The phospho-opsin is dephosphorylated by protein phosphatase 2A (PP2A) and opsin regenerated back to rhodopsin by the binding a new 11-*cis* retinal molecule. (See figure 7.4.)

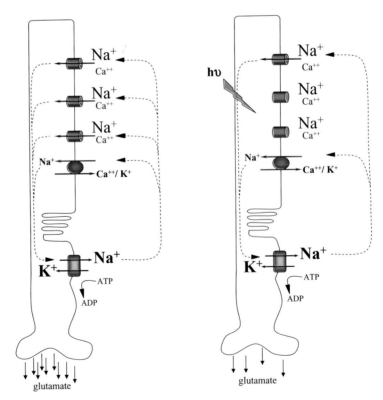

PLATE 8   Ion circulation across the photoreceptor membrane. In the dark photoreceptor, cGMP-gated channels are open, allowing influx of Na^+ and Ca^{2+} ions. Calcium balance is maintained by the action of a Na^+/Ca^{2+} exchanger, which uses the Na^+ gradient to extrude Ca^{2+}. The sodium balance is maintained by a Na^+/K^+ pump, which uses ATP to return Na^+ against its ionic gradient. In response to light, one or more cGMP-gated channels are closed, resulting in a hyperpolarization of the cell membrane, since the Na^+/K^+ pump continues to operate. Membrane hyperpolarization causes a decrease in glutamate release from the synaptic terminal. (See figure 7.5.)

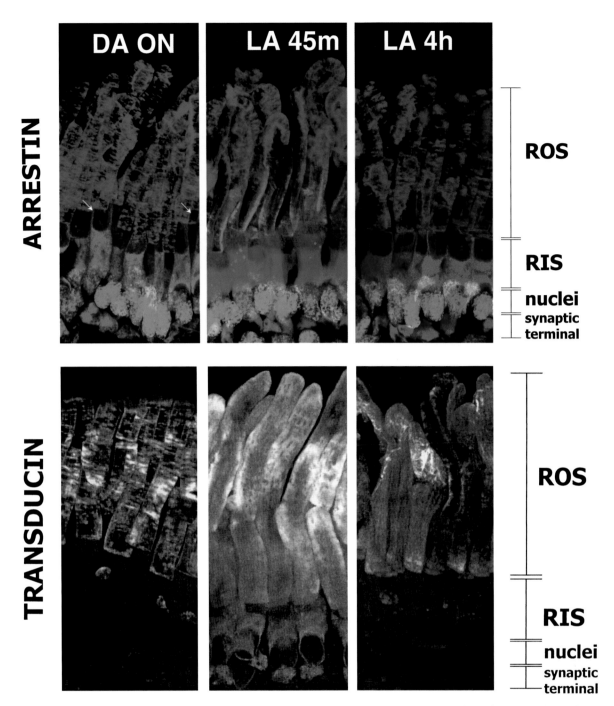

PLATE 9 Translocation of photoreceptor proteins in response to light. In a dark-adapted *Xenopus* retina, arrestin (upper panels) immunolocalizes to the inner segments, axonemes (arrows), and synaptic terminals. Transducin (lower panels) immunolocalizes to the outer segments. In response to 45 minutes of adapting light, there is a massive translocation of the proteins, with arrestin moving to the outer segments and transducin moving to the inner segments. In *Xenopus*, if the frog is maintained in the adapting light for an extended period of time (>2 hours), the proteins translocate back to their respective cellular compartments. (See figure 7.8.)

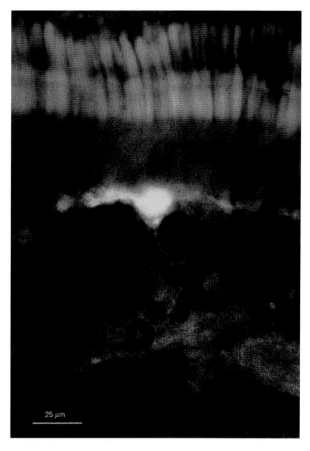

PLATE 10 Radial section of a dogfish retina viewed in a fluorescence microscope. In the center of the field is a rod bipolar cell injected with the fluorescent dye in situ after recording light responses, as in Figure 8.1. In the upper part of the photomicrograph, the autofluorescent rod outer segments can be seen. The larger bipolar cell dendrites extending through the outer plexiform layer have filled with fluorescent dye. The fine axon of the bipolar cell can be traced deep into the inner plexiform layer, terminating as a bulbous knob (calibration bar 25 μm). The large size of the cell body enabled stable recordings to be made. (Source: From Ashmore JF, Falk G: Responses of rod bipolar cells in the dark-adapt retina of the dogfish, *Scyliorhinus canicula. J Physiol (Lond)* 1980; 300:115–150. Used by permission.) (See figure 8.2.)

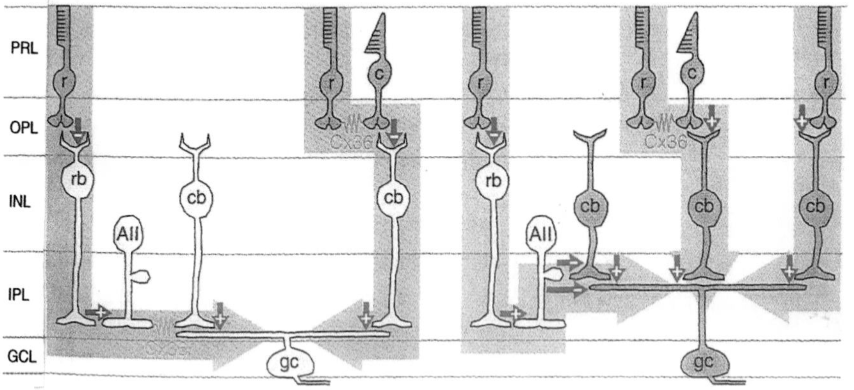

Rod signaling pathways

PLATE 11 Mammalian retinal signaling pathways. On-pathways are shown in green, off-pathways in blue (and are labeled ON or OFF above). Synapses are shown by arrows with (+) indicating sign conserving and (–) sign indicating reversing. Dark gray cells hyperpolarize in response to light. Gap junctions are indicated in red. Symbols: r, rod; c, cone; rb, rod bipolar cell; AII, amacrine cell; gc, ganglion cell; PRL photo-receptor layer; OPL, outer plexiform layer; INL, inner nuclear layer; GCL ganglion cell layer. Horizontal cells have been excluded from the diagram. (Source: Reproduced from Demb JB, Pugh EN: Connexin36 forms synapses essential for night vision. *Neuron* 2002; 336:551–553. Used by permission.) (See figure 8.7.)

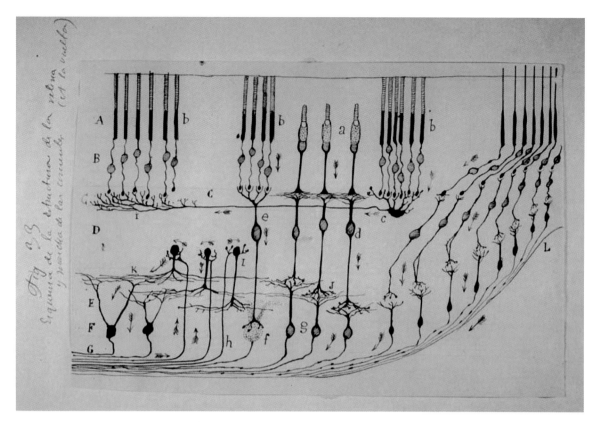

PLATE 12   Santiago Ramón y Cajal's schematic drawing of the parafoveal region of the vertebrate retina. In this illustration, Cajal demonstrates his insight into the connectivity of the retina and the dynamic polarization of retinal neurons and consequently information transfer from photoreceptors to bipolar cells and ganglion cells. In addition to vertical organization, Cajal illustrates the lateral pathways. A, Inner and outer segments. B, Outer nuclear layer. C, Outer plexiform layer. D, Inner nuclear layer. E, Inner plexiform layer. F, Ganglion cell layer. G, Nerve fiber layer. b, rods; a, cones; c, horizontal cell; d, cone bipolar cells; e, rod bipolar cell; g, ganglion cell; h, centrifugal fiber. (Note: Not all suggestions implicit in this prescient drawing have been found correct. For example, rod bipolars do not make direct contact with ganglion cells—see text.) (Source: The original figure is in the collection of the Cajal Institute, CSIC, Madrid.) (See figure 9.1.)

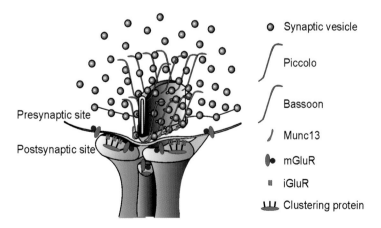

- ⊙ Synaptic vesicle
- ∫ Piccolo
- ∫ Bassoon
- / Munc13
- ⊩ mGluR
- ▥ iGluR
- � Clustering protein

PLATE 13   Diagrammatic scheme of the molecular organization of the photoreceptor synapse is shown. The ribbon (large, gray, saclike structure) is studded with synaptic vesicles; in association with the ribbon are cytomatrix molecules bassoon and piccolo; Munc13 is seen at the release site. Ribeye, not shown in this figure, labels the ribbon itself. Directly opponent to the release site are the molecules of the transmitter response cascade; these include both iontropic (IGluR) and metabotropic (mGluR) glutamate receptors and clustering molecules. Outside the release area, other molecules are expressed, including various cell adhesion molecules and, in the photoreceptor, glumate receptors. (Source: This figure was kindly supplied by Dr. J. H. Brandstätter for use in this chapter.) (See figure 9.4.)

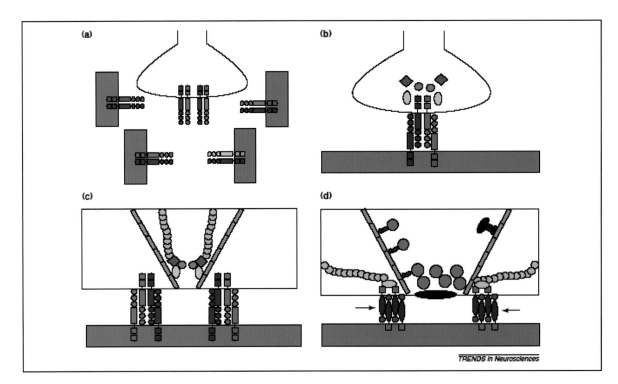

PLATE 14   The process of target recognition and synapse formation is idealized in this cartoon. Presynaptic terminals express certain target recognition molecules on their leading processes; here, these are conceived of as homophilic binding molecules (such as CAM, nectins, or sidekicks). Target selection is based on the expression of homophilic partners on the postsynaptic (A to B transition); on binding to the postsynaptic receptor pair, a variety of proteins are recruited to the synapse (B, colored circles and diamonds); these ele-ments produce a reorganization of the cytoskeleton (actin and micro-tubule, gray circles and rods, respectively) and assembly of the ele-ments of the release mechanism, including the synaptic vesicle (green circles), and proteins of the release cascade (black ovals). Homophilic molecules and other molecules (arrows) are recruited to stabilize the synapse. (Source: Figure 2 from Ackley BD, Jin Y: Genetic analysis of synaptic target recognition and assembly. *Trends Neurosci* 2004; 27:540–547.) (See figure 9.5.)

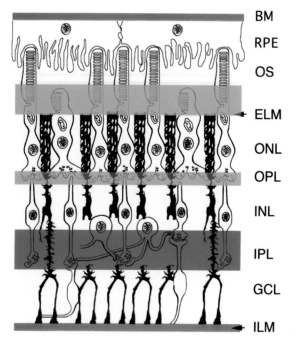

BM

RPE

OS

ELM

ONL

OPL

INL

IPL

GCL

ILM

PLATE 15   This cartoon illustrates the various cell adhesion compartments of the retina; two true basement membranes are illustrated (red): Bruch's (BM) and the inner limiting membrane (ILM). These basement membranes form the adhesion substrate for the basal side of the retinal pigmented epithelium (RPE) and the endfeet of the Müller cells (black cells). These are known to contain many elements of epithelial basement membranes, including collagen type IV, laminins (many), and nidogen. Cell adhesion molecules expressed here include integrins, CAMs, and cadherins. In green are the matrices surrounding the photoreceptor; these do not contain either collagen type IV or nidogen but do contain other critical ECM molecules, including laminins, usherin, crumbs, and various heparin sulfates. Recep-tor molecules in these compartments include various CAM such as side-kicks, integrins, and transmembrane collagens. Genetic disruptions of these molecules lead to photoreceptor dysmorphogenesis and degeneration. The blue indicates the matrix compartment in the IPL. The matrix components expressed here are not well established; on the other hand, some CAM mol-ecules, such as sidekicks, are found here. The mechanisms that control lam-ination and dendrite elongation are just coming under study (see the papers from the Masland and Wong laboratories). (Source: This figure is taken from the authors' work; it was published in Libby RT et al.: Laminin expres-sion in adult and develping retinae: Evidence of two novel CNS laminins. *J Neurosci* 2000; 20:6517–6528.) (See figure 9.6.)

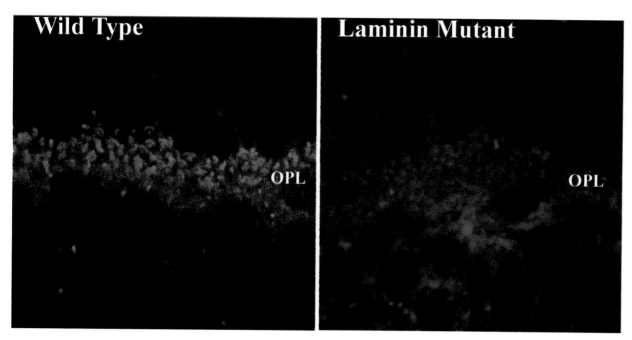

PLATE 16 Laminin deletion results in a disruption of the transsynaptic molecular organization of the photoreceptor synapse. Immunohistochemical localization of the bassoon (red) and mGluR6 (blue) in wild-type retina demonstrates the normal arrangement of molecules. Bassoon, associated with the ribbon, is directly opponent to mGluR6, the transmitter receptor that is expressed in invaginating bipolar cells. In the laminin-mutant (β2 null) mouse, both molecules are expressed by mGluR6 is delocalized and not concentrated at the synapse. (Source: This is taken from the author's unpublished work.) (See figure 9.9.)

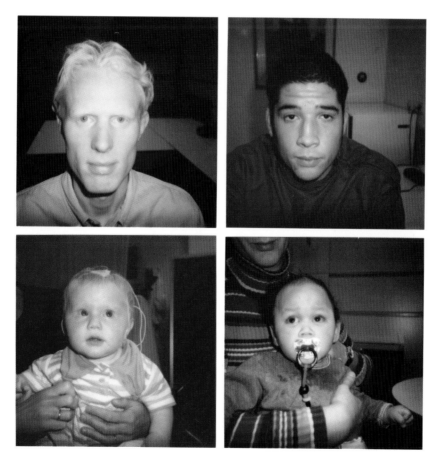

PLATE 17 Variable genotype and phenotype in a representative sample of albinos including autosomal-recessive oculocutaneous, tyrosinase-negative albinism (left column), X-chromosomal ocular albinism, and autosomal-recessive oculocutaneous, tyrosinase-positive albinism (right column). Foveal hypoplasia, reduced visual acuity, and VEP optic pathway misrouting are common features regardless of inheritance mode or phenotypic expression. (See figure 25.1.)

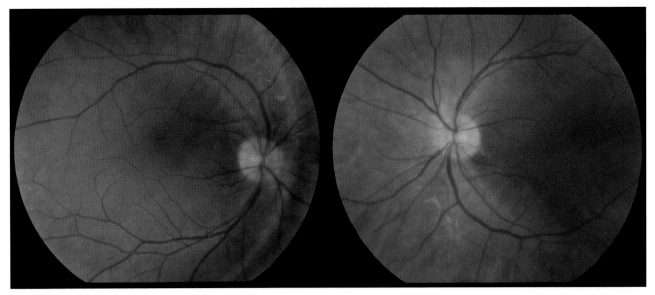

A

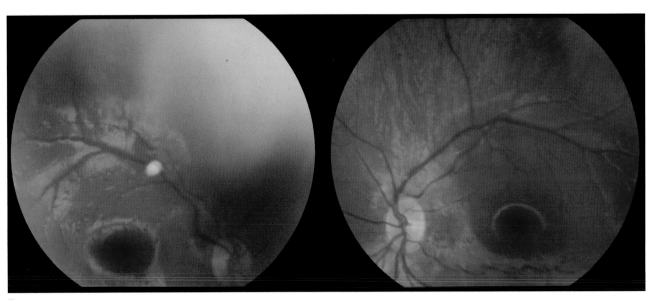

B

PLATE 18   Fundi of left and right eye (A) of an 18-year-old albino and (B) of a 16-year-old achiasmat. For comparison, note the presence of foveal hypoplasia only in the albino fundi; foveal hypoplasia, characteristic to albinism, is absent in the achiasmat. (See figure 25.2.)

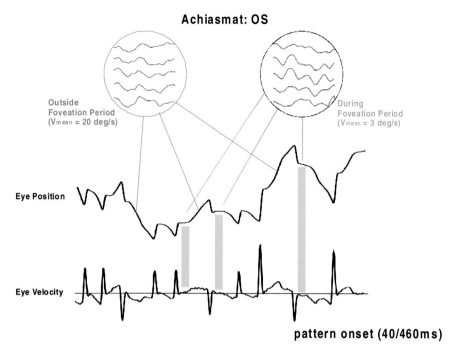

Achiasmat: OS

Outside
Foveation Period
(V_{mean} = 20 deg/s)

During
Foveation Period
(V_{mean} = 3 deg/s)

Eye Position

Eye Velocity

pattern onset (40/460ms)

PLATE 19 Schematic of an eye movement recording of a patient with CN. Vertical yellow bars indicate foveation periods when retinal velocity approaches zero. This can readily be observed from the lower velocity trace. Two sets of VEP averages are depicted: one obtained from VEP responses following visual stimulation outside foveation periods and another obtained from VEP responses following visual stimulation during foveation periods. The latter are significantly more robust. (See figure 25.14.)

Albino

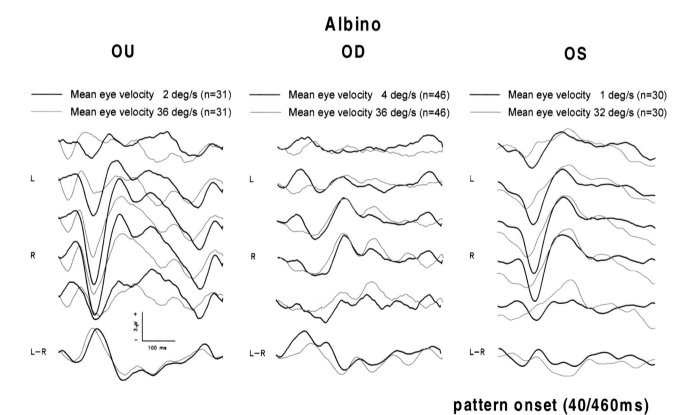

OU

── Mean eye velocity 2 deg/s (n=31)
── Mean eye velocity 36 deg/s (n=31)

OD

── Mean eye velocity 4 deg/s (n=46)
── Mean eye velocity 36 deg/s (n=46)

OS

── Mean eye velocity 1 deg/s (n=30)
── Mean eye velocity 32 deg/s (n=30)

L

R

L−R

pattern onset (40/460ms)

PLATE 20 Depicted are VEP averages (black traces) in an albino during OU, OD, and OS viewing extracted from periods with low mean ocular velocity (less than 5 degrees/second). Also depicted are VEP averages (red traces) extracted from responses to pattern-onset stimulation during high mean ocular velocity. Five channels positioned across the occiput and one difference channel (i.e., VEP channel 4 positioned at left occiput subtracted from VEP channel 2 positioned at right occiput) also are presented. (See figure 25.15.)

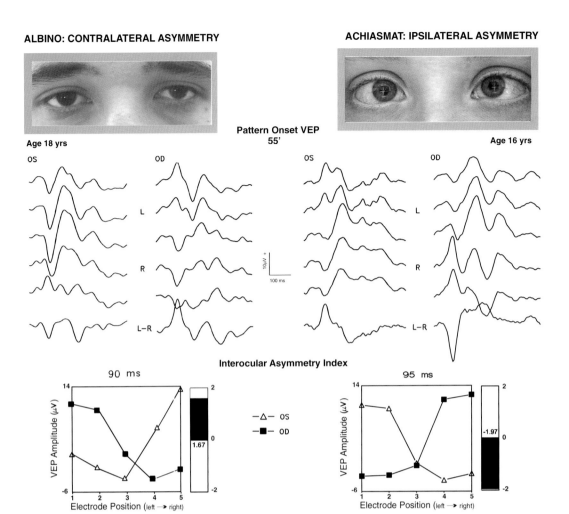

ALBINO: CONTRALATERAL ASYMMETRY

Age 18 yrs

ACHIASMAT: IPSILATERAL ASYMMETRY

Age 16 yrs

Pattern Onset VEP
55'

OS   OD   OS   OD

L

R

L-R

10μV +
100 ms

Interocular Asymmetry Index

90 ms   95 ms

PLATE 21 VEP misrouting test. Left eye (OS), and right eye (OD) pattern onset/offset (40 ms/460 ms) VEP responses (check size = 55′) from an X-chromosomal ocular albino (left panel) and a patient with nondecussating retinal-fugal fiber syndrome (right panel). Fundi of both patients are shown in figures 25.2A and 25.2B, respectively. VEP amplitude distribution across the electrode array for OD and OS stimulation is depicted below the VEP traces. In the case of contralateral asymmetry (left) in the albino, following left eye stimulation (OS), a major positive peak of the pattern onset response lateralizes to the right occiput, and with right eye stimu-

lation, a major positive peak lateralizes to the left occiput. This interocular occipital lateralization yields a highly significant interocular asymmetry index of 1.67 at 90 ms. For comparison, occipital lateralization in an achiasmat is also presented. In the case of ipsilateral asymmetry (right) in an achiasmat, following left eye stimulation (OS), a major positive peak of the pattern onset response lateralizes to the left occiput, and with right eye stimulation, a major positive peak lateralizes to the right occiput. This rare interocular ipsilateral VEP response lateralization results in a highly significant interocular asymmetry index of −1.97 at 90 ms. (See figure 25.18.)

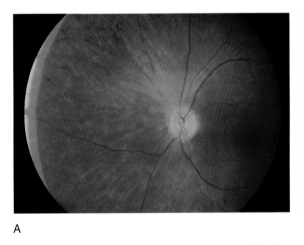

A

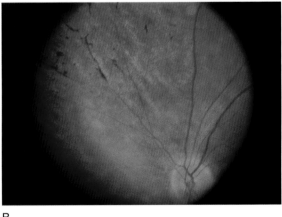

B

PLATE 22 Serial fundus photographs of the same patient dated 1986 (A) and 1994 (B) showing increased retinal pigmentation from salt-and-pepper retinopathy to frank bone spiculing. Note that the

magnification in part B is higher, showing more central encroachment of the pigmentary changes. Both images demonstrate substantial arterial attenuation. (See figure 55.2.)

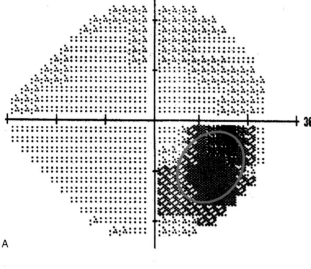

A

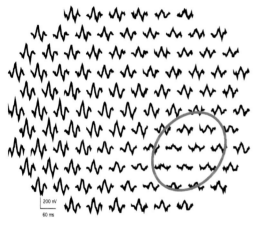

B

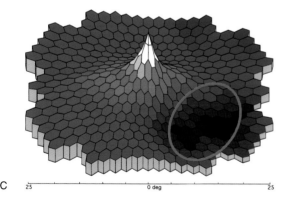

C

PLATE 23 Central serous chorioretinopathy. A, An eccentric serous detachment superior to the optic disk causes a localized visual field defect inferior to the physiologic blind spot. B,C: Attenuation of the multifocal ERG is seen in the region corresponding to the visual field defect. (Courtesy of Donald Hood, Ph.D.) (See figure 57.2.)

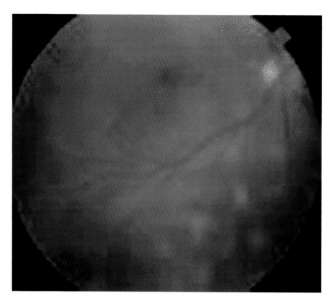

PLATE 24 Birdshot chorioretinitis. Pale fundus lesions are neither raised nor depressed relative to the surrounding retina. (Courtesy of Alan Friedman, M.D.) (See figure 57.3.)

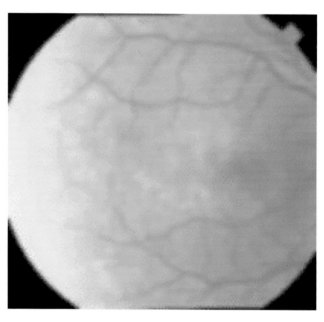

PLATE 25 Multiple evanescent white dot syndrome (MEWDS). Pale white dots are seen early in the course of the disorder. (Courtesy of Wayne Fuchs, M.D.) (See figure 57.4.)

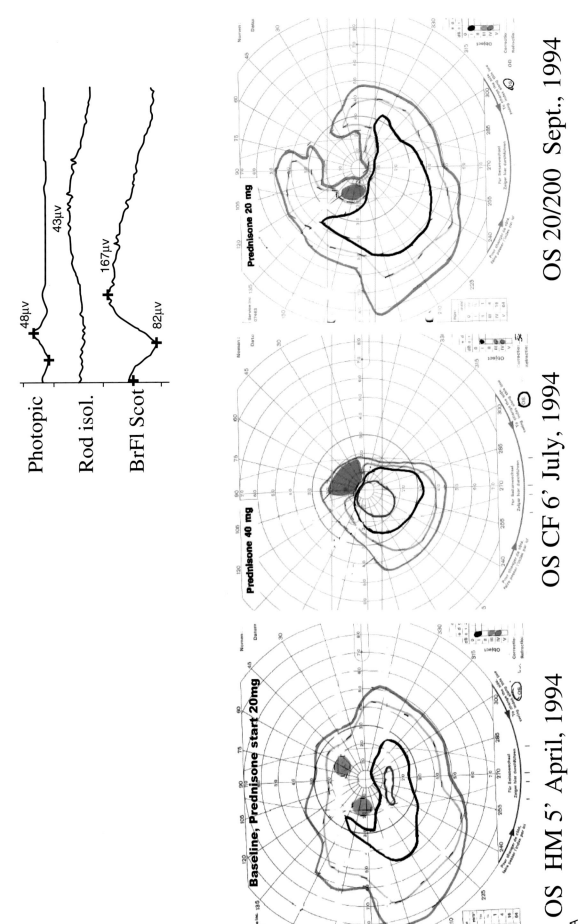

Electroretinogram April, 1994

Photopic 48μv 43μv

Rod isol. 167μv

BrFl Scot 82μv

Baseline, Prednisone start 20mg
OS HM 5' April, 1994

Prednisone 40 mg
OS CF 6' July, 1994

Prednisone 20 mg
OS 20/200 Sept., 1994

A

PLATE 26 Cases of CAR syndrome. A, Case 1. Eighty-four-year-old man who was found to have colon carcinoma in October 1994. No vision in OD from advanced glaucoma. Found to have CAR in April 1994. Relatively low doses of prednisone gave good visual recovery. Larger doses would be used today. (See figure 58.1A.)

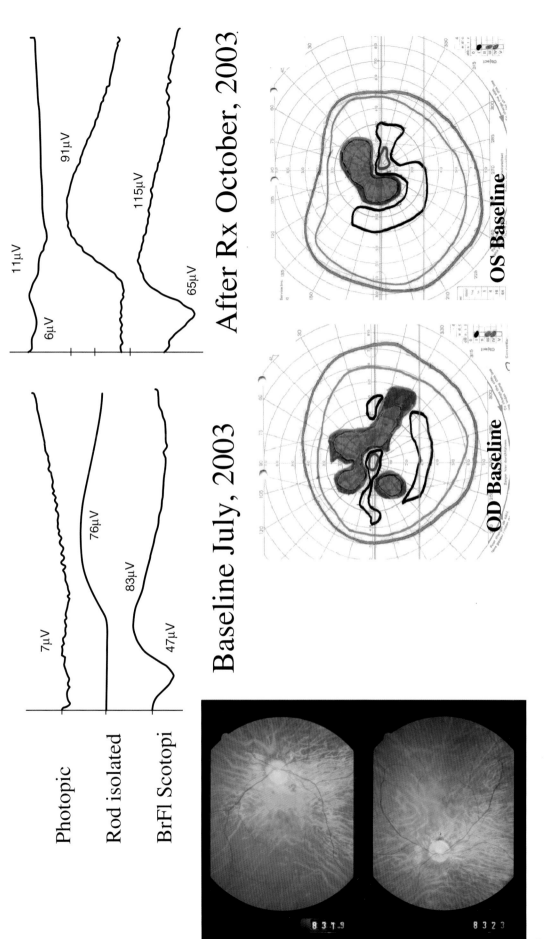

After Rx October, 2003

11μV

91μV

115μV

6μV

65μV

Baseline July, 2003

7μV

76μV

83μV

47μV

Photopic

Rod isolated

BrFl Scotopi

OS Baseline

OD Baseline

8 3 1 9

8 3 2 3

B

Plate 27   B, Case 2. Seventy-one-year-old woman with ovarian carcinoma found in October 2002. Vision was severely diminished six months later. She was placed on 60 mg prednisone, 100 mg Immuran, and 100 mg cyclosporine. ERG values increased, while Goldmann visual fields remained the same on follow-up visit. Fundus showed diffuse atrophy without pigment deposits. (See figure 58.1B.)

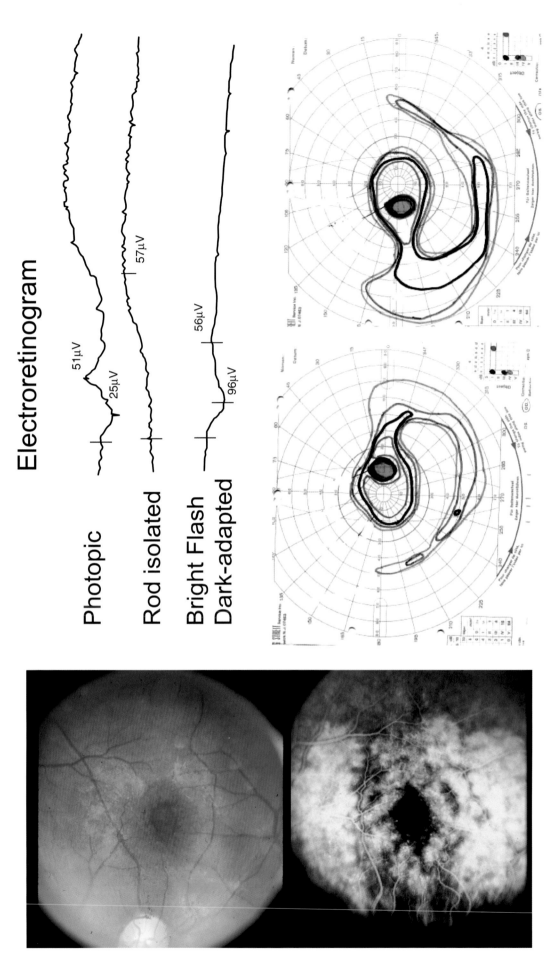

PLATE 28   Forty-two-year-old woman with CAR-like syndrome and severe cystic edema of the posterior pole and no pigment deposits in the periphery. This patient had antirecoverin antibodies with bands of activity to seven other retinal proteins. There was no history of cancer. (See figure 58.2.)

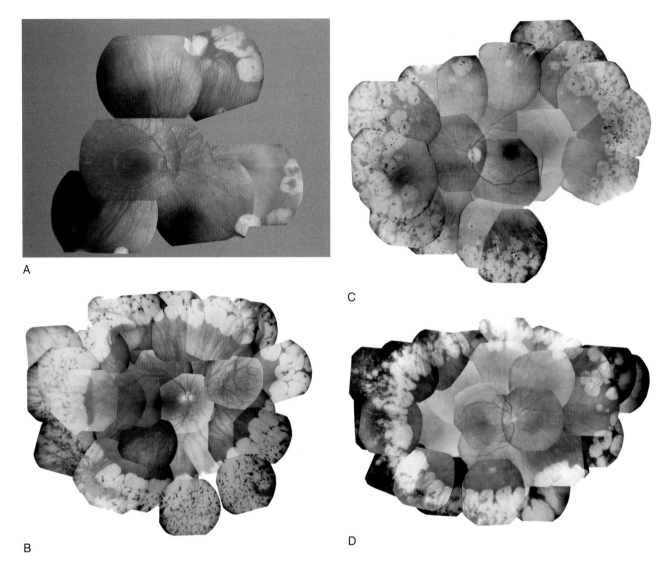

A

B

C

D

PLATE 29   Fundus appearance of right eye of a 12-year-old girl with early pyridoxine-nonresponsive gyrate atrophy (A) (same patient as in figure 12.1 in Weleber and Kennaway), a 28-year-old woman with pyridoxine-responsive gyrate atrophy (B) (patient 1), a 37-year-old woman with pyridoxine-responsive gyrate atrophy (C) (patient 3), and a 40-year-old man with pyridoxine-nonresponsive gyrate atrophy (D) (patient 4). (From Weleber RG, Kennaway NG: Gyrate atrophy of the choroid and retina. In Heckenlively JR (ed): *Retinitis Pigmentosa*. Philadelphia, JB Lippincott, 1988, pp 198–220. Used by permission.) (See figure 60.4.)

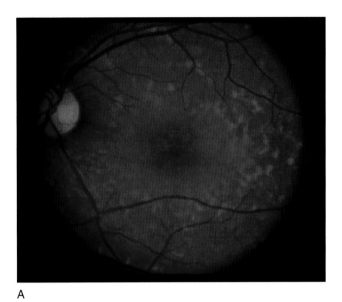

A

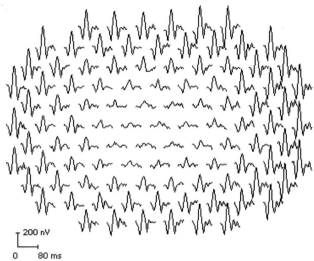

200 nV

0   80 ms

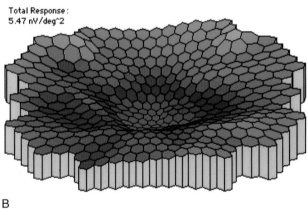

Total Response:
5.47 nV/deg^2

B

PLATE 30   A, Fundus photo from left eye showing lipofuscin accumulation within the posterior pole. B, mfERG from same patient showing selective loss of responses from the central 10 degrees. (See figure 62.2)

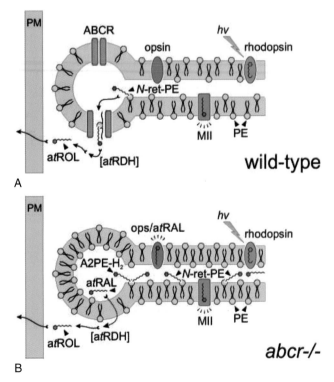

PLATE 31   Model for the function of RmP (ABCR) protein in disk membranes. A, Wild-type, in which ABCT is a transporter (flippase) for N-ret-PE. B, *abcr*−/− mouse (and patients with reduced flippase activity). N-ret-PE trapped in the disk combines with a second molecule of all-*trans*-retinal to produce A2PE-H₂. A2PE-H₂ is ultimately hydrolyzed to form A2E. Many of these reactions occur in the RPE after disks containing the excessive trapped A2PE-H₂ are shed as part of the normal phagocytotic process. The A2E accumulates as lipofuscin in the RPE and may ultimately damage intracellular membranes and destroy the overburdened RPE cells within the macula. A2E: N-retinylidene-N-retinyl-ethanolamine; A2PE-H₂: N-retinylidene-N-retinyl-PE; a*t*RAL: all-*trans*-retinal; a*t*RDH: all-*trans*-retinal dehydrogenase; a*t*ROL: all-*trans*-retinol; ops: opsin; PE: phosphatidylethanolamine; PM: plasma membrane. (From Weng J, Mata NL, Azarian SM, Tzekov RT, Birch DG, Travis GH: Insights into the function of Rim protein in photoreceptors and etiology of Stargardt's disease from the phenotype in abcr knockout mice. *Cell* 1999; 98:13–23.) (See figure 62.3.)

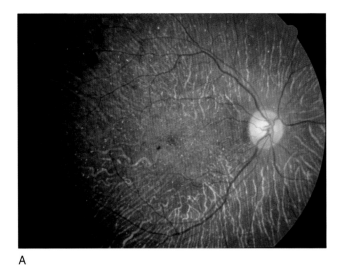
A

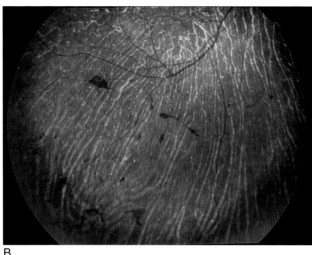
B

PLATE 32 Same patient as in figure 63.1 at 45 years of age (A and B). Note the further loss of pigment epithelium and choriocapillaris over the nine-year interval. (From Wilson DJ et al: Bietti's crystalline dystrophy: A clinicopathological correlative study. *Arch Ophthalmol* 1989; 107:213–221. Used by permission.) (See figure 63.2.)

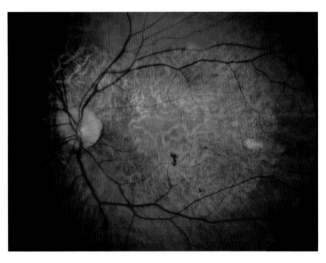

PLATE 33 Fundus appearance of a 61-year-old man with the regional form of Bietti's crystalline dystrophy (patient 3 in Wilson DJ et al: Bietti's crystalline dystrophy: A clinicopathological correlative study. *Arch Ophthalmol* 1989; 107:213–221.). The visual fields had not changed over those determined nine years previously, but the visual acuity had decreased from 20/30 J1 to 20/40 J2. (See figure 63.6A.)

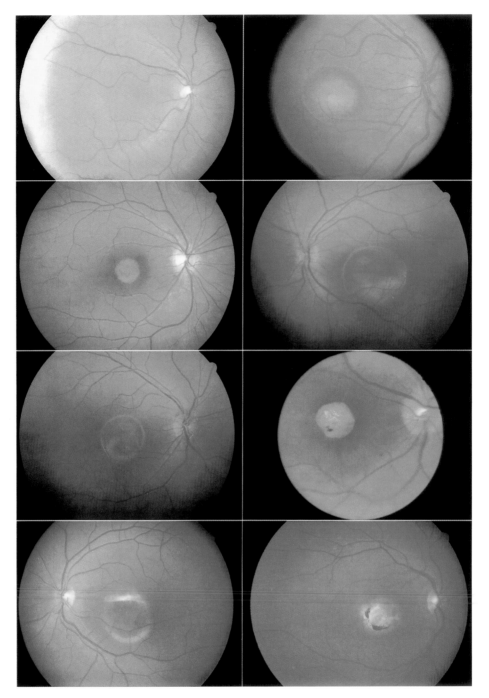

PLATE 34 Fundus photographs representing various stages of macular lesions that can be observed in patients with Best macular dystrophy. Top left, Stage I: mild degree of foveal pigment mottling and nonspecific hypopigmentation. Top right, Stage II: typical vitelliform or egg-yolk-like lesion. Second row left, Stage IIIa: scrambled or "fried egg" phase as the vitelliform lesion becomes diffusely more amorphous and diluted in appearance. Second row right, Stage IIIb: pseudohypopyon phase in which the yellow substance in the vitelliform cyst develops a layered appearance as a consequence of partial resorption. Third row left, Stage IIIc: only a sparse amount of yellowish substance remains as resorption of the vitelliform lesion is almost complete. Third row right, Stage IIId shows atrophic changes of both the retinal pigment epithelium and choriocapillaris vessels. Bottom, Stage IV: both less and more extensive examples are depicted. Characteristic feature is a fibrotic-gliotic-appearing scar in addition resorption of the vitelliform material. (See figure 66.1.)

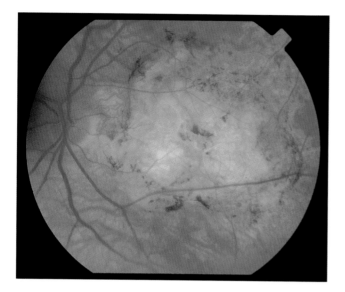

PLATE 35 Left fundus of a patient with SFD showing large disciform scar. (See figure 67.1.)

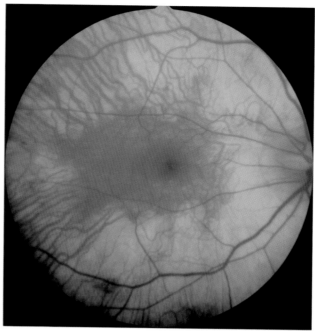

A

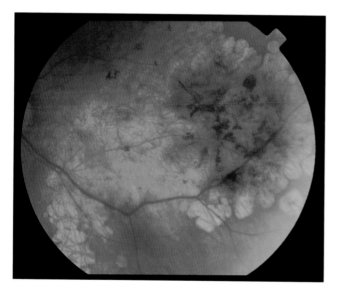

PLATE 36 Left fundus of a patient with SFD showing atrophy of the retinal pigment epithelium and choriocapillaris at the posterior pole. (See figure 67.2.)

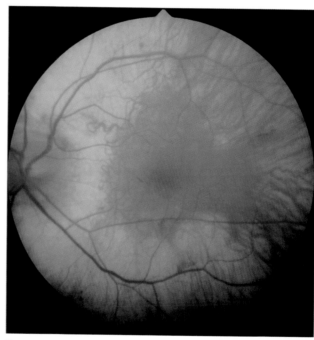

B

PLATE 37 Fundus photographs of a 17-year-old CHM affected male showing preserved deep choroidal vessels and central macula, normal-appearing retinal vessels and optic nerve, and no pigment dispersion. A, OD. B, OS. Vision: 20/20 OU. (See figure 68.1.)

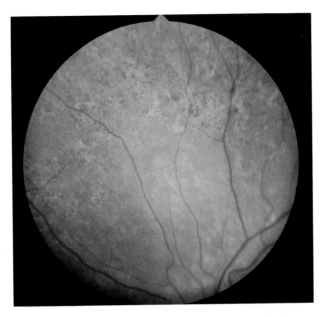

PLATE 38 Fundus photograph (nasal midperiphery) of a 29-year-old female carrier with patchy RPE changes. Vision: 20/20 OS. (See figure 68.2.)

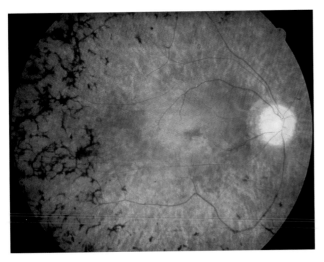

PLATE 39 Fundus photograph showing the posterior pole of a 42-year-old patient with XlRP. Note the "waxy disk," the attenuated retinal vessels, and the bone spicule–like pigmentary deposits throughout the midperiphery. (See figure 69.1.)

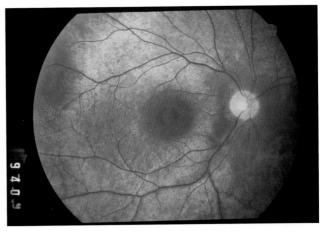

A

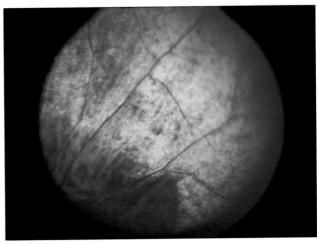

B

PLATE 40 Symmetric, round atrophy of fovea centralis is typically seen in a number of types of cone dystrophy or degeneration. A, In this case of X-linked cone dystrophy with tapetal sheen, the atrophy of the foveal centralis is highlighted by the surrounding sheen. This 54-year-old man had photosensitivity OU and a history of retinal detachment in his right eye; his visual acuity was 20/200 OU. B, While the sheen is seen as patches in the periphery. These patients exhibit the Mizuo-Nakamura effect on dark adaptation. (See figure 70.1.)

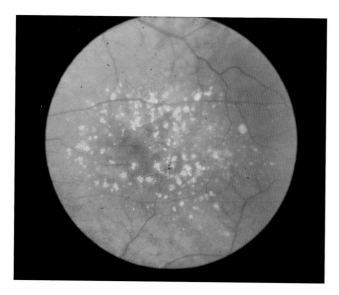

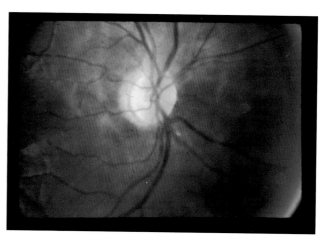

PLATE 41 Cone dystrophy with foveal crystals. Right eye of a 58-year-old woman with urban night blindness with nonrecordable photopic ERG and normal scotopic ERGs. Visual acuity was OD 20/40, OS 20/60, and Goldmann visual fields were full. (See figure 70.2.)

PLATE 43 Temporal optic nerve head atrophy is commonly seen in many cone degenerations; illustrated here by a 9-year-old boy with rod monochromatism with temporal pallor. Sometimes the temporal edge of the nerve is flattened or missing. (See figure 70.5.)

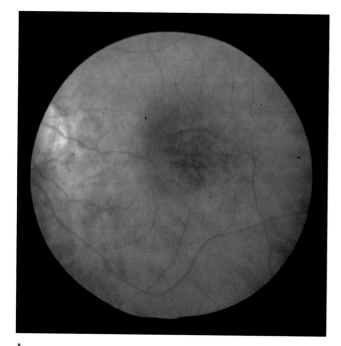

A

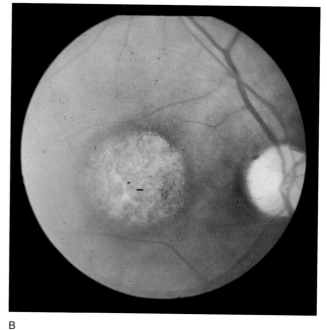

B

PLATE 42 Fundus photographs of patients with inherited cone dystrophies; A, A 60-year-old man with blue-cone monochromatism who recently noted some mild decreases in his central vision from 20/60 to 20/200, presumably from aging. B, A 54-year-old woman with 20/400 vision OU from a large dominant pedigree with cone dystrophy from a GUCY2D gene mutation, with foveal centralis atrophy giving a "cookie cutter" appearance to macula. This pattern is characteristic of many cone dystrophies. (See figure 70.4.)

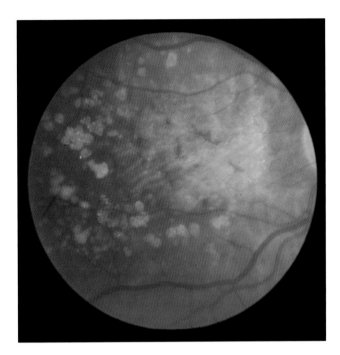

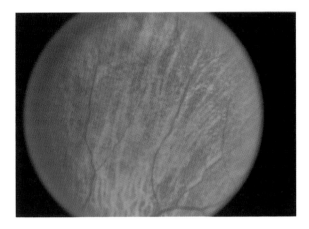

PLATE 46 Fundus photograph of a 53-year-old woman with documented vitamin A deficiency from complications secondary to bowel resection in Crohn's disease. Her barely recordable ERG and night vision became normal after parenteral vitamin A and E therapy. (Courtesy of John Heckenlively, M.D.) (See figure 71.1.)

PLATE 44 Senile cone degeneration in an 80-year-old woman with failing vision over ten years, who was found to have poor photopic ERGs with both eyes. Her right eye had a 45 uV b-wave amplitude while the left eye was barely recordable with count finger vision. Rod responses were abnormal. Visual fields were full with central scotomata. Many patients with senile cone degeneration have regional atrophy with crystallike drusen deposits. (See figure 70.7.)

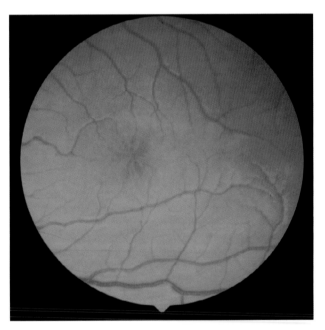

PLATE 47 Fundus photograph of XLRS-affected male with juvenile retinoschisis showing spoke-wheel pattern of foveal cysts covering an area of approximately one disk diameter. (See figure 73.1.)

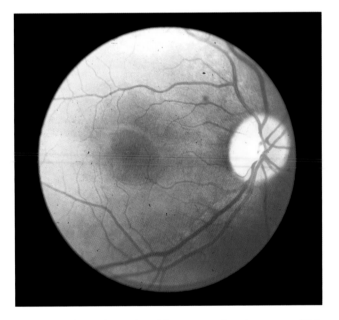

PLATE 45 Cone dystrophy with apparent foveal structure. This 22-year-old woman presented with a history of color blindness and photosensitivity for at least ten years. The family history was negative. Her vision was 20/200 OU, and her photopic ERG was nonrecordable, while her scotopic waveforms were within normal limits. Her Goldmann visual field was full OU. On fundus examination, she appeared to have some foveal structure; but on close inspection, the fovea centralis showed atrophy and mild granularity. (See figure 70.8.)

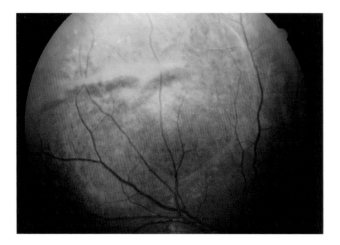

PLATE 48 Fundus photograph of XLRS-affected male with peripheral schisis cavity, which occurs in 50% of affected males. (See figure 73.2.)

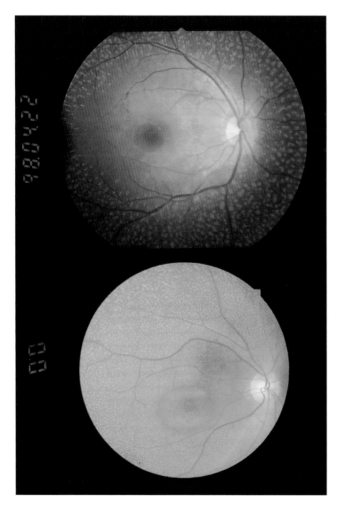

PLATE 49 Fundus photograph in fundus albipunctatus (upper) and fundus albipunctatus associated with cone dystrophy (lower). (See figure 74.9.)

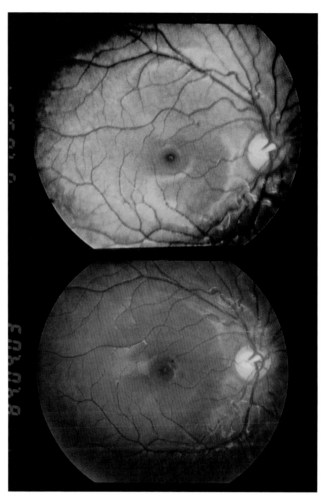

PLATE 50 Fundus photographs of Oguchi's disease in light adaptation (upper) and after a long period of dark adaptation (lower). (See figure 74.11.)

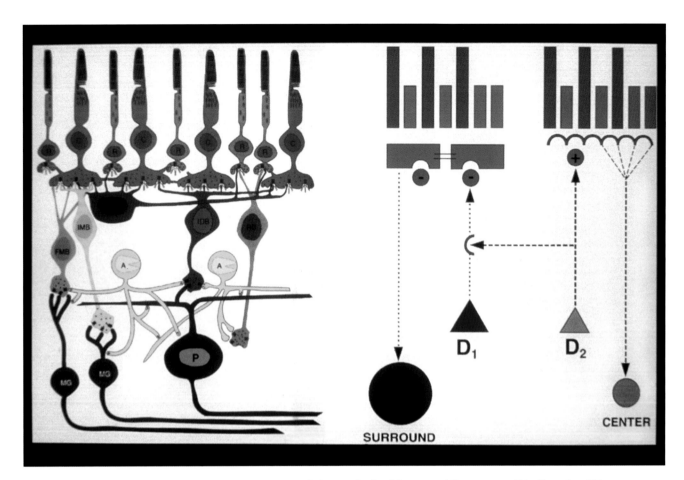

PLATE 51 Simplified schema of the D1–D2 interaction of the retina. The D1 DA pathway enhances the surround signal, while the D2 pathway enhances the center signal. Experimental results suggest that these two DA pathways are not independent of each other: D2 is involved in the D1 pathway participating in a negative feedback loop, providing a greater D1 effect when D2 receptors are blocked. (Adapted from Bodis-Wollner I, Tzelepi A: Push-pull model of dopamine's action in the retina. In Hung GK, Ciuffreda KC (eds): Models of the visual system. Kluwer Academic Publishers, 2002, pp 191–214; with permission.) (See figure 79.5.)

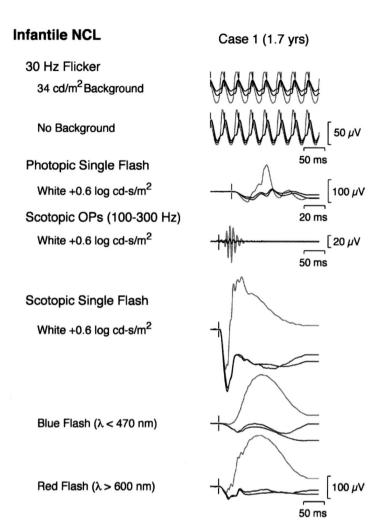

Infantile NCL

Case 1 (1.7 yrs)

30 Hz Flicker

34 cd/m^2 Background

No Background

50 µV

50 ms

Photopic Single Flash

White +0.6 log cd-s/m^2

100 µV

20 ms

Scotopic OPs (100–300 Hz)

White +0.6 log cd-s/m^2

20 µV

50 ms

Scotopic Single Flash

White +0.6 log cd-s/m^2

Blue Flash (λ < 470 nm)

Red Flash (λ > 600 nm)

100 µV

50 ms

PLATE 52   Computer-averaged ERGs, using intravenous propofol sedation, to a modified ISCEV protocol in a patient with infantile NCL from the Arg151 stop mutation of the *CLN1* gene that encodes PPT1. The tracings from the right and left eyes are shown in black; the red tracings show the average of both eyes from a normal subject age 1.6 years. The scotopic blue and red flash stimuli were matched in normal control subjects to produce equal rod amplitudes. Note the sizable rod a-wave and profoundly subnormal rod b-wave for the blue flash, the electronegative configuration of the scotopic ERG to the bright white flash, and the subnormal, prolonged photopic cone response. (Reproduced with permission from Weleber RG: The dystrophic retina in multisystem disorders: The electroretinogram in neuronal ceroid lipofuscinosis. *Eye* 1998; 12:580–590.) (See figure 80.2.)

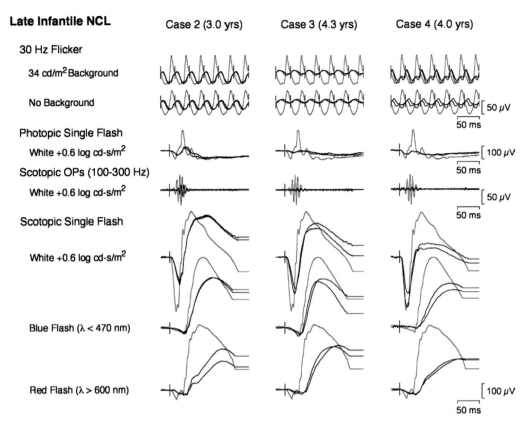

Late Infantile NCL

Case 2 (3.0 yrs) Case 3 (4.3 yrs) Case 4 (4.0 yrs)

30 Hz Flicker

34 cd/m^2 Background

No Background

50 µV

50 ms

Photopic Single Flash

White +0.6 log cd-s/m^2

100 µV

50 ms

Scotopic OPs (100-300 Hz)

White +0.6 log cd-s/m^2

50 µV

50 ms

Scotopic Single Flash

White +0.6 log cd-s/m^2

Blue Flash (λ < 470 nm)

Red Flash (λ > 600 nm)

100 µV

50 ms

PLATE 53   Computer-averaged ERGs to modified ISCEV protocol in three patients with late infantile NCL. The tracings from the right and left eyes are shown in black; the red tracings show the average of both eyes from an age-similar normal subject. Note the sizable but delayed rod responses, the prolongation of the scotopic oscillatory potentials, and the subnormal, prolonged cone responses. (Reproduced with permission from Weleber RG: The dystrophic retina in multisystem disorders: The electroretinogram in neuronal ceroid lipofuscinosis. *Eye* 1998; 12:580–590.) (See figure 80.3.)

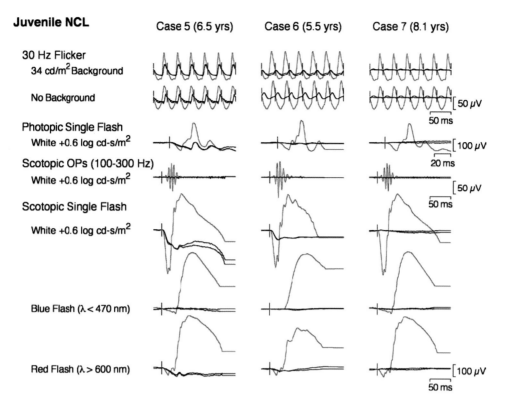

PLATE 54 Computer-averaged ERGs to a modified ISCEV protocol in three patients with juvenile NCL from mutation of the *CLN3* gene. The tracings from the right and left eyes are shown in black; the red tracings show the average of both eyes from an age-similar normal subject. All responses were elicited using the same Ganzfeld stimulator, but because a different computer system was used for recording the responses for Case 6, a different normal is shown.

Note the profoundly subnormal rod responses, the electronegative configuration of the scotopic ERG to the bright white flash for Cases 5 and 6, and the subnormal photopic responses, which were greater for the b-wave than the a-wave for Case 5. (Reproduced with permission from Weleber RG: The dystrophic retina in multisystem disorders: The electroretinogram in neuronal ceroid lipofuscinosis. *Eye* 1998; 12:580–590.) (See figure 80.4.)

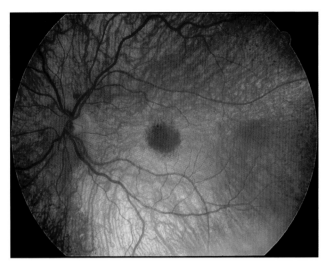

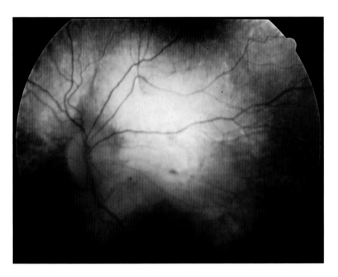

PLATE 55 Fundus appearance in 4-year-old patient with LCHAD deficiency and early retinal degeneration. Note the characteristic dark brown spot in the fovea, the early thinning and atrophy of the retinal pigment epithelium (RPE), and the early pigment dispersion with fine clumping. The ERG was still normal at this stage. (See figure 80.5.)

PLATE 56 Fundus appearance in a patient with later stage LCHAD deficiency and retinal degeneration. Note the more extensive atrophy of the RPE and choroid in the posterior pole. (See figure 80.6.)

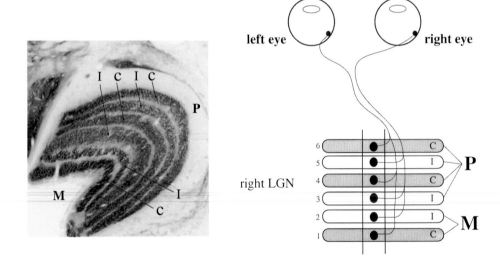

PLATE 57 Left, Vertical section of a macaque monkey LGN. Right, Interconnections with the retinas. (See text for details.) (LGN section courtesy of MLJ Crawford.) (See figure 84.2.)

mation provided by the PERG; in patient A, with "classical" RP, full-field ERGs are almost undetectable, but a normal PERG indicates macular sparing. The other two patients have variable degrees of macular involvement with a reduced and undetectable PERG, respectively; the severity of PERG P50 component reduction reflects the degree of macular involvement. Note the delayed 30-Hz flicker ERG implicit times, a common feature of generalized cone dysfunction. The mfERG is more difficult to quantify but can clearly demonstrate spared areas of macular function (figure 36.2). Patients with restricted loss of function such as may occur in sector RP or retinal detachment usually show ERGs of reduced amplitude but without implicit time shift.[1]

In one particular condition, enhanced S-cone syndrome (ESCS),[13] the predominant abnormality in the maximal ERG response can be that of implicit time and waveform change rather than amplitude. In this rare autosomal-recessive disorder, related to mutation in *NR2E3*, the retina is devoid of rods; there is an increased number of cones,[14] and the majority of those cones respond maximally to short-wavelength stimulation. The presentation is usually with life-long night blindness but may present with visual acuity loss due to foveal schisis. Goldman-Favre syndrome (GFS) has been used to describe a combination of foveal schisis and peripheral degeneration; the ERGs in GFS are usually very abnormal and may be undetectable. ESCS is characterized by pigmentary changes, maximal in relation to the arcades, but although the pigmentary deposition is nummular and at the level of the RPE rather than the intraretinal bone spicule pigment deposition of RP, the combination of pigment deposition and night blindness sometimes leads to the erroneous diagnosis of "atypical RP." There may be small areas of hyperpigmentation within the arcades that hyperfluoresce on fundus autofluorescence imaging. The ERG findings are pathognomonic (figure 36.3). The rod-specific ERG is undetectable, and the maximal ERG is both simplified and markedly delayed, with an altered waveform that shows minimal difference to the same stimulus under photopic and scotopic conditions. Additionally, the amplitude of the grossly delayed photopic 30-Hz flicker response is of lower amplitude than that of the photopic a-wave; in a normal subject, the 30-Hz amplitude falls between that of the single-flash photopic ERG a-wave and b-wave. Short-wavelength stimulation (blue on amber) elicits responses that are of much higher amplitude and altered waveform compared with normal; stimulation directed at L-/M-cone populations (long-duration orange on green) gives severely reduced responses. Note that some patients appear to show OFF-related activity with long-duration blue stimulation, not a feature usually associated with short-wavelength cones. This raises the possibility that the S-cones that predominate in the retina are atypical and/or may not have the intraretinal wiring anticipated for that type of photoreceptor. Some patients, particularly with increasing age, show the characteristic features described above, but there can be marked overall amplitude reduction. In common with other inherited disorders, there can be marked interindividual phenotypic variability in amplitude (figure 36.3).

Normal maximal ERG response, abnormal cone ERGs: cone dysfunction

Much less common than those conditions that affect both rod and cone photoreceptors, some disorders are confined to the cone system. In such cases, the rod-specific ERG is normal, and there is a normal or near-normal maximal ERG response, but the cone ERGs are profoundly abnormal. The cone dystrophies usually have abnormalities of flicker response implicit time (e.g., figure 36.4), although there are some exceptions,[3] and eventually, there may be mild rod system involvement. Two stationary inherited disorders of cone function may have no detectable cone flicker ERG at an early age. These are rod monochromacy and S-cone (blue cone) monochromacy. Although there may be clinical distinguishing features, the electrophysiological distinction is suggested by conventional ERG. The single-flash photopic ERG shows some preservation in S-cone monochromacy, and this can be confirmed by the use of short-wavelength stimulation (figure 36.4). Measures of central retinal function, such as the PERG, are profoundly abnormal. Many of these patients have involuntary eye movement disorders, and it may be difficult to obtain technically satisfactory mfERG or PERG recordings.

Abnormal rod-specific b-wave, (electro-) negative maximal ERG response: dysfunction postphototransduction

The presence of a negative maximal ERG response, in which a normal a-wave is accompanied by a markedly reduced b-wave, indicates dysfunction post-phototransduction. There are many causes of a negative ERG, including congenital stationary night blindness (CSNB), X-linked juvenile retinoschisis, and central retinal artery occlusion (CRAO) (see also chapter 72). The negative ERG in CRAO reflects the duality of the blood supply to the retina; the photoreceptors are supplied via choroidal circulation, whereas the inner nuclear layer of the retina is supplied via the central retinal artery. Thus, the ERG b-wave, which arises in the inner nuclear layer, is abnormal, but the a-wave of the maximal response, reflecting photoreceptor function, is spared. In the cone system, S-cones, similar to rods, connect to depolarizing (ON) bipolar cells, whereas L- and M-cones also have an OFF pathway via hyperpolarizing bipolar cells.

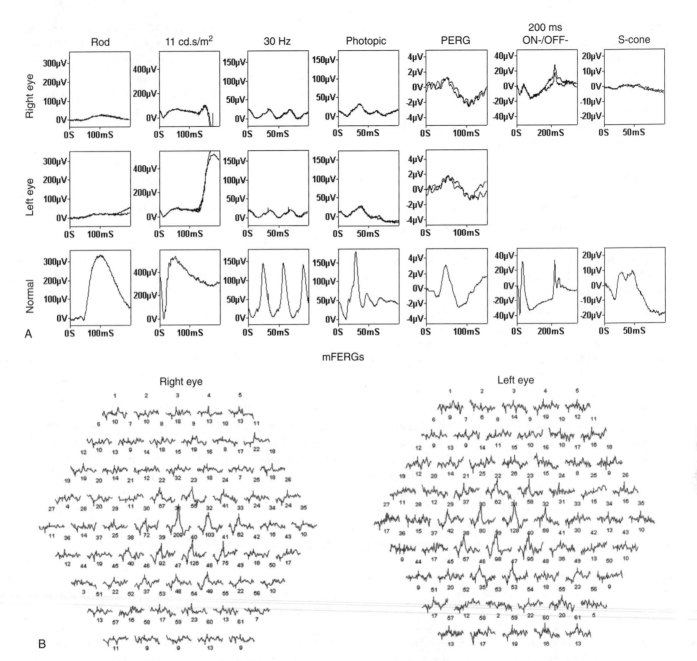

FIGURE 36.2 ERGs, PERGs, and mfERGs from a 44-year-old male with sporadic RP. Rod-specific ERGs are markedly subnormal, confirmed by the maximal response a-wave loss to reflect photoreceptor dysfunction. Cone single-flash and flicker ERGs are markedly reduced and delayed. ON/OFF responses and S-cone ERGs are attenuated. PERG is mildly subnormal from both eyes, and the mfERG demonstrates the spatial aspects of macular cone function.

FIGURE 36.3 Representative findings in four patients with enhanced S-cone syndrome. The data for the four patients (rows 1, 2, 3, and 4) are shown in relation to a typical normal control subject (row 5). A, Conventional ERGs. Note the undetectable rod-specific ERGs, the simplified waveform and delayed bright flash responses with a similar waveform to the same stimulus under photopic and scotopic conditions, and the amplitude of the grossly delayed 30-Hz flicker ERG lying below that of the photopic a-wave (see text for further details). The PERG, when detectable, is markedly delayed. B, S-cone-specific and ON/OFF ERG responses. Note the increased amplitude responses to short-wavelength stimulation and the markedly reduced responses to longer wavelength stimulation. Note also the presence of apparently OFF activity in patients 1 and 3 (with concomitant b-wave reduction going from 10-ms to 200-ms blue stimulation). Patient 1 is a 6-year-old male; patient 2 is a 16-year-old male; patient 3 is a 23-year-old male; patient 4 is a 42-year-old female. Note the differences in scale for some of the traces for patients 3 and 4 relative to the normal traces.

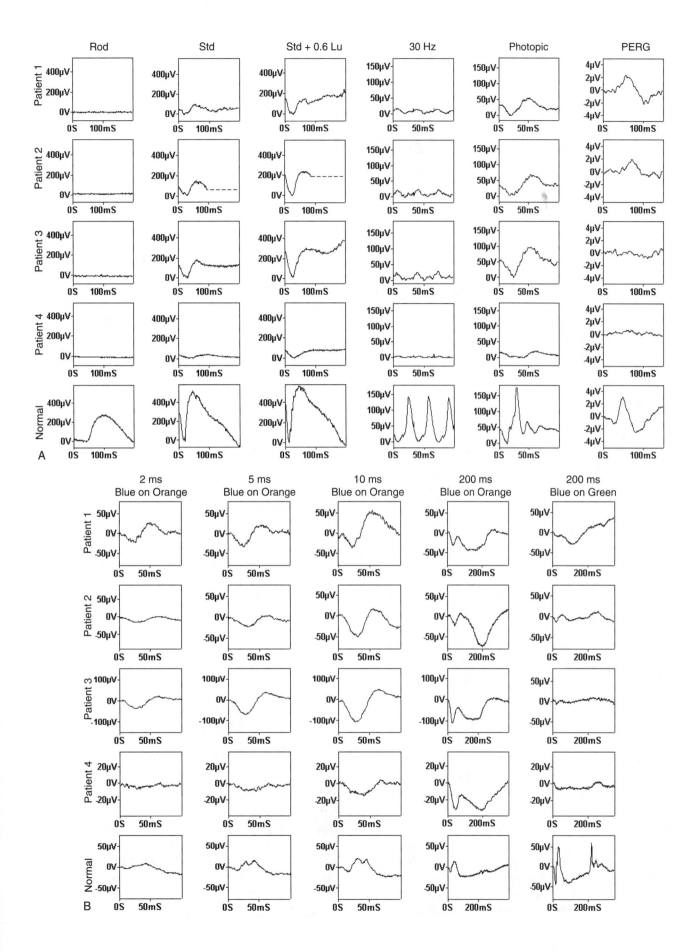

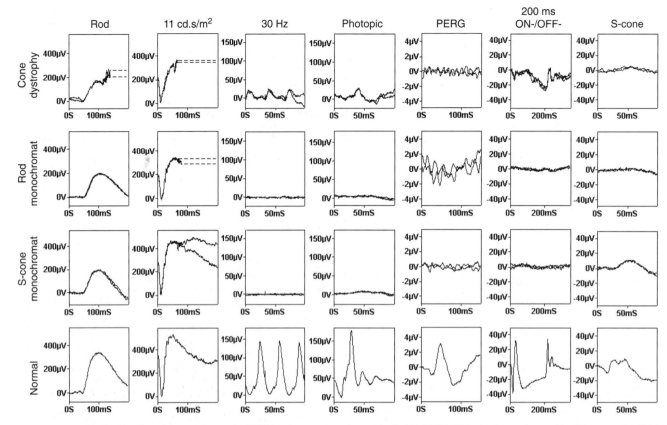

FIGURE 36.4   Typical findings in cone dystrophy (CD), rod mono-chromacy (RM), and S-cone monochromacy (SCM). Rod and maximal ERGs fall within the normal range. The patient with CD has markedly delayed and reduced 30-Hz cone flicker ERG; the patients with RM and SCM have no detectable flicker ERG. There is residual ON/OFF ERG in the patient with CD; not with RM and SCM. There is low-amplitude photopic ERG in the patient with SCM, suggested by S-cone-specific ERGs to arise in S-cones but not in RM. PERG is undetectable in all three patients but will not always be undetectable in CD.

These cone subsystems can be separately assessed using long-duration photopic stimulation.[16] Application of this technique to complete X-linked CSNB is shown in figure 36.5. The rod-specific ERG is undetectable, and the maximal response is profoundly negative. This combination indicates rod system dysfunction post-phototransduction. There are subtle but specific changes in the photopic ERGs: There is a broadened trough to the 30-Hz flicker response with minimal implicit time shift, and the single-flash photopic ERG shows a broadened a-wave followed by a sharply rising b-wave with no photopic oscillatory potentials. These appearances are characteristic of disruption of the ON-bipolar cell pathway but preservation of the OFF pathway. This is confirmed by using a 200-ms stimulus: The ON-response a-wave is normal, the ON-response b-wave is profoundly reduced, and the OFF-response (d-wave) is normal. S-cone-specific responses are undetectable (not shown). The findings in this type of CSNB therefore represent loss of ON pathway function in rods, L-/M- and S-cones, with sparing of OFF pathway function and sparing of photoreceptor phototransduction. PERGs are abnormal, reflecting the dependence of the PERG on ON pathway function. The necessity always to interpret ERG findings in the context of clinical examination and an accurate history are well illustrated by complete X-linked CSNB; identical electrophysiological findings occur in melanoma-associated retinopathy (MAR) (see chapter 58), but MAR is an acquired nyctalopia accompanied by shimmering photopsias that can occur in both females and males, is not associated with myopia, and almost invariably involves a history of cutaneous malignant melanoma. In incomplete CSNB, there is a subnormal but detectable rod-specific ERG and more markedly abnormal cone ERGs shown by the use of long-duration stimulation to involve both ON and OFF systems (figure 36.5).

Normal ERG, abnormal PERG P50 component (N95:P50 ratio not reduced) or mfERG—VEP usually abnormal, often delayed: macular dysfunction

An undetectable PERG or a subnormal PERG P50 component (N95:P50 ratio not reduced) or marked abnormality centrally in mfERG, combined with a normal full-field ERG, indicates dysfunction confined to the macula and eliminates

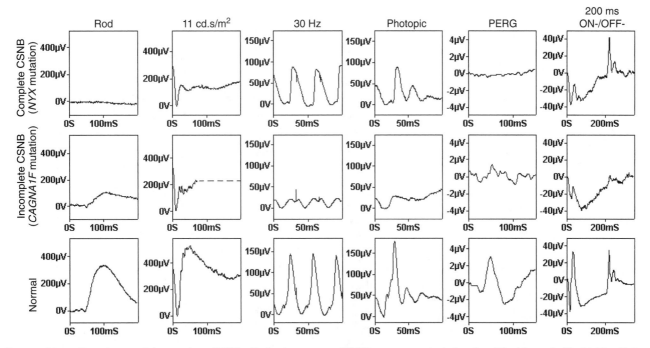

FIGURE 36.5 Complete and incomplete CSNB. Both show a profoundly electronegative bright flash ERG, with a normal a-wave confirming normal photoreceptor function. Cone system abnormalities are more pronounced in incomplete CSNB; note particularly the "double-peaked" 30-Hz flicker ERG that is characteristically present, in keeping with the involvement of both ON and OFF photopic systems. See text for further details.

significant generalized retinal dysfunction. A macular dystrophy or localized maculopathy displays this pattern of electrophysiological abnormality. The most common genetically determined macular dystrophy is Stargardt–fundus flavimaculatus (S-FFM), a usually autosomal-recessive disorder, some or all of which may be related to mutation in *ABCA4* (ABCR).

In a "pure" macular dystrophy, the (full-field) ERG is normal. However, a recent large prospective study of S-FFM[11] identified three groups of patients: group 1 with dysfunction confined to the macula (abnormal PERG, normal rod and cone ERGs), group 2 with abnormal PERG and abnormal photopic ERGs, and group 3 with abnormal PERG and abnormalities in both photopic and scotopic ERGs (figure 36.6). It was shown that although there was a highly significant relationship between the magnitude of the full-field ERG abnormality and the duration of disease in group 3 patients, no such relationship existed for groups 1 and 2. It had previously been reported[12] that sibling pairs with S-FFM could have markedly different fundus appearance, length of disease, or visual acuity but that the electrophysiological grouping was 100% concordant across sibling pairs. It therefore appears that the finding of a normal ERG at any stage during the course of the disorder is associated with continuing normal full-field ERGs. A similar analysis applied to patients with bull's-eye maculopathy (BEM)[10] failed to find similar results, and it cannot be concluded

that BEM is not an inexorably progressive disorder. It is remarkable that although BEM is widely perceived as being associated with cone dystrophy, only a small number of patients presented with that electrophysiological phenotype; most had either a pure macular dystrophy or cone-rod dystrophy.

Macular dysfunction, either inherited or acquired, is usually associated with a delayed pattern VEP. It is therefore of great diagnostic importance that such delay is invariably accompanied by a reduced-amplitude P50 component in the PERG, sometimes with additional latency increase, a finding not usually encountered in optic nerve or retinal ganglion cell dysfunction (see below, and figure 36.7). It is likely that the mfERG will also usually be abnormal under such circumstances, but data similar to those that have been accumulated over many years for the PERG have yet to be acquired for the mfERG, which, at the time of writing, remains in relative infancy.

Normal ERG, preserved PERG P50 component, abnormal N95 component—VEP usually abnormal, often delayed: retinal ganglion cell dysfunction

Disease of the retinal ganglion cells may be primary, such as in Leber hereditary optic neuropathy or dominant optic atrophy (DOA), or may be consequent on optic nerve dys-

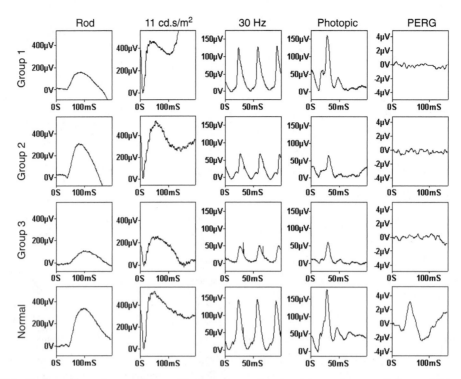

FIGURE 36.6 S-FFM. Findings from three patients with Stargardt–fundus flavimaculatus to demonstrate electrophysiological grouping. The PERG is characteristically undetectable. The group 1 patient shows normal full-field ERGs in keeping with dysfunction confined to the macula; group 2 shows additional cone ERG abnormalities but normal rod and bright-flash ERGs; the group 3 patient has both rod and cone ERG abnormalities in addition to the undetectable PERG.

function. The N95 component of the PERG directly relates to the function of the retinal ganglion cells and may be selectively affected in ganglion cell dysfunction. Usually, the pattern VEP is delayed, but in severe disease may be undetectable. The putative changes in the PERG that occur over time were deduced from patients with different disease stages in DOA[9] (figure 36.8), and can be related to the cellular origins of the PERG. All of N95 and much of P50 (approximately 70%) is thought to arise in the ganglion cells; the origins of the remainder of P50 have not been fully ascertained at the time of writing but are unrelated to spiking cells.[17] In the initial stages of DOA, there is usually amplitude reduction of the N95 component with a completely normal P50. In more advanced disease, N95 shows a greater degree of reduction. In severe disease, there is eventual involvement of P50, but unlike the P50 reduction that occurs in maculopathy, this reduction in P50 is accompanied by a *shortening* of P50 component latency. In this author's experience, extinction of the PERG does not occur in optic nerve disease, provided that technical factors are given adequate consideration during recording. It has been shown in severe longstanding optic nerve compression that the PERG can still be detected even when optic nerve disease is so longstanding that there is no light perception[8] (see also chapter 22). Similar observations have been described following human optic nerve section (see chapter 22).

Normal PERG or PERG abnormality confined to the N95 component—VEP abnormal, usually delayed: optic nerve dysfunction

The VEP is the investigation of choice in the detection and characterization of optic nerve disease, but given that blurring of vision, central field loss, color vision disturbance, and a relative afferent pupillary defect, usually associated with optic nerve disease, may also occur in macular disturbance, it is of crucial importance that the possibility of macular dysfunction not be overlooked. The different effects of optic nerve and macular disease on the PERG enable this distinction in the vast majority of cases (see figures 36.7A and 36.7B). Most optic nerve disorders are accompanied by delay in the pattern-reversal VEP, but there are some exceptions. For example, nonarteritic anterior ischemic optic neuropathy may show amplitude reduction in the absence of latency change (see chapter 59). In many patients, there will be insufficient retrograde degeneration to the retinal ganglion cells for an N95 abnormality to be evident. A large series of patients with optic nerve demyelination

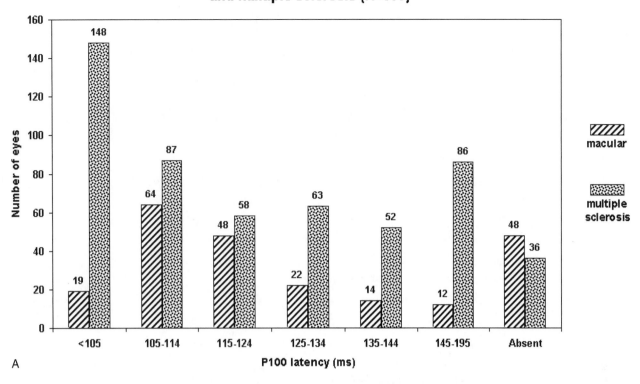

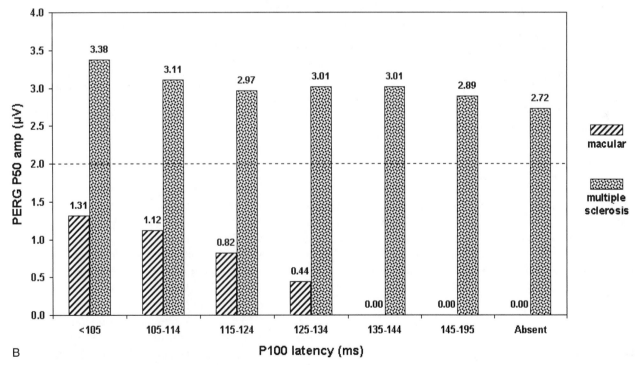

FIGURE 36.7   A, Histogram demonstrating the incidence of PVEP delay in macular dysfunction and multiple sclerosis. All values larger than 105 ms are abnormal. Note the high incidence of PVEP P100 delay in macular dysfunction, with more than 50% of eyes having a VEP delay greater than 10 ms. (From Holder GE: The pattern electroretinogram and an integrated approach to visual pathway diagnosis. *Prog Ret Eye Res* 2001; 20:531–561. Reproduced with permission.) B, PERG parameters in macular dysfunction and multiple sclerosis. No eye with macular disease and a P100 latency greater than 135 ms still had a detectable PERG. Mean P50 ampli-tude with a latency of 125–134 ms was less than 0.5 μV in macular disease, but approximately 3.0 μV in optic nerve demyelination. The normal latency values shown in the multiple sclerosis group reflect the "normal" eye in patients with monocular VEP delay. Note that even in eyes with no detectable PVEP, the P50 component remains well within the normal range in the patients with optic nerve dysfunction. (From Holder GE: The pattern electroretinogram and an integrated approach to visual pathway diagnosis. *Prog Ret Eye Res* 2001; 20:531–561. Reproduced with permission.)

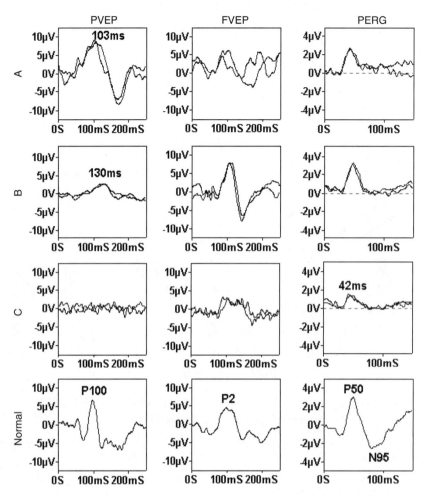

FIGURE 36.8 Findings from three patients with dominantly inherited optic atrophy. The first patient (A), despite the normal pattern VEP, shows significant loss of the N95 component of the PERG. The second patient (B) shows a delayed PVEP accompanied by N95 loss. P50 is normal in both those patients. The third patient (C) has severe end-stage disease with no detectable pattern VEP and a poorly formed low-amplitude flash VEP. In addition to N95 reduction, there is P50 amplitude reduction with shortening of P50 component latency. (From Holder GE: Electrophysiological assessment of optic nerve disease. *Eye* 2004; 18:1133–1143.)

and VEP conduction delay revealed an incidence of PERG abnormality of approximately 40%.[5] However, of those abnormalities, 85% were confined to the N95 component. Typical findings in a patient with multiple sclerosis and optic nerve demyelination are shown in figure 36.9. Note the ability of the VEP to detect subclinical demyelination.

Asymmetrical VEP distribution, crossed asymmetry: chiasmal dysfunction or misrouting

The majority of optic nerve dysfunction has a posterior distribution that is largely symmetrical across the two hemispheres. However, when the dysfunction is primarily at the level of the optic chiasm or in the presence of chiasmal misrouting, there is a crossed asymmetry whereby the findings obtained on stimulation of one eye show an asymmetrical distribution that is reversed when the other eye is stimulated. Great caution is needed when interpreting pattern-reversal VEPs because of the phenomenon of paradoxical lateralization that occurs with a large-field, large-check stimulus and common reference recording to Fz (see chapter 78). The most common cause of acquired chiasmal dysfunction is compression from a pituitary tumor, which gives characteristic VEP abnormalities that are described in detail elsewhere in this volume but that show predominance of the responses from the ipsilateral hemisphere. A congenital misrouting of chiasmal fibers occurs in association with ocular or oculocutaneous albinism such that the majority of fibers from each eye decussate to the contralateral hemisphere; this contralateral predominance is best revealed with

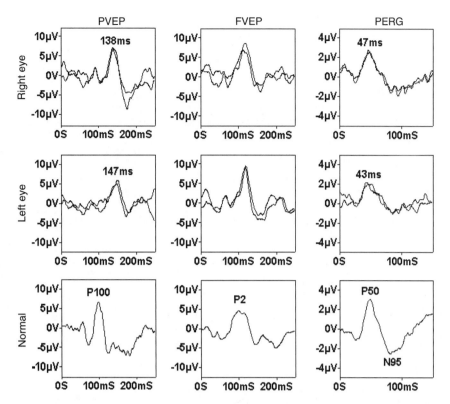

FIGURE 36.9 The findings in this patient demonstrate the ability of the PERG to detect subclinical optic nerve demyelination. The patient is a 35-year-old female with blurred vision following exercise or a hot bath (Uhthoff phenomenon). Although demyelination was suspected, visual acuity was 6/5 bilaterally, and there was no relative afferent pupillary defect. Note the profound delay present in the VEP both from the symptomatic and asymptomatic eyes. The left eye PERG shows some N95 loss and shortening of P50 latency. (From Holder GE: Electrophysiological assessment of optic nerve disease. *Eye* 2004; 18:1133–1143.)

pattern appearance stimulation in older patients or diffuse flash in children or infants (e.g., Dorey et al.,[2] Neveu et al.[15]; see also chapter 25). Typical findings are shown in figure 36.10.

Asymmetrical VEP distribution, uncrossed asymmetry: retrochiasmal dysfunction

Dysfunction posterior to the optic chiasm gives an uncrossed asymmetry such that the findings obtained on stimulation of each eye show an asymmetrical distribution across the two hemispheres that are similar when either eye is stimulated. As with chiasmal dysfunction, caution is needed when interpreting pattern-reversal VEPs owing to the phenomenon of paradoxical lateralization that occurs with a large-field, large-check stimulus and common reference recording to Fz. Retrochiasmal lesions are addressed elsewhere in this volume (see chapter 78).

Concluding remarks

It should be evident, from the nature of the electrophysiological changes described, that appropriate electrophysiological testing allows accurate localization of visual pathway dysfunction. Diagnostic flowcharts have been devised[6,7] to assist in ascertaining the cause of a delayed pattern VEP and further to demonstrate how to evaluate, commencing with PERG, the patient with unexplained visual acuity loss. These appear in figures 36.11A and 36.11B. It is possible partly to substitute mfERG for PERG, but the direct assessment of ganglion cell function that the PERG provides is not readily available in the mfERG. It is perhaps also more appropriate to examine macular function by using a stimulus similar to that used to evoke the PVEP. The evaluation of "functional" or nonorganic visual loss is fully addressed elsewhere (see chapter 51).

The flowchart in figure 36.11A can be applied to the patient illustrated in figure 36.12. This unfortunate person was involved in a road traffic accident and sustained a traumatic left optic neuropathy. During face-down surgery for a spinal injury that was sustained during the accident, a severe pressure retinopathy in the right eye occurred. Pattern VEPs are undetectable, and flash VEPs are severely abnormal from both right and left eyes. The PERG is undetectable from the right eye but in the left eye shows a normal P50 component with selective loss of N95, in keeping with

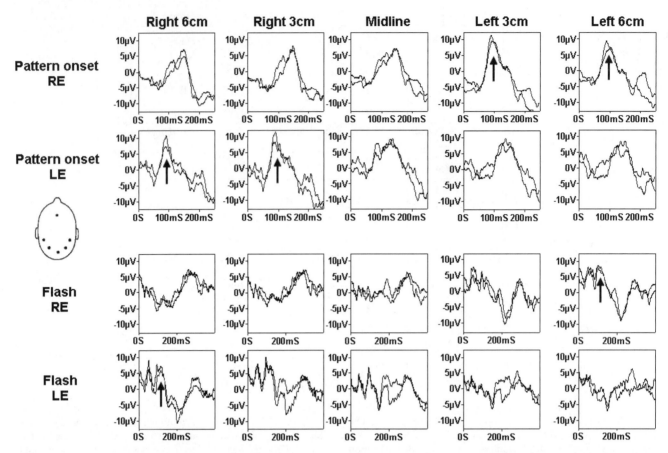

FIGURE 36.10   Pattern appearance (150-ms onset) and flash VEPs in a 7.5-year-old girl with ocular albinism. Note the pronounced contralateral predominance of the VEPs (arrows). Pattern appearance VEPs show only the positive component at 100 ms in the contralateral hemisphere traces. The flash VEPs show little activity in the first 100 ms in the ipsilateral hemisphere traces but a clear FVEP in the contralateral traces.

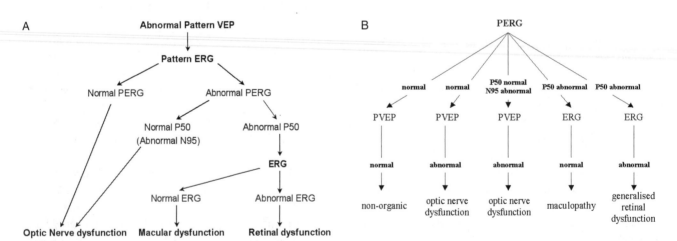

FIGURE 36.11   These diagnostic flowcharts detail the diagnostic strategy that can be applied to the improved assessment of an abnormal pattern VEP and the patient who presents with unexplained visual loss. Note the pivotal role played by the PERG. (A from Holder GE: The pattern electroretinogram in anterior visual pathway dysfunction and its relationship to the pattern visual evoked potential: A personal clinical review of 743 eyes. *Eye* 1997; 11:924–934. B from Holder GE: The pattern electroretinogram and an integrated approach to visual pathway diagnosis. *Prog Ret Eye Res* 2001; 20:531–561.)

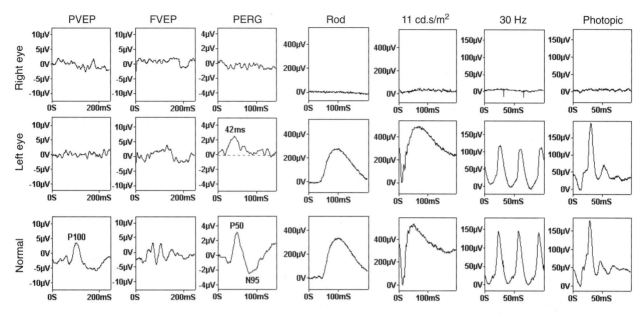

FIGURE 36.12   VEPs and ERGs in a patient with a pressure-induced retinopathy in the right eye and traumatic optic neuropathy in the left eye. See text for details.

retrograde degeneration to the retinal ganglion cells from the optic neuropathy. The ERGs are normal in the left eye but undetectable in the right eye, in keeping with severe generalized retinal dysfunction. The electrophysiological findings identify and localize the dual pathology.

REFERENCES

1. Berson EL, Gouras P, Hoff M: Temporal aspects of the electroretinogram. *Arch Ophthalmol* 1969; 81:207–214.

2. Dorey SE, Neveu MM, Burton L, Sloper JJ, Holder GE: The clinical features of albinism and their correlation with visual evoked potentials. *Br J Ophthalmol* 2003; 87:767–772.

3. Downes SM, Holder GE, Fitzke FW, Payne AM, Warren MJ, Bhattacharya SS, Bird AC: Autosomal dominant cone and cone-rod dystrophy with mutations in the GUCA 1A gene encoding guanylate cyclase activating protein-1. *Arch Ophthalmol* 2001; 119:96–105.

4. Fishman GA, Birch DG, Holder GE, Brigell MG: *Electrophysiologic Testing in Disorders of the Retina, Optic Nerve, and Visual Pathway*, 2 ed. Ophthalmology Monograph 2. San Francisco, The Foundation of the American Academy of Ophthalmology, 2001.

5. Holder GE: The incidence of abnormal pattern electroretinography in optic nerve demyelination. *Electroencephalogr Clin Neurophysiol* 1991; 78:18–26.

6. Holder GE: The pattern electroretinogram in anterior visual pathway dysfunction and its relationship to the pattern visual evoked potential: A personal clinical review of 743 eyes. *Eye* 1997; 11:924–934.

7. Holder GE: The pattern electroretinogram and an integrated approach to visual pathway diagnosis. *Prog Ret Eye Res* 2001; 20:531–561.

8. Holder GE: The pattern electroretinogram. In Fishman GA, Birch DG, Holder GE, Brigell MG (eds): *Electrophysiologic Testing*

in *Disorders of the Retina, Optic Nerve, and Visual Pathway*, 2 ed. Ophthalmology Monograph 2. San Francisco, The Foundation of the American Academy of Ophthalmology, 2001.

9. Holder GE, Votruba M, Carter AC, Bhattacharya SS, Fitzke FW, Moore AT: Electrophysiological findings in dominant optic atrophy (DOA) linking to the OPA1 locus on chromosome 3q 28-qter. *Doc Ophthalmol* 1999; 95:217–228.

10. Kurz-Levin M, Halfyard AS, Bunce C, Bird AC, Holder GE: Clinical variations in assessment of bull's eye maculopathy. *Arch Ophthalmol* 2002; 120:567–575.

11. Lois N, Holder GE, Bunce C, Fitzke FW, Bird AC: Stargardt macular dystrophy–fundus flavimaculatus: Phenotypic subtypes. *Arch Ophthalmol* 2001; 119:359–369.

12. Lois N, Holder GE, Fitzke FW, Plant C, Bird AC: Intrafamilial variation of phenotype in Stargardt macular dystrophy–fundus flavimaculatus. *Invest Ophthalmol Vis Sci* 1999; 40:2668–2675.

13. Marmor MF, Jacobson SG, Foerster MH, Kellner U, Weleber RG: Diagnostic clinical findings of a new syndrome with night blindness, maculopathy, and enhanced S cone sensitivity. *Am J Ophthalmol* 1990; 110:124–134.

14. Milam AH, Rose L, Cideciyan AV, Barakat MR, Tang WX, Gupta N, Aleman TS, Wright AF, Stone EM, Sheffield VC, Jacobson SG: The nuclear receptor NR2E3 plays a role in human retinal photoreceptor differentiation and degeneration. *Proc Natl Acad Sci U S A* 2002; 99:473–478.

15. Neveu MM, Jeffery G, Burton LC, Sloper JJ, Holder GE: Age-related changes in the dynamics of human albino visual pathways. *Eur J Neurosci* 2003; 18:1939–1949.

16. Sieving PA: Photopic ON- and OFF-pathway abnormalities in retinal dystrophies. *Trans Am Ophthalmol Soc* 1993; 91:701–773.

17. Viswanathan S, Frishman LJ, Robson JG: The uniform field and pattern ERG in macaques with experimental glaucoma: Removal of spiking activity. *Invest Ophthalmol Vis Sci* 2000; 41:2797–2810.

37 Paired-Flash ERG Analysis of Rod Phototransduction and Adaptation

DAVID R. PEPPERBERG

IT HAS BEEN WELL established that the rising phase of the scotopic electroretinogram (ERG) a-wave largely represents the massed electrical response of the rod photoreceptors.[9,11,17,19,20,36,45] This has motivated wide use of the ERG to study fundamental and clinically relevant aspects of rod function in the living eye. However, a severe constraint associated with conventional (i.e., single-flash) ERG recording is that intrusion by the b-wave and other postreceptor ERG components begins to mask the a-wave shortly after test flash presentation and thus obscures all but the initial portion of the photoreceptor flash response. The constraint is especially pronounced in the case of rods in the mammalian eye. That is, intrusion by the b-wave in the mammalian ERG becomes substantial at ~25 ms or less after test flash presentation, while photocurrent data from mammalian rods in vitro indicate a flash response duration of at least several hundred milliseconds.[2,26,33] Recently, however, we and others have developed a paired-flash ERG technique that allows approximate determination of the rod response's full time course.[3,14,16,29,37,39,41] The aim of this chapter is to describe the measurement of rod phototransduction and adaptation properties using the paired-flash ERG method. The work to be highlighted is drawn from recent studies conducted on human subjects and on wild-type (C57BL/6J) mice.

Concept and methodology

Numerous studies of rods in vitro have described the property of *photocurrent saturation*, a condition of essentially zero circulating current and thus maximal photocurrent response amplitude, produced transiently by a bright flash. Photocurrent saturation reflects the flash generation of a large quantity of activated cGMP phosphodiesterase (PDE*) on the disk membranes of the rod outer segment (for recent reviews, see Arshavsky et al.[1] and Burns and Baylor[6]). The resulting large burst of PDE*-mediated cGMP hydrolysis produces a drop in the intracellular level of free cGMP to near zero, a resulting closure of virtually all of the cGMP-gated channels in the plasma membrane of the outer segment, and rapid development of an ERG a-wave of near-maximal amplitude.

The paired-flash method is based on the notions that (1) a bright flash, by rapidly driving the rods to saturation, generates a rapidly developing ERG a-wave that essentially titrates the prevailing level of circulating current, and (2) rod saturation (closure of essentially all of the cGMP-gated channels) is a fixed reference condition that is presumably independent of simultaneously occurring, postreceptor ERG potentials. In this method, the full time course of the rod response to a test flash of arbitrary strength is reconstructed, that is, "derived," from results obtained in a series of paired-flash trials. Each trial involves presentation of the test flash at time zero in the experimental run and subsequent presentation of a bright probe flash of fixed strength. The interval between the test and probe flashes (termed t_{probe} below) is varied among trials, and the rod-mediated a-wave response to the probe flash of each trial is analyzed for amplitude. As referenced to the probe response obtained in the absence of recent test flash presentation ("probe-alone" response), the family of probe response amplitudes yields the test flash response (figure 37.1). $A(t)$, the full time course of the derived response to the test flash, is obtained through the relation

$$A(t) = A_{mo} - A_m(t) \tag{1}$$

where A_{mo} is the amplitude of the probe-alone response and $A_m(t)$ is the probe response amplitude determined in a paired-flash trial at time t after the test flash. With a fixed interflash interval and varying test flash strength, the paired-flash method can similarly be used to determine the amplitude-intensity function of the rod response at a fixed time after test flash presentation.

Paired-flash ERG experiments utilize a Ganzfeld (i.e., full-field) photostimulator equipped with short-duration (~2 ms or less) flash lamps. The short duration of the probe flash specifically permits delivery of this stimulus within an interval that is small by comparison with that of the time-to-peak of the probe-generated a-wave. In the mouse,

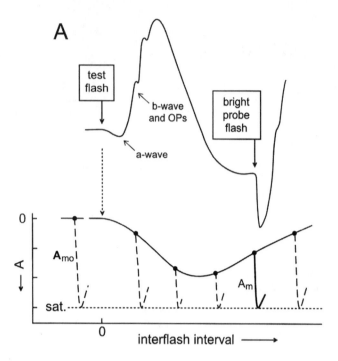

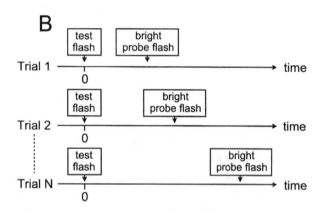

FIGURE 37.1 Diagram describing the paired-flash method. A, Hypothetical ERG response obtained in a paired-flash trial, with test flash presentation at time zero and subsequent presentation of a bright probe flash. Lower part shows hypothetical responses to probe flashes presented in paired-flash trials of differing interflash intervals, the vertical alignment of these probe responses to match their peak amplitudes, and representation of the preprobe baselines (solid circles) as the amplitudes of the derived rod response (solid curve). For simplicity, the diagram ignores the correction of probe responses to remove the cone contribution to these responses. B, Variation of the test-probe interval among paired-flash trials. (Reproduced from Pepperberg et al.[40] with permission from Elsevier Science.)

the time-to-peak of the a-wave generated with our standard probe flash (~300–400 scotopic candela second per square meter ($sc\,cd\,s\,m^{-2}$)) is typically ≈ 7–$8\,ms$, and probe responses are routinely analyzed for amplitude at $6\,ms$ after probe flash presentation (determination time $t_{det} = 6\,ms$).[16,46] However, analyses of probe responses that are obtained after

substantial rhodopsin bleaches have employed a t_{det} of $7\,ms$[24] (see below). In the mouse experiments highlighted below, values of the post-test-flash time t quoted in determinations of the derived response $A(t)$ represent the sum of the test probe interval and the probe response determination time ($t = t_{probe} + t_{det}$). In experiments on human subjects, in which the probe flash strength is typically $\sim 1.2 \times 10^4$ to 1.6×10^4 scotopic troland seconds ($sc\,td\,s$), the time-to-peak of the probe response is about 8–9 ms, and probe responses obtained in a given session are analyzed for amplitude at a fixed near-peak time. For the experiments on human subjects highlighted below, quoted values of the post-test-flash time t ignore the determination time t_{det} (i.e., $t = t_{probe}$). Raw probe responses recorded from human subjects furthermore contain a significant contribution from the cone photoreceptors, necessitating determination and computational subtraction of the cone-mediated component to obtain the rod-only component (see below). Full details of this cone subtraction technique, as well as other procedures for recording and data analysis in paired-flash ERG experiments on human subjects and mice, have been described.[16,23,24,39,40,46]

Dark-adapted flash response

Figure 37.2 illustrates data obtained from a human subject and describes the approach used to derive the rod response to fixed, relatively weak test flash (test flash strength $I_{test} = 11$ $sc\,td\,s$). Figure 37.2A shows raw responses to a fixed, short-wavelength probe flash delivered at varying times after the $11\,sc\,td\,s$ test flash in a series of paired-flash trials. Also shown in figure 37.2A is response C, the presumed cone-mediated response to a long-wavelength probe flash that is photopically matched to the nominally used short-wavelength probe (cf. figures 1–3 and accompanying text of Pepperberg et al.[39]). Shown in figure 37.2B are rod-only probe responses obtained after computational subtraction of response C from the raw probe responses. Figure 37.2C shows the derived response to the test flash determined from the rod-only probe responses; here, these probe responses are vertically positioned to achieve a match of their negative peaks at a fixed value (labeled A_{mo}) that represents the presumed fixed condition of photocurrent saturation (see figure 37.1). These probe responses, which are positioned horizontally according to the time of probe flash presentation, define a family of preprobe baselines (solid circles) that together represent the derived response to the test flash. The derived response exhibits a peak at $t \approx 170\,ms$ and a falling phase that lasts several hundred milliseconds. Support for the notion that this derived response approximates the in vivo massed response of the rods comes from the response's similarity to photocurrent flash responses recorded from human rods in vitro.[26]

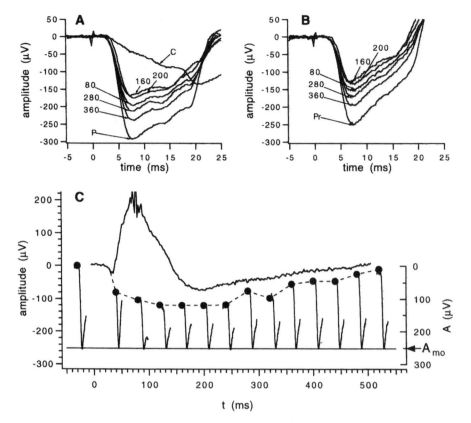

FIGURE 37.2   Derived rod response of human rods to a fixed weak test flash (I_{test} = 11 sc td s). A, Raw probe flash responses obtained with differing interflash intervals. Labels accompanying the waveforms identify the test-probe intervals in milliseconds. B, Rod-only (i.e., cone-corrected) probe responses obtained after computational subtraction of the putative cone contribution (response C in part A) from each raw probe response. C, Derived rod response to the test flash. See text for further details. (Reproduced from Pepperberg et al.[39] with permission from Cambridge University Press and Elsevier Science.)

Paired-flash ERG experiments on mice indicate that shortly after a bright (i.e., rod-saturating) conditioning flash, the small a-wave response that is produced by the bright probe flash largely reflects the activity of cone photoreceptors (see figure 9 of Hetling and Pepperberg[16]). However, at the early times that are used to determine the probe response amplitude in mouse (6 or 7 ms), the size of this cone contribution is tiny by comparison with that of the dark-adapted probe response and ordinarily can be ignored in deriving the flash response of the rods.[16,24,28,46] Figure 37.3 shows the paired-flash-derived rod response to a weak test flash (I_{test} = 0.12 ± 0.02 sc cd s m^{-2}), obtained with use of a 6-ms determination time for the probe response amplitude. The derived response resembles those of photocurrent recordings obtained from mouse rods in vitro[7,49,53] and is well described by the nested exponential relation (solid curve)

$$A(t)/A_{mo} = 1 - \exp[-k_{86}I_{test}u(t)] \tag{2a}$$

$$u(t) = \gamma\{1 - \exp[-\alpha(t - t_d)^2]\}\exp(-t/\tau_\omega) \tag{2b}$$

where k_{86} = 7.0 (sc cd s m^{-2})$^{-1}$ is a sensitivity parameter determined from the amplitude-intensity relation at the near-peak time of t = 86 ms (test probe interval of 80 ms and t_{det} = 6 ms; see figure 2 of Hetling and Pepperberg[16]), α = 2.32 × 10^{-4} (ms)$^{-2}$ describes the acceleration of the response (counterpart of the amplification constant used by Lamb and Pugh[27] and Breton et al.[5]), t_d = 3.1 ms is a fixed delay (see, e.g., Birch et al.[3]), τ_ω = 132 ms is an exponential decay constant, γ = 2.21 is a dimensionless scaling factor, and the time-dependent function $u(t)$ represents a unit (i.e., elemental) contribution to the dark-adapted response.[16,46,47] Equation (2) accounts well for the approximately exponential behavior of the amplitude-intensity relation that is obtained at a fixed time in the weak-flash response, and for the overall time course of the response to brighter flashes, including the progressively longer period of rod saturation that is produced with increasing test flash strength (see figures 2, 3, and 8 of Hetling and Pepperberg[16]). However, equation (2) does not capture the progressive slowing of the derived response's recovery phase that occurs with increases in test flash strength well above saturation. Furthermore, with the fixed delay t_d, this equation does not account for the advance of the rising phase to shorter times that is observed with very bright flashes.[42]

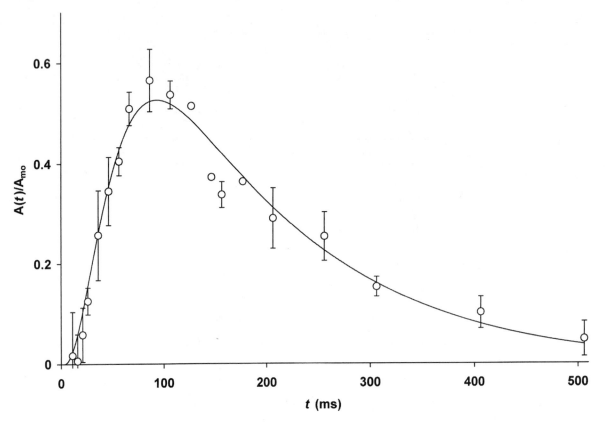

FIGURE 37.3   Derived normalized response $A(t)/A_{mo}$ of mouse rods to a weak test flash ($I_{test} = 0.12 \pm 0.02\,\mathrm{sc\,cd\,s\,m^{-2}}$). (Adapted from Hetling and Pepperberg[16] with permission from The Physiological Society and Elsevier Science.)

Light adaptation

It is well established that in the presence of steady background illumination, rod photoreceptors in vitro exhibit a maintained response to the background as well as a reduced sensitivity and duration of their response to a superimposed test flash (reviewed by Burns and Baylor[6] and Fain et al.[12]). Figure 37.4 shows the effect of steady background light on the maintained derived response of mouse rods. In each of a group of experiments, the probe-alone response that was obtained in darkness was analyzed to yield the dark-adapted maximal amplitude A_{moD}. The same probe flash was presented during background illumination of fixed intensity (background strength I_b ranging from 0 to $21\,\mathrm{sc\,cd\,m^{-2}}$; background on for at least 2 minutes before probe flash presentation), and the probe-alone response was similarly analyzed to yield A_{moL}, the light-adapted maximal amplitude. A_b, the maintained derived response to the background, was then determined from the relation (cf. equation [1] above)

$$A_b = A_{moD} - A_{moL} \qquad (3)$$

It is of interest to compare the background dependence of the maintained normalized response (A_b/A_{moD} versus $\log I_b$) with the amplitude-intensity relation obtained under dark-adapted conditions. Curve 1 in figure 37.4 ($A(86)/A_{moD}$ versus $\log I_{test}$) shows the normalized amplitude-intensity function for the dark-adapted flash response at the near-peak time $t = 86\,\mathrm{ms}$ determined in separate experiments (not illustrated; see figure 2 of Hetling and Pepperberg[16]). Curve 2 represents the background dependence of the normalized maintained response (A_b/A_{moD} versus $\log I_b$) that is expected in the absence of light adaptation, that is, if this maintained response reflected the superposition of nonadapting elemental responses; this curve is related to curve 1 by an integration time ($\tau_{int} = 235\,\mathrm{ms}$) determined for the dark-adapted weak-flash response (see figure 1 of Silva et al.[46]). Curve 2 approximates the behavior of the maintained response A_b/A_{moD} determined experimentally with weak backgrounds but becomes a progressively poorer description of the data at higher values of A_b/A_{moD} (i.e., at higher background strengths), consistent with the action of light adaptation in reducing the amplitude of the maintained response.

Accurate determination of the paired-flash-derived response requires the probe flash to be bright enough to rapidly saturate the rods even in the presence of background light. Figure 37.5, which shows results obtained from mouse, describes a test of the extent to which backgrounds alter the dependence of the probe response amplitude on the strength

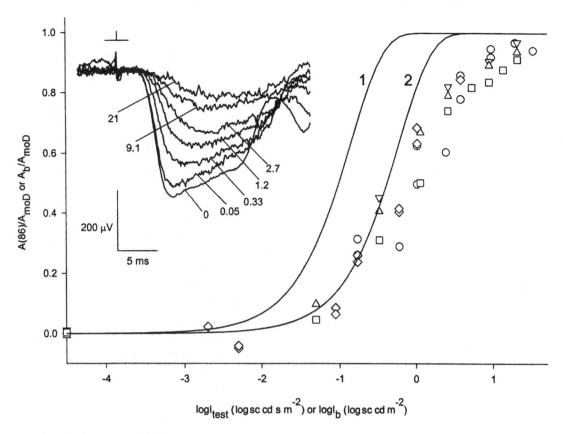

FIGURE 37.4 Effect of steady background light on the maintained derived rod response of mouse rods. Data points plot determinations of the normalized maintained response A_b/A_{moD} as a function of $\log I_b$, the log value of the background strength in scotopic candela per square meter (sc cd m^{-2}). Curve 1 plots the amplitude-intensity relation at $t = 86\,\text{ms}$ for dark-adapted mouse rods determined in separate experiments as a function of $\log I_{test}$, the log value of test flash strength in scotopic candela seconds per square meter (sc cd s m^{-2}). Curve 2, derived from the function plotted as curve 1, is the dependence of A_b/A_{moD} on $\log I_b$ predicted in the absence of light adaptation. (Reproduced from Silva et al.[46] with permission from The Physiological Society.)

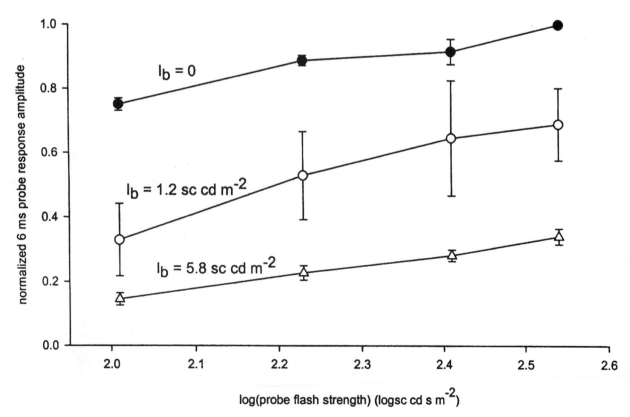

FIGURE 37.5 Dependence of normalized probe response amplitude on probe flash strength under dark-adapted conditions (solid circles) and in background light of 1.2 and 5.8 sc cd m^{-2} (open circles and open triangles, respectively). (Adapted from Silva et al.[46] with permission from The Physiological Society.)

of the probe flash. Here, probe flashes of differing strength were presented in darkness ($I_b = 0$) and in the presence of backgrounds of 1.2 and 5.8 sc cd m^{-2}. The data indicate a relatively modest dependence of the normalized probe response amplitude on probe flash strength under dark-adapted conditions and relatively little effect of the tested backgrounds on the slope of the illustrated functions. These results indicate that over the investigated range of background strength, the strength of the routinely used probe flash (~300 sc cd s m^{-2} or greater) is sufficient

to permit accurate determination of derived rod responses.

A central property of rod light adaptation is the reduction in peak amplitude and duration of the response to a superimposed test flash. Figure 37.6 illustrates the effect of steady background light on the flash response of mouse rods. Here, dashed curve *DA* is the function that was previously shown to describe the normalized dark-adapted response ($A(t)/A_{moD}$ versus t) to a test flash of 0.12 sc cd s m^{-2} (equations (2a) and (2b) with $I_{test} = 0.12$ sc cd s m^{-2}). Open circles show paired-flash determinations of the normalized response ($A(t)/A_{moL}$ versus t) to a test flash of 0.30 sc cd s m^{-2} superimposed on a background of 0.63 sc cd s m^{-2}. Note that the peak amplitude of the normalized light-adapted response to the 0.30 sc cd s m^{-2} test flash is similar to that of the normalized dark-adapted response to the 0.12 sc cd s m^{-2} test flash, and that the light-adapted response falls to preflash baseline more rapidly than the dark-adapted response does. An accelerated recovery of the flash response is indicated also by the integration time τ_{ref} determined for the derived response (see table 1 and accompanying text in Silva et al.[46]). By contrast with the 234-ms value of τ_{ref} obtained under dark-adapted conditions, τ_{ref} for the derived flash response in the presence of the 0.63 sc cd s m^{-2} background was 71 ms. Backgrounds of 1.2 and 2.5 sc cd s m^{-2} further reduced this integration time to 65 and 54 ms, respectively.

Figure 37.7 illustrates the effect of steady background light on the flash response of human rods. Figure 37.7A shows the derived rod response to a fixed test flash (44 sc tds) determined in the absence and presence of a 32 sc td background (solid and open circles, respectively) and with use of a nominal probe flash strength of 1.2×10^4 sc tds. The dashed

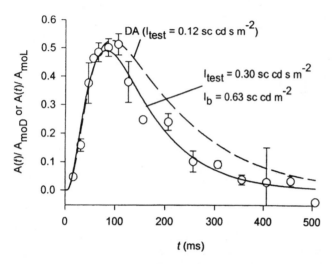

FIGURE 37.6 Open circles: Normalized response of mouse rods to a test flash (0.30 sc cd s m^{-2}) superimposed on steady background illumination (0.63 sc cd m^{-2}). Dashed curve: Normalized dark-adapted response to a test flash of 0.12 sc cd s m^{-2}, based on data obtained in separate experiments. (Adapted from Silva et al.[46] with permission from The Physiological Society.)

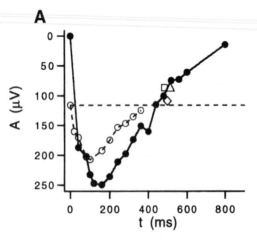

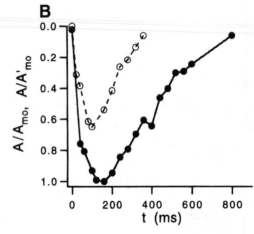

FIGURE 37.7 Effect of background light (32 sc td) on the derived response of human rods to a 44-sc tds test flash. Solid and open circles: Dark- and light-adapted responses, respectively. Data obtained from a single subject. A, Derived amplitudes *A*, in microvolts. B, Dark- and light-adapted derived responses

normalized to prevailing maximal amplitudes of the flash-generated response (A_{mo} and A'_{mo}, respectively). See text for further details. (Adapted from Pepperberg et al.[39] with permission from Cambridge University Press and Elsevier Science.)

line represents the amplitude of the derived rod response maintained by the background itself. In background light, the derived response to the test flash exhibits a shortened duration, that is, the response recovers more quickly than does the dark-adapted response to the prevailing baseline. This shortening of time scale by the background is evident also when the dark- and light-adapted derived responses are plotted on normalization to the prevailing maximal amplitude (figure 37.7B). The open diamond, open triangle, and open square in figure 37.7A show results obtained under dark-adapted conditions at $t = 500\,ms$ with probe flash strengths of 2.5×10^3, 5.0×10^3, and $2.4 \times 10^4\,sc\,td\,s$, respectively. That these differing probe strengths yielded derived amplitudes similar to that obtained with the nominal ($1.2 \times 10^4\,sc\,td\,s$) probe flash is consistent with the notion that the response to the nominal probe flash was not subject to substantial desensitization by the test flash itself.

The decrease in rod responsiveness that is observed in steady background light motivates interest in understanding the time course of the change produced by stepped onset of a background. The derived response to a background step can be determined in a series of experimental runs, each of which involves background onset at time zero and presentation of the probe flash at defined times after this onset. Because this series of runs requires repeated presentation of the background step, it is important to limit the intensity and duration of the background to conditions that permit full dark adaptation between runs, to avoid a cumulative adapting effect of the measurement procedures. Figure 37.8A shows results obtained in mouse for the derived response to step onset of a $1.2\,sc\,cd\,m^{-2}$ background. Here, each experimental run involved a 1-s exposure to the background, and consecutive runs were separated by a 2-min period of dark adaptation. Consistent with results obtained in vitro for backgrounds that are approximately half-saturating in steady state,[30,50] the response to the $1.2\,sc\,cd\,m^{-2}$ background step suggests a slight sag from initial peak within the first 1s after background onset. Figure 37.8B presents evidence that this stepped $1.2\,sc\,cd\,m^{-2}$ background furthermore desensitizes the flash response within a 1-s period. Here, a fixed test flash (T) of $0.98\,sc\,cd\,s\,m^{-2}$ was presented in darkness, or at 50 or 700 ms after background (B) onset (conditions termed "Dark-adapted," "B50T," and "B700T," respectively, in figure 37.8B). Under each condition, experimental runs were conducted in which presentation of the probe flash occurred at 20 ms or 250 ms after the test flash. The use of these two test probe intervals was designed to yield information about the test flash response at relatively early and late times, respectively, in this response. The illustrated data show the effect of the background on normalized amplitudes of the derived response to the test flash. The similarity of normalized amplitudes obtained with the 20-ms test-probe interval (open bars) indicates that there was no substantial effect of

the background at this very early time in the test flash response. However, results obtained with the 250-ms test probe interval (solid bars) indicated a substantial effect of the background. That is, as is noted by the asterisk above the bar representing the B700T results with the 250 ms test probe interval, background desensitization led to a significant reduction in the derived response to the test flash presented at 700 ms after background onset (see figure 8 and accompanying text of Silva et al.[46]).

Recovery following bright illumination

Recovery of the rod response from the condition of photocurrent saturation produced by a bright test flash can be determined in paired-flash trials involving variation of the test probe interval, as in measurement of the weak-flash response.[3,15,22,29] Determining the time course of recovery from the bright-flash-induced condition of rod saturation can provide information on the relationship between the strength of the bright test flash and the progress of reactions that terminate excitation in the phototransduction cascade. Figure 37.9 shows results obtained from a human subject in an experiment that involved presentation of a fixed bright flash ($2.0 \times 10^3\,sc\,td\,s$). Figures 37.9A and 37.9B show rod-only probe responses and amplitudes of these responses, respectively, determined at defined times after this bright flash. These data indicate the occurrence of rod saturation (near-zero amplitude of the probe response) for a period of about 1s and a subsequent recovery of the response. Figure 37.9C shows determinations of the rod saturation period as a function of the bleaching strength of the test flash. Over a range corresponding with up to $\sim4 \times 10^5$ rhodopsin photoisomerizations (R_o^*) per rod, the saturation function (saturation period T versus the natural logarithm (ln) of R_o^*) is approximately described by a line (not illustrated) of slope $\approx 0.3\,s$. ERG and photocurrent data from mouse rods have yielded generally similar values of slope of the saturation function over a corresponding test flash range.[7,8,16,29] Above this range, there occurs an acceleration of the saturation function to a regime of higher slope, a result implicating rate limitation of recovery by a process that is distinct from that responsible for the slope of the function's lower branch.[3,38] Birch et al.,[3] in a paired-flash ERG study of normal subjects and of patients with retinitis pigmentosa (RP) and the pro-23-his rhodopsin mutation, observed in the RP patients an abnormally slow recovery from rod saturation that is describable by an abnormally high slope of the upper branch of the saturation function (their figure 10).

Properties of the rod weak-flash response during recovery from bright adapting light can also be determined. Hetling and Pepperberg[16] investigated the recovery of mouse rods from a brief adapting flash of high intensity. In each of a series of three-flash trials, the eye was exposed to the bright

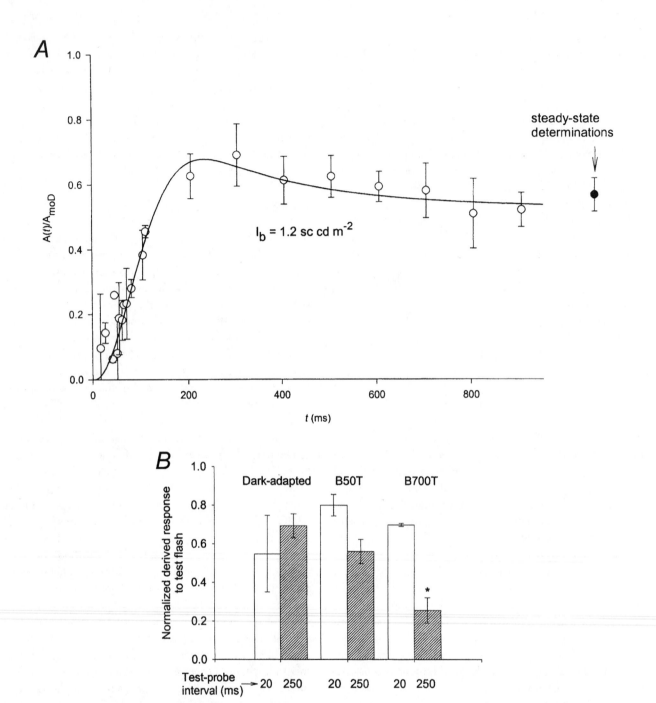

FIGURE 37.8   A, Derived response of mouse rods to a step of light (1.2 sc cd m^{-2}). Background onset was at time zero. B, Normalized amplitudes of the derived response to a test flash (0.98 sc cd s m^{-2}) presented at differing times after onset of a 1.2 sc cd m^{-2} background. Pairs of histograms indicate data obtained under dark-adapted conditions (left) and with test flash presentation at 50 ms (middle) and 700 ms (right) after step onset. See text for further details. (Adapted from Silva et al.[46] with permission from The Physiological Society.)

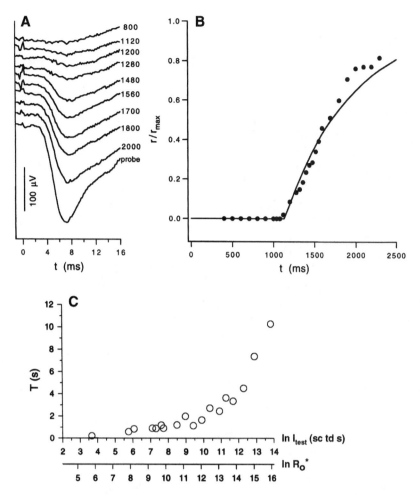

FIGURE 37.9 Recovery of human rods following a bright test flash. Data in parts A and B obtained from a single subject in response to a 2×10^3 sc td s test flash. A, Rod-only probe response waveforms. Labels indicate the test-probe interval in ms. B, Recovery of r/r_{max}, the normalized probe response amplitude. Here, r/r_{max} corresponds with A_m/A_{mo} in equation (1). The fitted curve plots the relation, $r/r_{max} = \{1 - \exp[-(t - T)/\tau_r]\}$, with T = 1.2 s and $\tau_r = 0.82$ s. C, Dependence of the saturation period T on the natural logarithm of the test flash strength ($\ln I_{test}$), and on the natural logarithm of R_o^* ($\ln R_o^*$). R_o^*, the number of rhodopsin photoisomerizations per rod produced by the test flash, was determined by equating 1 sc td s with 8.6 R_o^*.[5] (Adapted from Pepperberg et al.[38] with permission from the Optical Society of America and Elsevier Science.)

adapting flash, a relatively weak test flash at $t = 10$ s or 12 s, and a bright probe flash at varying times after the test; the test flash presentation times were chosen to correspond with partial recovery from the adapting flash. Analysis of the probe responses yielded the time course of derived responses to the test flash delivered at 10 or 12 s. The relatively short duration that was observed for these derived weak-flash responses (figure 10 of Hetling and Pepperberg[16]) suggests that under the investigated conditions, photocurrent recovery from the bright-adapting flash was rate-limited by the deactivation of an excitatory transduction intermediate rather than by the resynthesis of cGMP.

Adapting illumination of sufficient bleaching strength is associated with robust operation of the series of metabolic and transport reactions, collectively termed the *retinoid visual*

cycle, that support the regeneration of rhodopsin (reviewed by McBee et al.[31] and Saari[43]). The relatively long periods that are required for rod recovery after substantial rhodopsin bleaches preclude the experimental design used in the experiment of figure 37.9, in which each run involved presentation of the bleaching light. Rather, analyses are carried out over the course of recovery from a single adapting (bleaching) illumination terminated at time zero in the experiment. A striking feature of results obtained from mouse rods following substantial bleaching is a change in the rising-phase kinetics of the probe flash response (figure 37.10). The experiment described in figures 37.10A and 37.10B involved a 45-s exposure to bright light (referred to below as the "standard" adapting illumination) that, as determined at 5, 10, and 20 min after the illumination (extraction and analysis of retinoids contained in the eye tissues), produced average rhodopsin bleaching extents of 25%, 14%, and 9%, respectively (table 1 of Kang Derwent et al.[24]). Waveforms labeled PA_D in figure 37.10A are probe-alone responses recorded under dark-adapted conditions. Those labeled PA_1–PA_{40} are probe responses obtained at 1–40 min after the standard adapting illumination. Figure 37.10B shows the responses from figure 37.10A in peak-normalized form and illustrates a similarity among the rising-phase kinetics of the postbleach responses, the key feature of which is a slight delay in onset of the rising phase. This bleach-induced delay resembles the delay that is evident in responses to probe flashes of reduced strength obtained in a separate experiment (figure 37.10C) and thus indicates, for the experiment of figures 37.10A and 37.10B, a bleach-induced desensitization of the response to the probe flash. To compensate for this delay, Kang Derwent et al.[24] employed a determination time t_{det} of 7 ms (rather than 6 ms; see above) to obtain amplitudes of responses to probe flashes presented after bleaching. This analysis yielded the data of figure 37.11A, which shows determinations of the normalized probe response amplitude $A_{moL}(t_{da})/A_{moD}$ as a function of dark-adaptation time t_{da} following a standard bleaching illumination. Here, rod recovery was 80% complete at 13.5 min, on average, after the adapting exposure. Furthermore, for a given extent of recovery (i.e., at a given value of $A_{moL}(t_{da})/A_{moD}$), results obtained from different mice differed primarily with respect to the time required to achieve this recovery extent, rather than to the instantaneous absolute rate of recovery at the given value of $A_{moL}(t_{da})/A_{moD}$ (figure 37.11B).

The data of figure 37.11A and results obtained in steady background light (figure 37.4, reproduced in figure 37.11C) allow determination of the "excitation-equivalent background (I_e)," a time-dependent parameter with units of background strength that can be associated with a given extent of rod recovery (see, e.g., Kennedy et al.[25] and Thomas and Lamb[51]). Figures 37.11D and 37.11E show the transform that links I_e with a given extent of rod recovery, and figure 37.11F illustrates determination of the decay kinetics of I_e ($\log I_e$ versus t_{da}). The plot in figure 37.11F yields an exponential time constant of 5.2 min for decay of the excitation-equivalent background associated with the bleaching experiments of figure 37.11A. Kennedy et al.[25] investigated recovery of the rod ERG a-wave in mouse following a similar extent of rhodopsin bleaching, and determined the course of rod recovery by analysis employing a model of the a-wave rising phase.[5,27] They observed a biphasic recovery of the rod response characterized by exponential decay constants of 2.4 min (accounting for the major portion of recovery) and 56 min. Kennedy et al.[25] furthermore determined the time course of enzymatic reduction of all-*trans* retinal, the immediate retinoid product of rhodopsin bleaching and a component that has been hypothesized to

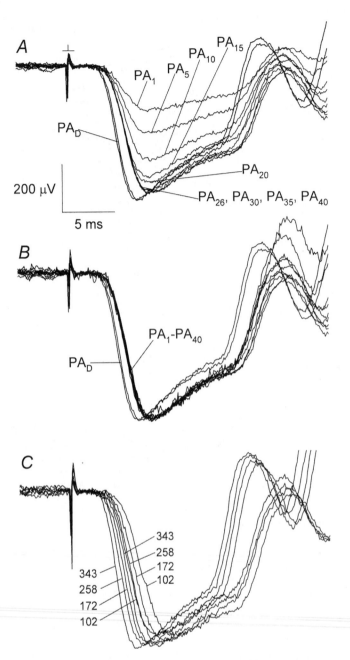

FIGURE 37.10   Effect of bright adapting light on probe responses of mouse rods. A–B, Responses PA_D were obtained under dark-adapted conditions; PA_1–PA_{40} were obtained at 1–40 min after a standard adapting illumination. In part B, PA_1–PA_{40} are rescaled to achieve a match of the peak amplitudes with the average peak amplitude of PA_D. C, Delay in response rising phase obtained with attenuation of the probe flash. Data obtained in an experiment separate from that of parts A and B. Labels indicate the strengths (in sc cd s m^{-2}) of flashes presented before (left-hand labels) and after (right-hand labels) a standard adapting illumination. (Reproduced from Kang Derwent et al.[24] with permission from The Physiological Society.)

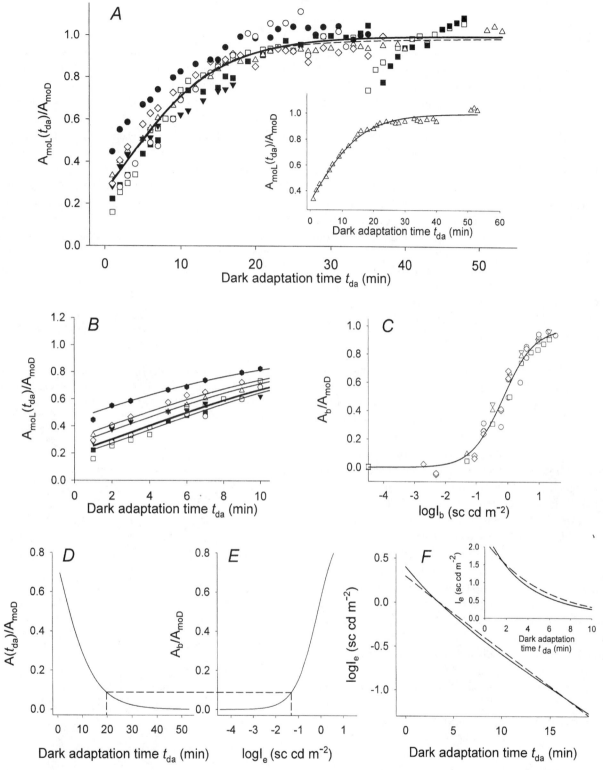

FIGURE 37.11　Recovery of mouse rods following a standard adapting illumination. A–B, Recovery of $A_{moL}(t_{da})/A_{moD}$, the normalized probe response amplitude, as a function of dark-adaptation time t_{da}. C–F, Determination of decay kinetics of the excitation-equivalent background I_e. See text for further details. (Reproduced from Kang Derwent et al.[24] with permission from The Physiological Society.)

maintain excitation during dark adaptation by continued interaction with opsin (cf. Hofmann et al.[18] and Sachs et al.[44]). For the decay of all-*trans* retinal, Kennedy et al.[25] determined a decay time constant of 14 min under bleaching conditions similar to that of the experiments in figure 37.11A. Because the exponential decay constant for I_e described above (5.2 min) is considerably less than 14 min, the ERG data in figure 37.11 suggest that a reaction that occurs before all-*trans* retinal reduction, perhaps removal of all-*trans* retinal from opsin or the translocation of this retinal across the outer segment disk membrane, is the origin of the 5.2-min time constant. Consistent with this possibility, Weng et al.[52] have reported a marked impairment of postbleach rod recovery in *abcr* mice, which lack the transporter that facilitates the translocation of all-*trans* retinal photoproduct from the disk lumen to the cytosol.

Paired-flash determinations of rod response amplitudes after bright adapting illumination have yielded information specifically on the extent of bleach-induced rod desensitization. Using test-probe intervals of 80 ms and 250 ms, Kang Derwent et al.[24] determined amplitudes of the derived response of mouse rods to a weak test flash ($0.11 \, \mathrm{sc\,cd\,s\,m^{-2}}$) presented at varying times after a standard adapting illumination. Figures 37.12A and 37.12B show probe responses recorded in a single experiment of this type. Waveform $\mathrm{PA_D}$ in figure 37.12A is the dark-adapted probe-alone response, and waveforms $\mathrm{T80P_D}$ and $\mathrm{T250P_D}$ are probe responses obtained in paired-flash trials with test-probe intervals of 80 ms and 250 ms, respectively, under dark-adapted conditions. Figure 37.12B shows probe responses obtained at defined times after the standard adapting illumination (subscripts identify dark-adaptation times, in minutes). These data provide evidence for a lingering desensitization, that is, a reduction in amplitude of the derived response to the $0.11 \, \mathrm{sc\,cd\,s\,m^{-2}}$ test flash, produced by the adapting exposure. For example, with the 80-ms test-probe interval, the derived amplitude at ≈ 25–26 min after the adapting illumination (in figure 37.12B, the difference between waveforms $\mathrm{PA_{25}}$ and $\mathrm{T80P_{26}}$ at $t_{det} = 7 \, \mathrm{ms}$) is considerably smaller than the dark-adapted derived amplitude (in figure 37.12A, the difference between waveforms $\mathrm{PA_D}$ and $\mathrm{T80P_D}$ at $t_{det} = 6 \, \mathrm{ms}$) (cf. equation (1)) despite the essentially full recovery of the probe-alone response (in figure 37.12B, the similarity in amplitudes of waveform $\mathrm{PA_{25}}$ at $t_{det} = 7 \, \mathrm{ms}$ and waveform $\mathrm{PA_D}$ at $t_{det} = 6 \, \mathrm{ms}$). Data obtained in a group of experiments of this type indicate a lingering desensitization of about fourfold at 5 min and about twofold at 20 min following the standard adapting illumination. As discussed by Kang Derwent et al.,[24] a possible basis for this lingering desensitization is the light-dependent translocation of transducin from the outer to the inner segment, that is, the removal of a key signaling component in the amplifying chain of disk-based transduction reactions.[4,32,34,48]

Summary

The paired-flash ERG method provides a means by which to determine in vivo the full time course of the dark-adapted rod flash response and to track changes in rod response properties produced by light and dark adaptation. This noninvasive method is likely to be of increasing significance for clinical vision electrophysiology—in particular, for determining the effects of photoreceptor and other retinal diseases on specific properties of the rod electrical response (for an example, see Kang Derwent et al.[23]). The method can furthermore be extended to the study of cone photoreceptors, and several studies examining paired-flash-derived cone responses have already appeared.[10,13,21,35] In combination with in vitro and ERG-based studies of postreceptor neurons, paired-flash ERG analyses of photoreceptor function should prove helpful in advancing the understanding of visual signal generation and processing in the retina.

ACKNOWLEDGMENTS The studies highlighted in this chapter were conducted in close collaboration with Drs. David G. Birch (Retina Foundation of the Southwest), Donald C. Hood (Columbia University), John R. Hetling (University of Illinois at Chicago), Gabriel A. Silva (University of California, San Diego), Jennifer J. Kang Derwent (Illinois Institute of Technology), and Nasser M. Qtaishat (University of Illinois at Chicago). I acknowledge with many thanks the major contributions to these studies made by these colleagues.

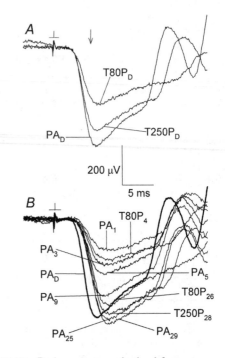

FIGURE 37.12   Probe responses obtained from mouse rods before and after a standard adapting illumination. Results obtained in a single experiment, before (A) and after (B) the adapting illumination. See text for further details. (Adapted from Kang Derwent et al.[24] with permission from The Physiological Society.)

ERG research in my laboratory is supported by NIH Grants EY-05494 and EY-01792, by the Foundation Fighting Blindness (Owings Mills, MD), by a Senior Scientific Investigator award from Research to Prevent Blindness (New York, NY), and by a departmental award from Research to Prevent Blindness.

REFERENCES

1. Arshavsky VY, Lamb TD, Pugh EN Jr: G proteins and phototransduction. *Ann Rev Physiol* 2002; 64:153–187.

2. Baylor DA, Nunn BJ, Schnapf JL: The photocurrent, noise and spectral sensitivity of rods of the monkey *Macaca fascicularis*. *J Physiol* 1984; 357:575–607.

3. Birch DG, Hood DC, Nusinowitz S, Pepperberg DR: Abnormal activation and inactivation mechanisms of rod transduction in patients with autosomal dominant retinitis pigmentosa and the pro-23-his mutation. *Invest Ophthalmol Vis Sci* 1995; 36:1603–1614.

4. Brann MR, Cohen LV: Diurnal expression of transducin mRNA and translocation of transducin in rods of rat retina. *Science* 1987; 235:585–587.

5. Breton ME, Schueller AW, Lamb TD, Pugh EN Jr: Analysis of ERG a-wave amplification and kinetics in terms of the G-protein cascade of phototransduction. *Invest Ophthalmol Vis Sci* 1994; 35:295–309.

6. Burns ME, Baylor DA: Activation, deactivation, and adaptation in vertebrate photoreceptor cells. *Ann Rev Neurosci* 2001; 24:779–805.

7. Calvert PD, Govardovskii VI, Krasnoperova N, Anderson RE, Lem J, Makino CL: Membrane diffusion sets the speed of rod phototransduction. *Nature* 2001; 411:90–94.

8. Chen C-K, Burns ME, He W, Wensel TG, Baylor DA, Simon MI: Slowed recovery of rod photoresponse in mice lacking the GTPase accelerating protein RGS-9. *Nature* 2000; 403:557–560.

9. Cideciyan AV, Jacobson SG: An alternative phototransduction model for human rod and cone ERG a-waves: Normal parameters and variation with age. *Vision Res* 1996; 36:2609–2621.

10. Cideciyan AV, Zhao X., Nielsen L, Khani SC, Jacobson SG, Palczewski K: Null mutation in the rhodopsin kinase gene slows recovery kinetics of rod and cone phototransduction in man. *Proc Natl Acad Sci USA* 1998; 95:328–333.

11. Dowling JE, Ripps H: Adaptation in skate photoreceptors. *J Gen Physiol* 1972; 60:698–719.

12. Fain GL, Matthews HR, Cornwall MC, Koutalos Y: Adaptation in vertebrate photoreceptors. *Physiol Rev* 2001; 81:117–151.

13. Friedburg C, Allen CP, Mason PJ, Lamb TD: Contribution of cone photoreceptors and post-receptoral mechanisms to the human photopic electroretinogram. *J Physiol* 2004; 556:819–834.

14. Friedburg C, Thomas MM, Lamb TD: Time course of the flash response of dark- and light-adapted human rod photoreceptors derived from the electroretinogram. *J Physiol* 2001; 534:217–242.

15. Goto Y, Peachey NS, Ziroli NE, Seiple WH, Gryczan C, Pepperberg DR, Naash MI: Rod phototransduction in transgenic mice expressing a mutant opsin gene. *J Opt Soc Am A* 1996; 13:577–585.

16. Hetling JR, Pepperberg DR: Sensitivity and kinetics of mouse rod flash responses determined *in vivo* from paired-flash electroretinograms. *J Physiol* 1999; 516:593–609.

17. Heynen H, van Norren D: Origin of the electroretinogram in the intact macaque eye: I. Principal component analysis. *Vision Res* 1985; 25:697–707.

18. Hofmann KP, Pulvermüller A, Byczyłko J, Van Hooser P, Palczewski K: The role of arrestin and retinoids in the regeneration pathway of rhodopsin. *J Biol Chem* 1992; 267:15701–15706.

19. Hood DC, Birch DG: A quantitative measure of the electrical activity of human rod photoreceptors using electroretinography. *Visual Neurosci* 1990; 5:379–387.

20. Hood DC, Birch DG: Light adaptation of human rod receptors: The leading edge of the human a-wave and models of rod receptor activity. *Vision Res* 1993; 33:1605–1618.

21. Hood DC, Pepperberg DR, Birch DG: The trailing edge of the photoresponse from human cones derived using a two-flash ERG paradigm. *Opt Soc Am 1996 Tech Digest Series* 1996; 1:64–67.

22. Jeffrey BG, Mitchell DC, Gibson RA, Neuringer M: n-3 fatty acid deficiency alters recovery of the rod photoresponse in rhesus monkeys. *Invest Ophthalmol Vis Sci* 2002; 43:2806–2814.

23. Kang Derwent JJ, Derlacki DJ, Hetling JR, Fishman GA, Birch DG, Grover S, Stone EM, Pepperberg DR: Dark adaptation of rod photoreceptors in normal subjects, and in patients with Stargardt disease and an *ABCA4* mutation. *Invest Ophthalmol Vis Sci* 2004; 45:2447–2456.

24. Kang Derwent JJ, Qtaishat NM, Pepperberg DR: Excitation and desensitization of mouse rod photoreceptors *in vivo* following bright adapting light. *J Physiol* 2002; 541:201–218.

25. Kennedy MJ, Lee KA, Niemi GA, Craven KB, Garwin GG, Saari JC, Hurley JB: Multiple phosphorylation of rhodopsin and the in vivo chemistry underlying rod photoreceptor dark adaptation. *Neuron* 2001; 31:87–101.

26. Kraft TW, Schneeweis DM, Schnapf JL: Visual transduction in human rod photoreceptors. *J Physiol* 1993; 464:747–765.

27. Lamb TD, Pugh EN Jr: A quantitative account of the activation steps involved in phototransduction in amphibian photoreceptors. *J Physiol* 1992; 449:719–758.

28. Lyubarsky AL, Falsini B, Pennesi ME, Valentini P, Pugh EN Jr: UV- and midwave-sensitive cone-driven retinal responses of the mouse: a possible phenotype for coexpression of cone photopigments. *J Neurosci* 1999; 19:442–455.

29. Lyubarsky AL, Pugh EN Jr: Recovery phase of the murine rod photoresponse reconstructed from electroretinographic recordings. *J Neurosci* 1996; 16:563–571.

30. Matthews HR: Incorporation of chelator into guinea-pig rods shows that calcium mediates mammalian photoreceptor light adaptation. *J Physiol* 1991; 436:93–105.

31. McBee JK, Palczewski K, Baehr W, Pepperberg DR: Confronting complexity: The interlink of phototransduction and retinoid metabolism in the vertebrate retina. *Progr Ret Eye Res* 2001; 20:469–529.

32. McGinnis JF, Matsumoto B, Whelan JP, Cao W: Cytoskeleton participation in subcellular trafficking of signal transduction proteins in rod photoreceptor cells. *J Neurosci Res* 2002; 67:290–297.

33. Nakatani K, Tamura T, Yau K-W: Light adaptation in retinal rods of the rabbit and two other nonprimate mammals. *J Gen Physiol* 1991; 97:413–435.

34. Organisciak DT, Xie A, Wang H-M, Jiang Y-L, Darrow RM, Donoso LA: Adaptive changes in visual cell transduction protein levels: effect of light. *Exper Eye Res* 1991; 53:773–779.

35. Paupoo AAV, Mahroo OAR, Friedburg C, Lamb TD: Human cone photoreceptor responses measured by the electroretinogram a-wave during and after exposure to intense illumination. *J Physiol* 2000; 529:469–482.

36. Penn RD, Hagins WA: Signal transmission along retinal rods and the origin of the electroretinographic a-wave. *Nature* 1969; 223:201–205.

37. Pepperberg DR: The flash response of rods in vivo. In Kolb H, Ripps H, Wu S (eds): *Concepts and Challenges in Retinal Biology: A Tribute to John E. Dowling.* Amsterdam, Elsevier Science, *Progr Brain Res* 2001; 131:369–381.

38. Pepperberg DR, Birch DG, Hofmann KP, Hood DC: Recovery kinetics of human rod phototransduction inferred from the two-branched a-wave saturation function. *J Opt Soc Am A* 1996; 13:586–600.

39. Pepperberg DR, Birch DG, Hood DC: Photoresponses of human rods *in vivo* derived from paired-flash electroretinograms. *Vis Neurosci* 1997; 14:73–82.

40. Pepperberg DR, Birch DG, Hood DC: Electroretinographic determination of human rod flash response *in vivo*. In Palczewski K (vol. ed.): *Methods in Enzymology, vol. 316: Vertebrate Phototransduction and the Visual Cycle, Part B.* San Diego, Academic Press, 2000, pp 202–223.

41. Robson JG, Frishman LJ: Dissecting the dark-adapted electroretinogram. *Doc Ophthalmologica* 1999; 95:187–215.

42. Robson JG, Saszik SM, Ahmed J, Frishman LJ: Rod and cone contributions to the a-wave of the electroretinogram of the macaque. *J Physiol* 2003; 547:509–530.

43. Saari JC: Biochemistry of visual pigment regeneration: The Friedenwald Lecture. *Invest Ophthalmol Vis Sci* 2000; 41:337–348.

44. Sachs K, Maretzki D, Meyer CK, Hofmann KP: Diffusible ligand all-*trans*-retinal activates opsin via a palmitoylation-dependent mechanism. *J Biol Chem* 2000; 275:6189–6194.

45. Sillman AJ, Ito H, Tomita T: Studies on the mass receptor potential of the isolated frog retina: I. General properties of the response. *Vision Res* 1969; 9:1435–1442.

46. Silva GA, Hetling JR, Pepperberg DR: Dynamic and steady-state light adaptation of mouse rod photoreceptors *in vivo J Physiol* 2001; 534:203–216.

47. Silva GA, Pepperberg DR: Step response of mouse rod photoreceptors modeled in terms of elemental photic signals. *IEEE Trans Biomed Eng* 2004; 51:3–12.

48. Solokov M, Lyubarsky AL, Strissel KJ, Savchenko AB, Govardovskii VI, Pugh EN Jr, Arshavsky VY: Massive light-driven translocation of transducin between the two major compartments of rod cells: a novel mechanism of light adaptation. *Neuron* 2002; 34:95–106.

49. Sung C-H, Makino C, Baylor D, Nathans J: A rhodopsin gene mutation responsible for autosomal dominant retinitis pigmentosa results in a protein that is defective in localization to the photoreceptor outer segment. *J Neurosci* 1994; 14:5818–5833.

50. Tamura T, Nakatani K, Yau K-W: Light adaptation in cat retinal rods. *Science* 1989; 245:755–758.

51. Thomas MM, Lamb TD: Light adaptation and dark adaptation of human rod photoreceptors measured from the a-wave of the electroretinogram. *J Physiol* 1999; 518:479–496.

52. Weng J, Mata NL, Azarian SM, Tzekov RT, Birch DG, Travis GH: Insights into the function of Rim protein in photoreceptors and etiology of Stargardt's disease from the phenotype in *abcr* knockout mice. *Cell* 1999; 98:13–23.

53. Xu J, Dodd RL, Makino CL, Simon MI, Baylor DA, Chen J: Prolonged photoresponses in transgenic mouse rods lacking arrestin. *Nature* 1997; 389:505–509.

38 Hyperabnormal (Supranormal) Electroretinographic Responses

JOHN R. HECKENLIVELY AND STEVEN NUSINOWITZ

THE ELECTRORETINOGRAM (ERG) is widely used to diagnose various disorders with panretinal dysfunction. Changes in the photopic, rod-isolated, and bright flash scotopic ERG are compared and analyzed to arrive at more specific diagnoses.[12] (See also chapter 49.) Almost uniformly, poor or less than normal responses are used to determine abnormality, and larger-than-normal responses fall into a conceptual category that "bigger is better" and therefore they must be normal. To examine the question of what is really normal, it is essential to establish good normal controls for a laboratory. Standardized testing is essential, such that the electroretinogram methodology tests isolated cone and rod responses as well as both cone and rod responses together. Flicker and dark-adapted red and blue stimuli give added information. The International Society for Clinical Electrophysiology of Vision (ISCEV) ERG standard establishes protocols for achieving reproducible results that are easily interpreted by experienced ophthalmic electrophysiologists. (See the ISCEV Electrophysiologic standard in chapter 20 or at www.iscev.org.)

The concept of what is "normal" may be more difficult to establish than might be expected, since physiologic measurements have innate variability and setting protocols with multiple variables, such as light flashes that are uniform, pupil dilation that is adequate, standard lengths of dark and light adaptation, and accounting for age, gender, and generalized health and eye status, are all confounding factors in assessing "normality." To establish normal values, most laboratories run tests on a set of subjects who have had normal eye examinations through a standardized protocol, recording the amplitudes and implicit times of the a- and b-waves for each test parameter. (Rod-isolated ERGs have minimal a-waves.)

What is a normal value?

To examine the issue of normal electroretinographic values, we tested 242 normal subjects with a standardized electroretinographic protocol between the years 1979 and 1992. All patients had dilated eye examinations to ensure that there were no discernible retinal abnormalities.[11] These ERG values consisted initially of those from normal subjects who were recruited to establishing normal laboratory values; because there were patients who had ERGs on referral that were normal by these initial standards, they were included after a fundus examination was normal. Similarly, some patients with unilateral conditions had the other good eye's data included after the eye was inspected. While these additions did not provide as rigorous normal control data as a prospectively derived study would, they still provided reasonably normal data that were within the standards that are employed at large numbers of universities around the world.

The data were analyzed, and distribution curves, means, normal ranges, and standard deviations were calculated for the group and by gender. Ranges and maximum values were established for b-wave amplitudes, which were equal to or great than two standard deviations by age group (table 38.1, figure 38.1). These values are subjected to analysis to ensure that there is a bell-shaped distribution curve common to population study measurements, and values two standard deviations above and below the mean are taken to be abnormal. Because normal ERG studies have demonstrated some amplitude and implicit time changes with age, age-adjusted values are commonly used (table 38.1).

The maximum value can be identified on the right-hand side of each range for b-wave amplitudes. As examples, an 18-year-old man would have to show a photopic b-wave amplitude of $\geq 244\,\mu V$, and a 43-year-old woman would need a bright-flash dark-adapted b-wave amplitude of $\geq 666\,\mu V$ to be included in the study.

Between 1979 and 1993, over 5000 diagnostic ERGs were performed on patients who had been referred to the UCLA Visual Physiology Laboratory. These ERGs were screened by gender and age bracket for patients who had hyperabnormal b-wave amplitudes that were more than two standard deviations from the mean. The photopic, scotopic rod-isolated, and dark-adapted bright-flash ERGs were all included as parameters for study. The minimum qualification for patient selection was a single amplitude in one eye that was hyperabnormal (>2 standard deviations). Once suitable patients were identified, their records were evaluated to ensure that there was adequate information, including fundus photographs, for the retrospective analysis.[11] As part of this study, we were interested in whether

TABLE 38.1

ERG normal ranges* (determined by normal ±2 standard deviations of each parameter)

Photopic a-Wave Amplitude (μV)			Photopic b-Wave Amplitude (μV)		
Age	Male	Female	Age	Male	Female
0–20	30–94	36–109	0–20	96–244	95–282
21–40	33–91	37–94	21–40	85–223	95–225
41–60	29–78	33–89	41–60	86–186	85–212
61+	19–105	30–78	61+	75–217	109–178

Photopic a-Wave Implicit Time		Photopic b-Wave Implicit Time	
Age	Implicit Time (ms)	Age	Implicit Time (ms)
0–20	12.2–14.3	0–20	28.8–34.4
21–40	12.0–14.8	21–40	28.9–33.5
41–60	12.7–14.9	41–60	29.6–35.6
61+	12.7–15.4	61+	29.6–37.2

Scotopic b-Wave Amplitude (μV)		
Age	Male	Female
0–20	213–515	240–512
21–40	205–463	232–575
41–60	187–449	220–565
61+	156–432	181–443

Scotopic b-Wave Implicit Time	
Age	Implicit Time (ms)
0–20	63.0–86.9
21–40	61.5–96.6
41–60	69.3–97.5
61+	71.1–100.9

Bright-Flash, Dark-Adapted a-Wave Amplitude (μV)			Bright-Flash, Dark-Adapted b-Wave Amplitude (μV)		
Age	Male	Female	Age	Male	Female
0–20	156–336	176–387	0–20	276–756	419–698
21–40	160–369	160–358	21–40	355–639	338–717
41–60	164–330	148–368	41–60	255–655	339–666
61+	118–340	132–327	61+	303–602	321–617

Bright-Flash, Dark-Adapted a-Wave Amplitude Implicit Times (ms)			Bright-Flash, Dark-Adapted b-Wave Implicit Times (ms)		
Age	Male	Female	Age	Male	Female
0–20	20.0–22.9	19.7–23.2	0–20	39.8–52.5	41.1–58.3
21–40	20.7–23.1	19.9–21.0	21–40	39.6–55.2	40.7–56.2
41–60	20.4–23.4	19.6–23.3	41–60	42.3–51.8	47.0–58.6
61+	21.5–24.4	20.6–24.3	61+	46.8–53.7	46.8–58.9

*Normal electroretinographic ranges for control male and females divided by age groups (see text for further selection methodology). The highest amplitude for each gender and age group was used as the cutoff value for inclusion in the hyperabnormal group. On the left center is a standard bell-shaped distribution curve illustrating the concept that 95% of population would be considered normal, while those outside the two standard deviations would be abnormal.

Photopic a-wave

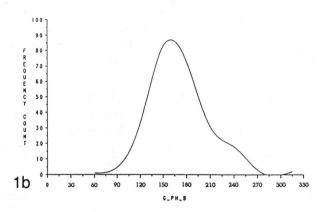

Photopic b-wave

Scotopic b-wave

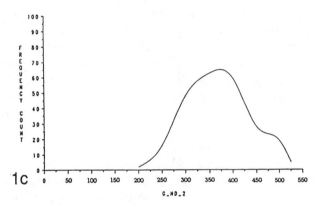

Dark-adapted bright blash b-wave

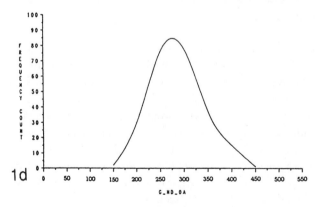

Dark-adapted bright flash a-wave

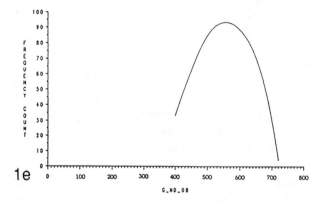

FIGURE 38.1   Distribution curves for 241 normal control subjects evaluating their photopic, rod-isolated, and bright-flash dark-adapted a- and b-wave amplitudes. Normal population distributions curves were generally seen (see results).

hyperabnormal (supernormal) responses should be interpreted as normal.

Once a patient was identified as having an amplitude greater than two standard deviations from the mean, the patient's chart was examined to identify aspects of the history or clinical findings that could be related to the associated finding of a hyperabnormal response. The pertinent findings were categorized by the most prominent feature. In particular, the fundus photographs and fluorescein angiogram were carefully evaluated for pathology.

The 242 normal control results were plotted on frequency distribution curves, which gave reasonably normal bell-shaped distributions (see figures 38.1A through 38.1E). There were 139 females and 103 males. The photopic and rod scotopic b-wave distribution appeared to be slightly bimodal (see figures 38.1B and 38.1C), with higher-amplitude values represented more frequently. The photopic a-wave distribution has a long tail on the high end; both these findings suggest that a few patients were marked as normal but had hyperabnormal responses that were not appreciated at the time of testing. If this were true and a correction had been made, it would only have moved the two-standard-deviation cutoff point lower than the one that was used in the second part of the study, in which patients with hyperabnormal responses were carefully evaluated for associated pathology. The normal ranges for the amplitudes and implicit times by gender and age are listed in table 38.1 for the photopic, scotopic, and bright-flash dark-adapted ERGs, all performed on the same equipment using a standardized protocol.

In searching our records, 381 patients were found to have a response more than two standard deviations from the mean in at least one ERG parameter. Because ours was a referral laboratory for testing, the number of patients with complete eye examinations was limited. However, 104 patients with hyperabnormal responses were found to have adequate information to allow a full review of their clinical findings. Representative examples can be viewed in figure 38.2. In classifying their ophthalmologic findings, the following categories and numbers of patients were found (table 38.2): maculopathies, twenty-two patients (22%) of all types, including four patients with Best's vitelliform dystrophy; optic neuropathies, nineteen (19%); retinitis pigmentosa suspect or carriers, twenty (20%), including five who were known carriers and two patients with family histories of retinitis pigmentosa; panretinal degenerations (other than maculopathy), seven (7%); color blindness or cone dysfunction, seven (7%); drug toxicity, six (6%); neurologic referrals of ataxic patients, six (6%); posttrauma, five (5%); aniridia, three (3%); and miscellaneous findings, thirteen (13%), including two patients with congenital nystagmus.

In looking at the categories, no particular hyperabnormal component of the ERG was predominant. Optic neuropa-thy and maculopathy patients had representation from hyperabnormal photopic, scotopic, and bright-flash dark-adapted ERGs, although there was only one patient with optic neuropathy and a hyperabnormal rod response. Hyperabnormal responses were also underrepresented in the drug toxicity and trauma categories.

In correlating fluorescein angiographic changes in the hyperabnormal group, fourteen patients had bright temporal disk staining on late phases of the angiogram (see figures 38.4B, 38.5, and 38.7), which was not easily explained, since the majority (ten) were in cases of maculopathy or retinal degeneration (table 38.3). While temporal optic nervehead staining was found in only 14% of the hyperabnormal ERG cases, it was distinctive and suggests that there may be an association between temporal disk staining on the fluorescein and hyperabnormal ERGs.

Illustrative case reports

CASE 1   A 55-year-old Hispanic man presented with complaints in the right eye of decreasing visual acuity. History revealed an alcohol consumption of seven scotches a day for about 20 years. On examination, his best-corrected visual acuity was 20/70 O.U. Fundus examination revealed multiple round yellow-white deposits at the level of the retinal pigment epithelium in the foveae (figure 38.3A). The fluorescein angiogram demonstrated numerous basilar deposits in the posterior pole as well as foveal edema (figure 38.3B). On late phases, both optic nerveheads had a sliver of intense temporal disk staining. His ERG demonstrated hyperabnormal scotopic b-wave amplitudes and dark-adapted bright flash a- and b-waves amplitudes (see figure 38.2 composite). The diagnosis was macular degeneration with basilar laminar drusen.

CASE 2   A 25-year-old college student complained of intermittent blurry vision. Family history was negative for any other affected persons with eye problems. On examination, her visual acuity was 20/25 O.U. Ophthalmoscopy demonstrated focal areas of RPE dropout in the perifoveal regions with some flecklike deposition. The fluorescein angiogram showed a dark choroids effect and window defects in the perifoveal regions; and on late phases, an intense staining of the temporal optic nervehead was seen (figure 38.4). Her ERG showed hyperabnormal scotopic and bright-flash dark-adapted b-wave amplitudes (see figure 38.2). Although the ERG is not typical of Stargardt's disease, which typically shows a cone-rod dysfunction pattern), the fundus findings were consistent with Stargardt's disease. Molecular testing was not performed in this patient.

CASE 3   A 27-year-old woman had a 1.5-year history of blurred vision and related having headaches and

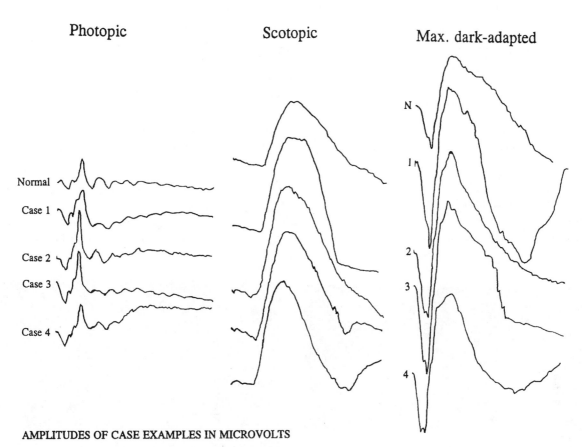

| Photopic | Scotopic | Max. dark-adapted |

AMPLITUDES OF CASE EXAMPLES IN MICROVOLTS

Case	Photopic a-wave	Photopic b-wave	Scotopic b-wave	Max. dark-adapted a-wave	Max. dark-adapted b-wave
Normal	51	141	385	207	422
Case 1	74	164	<u>450</u>	<u>402</u>	<u>753</u>
Case 2	57	<u>271</u>	<u>496</u>	308	<u>773</u>
Case 3	<u>94</u>	230	<u>527</u>	414	809
Case 4	62	<u>191</u>	<u>476</u>	253	<u>648</u>

Out of 2 standard deviation range (age-matched) values are underlined.

FIGURE 38.2   Composite illustration of normal and four case examples of hyperabnormal electroretinograms; amplitudes are listed below the waveforms by case.

TABLE 38.2

Distribution of hyperabnormal responses by category

Category	Number of Patients	Photopic	Rod	Bright Flash
Maculopathy	22	15	6	11
Optic neuropathy	19	12	1	9
RP Suspect/carrier	20	14	6	12
RPE/retinal degeneration	7	1	2	4
Cone dysfunction	6	1	2	4
Drug toxicity	6	5	0	2
Neurology referral	3	1	2	2
Posttrauma	5	2	0	4
Aniridia	3	2	0	2
Miscellaneous	13	3	3	10

TABLE 38.3

Diagnoses in hyperabnormal ERG patients with temporal disk staining on late phases of the fluorescein angiogram

Retinal pigment epitheliopathy
Optic neuropathy
Chronic macular edema and degeneration
Macular degeneration
Idiopathic foveal dysfunction
Suspected retinitis pigmentosa (mother had)
Macular degeneration
Optic neuropathy
Optic neuritis
Behr's syndrome (optic atrophy)
Early macular degeneration
Macular degeneration

photosensitivity. On examination, the visual acuity was 20/200 in each eye. Fundus examination revealed a blond fundus and optic pallor O.U. There were some granular changes and atrophy in the foveae, and fluorescein angiograms showed minor window defects in the maculae and an intense late staining of the temporal optic nervehead O.U. (figure 38.5). The ERG demonstrated hyperabnormal photopic, scotopic, and bright-flash dark-adapted responses (see figure 38.2).

CASE 4   A 72-year-old woman with regional atrophic macular degeneration had been followed routinely for eight years. An electroretinogram had been ordered to rule out a senile cone dystrophy because of the distribution of macular

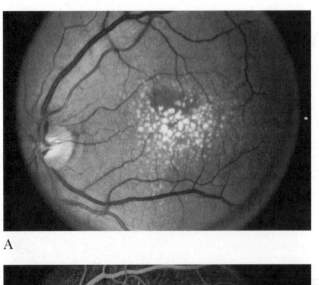

A

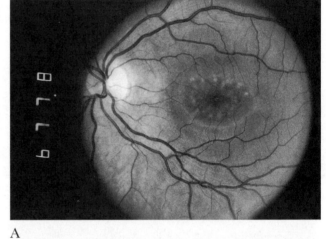

A

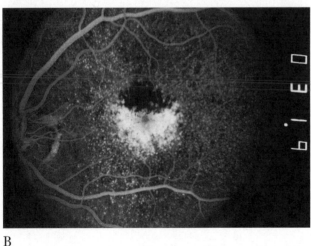

B

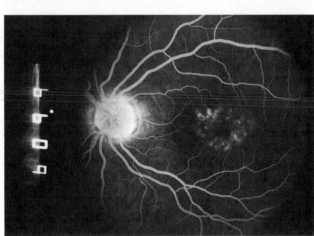

B

FIGURE 38.3   Case 1: fundus photograph (A) and fluorescein angiogram (B) of left eye of a 55-year-old man with macular degeneration and basilar laminar drusen in posterior pole. Late phases of the fluorescein angiogram show diffuse small drusen throughout the posterior pole and intense hyperfluorescence of the fovea. (Adapted from Heckenlively JR, Tanji T, Logani S: Retrospective study of hyperabnormal (supranormal) electroretinographic responses in 104 patients. *Trans Am Ophthalmol Soc* 1994; 92:217–231. Reprinted with permission.)

FIGURE 38.4   Case 2: fundus photograph (A) and fluorescein angiogram (B) of left eye of a 25-year-old woman with Stargardt's disease. The patient had flecklike lesions in the parafoveal regions, and on the fluorescein angiogram, a dark choroid effect was seen. Minor window defects were present in the area of the flecks. There was notable late staining of the temporal optic nervehead O.U. The ERG b-wave amplitudes were all hyperabnormal (see figure 38.2).

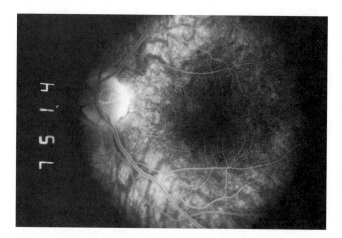

FIGURE 38.5   Case 3: left eye, fluorescein angiogram of a 27-year-old woman with optic neuropathy with a history of headaches and photosensitivity. Optic pallor was evident on funduscopy, while on late phases of the fluorescein aniogram, intense temporal staining was seen in the optic nervehead. Her ERG amplitudes were hyperabnormal for all modalities tested (see figure 38.2).

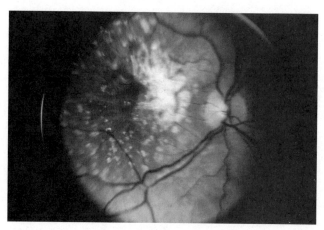

FIGURE 38.6   Case 4: fundus photograph of the left eye of a 72-year-old woman with geographic macular degeneration with crystalline drusen scattered in the posterior pole. One late phases of the fluorescein angiogram, there was a distinct edge of temporal disk staining O.U. Her hyperabnormal photopic ERG values were particularly surprising in light of the macular atrophy.

loss and complaints of photosensitivity. The visual acuity was 20/20 O.U., owing to intact foveal islands. Fundus examination showed scalloped loss of the retinal pigment epithelia in the perifoveal region and hyperpigmented intact foveolar tissue, with scattered crystallinelike drusen in the posterior pole (figure 38.6). The fluorescein angiogram showed window defects in the perifoveal region and an edge of temporal staining in each optic nerve. The ERG demonstrated hyperabnormal photopic, scotopic, and bright-flash dark-adapted b-waves (see figure 38.2), an unexpected finding in this elderly woman with atrophic macular degeneration.

CASE 5   A 41-year-old woman presented with visual loss over the previous month in her left eye. Her medical history revealed that the year before, she had undergone a kidney transplant and a parathyroidectomy. She had been on dialysis 1.5 years before her renal transplant. There was no family history of eye disease. On examination, her visual acuity was O.D. 20/20, O.S. 20/200, with scattered drusen in her fundus and macular atrophy OS (figure 38.7). The Goldmann visual field was normal O.U. Her b-wave amplitudes O.D. 277, O.S. 304 for the photopic ERG, were O.D. 531, O.S. 585 for the rod-isolated ERG, and O.D. 781, O.S. 851 microvolts for her bright-flash dark-adapted ERG, all nearly double normal values.

Hyperabnormal responses suggest a pathologic process

Less than normal ERG responses have been useful in diagnosing a large number of clinical disorders and, in patients with minimal to no retinal findings, can be very important in proving that a disorder exists. Generally, however, when

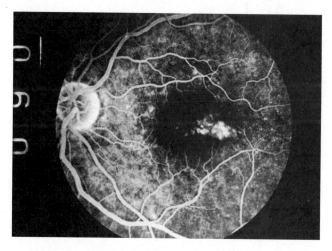

FIGURE 38.7   Case 5: fluorescein angiogram of a 41-year-old woman who had noted visual loss the previous month with 20/200 vision O.S. She had scattered drusen and macular atrophy O.S. The Goldmann visual field was normal O.U. Her b-wave amplitudes were all nearly double normal values (see text).

an electroretinographic response was found to be bigger than normal (more than two standard deviations from the mean), the finding has been ignored and thought to be part of "normal." The analysis of these 104 patients with hyperabnormal ERG responses suggests that hyperabnormal responses need to be considered in a more critical fashion, as they likely reflect a disease process or possibly a disorder in which inhibitory circuits are suppressed or underrepresented,[9,15] albinism,[16] atypical cone dystrophies,[1,10,22] optic nerve sectioning,[8,14] optic neuropathies (e.g., optic nerve hypoplasia, optic atrophy),[6,7,20] vascular occlusions and ischemia,[2,13,19] uveitis,[3,17,18,21] cortical steroids,[24] low-dose barbiturates,[23] and carbon disulphide poisoning.[4,5] In some of these examples, it is easy to intuitively comprehend that metallosis, chronic inflammation, and ischemia are physiologically irritating to the retina and may result in larger-than-normal responses. Similarly, in our cases of aniridia and albinism, more light is reaching the photoreceptors, and larger responses can be expected.

The mechanism of higher electroretinographic amplitudes in optic neuropathies is unknown, and it can be speculated that inhibitory components within the retina may be affected during the course of transsynaptic degeneration, resulting in higher ERG amplitudes. It can be speculated that the temporal optic atrophy and staining that are seen in some of the patients with hyperabnormal responses may be related to degeneration of inhibitory neurons.

Perhaps the most puzzling group of patients with hyperabnormal responses were those with macular degeneration. Generally, any patient who exhibits retinal degeneration, whether in the posterior pole or more diffusely, would be expected to have a reduced ERG. Yet in a number of our patients, there were thirteen hyperabnormal photopic and eleven with dark-adapted bright-flash hyperabnormal values. (Some eyes were affected bilaterally.) These findings might imply that these patients are experiencing a panretinal process in which the demonstrable sign is macular degeneration. Certainly, it appears that the ERG might be more useful than was previously thought in differentiating types of macular degeneration.

The correlation of pathologic findings and visual symptoms in these patients with hyperabnormal ERG responses strongly suggests that patients who show hyperabnormal responses need a careful evaluation for diseases which will explain their findings and that a hyperabnormal response should not automatically be treated as normal. Even in the face of no obvious ocular pathology, it might be an indication that the patient should be followed more closely and have a repeat ERG in the future to further evaluate the patient.

Identification of hyperabnormal ERGs is contingent on each electrophysiology laboratory's having carefully maintained standardized testing with normal control values by age and gender. Inherent in this methodology are the use of Ganzfeld stimulation and a Burian-Allen-style contact lens electrode for recording to reduced the variability in testing methodology. Furthermore, maintenance of light stimuli and background light calibration must be checked on a regular basis.

REFERENCES

1. Alexander KR, Fishman GA: Supernormal scotopic ERG in cone dystrophy. *Br J Ophthalmol* 1984; 68:69–78.
2. Brunnette JR, Olivier P, Galeano C, et al: Hyperresponse and delay in the electroretinogram in acute ischemia. *Can J Ophthalmol* 1989; 107:1459–1462.
3. Burian HM: Electroretinography in temporal arteritis. *Am J Ophthalmol* 1963; 56:796–800.
4. Delaey JJ, de Rouck A, Priem H, et al: Ophthalmological aspects of chronic CS_2 intoxication. *Int Ophthalmol* 1980; 1:51–56.
5. De Rouck A, De Lae JJ, van Hoorne M, et al: Chronic carbon disulphide poisoning: A 4 year follow-up study of the ophthalmological signs. *Int Ophthalmol* 1986; 9:17–27.
6. Feinsold M, Howe H, Auerbach E: Changes in the electroretinogram in patients with optic nerve lesions. *Doc Ophthalmol* 1971; 29:169–200.
7. Francois J, deRouck A: Electroretinographical study of hypoplasia of the optic nerve. *Ophthalmologica* 1976; 172:308–330.
8. Gills JP: The electroretinogram after section of optic nerve in man. *Am J Ophthalmol* 1966; 62:287–291.
9. Good P, Gross K: Electrophysiology and metallosis: Support for an oxidative (free radical) mechanism in the human eye. *Ophthalmologica* 1988; 196:204–209.
10. Gouras P, Eggers HM, MacKay CJ: Cone dystrophy, nyctalopia, and supernormal rod responses: A new retinal degeneration. *Arch Ophthalmol* 1983; 101:718–724.
11. Heckenlively JR, Tanji T, Logani S: Retrospective study of hyperabnormal (supranormal) electroretinographic responses in 104 patients. *Trans Am Ophthalmol Soc* 1994; 92:218–233.
12. Heckenlively JR, Weleber RG, Arden GB: Testing levels of the visual system. In Heckenlively JR, Arden GB (eds): *Principles and Practice of Clinical Electrophysiology of Vision*. St. Louis, Mosby Yearbook, 1991, pp 485–493.
13. Henkes HE: Electroretinogram in circulatory disturbances of the retina. *Arch Ophthalmol* 1954; 52:30–41.
14. Jacobson JH, Suzuki TA: Effects of optic nerve section on the ERG. *Arch Ophthalmolol* 1962; 667:791–801.
15. Knave B: Electroretinographic in eyes with retained intraocular metallic foreign bodies. *Acta Ophthalmol Suppl* 1969; 100:1–63.
16. Krill AE, Lee GB: The electroretinogram in albinos and carriers of the ocular albino trait. *Arch Ophthalmol* 1963; 69:32–38.
17. Kurachi Y, Hirose T, Yonemura D: ERG in pulseless (Takayasu's) disease. Proceedings of 4th ISCERG symposium. *Jpn J Ophthalmol Suppl* 1966; 10:106–112.
18. Lawwill T, Wacker W, MacDonald H: The role of electroretinography in evaluating posterior uveitis. *Am J Ophthalmol* 1972; 74:1086–1090.
19. Sakaue H, Katsumi O, Hirose T: Electroretinographic findings in fellow eyes of patients with central retinal vein occlusion. *Arch Ophthalmol* 1989; 107:1459–1462.
20. Sprague JB, Wilson B: Electrophysiologic findings in bilateral optic nerve hypoplasia. *Arch Ophthalmol* 1981; 99:1028–1029.
21. Standord MB, Robbins J: Experimental posterior uveitis: II. Electroretinographic studies. *Br J Ophthalmol* 1988; 72:88–96.
22. Yagasaki K, Miyake Y, Litao RE, et al: Two cases of retinal degeneration with an unusual forms of electroretinogram. *Doc Ophthalmol* 1986; 63:73–82.
23. Yonemura D, Kawasaki K, Tsuchida Y: 3–4 Differential vulnerability of the ERG components to pentobarbital. Proceedings of the 4th ISCERG Symposium. *Jpn J Ophthalmol Suppl* 1966; 10:155–166.
24. Zimmerman TJ, Dawson WW, Fitzgerald CR: I: Electroretinographic changes in normal eyes during administration of prednisone. *Ann Ophthalmol* 1973; 5:757–765.

39 Technical Issues in Evaluating Patients for Therapeutic Trials

BETH EDMUNDS, PETER J. FRANCIS, AND RICHARD G. WELEBER

THE RETINAL DYSTROPHIES are an individually rare but collectively common cause of progressive visual loss in children and adults.[6,7,12] Treatment is currently limited to visual aids and rehabilitation. In light of recent advances in understanding these conditions at the molecular level, there is a realistic prospect that soon, gene therapies and novel pharmaceutical agents will become available that will purport to prevent, arrest, or ameliorate retinal degeneration.[1,36] In addition, it has been suggested that dietary or vitamin supplements might be useful in working against disease progression in certain individuals.[5]

Study design

It is therefore incumbent on those who are interested in exploring this potentially exciting area to design treatment trials that examine the efficacy of new interventions. The randomized controlled trial (RCT) is the gold standard method for interventional studies, and guidelines for the conduct of such studies have been published in the CONSORT statement.[24] Factors specifically relating to studies of therapeutic intervention in retinal dystrophies will be discussed further.

Outcome measures

Outcome measures should be carefully chosen to optimize the likelihood of demonstrating a treatment effect (beneficial, not beneficial, or even harmful). Because vision is a complex function, outcome measures should ideally provide information about both the status of retinal function as close as possible to the cellular disturbance that is created by the disease and the status of retinal function as is meaningful and important for the patient. The treatment, for example with a growth or survival factor, may be able to rescue or preserve the anatomical number of cells within the retina, but if rescue or preservation of functional sight is not achieved, then no true benefit has been derived.

In human studies, the most important clinical outcomes are functional capabilities in real-life situations, such as reading, recognizing family and friends, driving, participating in sports and recreational activities, and other visually oriented tasks. These aspects of vision are subject to personality variables

and the influence of other physical, social, and psychological factors that argue for more objective outcomes for treatment trials, such as those given by optotype acuity testing and standardized visual field algorithms. Even these measures, however, are subject to performance factors and, because of their contrived nature, might not reflect the patient's real-life experience. Furthermore, these tests might not evaluate visual symptoms specific to patients with retinal dystrophies, limiting their ability to quantify disease and response to treatment. Despite these limitations, however, it is advisable in designing an intervention study, to use previously validated methods of assessing visual function. This not only ensures that the tool measures its purported substrate, but also allows comparison with other trials and research outcomes.

Visual acuity measures

Snellen visual acuities are often used for distance vision testing in the clinical setting, but in a trial, logarithmic-based acuities, such as those used in the Early Treatment for Diabetic Retinopathy Study (ETDRS),[11] are preferable, as they are more standardized and offer greater precision of measurement. Additionally, geometric progression in letter height allows analysis of acuity as a continuous variable with the advantage of greater statistical flexibility. One solution that the National Eye Institute of the United States of America is supporting for clinical trials is to use a computerized method of visual acuity determination, such as the electronic vision acuity (EVA) based on the standard ETDRS testing protocol, or EVA E-ETDRS, developed by the Jaeb Center for Health Research in Tampa, Florida.[3] There are many methods of near vision testing, but once again, a logarithmic-based chart has distinct advantages. Identification of single optotypes at near, however, is different from reading words and sentences, which is a much more complex task. Some trials have therefore included reading speed as an outcome measure that is more representative of patients' daily reading activity.[19,28]

Visual field measures

Goldmann kinetic visual field testing is a convenient, reproducible method for the assessment of field defects in peripheral retinal degenerations, such as retinitis pigmentosa (RP).[29] Here, perimetry provides the opportunity to use a wide variety of stimulus sizes and intensities. For progressive retinal degenerations, an intermediate test target, for example, the I-4e, would be predicted to be the best choice, as it is likely to provide data for the largest number of individuals.[25] Overall, visual field size can then be calculated from the solid angle in steradians of seeing field minus scotomas.[26,37]

Currently, the static visual field programs that exist for commercial perimeters, such as the Humphrey Field Analyzer, are optimized for algorithms that are designed to detect visual field loss from glaucoma and neuro-ophthalmologic disease. Visual field programs need to be developed and optimized for the type of progressive visual field loss that is seen in the various types of inherited retinal degenerations, such as RP. Visual field testing in RP often is very time consuming and stressful for the patient, who might be unable to see many, if not most, of the test target presentations. The time needed to reliably assess the visual field in patients with retinal dystrophies can be decreased by using Bayesian probability algorithms rather than the lengthier full threshold staircase methods. Also, attention must be directed toward standardizing instructions that are given to patients who are undergoing testing, since these instructions can dramatically influence the resulting findings on static perimetry.[17]

When all of the peripheral visual field has been lost but significant visual retinal function persists centrally, as, for example, in gyrate atrophy of the retina,[10] a useful measure for following patients is the sum of all thresholds measured with a program such as the 30-2, the 24-2, or even the 10-2 static perimetry program of the Humphrey Field Analyzer. Such programs have also been used to follow patients with advanced RP.[13] The advantage of such measurements is that a single variable is derived that correlates relatively well with overall remaining retinal sensitivity. Other perimetric techniques, such as two-color scotopic threshold perimetry,[16] that are currently available only as custom-made research instruments may become commercially available in due course, but these devices and their protocols will require the same validation as has been undertaken for Humphrey field testing.

Electrophysiology

Retinal electrophysiology, principally the electroretinogram (ERG), is commonly used for the assessment of retinal dystrophies because it provides objective measures of retinal function and correlates well with anatomic preservation, restoration of cellular function, and subjective aspects of vision, such as acuity and visual field. Parameters such as implicit times and peak amplitudes can be compared between treated and control eyes and over time in the same

eye. Because ERG amplitudes and implicit times exhibit skewed distribution among normal subjects, transformation of the data by conversion to the log or square root is usually performed before statistical analysis.[4,7,26] Assessment of PIII function through a-wave analysis using bright-flash ERG has allowed investigators to infer mechanisms of photoreceptor dysfunction in retinal degenerations.[8,9,14,27,34] The multifocal ERG (mfERG), developed by Sutter and his colleagues,[30] has become a valuable tool to evaluate the topography of residual central ERG responses in patients with RP and the carrier state for X-linked RP.[15,35]

In recent years, an international effort has been made to standardize electrophysiological measures[2,21–23] that will prove critical for future treatment trials of rare diseases in which multicenter collaboration is essential. Variability among subjects across one or more testing sessions and between eyes tested, with possible differences in the degree of variability between normals and affecteds, exists for all of these electrophysiological measurements. Quantification of these variabilities is important for estimations of power calculations in designing clinical trials. Furthermore, although the testing protocols can be standardized, normal values for electrophysiological responses will vary from laboratory to laboratory. This presents problems for analysis of tests that are performed in more than one center. One method that copes with this is the response ratio, which uses the lower limit of normal for a particular laboratory as the denominator and patient response as the numerator.[25]

Other psychophysical tests

Other measures of macular function, such as contrast sensitivity and color vision, may also contribute to the assessment of the visual impact of an intervention but are not usually the main study outcome of interest. The Pelli-Robson chart has proven robust in varying clinical conditions and is the most frequently used test of contrast sensitivity in clinical trials. There are numerous color vision tests; some of these, for example, the Ishihara plates, are designed to detect congenital color defects, and others, such as the A.O.H.R.R. series, are more appropriate for acquired disease. The choice of chart may depend on the dystrophy that is under investigation. For clinical trials, arrangement tests, such as the Farnsworth-Munsell 100-hue color discrimination test, are preferable to plate tests, as they allow better quantification of the color deficiency and have normative databases for comparison.[20] (See also chapter 47.)

Questionnaires and assessment of activities of daily living

Increasingly, we are aware of the need to assess the functional aspects of disease on patients' lives and the impact of treatment interventions on patient's quality of life (QOL). Once again, in examining the impact of an intervention, this is best done as an RCT. Ideally, QOL and objective measures of visual function would be the same; but more often, they are not and need to be evaluated separately. Several questionnaires have been developed to assess general QOL issues, as well as vision-specific QOL issues. However, these visually orientated questionnaires, based mainly on studies of cataract and glaucoma,[18] might not be relevant or appropriately sensitive to the visual disabilities that are experienced by patients with retinal dystrophies. The development of valid QOL questionnaires for the future study of interventions in retinal dystrophies would therefore be useful.

Statistical considerations

The main outcome measures that are chosen currently for most clinical trials are derived from acuity, visual field, and electroretinographic testing. Often, one of these is chosen as the main outcome measure, which is used to calculate the required sample size to provide statistical significance to a clinically significant treatment effect. If more than one outcome measure is chosen, power calculations should be adjusted accordingly, or a stricter level of statistical significance should be used to overcome the increased likelihood of finding an effect by chance. Ideally, methods of analysis that take into consideration the complex nature of vision should be developed so that results of studies are not clouded by a seemingly significant benefit for one measure, for example, the ERG, but no benefit when other variables are examined. For example, a retinal dystrophy treatment could result in a significant beneficial effect on the ERG, through a buoying effect on retinal cell function that results in either a temporary increase in the ERG amplitude or an increase in the ERG that is not associated in any way with improved visual function as determined by other measures. Fortunately, in the majority of treatment interventions, improvement in the ERG will be correlated with improvement in visual acuity, field, and other, more subjective measures, but the characterization of the visual impact of the disease and the effects of treatment remain complex.

Continuous versus categorical variables as endpoints

Some variables, for example, the ERG implicit times and wave amplitudes and Humphrey visual field parameters, may be expressed as continuous variables. When numbers are small or distributions are skewed, nonparametric analyses should be used. Other measures, for example, the abnormalities that are seen on fundus examination in RP (vessel attenuation, retinal pigmentation, optic atrophy, and macular changes) might not easily be scaled continuously but instead might be classified into stages or degrees of severity

based on prior agreement among the investigators. These different data types must be analyzed in different fashions but will still provide valuable insight into the effects of therapeutic interventions.

Ceiling and floor effects

The choice of outcome measure must take into consideration the natural history of the disease. A good example of this is the choice of visual field parameter that is used to detect change in RP. For some of the late adult onset forms of RP, the Goldmann V-4e isopter (the area of field defined by the isopter using the largest, brightest test target) will be too crude a measure if the intervention study is conducted during the early phase of disease. A smaller, dimmer test target, such as the I-4e test target, might be a much better choice. As the disease progresses, retinal function might become so disturbed that finer measures of visual function are no longer readily and accurately measurable. Using the example of RP, in the late stage of disease, the peripheral visual field might be entirely lost to the I-4e test target, and larger test targets, such as the III-4e or V-4e targets, might be more appropriate.

The choice of outcome measure must therefore take into consideration the natural history of the disease for the enrolled subjects during the entire course of the intervention study. The parameters that are chosen must reflect the expected spectrum of retinal function to avoid ceiling and floor effects and to give an even spread of data, which will improve the likelihood of meaningful statistical analysis.

Strategies to overcome small sample sizes

Studies should be sufficiently powered to show a treatment effect, if there is one. All too often, failure to show an effect from an intervention is due to inadequate sample size rather than genuine lack of effect. In rare diseases, such as the retinal dystrophies, achieving adequate sample sizes can be difficult and may require multicenter collaborations or outcome measures that yield large magnitudes of effect to show statistical significance between treatment and control groups. One advantage of the retinal dystrophies, if there can be said to be any, is that both eyes tend to be involved, most often in a symmetrical fashion. For intervention strategies in which only one eye is treated, this gives the opportunity for between-eye comparisons with one eye acting as the control. There is thus automatic matching for many variables such as age and sex and other constitutional prognostic factors. Because both eyes contribute to the study, fewer patients are required to achieve adequate sample size. For studies of interventions that would affect both eyes, such as pharmaceuticals or supplements given systemically, more subjects will be needed. For some interventions, the expected result will be a notable improvement in function; for others, only a slowing of the process might be expected. One method that can reduce the number of patients required is to employ a crossover design in which the same groups of patients are given both treatments in random order. This method is best for interventions that take effect quickly and have little carryover effect to interfere with the second treatment outcome.[38]

Although the RCT is the gold standard method for investigating an intervention and should be used whenever possible, two other methods are described that may offer adequate control of bias in studying rare diseases with small sample sizes. The first is minimization, in which cases are allocated to the intervention and control arm of the study according to predetermined allocation variables.[32,33] These variables reflect factors that are already known to affect outcome. By balancing the two groups with sequential addition of cases in a way to minimize the differences between the two groups, two groups are formed that have very similar characteristics except for the treatment allocation. The second method involves using a Bayesian approach, in which a prior probability distribution of outcome is calculated from previously conducted studies in the literature and combined with trial data to give a posterior distribution of outcome.[31]

Case selection

The retinal dystrophies are a heterogenous group of disorders, many inherited, that present at various stages of life with varying severity. In designing an intervention trial, it is important to characterize the target patient population. By application of inclusion and exclusion criteria, patients should be admitted to the trial only if they have the disease characteristics of interest. To make analysis cleaner, exclusion criteria often eliminate factors that might confound the analysis, such as eyes with multiple pathologies (e.g., trauma, glaucoma, and uveitis). Early clinical trials may be helped in their demonstration of efficacy by exclusion of patients with confounding secondary changes, such as severe, advanced atrophy of the choroid or of the optic nerve. However, restriction of cases limits study generalizability, meaning that the study findings are directly applicable only to patients who have the same disease characteristics as those who were included in the trial. Quite often, a balance between the two needs to be struck. In reporting trial methodology, it is also important to indicate which eligible patients did not participate, because nonparticipation can also introduce bias.

Masking

In studies of ophthalmic disease, it is considered polite to use the term *masking* rather than *blinding* to indicate the degree of concealment of treatment allocation from participants. Although bias is limited by randomization, it can nonetheless be introduced during the trial by study participants' awareness of the treatment allocation of a patient. Awareness of treatment allocation may influence, consciously or not, the researcher's measurement of exposure and outcome variables. Similarly, the patients' perception of treatment may affect their behavior and responses. Ideally, double masking, in which neither patient nor researcher knows the treatment status at any stage of the trial until the code is broken, is ideal. But where double masking is not possible, single masking, in which the patients are unaware of their treatment status, should be used as much as possible.

Interventions

Although there are currently no treatments for the majority of the retinal dystrophies, there are conditions, such as Refsum's disease and abetalipoproteinemia, for which there are established treatments, such as dietary restriction and supplementations. In these cases, the established treatment should be used in the control arm. In most cases, however, placebo or sham treatment should be used in the controls to maintain concealment of treatment allocation. This can prove difficult when the intervention involves a subretinal or intravitreal injection, as might be the case in gene therapy, since it might be considered unethical to subject patients to sham intraocular procedures.

Ethical issues

Randomized controlled trials for retinal dystrophies are subject to all the ethical considerations that are normally encountered in medical research. However, one further issue, particularly pertinent to inherited diseases such as the dystrophies, concerns gene therapy interventions. Gene therapy, unlike many other treatments, results in permanent alteration of the subject's DNA and cannot be repeated. This means that a trial involving an extremely rare dystrophy, perhaps a trial in which patients have been collected from all over the world, may alter the entire cohort for a generation, not allowing the possibility of subsequent trials for improved therapies until a later generation. At our current early stage of gene therapy research, there are therefore both ethical and practical justifications for conducting trials in the commoner dystrophies first and refining treatments in these populations before attempting treatment of the extremely rare diseases.

ACKNOWLEDGMENTS Supported by The Foundation Fighting Blindness, Research to Prevent Blindness, and The Frost Charitable Trust.

REFERENCES

1. Acland GM, Aguirre GD, Ray J, Zhang Q, Aleman TS, Cideciyan AV, Pearce-Kelling SE, Anand V, Zeng Y, Maguire AM, Jacobson SG, Hauswirth WW, Bennett J: Gene therapy restores vision in a canine model of childhood blindness. *Nat Genet* 2001; 28:92–95.

2. Bach M, Hawlina M, Holder G, Marmor M, Meigen T, Vaegan T, Miyake Y: Standard for pattern electrophysiology. International Society for Clinical Electrophysiology of Vision. *Doc Ophthalmol* 2000; 101:11–18.

3. Beck RW, Moke PS, Turpin AH, Ferris FL 3rd, SanGiovanni JP, Johnson CA, Birch EE, Chandler DL, Cox TA, Blair RC, Kraker RT: A computerized method of visual acuity testing: Adaptation of the early treatment of diabetic retinopathy study testing protocol. *Am J Ophthalmol* 2003; 135:194–205.

4. Berson EL, Rosner B, Sandberg MA, Dryja TP: Ocular findings in patients with autosomal dominant retinitis pigmentosa and a rhodopsin gene defect (Pro-23-His). *Arch Ophthalmol* 1991; 109:92–101.

5. Berson EL, Rosner B, Sandberg MA, Hayes KC, Nicholson BW, Weigel-DiFranco C, Willett W: A randomized trial of supplemental vitamin A and vitamin E supplementation for retinitis pigmentosa. *Arch Ophthalmol* 1993; 111:761–772.

6. Berson EL, Sandberg MA, Rosner B, Birch DG, Hanson AH: Natural course of retinitis pigmentosa over a three-year interval. *Am J Ophthalmol* 1985; 99:240–251.

7. Birch DG, Anderson JL, Fish GE: Yearly rates of rod and cone functional loss in retinitis pigmentosa and cone-rod dystrophy. *Ophthalmology* 1999; 106:258–268.

8. Birch DG, Hood DC, Locke KG, Hoffman DR, Tzekov RT: Quantitative electroretinogram measures of phototransduction in cone and rod photoreceptors: Normal aging, progression with disease, and test-retest variability. *Arch Ophthalmol* 2002; 120:1045–1051.

9. Birch DG, Hood DC, Nusinowitz S, Pepperberg DR: Abnormal activation and inactivation mechanisms of rod transduction in patients with autosomal dominant retinitis pigmentosa and the Pro-23-His mutation. *Invest Ophthalmol Vis Sci* 1995; 36:1603–1614.

10. Caruso RC, Nussenblatt RB, Csaky KG, Valle D, Kaiser-Kupfer MI: Assessment of visual function in patients with gyrate atrophy who are considered candidates for gene replacement. *Arch Ophthalmol* 2001; 119:667–669.

11. Ferris FL 3rd, Kassoff A, Bresnick GH, Bailey I: New visual acuity charts for clinical research. *Am J Ophthalmol* 1982; 94:91–96.

12. Fishman GA, Farber M, Patel BS, Derlacki DJ: Visual acuity loss in patients with Stargardt's macular dystrophy. *Ophthalmology* 1987; 94:809–814.

13. Hirakawa H, Iijima H, Gohdo T, Imai M, Tsukahara S: Progression of defects in the central 10-degree visual field of patients with retinitis pigmentosa and choroideremia. *Am J Ophthalmol* 1999; 127:436–442.

14. Hood DC, Birch DG: Assessing abnormal rod photoreceptor activity with the a-wave of the ERG: Applications and methods. *Doc Ophthalmol* 1996–7; 92:253–267.

15. Hood DC, Holopigian K, Greenstein V, Seiple W, Li J, Sutter EE, Carr RE: Assessment of local retinal function in patients with retinitis pigmentosa using the multi-focal ERG technique. *Vision Res* 1998; 38:163–179.

16. Jacobson SG, Apáthy PP, Parel J-M: Rod and cone perimetry: Computerized testing and analysis. In Heckenlively JR, Arden GB (eds): *Principles and Practice of Clinical Electrophysiology of Vision*. St. Louis, Mosby Yearbook, 1991, pp 475–482.

17. Kutzko KE, Brito CF, Wall M: Effect of instructions on conventional automated perimetry. *Invest Ophthalmol Vis Sci* 2000; 41:2006–2013.

18. Lee BL, Wilson MR: Health-related quality of life in patients with cataract and glaucoma. *J Glaucoma* 2000; 9:87–94.

19. Macular Photocoagulation Study Group: Visual outcome after laser photocoagulation for subfoveal choroidal neovascularization secondary to age-related macular degeneration. The influence of initial lesion size and initial visual acuity. *Arch Ophthalmol* 1994; 112:480–488.

20. Mantyjarvi M: Normal test scores in the Farnsworth-Munsell 100 hue test. *Doc Ophthalmol* 2001; 102:73–80.

21. Marmor MF, Hood DC, Keating D, Kondo M, Seeliger MW, Miyake Y: Guidelines for basic multifocal electroretinography (mfERG). *Doc Ophthalmol* 2003; 106:105–115.

22. Marmor MF, Zrenner E: Standard for clinical electro-oculography. International Society for Clinical Electrophysiology of Vision. *Arch Ophthalmol* 1993; 111:601–604.

23. Marmor MF, Zrenner E: Standard for clinical electroretinography (1999 update). International Society for Clinical Electrophysiology of Vision. *Doc Ophthalmol* 1998; 97:143–156.

24. Moher D, Schulz KF, Altman DG: The CONSORT statement: Revised recommendations for improving the quality of reports of parallel-group randomised trials. *Clin Oral Invest* 2003; 7:2–7.

25. Oh KT, Longmuir R, Oh DM, Stone EM, Kopp K, Brown J, Fishman GA, Sonkin P, Gehrs KM, Weleber RG: Comparison of the clinical expression of retinitis pigmentosa associated with rhodopsin mutations at codon 347 and codon 23. *Am J Ophthalmol* 2003; 136:306–313.

26. Oh KT, Weleber RG, Lotery A, Oh DM, Billingslea AM, Stone EM: Description of a new mutation in rhodopsin, Pro23Ala, and comparison with electroretinographic and clinical characteristics of the Pro23His mutation. *Arch Ophthalmol* 2000; 118:1269–1276.

27. Pepperberg DR, Birch DG, Hofmann KP, Hood DC: Recovery kinetics of human rod phototransduction inferred from the two-branched a-wave saturation function. *J Opt Soc Am A Opt Image Vis Sci* 1996; 13:586–600.

28. Pesudovs K, Patel B, Bradbury JA, Elliott DB: Reading speed test for potential central vision measurement. *Clin Exp Ophthalmol* 2002; 30:183–186.

29. Ross DF, Fishman GA, Gilbert LD, Anderson RJ: Variability of visual fields measurements in normal subjects and patients with retinitis pigmentosa. *Arch Ophthalmol* 1984; 102:1004–1010.

30. Sutter EE, Tran D: The field topography of ERG components in man: I. The photopic luminance response. *Vision Res* 1992; 32:433–446.

31. Tan SB, Dear KB, Bruzzi P, Machin D: Strategy for randomised clinical trials in rare cancers. *Br Med J* 2003; 327:47–49.

32. Taves DR: Minimization: A new method of assigning patients to treatment and control groups. *Clin Pharmacol Ther* 1974; 15:443–453.

33. Treasure T, MacRae KD: Minimisation: The platinum standard for trials? Randomisation doesn't guarantee similarity of groups; minimisation does. *Br Med J* 1998; 317:362–363.

34. Tzekov RT, Locke KG, Hood DC, Birch DG: Cone and rod ERG phototransduction parameters in retinitis pigmentosa. *Invest Ophthalmol Vis Sci* 2003; 44:3993–4000.

35. Vajaranant TS, Seiple W, Szlyk JP, Fishman GA: Detection using the multifocal electroretinogram of mosaic retinal dysfunction in carriers of X-linked retinitis pigmentosa. *Ophthalmology* 2002; 109:560–568.

36. Van Hooser JP, Aleman TS, He YG, Cideciyan AV, Kuksa V, Pittler SJ, Stone EM, Jacobson SG, Palczewski K: Rapid restoration of visual pigment and function with oral retinoid in a mouse model of childhood blindness. *Proc Natl Acad Sci U S A* 2000; 97:8623–8628.

37. Weleber RG, Tobler WR: Computerized quantitative analysis of kinetic visual fields. *Am J Ophthalmol* 1986; 101:461–468.

38. Woods JR, Williams JG, Tavel M: The two-period crossover design in medical research. *Ann Intern Med* 1989; 110:560–566.

VIII OTHER PROTOCOLS FOR RECORDING OF ERG AND SLOWER POTENTIALS, TECHNICAL ISSUES, AND AUXILIARY TESTING TECHNIQUES

40 Early Receptor Potential

GORDON L. FAIN

THE EARLY RECEPTOR POTENTIAL (ERP) was first discovered by Brown and Murakami,[3] who were recording a local electroretinogram (ERG) with an electrode placed within the photoreceptor layer of the monkey retina and were stimulating with a very bright light. What they saw (figure 40.1) was a rapid response having no detectable latency, which they called the *early receptor potential*, or *early RP*, followed by the a-wave of the ERG. The polarity of the ERP was the same as that of the a-wave of the ERG, which in their experiments was positive-going. They then showed that the ERP was remarkably resistant to anoxia, suggesting that it was produced not by activation of the transduction cascade, but rather by some other movement of charge within the photoreceptor.

Richard Cone[4] subsequently demonstrated that the ERP could be detected with the same configuration of electrodes and amplifier used to measure the ERG. The polarity of the major component of the ERP was again the same as that of the a-wave, but when the active electrode was placed at the cornea or in the vitreous, both the ERP and the a-wave were negative-going (figure 40.2). Cone also demonstrated that in the rat, the spectral sensitivity of the ERP matched that of the rod pigment and that the amplitude of the major component of the ERP increased nearly linearly with the intensity of the stimulus and saturated at about the light level required to bleach all of the pigment in the photoreceptor. These observations showed that the ERP is produced directly by the photopigment, probably by the movement of charge within the rhodopsin molecule that is triggered by the changes in conformation produced by bleaching.

Once it became feasible to make intracellular recordings routinely from vertebrate photoreceptors, it was possible to show that the electrical events that are responsible for the ERP can be produced in both rods[15] and cones[11] and that they have properties in single receptors identical to those originally inferred from measurements of whole retina. In most recordings, the ERP can be seen to have two components, usually called R1 and R2 (figure 40.3). The R1 component is an initial depolarization with a latency less than $0.5\,\mu s$[5] or perhaps even smaller.[19] The R2 component is hyperpolarizing, develops with a longer latency, and is usually considerably larger in amplitude. It is this R2 component that is responsible for the signal that Brown and Murakami originally recorded (see figure 40.1).

Since the ERP can be detected intracellularly from single photoreceptors as a change in membrane potential (as in figure 40.3) or as a membrane current from cells that have been voltage clamped,[10,12,13] we may conclude that it is caused by the movement of charge with some component perpendicular to the plane of the plasma membrane. Because the size of the ERP is proportional to the number of pigment molecules bleached by the stimulus, it is apparently produced by changes in the conformation of the rhodopsin molecule that move either charged amino acids or associated bound charges (such as H^+) across the plasma membrane. A simple calculation shows that the amplitude of the R2 component can be accounted for by the movement of a single charge a distance of a few angstroms.[7,10,11,13] The amplitude of the ERP would be expected to be larger in cones than in rods, since all of the photopigment in a cone is embedded in the plasma membrane, whereas for rods, only a small fraction of the rhodopsin lies in the plasma membrane or in the few basal disks that are continuous with the plasma membrane. This would explain why, in humans, the rods make a smaller contribution to the ERP of the whole retina (see, e.g., Goldstein and Berson[9] and Sieving and Fishman[17]), even though rods are nearly 20 times more numerous than cones.

Because the R1 and R2 components have different time courses and are of opposite polarity, they are likely to be produced by different conformational changes of the rhodopsin molecule. They are easily separated from one another by reducing temperature, which blocks R2 (see, e.g., Pak and Ebrey[16]), and they have been extensively studied.[7] The R1 component is probably produced by some change that occurs between the absorption of a photon and the formation of the pigment intermediate metarhodopsin I.[5,6,16] The R2 component, on the other hand, probably reflects the movement of charge during the transition from metarhodopsin I to the active intermediate metarhodopsin II or R*. These charge movements are reversible.[2,5] That is, one flash of light can be used to convert rhodopsin to metaI, producing R1, and another can then be given to photoreverse the metaI back to rhodopsin, producing a charge movement that is identical in waveform to R1 but opposite in sign.

Clinical application of ERP

The ERP has been used for the most part in basic research, to study aspects of photopigment function. Because the

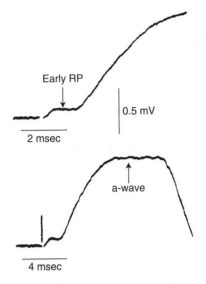

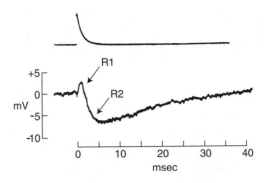

FIGURE 40.3 Intracellular recording of ERP from turtle cone stimulated with xenon flash. The upper trace shows the waveform of the flash. Note the two components of the ERP labeled R1 and R2. (Modified and reprinted with permission from Hodgkin and O'Bryan.[11])

FIGURE 40.1 Discovery of ERP. The traces give same recording at two different sweep speeds. The records show potential recorded from the retina of a cynomolgus monkey (*Macaca irus*) with a tungsten microelectrode inserted into the layer of the photoreceptors. The reference electrode was placed in the vitreous. Notice that with this configuration, the a-wave is positive-going, opposite in polarity to the a-wave of the ERG recorded conventionally with a corneal electrode (see figure 40.2). Photoreceptors were stimulated with bright light from a condenser-discharge lamp. Stimulus artifact appears as break in record in upper trace. (Modified and reprinted with permission from Brown and Murakami.[3])

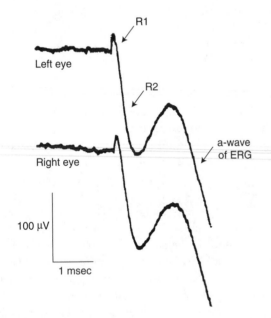

FIGURE 40.2 ERP recorded from a 38-year-old man with ocular siderosis. The recording was made with monopolar corneal contact lens. The patient had sustained traumatic injury to his right eye by penetration of a metal fragment containing a high iron concentration. Even though the a- and b-waves of the involved eye were substantially reduced (not shown), the amplitude of the ERP in the right eye was approximately the same as that in the left (uninjured) eye. (Modified and reprinted with permission from Sieving et al.[18])

amplitude of the ERP is proportional to pigment concentration, measurement of ERP provides a convenient way to quantitate pigment concentration in the living retina and can, for example, be used to determine the photosensitivity of the visual pigment.[12,13]

Because the ERP can be measured with the same apparatus that is used to measure the ERG, it is possible to record the ERP from patients in a clinical setting (see, e.g., Goldstein and Berson,[9] Sieving and Fishman,[17] and Walther and Hellner[20]). The proportionality of ERP amplitude with the amount of photopigment makes possible the use of the ERP to assess the general health of the photoreceptors. Several groups have reported, for example, a decrease in the size of the ERP in humans affected with inherited retinal disease (see, e.g., Goldstein and Berson[9] and Muller and Topke[14]). It is unclear, however, whether measurements of ERP are more accurate or more informative in the assessment of retinal function than is the ERG or even simpler tests, such as tests of visual acuity.

There are, however, two circumstances for which the ERP could be particularly useful in a clinical setting. Suppose, for example, that a patient exhibited a decrease in visual acuity and ERG amplitude with no evidence of degeneration or other anatomical lesion. One possible explanation might be that the photoreceptor outer segments were undamaged but that the patient was experiencing some difficulty either with the mechanism of transduction by the rods and cones or with synaptic processing by interneurons in the retina. The measurement of ERP might then be useful, since if the ERP amplitude were normal, it would indicate that no impairment of distribution of photopigment in the outer segment plasma membrane had occurred. The ERP was used in just this way by Sieving et al.[18] in a study of human ocular siderosis (see figure 40.2).

The ERP might also be helpful in assessing the general health of the photoreceptors in selecting patients for genetic therapy. Imagine a future in which all of the difficulties of molecular gene therapy had been solved, so it had become possible to introduce foreign genes into the eyes of patients who had lost or were losing visual function from genetically inherited retinal degeneration. Recent experiments on a canine model for RPE65-related retinal degeneration[1] suggest that such a future might arrive sooner than anyone previously thought possible.

It would, of course, be pointless to inject a novel gene into the eye of a patient for whom the photoreceptor cells had already completely degenerated. The ERP might then provide a helpful index of the morphological state of the rods and cones. This might be particularly useful for mutations that do not affect rhodopsin itself but affect some other protein that is essential for visual function.[8] In such cases, the ERP may provide a simple test of the integrity of the photoreceptors when other measures such as acuity or ERG amplitude are uninformative.

REFERENCES

1. Acland GM, Aguirre GD, Ray J, et al: Gene therapy restores vision in a canine model of childhood blindness. *Nat Genet* 2001; 28:92–95.
2. Arden GB, Ikeda H: A new property of the early receptor potential of rat retina. *Nature* 1965; 208:1100–1101.
3. Brown KT, Murakami M: A new receptor potential of the monkey retina with no detectable latency. *Nature* 1964; 201:626–628.
4. Cone RA: Early receptor potential of the vertebrate retina. *Nature* 1964; 204:736–740.
5. Cone RA: Early receptor potential: Photoreversible charge displacement in rhodopsin. *Science* 1967; 155:1128–1131.
6. Cone RA, Cobbs WH 3rd: Rhodopsin cycle in the living eye of the rat. *Nature* 1969; 221:820–822.
7. Cone RA, Pak WL: The early receptor potential. In Lowenstein WR (ed): *Handbook of Sensory Physiology, vol. 1: Principles of Receptor Physiology.* Berlin, Springer Verlag, 1971, pp 345–365.
8. Fain GL, Lisman JE: Light, Ca^{2+}, and photoreceptor death: New evidence for the equivalent-light hypothesis from arrestin knockout mice. *Invest Ophthalmol Vis Sci* 1999; 40:2770–2772.
9. Goldstein EB, Berson EL: Rod and cone contributions to the human early receptor potential. *Vision Res* 1970; 10:207–218.
10. Hestrin S, Korenbrot JI: Activation kinetics of retinal cones and rods: Response to intense flashes of light. *J Neurosci* 1990; 10:1967–1973.
11. Hodgkin AL, O'Bryan PM: Internal recording of the early receptor potential in turtle cones. *J Physiol* 1977; 267:737–766.
12. Makino CL, Dodd RL: Multiple visual pigments in a photoreceptor of the salamander retina. *J Gen Physiol* 1996; 108:27–34.
13. Makino CL, Taylor WR, Baylor DA: Rapid charge movements and photosensitivity of visual pigments in salamander rods and cones. *J Physiol* 1991; 442:761–780.
14. Muller W, Topke H: The early receptor potential (ERP). *Doc Ophthalmol* 1987; 66:35–74.
15. Murakami M, Pak WL: Intracellularly recorded early receptor potential of the vertebrate photoreceptors. *Vision Res* 1970; 10:965–975.
16. Pak WL, Ebrey TG: Visual receptor potential observed at sub-zero temperatures. *Nature* 1965; 205:484–486.
17. Sieving PA, Fishman GA: Rod contribution to the human early receptor potential (ERP) estimated from monochromats' data. In Niemeyer G, Huber C (eds): *Techniques in Clinical Electrophysiology of Vision. Documenta Ophthalmologica Proceedings Series, vol. 31.* The Hague, Dr. W. Junk Publishers, 1982, pp 95–102.
18. Sieving PA, Fishman GA, Alexander KR, Goldberg MF: Early receptor potential measurements in human ocular siderosis. *Arch Ophthalmol* 1983; 101:1716–1720.
19. Trissl HW: On the rise time of the R1-component of the "early receptor potential": Evidence for a fast light-induced charge separation in rhodopsin. *Biophys Struct Mech* 1982; 8:213–230.
20. Walther G, Hellner KA: Early receptor potential recordings for clinical routine. *Doc Ophthalmol* 1986; 62:31–39.

41 Nonphotic Standing Potential Responses: Hyperosmolarity, Bicarbonate, and Diamox Responses

KAZUO KAWASAKI, JHOJI TANABE, AND KENJI WAKABAYASHI

THE LIGHT PEAK/DARK trough ratio (L/D) (Arden ratio[1]) is widely accepted as useful for evaluating retinal pigment epithelium (RPE) activity since the light peak and dark trough represent mainly the changes of the RPE membrane potentials. It also depends on the photoreceptor activity and RPE-receptor attachment, because the photoreceptors and their attachment with the RPE are essential for evoking the light peak. The L/D is also changed by occlusion of the central retinal artery, which nourishes the middle and inner layers of the retina. Therefore, abnormal L/D alone does not necessarily indicate RPE disorders. So far as a photic stimulus to the photoreceptors is used, the response obtained is not solely specific to the RPE.

The ocular standing potential, which mainly comes from the transepithelial potential (TEP) of the RPE, can be changed by nonphotic stimuli. For example, hyperosmolarity,[5,8,10] bicarbonate,[11,12] and acetazolamide[3] (Diamox) decrease the TEP in vitro and the ocular standing potential in vivo. We call these responses the hyperosmolarity response, bicarbonate response, and Diamox response, respectively. The standing potential is changed by breathing a hypoxic mixture of oxygen and nitrogen.[9] These responses are recordable by conventional electro-oculographic (EOG) technique in the dark.

Figure 41.1 shows these three responses in normal human subjects. The EOG amplitude is virtually stabilized (V_0) usually about in 30 minutes in the dark. Then, a hypertonic solution (e.g., 20% mannitol or Fructmanit, see legend for figure 41.1), 7% sodium bicarbonate solution (Meylon), or Diamox is given intravenously. These procedures decrease the EOG amplitude in the dark down to the minimum (V_{min}) approximately 8 to 20 minutes after the onset of administration. The amplitude of the response is defined as the percent amplitude change of the EOG: $100 \times (V_0 - V_{min})/V_0$. The distribution of the amplitudes of these responses in the normal subjects is approximated by the normal distribution. Thus, their normal range is the mean ± 2 SD of the amplitude in the normal subjects; 22.8% to 45.2% for the hyperosmolarity response, 15.2% to 28.6% for the bicarbonate response, and 32.1% to 52.9% for the Diamox response (the dose of each stimulant is described in the legend for figure 41.1).

The amplitudes of the hyperosmolarity response and bicarbonate response are frequently decreased in retinitis pigmentosa,[15] rhegmatogenous retinal detachment even in a localized area,[2] diabetic retinopathy[4] (occasionally abnormal even in diabetics without visible retinopathy), angioid streaks, Stargardt's disease-fundus flavimaculatus,[14,16] vitelliform macular dystrophy (Best's disease[13]), Vogt-Harada-Koyanagi disease,[7] and temporarily after cataract extraction[6] (especially after intracapsular extraction) (Table 41.1). The hyperosmolarity response is more frequently abnormal than the L/D in the aforementioned diseases. The Diamox response remains within the normal range in most of the diseases described above and predominantly depends on the RPE in the posterior region of the ocular fundus since this response is suppressed in patients with severe macular atrophy (e.g., advanced stage in Stargardt's disease).[14]

TABLE 41.1

Characteristics of responses related to the retinal pigment epithelium

Characteristic	Hyperosmolarity Response	Bicarbonate Response	Diamox Response	Light Rise	C-Wave
	Nonphotic Stimulus			*Photic Stimulus*	
	Hyperosmolarity	*HCO₃⁻*	*Diamox*		
Origin	Mainly hyperpolarization of RPE basal membrane	Mainly depolarization of RPE apical membrane		Mainly depolarization of RPE basal membrane	Hyperpolarization of RPE apical membrane modified by slow PIII from Müller cell
By hyperosmolarity				Suppressed to abolished	Enhanced
By Diamox				Not suppressed	
By ketamine hydrochloride	Suppressed to abolished	Suppressed to abolished	Suppressed to abolished		Suppressed
Retinitis pigmentosa	Suppressed		Not suppressed		Suppressed
Pigmented paravenous retinochoroidal atrophy	Suppressed				
Fundus albipunctatus	Suppressed		Not suppressed	Suppressed in some cases	
Familial drusen	Suppressed				
Stargardt's disease and fundus flavimaculatus	Suppressed in some cases	Suppressed in some cases			
Angioid streaks					
Vitelliform macular dystrophy	Suppressed		Suppressed in some cases	Suppressed	
Carrier of vitelliform macular dystrophy	Suppressed in some cases		Not suppressed	Suppressed	
Cone dystrophy	Not suppressed		Not suppressed	Not suppressed	
Diabetic retinopathy	Frequently suppressed				
Rhegmatogenous retinal detachment	Suppressed	Suppressed	Not suppressed	Suppressed	Suppressed
Harada's disease	Occasionally suppressed	Occasionally suppressed		Occasionally suppressed	
X-linked juvenile retinoschisis	Not suppressed in cases without peripheral schisis		Not suppressed in cases without peripheral schisis	Not suppressed in cases without peripheral schisis	
After cataract extraction	Temporarily suppressed	Temporarily suppressed			
Occlusion of the central retinal artery	Suppressed			Suppressed in some cases	
Choroideremia	Suppressed		Not suppressed	Suppressed	

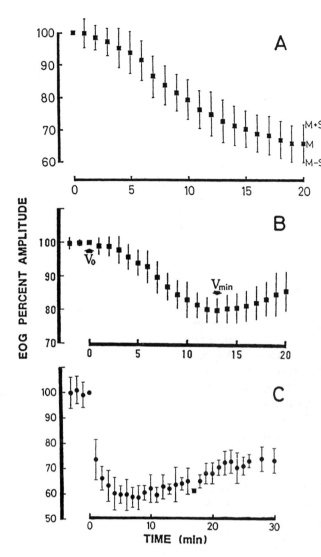

FIGURE 41.1 Hyperosmolarity response (A), bicarbonate response (B), and Diamox response (C) in normal human subjects. The mean and standard deviation of the EOG amplitude as a percentage of the stabilized amplitude (so-called base value) after dark adaptation of 30 minutes are shown. The hyperosmolarity response was recorded in 50 eyes of 30 subjects, bicarbonate response in 70 eyes of 45 subjects, and Diamox response in 36 eyes of 24 subjects. To evoke the hyperosmolarity response, Fructmanit (10% fructose, 15% mannitol) was given intravenously. The solution was administered for 15 to 20 minutes at a rate of 11% of the subject's total blood volume per hour. The total blood volume (liters) was calculated by the following formulas: $0.168 H^3 + 0.05 W + 0.444$ in males or $0.25 H^3 + 0.063 W - 0.662$ in females, where H is the height in meters and W is weight in kilograms. To evoke the bicarbonate response, $0.83 \, \text{mL/kg}$ of 7% sodium bicarbonate (Meylon) was intravenously given in 5 minutes. To evoke the Diamox response, $500 \, \text{mg}$ of Diamox was given intravenously in 1 minute. No light was used except for two dim miniature lamps to alternatively fixate the eye for the conventional EOG procedure. The onset of stimulant application was at 0 minutes on the abscissa.

1. Arden GB, Barrada A, Kelsey JH: New clinical test of retinal function based upon the standing potential of the eye. *Br J Ophthalmol* 1962; 46:449–467.

2. Kawasaki K, Madachi-Yamamoto S, Yonemura D: Hyperosmolarity response of ocular standing potential as a clinical test for retinal pigment epithelium activity—Rhegmatogenous retinal detachment. *Doc Ophthalmol* 1984; 57:175–180.

3. Kawasaki K, Mukoh S, Yonemura D, Fujii S, Segawa Y: Acetazolamide-induced changes of the membrane potentials of the retinal pigment epithelial cell. *Doc Ophthalmol* 1986; 63:375–381.

4. Kawasaki K, Yonemura D, Madachi-Yamamoto S: Hyperosmolarity response of ocular standing potential as a clinical test for retinal pigment epithelium activity—Diabetic retinopathy. *Doc Ophthalmol* 1984; 58:375–384.

5. Kawasaki K, Yonemura D, Mukoh S, Tanabe J: Hyperosmolarity-induced changes in the transepithelial potential of the human and frog retinae. *Doc Ophthalmol* 1983; 37:29–33.

6. Kawasaki K, Yonemura D, Yanagida T, Segawa Y, Wakabayashi K, Mukoh S, Ishida H, Fujii S, Takahara Y: Suppression of the hyperosmolarity response after cataract surgery. *Doc Ophthalmol* 1986; 63:367–373.

7. Madachi-Yamamoto S, Kawasaki K, Yonemura D: Retinal pigment epithelium disorder in Vogt-Koyanagi-Harada disease revealed by hyperosmolarity response of ocular standing potential. *Jpn J Ophthalmol* 1984; 28:362–369.

8. Madachi-Yamamoto S, Yonemura D, Kawasaki K: Hyperosmolarity response of ocular standing potential as a clinical test for retinal pigment epithelium activity—Normative data. *Doc Ophthalmol* 1984; 57:153–162.

9. Marmor MF, Donovan WJ, Gaba DM: Effects of hypoxia on the human standing potential. *Doc Ophthalmol* 1985; 60:347–352.

10. Mukoh S, Kawasaki K, Yonemura D: Hyperosmolarity-induced hyperpolarization of the membrane potential of the retinal pigment epithelium. *Doc Ophthalmol* 1985; 60:369–374.

11. Segawa Y, Mukoh S, Tanabe J, Kawasaki K: Bicarbonate-induced response from the retinal pigment epithelium for electrodiagnosis. Presented at the 26th International Symposium on Clinical Electrophysiology of Vision, Estoril, Portugal, May 23, 1988.

12. Steinberg RH, Miller SS: Transport and membrane properties of the retinal pigment epithelium. In Marmor MF, Zinn KH (eds): *The Retinal Pigment Epithelium.* Cambridge, Mass, Harvard University Press, 1979, pp 205–225.

13. Wakabayashi K, Yonemura D, Kawasaki K: Electrophysiological analysis of Best's macular dystrophy and retinal pigment epithelial pattern dystrophy. *Ophthalmic Paediatr Genet* 1983; 3:13–17.

14. Wakabayashi K, Yonemura D, Kawasaki K: Electrophysiological analysis of Stargardt's disease fundus flavimaculatus group. *Doc Ophthalmol* 1985; 60:141–147.

15. Yonemura D, Kawasaki K, Madachi-Yamamoto S: Hyperosmolarity response of ocular standing potential as a clinical test for retinal pigment epithelium activity—Chorioretinal dystrophies. *Doc Ophthalmol* 1984; 57:163–173.

16. Yonemura D, Kawasaki K, Wakabayuashi K, Tanabe J: EOG application for Stargardt's disease and X-linked juvenile retinoschisis. *Doc Ophthalmol Proc Ser* 1983; 37:115–120.

42 Direct Current Electroretinogram

SVEN ERIK G. NILSSON

THE A- AND B-WAVE electroretinogram (ERG) represents the initial events of a fairly long series of potential changes in the retina and the retinal pigment epithelium (PE) that are evoked by light. When the dark-adapted eye is stimulated by turning on a continuous light, the fast a- and b-waves are followed by the slow c-wave of the ERG and by fast and slow (light peak) oscillations, which are still much slower (figure 42.1). If the light is turned off, a series of off-effects arise, including the "off c-wave," the "off fast oscillation," and the "off slow oscillation" (the dark trough). These off-potentials are of opposite polarity as compared with the corresponding on-potentials (figure 42.1). Whereas the a- and b-waves represent the photoreceptor potential[2,4] and interactions between the neural elements and the Müller cells in the inner retina[6,30,34] respectively, the slower potential changes reflect mainly PE changes in response to neuroretinal activity. It is of interest to study these PE responses clinically. The slow oscillations are generally investigated indirectly by means of the electro-oculogram (EOG).[3,14,16] For the c-wave of the ERG, however, a setup for corneal direct current (dc) recordings must be used. Such equipment allows us to record the fast and slow oscillations as well. This section will provide a brief background regarding the generation of the three PE potential changes mentioned above as well as a description of equipment for corneal dc recordings of such slow responses in patients.

Slow pigment epithelium responses

The standing potential (SP) of the eye is a transocular potential built up by several components, e.g., from the cornea. The major contribution (approximately 10 mV) comes from the PE, however.[30,31] In the dark, the apical PE membrane is more hyperpolarized than the basal one is.[19,46] This voltage across the eye may be altered by several events in the retina and PE such as the ERG potentials, the fast oscillation, and the slow oscillation (the light peak).

The c-wave of the ERG (figure 42.2) originates to a large extent in the PE.[31] It represents the sum of a positive component from the PE (PI) and a simultaneous negative (and generally smaller) component from the Müller cells (slow PIII). The positive component is generated as PE cell hyperpolarization (the difference in hyperpolarization between the apical and basal membranes) in response to the decrease in extracellular potassium concentration that occurs in the photoreceptor layer during light stimulation, and the negative component arises as Müller cell hyperpolarization in response to the same potassium change.[6,11,12,19,32,33,49,59] Since the positive response is generally the larger one, the c-wave of the ERG provides information on the health of the PE.

A direct corneal dc recording of the fast oscillation and the light peak (slow oscillation) from a normal, dark-adapted subject in response to continuous light stimulation is demonstrated in figure 42.3. (With this slow time course, the ERG is seen only as a small upward deflection at light onset that represents the c-wave.) We showed long ago that these slow amplitude variations of the transocular potential can be recorded in the human without general anesthesia.[26,28] The negative fast oscillation, peaking at 45 to 60 seconds in humans, is caused by a delayed hyperpolarization of the basal PE membrane. This response is related to the light-induced decrease in potassium concentration in the subretinal space mentioned above.[8,17] The positive light peak has a maximum at 10 to 12 minutes in humans. It represents a depolarization of the basal PE membrane. It is not related to the potassium changes in the subretinal space but seems to depend on a "light peak substance" or a transmitter substance originating in the photoreceptors.[9,18,38,47,56] A dependence of the light peak on the neuroretina was demonstrated long ago when it was found that it was abolished by experimental occlusion of the retinal circulation in the monkey.[54] Melatonin,[20,52] synthesized in the photoreceptors, and dopamine[5,35,44,53] have been thought of as tentative candidates for transmitter substances.

Equipment and procedure for recording and light stimulation

RECORDING EQUIPMENT There is no equipment commercially available for dc recordings of slow ocular potentials in patients. Each laboratory has to build its own equipment. Our setup and procedure, which have been improved throughout the years,[24,26,28,55] are described here.

The pupils of the patient's eyes are dilated with 0.5% tropicamide and 10% phenylephrine hydrochloride. Topical tetracaine anesthesia is used. A polymethylmethacrylate (PMMA) contact lens is placed on one of the eyes (figure 42.4). The eyelids are held apart by means of a groove and a ridge along the edge of the contact lens. A chamber made

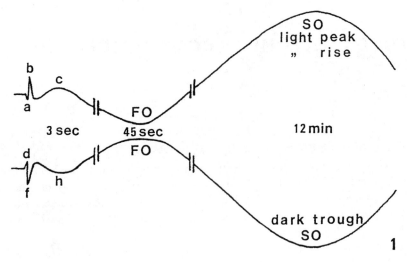

FIGURE 42.1 Schematic representation of the light-induced changes in the voltage across the eye. In response to a prolonged light stimulus (upper curve), the ERG with the a-, b-, and c-waves is first elicited. At about 45 seconds the negative "fast oscillation" is maximal, and at about 12 minutes the positive "slow oscillation" (light peak, light rise) reaches its peak. After light adaptation when the light is turned off (lower curve), a series of off-effects occur. The "off-ERG" includes the h-wave or "off c-wave." The fast oscillation is now positive, and the slow oscillation (dark trough) is negative. The response is to a large extent a mirror image of the response to light. (From Nilsson SEG.[25] Used by permission.)

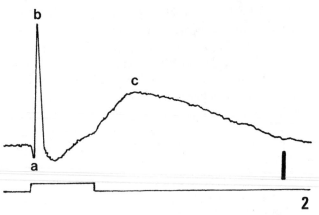

FIGURE 42.2 The human dc recorded ERG. A 1-second light stimulus is indicated on the lower line (amplitude calibration, 100 μV).

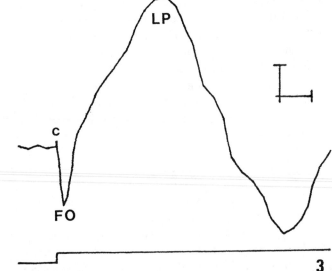

FIGURE 42.3 Direct corneal dc recording of the ERG (c-wave only is seen), the fast oscillation (FO), and the light peak (LP) in a normal patient (light stimulus, 16 lux; amplitude calibration, 1 mV; time calibration, 3 minutes).

of PMMA is attached to the forehead above the eye by means of a piece of ring-shaped, double-sided adhesive tape. Both the chamber and the contact lens are filled with a solution containing 2% sterile methyl-cellulose and 0.9% sodium chloride. If the recording session is intended to be long in duration, a few drops of tetracaine are added to the solution. Saline-agar bridges in polyethylene tubes are used to connect the contact lens and the chamber to matched calomel half-cells, which serve as recording and reference electrodes, respectively (see figure 42.4). Both electrodes are plugged into a preamplifier (impedance, $10^9 \Omega$). The saline-agar bridges are replaced with new ones for each patient to make certain that mercury ions will not reach the eye. The calomel half-cells are filled, from top to bottom, with saline, mercury chloride powder, metallic mercury and mercury

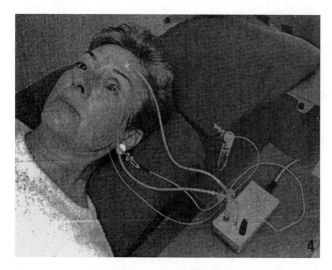

FIGURE 42.4   A contact lens on the eye and a plastic chamber on the forehead are connected by means of saline-agar bridges to matched calomel half-cells (recording and reference electrodes) plugged into a preamplifier. To provide a well-defined suction the contract lens is equipped with a second tube ending in a test tube with saline, the surface of which is located 20 cm below the eye. The earlobe is grounded. (From Nilsson SEG, Andersson BE.[26] Used by permission.)

chloride powder (mixed thoroughly by stirring in a mortar), and metallic mercury. The contact lens is prevented from sliding on the eye by means of a negative pressure of 20 cm of water that is created by connecting the lens through a saline-filled second polyethylene tube to a test tube with saline (see figure 42.4). The surface of this solution is placed 20 cm below the level of the eye. One earlobe is grounded. Silver–silver chloride electrodes, in the form of a freshly chlorinated silver rod in a contact lens and an electrocardiographic (ECG) electrode on the forehead, were tried for dc recordings. They were found to be less stable than calomel electrodes for long recording sessions.

From the preamplifiers, the signals pass to a two-channel, low-drift, differential-input dc amplifier built in our own department to meet very high demands regarding high impedance, low drift, and low noise. The common-mode rejection ratio (CMRR) is approximately 100 dB, which means that disturbing 50 Hz is attenuated sufficiently to allow us to record without the use of a shielding cage. Coarse offset adjustment is performed manually. Both amplifier channels are provided with low-pass filters, 12 dB per octave, with the high-frequency cutoff set to 300 Hz (with 100 Hz as an option). Each channel is in turn divided into two branches, one of which (gain set to 100) is used for recording very slow potential changes such as the fast oscillation and the light peak. The second branch, the gain of which is set to 1000 (with 100, 200, and 500 as options), is used for ERG recordings. This second branch is equipped with an internal balance for final offset adjustment. It may be con-

trolled manually, but it is generally controlled automatically from the computer. In such a case, the computer orders the amplifier just before each flash to balance the potential level against zero level.

On their way from the amplifier to a Hewlett-Packard (HP) 9826 computer, the signals pass an oscilloscope (showing the noise level) and an analogue to digital (A/D) converter (in an HP 6940B multiprogrammer). The computer analyzes ERG a-, b-, and c-wave amplitudes and implicit times and displays them digitally on the screen together with the curve. Selected recordings may be averaged. When the fast and slow oscillations are recorded via one of the channel branches, the computer samples the signal four times per minute during the first 2 minutes and then once per minute. The potential variations are displayed on the screen. The light peak may be elicited not only by turning on continuous light but also by using repeated flashes. In such a way, the ERG may be recorded repeatedly and simultaneously with the light peak. The computer analyzes the potential level just before every stimulus flash and displays the ERG traces superimposed on the light peak.

LIGHT STIMULATION   A 150-W halogen lamp (Osram) provides the stimulus light, which is first focused upon the entrance to fiber optics (Fiberoptic-Heim AG).[26] Neutral-density filters (Balzers) in a rotating mount (moved by a Philips stepping motor controlled by the computer via the multiprogrammer) allowing changes in light intensity over a total range of 7 log units in steps of 0.5 log units are interposed between the light source and the fiber optics. An electronic shutter (Uniblitz, Vincent Associates, Inc.), which is computer and multiprogrammer controlled, permits continuous variations in flash durations from 10 ms to infinity and in flash intervals from about 30 ms (flicker) to infinity. The exit of the fiber optics is connected to a hemisphere half a tennis ball in size that is approximately evenly illuminated by the stimulus light. In this way, Ganzfeld stimulation of one eye can be obtained (figure 42.5).

RECORDING PROCEDURE   For stable recordings of 5 seconds' duration (dc ERG with a-, b-, and c-waves), it is essential to ensure a steady eye position. This can be achieved by investigating one eye at a time and having the free eye fixate on a deep red light-emitting diode (LED) located about 1 m above the eye.[26] Five seconds before each flash, the computer tells the patient by means of an acoustic signal and by turning on the LED that a flash is to come. In this way, the patient is given sufficient time to fixate on the LED before light stimulation and thus obtain and maintain a steady eye position just before and during the recording. When the sweep is completed, the LED is turned off, and the patient can close the free eye and rest until the next signal comes (often 1- to 3-minute intervals between 1-second stimuli for

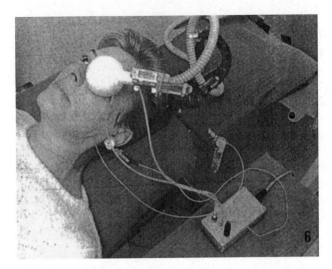

FIGURE 42.5   Ganzfeld stimulation of the left eye. (From Nilsson SEG, Andersson BE.[26] Used by permission.)

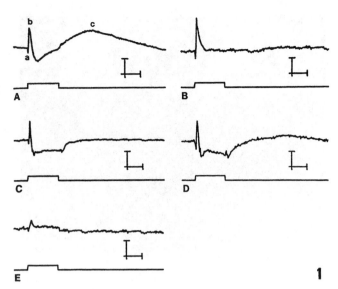

FIGURE 42.6   dc recorded human ERGs (a-, b-, and c-waves indicated) in response to a 1-second light stimulus (*lower line*) 4.0 log relative units above the b-wave threshold (amplitude calibration, $200\,\mu V$ [A, C, D] or $100\,\mu V$ [B, E]; time calibration, 0.5 seconds). A, normal subject. B, Best's disease. C and D, choriocapillaris atrophy, right and left eye, respectively. E, retinitis pigmentosa (for details, see the text). (From Nilsson SEG, Andersson BE.[26] Used by permission.)

dc ERGs). When general anesthesia is used for small children, it is possible to record from both eyes at the same time.

We have written programs for several kinds of recordings (a- and b-wave ERG; a-, b-, and c-wave ERG; 30-Hz flicker ERG; EOG; direct corneal recordings of the fast oscillation, the light peak, or the dark trough; light peak with ERGs superimposed), as well as for analysis and graphic plotting of information such as intensity-amplitude curves.

By using the technique described above it is possible to obtain stable dc recordings in most patients. Averaging is generally necessary for patients, whereas in volunteers with some previous experience, single recordings are sufficiently stable.

Clinical applications

As previously discussed, the c-wave of the electroretinograms (ERG) represents the sum of a cornea-positive potential (P_I) generated in the pigment epithelium (PE) and a cornea-negative potential (slow P_{III}) originating in the Müller cells, both arising as responses to a light-evoked decrease in extracellular potassium concentration in the photoreceptor layer. The PE response is generally the bigger one and gives rise to a positive c-wave (figure 42.6A). There is a sizable interindividual variation, however, and it is known that a few individuals with seemingly healthy eyes have a "flat" c-wave, i.e., the two components appear to be equal in size. The reason may possibly be variations in membrane surface area of the PE and Müller cells. Thus, c-wave amplitudes must be judged with some caution. The safest conclusions can be drawn from comparisons of the right and the left eye in an individual with a uniocular disease.

The still slower variations of the voltage across the eye, the fast and slow (light peak) oscillations, also represent PE activity, the first on being potassium dependent and the second one being dependent upon a transmitter substance (a light peak substance) from the neuroretina. Instead of recording the light peak (the response to continuous light following dark adaptation) and dark trough (the response to darkness following light adaptation) indirectly as the electro-oculogram (EOG), both potential changes can be recorded directly from the cornea together with the fast oscillation (see below) by using the direct coupled (DC) technique employed for c-wave recordings.[28,38] This is particularly advantageous in patients who cannot cooperate in ERG and EOG recordings but must be anesthetized, such as small children. Furthermore, such dc recordings are necessary in animal experiments.

The dc recordings of the ERG c-wave and of the fast and slow oscillations may be valuable in clinical diagnostic work regarding PE disease. The Arden index[3] used for EOG evaluation may also be calculated from DC recordings.

The c-wave of the human electroretinogram

THE NORMAL c-WAVE   The c-wave amplitude is linearly related to the stimulus intensity in humans, at least within the range of intensities studied (3.5–5.5 log relative units above the b-wave threshold).[40] With increasing stimulus duration, the c-wave amplitude and implicit time both increase.[51] The c-wave amplitude shows cyclic variations with time[41] in such a way that the c-wave amplitude follows that of the slow oscillations, that is, the c-wave amplitude is largest at a time that coincides with the maximum of the light peak and is smallest when the transocular potential (standing potential) thereafter goes negative.[28] This is best demonstrated when the ERG is superimposed upon the slow oscillation of the transocular potential (monkey).[54] Such a recording from a human subject is shown below. Solvents such as ethanol,[37] toluene, styrene,[39] trichlorethylene, methylchloroform, and halothane[10] have been shown to influence the c-wave amplitude.

The c-Wave in Some Diseases Affecting the Pigment Epithelium Best's disease (vitelliform or vitelliruptive macular degeneration) is now known to be a disease affecting the PE across the entire fundus, with the most advanced changes located in the macula.[34] It seems that the PE is the primary site of the changes and that the photoreceptors degenerate over the areas with the most pronounced PE lesions. The a- and b-waves are normal,[7] whereas the EOG is highly pathological.[15] In accordance with these findings, we[24,29] found that in the families we studied the a- and b-waves were within normal limits but the c-wave was missing (figure 42.6B) or, in a few cases, extremely small and present only under certain stimulus conditions.

Choriocapillaris atrophy may be regional or diffuse and involves degeneration of the PE and the choroidal capillaries as well as the overlying photoreceptors. Figures 42.6C and 42.6D show the dc ERGs of the right and left eye, respectively, of a patient with a fairly early stage of choriocapillaris atrophy.[26] The a- and b-waves are larger in amplitude for the left eye, but they are also within normal limits for the right eye. There is no c-wave for the right eye, but the left eye shows a small c-wave. These ERG findings agree very well with the EOG results (Arden index 140 and 183 for the right and left eye, respectively) and with the clinical findings (right eye ophthalmoscopically more affected than the left eye; visual acuity 0.9 [18/20] for the right eye and 1.0 [20/20] for the left eye).

Retinitis pigmentosa (RP) in its classic form is characterized by early rod degeneration followed later by cone degeneration. The PE does not seem to be affected primarily. Figure 42.6E demonstrates a dc ERG from a patient with RP. Small a- and b-waves are often found at early stages, at least in the dominantly inherited forms. In our RP patient data, we have never seen a c-wave.[26]

Central retinal artery occlusion was shown to reduce not only the ERG b-wave but also the c-wave in humans (figure 42.7)[50] as well as experimentally in monkeys.[54] This was surprising, since vascular support for the PE is from the choriocapillaris. Thus, the positive PE component of the c-wave

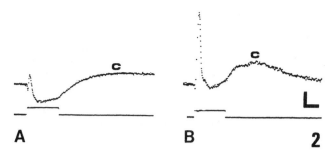

Figure 42.7 dc ERG recordings from a human eye with occlusion of the central retinal artery (A) and from the healthy fellow eye (B). The b-wave and the c-wave (indicated) are both reduced in the eye with central retinal artery occlusion (stimulus duration, 1 second [indicated on lower line]; stimulus intensity, 130 cd/m²; amplitude calibration, 100 μV; time calibration, 0.5 seconds). (Adapted from Textorius O.[50])

ought to be normal. Furthermore, blocking of the retinal circulation should damage Müller cells, which would reduce the negative Müller cell component of the c-wave. As a consequence, one would expect the c-wave to be increased. The reduction in the c-wave may possibly reflect changes in neuroretinal extracellular potassium concentration that are caused by inner retinal damage.

Clinical use of the c-wave amplitude is limited to a certain extent by its fairly large interindividual variability, also in normal subjects, which seems to be due to the fact that the c-wave is built up by two components from two different cell types. The question is whether there are ways of testing the PE component of the c-wave alone without involving the Müller cells. Experimental work on an isolated retina-PE-choroid preparation[36] showed that choroidal hyperosmolarity hyperpolarized the basal PE membrane and decreased the amplitude of the light-evoked c-wave. Further work will show whether this hyperosmolarity response of the c-wave can be of clinical use.

The "off c-wave"

After light adaptation or light stimulation and when the light is turned off, the extracellular potassium concentration in the photoreceptor layer increases,[47,48] which gives rise to the "off c-wave."[6,30] The off c-wave (named the h-wave by us) was studied further in our laboratory in normal humans (figure 42.8) and in monkeys.[42,43,57,58] The off c-wave (h-wave) was found to behave in exactly the same way as the c-wave regarding stimulus intensity-amplitude relationship, cyclic variations with time, and response to ethanol.

Fast and slow (light peak) oscillations

The dark trough and light peak are generally recorded indirectly as the EOG.[1,3,14,16] However, these slow oscillations,

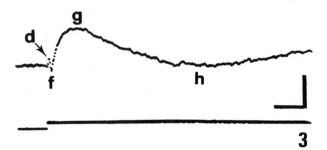

FIGURE 42.8   Off-responses of the human dc recorded ERG after the termination of an illumination of 60 lux (average of two recordings). The "h-wave" in our terminology corresponds to the "off c-wave" (amplitude calibration, 100 μV; time calibration, 1 second). (From Skoog K-O, Welinder E, Nilsson SEG.[43] Used by permission.)

together with the fast oscillations, may very well be recorded directly from the cornea with a dc technique, which is basically the same as the one used for c-wave recordings.[28,38] This is valuable, especially in patients who require general anesthesia (e.g., small children) for electrophysiological tests. In addition, dc recordings of this kind are necessary for the evaluation of PE health in animal models of hereditary diseases of the PE and retina.[10,13]

Figure 42.9 shows a direct recording of the fast oscillation and the light peak in a normal subject as compared with a recording from a patient with RP. The latter recording, which shows almost no response, corresponds to an almost flat EOG.

The light peak can be evoked not only by continuous light but also by repeated flashes of light. In such a recording, the a- and b-waves of the ERGs are too fast to show up, but the ERG c-waves are superimposed upon the light peak (figure 42.10). In this way, it is easily seen that the c-wave amplitude follows that of the light peak, that is, it is largest at the time of the maximum of the light peak. (The fast oscillation does not show up with 2-minute intervals between recordings.)

The hyperosmolarity response mentioned above has been used clinically regarding the effect on the transocular potential (standing potential), as reflected in the EOG or in direct dc recordings of the transocular potential. Intravenous administration of a hypertonic solution decreases the transocular potential.[60] The hyperosmolarity response was reported to be suppressed or absent in eye diseases involving the PE (e.g., RP and advanced diabetic retinopathy with breakdown of the blood-retinal barrier). The explanation was given by Shirao and Steinberg.[36] Choroidal hyperosmolarity hyperpolarized the basal membrane of the PE and decreased the transtissue potential in an isolated retina-PE-choroid preparation (corresponding to the transocular potential in the intact eye). Yonemura and Kawasaki[60] also found that acetazolamide given intravenously decreased the

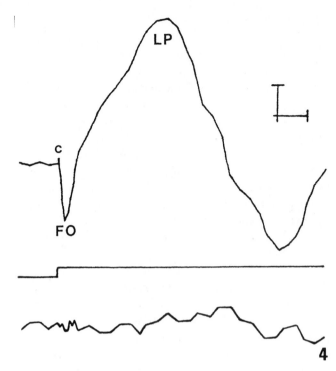

FIGURE 42.9   The upper trace shows a direct corneal dc recording of the ERG (only the c-wave is seen), the fast oscillation (FO), and the light peak (LP) (slow oscillation) in a normal subject. The bottom trace shows the same kind of recording from a patient with RP. The latter response is essentially flat. The onset of a 16-lux light stimulus is indicated between the two recordings (amplitude calibration, 1 mV; time calibration, 3 minutes).

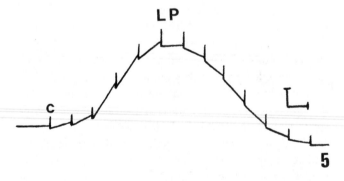

FIGURE 42.10   Light peak (LP) evoked by repeated light flashes. The ERG c-waves are seen to be superimposed upon the LP. The c-wave amplitude is largest at the time of the maximum of the LP (amplitude calibration, 0.5 mV; time calibration, 2 minutes).

transocular potential in EOG studies or in direct dc recordings. The acetazolamide response was normal in RP, however. Kawasaki et al.[13] reported that acetazolamide on the choroidal side of an isolated PE-choroid preparation hyperpolarized both the basal and apical PE membrane, the basal more than the apical one, thus decreasing the transepithelial potential.

Conclusions

The ERG c-wave can be dc recorded clinically and, when using averaging technique, with fairly stable results. The c-wave amplitude is one of a number of valuable parameters regarding PE health. However, it should be used with some caution since the interindividual variability is fairly large and since a few individuals with healthy eyes actually do not show a c-wave. It is possible that the hyperosmolarity response of the c-wave may be a way of getting away from this problem in the future.

Direct dc recordings of the fast and slow (light peak, dark trough) oscillations can be obtained clinically without difficulty. Such recordings are of particular value when general anesthesia has to be used and when the EOG cannot be employed.

ACKNOWLEDGMENTS This investigation was supported by the Swedish Medical Research Council (Project No. 12X-734).

REFERENCES

1. Arden GB, Barrada A, Kelsey JH: New clinical test of retinal function based upon the standing potential of the eye. *Br J Ophthalmol* 1962; 46:449–467.
2. Arden GB, Brown KT: Some properties of components of the cat electroretinogram revealed by local recording under oil. *J Physiol (Lond)* 1965; 176:429–461.
3. Arden GB, Kelsey JH: Changes produced by light in the standing potential of the human eye. *J Physiol (Lond)* 1962; 161:189–204.
4. Brown KT, Wiesel TN: Localization of origins of electroretinogram components by intraretinal recordings in the intact cat eye. *J Physiol (Lond)* 1961; 158:257–280.
5. Dawis SM, Niemeyer G: Dopamine influences the light peak in the perfused mammalian eye. *Invest Ophthalmol Vis Sci* 1986; 27:330–335.
6. Faber DS: *Analysis of the Slow Transretinal Potentials in Response to Light* (thesis). State University of New York at Buffalo, 1969.
7. François J, Gallet G, Blervacque A: La dégénérescence vitelliforme de la macula. *Bull Soc Ophthalmol Fr* 1963; 63:450–451.
8. Griff ER, Steinberg RH: Changes in apical [K$^+$] produce delayed basal membrane responses of the retinal pigment epithelium in the gecko. *J Gen Physiol* 1984; 83:193–211.
9. Griff ER, Steinberg RH: Origin of the light peak: *In vitro* study of *Gekko gekko*. *J Physiol (Lond)* 1982; 331:637–652.
10. Jarkman S, Skoog K-O, Nilsson SEG: The c-wave of the electroretinogram and the standing potential of the eye as highly sensitive measures of effects of low doses of trichloroethylene, methylchloroform, and halothane. *Doc Ophthalmol* 1985; 60:375–382.
11. Karwoski CJ, Proenza LM: Relationship between Müller cell responses, a local transretinal potential, and potassium flux. *J Neurophysiol* 1977; 40:244–259.
12. Karwoski CJ, Proenza LM: Spatio-temporal variables in the relationship of neuronal activity to potassium and glial responses. *Vision Res* 1981; 21:1713–1718.
13. Kawasaki K, Mukoh S, Yonemura D, Fujii S, Segawa Y: Acetazolamide-induced changes of the membrane potentials of the retinal pigment epithelial cell. *Doc Ophthalmol* 1986; 63:375–381.
14. Kolder H: Spontane und experimentelle Änderungen des Bestandpotentials des menschlichen Auges. *Pflügers Arch Gesamte Physiol* 1959; 268:258–272.
15. Krill AE, Morse PA, Potts AM, Klein BA: Hereditary vitelliruptive macular degeneration. *Am J Ophthalmol* 1966; 61:1405–1415.
16. Kris C: Corneo-fundal potential variations during light and dark adaptation. *Nature* 1958; 182:1027–1028.
17. Linsenmeier RA, Steinberg RH: Delayed basal hyperpolarization of cat retinal pigment epithelium and its relation to the fast oscillation of the DC electroretinogram. *J Gen Physiol* 1984; 83:213–232.
18. Linsenmeier RA, Steinberg RH: Origin and sensitivity of the light peak of the intact cat eye. *J Physiol (Lond)* 1982; 331:653–673.
19. Miller SS, Steinberg RH: Passive ionic properties of frog retinal pigment epithelium. *J Membr Biol* 1977; 36:337–372.
20. Nao-i N, Nilsson SEG, Gallemore R, Steinberg RH: Effects of melatonin on the chick retinal pigment epithelium: Membrane potentials and light-evoked responses. *Exp Eye Res* 1989; 49:573–589.
21. Narfström KL, Nilsson SE, Andersson BE: Progressive retinal atrophy in the Abyssinian cat: Studies of the DC-recorded electroretinogram and the standing potential of the eye. *Br J Ophthalmol* 1985; 69:618–623.
22. Newman EA: B-wave currents in the frog retina. *Vision Res* 1979; 19:227–234.
23. Newman EA: Current source-density analysis of the b-wave of frog retina. *J Neurophysiol* 1980; 43:1355–1366.
24. Nilsson SEG: Electrophysiological responses related to the pigment epithelium and its interaction with the receptor layer. *Neurochemistry* 1980; 1:69–80.
25. Nilsson SEG: Electrophysiology in pigment epithelial changes. *Acta Ophthalmol* 1985; 63 (suppl 173):22–27.
26. Nilsson SEG, Andersson BE: Corneal D.C. recordings of slow ocular potential changes such as the ERG c-wave and the light peak in clinical work. Equipment and examples of results. *Doc Ophthalmol* 1988; 68:313–325.
27. Nilsson SEG, Armstrong D, Koppang N, Persson P, Milde K: Studies on the retina and the pigment epithelium in hereditary canine ceroid lipofuscinosis: IV. Changes in the electroretinogram and the standing potential of the eye. *Invest Ophthalmol Vis Sci* 1983; 24:77–84.
28. Nilsson SEG, Skoog K-O: Covariation of the simultaneously recorded c-wave and standing potential of the human eye. *Acta Ophthalmol* 1975; 53:721–730.
29. Nilsson SEG, Skoog K-O: The ERG c-wave in vitelliruptive macular degeneration (VMD). *Acta Ophthalmol* 1980; 58:659–666.
30. Noell WK: *Studies on the Electrophysiology and the Metabolism of the Retina.* Randolph Field, Tex, US Air Force, SAM Project 21-1201-004, 1953.
31. Noell WK: The origin of the electroretinogram. *Am J Ophthalmol* 1954; 38:78–90.
32. Oakley B II, Green DG: Correlation of light-induced changes in retinal extracellular potassium concentration with c-wave of the electroretinogram. *J Neurophysiol* 1976; 39:1117–1133.
33. Oakley B II, Steinberg RH, Miller SS, Nilsson SEG: The in vitro frog pigment epithelial hyperpolarization in response to light. *Invest Ophthalmol Vis Sci* 1977; 16:771–774.

34. O'Gorman S, Flaherty WA, Fishman GA, Berson EL: Histopathologic findings in Best's vitelliform macular dystrophy. *Arch Ophthalmol* 1988; 106:1261–1268.

35. Sato T, Yoneyama T, Kim HK, Suzuki TA: Effect of dopamine and haloperidol on the c-wave and light peak of light-induced retinal responses in chick eye. *Doc Ophthalmol* 1987; 65:87–95.

36. Shirao Y, Steinberg RH: Mechanisms of effects of small hyperosmotic gradients on the chick RPE. *Invest Ophthalmol Vis Sci* 1987; 28:2015–2025.

37. Skoog K-O: The c-wave of the human d.c. registered ERG: III. Effects of ethyl alcohol on the c-wave. *Acta Ophthalmol* 1974; 52:913–923.

38. Skoog K-O: The directly recorded standing potential of the human eye. *Acta Ophthalmol* 1975; 53:120–132.

39. Skoog K-O, Nilsson SEG: Changes in the c-wave of the electroretinogram and in the standing potential of the eye after small doses of toluene and styrene. *Acta Ophthalmol* 1981; 59:71–79.

40. Skoog K-O, Nilsson SEG: The c-wave of the human D.C. registered ERG: I. A quantitative study of the relationship between c-wave amplitude and stimulus intensity. *Acta Ophthalmol* 1974; 52:759–773.

41. Skoog K-O, Nilsson SEG: The c-wave of the human D.C. registered ERG: II. Cyclic variations of the c-wave amplitude. *Acta Ophthalmol* 1974; 52:904–912.

42. Skoog K-O, Welinder E, Nilsson SEG: Off-responses in the human d.c. registered electroretinogram. *Vision Res* 1977; 17:409–415.

43. Skoog K-O, Welinder E, Nilsson SEG: The influence of ethyl alcohol on slow off-responses in the human d.c. registered electroretinogram. *Vision Res* 1978; 18:1041–1044.

44. Steinberg RH, Gallemore RP: Effects of dopamine on RPE membrane potentials and light-evoked responses in chick. *Invest Ophthalmol Vis Sci* 1988; 29 (suppl):100.

45. Steinberg RH, Gallemore RP, Griff E: Origin of the light peak: Contribution from the neural retina. *Invest Ophthalmol Vis Sci* 1987; 28 (suppl):402.

46. Steinberg RH, Linsenmeier RA, Griff ER: Retinal pigment epithelial cell contribution to the electroretinogram. In Osborne NN, Chader GJ (eds): *Progress in Retinal Research, vol 4.* New York, Pergamon Press, 1985, pp 33–66.

47. Steinberg RH, Niemeyer G: Light peak of cat DC electroretinogram: Not generated by a change in $[K^+]_O$. *Invest Ophthalmol Vis Sci* 1981; 20:414–418.

48. Steinberg RH, Oakley B II, Niemeyer G: Light-evoked changes in $[K^+]_O$ in retina in intact cat eye. *J Neurophysiol* 1980; 44:897–922.

49. Steinberg RH, Schmith R, Brown KT: Intracellular responses to light from cat pigment epithelium: Origin of the electroretinogram c-wave. *Nature* 1970; 227:728–730.

50. Textorius O: The c-wave of the human electroretinogram in central retinal artery occlusion. *Acta Ophthalmol* 1978; 56:827–836.

51. Textorius O: The influence of stimulus duration on the human D.C. registered c-wave. A quantitative study. *Acta Ophthalmol* 1977; 55:561–572.

52. Textorius O, Nilsson SEG: Effects of intraocular irrigation with melatonin on the c-wave of the direct current electroretinogram and on the standing potential of the eye in albino rabbits. *Doc Ophthalmol* 1987; 65:97–111.

53. Textorius O, Nilsson SEG, Andersson B-E: Effects of intravitreal perfusion with dopamine in different concentrations on the DC electroretinogram and the standing potential of the albino rabbit eye. *Doc Ophthalmol* 1989; 73:149–162.

54. Textorius O, Skoog K-O, Nilsson SEG: Studies on acute and late stages of experimental central retinal artery occlusion in the cynomolgus monkey: II. Influence on the cyclic changes in the amplitude of the c-wave of the ERG and in the standing potential of the eye. *Acta Ophthalmol* 1978; 56:665–676.

55. Textorius O, Welinder E, Nilsson SEG: Combined effects of DL-α-aminoadipic acid with sodium iodate, ethyl alcohol, or light stimulation on the ERG c-wave and on the standing potential of albino rabbit eyes. *Doc Ophthalmol* 1985; 60:393–400.

56. Valeton JM, van Norren D: Intraretinal recordings of slow electrical responses to steady illumination in monkey: Isolation of receptor responses and the origin of the light peak. *Vision Res* 1982; 22:393–399.

57. Welinder E: Cyclic amplitude variations of a slow ERG off-effect, the h-wave, in the Cynomolgus monkey. *Vision Res* 1981; 21:1159–1163.

58. Welinder E, Textorius O: Early effects of sodium iodate on the slow off-effects, particularly the h-wave, and on the c-wave of the DC recorded electroretinogram in rabbit. *Acta Ophthalmol* 1982; 60:305–312.

59. Witkovsky P, Dudek FE, Ripps H: Slow PIII component of the carp electroretinogram. *J Gen Physiol* 1975; 65:119–134.

60. Yonemura D, Kawasaki K: New approaches to ophthalmic electrodiagnosis by retinal oscillatory potential, drug-induced responses from retinal pigment epithelium and cone potential. *Doc Ophthalmol* 1979; 48:163–222.

43 The Oscillatory Potentials of the Electroretinogram

PIERRE LACHAPELLE

THE OSCILLATORY POTENTIALS (OPs) of the electroretinogram (ERG), first demonstrated by Cobb and Morton,[11] and subsequently named by Yonemura et al.,[65] identify the low-voltage, high-frequency components, sometimes referred to as ERG wavelets, which are often seen indenting the rising phase of the b-wave. This is best exemplified with the ERG tracings shown in figure 43.1A, where two OPs (identified as 2 and 3 in the figure) are seen riding on the ascending limb of the b-wave. Although the true oscillatory nature of the OPs was previously questioned,[12] what singles them out is really the difference in frequency domain between the OPs and the other components of the ERG. This prompted Dawson and Stewart[12] to suggest the term *fast retinal potential* as a more appropriate descriptor of these low-voltage, high-frequency ERG components. As we will see, the OPs are not oscillations in the true sense of the word and are most probably not generated by the same retinal structure or pathway. In this chapter, I will focus mostly on oscillatory potentials (and therefore on the ERG) evoked to full-field (Ganzfeld) brief flashes of white light delivered in light- and dark-adapted conditions because this remains, to date, the most universally used method to elicit clinical electroretinograms. It should be noted, however, that OPs can be obtained by using long flashes (i.e., >100 ms) to separate ON-OPs and OFF-OPs[23] or colored flashes.[54] Finally, OPs can also be evoked to localized spots of light, either projected directly on the retina,[46] such as in the technique that is used to obtain focal ERGs, or viewed on a screen, as is the case with multifocal ERG techniques (mfERG).[64]

Extracting the OPs from the raw ERG signal

The electroretinogram is normally recorded by using a bandwidth as wide as possible (low-frequency cutoff: ≤1 Hz, high-frequency cutoff: ≥300 Hz) to include all the frequency components that compose the retinal biopotential. As is shown in figure 43.1C and previously reported elsewhere,[1,17] fast Fourier transform (FFT) of the broadband ERG signal indicates that this biopotential is composed of at least three major frequency components, which, for the photopic ERG shown in figure 43.1A, peak at approximately 35, 70, and 130 Hz. This segregation in high (>100 Hz) and low

(<100 Hz) ERG components is what distinguishes the slow (mainly the a- and b-waves) from the fast (the oscillatory potentials) ERG components. This difference in frequency range is at the basis of the different techniques used to separate the OPs from the raw ERG signal to facilitate their analysis. It should be noted, however, that the exact values of the frequency domain of the OPs may change depending on the intensity of the stimulus that is used to generate the response and, more important, on the state of retinal adaptation; the frequency domain of the scotopic OPs is usually higher (about 150–160 Hz) than that of the photopic OPs (≈125 Hz).[1,17] This point should be taken into consideration in determining the limits of the recording bandwidth, especially the low-frequency cutoff.

Currently, the method that is most often used in order to extract the OPs from the raw ERG is that of bandwidth restriction, where the low-frequency cutoff of the recording bandwidth (of analog or digital amplifiers) is raised from 1 Hz (normally used to record the broadband a- and b-wave ERG signals) to 70–100 Hz, while the high-frequency cutoff is maintained at >300 Hz.[42] The resulting waveforms look somewhat like those shown in figure 43.1B. What stands out immediately is that while in the raw waveforms (figure 43.1A), one can identify only two major OPs on the rising phase of the b-wave (identified as 2 and 3 in figure 43.1A), three major OPs (identified as 2, 3, and 4) are evidenced when the recording bandwidth is restricted to the OP frequency domain. Other, more minor oscillations (identified as 1, 5, 6, and 7) are also observed. It should be noted that other investigators will neglect the small OP (identified as OP_1) that is seen prior to OP_2 and will identify as OP_1 the first major OP (here identified as OP_2).[50]

It is also of interest to note that the peak times of the bandwidth-filtered OPs are slightly faster (by about 2 ms) than the peak times of the corresponding OPs on the ascending limb of the broadband ERG b-wave, a feature that was also previously reported elsewhere.[58] This is best illustrated in figure 43.2, in which the timing of the bandwidth-filtered OPs (tracing 2) is compared to that of the OPs found on the rising phase of the b-wave (tracing 1). However, in the past 20 years or so, the progress that has been made in digital amplifier technologies has allowed us to use new means to

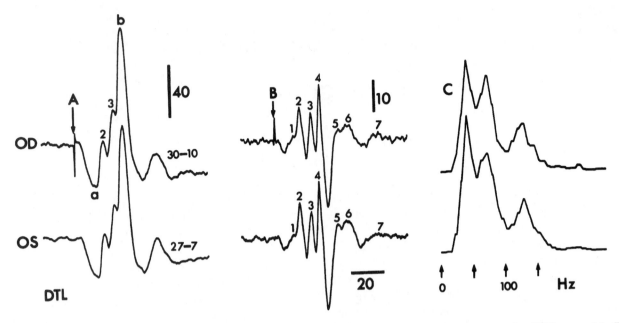

FIGURE 43.1 Representative broadband photopic ERGs (1- to 1000-Hz bandwidth; column A) and oscillatory potentials (100- to 1000-Hz bandwidth; column B) recorded simultaneously from the two eyes of a normal human subject. C shows the fast Fourier transform obtained from the two broadband ERG responses. Note the three major power peaks at approximately 35, 72, and 132 Hz, the latter component representing the oscillatory potential contribution to the ERG potential. The signals were recorded with DTL fiber electrodes (30 deniers/10 filaments in OD and 27 deniers/7 filaments in OS for comparison). Calibration: vertical, 40 μV (A) and 10 μV (B); horizontal, 20 ms (A, B) and hertz (C). Vertical arrows identify flash onset. Tracings in A and B are preceded by a 20-ms prestimulus baseline.

extract the OPs on the basis of FFT analysis of the raw ERG signal in which the low-frequency components (derived from FFT analysis) are software-subtracted from the raw signal to yield the OP signal. An example of the resulting OP signal is illustrated in figure 43.2 (tracing 3). A simple inspection of the resulting OP response reveals, as was previously pointed out,[21] major differences between the bandwidth-filtered OPs (tracing 2) and the software-filtered OPs (tracing 3). The peak times of the software-filtered OPs (tracing 3) are identical to those measured for the raw ERG OPs (tracing 1) and consequently are delayed in comparison to the bandwidth-filtered OPs (tracing 2). Also, the shapes of the two waveforms differ substantially, as if one were the inverted version of the other. This is best exemplified with the OP response illustrated in tracing 4, which is in fact the inverted version of tracing 3. The troughs and peaks in tracing 4 now seem to be in better synchrony with those of tracing 2, suggesting that what is measured as peaks in the software-filtered OPs (tracing 3) actually correspond to the troughs of bandwidth-filtered OPs (tracing 2) and vice versa. Although theoretical at this point, the above differences between bandwidth-filtered (analog or digital) and software-extracted OPs could potentially become clinically significant, should the troughs and peaks of the OPs be independently generated or differently affected by a given disease process. As we will see later on, there are some suggestions that this might be the case.

The OPs were initially considered to be hard-to-record and consequently highly variable components of the ERG that required extreme precautions as well as special stimulating conditions to be recorded reproducibly. There is now enough evidence to suggest that OPs are most probably present in all ERGs, irrespective of the strength of the stimulus that is used or the state of retinal adaptation. Furthermore, although the OPs are of significantly smaller voltage than is the b-wave, it is not always necessary to use averaging techniques to visualize them. This is best exemplified in figure 43.3, in which single-sweep and averaged OPs are compared. The OP responses illustrated on the left-hand side were photographed directly from the screen of an oscilloscope. Each tracing actually includes two superposed single-sweep OP responses evoked, in photopic condition, to flashes of white light of progressively dimmer intensities (tracings 1 to 3) and after 20 minutes of dark adaptation (tracing 4). On the right-hand side are shown the corresponding averaged OP responses, in which each tracing represents an average of 16 flashes. Of course, the purpose of this figure is not to demonstrate that averaging will augment the signal-to-noise ratio, as this is a predictable (and quite visible in figure 43.3) outcome of signal averaging. However, despite noisier tracings (noise level purposely enhanced with the use of DTL fiber instead of contact lens as the active electrode[35]), one can easily identify on the single-sweep trac-

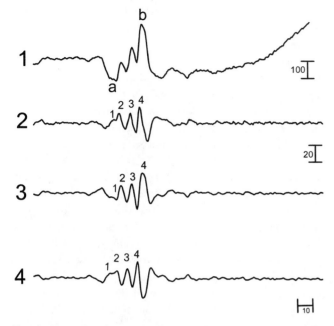

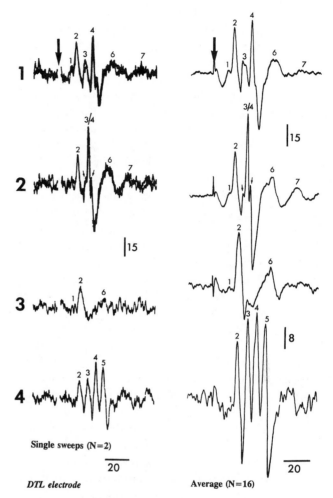

FIGURE 43.2 Comparison between the broadband photopic ERG waveform (0.3–500 Hz; tracing 1), the online bandwidth-filtered oscillatory potential (bandwidth: 75–500 Hz; tracing 2), and software-filtered OPs (bandwidth: 75–500 Hz; tracing 3). The response in tracing 2 was obtained by recording online the ERG signal within a restricted bandwidth, while the waveform in tracing 3 was obtained by using the "extract OP" software option of the LKC UTAS-E 3000 system (LKC Technologies Inc., Gaithersburg, Maryland, USA. Website: www.lkc.com). Note that the OPs of waveforms 2 and 3 appear to be slightly out of phase. However, inverting the waveform in tracing 3 restores the synchrony as well as the similarity in shape, suggesting that the peaks in tracing 2 correspond to the troughs in tracing 3. Calibration: horizontal, 10 ms; vertical, 20 µV.

ings all the major features seen in the average response and vice versa (such as the indentations on the $OP_{3/4}$ complex, which are equally visible on the single-sweep and averaged OP waveforms). These results confirm that, provided that care is taken to ascertain a good electrode contact, recording of the OPs should not represent a greater technical challenge than does the recording of the broadband a- and b-wave ERGs.

Origin of the oscillatory potentials

The oscillatory potentials were first found in ERGs evoked to very strong flashes of light delivered to a fully dark-adapted retina.[11] This combination, which literally dazzled the retina, most probably led some to believe that the OPs represented the oscillation of some retinal structure (or membrane) triggered by the powerful flash of light, thus explaining the choice of the term used to describe these components of the ERG. However, the OPs are not distributed at random, as their name would suggest. Rather, the OPs are, like the other ERG components, time-locked to the

FIGURE 43.3 Comparing single-sweep and averaged oscillatory potentials. On the left-hand side are illustrated OPs recorded by using an oscilloscope. Each tracing shows two responses, which are superposed to demonstrate the reproducibility and the strength of this potential. On the right-hand side are illustrated the corresponding averaged responses ($N = 16$ sweeps averaged). Note that all the OPs identified in the single-sweep responses are also seen in the averaged responses and vice versa. Similarly, the small indentations that are seen in some responses (particularly in tracing 2) are seen with the same accuracy in the single-sweep and averaged responses. Responses were evoked to flashes of white light of 8, 2, and 0.5 cd s m⁻² (tracings 1, 2, and 3) delivered in photopic condition (background: 30 cd m⁻²) and 0.5 cd s m⁻² delivered after 20 minutes of dark adaptation (tracing 4). Single sweeps and averages were recorded simultaneously with a DTL fiber electrode. Calibration: horizontal, 20 ms; vertical, 15 µV (all single-sweep responses and tracings 1 and 2 of averaged responses) and 8 µV (tracings 3 and 4 of averaged responses). Vertical arrows identify flash onset. All tracings are preceded by a 20-ms prestimulus baseline.

onset of the stimulus. Furthermore, previous studies have shown that each OP can be specifically attenuated and even abolished by experimental conditions or pathologies, suggesting that each of them could represent a separate electrical entity, most probably generated by a distinct retinal structure or pathway and consequently no longer fitting the behavior that one would predict for an oscillation.

Although the retinal structures at the origin of the OPs is still being debated, several clinical and experimental observations suggest that the OP generators are postsynaptic to the photoreceptors. This hypothesis initially arose from the pioneering work of Wachtmeister and Dowling,[61] who showed, with intraretinal recordings of oscillatory potentials in isolated retina of mud puppies, that the electrical dipole of each OP was situated at a different retinal depth. Their study revealed that the short-latency OPs were generated in the proximal retina (i.e., near the retinal ganglion cells), while the longer-latency OPs were generated in the distal retina (i.e., nearer the photoreceptors). To explain the apparent discrepancy between the chronological sequence of events (i.e., OP_2 occurs at a shorter latency than OP_5) and retinal distribution of each OP (the suggested generator of OP_2 being closer than that of OP_5 to the photoreceptors, which are at the origin of the retinal response), they suggested that the longer-latency OPs were produced through some inhibitory feedback loop traveling from the inner to the outer retinal layers. Although their findings could not be replicated in the macaque retina,[19] Wachtmeister and Dowling[61] were first to suggest that each OP had a different retinal origin and therefore possibly represented a different physiological entity. To date, experimental and clinical studies have ruled out the photoreceptors,[8] the horizontal cells,[19,48] and the Muller cells[44] as possible contributors to their genesis. There is still some controversy as to a possible contribution from the retinal ganglion cells (RGC). Wachtmeister and el Azazi[62] have reported normal OPs in patients with optic atrophy, while Lachapelle[26] has shown a near extinction of the long-latency photopic OPs in a patient who suffered an accidental section of the optic nerve. Interestingly, the study of Fortune et al.[13] on the mfERG in glaucoma also revealed the selective loss of an oscillation of the long-latency-induced component (IC), which was most prominent in recordings originating from the temporal retina. Of interest, this oscillation peaked at approximately 70 ms, that is, at a latency similar to that of the abolished OPs of Lachapelle's study.[26] According to Fortune et al.,[13] the alleged pathophysiology of glaucoma combined with the retinal mechanisms that are believed to be at the origin of the mfERG response would situate the origin of this mfERG IC oscillation most probably at the level of the inner plexiform layer of the retina or at the optic nerve level. Similar controversial evidences came from the pharmacological blockage of the retinal ganglion cells' activity. Intravitreal injection of tetrodotoxin in monkeys[48] or lidocaine in rabbits[47] did not significantly modify the OPs in the former, while in the latter, it minimally reduced their amplitude and delayed their timing, adding again to the controversy. To date, the most probable generators would appear to be the bipolar cells (depolarizing and hyperpolarizing), the amacrine cells, and the interplexiform cells.[55,60] However, despite our inability to more accurately identify the retinal site where the OPs are generated, it is most probable that more than one site is involved and that the normal functioning of these loci can be independently modified either experimentally (stimulus manipulation, pharmacology, etc.) or clinically and consequently affect the genesis of one or more OPs. This claim cannot be better supported than with the concept of physiologically grouping the OPs into early and late (as per latency), as Wachtmeister and Dowling originally suggested.[61] For example, in a study conducted in newborn rabbits, the early OPs were shown to mature earlier than the long-latency OPs.[14] Similarly, use of a slow-flickering stimulus (in humans) selectively abolished the short-latency OPs from the photopic response, while the longer-latency OP remained almost intact.[27] Use of stimuli of long duration (>100 ms) revealed that the short-latency OPs were triggered through the ON retinal pathway, while the longer-latency OPs were linked to the OFF retinal pathway.[23] Pharmacological experiments showed that the earlier OPs were more susceptible to GABA antagonists,[60] haloperidol (a dopamine antagonist),[60] 2-amino-4-phosphonobutyric acid (a glutamate analogue),[16] and low doses of inspired trichloroethylene,[6] to name a few, while longer-latency OPs were shown to be more susceptible to ethanol,[60] strychnine,[60] iodoacetic acid (a blocker of glycolysis),[33] and the anticonvulsive diphenylhydantoin (effect observed in humans and rabbits).[37] Also of interest is the report that showed that retinal cooling, obtained by circulating cold water in a tube glued to the sclera of rabbits, abolished the long-latency OPs first when the cold water circulated from the peripheral to the central retina and abolished the short-latency OPs first when it circulated from the central to the peripheral retina, suggesting that the dipoles of individual OPs also differed in their topographical distribution.[32] In their study on the focal macular OPs, Miyake et al.[45] also evidenced topographical disparity in the distribution of retinal OPs, where OPs that were evoked to the focal stimulation of discrete loci of the temporal retina were significantly larger than those evoked following the activation of an equivalent area of the nasal retina. As was discussed above, a similar nasotemporal asymmetry in OP distribution was also demonstrated with the mfERG technique.[4,13,64] Similarly, using an imaginative approach, Tremblay and Lam[56] showed that the relative amplitude of each of the photopic OPs varied as the subjects shifted their gaze from nasal to temporal, suggesting that the dipoles of OP_2 and OP_3 were at a different location than that of OP_4. Clearly, although a great deal of information has been gathered to better understand the origin and functional significance of the OPs, more is needed to better grasp what they really signal.

Relationship between the b-wave and the OPs

As was stated above, the oscillatory potentials were originally presented as small, high-frequency components, seen on the ascending limb of the b-wave and most probably generated by retinal structures that were not closely, if at all, involved in the genesis of the b-wave. It was originally believed that special stimulating conditions were required for their demonstration and, more important, that they could be specifically abolished by pharmacological agents or pathologies while the b-wave remained intact. This was the case for the ERG in diabetic retinopathy (DR), in which the absent OPs in an otherwise normal ERG response became almost pathognomonic for the early stage of this retinopathy.[7,9] This is best exemplified in figure 43.4, in which normal photopic ERGs (tracing 1, 12 normal responses superposed) and OPs (tracing 3, 12 normal responses superposed) are compared to the photopic ERG (tracing 2) and OPs (tracing 4) obtained from a patient with documented background diabetic retinopathy (DR). Compared to the normal ERG, that of the DR patient shows an ascending limb of the b-wave that is almost entirely devoid of the typical OP indentation; there is only the suggestion of one, as indicated by the arrowhead. The specific attenuation of the OPs in DR is confirmed by the analysis of the oscillatory potential recordings shown in tracings 3 and 4. One notes that in normal, the filtered ERG (tracing 3) is composed of three major OPs identified as 2, 3, and 4, and each of them is composed of an ascending and a descending segment with the troughs descending to deep below the baseline portion of tracing prior to flash. This contrasts with the DR response, in which all (but that following OP_4) the troughs of the OPs peak above the baseline resulting in OP amplitudes that are significantly smaller than normal. It is interesting to note that the more pronounced attenuation of the OPs (compared to the b-wave) reported in the preproliferative phase of diabetic retinopathy was also evidenced using the mfERG technique.[49] The exact mechanisms at the origin of the (near) selective abolition of the OPs in diabetic retinopathy (especially in the early phase) remains unknown.

Pharmacological manipulation was also shown to produce a similar selective abolition of the OPs while preserving the slower ERG components.[43] This is best exemplified in figure 43.5, in which an intravitreal injection of glycine (in rabbits), a known inhibitory neurotransmitter that is used mainly by amacrine cells, gradually abolished the long-latency OP_3 and OP_4 and slightly reduced the amplitude of OP_2. This resulted in a broadband ERG in which the ascent of the b-wave is devoid of OPs in a way similar to the DR ERG waveform (see figure 43.4). The above would therefore support the claim that the genesis of the OPs is dissociated from that of the slower ERG components, since the OPs can be selectively abolished without significantly modifying the ERG

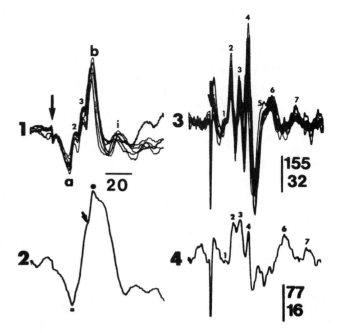

FIGURE 43.4 Comparing the photopic broadband ERGs (tracings 1 and 2) and OPs (tracings 3 and 4) of normal human subjects (tracings 1 and 2) with the responses obtained from a patient with diabetic retinopathy (tracings 2 and 4). In tracings 1 and 3 are superposed on the responses obtained from 12 different normal subjects to illustrate the reproducibility of the OP signal compared to the broadband ERG one. Note that the broadband ERG waveform of the diabetic patient has only one small inflection (arrowhead) on the ascending limb of the b-wave, while in the normal patient, two OPs are seen (corresponding to OP_2 and OP_3 in the filtered response). The filtered OP response recorded from our DR patient confirms the selective attenuation of the OPs compared to the broadband ERG components. Calibration: horizontal, 20 ms; vertical: 155 μV (tracing 1), 77 μV (tracing 2), 32 μV (tracing 3), and 16 μV (tracing 4). Vertical arrows identify flash onset. All tracings are preceded by a 20-ms prestimulus baseline.

a- and b-waves. There are, however, other published experimental and clinical evidences that could support the opposite view. For example, we have previously shown that a systemic injection of iodoacetic acid (IAA) in rabbits, a blocker of glycolysis, caused the gradual attenuation of the long-latency OPs (OP_3 and OP_4) while leaving OP_2 almost intact, an effect that is almost identical to that obtained following the intravitreal injection of glycine.[33] However, like glycine, IAA also reduced the amplitude of the b-wave (see figure 43.5). The latter is accomplished in a very structured fashion, in which the earlier segments of the ERG (i.e., a-wave and first step [identified as 2] of the b-wave) are basically unaltered, while the later components (second step [identified as 3] of the b-wave and b-wave peak [identified as 4]) are abolished. A similar picture is observed following the intravitreal injection of 2-amino-4-phosphonobutyric acid (APB),[16,43] a glutamate analog that blocks the synapse

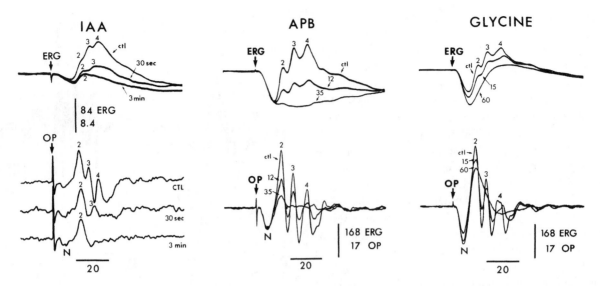

FIGURE 43.5 Pharmacological dissection of the broadband ERG and simultaneously recorded OPs in rabbits. The effects were obtained following the systemic injection of iodoacetic acid (IAA) and intravitreal injections of 2-amino-4-phosphonobutyric acid (APB) and glycine. All recordings were obtained in photopic condition (background: $30\,cd\,m^{-2}$; flash: $8\,cds\,m^{-2}$). Calibration: horizontal, 20 ms; vertical, $168\,\mu V$ (broadband ERG tracings) and $17\,\mu V$ (filtered OP responses). Waveforms are identified as control (CTL: response obtained prior to injection) and, unless otherwise indicated, in minutes following the injection. Vertical arrows identify flash onset. All tracings are preceded by a 20-ms prestimulus baseline.

between the photoreceptors and the ON-depolarizing bipolar cells. Again one notices (see figure 43.5) the gradual reduction in the amplitude of all the OPs. At maximal effect, only remnants of OP_2 and OP_4 are seen. Similarly, the broadband ERG response was significantly modified, and at maximal effect, obtained at 35 minutes postinjection, the response included only an a-wave and no evidence of a b-wave. From the above, it would therefore appear that it is possible to simultaneously impair the normal functioning of the b-wave and OP generators. The results that are probably most supportive of the latter claim came with the previously published comparison between the photopic ERGs obtained from two different but complementary retinopathies: congenital stationary night blindness (CSNB) and cone dystrophy.[36] Figure 43.6 shows the typical broadband photopic ERG (tracing A3) and OPs (tracing B3) obtained from a patient affected with CSNB. The ERG and OP responses are easily identified by their almost pathognomonic features, namely, a square wave–like broadband ERG waveform with truncated b-wave resulting from the absence of the initial segment of the rising phase of the b-wave (compare with normal ERG: tracing A1) and a complete abolition of OP_2 and OP_3 with relative preservation of OP_4 (compare with normal OPs: tracing B1).[18,38,57] This contrasts with the retinal signals that were recorded from our patient who was affected with a familial form of cone dystrophy.[36] Once again, the broadband ERG waveform is truncated, but this time, it is the later parts of the b-wave that are selectively removed. This corresponds, in the OP

response, to the marked attenuation and delay of OP_4 and, to a lesser extent, of OP_3, while OP_2 is of normal amplitude with a slight peak time delay. Results obtained from these two pathologies would again suggest that the OPs and the b-wave are intimately tied; each OP in fact corresponding to one of the three steps (or building blocks) that compose the ascent of the b-wave, a concept that was previously advanced elsewhere.[40] In fact, as was previously demonstrated, when filtering (by raising the low-frequency cutoff) the ERG response to retrieve the OPs, we are taking a derivative (dV/dT) of the broadband ERG. Consequently, the OP signal is nothing more (or less) than another way of representing the ERG response.[40] Clearly, the relationship between the b-wave and the OPs is not as close a case as some would like to think, and more research will be needed before this enigma is once and for all resolved to the satisfaction of all.

The photopic oscillatory potentials

As was alluded to above, one does not require special stimulating conditions to reveal the OPs. The only real requirement is that of limiting the recording bandwidth (analog filtration or software that subtracts the slow components from the raw ERG waveform) to eliminate the slow ERG components and thus relatively amplify the high-frequency components that are the OPs. Consequently, OPs can be obtained in most if not all the recording conditions that normally yield an ERG response, provided that an appropriate

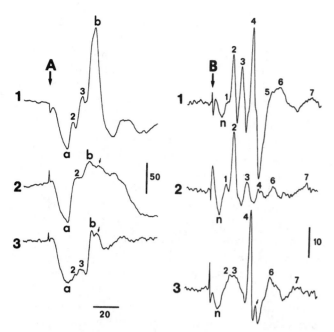

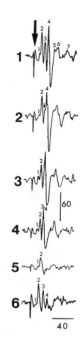

FIGURE 43.6 Photopic broadband ERGs (column A) and corresponding OPs (column B) recorded from a normal subject (tracings A–B 1), a patient affected with a familial form of congenital cone dystrophy (tracings A–B 2), and a patient affected with congenital stationary night blindness (CSNB) (tracings A–B 3). Note that in both patients, the a-wave is of normal amplitude, while the b-wave is truncated—in the later phase for the patient with cone dystrophy and in the early phase for the patient with CSNB. This corresponds to the marked reduction to an almost complete abolition of OP_3 and OP_4 in the signal obtained from our patient with cone dystrophy and to the absence of OP_2 and OP_3 in that obtained from our CSNB patient. Calibration: horizontal, 20 ms; vertical, 50 μV (column A) and 10 μV (column B). Vertical arrows identify flash onset. All tracings are preceded by a 20-ms prestimulus baseline.

FIGURE 43.7 Photopic OPs recorded from a normal subject in response to flashes of white light of decreasing intensity (in 0.3 log unit step; maximum intensity: $8\,cd\,s\,m^{-2}$) delivered against a photopic background of $30\,cd\,m^{-2}$. Tracing 6 illustrates the photopic response obtained at the onset of light adaptation (i.e., immediately following the 20-minute period of dark adaptation). The response was thus evoked to a flash of light of $8\,cd\,sec\,m^{-2}$ delivered against a background of $30\,cd\,m^{-2}$, that is, recording conditions identical to those needed to record the response illustrated in 1. Note the marked attenuation of OP_4, which is typical of the light adaptation effect of the OPs. OP_4 will require some 10 minutes of light adaptation to reach its control amplitude. Calibration: horizontal, 40 ms; vertical: 60 μV. Vertical arrow identifies flash onset. All tracings are preceded by a 20-ms prestimulus baseline.

method is used to enhance their presence. For example, oscillatory potentials that are extracted (bandwidth or software) from ERGs evoked to flashes of light (white or colored) presented against a rod-desensitizing background light are identified as photopic OPs, while those obtained following a prolonged period of dark adaptation are identified as scotopic OPs (see below). Figure 43.7 illustrates the photopic OPs obtained from a normal subject in response to progressively brighter flashes. As the strength of the flash stimulus grows (from tracings 5 to 1), there is a gradual increase in the number of OPs from one (namely, OP_2: tracing 5) to a maximum of three major OPs (OP_2, OP_3, and OP_4: tracing 1). Smaller OPs are also seen: the short-latency OP_1 (which is often difficult to accurately identify) and the longer-latency OP_5, OP_6, and OP_7, which were previously suggested to arise at the level of (or near) the retinal ganglion cells and/or the optic nerve.[26]

What stands out when one examines the OP responses shown in figure 43.7 is the difference in threshold (also seen with the results shown in figure 43.8) of the different OPs.

At threshold (tracing 5), the OP response only includes one major component: OP_2. With the gradual increase in intensity of the flash stimulus, the amplitude of OP_2 increases, and its peak time shortens. At the same time, a new OP (identified as OP_{3-4}) is added to the original OP_2, thus increasing the length (or duration) of the OP response. With brighter stimuli, this new OP will eventually break into two new OPs, identified as OP_3 and OP_4, and thus further increase the duration of the OP response. This is best illustrated with the OP response shown in tracing 2, in which the onset of the split of OP_{3-4} into OP_3 (arrowhead) and OP_4 is shown. This method of OP multiplication is also observed with the scotopic OPs. Not illustrated here but previously reported elsewhere, a further increase in the strength of the stimulus, beyond that used to generate the OP response shown in tracing 1, will continue to augment the amplitude of OP_2 and OP_3 but at the same time decreases that of OP_4.[41,50] This dichotomy further suggests that the early and late OPs are probably generated by different retinal structures. As we will see below, a similar conclusion is reached

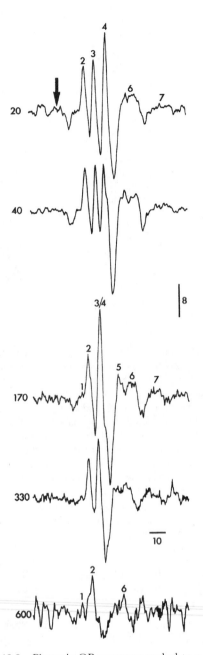

FIGURE 43.8 Photopic OP responses evoked to a flash of white light of $8\,cd\,s\,m^{-2}$ delivered against a background of 20, 40, 170, 330, and $600\,cd\,m^{-2}$. Note that with the gradual increase in strength of the background light, there is a progressive removal of the long-latency OPs (starting with OP_4). The response gathered against the brightest background includes only OP_2, whose amplitude and timing were not significantly modified throughout the entire procedure. The sequence illustrated here is similar to that shown in figure 43.7, the only major difference being that the amplitude of OP_2 is gradually reduced and its timing increased with progressively dimmer flashes, while both parameters are not significantly modified when the background is changed provided that the intensity of the flash is kept constant. The latter best illustrates the intensity-coding properties of OP_2. Calibration: horizontal, 10 ms; vertical, $8\,\mu V$. Vertical arrow identifies flash onset.

in comparing the physiology of early- and late-latency scotopic OPs.

A similar picture arises when the intensity of the flash stimulus is kept constant at maximum strength while the luminance of the background light is gradually enhanced. This is best exemplified with the result shown in figure 43.8, which illustrates the photopic OP response evoked to a flash of light of $8\,cd\,s\,m^{-2}$ presented against progressively brighter backgrounds (from 20 (top tracing) to 600 (bottom tracing) $cd\,m^{-2}$). With the gradual increase in luminance of the background light, there is a progressive reduction in the number of OPs generated to end, at maximal background luminance (tracing 600), with only one major OP, namely, OP_2, a sequence reminiscent of that obtained when the strength of the stimulus is decreased while the luminance of the background is kept constant (such as is illustrated in figure 43.7). There is one major difference, however. While the amplitude of OP_2 grows and its timing shortens as the strength of the stimulus increases and the background light is kept constant (see figure 43.7), OP_2 does not budge (in amplitude or timing) when the background light is gradually enhanced, provided that the intensity of the flash stimulus is kept constant (see figure 43.8). These results were previously interpreted as evidence that OP_2 coded the absolute intensity of the flash (i.e., intensity of flash irrespective of retinal adaptation) while the longer-latency OPs were generated in response to the relative intensity of the stimulus, which took the intensity of the flash as well as the state of retinal adaptation into consideration.[5,28,31,34] As we will see later on, this (stimulus) intensity-coding property of OP_2 can be verified with scotopic recordings.

Two other features of the photopic ERG signal also affect the oscillatory potentials, namely, a flickering stimulus and the light-adaptation effect (LAE).[25,27,50] The flickering light stimulus,[27] especially beyond 30 Hz, is suggested as the best method to isolate the cone ERG response, since rods cannot follow such a rapid rate of stimulation. As is shown in figure 43.9, one notes that with the gradual increase in the rate of presentation of the flash stimulus (from 1 Hz in the top tracing to 15 Hz in the bottom tracing), there is a gradual attenuation in amplitude of OP_2 and OP_3, while the amplitude of OP_4 is slightly enhanced. At maximal effect, OP_3 is completely abolished, while OP_2 is significantly reduced and delayed. It is of interest to note that a method that is suggested to enhance the cone contribution to the ERG (and by extension to the OPs as well) selectively attenuated (and removed in the case of OP_3) the same OPs that are specifically absent from the photopic OP response of patients who are affected with congenital stationary night blindness.[18,36,38,57] (Compare the OP responses shown in tracing 3 of figure 43.6B (CSNB) with that shown in figure 43.9 (15-Hz flicker).) This further supports the concept, as previously advanced, that the photopic OP_2 and OP_3 are intimately tied to the rod pathway (most proba-

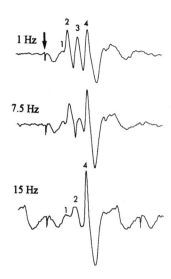

FIGURE 43.9 Photopic OPs (background: 30 cd m⁻²; flash: 8 cd sec m⁻²) recorded from a normal subject. Flashes were delivered at the rate of 1, 7.5, and 15 Hz. Note that with progressively faster flickers, the amplitude of OP_2 and OP_3 goes down while that of OP_4 increases. At 15 Hz, OP_3 is abolished, and OP_2 is reduced in amplitude and delayed in timing. Vertical arrow identifies flash onset. All tracings are preceded by a 20-ms prestimulus baseline.

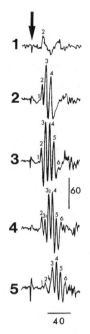

FIGURE 43.10 Representative OPs recorded from a normal subject in response to flashes of white light of 0.5 cd s m⁻² delivered in photopic condition (tracing 1: conditions similar to those used to generate the OP response shown in tracing 5 in figure 43.7), at the onset of dark adaptation (tracing 2), and after 20 minutes of dark adaptation (tracing 3). The response illustrated in tracing 4 was recorded from a different subject under the same experimental conditions as in tracing 3 (i.e., 20 minutes of dark adaptation; flash: 0.5 cd sec m⁻²). Note that in the latter case, OP_3 splits into two OPs identified as OP_{3-1} and OP_{3-2}, a feature often seen in normal subjects. Tracing 5 illustrates the OP response obtained after 20 minutes of dark adaptation in response to a flash of white light 1.5 log-unit dimmer than that used in tracing 1. Note the indentation on the rise of OP_3, which is suggestive of a near split into OP_{3-1} and OP_{3-2}, similar to what is seen in tracing 4. At this intensity, the broadband ERG is of a morphology typical of a rod response (i.e., no measurable a-wave). Calibration: horizontal, 40 ms; vertical, 60 μV. Vertical arrows identify flash onset.

bly at the level of the ON-depolarizing bipolar cells, where signals from cones and rods converge)[36,38] and consequently further supports the physiological distinction between early- and late-latency OPs presented above. This temporal dichotomy also received support from the findings that are obtained with the light-adaptation effect.[15,25,50,53] The latter describe the ERG amplitude and peak time changes measured as the cone ERG gradually adapts to a photopic environment following a prolonged period of dark adaptation. Previous studies have shown that the amplitude of the ERG b-wave almost doubles (and its peak time shortens by nearly 5 ms) in the first 10 minutes or so following the opening of the photopic background light, while the a-wave is minimally altered. Similarly, of all the major photopic OPs, only OP_4 demonstrates a similar effect.[25,50,53] This is best exemplified by comparing, in figure 43.7, the OP response illustrated in tracing 6 (obtained in response to a flash of white light of 8 cd s m⁻² in intensity presented against a photopic background of 30 cd m⁻² lit immediately after a period of 20 minutes of dark adaptation) with that shown at tracing 1 (obtained with the same background and flash but prior to the dark-adaptation period). One notes that of all the major OPs, OP_4 is the one that shows the most dramatic effect, its amplitude measured at the onset of light adaptation (figure 43.7, tracing 6) being significantly smaller (50% smaller on average[25]) than that measured prior to the dark-adaptation period (figure 43.7, tracing 1).

The scotopic oscillatory potentials

As was stated above, OPs can be recorded in most, if not all, conditions that will yield an ERG response. Scotopic OPs are thus obtained in response to flashes of light (white or blue) delivered to a dark-adapted retina. Figure 43.10 shows the OP responses evoked to flashes of white light of 0.5 cd sec m⁻² delivered in photopic condition (tracing 1; conditions identical to those used to evoke the OP response shown in tracing 5 of figure 43.7) and following 1 minute (tracing 2) and 20 minutes (tracing 3) of dark adaptation. Again, one notes that there is no significant modification in the amplitude or peak time of OP_2 whether measured in the photopic response or in that obtained after some 20 minutes of dark adaptation, suggesting that the two OP_2 are one and the same. The latter also further exemplifies the (flash) intensity-coding property of OP_2, which was presented above. It is also of interest to note that as soon as the photopic background closes, two new OPs (identified as OP_3 and OP_4) are added to OP_2, and another two (OP_5 and OP_6) will join after 20 minutes of dark adaptation. This gradual addition of long-latency OPs with progressive dark adaptation is reminiscent of what was observed in photopic condition following an increase in flash intensity (see figure 43.7) or dimming of the background luminance (see figure 43.8). The above would also suggest that the long-latency OPs that add to the (photopic) OP_2 are generated via the rod pathway, given that their amplitude increases as the duration in dark adaptation augments. (Compare the amplitudes of OP_3 and OP_4 in tracing 2 with those of tracing 3.) Consequently, it is most likely that the scotopic OP_3 and OP_4 are of a different origin than the OP_3 and OP_4 of the photopic response (i.e., figure 43.7, tracing 1). This discrepancy in the photoreceptoral origin of the dark-adapted OPs was previously addressed by King-Smith et al.,[22] who suggested that the short-latency scotopic OPs originated via the cone pathway while the long-latency scotopic OPs were generated following the activation of the rod pathway. This was confirmed in a series of experiments that showed that prior exposure to a progressively brighter photopic environment gradually abolished OP_4 and approximately 50% of OP_3 in the OP response recorded at the onset of dark adaptation, such as that shown at tracing 2 of figure 43.10, while OP_2 remained unaffected.[52] This finding again supported the claim that the (abolished) long-latency OPs were most probably generated via the rod pathway, while the (resistant) shorter-latency OPs were most probably generated through the cone pathway. These results also suggested that the large OP_3 that is seen in scotopic responses (in fact, significantly larger than its photopic counterpart) was probably made of two OPs (i.e., superposed cone and rod-driven OPs) that were fused in a way similar to that of the photopic OP_{3-4} (tracing 2 of figure 43.7).

The splitting of OP_3 into OP_{3-1} and OP_{3-2} can, in some instances, occur naturally, as is illustrated in tracing 4 in figure 43.10. This OP response was obtained from a normal subject in response to a flash of white light of $0.5\,cd\,sec\,m^{-2}$ delivered after 20 minutes of dark adaptation and thus the same stimulus and recording conditions as for the response shown in tracing 3. Approximately 50% of our normal subjects generated scotopic OP responses with a split OP_3. As was suggested above, the short-latency OP_2 and OP_{3-1}, which are almost of the same amplitudes, are most probably generated through the cone pathway. The latter claim is not only supported by the fact that they are most resistant to preexposure to a bright photopic environment,[52] but also by the fact that they were shown to be specifically abolished in scotopic responses recorded from achromates and selectively enhanced in scotopic responses recorded from affected

members of a pedigree of cone dystrophy.[36] Also supportive of the above dichotomy is the suggested origin of the conditioning flash effect (CFE). In a study published in 1972, Algvere and Westbeck[1] showed that the first flash of a series of flashes that were delivered in dark adaptation always evoked the smallest OPs. This effect, subsequently identified as the CFE, was shown to be optimal (i.e., smallest initial OPs) when the flashes were spaced by less than 15 s and disappeared with intervals greater than 60 s. A strong flash, well above photopic threshold, is also required to generate a measurable CFE, as it was previously shown that dim flashes of light (but still within the photopic range) did not yield a CFE.[30] As a possible explanation, it was suggested that the initial flash removed the rod system contribution to the OPs generated by the later flash, thus enhancing the cone-mediated OPs.[51] Interestingly, it is the long-latency OPs, those that are suggested above to arise from the activation of the rod pathway, that are most susceptible to the CFE.

As is exemplified by the photopic OP response, a regular increase in strength of the flash stimulus gradually augments the amplitude and shortens the peak time of OP_2. A similar relationship is observed in scotopic condition. This is best illustrated with the OP responses shown in tracings 3 and 5 of figure 43.10, which were obtained from the same individual but the latter was evoked to a flash of light 1.5 log unit dimmer than the former. One notes that in response to the dimmer flash, all the OPs are reduced in amplitude, and the entire OP sequence is displaced to the right. The shift in timing of OP_2 (approximately 7.5 ms for a 1.5 log unit shift) is similar to that measured in photopic condition (approximately 5.0 ms for a 1.0 log unit shift). These results are in line with a previous report that showed that the peak time of OP_2 lengthened by more than 15 ms for 2.5 log unit of attenuation in the strength of the stimulus (from the brightest photopic to the dimmest scotopic flashes).[28] These results further exemplify the general applicability of the intensity-coding property of OP_2, which confers to this OP, as was previously documented elsewhere, unique diagnostic properties.[34] However, unlike what was observed with the photopic OPs (figure 43.7), there is no suggestion of a gradual reduction in the number of scotopic OPs with dimmer flashes. In fact, the responses shown in tracings 3 and 5 of figure 43.10 include the same number of OPs (albeit of smaller amplitude in tracing 5), despite the fact that in tracing 5, the OPs were evoked to a flash of light 1.5 log unit dimmer than that used to generate the response shown in tracing 3. In comparison, 1 log unit of attenuation of the stimulus in photopic condition reduced the number of OPs from three to one (figure 43.7). Finally, it should be noted that the OP response shown in tracing 5 was evoked at an intensity near the rod V_{max} as per the International Society for Clinical Electrophysiology of Vision (ISCEV) standard (i.e., a pure rod ERG made only of a b-wave) and consequently well below the intensity suggested by the ISCEV to be optimal for the recording of OPs.[42] The latter further exemplifies, as was stated above, that OPs are present in all ERG responses.

Suggested method of analysis of the OP response

Two major techniques are suggested to quantify the OPs of the ERG. The first one makes use of bandwidth restriction (analog or digital filtration) to filter out the slow components of the ERG and thus enhance the high-frequency OPs.[24,30,51] It is probably the most widely used method to isolate the OPs. The OPs that are included in the resulting signal can be analyzed either separately, where the amplitude and peak time of each OP are reported individually, or collectively, where the amplitudes of each OP are added together to yield the artificial variable sum OP amplitude (or SOP).[29] An alternative method of analysis that combines both approaches was also previously suggested. In the latter method, the amplitude of each OP is measured individually (from the preceding trough to the peak) and is reported as a percentage of the summed amplitude of all the OPs that compose the response (i.e., amplitude of OP_x/sum of all OPs).[29] The latter method was shown to yield highly reproducible intersubject and intrasubject amplitude measurements and thus potentially facilitate the clinical use as well as the interlaboratory comparisons of the OPs. However, for this to occur, one needs to standardize the OP response to be used, and as is shown in figures 43.7, 43.8, and 43.10, the OP content of an ERG will vary considerably depending on the intensity of the stimulus as well as the state of retinal adaptation. For that reason, it was suggested,[41] as the ISCEV standard flash definition, to standardize the OP response rather than the flash intensity required to produce this response. Thus, the standard photopic OP response would be one in which the amplitudes of OP_2, OP_3, and OP_4 represent 25%, 25%, and 50%, respectively, of the sum OP amplitude (such as is shown in tracing 1 in figure 43.7).

It is claimed by some that analysis of the OP response in the time domain (i.e., peak time and amplitude measurements on the filtered OP response), whether individually or collectively, is prone to include some artifacts that result from the filters themselves—artifacts that can often be mistaken for OPs. Similarly, it was previously shown that use of strictly applied bandwidth limits can yield erroneous conclusions. For example, in a study on the maturation of the OPs in rabbit pups,[14] it was shown that while the 100- to 1000-Hz bandwidth was quite adequate to record the OPs in adult rabbits, it was not at all appropriate for younger rabbits, since their OPs were of a significantly lower frequency domain and therefore were completely eliminated by the 100-Hz cutoff. This resulted in a filtered ERG that was devoid of OPs and in the false conclusion that the slow ERG

components matured earlier than the fast ERG components. The presence of OPs in the young rabbit's ERG could, however, be demonstrated by lowering the low-frequency cutoff to 70 Hz. This suggested that use of a universal method of OP extraction, based on rigid bandwidth restrictions, will be adequate, provided that the OPs remain in the frequency domain for which the limits were originally set (i.e., approximately 130 Hz). Any situations (experimental or pathological) in which the frequency domain of the OPs is prone to be lowered may (and most probably will) have an impact on the amplitude of the resulting signals. This will complicate the interpretation of the results, as it will be difficult to determine which of the two (pathology experiment or low-frequency cutoff) will have been the most important contributor to the effect. To overcome this type of situation, some investigators have suggested evaluating the OP response in the frequency domain rather than in the time domain.[2,3,10,59] The method that they suggest examines the power spectrum of the ERG, using an FFT analysis approach and concentrates on the higher (>120 Hz) frequency domain and how this frequency component is altered with pathology or experiments. The results are therefore reported in frequency (hertz), and the magnitude of the frequency component is usually reported in units of power (watts). Another approach makes use of the FFT technique to extract the frequency domain of the OPs and then makes use of this information to condition the ERG signal prior to OP extraction.[10] Supporters of the latter approach claim that in doing so, they remove from the raw ERG signal all the components that are not within the OP frequency domain, thus permitting a more precise and reproducible extraction of the oscillatory potentials.

Both methods of analyzing the OPs have their strengths and drawbacks. While it is possible to separately assess each OP individually with the restricted bandwidth approach (time domain approach), an approach that was shown to yield valuable experimental and clinical information, this technique is also prone to artifactual biases. In contrast, the more holistic approach that the frequency domain analysis offers will limit the analysis, since it considers the OPs as a whole, irrespective of the number of OPs that make the response. As has been shown on numerous occasions, specific OPs can be abolished by experiments or pathologies, while others remain intact, a feature of the OP response that would be missed or underestimated with the frequency domain approach. However, given that a change in the frequency domain of the OPs (by disease or experiments) could affect the resulting filtered signal, it might be advisable to use both approaches and perform an FFT of the raw ERG signal before filtering. With the technology that is now available to most ERG laboratories, it is possible to record the raw ERG, perform an FFT analysis to accurately determine the frequency domain of the OPs, and then apply a better delimited filter to more precisely isolate the OPs. Use of this combined approach should undoubtedly augment the reproducibility, and consequently the clinical utility, of the OPs.

The diagnostic use of the OPs

As was suggested above, each OP (photopic or scotopic) appears to be generated by a distinct and possibly independent retinal pathway. Although the exact origin of each OP remains to be determined, the fact that each of them most probably represents a distinct and possibly independent retinal event generated by a distinct retinal structure or pathway becomes of prime importance in the diagnostic application of this retinal signal. Figures 43.11 to 43.15 show OP responses obtained from patients affected with different retinopathies (solid tracings), which are compared to those obtained from normal subjects (background dotted tracings). In these examples, the numeral identification of the remaining OPs that compose the pathological recordings was based on known properties that were previously shown, as presented above, to single out individual photopic OPs, namely, threshold, flicker, and intensity coding property, to name a few. A more detailed account can be found elsewhere.[29] It should be noted that all the responses shown here were obtained in photopic conditions at optimal flash intensity (see above). This is not to say that OP-specific diseases can be demonstrated only with the photopic response. In fact,

previous studies have reported OP-specific anomalies with the scotopic signal as well.[37,52] However, the photopic OP response is more easily reproduced throughout laboratories (especially the optimal OP response), a claim that one can easily verify by comparing the normal waveform of figure 43.11 (dotted tracings) with those published elsewhere.[18,39,50]

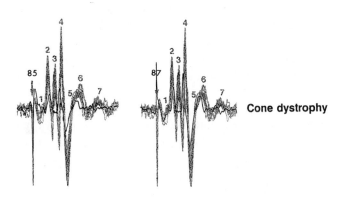

Selective attenuation of OP₃

Cone dystrophy

FIGURE 43.12 Representative photopic OP (background: 30 cd m⁻², flash: 8 cd s m⁻²) responses taken from normal subjects (dotted waveforms in background are composed of superposed responses taken from 12 normal subjects) compared to that obtained from a patient affected with cone dystrophy in two consecutive exams (1985, 1987). Note that OP₃ is the only OP that is systematically absent from the two recordings. Vertical arrows indicate flash onset. All tracings are preceded by a 20-ms prestimulus baseline.

Non OP selective ERG abnormality

X-R.P.

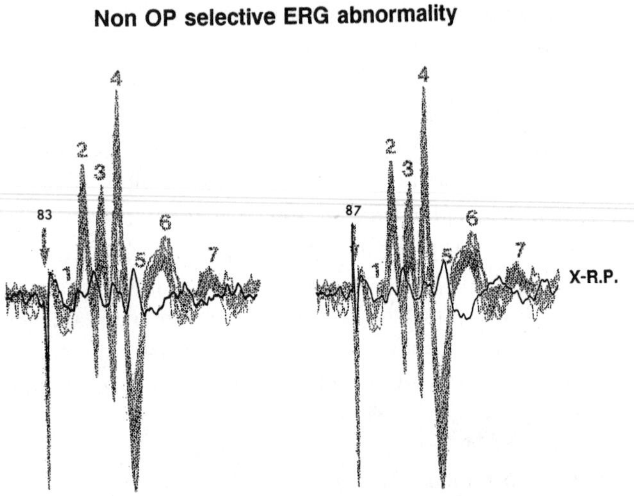

FIGURE 43.11 Representative photopic OP (background: 30 cd m⁻², flash: 8 cd s m⁻²) responses taken from normal subjects (dotted waveforms in background are composed of superposed responses taken from 12 normal subjects) compared to that obtained from a patient affected with X-linked retinitis pigmentosa at two consecutive examinations (1983, 1987). Note that all the major OPs (i.e., OP₂, OP₃, and OP₄) are present, though significantly reduced in amplitude and delayed in timing. Vertical arrows indicate flash onset. All tracings are preceded by a 20-ms prestimulus baseline.

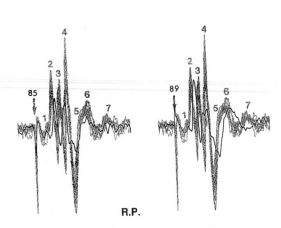

Selective attenuation of OP₃ and OP₄

R.P.

FIGURE 43.13 Representative photopic OP (background: 30 cd m⁻², flash: 8 cd s m⁻²) responses taken from normal subjects (dotted waveforms in background are composed of superposed responses taken from 12 normal subjects) compared to that obtained from a patient affected with retinitis pigmentosa in two consecutive exams (1985, 1989). Note that OP₄ was the only OP that was absent in the 1985 recording, while OP₃ was reduced substantially in the follow-up recording (1989). Vertical arrows indicate flash onset. All tracings are preceded by a 20-ms prestimulus baseline.

Relative preservation of OP$_4$

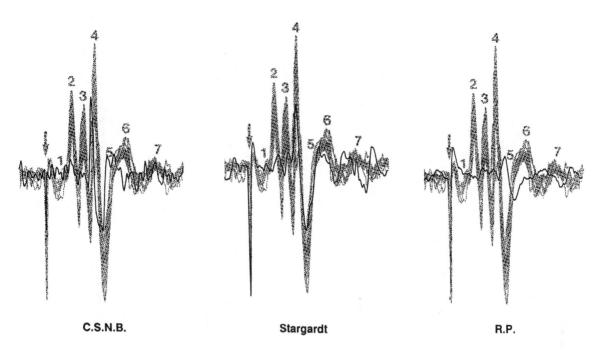

C.S.N.B.	Stargardt	R.P.

FIGURE 43.14 Representative photopic OP (background: 30 cd m^{-2}; flash: 8 cd s m^{-2}) responses taken from normal subjects (dotted waveforms in background are composed of superposed responses taken from 12 normal subjects) compared to that obtained from a patient affected with congenital stationary night blindness, Stargardt's disease, and retinitis pigmentosa. Note that in all three cases, OP$_4$ is relatively better preserved than OP$_2$ and OP$_3$, which are equally markedly attenuated. Also, it is only in our patient with RP that OP$_4$ is significantly delayed. Vertical arrows indicate flash onset. All tracings are preceded by a 20-ms prestimulus baseline.

As is shown in figure 43.11, the OP response does not always show OP-specific anomalies. As this example, taken from a patient affected with X-linked retinitis pigmentosa (RP), reveals, at the first ERG evaluation (1983), a significant reduction in amplitude and delay in timing of all three major OPs (OP$_2$, OP$_3$, and OP$_4$). On a subsequent evaluation, four years later (1987), the peak times of OP$_3$ and OP$_4$ had increased (compared to the 1983 measurement), while that of OP$_2$ had not budged, and only the amplitude of OP$_3$ had diminished. In the second example (see figure 43.12), taken from a patient affected with a cone dystrophy, consecutive assessments at a two-year interval showed, on both occasions, an OP response with a completely abolished OP$_3$. Figure 43.13 shows the OP responses taken from a patient affected with RP (of unknown etiology) at two ERG evaluations four years apart. In the first examination (1985), the OP response included an OP$_2$ and an OP$_3$ of almost equal amplitude (as in a normal response) and a minimal (if any) OP$_4$ presenting as a small bump following the trough of OP$_3$. On subsequent ERG evaluation, the amplitude of OP$_3$ was found to be significantly smaller than that of OP$_2$, a finding suggesting that there was significant progression in the disease process and that the OP response had evolved from one in which there was a selective removal of OP$_4$ to one

with a selective attenuation of OP$_3$ and removal of OP$_4$. Finally, the examples shown in figure 43.14 illustrate the complementary situation in which OP$_2$ and OP$_3$ are selectively abolished and OP$_4$ is relatively better preserved. Such an OP anomaly was repeatedly reported in CSNB. It is not, however, pathognomonic for the condition, as it was also observed in Stargardt's disease and in some forms of RP.[39] Therefore, while a careful analysis of the OP that takes into consideration each OP individually may eventually add to the diagnostic potential of the ERG, the diagnostic categories that are obtained clearly cannot be considered pathognomonic for a given retinopathy. This cannot be better illustrated than with the OP responses shown in figure 43.15, all of which were obtained from patients affected with different forms of RP and showing differences in the OPs that are specifically affected by the disease process. Rather, once the origin of each OP that composes the photopic response, for example, can be firmly established, a careful analysis of the OP signal and, more important, how this response is modified with time will help us to distinguish one disease process from another one, for example, a form of RP that would progress from an OP$_4$-specific retinopathy to one in which only OP$_2$ remains. Another way might be one in which OP$_3$ would be initially abolished to yield, with

Retinitis pigmentosa

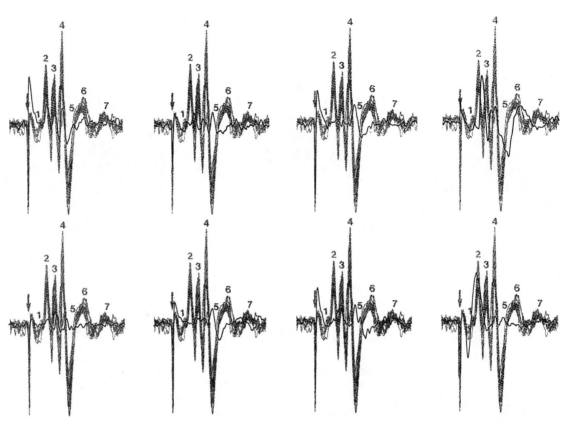

FIGURE 43.15 Representative photopic OP (background: $30\,cd\,m^{-2}$; flash: $8\,cd\,s\,m^{-2}$) responses taken from normal subjects (dotted waveforms in the background are composed of superposed responses taken from 12 normal subjects) compared to those obtained from patients affected with retinitis pigmentosa (RP). Note that RP can yield photopic responses where all three major OPs are present, albeit of reduced amplitude and normal timing, reduced amplitude and delayed timing, OP_2 and OP_3 are abolished and OP_4 delayed, selective attenuation of OP_4 and partly of OP_3 (top row, from left to right) and OP_2 and OP_4 are selectively attenuated, OP_2 and OP_3 are selectively attenuated and OP_4 delayed, OP_3 is selectively attenuated, and OP_3 and OP_4 abolished (bottom row, from left to right). Vertical arrows indicate flash onset. All tracings are preceded by a 20-ms prestimulus baseline.

progression, an OP response that includes only OP_4. Only time will tell whether a more detailed analysis of the OP signal can offer this quality of discrimination.

Concluding remarks

After more than 50 years of research, the oscillatory potentials remain mysterious not only in their origin, but also in their significance and their clinical use. Most of the confusion, I believe, comes from significant interlaboratory differences in stimulating and recording parameters that are important enough to yield inconsistent and/or irreproducible results. Once we recognize the possibility that each photopic and scotopic OP is a separate entity, which is most probably generated by a distinct retinal structure or pathway, we will rapidly progress toward a sound understanding of what retinal event(s) the OPs signal and, consequently, what clinical information they can provide.

ACKNOWLEDGMENTS This work was supported by grants from the McGill University–Montreal Children's Hospital Research Institute, the Canadian Institute for Health Research, and the Vision Network of the Fonds de la Recherche en Santé du Québec.

REFERENCES

1. Algvere P, Westbeck S: Human ERG in response to double flashes of light during the course of light adaptation: A Fourier analysis of the oscillatory potentials. *Vision Res* 1972; 12:145–214.
2. Asi H, Leibu R, Perlman I: Frequency-domain analysis of the human corneal electroretinogram. *Clin Vis Res* 1992; 7:9–19.
3. Asi H, Perlman I: Relationships between the electroretinogram a-wave, b-wave and oscillatory potentials and their application to clinical diagnosis. *Doc Ophthalmol* 1992; 79:125–139.
4. Bearse MA, Shimada Y, Sutter EE: Distribution of oscillatory components in the central retina. *Doc Ophthalmol* 2000; 100:185–205.

5. Benoit J, Lachapelle P: Temporal relationship between ERG components and geniculate unit activity in rabbits. *Vision Res* 1990; 30:797–806.

6. Blain L, Lachapelle P: Comparative effects of chronic trichloroethylene exposure on the electroretinogram components and oscillatory potentials. *Neurotoxicology* 1994; 15:627–632.

7. Bresnick GH, Palta M: Oscillatory potential amplitudes: Relation to severity of diabetic retinopathy. *Arch Ophthalmol* 1987; 105:810–814.

8. Brown KT: The electroretinogram, its components and their origins. *Vision Res* 1968; 8:633–677.

9. Brunette JR, Lafond G: Electroretinographic evaluation of diabetic retinopathy: Sensitivity of amplitude and time course. *Can J Ophthalmol* 1983; 18:285–289.

10. Bui BV, Armitage JA, Vingrys AJ: Extraction and modeling of oscillatory potentials. *Doc Ophthalmol* 2002; 104:17–36.

11. Cobb WA, Morton HB: A new component of the human electroretinogram. *J Physiol (Lond)* 1954; 123:36–37.

12. Dawson WW, Stewart HL: Signals within the electroretinogram. *Vision Res* 1968; 8:1265–1270.

13. Fortune B, Bearse MA, Cioffi GA, Johnson CA: Selective loss of an oscillatory component from temporal retinal multifocal ERG responses in glaucoma. *Invest Ophthalmol Vis Sci* 2002; 43:2638–2647.

14. Gorfinkel J, Lachapelle P: Maturation of the photopic b-wave and the oscillatory potentials of the electroretinogram in the neonatal rabbit. *Can J Ophthalmol* 1990; 25:138–144.

15. Gouras P, MacKay CJ: Growth in amplitude of the human cone electroretinogram with light adaptation. *Invest Ophthalmol Vis Sci* 1989; 30:619–624.

16. Guité P, Lachapelle P: The effect of 2-amino-4-phosphonobutyric acid on the oscillatory potentials of the electroretinogram. *Doc Ophthalmol* 1990; 75:125–133.

17. Gur M, Zeevi Y: Frequency-domain analysis of the human electroretinogram. *J Opt Soc Am* 1980; 70:53–59.

18. Heckenlively JR, Martin DA, Rosenbaum AL: Loss of electroretinographic oscillatory potentials, optic atrophy and dysplasia in congenital stationary night blindness. *Am J Ophthalmol* 1983; 96:526–534.

19. Heynen H, Wachtmeister L, van Norren D: Origin of the oscillatory potentials in the primate retina. *Vision Res* 1985; 25:1365–1373.

20. Kergoat H, Lovasik JV: The effects of altered retinal vasculature perfusion pressure on the white flash scotopic ERG and oscillatory potentials in man. *Electroencephalogr Clin Neurophysiol* 1990; 75:306–322.

21. Khani-Oskouee K, Sieving P: A digital band-pass filter for electrophysiology recording system, in Heckenlively JR, Arden GB (eds): *Principles and Practice of Clinical Electrophysiology of Vision*. St. Louis, Mosby Year Book, 1991, pp 205–211.

22. King-Smith PE, Loffing DH, Jones R: Rod and cone ERGs and their oscillatory potentials. *Invest Ophthalmol Vis Sci* 1986; 27:270–273.

23. Kojima M, Zrenner E: OFF-components in response to brief light flashes in the oscillatory potentials of the human electroretinogram. *Graefes Arch Clin Ophthalmol* 1978; 206:107–120.

24. Lachapelle P: Impact of the recording bandwidth on the electroretinogram. *Can J Ophthalmol* 1985; 20:211–215.

25. Lachapelle P: Analysis of the photopic electroretinogram recorded before and after dark-adaptation. *Can J Ophthalmol* 1987; 22:354–361.

26. Lachapelle P: A possible contribution of the optic nerve to the photopic oscillatory potentials. *Clin Vis Res* 1990; 5:412–426.

27. Lachapelle P: The effect of a slow flicker on the human oscillatory potentials. *Vision Res* 1991; 31:1851–1857.

28. Lachapelle P: Evidence for an intensity-coding oscillatory potential in the human electroretinogram. *Vision Res* 1991; 31:767–774.

29. Lachapelle P: The human suprathreshold photopic oscillatory potentials: Method of analysis and clinical illustration. *Doc Ophthalmol* 1994; 88:1–25.

30. Lachapelle P, Benoit J, Blain L, Guité P, Roy MS: The oscillatory potentials in response to stimuli of photopic intensities delivered in dark-adaptation: An explanation for the conditioning flash effect. *Vision Res* 1990; 30:503–513.

31. Lachapelle P, Benoit J, Cheema D, Molotchnikoff S: Temporal relationship between the ERG and geniculate unit activity in rabbits: Influence of background luminance. *Vision Res* 1991; 31:2033–2037.

32. Lachapelle P, Benoit J, Guité P: The effect of in vivo retinal cooling on the electroretinogram of rabbits. *Vision Res* 1996; 36:339–344.

33. Lachapelle P, Benoit J, Guité P, Cuong TN, Molotchnikoff S: The effect of iodoacetic acid on the electroretinogram and oscillatory potentials in rabbits. *Doc Ophthalmol* 1990; 75:7–14.

34. Lachapelle P, Benoit J, Little JM, Faubert J: The diagnostic use of the second oscillatory potential in clinical electroretinography. *Doc Ophthalmol* 1990; 73:327–336.

35. Lachapelle P, Benoit J, Little JM, Lachapelle B: Recording the oscillatory potentials with the DTL electrode. *Doc Ophthalmol* 1993; 83:119–130.

36. Lachapelle P, Benoit J, Rousseau S, McKerral M, Polomeno RC, Little JM, Koenekoop R: Evidence supportive of a functional discrimination between photopic oscillatory potentials as revealed with a cone and rod mediated retinopathies. *Doc Ophthalmol* 1998; 95:35–54.

37. Lachapelle P, Blain L, Quigley MG, Polomeno RC, Molotchnikoff S: The effect of diphenylhydantoin on the electroretinogram. *Doc Ophthalmol* 1990; 73:327–336.

38. Lachapelle P, Little JM, Polomeno RC: The photopic electroretinogram in congenital stationary night blindness with myopia. *Invest Ophthalmol Vis Sci* 1983; 24:442–450.

39. Lachapelle P, Little JM, Roy MS: The electroretinogram in Stargardt's disease and fundus flavimaculatus. *Doc Ophthalmol* 1990; 73:395–404.

40. Lachapelle P, Molotchnikoff S: Components of the electroretinogram: A reappraisal. *Doc Ophthalmol* 1986; 63:337–348.

41. Lachapelle P, Rufiange M, Dembinska O: A physiological basis for definition of the ISCEV ERG standard flash (SF) based on the photopic hill. *Doc Ophthalmol* 2001; 102:157–162.

42. Marmor M, Zrenner E: Standard for clinical electroretinography. *Doc Ophthalmol* 1999; 97:143–156. (Consult also the current update found at the ISCEV Website at www.iscev.org.)

43. Matthews GP, Crane WG, Sandberg MA: Effects of 2-amino-4-phosphonobutyric acid (APB) and glycine on the oscillatory potentials of the rat electroretinogram. *Exp Eye Res* 1989; 49:777–787.

44. Miller RF, Dowling JE: Intracellular responses of the Müller (glial) cells of the mudpuppy retina: Their relationship to the b-wave of the electroretinogram. *J Neurophysiol* 1970; 33:323–341.

45. Miyake Y, Shiroyama N, Horiguchi M, Ota I: Asymmetry of focal ERG in human macular region. *Invest Ophthalmol Vis Sci* 1989; 30:1743–1749.

46. Miyake Y, Shiroyama N, Ota I, Horiguchi M: Oscillatory potentials in electroretinograms of the human macular region. *Invest Ophthalmol Vis Sci* 1988; 29:1631–1635.

47. Molotchnikoff S, Lachapelle P, Casanova C: Optic nerve blockade influences the retinal responses to flash in rabbits. *Vision Res* 1989; 29:957–963.

48. Ogden TE: The oscillatory waves of the primate electroretinogram. *Vision Res* 1973; 13:1059–1074.

49. Onozu H, Yamamoto S: Oscillatory potentials of multifocal electroretinogram in diabetic retinopathy. *Doc Ophthalmol* 2003; 106:32–332.

50. Peachey NS, Alexander KR, Derlacki DJ, Bobak P, Fishman GA: Effects of light adaptation on the response characteristics of human oscillatory potentials. *Electroencephalogr Clin Neurophysiol* 1991; 78:27–34.

51. Peachey NS, Alexander KR, Fishman GA: Rod and cone system contributions to oscillatory potentials: An explanation for the conditioning flash effect. *Vision Res* 1987; 27:859–866.

52. Rousseau S, Lachapelle P: The electroretinogram recorded at the onset of dark-adaptation: Understanding the origin of the scotopic oscillatory potentials. *Doc Ophthalmol* 1999; 99:135–150.

53. Rousseau S, Lachapelle P: Transient enhancing of cone electroretinograms following exposure to brighter photopic backgrounds: A new light adaptation effect. *Vision Res* 2000; 40:1013–1018.

54. Rufiange M, Champoux F, Dumont M, Lachapelle P: Spectral sensitivity of the photopic luminance-response function in humans. *Invest Ophthalmol Vis Sci* 2000; 41(suppl):S498.

55. Shirao Y, Kawasaki K: Electrical responses from diabetic retina. *Prog Retin Eye Res* 1998; 17:59–78.

56. Tremblay F, Lam SR: Distinct electroretinographic oscillatory potential generators as revealed by field distribution. *Doc Ophthalmol* 1993; 84:279–289.

57. Tremblay F, Laroche RG, De Becker I: The electroretinographic diagnosis of the incomplete form of congenital stationary night blindness. *Vision Res* 1995; 35:2383–2393.

58. Tsuchida Y, Kawasaki K, Fujimura K, Jacobson JH: Isolation of faster components in the electroretinogram and visual evoked responses in man. *Am J Ophthalmol* 1973; 75:846–852.

59. van der Torren K, Groeneweg G, van Lith G: Measuring oscillatory potentials: Fourier analysis. *Doc Ophthalmol* 1988; 69:153–159.

60. Wachtmeister L: Oscillatory potentials in the retina: What do they reveal? *Prog Retin Eye Res* 1998; 17:485–521.

61. Wachtmeister L, Dowling JE: The oscillatory potentials of the mudpuppy retina. *Invest Ophthalmol Vis Sci* 1978; 17:1176–1188.

62. Wachtmeister L, el Azazi M: The oscillatory potentials of the electroretinogram in patients with unilateral optic atrophy. *Ophthalmologica* 1985; 191:39–50.

63. Weleber RG, Eisner A: Retinal function and physiological studies, in Newsome DA (ed): *Retinal Dystrophies and Degeneration.* New York, Raven Press, 1988, pp 21–69.

64. Wu S, Sutter EE: A topographic study of oscillatory potentials in man. *Vis Neurosci* 1995; 12:1013–1025.

65. Yonemura D, Masuda Y, Hatta M: The oscillatory potentials in the electroretinogram. *Jpn J Physiol* 1963; 13:129–137.

44 Flicker Electroretinography

DAVID G. BIRCH

VIRTUALLY ALL CLINICAL electroretinogram (ERG) protocols, including that endorsed by the International Society for Clinical Electrophysiology of Vision and the National Retinitis Pigmentosa, Inc., utilize a 30-Hz flickering stimulus to elicit an isolated cone response. Because of their low temporal sensitivity, rods are unable to follow frequencies above approximately 15 Hz.[9] Typical flicker responses from a normal subject are shown in figure 44.1A. Vertical spikes indicate each 10-µs flash. Cone b-wave implicit time is the time interval between flash onset and the major cornea-positive peak (horizontal arrow). Peak-to-peak amplitude is measured from the cornea-negative peak to the succeeding cornea-positive peak (vertical arrow). Implicit time and amplitude can vary independently. As shown in figure 44.1B, progressive forms of retinal degeneration such as retinitis pigmentosa typically lead to a substantial delay in cone b-wave implicit time.[3–5] Diseases that affect regional or localized areas of retina typically lead to decreased amplitude without necessarily affecting the cone b-wave implicit time (figure 44.1C).[5,6]

Flickering stimuli and the resulting "steady-state" ERG permit extensive use of analog and digital flickering techniques. As shown in figure 44.1D, many patients with retinitis pigmentosa show no response to flicker with traditional computer-averaging techniques. Band-pass amplification (tuned to the stimulus frequency) or digital filtering can be used to enhance the signal-to-noise ratio of very small signals.[1] When only that portion of the response that is time locked to the stimulus is amplified (figure 44.1E), the noise level drops to approximately 0.1 µV as compared with a noise level of approximately 2.0 µV without band-pass amplification.

The ERG to stimuli flickering at 30 Hz is an important diagnostic indicator, with two protocols in common use. Some laboratories obtain the response following 45 minutes of dark adaptation. The response is obtained with a medium-intensity white stimulus (i.e., Grass setting 4 or 8) to minimize patient discomfort and avoid the irregular behavior of the photostimulator at the highest setting. Since cone responses typically grow in amplitude during the first few minutes of light adaptation,[8] the patient should be pre-exposed to the flickering stimulus before recording the flicker response. The second protocol involves recording the flicker response in the presence of a steady background (typically 10 foot-lamberts [ft-L]) after at least 10 minutes of light adaptation. The two protocols differ primarily in the degree of light adaptation. The time-average retinal illuminance of 30-Hz flicker without a steady background is typically about 2.8 log photopic troland seconds (phot td s). The addition of a steady background of 10 ft-L raises the mean retinal illuminance to 3.4 log phot td s. We compared the two protocols in 10 normal subjects and 33 consecutive patients with retinitis pigmentosa (unpublished observations). In both normals and patients, the addition of a steady background lead to a shortening of cone b-wave implicit time of approximately 4.0 ms over that in the dark (figure 44.2). The degree to which implicit time decreased was not significantly different between normals and patients ($t = .16$, NS). Similarly, the steady background decreased the peak-to-peak amplitude by approximately the same percentage in patients and normals. Thus both protocols should be comparably sensitive in detecting an abnormal flicker response. A practical advantage of the lower background level is that it is more likely to yield a detectable response in patients.

The sensitivity of cone b-wave implicit time to retinal degeneration is evident in figure 44.3. Distributions are shown for 175 normal subjects and 250 patients with retinitis pigmentosa, excluding autosomal dominant individuals, who frequently have normal b-wave implicit times to flicker.[2] Since there is minimal overlap between distributions, 243 of 250 (97%) patients in this sample had significantly ($P < .05$) delayed cone b-wave implicit times to flicker.

Cone b-wave implicit time is delayed in many young patients at a time when the amplitude may be near normal. While much of the delay is undoubtedly due to intrinsic cone abnormalities, at least part of the delay may result from abnormal rod function. Cone b-wave implicit time in normal subjects varies with the state of rod adaptation.[10] It has been suggested that delayed cone b-wave times in retinitis pigmentosa are due, at least in part, to an absence or functional impairment of rods.[7,10] As shown in figure 44.4, there is a significant inverse correlation between cone b-wave implicit time and log rod b-wave amplitude. Among patients with retinitis pigmentosa, the variation in cone loss is not as significant a determinant of cone b-wave implicit time as is the degree of rod loss.[7] These results suggest that progressive rod degeneration leads to the loss of a rod-mediated mechanism that normally acts to shorten cone b-wave implicit time under light adaptation conditions.

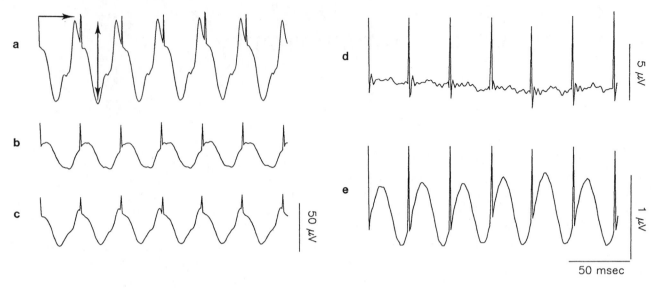

FIGURE 44.1 Flicker responses to 30-Hz stimulation. The spike artifact indicates stimulus flash. A normal subject has a b-wave implicit time of 29 ms (A). The response is reduced in amplitude and delayed in retinitis pigmentosa (B) but reduced with normal timing in presumed histoplasmosis (C). Even with extensive averaging, the response is nondetectable in many patients with retinitis pigmentosa (D). A band-pass amplifier tuned to the stimulus frequency selectively enhances time-locked activity to reveal a small response (E).

Effect of background on flicker parameters

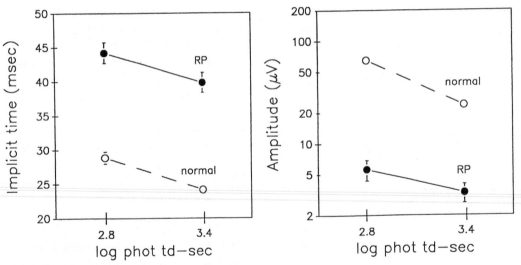

FIGURE 44.2 Cone b-wave implicit time (±1 SE) and cone b-wave amplitude (±1 SE) at two background levels in 10 normal subjects and 33 consecutive patients with retinitis pigmentosa. The lower background level is the time-average retinal illuminance of the 30-Hz white flashes. The higher background level is the mean retinal illuminance of the flicker superimposed on a steady (10 ft-L) background. Both normals and patients show a decrease in implicit time of approximately 4 ms and a decrease in amplitude of approximately 50% at the higher adaptation level.

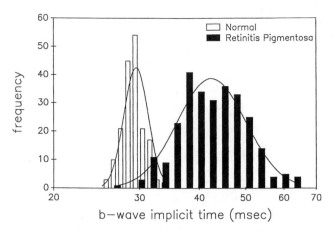

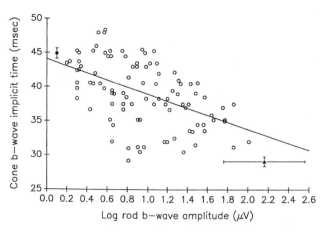

FIGURE 44.3　Cone b-wave implicit time distributions for 30-Hz flicker in 175 normal subjects and 250 patients with retinitis pigmentosa (excluding autosomal-dominant disease). Both distributions are plotted in logarithmic units and are normally distributed.

FIGURE 44.4　Scatter plot (open circles) and linear regression (solid line) for cone b-wave implicit time as a function of log b-wave rod amplitude in 100 patients with retinitis pigmentosa and detectable (>1 μV) rod and cone ERGs. Cone ERGs were elicited with 30-Hz white full-field flashes, and rod ERGs were elicited with single-flash short-wavelength flashes. All responses were computer averaged. The regression line ($r = -0.49$, $P < .001$) is $y = 44.2 - 5.3x$. The solid circle shows the mean b-wave implicit time (± 1 SE) for 109 patients with nondetectable rod responses. The solid triangle shows the mean implicit time (± 1 SE) for 178 normal subjects.

REFERENCES

1. Andréasson SOL, Sandberg MA, Berson EL: Narrowband filtering for monitoring low-amplitude cone electroretinograms in retinitis pigmentosa. *Am J Ophthalmol* 1988; 105:500.
2. Berson EL: Hereditary retinal diseases; classification with the full-field electroretinogram. *Doc Ophthalmol Proc Ser* 1977; 13:149.
3. Berson EL, Gouras P, Gunkel RD, Myrianthropoulis NC: Dominant retinitis pigmentosa with reduced penetrance. *Arch Ophthalmol* 1969; 81:226.
4. Berson EL, Gouras P, Gunkel RD, Myrianthropoulis NC: Rod and cone responses in sex-linked retinitis pigmentosa. *Arch Ophthalmol* 1969; 81:125.
5. Berson EL, Gouras P, Hoff M: Temporal aspects of the electroretinogram. *Arch Ophthalmol* 1969; 81:207.
6. Berson EL, Howard J: Temporal aspects of the electroretinogram in sector retinitis pigmentosa. *Arch Ophthalmol* 1971; 86:653.
7. Birch DG, Sandberg MA: Dependence of cone b-wave implicit time on rod amplitude in retinitis pigmentosa. *Vision Res* 1987; 27: 1105.
8. Gouras P, Mackay CJ, Ivert L, Mittl RN, Neuwirth J, Eggars H: Computer-assisted spectral electroretinography in vitrectomy patients. *Ophthalmol* 1985; 92:83.
9. Hecht S, Schlaer S: Intermittent stimulation by light: V. The relation between intensity and critical frequency for different parts of the spectrum. *J Gen Physiol* 1936; 19: 965.
10. Sandberg MA, Berson EL, Effron MH: Rod-cone interactions in the distal human retina. *Science* 1981; 212:829.

45 Chromatic Recordings of Electroretinograms

KAZUO KAWASAKI, JHOJI TANABE, KENJI WAKABAYASHI, AND YUTAKA SHIRAO

THE ELECTROPHYSIOLOGICAL investigation of chromatic responses is not a routine part of clinical ophthalmology, for better diagnostic methods exist. The interest lies in the information about intraretinal processing that is revealed by such recordings, mostly studied in congenital red-green color deficiency, as reviewed by Armington.[1] Most of the previous publications along this line dealt with the b-wave, flicker electroretinogram (ERG), or early receptor potential (ERP).[6–8,11,13,14,18–20,22,23] The spectral sensitivity of the b-wave and the flicker ERG were reported to be reduced at long wavelength in protans.[6,7] Yokoyama and his coworkers[20,22,23] demonstrated in protans and deutans abnormal spectral response curves of the b-wave and abnormal ERG responses to a mixture of red and green stimuli sinusoidally flickering in counterphase. The b-wave or flicker ERG is not solely indicative of the receptor activity.

Two kinds of electrical responses have been reported as being generated in photoreceptor cells: the early and late receptor potentials.[2,3] The major difference in waveform of the late receptor potential between the cones and rods lies in the off-response (response to a cessation of stimulus light); the off-response is rapid in the cones and slow in the rods.[2,3] (The off-response of blue cones is slow,[20,22,25] but blue cones are not concerned, insofar as we know, with red-green color deficiency.)

In the human ERG the off-response begins with a rapid positive-going deflection (the rapid off-response) at a stimulus intensity above about 6 lux at the retina.[24] The rapid off-response in humans follows flickering stimuli of high frequency (not less than 34 Hz)[24] and is resistant to light adaptation,[24] and the relative spectral sensitivity function curve approximates the psychophysical photopic curve.[10] This ERG rapid off-response is unchanged in congenital stationary night blindness,[9] but no rapid off-responses can be obtained in rod monochromatism.[9] The rapid off-response is preserved in vitro after treatment of the retina with aspartate or glutamate,[24] which is known to abolish the postsynaptic responses of the retina without abolishing the receptor potential. Thus, the rapid off-response is photopic in nature and is useful for an objective examination of the photopic function at the photoreceptor level.

Rapid off-response in protans and deutans

The method used is to employ a monochromatic, 4-Hz square-wave (50-duty cycle) flickering light. The maximum stimulus intensity was 1.0×10^{15} quanta $\cdot$ cm^{-2} $\cdot$ sec^{-1} at each wavelength at the position of the cornea of the eye to be examined. The pupil was fully dilated. Averaged responses to 40 stimuli were measured. Twenty-four protan patients (10 protanopes and 14 protanomalous aged 9 to 22 years with a mean age of 15.3 years) and 23 deutan patients (7 deuteranopes and 16 deuteranomalous aged 9 to 25 years with a mean age of 15.7 years) were studied. All were males except for one protanomalous female. The normal control group consisted of 24 men with ages ranging from 15 to 29 years (mean, 23.5 years).

The inset in figure 45.1A' shows a typical example of the ERG evoked by a monochromatic rectangular stimulus (550 nm) in a normal control subject. The onset of the stimulus light evoked the a-wave, the b-wave, and the oscillatory potential. The termination of the stimulus elicited an upward (positive-going) deflection, which is referred to as the rapid off-response. The relationship between the stimulus intensity and the amplitude of the rapid off-response was plotted at each wavelength of stimulus light. The reciprocal of the stimulus intensity needed to evoke a response of a constant criterion voltage (20 μV), i.e., the sensitivity, was obtained at each wavelength from the graphs depicting the amplitude-intensity relationship. The spectral sensitivity curves thus obtained for the rapid off-response showed a maximum sensitivity around 550 nm in all normal subjects studied and were approximated by the human photopic visibility curve (Commission Internationale de l'Eclairage [CIE] 10) (figure 45.1A).

The peak of the spectral sensitivity curve shifted toward the short wavelength (520 to 530 nm) in protans (figure 45.1B). The peak of the sensitivity curve in deutans was at 550 nm or its vicinity (figure 45.1C), as in normal subjects (figure 45.1A). The shape of the spectral sensitivity curves, however, clearly differed between normals and deutans; the sensitivity at 480 nm was definitely higher than the sensitivity at 620 nm in all normal subjects tested, whereas the

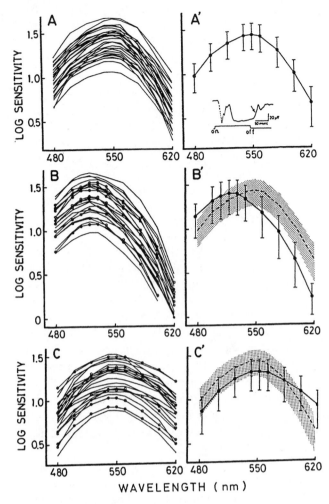

FIGURE 45.1 Spectral sensitivity of the rapid off-response in normal subjects (A and A′), protans (protanopes, protanomals) (B and B′) and deutans (deuteranopes, deuteranomals) (C and C′). The left graphs show sensitivity curves in each individual tested. Curves with small circles indicate protanopes (B) or deuteranopes (C). The remainder of the curves pertain to protanomals (B′) or deuteranomals (C′). Right graphs show means and standard deviations of spectral sensitivity. The dotted curve and shaded area in B′ and C′ indicate the mean and standard deviation in normal subjects, respectively. Averaged waveforms of 40 responses to repetitive monochromatic stimuli of 4 Hz were analyzed in figures 45.1 and 45.3 to 45.6. Ordinates indicate logarithms of the reciprocal of the quantal number of stimulus light to evoke the rapid off-response of the 20-μV criterion amplitude. Sensitivity at 0 log units on the ordinate corresponds to the sensitivity of 1.0×10^{15} quanta·cm^{-2} at the cornea. The inset in A′ illustrates a typical example of an ERG at 550 nm in a normal subject. The arrow indicates the rapid off-response.

tivity of the rapid off-response in normals, protans, and deutans, respectively. As compared with the normal control, in protans the mean of the sensitivity of the rapid off-response was higher at short wavelengths (480, 500 nm) ($P <$ .005) and lower at long wavelengths (560 nm and longer) ($P < .005$). The mean sensitivity in deutans was lower than normal between 480 and 560 nm ($P < .005$) and higher than normal at long wavelengths (620 nm) ($P < .001$) (figure 45.1). Reflection fundus densitometry has demonstrated a decrease or loss of the visual pigment at long wavelengths in protans and at medium wavelengths in deutans.[16,17] The reduction in sensitivity of the rapid off-response at long wavelengths in protans and at medium wavelengths in deutans (figure 45.1) is in agreement with such densitometric results. It is noteworthy that the sensitivity of the rapid off-response is higher than normal at short wavelengths in protans and at long wavelengths in deutans (figure 45.1). In this regard, we should refer to Wald's finding[21] that the psychophysical sensitivity was higher than normal at short wavelengths in protans and at long wavelengths in deutans. Wald[21] hypothesized that the red-absorbing cones lost in protans are replaced mainly by increased numbers of green-absorbing cones and that the green-absorbing cones lost in deutans are replaced mainly by added red-absorbing cones. This hypothesis is consistent with the high sensitivity of the rapid off-response at 480 to 500 nm in protans and at 620 nm in deutans (figure 45.1). Although the spectral characteristics of the rapid off-response differed among normals, protans, and deutans (figure 45.1), the amplitude of the rapid off-response to white stimulus light was not significantly different among these three groups (figure 45.2). This finding is also compatible with Wald's hypothesis mentioned above.

The difference in shape of the spectral sensitivity curve among normals, protans, and deutans can be described in a quantitative manner by the sensitivity ratio at short and long wavelengths. The number of quanta (reciprocal of the sensitivity) in the stimulus light that is required to evoke a rapid off-response of 20 μV was calculated from the amplitude-intensity curve in each subject at 480 and 620 nm. The ratio of the quantal numbers at 620 nm to those at 480 nm (ratio of the sensitivity at 480 nm to the sensitivity at 620 nm, S_{480}/S_{620}) is plotted on the ordinate in figure 45.3. This ratio was greater in all protans and smaller in all deutans than in normal control subjects (figure 45.3). It should be emphasized that we are able to differentiate protans and deutans from normals by recording the rapid off-response only at two different wavelengths of stimulus light. This would be a new method of diagnosing protans and deutans in an objective and quantitative manner.

The spectral sensitivity curve and the sensitivity ratio (S_{480}/S_{620}) of the rapid off-response showed no significant difference between protanopic and protanomalous or between

sensitivities at 480 and 620 nm were nearly equal in deutans (figures 45.1A and 45.1C). This difference is clearly illustrated in figure 45.3, which will be referred to in detail later.

The right-hand graphs (A′, B′, and C′) in figure 45.1 show the mean and the standard deviation of the spectral sensi-

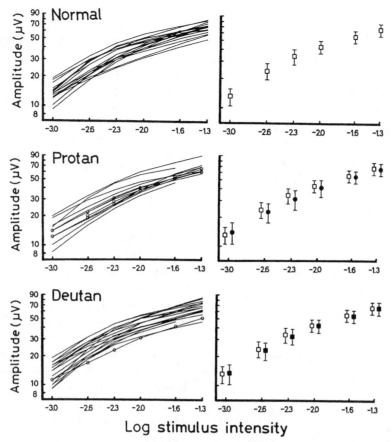

FIGURE 45.2 Amplitude of the rapid off-response in 20 normal subjects (10- to 27-year-old males, upper graph), in 13 protans (12- to 22-year-old males, middle graph), and in 19 deutans (12- to 22-year-old males, lower graph) as a function of the intensity of white stimulus light. Zero log unit of stimulus intensity was 1.0×10^5 lux at the cornea. Left graphs are amplitude-intensity curves of indi-

vidual subjects. Right graphs are means and standard deviations. Curves with open circles in the left graphs indicate dichromats. The rest of the curves indicate abnormal trichromats. Open squares in the right graphs indicate the mean amplitude in normal subjects. Solid circles and solid squares indicate the mean amplitudes in protans and deutans, respectively.

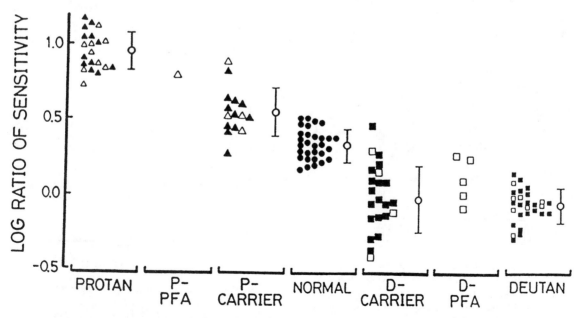

FIGURE 45.3 Log ratio of sensitivity of the rapid off-response at 480 nm to its sensitivity at 620 nm in protans, Pigmentfarbenamblyopie of the protan type (P-PFA), protan carriers (P-carrier), normal control subjects, deutan carriers (D-carrier), Pigmentfarbenamblyopie of the deutan type (D-PFA), and deutans. Sensitivity was defined here as the reciprocal of the quantal number of stimulus light that is needed to evoke a rapid off-response of 20-μV criterion amplitude. Open and solid triangles in protans

indicate protanopes and protanomals, respectively. Open and solid squares in deutans indicate deuteranopes and deuteranomals, respectively. Open and solid triangles in protan carriers indicate mothers of protanopes and those of protanomals, respectively. Open and solid squares in deutan carriers indicate mothers of deuteranopes and those deuteranomals, respectively. Open circles and vertical bars indicate the mean and standard deviation in figures 45.3, 45.4, and 45.7 to 45.9, respectively.

deuteranopic and deuteranomalous patients (figures 45.1 and 45.3). This result is not unexpected because Pokorny and Smith[15] demonstrated that dichromats diagnosed by anomaloscopy with a small test field show trichromacy by anomaloscopy with a large test field. The stimulus field used in the present study subtended about 60 degrees in visual angle. Therefore, it would be reasonable that no difference in the rapid off-response was found between dichromats and anomalous trichromats in the present study using a large stimulus field.

Majima[12] classified red-green color deficiency into four grades by routine psychophysical examinations: (1) very mild, (2) mild, (3) moderate, and (4) strong. We studied the ratio of the sensitivity of the rapid off-response at 500 nm to its sensitivity at 600 nm (S_{500}/S_{600}) in protans and deutans at each of the four grades described above. The sensitivity ratio did not differ among the four grades both in protans and deutans (figure 45.4). It should be emphasized that the sensitivity ratio of the rapid off-response is definitely abnormal even in protans or deutans with minimal anomaly detected by routine psychophysical examinations.

Rapid off-response in genetic carriers

ERG sensitivity was studied in only one protan carrier in the literature, the sensitivity to 32 Hz flickering stimuli being low at long wavelengths in a mother of protanopes.[6] We investigated the rapid off-response in mothers of protans (protan carriers) and in mothers of deutans (deutan carriers). The mean sensitivity curve of the rapid off-response in protan carriers was lower than normal at long wavelengths ($P < .05$ at 560 and 580 nm, $P < .01$ at 600 nm, $P < .001$ at 620 nm) and deviated upward toward the sensitivity curve of protans at the wavelengths of 480 to 520 nm. The mean sensitivity curve in deutan carriers was higher than normal at long wavelengths ($P < .005$ at 600 nm, $P < .001$ at 620 nm) and deviated downward toward the curve in deutans at 560 nm and shorter wavelengths. In brief, the mean sensitivity curve in protan carriers was situated between the mean sensitivity curves of normals and protans. The mean sensitivity curve in deutan carriers was between the mean sensitivity curves of normals and deutans (figures 45.5 and 45.6). The mean of the ratio S_{480}/S_{620} was larger in protan carriers than in normals ($P < .001$) (see figure 45.3). The ratios were not significantly different between carriers of protanopes and those of protanomals or between carriers of deuteranopes and those of deuteranomals (see figure 45.3).

We studied the rapid off-response in a mother who had three sons; two of them were deutans, and one was a protan. The ratio of the sensitivity of the rapid off-response at 480 nm to its sensitivity at 620 nm (S_{480}/S_{620}) in these sons was typical for their diagnosis: large in the protan and small in the deutans. Their mother, who was most likely a compound heterozygote, showed normal color discrimination by routine examinations. The ratio of the sensitivity of the rapid off-response at the two different wavelengths (S_{480}/S_{620})

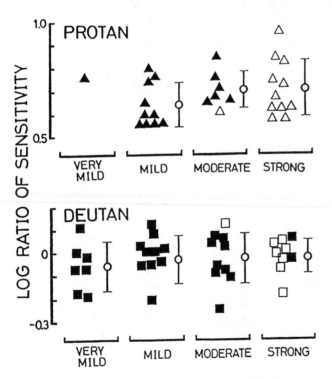

FIGURE 45.4 Log ratio of the sensitivity of the rapid off-response at 500 nm to its sensitivity at 600 nm in protans (upper graph) and in deutans (lower graph). Protans and deutans were classified into four grades (very mild, mild, moderate, strong) by Majima's criterion.[12] Open and solid symbols indicate protanopes and protanomals in the upper graph and deuteranopes and deuteranomals in the lower graph, respectively. The criterion amplitude was 20 μV in figures 45.4 to 45.6.

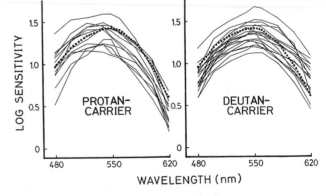

FIGURE 45.5 Spectral sensitivity of the rapid off-response in protan carriers (mothers of protans) aged 30 to 46 years with a mean age of 40.4 years) and in deutan carriers (mothers of deutans) aged 32 to 50 years with a mean age of 39.7 years. All of these mothers showed no anomaloscopic abnormality. Dotted curves indicate the mean sensitivity in normal control subjects.

was also within the normal range in this mother ($\log S_{480}/S_{620}$ was 0.39).

Early receptor potential in protan and deutan patients

A study of the ERP in congenital color deficiency would be pertinent because the ERP is closely related to photo-bleaching of visual pigments of the photoreceptors,[2,3,5] particularly of cones in humans.[4] We recorded the ERP in 27 eyes of 26 normal male subjects aged 19 to 24 years with a mean age of 20.9 years in response to monochromatic stimuli having equal quanta. The method of recording the ERP was previously described.[19] Briefly, the stimulus source was a 1.2×10^3-J xenon discharge tube. Interference filters (460 to 600 nm, half-width of 26 to 38 nm) and neutral-density filters were placed in the light path to obtain a mono-chromatic flash having equal numbers of quanta (1.08×10^{15} quanta·cm^{-2} per flash at the cornea). The spectral response curve (amplitude versus wavelength) showed the maximum amplitude of the R_2 at 520 to 540 nm in all these normal subjects. The mean spectral sensitivity curve of the R_2 closely followed a curve composed of the summation of the photopic and scotopic psychophysical curves at a ratio of $3:2$ (figure 45.7). The stimulus flash illuminated the posterior area of the ocular fundus, measuring approximately 60 degrees in the visual angle. The number of rods within this posterior fundus surpasses that of cones within the same retinal area (approximately $24:1$). In humans, the R_2 from a single cone is assumed to be much larger than the R_2 from a single rod, which agrees with this result.

Lapp and Tanabe[11] demonstrated a low sensitivity of R_2 at long wavelengths in protanomalous subjects. Okamoto et al.[13] reported that the mean amplitude of the R_2 evoked by a white flash was smaller than normal in protans and deutans. Tamai et al.[18] reported that the ERP evoked by a colored flash in protanopes was abnormal. We studied the ERP in 10 protans (5 protanopes and 4 protanomals aged 9 to 18 years with a mean age of 14.9 years) and 26 deutans (6 deuteranopes and 20 deuteranomals aged 10 to 20 years). Anomaloscopic examination could not be performed in one protan patient because of his lack of cooperation. The mean R_2 amplitude was smaller at long wavelengths (580 and 600 nm) in protans ($P < .01$) and at 520 nm in deutans ($P < .05$) as compared with the mean amplitude in normal subjects (figure 45.8). These results are consistent with the spectral sensitivity of the rapid off-response in protans and deutans (see figure 45.1). Neither group differed significantly

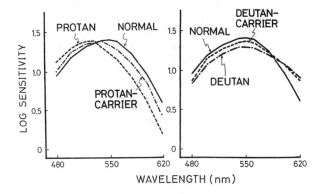

FIGURE 45.6 Mean sensitivity of the rapid off-response in protans, protan carriers (left graph), deutans, and deutan carriers (right graph). Solid curves pertain to normal control subjects.

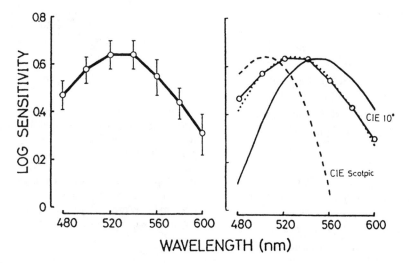

FIGURE 45.7 Left, mean and standard deviation of the spectral sensitivity curve of the ERP (R_2) in 54 eyes of normal subjects (criterion amplitude, 10 μV). Right, approximation of the spectral sensitivity curve between the ERP (solid curve with circles, from the left graph) and psychophysical measurement. The dotted curve was composed of the summation of the photopic (solid curve) and scotopic (dashed curve) psychophysical curves in the ratio of $3:2$. The ordinate indicates log relative sensitivity in arbitrary units. The top of each curve was at the same scale on the ordinate.

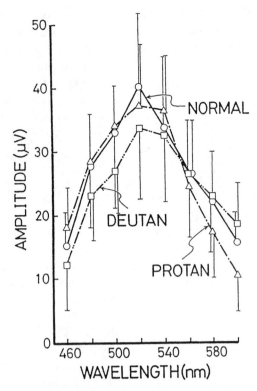

FIGURE 45.8   Mean and standard deviation of the amplitude of the ERP (R_2) evoked by monochromatic stimuli having equal quanta (1.08×10^{15} quanta·cm^{-2} per flash) in 18 normal (circles), 15 protan (triangles), and 31 deutan (squares) subjects.

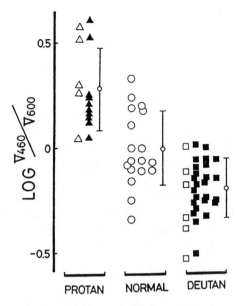

FIGURE 45.9   Log ratio of the ERP (R_2) amplitude at 460 nm to the amplitude at 600 nm. Open triangles and squares indicate dichromats. Solid triangles and squares indicate abnormal trichromats.

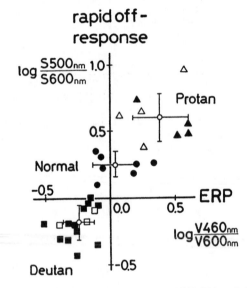

FIGURE 45.10   Relationship between the ERP (R_2) and the rapid off-response. The log ratio of the ERP (R_2) amplitudes at 460 nm to that at 600 nm (abscissa) is plotted against the log ratio to the sensitivity (criterion amplitude, 20 µV) of the rapid off-response at 500 nm to that at 600 nm (ordinate). Solid circles indicate normal subjects. Open and solid triangles indicate protanopes and protanomals, respectively. Open and solid squares indicate deuteranopes and deu-teranomals, respectively. Open circles and crosses indicate the mean and standard deviation in normal, protan, and deutan groups.

from normal controls at short wavelengths. Since the rods as well as cones participated in producing the ERP in our stimulus parameters, possible abnormalities of the ERP at short wavelengths would be masked by the response from the rods.

The ratio of the R_2 amplitude at 460 nm to its amplitude at 600 nm (V_{460}/V_{600}) was larger in all protans than in all deutans thus far tested (figure 45.9). Therefore, the protan and deutan groups were differentiated by this ratio. This indicates that protans and deutans differ from each other at the level of visual pigments. This ratio (V_{460}/V_{600}) is useful for the differentiation of protans and deutans in an objective manner at the level of the visual pigments in the photoreceptor cells.

No significant difference in the R_2 amplitude or the ratio V_{460}/V_{600} was found between protanopes and protanomalous or between deuteranopes and deuteranomal persons. This may be accounted for by the large stimulus field (approximately 60 degrees in the visual angle) in our ERG recordings, as already discussed in this chapter.

After recording the ERP, the eye was dark adapted for 1 hour. The rapid off-response was then recorded in the same subjects (7 normals, 8 protans, 15 deutans) to study the relationship between the ERP and the rapid off-response. The

log ratio of the R_2 amplitude at 460 nm to its amplitude at 600 nm (V_{460}/V_{600}) was significantly correlated with the log ratio of the sensitivity of the rapid off-response at 500 nm to its sensitivity at 600 nm (correlation coefficient, 0.823; $P < .001$) (figure 45.10). Thus, the present study electrophysiologically demonstrates that the anomaly in congenital red-green color deficiency is initiated in the outer segment of the photoreceptor cells.

REFERENCES

1. Armington JC: *The Electroretinogram*. New York, Academic Press, Inc, 1974.
2. Brown KT: The electroretinogram. Its components and their origins. *Vision Res* 1968; 8:633–677.
3. Brown KT, Watanabe K, Murakami M: The early and late receptor potentials of monkey cones and rods. *Cold Spring Harb Symp Quant Biol* 1965; 30:457–482.
4. Carr RE, Siegel IM: Action spectrum of the human early receptor potential. *Nature* 1970; 225:88–89.
5. Cone RA: The early receptor potential of the vertebrate retina. *Nature* 1964; 204:736–739.
6. Copenbaver RM, Gunkel RD: The spectral sensitivity of color-defective subjects determined by electroretinography. *Arch Ophthalmol* 1959; 62:55–68.
7. Dodt E, Copenhaver RM, Gunkel RD: Photopischer Dominator und Farbkomponenten im menschlichen Elektroretinogramm. *Pflugers Arch Gesamte Physiol* 1958; 267:497–507.
8. François J, Verriest G, De Rouck A: New electroretinographic findings obtained in congenital forms of dyschromatopsia. *Br J Ophthalmol* 1960; 44:430–435.
9. Kawasaki K, Tsuchida Y, Jacobson JH: Positive and negative deflections in the off-response of the electroretinogram in man. *Am J Ophthalmol* 1971; 72:367–375.
10. Kawasaki K, Yonemura D, Nakazato H, Kawaguchi I: Abnormal spectral sensitivity of the electroretinographic off-response in protanopia and protanomalia. *Doc Ophthalmol* 1982; 53:51–60.
11. Lapp ER, Tanabe J: Das frühe Rezeptorpotential (ERP): Aktionsspektren bei normal farbtüchtigen und Farbblinden. *Ber Dtsch Ophthalmol Ges* 1981; 78:727–731.
12. Majima A: Diagnostic criteria of defective color vision, The 3rd report. Majima's classification for social adaptability. *Folia Ophthalmol Jpn* 1972; 23:170–175.
13. Okamoto M, Okajima O, Tanino T: The early receptor potential in human eyes: II. ERP in dichromats. *Acta Soc Opthalmol Jpn* 1981; 85:296–299.
14. Padmos P, van Norren D: Cone spectral sensitivity and chromatic adaptation as revealed by human flicker-electroretinography. *Vision Res* 1971; 11:27–42.
15. Pokorny J, Smith VC: New observations concerning red-green color defects. *Color Res Appl* 1982; 7:159–164.
16. Rushton WA II: A cone pigment in the protanope. *J Physiol* 1963; 168:345–359.
17. Rushton WA II: A foveal pigment in the deuteranope. *J Physiol* 1965; 176:24–37.
18. Tamai A, Wada H, Kitagawa K, Wariishi S, Wariishi V, Sasaki T, Takemura M, Ueno H: Monochromatic flash ERP (early receptor potential) in dichromats. Presented at the 23rd Symposium of the International Society of Clinical Electrophysiology Vision, Mie, Japan, May 22, 1985.
19. Tanabe J, Yonemura D, Kawasaki K, Fujii S, Sakai N: Spectral sensitivity of the early receptor potential in man. *Acta Soc Ophthalmol Jpn* 1983; 87:1017–1021.
20. Uji Y: Spectral characteristics of electroretinography in congenital red-green color blindness. *Jpn J Ophthalmol* 1987; 31:61–80.
21. Wald G: Defective color vision and its inheritance. *Proc Natl Acad Sci U S A* 1966; 55:1347–1363.
22. Yokoyama M: Blue sensation in eye disease. *Jpn J Clin Ophthalmol* 1979; 33:111–125.
23. Yokoyama M, Yoshida T, Ui K: Spectral responses in the human electroretinogram and their clinical significance. *Jpn J Ophthalmol* 1973; 17:113–124.
24. Yonemura D, Kawasaki K: New approaches to ophthalmic electrodiagnosis by retinal oscillatory potential, drug-induced responses from retinal pigment epithelium and cone potential. *Doc Ophthalmol* 1979; 48:163–222.
25. Zrenner E, Gouras P: Blue sensitive cones of the cat produce a rodlike electroretinogram. *Invest Ophthalmol Vis Sci* 1979; 18:1076–1081.

46 Adaptation Effects on the Electroretinogram

PETER GOURAS AND CYNTHIA MACKAY

STUDYING VISUAL adaptation of the human retina by using the electroretinogram (ERG) provides insights into the function of the photoreceptors and probably the retinal pigment epithelium, both likely candidates for containing the genetic defect in a large variety of different hereditary retinal degenerations. Visual adaptation depends on a number of different processes working together. They can be broadly grouped into those involving the transduction machinery of the photoreceptor and those involving regeneration of the photopigment. The former has been called the "neural" and the latter the "photochemical" components of adaptation.[7,8]

Growth of the cone electroretinogram during light adaptation

The cone ERG increases gradually in amplitude during light adaptation an average of 75% over a period of 20 minutes. This increase is initially fast and later slower so that after 20 minutes little further change is apparent. This increase involves both the a- and b-wave components of the ERG, and both waves follow a similar time course. This involvement of the a-wave strongly suggests that the photoreceptors are responsible for the effect. The action spectrum for the effects of light adaptation on the ERG parallels the cone action spectrum. The phenomenon is greatest at suprathreshold levels of stimulation and fails to occur at threshold levels, which suggests a significant change in the relationship between light absorbed and response produced during the course of light adaptation, i.e., the input/output function. An increase in the intensity of the adapting light shortens the time course of the ERG, measured as b-wave implicit time, but this occurs almost immediately, and the implicit time then remains constant during the subsequent slow increase in response amplitude. The stronger the adapting light, the smaller the overall ERG amplitude, but the percent growth during light adaptation appears to be the same. This slow increase in amplitude is thought to reflect the redepolarization of the cones after their initial hyperpolarization to the adapting field. It does not resemble light rise of the electro-oculogram.[9]

This is a somewhat surprising effect because psychophysical studies of sensitivity changes during light adaptation indicate that there may be a slight decrease or no change in sensitivity over comparable time periods and certainly no progressive increase in responsiveness.[2,3] However, all these measurements were taken at threshold, and the ERG changes are also nonexistent at threshold but become quite large at suprathreshold levels. Granit and Therman[10] in 1935 indicated that the ERG response to flicker increased during the course of light adaptation. Previous workers have made observations that are in agreement with our observations (see chapter 44). Burian[6] appears to have been the first to have noticed this effect in the single-flash ERG. Armington and Biersdorf[2] examined it quantitatively. They found a relatively small effect that involved only the b-wave and not the a-wave, but they only used a 22-degree field and did not separate cone from rod responses. The introduction of the Ganzfeld test and adapting fields greatly facilitates isolation of the cone ERG and dramatically exposes the large magnitude of this effect. Hood[11] reexamined this flicker effect in the frog retina and concluded that it involved cone adaptation and the a- as well as the b-wave, both of which conclusions are in complete agreement with our own results on the low-frequency, that is, nonflickering, cone ERG. Recently Miyake et al.[12] have used this growth in the cone flicker ERG with light adaptation clinically and discovered an exaggerated growth of this response in an incomplete form of hereditary stationary nyctalopia.

This area of research is important in several respects. First it provides a means of minimizing variability between measurements of the cone ERG obtained by different laboratories or even within the same laboratory. Understanding this nonstationary nature of the light-adapted cone ERG enables one to take measures to control it. Second, the response itself provides a new insight into the physiology of cone adaptation and into certain forms of retinal degenerations.

Effect of background illumination on the cone electroretinogram

Increasing the level of background illumination decreases the amplitude and the implicit time (b-wave) of the cone ERG. There is a monotonic relationship between the strength of the adapting field and the percent reduction of

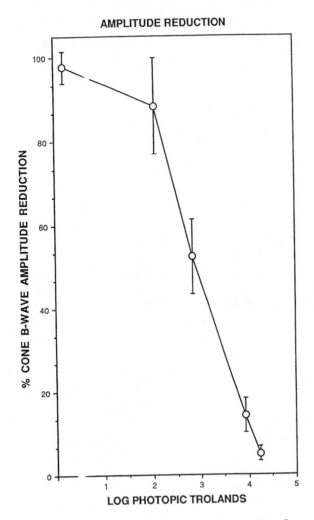

FIGURE 46.1 The relationship between the percentage of cone ERG b-wave amplitude reduction and Ganzfeld fields of different photopic luminances. These results were obtained from 20 normal subjects except for the highest luminance, which represents only three subjects. The vertical lines are the standard deviations. The response is obtained with a red (Wratten 29) filter that produces an identifiable cone ERG at all background fields.

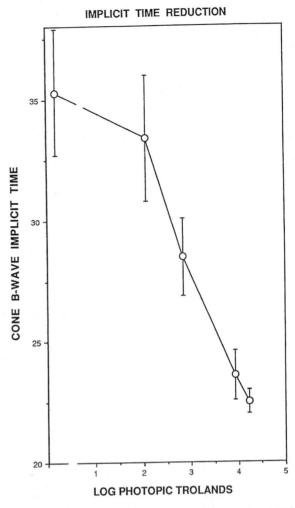

FIGURE 46.2 The relationship between cone b-wave implicit time in milliseconds and Ganzfeld fields of different photopic luminances. Otherwise, everything is the same as figure 46.1.

the ERG and the decrease in implicit time (figures 46.1 and 46.2). We have examined these changes in normal subjects and in subjects with various forms of retinal degeneration by using near-threshold cone stimuli to elicit the ERG, thus eliminating the growth that occurs with light adaptation (just discussed). Table 46.1 shows our current results.

Although the sample is still small, it seems that all retinitis pigmentosa (RP) patients, including Usher's syndrome and Leber's amaurosis, are less affected by the adapting field than are normals. This is true for the reduction both in b-wave amplitude and in b-wave implicit time. The most striking finding is that patients with Leber's amaurosis have implicit times that are unaffected by our brightest adapting lights. This is most remarkable considering that their ERG

amplitudes at high levels of background illumination are similar to many of the other RP patients. Our tentative interpretation of this is that they have a relatively large number of functioning cones but these cones have virtually no photopigment. This is what one might expect to find under such circumstances: normal implicit times in the dark but prolonged ones in the light because the adapting light is being absorbed ineffectively and therefore these cones remain relatively dark-adapted. The implicit times of test flashes on a zero background are larger in other forms of RP than in normal individuals. This implies that other differences occur in these conditions. We have also found that older normal subjects' ERGs are less changed by adapting lights than are those of younger ones. This occurs for both implicit time and amplitude reduction. Again the implicit times of older normals are longer than younger normals even in the dark. Again this implies that another factor than cone pigment density alone may be operating here to produce these changes, perhaps media transparency.

TABLE 46.1

Results of background illumination on normal subjects and those with various forms of retinal degeneration

Subjects	No.*	Dark %B	ms	Log Photopic Trolands 1.7 %B	ms	2.8 %B	ms	4.1 %B	ms
Normals <40 years	11	98	34	87	32	51	28	13	23
Normals >40 years	9	97	37	90	35	54	29	15	24
RP simplex	7	97	43	85	39	76	38	37	33
RP dominant	5	97	48	93	46	70	41	27	35
Cone/rod	2	93	41	97	40	82	38	19	31
Leber's amaurosis	3	92	35	95	35	91	35	73	35
Usher's syndrome	1	87	37	74	43	100	35	74	27

*No. = number of subjects; %B = percent maximum b-wave amplitude; ms = implicit time; RP = retinitis pigmentosa.

Using the Ganzfeld adapting field as the independent variable and leaving the deep red stimulus flash constant provide a new dimension to studying the electrophysiology of retinal disease: it can be examined independently of absolute ERG amplitude. The amplitude of the ERG to a first approximation reflects the number of functioning photoreceptors and diminishes with the progression of the disease. The change in amplitude and implicit time that is produced by light adaptation is presumably independent of the number of photoreceptors, depending on the ability of each photoreceptor itself to adapt. Therefore early and advanced forms of degeneration become more comparable. These changes reflect unique physiological aspects of the retina that can now be studied. It is very conceivable that the percent reduction in b-wave amplitude varies independently of the reduction in implicit time so that some degenerations may be distinguishable by comparing these two parameters. For example, the one case of Usher's syndrome we have now studied (table 46.1) shows a very slight reduction in response amplitude that is comparable to subjects with Leber's amaurosis, but with Usher's syndrome the patient has a significant reduction in his implicit time that none of the patient with Leber's amaurosis have. Larger sampling of these and other forms of RP may more clearly demonstrate whether this new method can distinguish different forms of RP by differences in the way the cone photoreceptor light-adapts.

Dark adaptation of the cone electroretinogram

It is necessary to understand prior light adaptation before beginning to examine what would happen in the dark. For example, if RP cones are not absorbing as well as normal cones, then it would be misleading to measure dark adaptation following exposure to the same physical adapting light. Such a light might not adapt RP cones as much as normal cones, and their recovery might occur more rapidly than normal. Such a result has in fact been reported.[4] Other authors[1,5] have reported that some RP patients adapt more

slowly than normal. These observations were made on rod rather than cone adaptation, however, but the cones might also dark-adapt slowly.

Our own attempts to examine cone ERG dark adaptation were influenced by reports[13] that there was a slow rod influence that increased the amplitude of the dark-adapting cone ERG, a sort of rod/cone inhibition that was turning off. We now have repeatedly studied the dark-adapting cone ERG by using a deep red flash, and we do not find any slow increase in amplitude that follows the time course of rhodopsin regeneration. If, however, we use a stimulus that also affects the rods, we do see a gradual increase in amplitude that parallels the slower adaptation of the rods. We have concluded that dark adaptation of the cone ERG does not result in a change in amplitude after the first few minutes when using 10^4 photopic trolands of prior Ganzfeld light adaptation. The major change in the cone ERG occurs within the first 2 minutes of dark adaptation. Following our strongest Ganzfeld light-adapting field (17,000 photopic trolands), the cone b-wave of both a normal and an RP simplex subject increases rapidly during the first 100 seconds in the dark, with a slight suggestion of an "overshoot." The same relative amplitude intensity relationship and time course holds for both, although the RP response is only $\frac{1}{10}$ of the normal amplitude. With this adapting light (11,000 photopic trolands) we are mainly studying neural rather than photochemical adaptation.

Dark adaptation of the rod electroretinogram

Dark adaptation of the rod ERG is a slow process, and because of this, rod adaptation has seldom been examined clinically by means of the ERG.

Figure 46.3 shows the time course of adaptation of the rod ERG in a rhesus macaque following a 5-minute exposure to 7,000 photopic trolands. Results are shown for two different test lights, both blue, but one is $\frac{1}{10}$ the strength of the other. The greatest changes occur within the first 10 to 15 minutes, especially with the brighter light. The time

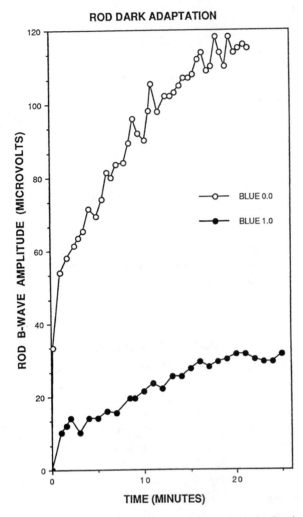

ROD DARK ADAPTATION

FIGURE 46.3 The change in rod b-wave amplitude in the dark after exposure to a Ganzfeld field of 500 photopic trolands. The test light is blue (Wratten 98), of two different intensities (maximum and $^1/_{10}$ of this), 10 µs in duration, and presented every second.

We have been determining the time that it takes for the response obtained at 1 minute to double in amplitude. This doubling time is about 10 minutes in normal subjects. This strategy has the advantage of limiting the study of rod dark adaptation to a more reasonable amount of time, and it leads to a number that reflects the kinetics of rod dark adaptation.

ACKNOWLEDGMENTS This research supported by NIH grant EY 04138 and an RP Center grant from The Retinitis Pigmentosa Foundation Fighting Blindness.

REFERENCES

1. Alexander KR, Fishman GA: Prolonged dark adaptation in patients with retinitis pigmentosa. *Br J Ophthalmol* 1984; 68:561–569.
2. Armington JC, Biersdorf WR: Long term light adaptation of the human electroretinogram. *J Comp Physiol Psychol* 1958; 51:1–5.
3. Baker HD: The course of foveal light adaptation measured by the threshold intensity increment. *J Opt Soc Am* 1949; 39:172–179.
4. Berson EL, Goldstein EB: Recovery of the human early receptor potential during dark adaptation in hereditary retinal disease. *Vision Res* 1970; 10:219–226.
5. Berson EL, Gouras P, Gunkel RD: Rod responses in retinitis pigmentosa, dominantly inherited. *Arch Ophthalmol* 1968; 80:58–67.
6. Burian H: Electric responses of the human visual system. *Arch Ophthalmol* 1954; 51:509.
7. Dowling JE: Neural and photochemical mechanisms of visual adaptation in the rat. *J Gen Physiol* 1963; 46:459–474.
8. Dowling JE, Ripps H: Adaptation in skate photoreceptors. *J Gen Physiol* 1972; 60:698–719.
9. Gouras P, MacKay CJ: Growth in amplitude of the human electroretinogram with light adaptation. *Invest Ophthalmol Vis Sci* 1989; 30:625–630.
10. Granit R, Therman PO: Excitation and inhibition in the retina and in the optic nerve. *J Physiol (Lond)* 1935; 83:359.
11. Hood DC: Adaptational changes in the cone system of the isolated frog retina. *Vision Res* 1972; 12:875.
12. Miyake Y, Hariguchi M, Ora I, Shiroyama N: Characteristic ERG flicker anomaly in incomplete congenital stationary night blindness. *Invest Ophthalmol Vis Sci* 1987; 28:1816–1823.
13. Sandberg MA, Berson EL, Effron MH: Rod cone interactions in the distal human retina. *Science* 1981; 212:829–831.

course at which the dark-adapted response is approached seems similar for both tests light, which implies that the brighter light is not itself producing any significant degree of light adaptation.

47 Clinical Electrophysiological and Psychophysical Investigations into Color Defects

GEOFFREY B. ARDEN AND THOMAS BERNINGER

THE HISTORY OF COLOR vision is closely linked to the Greeks' view of vision. In his late works (about 360 B.C.), Plato explained vision as a combined action of light from inside the eye and light from outside.[95] Thus, vision was for Plato a combination (*synaugeia*) of "outside" and "inside" light. Plato had the idea of a corpuscular emanation of light. Plato's theory can be abstractly explained as a close connection between the sensory organ (the eye) and the object. More than 2000 years later, Goethe, who was also very interested in color vision, wrote a poem based on Plato's theory:[41]

If the eye were not similar to the sun
It could not view the sun

Plato's theory is based on black, white, red and a quality best translated as "dazzling" or "sheen" (το λαμπρον), from which he believed all colors could be made. If you try to copy his mixtures, you will produce a result that is less multicolored than specified by Plato. Plato had most likely foreseen this and stated, "Who experiments in such a way, misjudges the difference between human and divine nature" and "to mix many into one and one back into many: for that only God has the wisdom. . . ."[95] We can perhaps see in that sentence a foreshadowing of Newton's realization that light exhibits many rays. But if we examine Plato's whole work, it becomes apparent that Plato believed that it is not the task of humans to examine nature and that no human will ever be able to understand nature. Aristotle[3] strongly opposed Plato's attitude. For him, research into nature was very important. Aristotle defined color as the passive reception by the eye of an action originating in the object viewed. Thus, we can see Aristotle as the originator of scientific optics. Examining nature had for Aristotle and his successors the same value as thinking about God and the sky and was an abstract philosophy similar to discussion about the human soul. Aristotle mentions color when he speaks about the analysis of sensory perceptions. For him, the color on the surface of objects is an actual object of the sensory perception. He stated, "What can be seen in light is color." Furthermore, Aristotle points to the white sun, which seems red

if seen through the fog and smoke; thus, he addresses a feature that more than 2000 years later became for Goethe the elemental phenomenon of his "Farbenlehre."[41]

Two thousand years after Aristotle, Newton experimented with the production and optimization of optical glasses. While doing this, he observed colored phenomena. These observations were for him the start of a research project about color that finally led to the *experimentum cruces*. On February 6, 1672, Newton wrote a letter to the Royal Society in London explaining his theories about light and color.[91] He wrote, "Light consists of Rays differently refrangible. Colors are not qualifications of light, derived by refraction, or reflections of natural bodies (as generally believed), but original and cognate properties, which in divers rays are diverse." His final point was "The color of natural bodies only shows the ability to light of a special ray more than others." For Newton, white light in reality was the "most surprising and wonderful composition." Further, he wrote that "white light is the usual color of light. For light is a confused aggregate of rays induced with all sorts of colors, as they are promiscuously darted from various parts of luminous bodies." So "pure" white light, was an unordered mixture of colored rays! This epochal scientific approach was an enormous reversal of the direct sensory experiences. More than 100 years later, Goethe and Schopenhauer could not accept such ideas.[62,118]

The developing of the physiological aspect of color vision: Schopenhauer's theory of color vision in comparison to Goethe's and Newton's theory

Schopenhauer (1788–1860), the philosopher of "Pessimism," was born in Danzig. He studied science and philosophy in Göttingen and Berlin. Between 1813 and 1814, Schopenhauer spent much time with Goethe (1749–1835), who introduced him to his color theory, which Goethe regarded as his most important research. It is reported that even on the day of his death, Goethe planned a color experiment with his daughter-in-law. Schopenhauer's color theory was based on Goethe's work. He also opposed the theories of Newton. To Goethe's displeasure, Schopenhauer's color theory differs in substantial points from Goethe's. Schopenhauer wrote to Goethe, "I am absolutely convinced that I developed the first true theory about color vision, the first in the history of science. If I compare my theory with yours, then yours represents the pyramid and mine the apex of the pyramid." Despite this—for Schopenhauer, a quite obliging statement—Goethe refused to write a preface to Schopenhauer's work *On Vision and Color*, which was published 1816.

Schopenhauer's first contribution corresponded to the part of Goethe's color theory that he described in his chapter about the "physiological colors." Goethe explained in detail how an eye, which is adapted to a color for some time, afterward recognizes an afterimage with a complementary color. Goethe (and Schopenhauer as well) identified three pairs of complementary colors: red-green, orange-blue, and yellow-blue. With these colors, Goethe arranged a color ring on which the complementary colors were just opposite each other.

On the other hand, Schopenhauer did not agree with the second point of Goethe's color theory. Goethe regarded color as an objective reality with the exceptions of the "physiological colors." By contrast, Schopenhauer regarded color not only as a product of the stimulated retina, but also as containing a subjective factor. Color vision thus became a physiological problem. To explain his theories, Schopenhauer turned back to the color theory of Aristotle. Each color was regarded as a mathematically calculable balance between light and darkness. Depending on the mixture of light and darkness, either gray or—with the correct choice of mixture—different colors developed. This theory survived 2000 years and until 1613, only approximately 50 years before Newton's discoveries, was spread by the scholar Aguilonius. Schopenhauer arranged the colors in such a way that the sum of the complementary colors resulted in 1. His theory was that the entire maximal activity of the retina should result in the color impression white. The part of the retina, however, that was not stimulated by a color should produce an afterimage with a complementary color. He proposed that the retina tries to reach this result by replacing the missing part. Color and complementary color produce white and are therefore in the modern sense complementary colors too. The accurate position on the color line was determined by the brightness of the color (as had been postulated by Aristotle). Thus, Schopenhauer's arrangement was different from the chromatic spectrum, in which yellow lies between orange and green. Schopenhauer's yellow was closer to white, while the complementary color violet lay close to darkness. He proposed that red and green would be equally bright and would therefore produce an equal amount of brightness, shade, or darkness. Schopenhauer's concept of evidence, showed how far he had departed from modern science, which already existed in his time and had

even been enunciated by Aristotle and Plato. According to Schopenhauer, there is a quantitative "mechanical" mixture beside the color-activating qualitative activity of the retina.

Schopenhauer's theory, however, still has two valid elements: on the one hand, the recognition of complementary colors and, on the other hand, the realization that color vision has a physiological basis. Schopenhauer was affected by Aristotle's linear arrangement of the colors and the numeric-mathematical speculation influenced by Pythagoras; therefore, he did not develop a durable theory. He was thereby a victim of the Neo-Hellenism and ignored the clearly better color arrangement of Newton (1642–1727).[118]

Newton arranged the colors in a circle and differentiated among seven colors (orange, yellow, green, blue, indigo, violet, and red). In the center was white, and between white and the spectral borders were unsaturated colors. Thus, Newton, in contrast to Aristotle, arranged the colors in two dimensions, and if we add the light intensity perpendicularly to the color surface, we will get the well-known three-dimensionality of color space (which Newton had not recognized). This was not recognized until Grassman and Maxwell in the nineteenth century.[43]

Schopenhauer also discussed the theory of perception. Schopenhauer, who regarded himself as a Kantian, called the world as we see it "a feeling of recognizing humans." For Newton, each diffraction of a white light corresponded to a completely determined color.[118] All other color perceptions, such as colored afterimages, contrasting colors, or the colors of dazzlingly bright lights, were regarded as a malfunction of the eye. By contrast, for Schopenhauer, the origin of color vision was within the eyes and presupposes a physiological basis for color recognition. Indeed, he was correct in that Newton's experiments said little about percepts. Is everyone's sensory impression of the same color—defined by a wavelength and a light intensity—similar? Today, we know that colors perceived by dichromats may be fundamentally different from those that are seen by normal trichromats. A good example is a pink sweater, which to a protanope seems a dark wine red. Recently, Mollon[82] has suggested that there are even women who are tetrachromats and have an additional cone type between the long and middle wavelengths of trichromatic observers. He mentions a woman who constantly complained that neighbors dressed in "impossible" color combinations. The fourth receptor (and the associated neural circuitry) could give the tetrachromats the possibility of recognizing and assigning distinguishing "clashing" color combinations that appear identical to "normal" trichromats. Perhaps Schopenhauer and Goethe were not entirely wrong to reject parts of Newton's theory. Color is not only a firm physical unit that can be described and defined by wavelength and light intensity. It is a property developed in the eye and in the brain. Livingstone and Hubel[9] described cells that responded only to stimuli of a given hue, subjectively defined by the experimenters. It did not matter whether this was produced by a monochromatic radiation or by spectral mixtures on a TV screen. What was important was not the individual cone absorptions but the resulting brain activity.

The history of trichromaticity and inherited color vision defects

Historically, the first account of color vision deficiency, unrelated to loss of visual acuity, was published by the chemist Robert Boyle (who originated Boyle's Law) in 1688,[20] and Mollon[81] has pointed out that Boyle also described a specific loss of blue vision: tritanopia. Huddart, in 1777, was the first who described inherited color vision defects.[52] He examined two brothers and recognized a red-green deficiency in both of them. The famous observations of the English chemist and physicist John Dalton (1766–1844) on his own vision[25] described not only his difficulty in detecting colors and naming colors, but also his development of a color test. He was sure that he himself had a red-green deficiency. In his will, he donated his eyes after his death for examinations. More than 200 years later, molecular geneticists were able to show that Dalton was deuteranopic and thus had only two types of functional cones. In English-speaking countries, color vision deficiencies are sometimes called Daltonism in his honor. In 1837, August Seebeck reported his examination of 14 color-defective subjects.[117] He observed that six had a shortened spectrum, which led to his suggestion that there are two different classes of color vision defects. From these results, Helmholtz concluded that two different red-green deficiencies existed and used this conclusion as a major explanation for his color theory.[49] His pupil Johannes von Kries was the first to name these color defects *protanopia*, *deutanopia*, and *tritanopia*.[65] Rayleigh (1881/1882) discovered that people who were asked to mix red and green to match yellow do not always use the same amount of each color. He described the technique of determining red:green ratios.[101] Johannes von Kries named anomalous trichromacy, recognizing that abnormal color vision could occur in people who required three primaries for color mixing.[65] Rayleigh's insight was so useful that equipment based on it is still in use. On the basis of Rayleigh's equation, Nagel (1907) constructed his anomaloscope,[85] which is still the best instrument to examine and classify congenital red-green color defects. Side by side with the development of spectral color tests, pseudoisochromatic plates were introduced by Stilling in 1878,[124] and fourteen editions were published before 1913. Various pseudoisochromatic plates followed all over the world. The most common are the Ishihara plates, which are quite useful for screening. (For a historical overview, see Fletcher and Voke[33]).

Normal human color vision depends on three cone mechanisms, in contrast to many primates that are dichromats. The three classes of pigment differ in their relative spectral sensitivities and are commonly referred to as the blue (short-wavelength or S-cones), green (middle-wavelength or M-cones) and red (long-wavelength or L-cones). The splitting of the longer-wavelength system into the L- and M-cones (red and green cone) occurred relative recently in the evolution. Thus, only humans and some primates, such as chimpanzees, have trichromatic vision. This evolutionary step provided important information; for example, trichromats are able to distinguish between ripe and unripe fruit on a tree.

The absorption of cone pigments depends on the precise structure of the protein opsin (figure 47.1). The chromophore 11-*cis*-retinal is identical in all mammalian photoreceptors. Up to 98% of the L- and M-cone opsins are

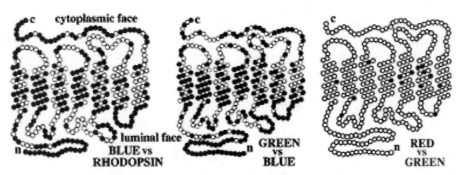

FIGURE 47.1 Homologies between the opsins of rods and short-, medium-, and long-wavelength human visual pigments. The amino acids that differ are shown by black dots. Blue versus rhodopsin and green versus blue have many differences, but green and red are very similar. Approximately 60% are most sensitive to light of 559 nm (L-cones), and approximately 30% are sensitive to 531 nm (M-cones). The genes coding for the protein (opsin) of the red and green cones lie on the X-chromosome. Ten percent of the cones are sensitive to 436-nm wavelength (S-cones). The gene coding for the (opsin) of the blue cone pigment lies on chromosome 7. The gene for rhodopsin is located on chromosome 3. (Adapted from Nathans J, Piantandia TP, Eddy RL, et al.[87])

identical. Only 19 amino acid dimorphisms are found, leading to a shift in spectral sensitivity of about 30 nm. The development of the third cone system added another dimension to color vision.[87] People with normal trichromatic color vision are able to name more than 100 different hues in addition to black, gray, and white and can distinguish among more than 1,000,000 colors. Although dichromats might say that they are able to differentiate among many colors, in truth they only become adept at using brightness and saturation differences as visual clues and learn to call these differences "colors."[89] We all, in our day-to-day clinical routine, have examined color-defective patients who were (according to the Nagel anomaloscope) true protanopes but who were perfectly able to correctly arrange all caps of a desaturated Panel D15 test. These color-defective subjects are able to array the caps correctly by arranging them according to minimal brightness differences.

The detection and the subjective experience of color depend on far more than the visual pigments. Thus, *chromatic constancy* is the term that is used to describe the ability of the human visual system to adjust itself in response to variation in the illuminant. For example, if white paper is illuminated by candlelight, the spectral emission determined by a spectrophotometer indicates that the light reflected is yellow. However, the visual system can automatically adjust for the yellowish light, and we see the paper as white. This ability is very important. It would be a very confusing world if the color of objects changed every time the surrounding light source changed. Ripe fruit must always look ripe, uninfluenced by the surrounding light situation at morning, noon, or evening. Chromatic constancy makes this possible. Again, the sensation of "red" that seems so unitary is derived from the differencing of L- and M-cone signals. The peak absorptions of these two pigments both occur at wavelengths that appear green to the normal observer.

The incidence of congenital color defects is approximately 8% in men and 0.4% in women. Understanding of the problems has been greatly advanced by molecular genetics.[87] Although in dichromats, who only require two primaries to match any color, one or the other of the cone pigments is absent or nonfunctional, genetic analysis has thrown new light on anomalous color vision (table 47.1).

How does congenital color vision deficiency develop?

During the process of meiosis, the paired chromosomes line up together, and LW and MW genes may exchange parts of their sequences. Thus, hybrid genes develop that contain L or M DNA sequences (figure 47.2). Neitz and Neitz[89] prefer to use the term *chimeric genes* for the variant forms of the human L and M pigment gene. The development of such chimeric genes also explains the huge amount of polymorphism in human L and M genes. This polymorphism is most

TABLE 47.1

Distribution of congenital color vision deficiencies for Caucasian males and females

Type	Male (%)	Female (%)
Protanopia	1.0	0.02
Protanomaly	1.0	0.02
Deuteranopia	1.1	0.01
Deuteranomaly	4.9	0.38
Tritanopia	0.002	0.001
Rod monochromatism	0.003	0.002
Totals	8.0	0.4

Modified after Rudolph G: Genetische und Klinische Aspekte des Farbensehens. *Orthoptik/Pleoptik* 2003; 27:63–72.

likely the explanation for the enormous range of different types of anomaly. Thus, protanomolous subjects can be nearly protanopic or nearly normal as shown by the huge range of the so-called AQ (anomaly quotient) determined with an anomaloscope. A protanopic subject has an AQ of 0, and a deuteranope has an AQ of ∞. The normal range lies between 0.66 and 1.33. Protanomalous values range from 0 to 0.66 and deuteranomalous from 1.34 to ∞. While almost all protanomalous subjects lack the normal gene for the L-cone, that is not true for deuteranomalous subjects. In about two thirds of them, the M-cone gene is present as well as the chimeric gene. Why the M-gene is not expressed is as yet unknown. Several hypotheses have been proposed.[88,120,136] More recently, it has been proposed that deuteranomalous subjects may have a mutation in the locus control region (LCR) that controls the point from which the gene is "read" (see figure 47.3).[137] If the LCR is normal (figure 47.2A), a LW sequence will be read. If the LCR causes a start at the second locus (figure 47.2B), a MW sequence will be read. If the second locus indicates the start of a chimeric gene (figure 47.2C), the subject will develop a deuteranomaly.

Investigation of chromatic mechanisms in acquired disease

Our perception of color is a very important aspect of our recognition and appreciation of the world around us. The aspect of the visual system that is peculiar to primates is the midget cell system, which is color coded. About 90% of all retinal ganglion cells fall into this class, and a similar proportion of the visual cortex is devoted to this afferent pathway. Moreover, the chromatic and achromatic visual systems are segregated in the retina, in the LGN, and even in V-1 and V-2. A special area of cortex (V-4) solely processes information about color and is involved in color constancy. It is therefore of interest to inquire whether there are special aspects of the electrical activity evoked in the brain that can be ascribed to color processing. Early experiments by Regan[102,103,105–110] showed that modulation of wavelength per se could evoke responses, but it has been difficult to demonstrate that responses to colored patches were different in

A. Deletion of the green pigment gene

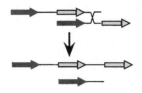

B. Formation of hybrid pigment genes

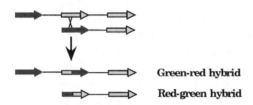

Green-red hybrid

Red-green hybrid

FIGURE 47.2 Diagram showing how the genes for red opsin (dark arrow) and green opsin (gray arrow) are arranged in an X-chromosome. During meiosis, the chromosomes line up and are later separated. Because the red and green genes are similar, they may line up improperly, and a recombination is possible between the two adjacent genes. In this example, one chromosome loses the green gene, and it is reduplicated in the other. The recombination can occur between complete genes as demonstrated in panel A and within genes as seen in panel B. If the recombination is within the gene, a hybrid or "chimeric" gene develops (Neitz and Neitz[89]). The site within the gene where the recombination has occurred determines whether the chimeric gene is closer to the M or the L gene and thus whether the subject is deuteranomalous or protanomalous. However, the recombination can lead to a chimeric gene in which the opsin is so close to normal that the subject will have normal color vision. All these possibilities lead to the huge variability of anomalous trichromats. (For further details, see references 87–89, 113, 120, 136, and 137.) (Modified from Nathans et al.[87])

A. Expression of the red pigment gene results in formation of a red cone.

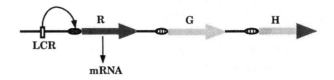

B. Expression of the green pigment gene gives rise to a green cone which confers <u>normal</u> color vision.

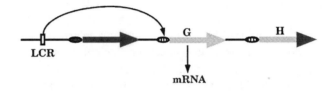

C. Expression of the <u>hybrid</u> pigment gene instead of the normal green gives rise to an anomalous "red-like" cone, resulting in <u>deuteranomaly</u>.

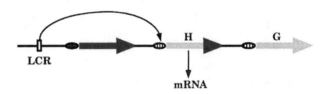

FIGURE 47.3 The locus control region (LCR) determines where the gene will start to be read. In panel A a red cone (dark arrow) and in panel B a green cone (gray arrow) will be formatted. If the LCR causes a start at a chimeric gene, an anomaly will develop (C). (Modified from Wissinger et al.[137])

nature from the responses to diffuse stimuli that stimulated luminance mechanisms. Even the application of techniques such as fMRI have proved ambiguous. The activity of the inferotemporal area can be excited, and its blood flow affected, by both chromatic and achromatic presentation of simple or complex objects. In most work on evoked potentials, responses have been evoked from V-1 by the use of achromatic patterns—gratings and checkerboards—because these were easier to generate. However, the introduction of computer graphics methods now allows the generation of colored stimuli that change in time only along a color dimension, and recent work has shown how such stimuli can be used to detect isolated lesions of magnocellular and parvocellular systems in psychophysical testing. Early accounts of the responses evoked by chromatic signals noted that they were of different waveform and timing compared to those of the achromatic pathway. In addition, such responses are

evoked by stimulation paradigms that are distinct from the stimuli that are commonly used to stimulate the electrical activity of the achromatic system. The subject has been confused because of the difficulty in handling colored stimuli; several different methods are employed. There has been a reluctance to employ stimuli that contain edges and sharp outlines in case responses from these aspects of the stimuli were independent of the responses to color. In the extreme, it has been suggested that because the optical power of the eye varies with wavelength, it is necessary in investigating color mechanisms to use systems in which each waveband is delivered to the eye by an optical system that compensates both for the differing refractive power of the eye for that wavelength, and also for the differing size of the retinal image thus caused.[109]

However, color testing is not generally employed in the investigation, diagnosis, and management of anything except congenital color anomalies. For a long time, it has been possible to obtain fairly simple equipment (color plates such as the HRR, color arrangement tests, anomaloscopes, and lanterns) that are adequate for detecting congenital anomalies and predicting the degree of disadvantage caused by them, but the use of such tests in acquired disease is problematic. This situation is now changing because of various technical developments. Chief among these is the immense power of graphics cards available for relatively inexpensive personal computers. In addition, the manufacture of light-emitting diodes (LEDs) has progressed to the point at which one can choose from a multiplicity of dies with differing spectral emissions. Thus, it is possible to construct new and powerful tests of the chromatic function of the retina and visual pathway that are equally able to analyze disease states. This chapter provides a summary of this information. It does not cover the photochemical or anatomical aspects of the subject. Nor is the subject of colorimetry dealt with in anything but the most superficial way, though it is important in understanding the principles behind the tests, which depend on detecting true chromatic mechanisms. A good general introduction into many of these topics is to be found in several textbooks, and there are several monographs (e.g., Mollon et al.[82]) covering recent advances. It is not sufficient in general to illuminate the eye with colored flashes (though there are exceptions) because these excite both chromatic and achromatic mechanisms.

Three methods of isolating chromatic color mechanisms are in use. Each is discussed below.

THE STILES TWO-COLOR TECHNIQUE   In this, the eye is exposed to a wide-angle intense chromatic background and tested with a smaller field of a particular wavelength. This probe is chosen so that in any particular situation, only one chromatic mechanism responds. An example is the blue-on-yellow paradigm.

SILENT SUBSTITUTION   In this technique,[121] the chromaticity (wavelength composition) and luminance of a stimulus are changed so that the excitation of one of the cone mechanisms is kept constant while those of the others change.

COLOR CONTRAST   In this technique, the color composition of a patterned stimulus is changed from a background. Almost invariably, the background is white, and the color of the stimulus changes along chromaticity coordinates as defined by the Committee Internationale d'Eclairage (CIE). The intensity of the colored stimulus (illuminance) is controlled so that it remains equiluminant with the background as the color changes. This technique was first employed with the Farnsworth-Munsell 100-hue test, but a true realization was possible only with very complex optics[74] until electronic generation of hue became simple with modern electronic techniques. The principle of such tests and the measurement units depend on the theory of colorimetry.

In the well-known color triangle, the center of gravity represents the location of "white," and the margins of the triangle represent the limit of possible color experience. The ordinate and abscissa of the triangle are in the artificial CIE (x, y) coordinates.[74] The three coordinates x, y, and z vary between 0 and 1, and the value of each coordinate represents the proportion of light that stimulates one of the three trichromatic mechanisms. It is impossible to stimulate only one mechanism, so the point $x = 1$, $y = 0$, $z = 0$ is outside the color triangle. When all three are equally stimulated ($x = y = z = 0.33$), the perceived color is white. (Note that the units of measurement are defined so that $z = 1 - (x + y)$ and thus three-dimensional color space can be precisely described in a two-dimensional color diagram.) If a hue is changed so that the proportion of x increases, the color appears to contain more red; if the proportion of y increases, the color will appear more green; and if the proportion of z increases (i.e., both x and y decrease), the color appears more blue. Nevertheless, the artificial primaries do not represent physical colors and have other properties that make them suitable for mathematical manipulation; for example, all luminance information is conveyed by y.

Within the color triangle, there are a number of different points with x and z values that have the same ratio but that differ in the quantity of y. These form a line on the color triangle called a *color confusion line*. Objects with colors that lie on points with the same x/z ratio can have different color appearance only because of the varying amount of y (of course, they may be distinguishable by virtue of brightness or the saturation of the color and on other grounds). If the color mechanism corresponding to y is absent (as it is in deuteranopes), all the colors on a line joining points on the same x/z ratio are confused. Such a line is called a *deuteranopic color confusion line*. Similarly, if the ratio x/y is fixed, colors are distinguished on the basis of the variation in z; such a line is a *tritan color confusion line*. Each congenital color defect has a number of different color confusion lines.

MacAdam[74] determined how far hue had to move from various points within the color triangle before a change in color could be detected. (He measured the standard deviation of the distance in color space.) Using these units, the region in space that appears to have the same color forms an ellipse, the *MacAdam ellipse*. When the ellipse is centered near the white point, its short axis is on a protan color confusion line. The major axis, at 90 degrees in color space, is on a tritan color confusion line. Hence, it is possible to assess color vision by measuring the length of these two axes, though greater precision can be obtained if the dimension of the ellipse is determined in subsidiary directions. In congenital color defects—protanopia and deuteranopia—the minor axis enlarges greatly and is limited only by the fact that at the end, the most extreme stimuli becomes monochromatic, that is, are found on the rim of the color triangle.[61] However, the length of the major (tritan) axis is unchanged. In acquired disease, it is common to find that especially in the first stages, the minor (protan) axis is unchanged but that the tritan major axis lengthens. Later, the entire ellipse enlarges and its axes rotate in color space.[22]

The tritan axis is most important because there are very few congenital causes of loss of blue vision (exceptions to this rule exist; see below). Because of macular pigmentation and changes in relative cone density across the retina, it is impossible to obtain strictly isoluminant stimuli that subtend large angles at the pupil. Tests of color vision that are independent of other visual functions must therefore employ additional technical modifications to the stimulus. The usual method is to split the stimulus into a number of parts with differing luminances but equal color coordinates. With complex software driving complex electronic systems, the relative luminance of adjacent small parts of the image can be modified rapidly so that a colored image is detected against a background of random dynamic luminance noise. Thresholds for color contrast are unaffected by the presence of "luminance noise," which can be made large with respect to the residual luminance change associated with equipment limitations, or the difference in the spectral sensitivity between normal individuals, or the difference between different retinal loci.[61]

The topic of colored stimuli intrudes into other chapters of this book (see chapters 6 and 7). The purpose of this chapter is to summarize new knowledge about the chromatic mechanisms in disease. The use of color is not without complications. The first is that the optics of the eye are not compensated for wavelength change, so various aberrations occur (mostly with blue light) that may complicate findings.[34] The second is that preretinal filters such as the lens and macular pigment have strong spectral characteristics, and these differ between individuals and with age. The result is that in one subject, luminance clues can occur with stimuli that are isoluminant for different subjects, and that it is impossible for any one circumscribed stimulus to be truly isoluminant both in the fovea and in the periphery. Again, the shorter wavelengths are mostly affected. The third is that the color system for blue-yellow (tritan) detects only low spatial frequencies. The maximum sensitivity of the low-pass spatial filter extends from very low frequencies up to no more than two cycles per degree, so any system that uses smaller stimuli is less sensitive and more subject to artifact.

Color ERGs

When extremely bright LEDs were developed, it became possible and convenient to study the responses to long stimuli (see chapter 19). As a result, the OFF response or d-wave of the human ERG could be studied in detail. The scotopic

system produces OFF responses that are large, slow, and of polarity to the rapid cone-generated OFF responses because rod bipolar cells are only of the ON variety (see chapters 6 and 7). Hence, cone OFF responses are studied on a rod-suppressing background. The early bright ERGs emitted red or green light, and OFF responses and ON responses could be seen with green-to-red transitions.[31,122,123]

Such studies can be carried out today with light of varying spectral composition, both in the rod-suppressing background and in the stimulus itself. Long-flash ERGs have been used to characterize congenital color defects, to detect retinal color processing, and to demonstrate selective loss of the ON or OFF systems in retinal diseases. Examples are shown in chapters 45 and 19.

S-cone responses in normals and disease states

Human S-cone ERGs were first described as very small slower components rising from the photopic b-wave after intense selective adaptation[42] but may be isolated by silent substitution.[29] However, simpler techniques may be used to obtain far larger responses.

The characteristic of the S-cone b-wave is that it arises and peaks later than when the long- and medium-wavelength cones are excited. When prolonged flashes are used, the OFF response, so prominent with longer-wavelength stimulation, is almost completely absent,[10] which in many observers give results equivalent to those of silent substitution.[23] The S-cone ERG is reported to be more severely reduced than other photopic ERGs in several conditions: retinitis pigmentosa,[142] after detachment surgery,[141] multiple evanescent white dot syndrome,[146] X-linked retinoschisis,[145] complete congenital stationary night blindness,[56] and Posner-Schlossman syndrome.[75] However, the retinal distribution of blue cones may involve a discrepancy between psychophysical and ERG measures.[102,110,126,137]

The loss of the S-cone system in acquired disease is also demonstrable with electrophysiology. In diabetic retinopathy, it is very evident before changes in photopic b-waves occur[148] (although oscillatory potentials may be affected early; see chapter 43). The selective loss of the S-cone b-wave is related not to age or degree of retinopathy but to insulin dependence and is evidence of the onset of the microvasculopathy. The S-cone response is also selectively reduced in glaucoma.[102] No loss of S-cones is seen in Oguchi's disease.[144] S-cones and L- and M-cones are equally affected in myopia.[147]

Enhanced S-cone syndrome

In 1990, a syndrome of retinal abnormality, reduced visual acuity, loss of color vision, and large, slow b-waves in light-adapted conditions was described.[77] There appeared to be very large blue cone responses[53] due to a larger than usual number of S-cones that apparently replace other cones. The condition is familial, and abnormalities in the gene *NR2E3*[48,49] are associated with the syndrome in mouse and in man. The cones develop abnormally at the stage of cellular differentiation when the visual pigment is specified.[135]

Other retinal degenerations

The ERG findings distinguish the enhanced S-cone syndrome from other mutations leading to juvenile macular disorders,[53] many of which produce small and delayed responses in response to long- and medium-wavelength stimuli that evoke responses in L- and M-cones.[129] The responses in congenital stationary night blindness have been shown to be postreceptoral, and detailed analysis indicates that there is a loss of the ON pathway.[14] In Stargardt's disease[115] there may be differential changes in the L and M pathway that, for example, are completely different from the results obtained from congenital dichromats.[63,130] The absolute amplitude of the photopic response decreases, but in addition, the relative amplitudes of L and M components change, and the timing of responses to different cone types is differentially affected. If rapid flicker is the stimulus, so that the response approximates to a sinusoid, the L-cone ERG may show a phase advance while the M-cone response shows a phase lag. These differences may be associated with different phenotypes; therefore, the cone ERG is also useful in analyzing different phenotypes of genetic disorders.[58,73]

Pattern stimulation and color

Pattern ERGs to black-and-white checkerboards are caused by stimulus contrast changing, and the very fact that they can be recorded at all implies that there is a nonlinearity: Black-to-white transitions cannot give an equal and opposite response to the transition from white to black. The achromatic system is extremely nonlinear, while the color system, with information carried in the midget ganglion cells, is more linear. Hence, pattern ERGs to red-and-green checkerboards produce small retinal responses, and even if the luminance of the checkerboard is very high, when the intensity of one set is changed to pass through equiluminance, at the equiluminant point, there is a minimum response. It is possible that the response to ordinary intensities produced by a monitor are due to residual luminance difference between some of the adjacent colored squares.[63,79,96,100,146] However, it has been shown that blue cone responses are superior in detection of glaucoma,[100] being more sensitive to changes in intraocular pressure.

Color visual evoked cortical potentials

The largest of evoked responses are those that are evoked by chromatic contrast. Responses evoked by activity in the yellow-blue system (involving S-cones) in general have longer latencies than those for the red-green pathway and different waveforms.[2,15,24,66–68,80,84,93,97,98,100,112,128] Achromatic responses have a very nonlinear amplitude/response voltage characteristic, which saturates at a relatively low contrast: this is characteristic of the magnocellular system. The colored evoked potentials (EPs) should be evoked by activity in the parvocellular system, and EPs evoked by nearly isoluminant color contrast have been shown to have linear contrast/amplitude relationships, longer latencies, and lack of frequency doubling, contrasting with the achromatic potentials (even when the stimuli are equalized so that they are similar multiples of the threshold contrast), which is consistent with this view.[2,66,67,80,84,97,98] They also have a waveform that is different from that of achromatic contrast. The first activity seen with black-and-white checkerboards is usually positive-going; with color contrast, it is negative. Therefore, either different groups of cells are responsive in the same cortical locations or, when black and white is substituted for color, the cortical locus of the appearance EPs changes. Despite several investigations of topography[21] and the fact that responses from V-4[40] can be characterized, it is not yet certain which of these two alternatives results in the waveform alterations shown in figure 47.4 with recording from Oz. In the cortex, visual evoked potentials (VEPs) evoked by isoluminant colored gratings in pattern appearance mode produce quite different responses to patterns in which there is luminance and no color contrast.

Chromatic responses have the peculiarity that the amplitude of the initial negative response depends dramatically on the presentation time of the stimulus. Figure 47.5 shows EPs evoked by a stimulus with a repetition rate of two per second. The upper row shows recordings with a 50% duty cycle, in which an early negative response followed by a positive Off response can be seen. Shortening the duty cycle to 10% produces a large response with a marked negativity by about 100 ms followed by a positivity at 150 ms. Figure 47.5 shows that this change in response amplitude is not just a function of the duration of the stimulus but depends on the interval between stimuli and the relationship being approximately constant over very prolonged periods.

A different response configuration was found in children and adults. In children (see figure 47.6A for protan and figure 47.6B for tritan), the response to isoluminant color stimuli is larger both for the early negativity and for the following positivity. The development of such responses has been studied in children. They are not seen before the age of 7 weeks[24,84] and mature more slowly than achromatic EPs, which assume adult configuration at age 2 to 3 years. At the

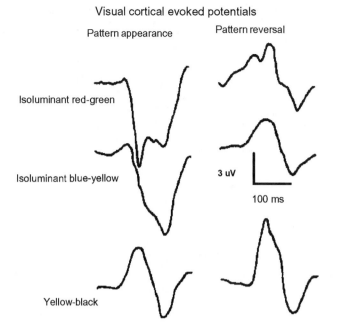

Visual cortical evoked potentials

Pattern appearance | Pattern reversal

Isoluminant red-green

Isoluminant blue-yellow

3 uV

100 ms

Yellow-black

FIGURE 47.4 Color versus luminance EPs. Stimuli (stripes) subtend 1.5 cycles per degree. Surface positivity gives an upward deflection. For isoluminant gratings, a significant difference between appearance and reversal mode can be seen. For both red-green and blue-yellow gratings (rows 1 and 2), a large negative response is found, with an early maximum for red-green and a late maximum for blue-yellow. Note that reversal of a colored pattern produces a VEP with an early positive component. Similar responses are also found for black-yellow stimuli.

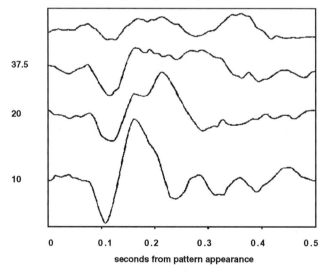

Percentage of period during which pattern is present

37.5

20

10

0   0.1   0.2   0.3   0.4   0.5

seconds from pattern appearance

FIGURE 47.5 Color VEP to isoluminant protan stimuli. The duty cycle was altered from 50% in the top row to 10% in the lowest row. The reduced duty cycle leads to a large response dominated by an early negativity at about 100 ms followed by a positivity at about 150 ms.

age of about 14 to 16 years, the response configurations of young people are indistinguishable from those of adults. Thus, the color evoked VEP seems to be the electrophysiological response of the visual system that develops most slowly.

Color evoked cortical potentials to reversal and motion

When motion EPs are recorded, a chromatic component has been noted,[65] though Regan[104] showed that the spectral sensitivity of EPs depended on the nature of the stimuli and very rarely corresponded to V_λ. By using multiple electrode arrays, it is possible to identify components that appear to arise from the fusiform area, corresponding to the V-4 region of monkey brain, which is known to be associated with discrimination of hue.[65,84] By contrast, when color contrast gratings have low spatial frequency and are used in the pattern-reversal mode, they produce the sensation of motion, like monochromatic patterns, and the VEPs that are evoked resemble the VEPs produced by achromatic patterns. It is known that the amplitude of responses to luminance contrast varies with spatial frequency, but a calculated spatial frequency for zero amplitude does not correspond to visual acuity. A much closer correlation is obtained with pattern appearance. Hence, it is often suggested that the pattern-reversal VEP evoked by coarse patterns is related to motion detection. This strongly suggests that the specific negative responses produced by the isoluminous colored patterns, in the appearance mode, may correspond to the operation of the parvocellular system. Consistent with this view is the finding that achromatic patterns with high spatial frequencies (10 cycles per degree and more) may also evoke surface-negative evoked potentials.

Clinical data

Regan[104] as well as Kulikowski et al.[65] examined a deuteranopic patient with red-green gratings and did not record any response when the gratings were isoluminant. Juraske[55] examined a deuteranopic subject and a tritanopic subject and observed normal VEP responses to achromatic stimulation and to stimulation by color contrast in a dimension of color space that was unaffected by the inherited defect. However, when blue-yellow stimuli were employed for the tritanope or red-green for the deutan observer, the EP evoked was abnormal and contained no initial negativity (figures 47.7 and 47.8). Since both subjects were young, the specific initial negativity of the chromatic EP would be expected to be prominent and easy to detect. Thus, these results are congruent with the findings of Regan[104] and Kulikowski et al.[65]

The color VEP is able to detect hereditary color vision defects. Detection of acquired color vision deficiency,

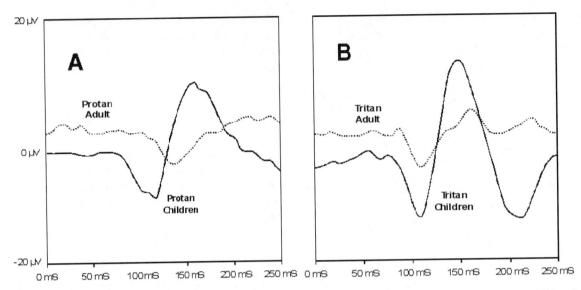

FIGURE 47.6   Color VEPs to isoluminant protan stimuli (A) and tritan stimuli (B). In children (solid line), an early negative component followed by a later positive component can be seen, while the response of adult subjects (dotted line) mainly exhibits a later negative response. Note that the adult tritan negative trough timing is nearer the children's timing than is the case for the protan stimuli.

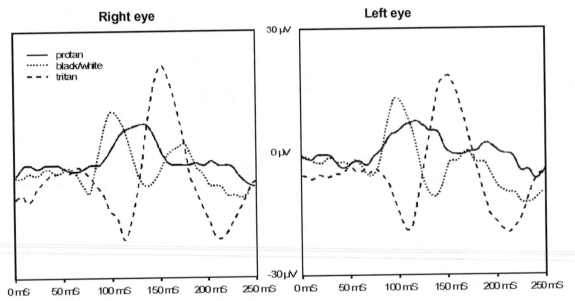

FIGURE 47.7   Right and left eyes of a 9-year-old female protanopic subject with visual acuity 1.0. The dotted line represents the response to luminance stimuli; the dashed line represents the response to tritan stimuli. Both responses are indistinguishable from those of normal subjects. By contrast, the responses to the red-green stimuli (solid line) exhibits only a positive component, while the early negative component is missing. The normal luminance and tritan results exclude a juvenile retinal cone degeneration.

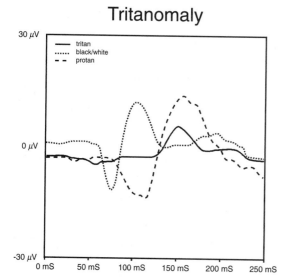

Tritanomaly

30 μV

- tritan
...... black/white
- - protan

0 μV

-30 μV

0 mS   50 mS   100 mS   150 mS   200 mS   250 mS

5 year old boy: visual acuity 1.0 /1.0

FIGURE 47.8   The color VEP recordings from a 5-year-old boy. The dotted line represents the response to luminance stimuli with a P100 at 106 ms; the dashed line represents the response to red-green stimuli. Both responses are indistinguishable from those of a normal subject. By contrast, the response to the tritan stimuli (solid line) exhibits only a positive component; the early negative component is missing. Thus, in both deuteranopic and tritanopic subjects, a marked difference between normal and color-deficient subjects can be detected. A loss of the early negative component is seen in the color VEP.

however, is of more importance. The ability of the color VEP for this purpose has to be shown in future research. However (see below), new psychophysical color vision tests have proved to be of value for detection and follow-up of acquired color vision defects.

Practical considerations

Thanks to new computer graphics systems, it is now simple to obtain color VEPs as a clinical routine. Strict isoluminance is needed to record color VEPs. This means that at each boundary in every stimulus and at each boundary between stimulus and background, the luminance of the monitor must not change. For example, if grating patterns of red/green or blue/yellow appear from a near-white blank screen, a casual observer will see a relatively light (desaturated) blue and red light, while the yellow and the green light may appear relatively more saturated at isoluminance. It is essential that the screen colors be carefully calibrated by using special equipment designed for use with monitor screens (e.g., a Minolta D3000 Photometer). Whenever there is any luminance difference between the colored patterns used, the very sensitive luminance detection system will dominate the VEP, and the response will be due only to

luminance contrast, and an early positive component will appear. In addition, reducing the ratio of the ON-duration/OFF duration leads to a larger stable negative response, which allows us to use the color VEP more frequently in our day-to-day routine. Thus, using equiluminous color contrast stimuli simplifies the visual evoked response, a finding that is of practical interest.

The use of patterns containing color or luminance contrast may distinguish between the two parallel visual systems. This raises the further possibility that the structural organization of parvocellular and magnocellular pathways or the different neurotransmitters account for the polarity differences in the EPs; the EPs produced by color may assist in understanding a variety of ophthalmological and neurological conditions. Chromatic VEPs have been used to monitor toxicity, cone dysfunction syndromes, glaucoma, Parkinson's disease, and dysthyroid eye disease.[12,40,51,59,99,127] Even though complex imaging equipment (e.g., the Heidelberg retinal tomograph HRT II, GdX form LDT, or autofluorescence measurements) demonstrates changes in retinal structure with great precision, information about the function of the parallel visual systems can be obtained only with electrophysiological and psychophysical techniques such as VEP, electroretinogram, pattern electroretinogram, and color contrast sensitivity testing.

New psychophysical tests of color defects

All routine clinical tests of color vision have been psychophysical tests. The fact that they are not frequently employed in the detection and management of acquired disease states indicates that they have deficiencies, but newer methods have proved more successful. Short-wavelength automated perimetry (SWAP) has been used to investigate the extent of loss of color mechanisms in glaucoma.[69] In night blindness, it has been shown that SWAP color discrimination is abnormal only near the fovea,[125] and SWAP functions as a check on multifocal techniques in centripetal cone dystrophy[64] where perimetry confirms the localized loss of cones.

Up to now, it has been difficult to quantify thresholds in most color vision tests, and this is especially the case for tritan hues, for which a strong-age related increase has been reported. Thus, for the Farnsworth-Munsell 100-hue test, the upper normal error score for a 20-year-old normal subject is 20, while it is over 200 for a normal 70-year-old subject.[60,134] However, the development of rapid methods of determining color contrast sensitivity has changed the situation. With the development of computer graphics, it has become possible to remove brightness clues caused by lens absorption. No correlation between age and central color vision thresholds was observed. By contrast, a significant but minor increase of peripheral color vision threshold was seen for the peripheral protan and tritan axis. The mean from 10-year-old subjects to 70-year-old subjects rises only from 16% to 17.5% for the protan axis and from 14.5% to 19% for the tritan axis.[19] Thus, the contrast sensitivity tests, by removing luminance clues from color vision tests, increase discrimination and also allows the determination of both central and peripheral color vision thresholds.

Several computer graphics systems have been described. The first, in continuous use since 1988,[6] briefly displays large optotype letters that the patient has to name. In the later version, the colored optotype appears on a dynamic luminance background. In another, an achromatic noise pattern develops color; this system allows a complete specification of the limits of color vision (the MacAdam ellipse) to be determined and can be used to probe both acuity and motion detected by pure color mechanisms.[13] Because of the design characteristics, this system also introduces luminance and chromatic noise. Another uses a familiar Landoldt C, composed of small disks of varying luminosity superimposed on a dark background, like the familiar Ishihara plates, but the hue discrimination can be made in various directions in color space.[83,133] All these systems are robust and rapid. The speed of testing increases with the reduction of directions in color space that are employed. The use of these systems has led to analysis and better understanding of a number of different clinical conditions. Color and form vision can be lost separately, indicating that magnocellular and parvocellular systems are selectively attacked[138] in rare conditions. Normative surveys on ophthalmologists[4,7,16–18,36,42,45] led to the finding that tritan vision is affected very early in hypertension and diabetes, even before fundus changes are apparent. Even exposure to intense blue laser light in ophthalmology can cause a long-lasting loss of tritan contrast sensitivity. Apparently, other users of blue argon lasers are not affected.[1] The sensitivity for detection of tritan changes is greater than that of other systems. Thus, changes have been noted with intraocular lenses.[94] In glaucoma, color vision tests can detect early peripheral losses even before scotomata can be detected by perimetry.[5,22,27,28,32,46,111,125]

In diabetic retinopathy, loss of tritan vision occurs in stage 0,[5–7,73,92,132] that is, before any vasculopathy can be detected. Thus, in a survey of 400 U.K. ophthalmologists,[7] the 15 people with diabetes had normal protan thresholds, but the tritan thresholds were three times higher than those of the remainder. All the surgeons had normal ocular fundi. The tritan loss can be partially and temporarily reversed by breathing oxygen from a face mask and therefore is apparently due to a mild degree of hypoxia in the diabetic retina that occurs before any significant vasculopathy.[26,54] Only later in the natural history of the condition does loss of color contrast for protan and deutan color contrast develop, but "blue" vision is lost within a few years of initial diagnosis, and the loss increases when background retinopathy develops (figure 47.9). It is not associated with any change in the transmittance of the lens. When macular edema develops, all color modalities suffer.

Selective loss of tritan color vision is associated with most retinal degenerations.[5,11,73,90,131,132] It is particularly marked in age-related maculopathy.[8,9,35,37–39] In one prospective randomized trial, it has been shown that light lasering in the

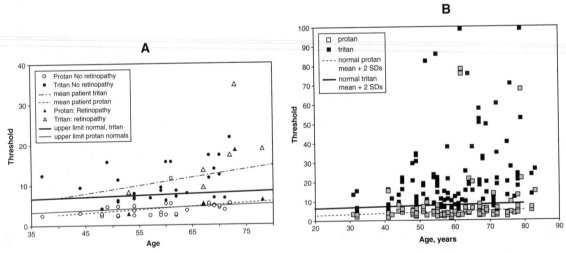

FIGURE 47.9   A, Thresholds of diabetics with no clinical retinopathy (small symbols) or mild background retinopathy (larger triangles). The upper limit of normal for protan and tritan thresholds (mean + 2 SDs) are shown as dashed and solid lines, respectively. (Arden GB, Wolf JE, Wood N, unpublished data.) B, Data for a number of patients with nonproliferative diabetic retinopathy who were referred to an ophthalmological clinic. Note the different ordinate scale. Almost every patient has abnormal tritan vision, and in many, the results are grossly abnormal. (Courtesy of V. Choong and R Wong, unpublished data.)

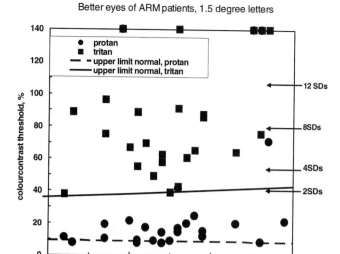

FIGURE 47.10   In age-related maculopathy, tritan vision within the central 1.5 degrees of the macula is greatly abnormal. By testing with smaller optotypes, discrimination between patients with early changes and normals is possible. It would be possible to set arbitrary criteria for detection of severe changes that require ophthalmological examination. (From Arden and Wolf.[9])

paramacular region (of one eye in each patient) causes drusen to disappear, and the color contrast of the macular remains normal; in the untreated eye, the drusen progress, and color vision declines. After eight years, the diminution of the incidence of "wet" macular degeneration in lasered eyes appeared to be significant.[35]

In a series of patients with age-related maculopathy, it has been shown that tritan color vision is reduced in people with even the least fundal changes, and there is a correlation between degree of fundus change and loss of vision. In patients with loss of visual acuity due to geographic atrophy or disciform, tritan vision is nearly absent throughout the macula. In patients with less advanced disease, thresholds rise (figure 47.10), and the degree of elevation is greater the smaller the optotype used to determine the threshold. For a letter of subtense corresponding to the 20/400 line (−1.3 Logmar), thresholds that are 6–8 standard deviations from the normal mean can be found even with visual acuity of 20/20. Because the loss is so great, and so selective, this test seems suitable for screening programs.[9] Similar though not so striking threshold elevations occur between the thresholds of normal patients, glancoma suspects, and patients with manifest glancoma (figure 47.11).

Köllner's rule, that in retinal diseases tritan defects are seen while in optic atrophies red-green defects are observed, remains a useful summary. However, there are many exceptions. Stargardt's disease (figures 47.12 and 47.13) is one.

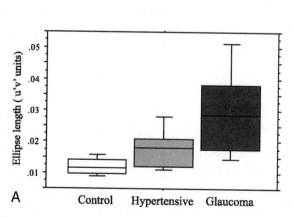

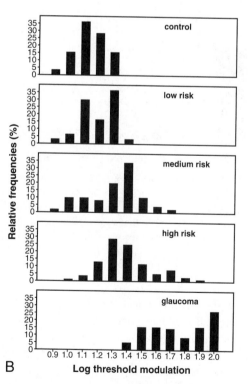

FIGURE 47.11   Color contrast in glaucoma. A, Tritan losses in controls, ocular hypertensives and glaucoma, using a technique that determined the MacAdam ellipse. Note the almost complete separation of patients with field defects from normals. (After Castelo-Branco et al.[22]) B, Tak-Yu et al.[125] obtained similar results by measuring color contrast along three color confusion axes.

STARGARDT DISEASE

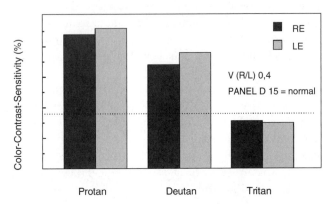

FIGURE 47.12 Color contrast sensitivity thresholds for a patient with Stargardt's disease. Note that a significant threshold increases in the protan and deutan axes were observed, while the tritan axis was within the normal range. A loss of red sensitivity is pathognomonic for Stargardt's disease. In many optic atrophies (for example, Leber's optic atrophy; see figure 47.13) and optic neuritis, there may be no selective loss of red-green but also loss of tritan. By contrast, in autosomal-dominant optic atrophy (see figure 47.14), a tritan color defect is a key sign for the diagnosis. In optic neuritis, the color test is especially useful for the follow-up of the disease because color deficiencies remain after visual acuity has improved.

LEBER'S OPTIC ATROPHY

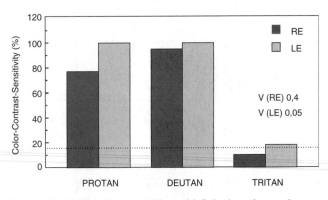

FIGURE 47.13. This 18-year-old boy with Leber's optic atrophy was tested shortly after the onset of the disease. While the visual acuity of the left eye had already dropped significantly, the loss of vision had just started in the right eye. At that stage of the disease, typical color defects for an optic nerve disease can be observed. The patient had a significant loss of protan and deutan color vision, while the tritan axis was only mildly raised.

The value of the new color test has been seen not only in inherited retinal and optic nerve diseases, but also in conditions as diverse as systemic hypertension,[116] mercury poisoning,[119] nutritional/alcohol amblyopia,[114,139] macular holes, central serous chororetinopathy,[38] and drug retinopathies (figure 47.14).[30,70,76,114,116,119,139]

In patients with chloroquin therapy, a tritan defect was the earliest sign of toxicity. None of the patients with normal

AUTOSOMAL DOMINANT OPTIKUSATROPHY

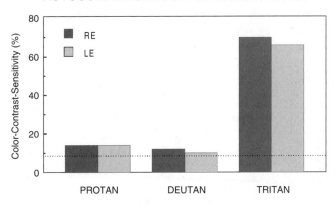

FIGURE 47.14 Typical color contrast sensitivity result of a 27-year-old subject with autosomal-dominant optic atrophy. A tritan defect is the diagnostic key for the diagnosis.[54] With the progress of the disease, thresholds in the protan and deutan axis may also be raised.

Chloroquine Retinopathy

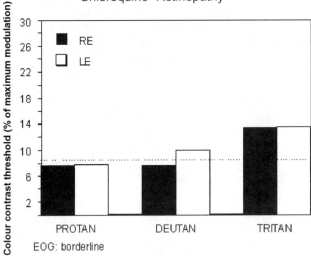

FIGURE 47.15 Chloroquin retinopathy. Color contrast sensitivity threshold of a patient with a one-year intake of chloroquine for treatment of rheumatoid arthritis. While all routine ophthalmological examinations revealed no changes, an increased tritan threshold was found as the earliest sign of chloroquine retinopathy.

color vision had any sign of retinal damage. Color contrast sensitivity was the most sensitive test for detecting early retinal damage.[90] In all cases in which clinical or electrophysiological examination revealed an abnormality, there was a marked impairment of tritan vision, and this also occurred in some cases in which there were no symptoms or signs (figure 47.15), strongly suggesting simple routine testing could provide early warning of this type of iatrogenic retinopathy. Determining color contrast sensitivity has proved to be an important and powerful tool for follow-up in acquired color vision defects in many diseases such as inherited maculopathies, optic atrophies, diabetes, glaucoma, age-related macular degeneration, and—last but not least—drug toxicities.

REFERENCES

1. Allen LE, Luff AJ, Canning CR: Survey of colour contrast sensitivity in non-ophthalamic users of blue-green wavelength argon lasers. *Br J Ophthalmol* 1995; 79:332–334.

2. Arakawa K, Tobimatsu S, Tomoda H, Kira J, Kato M: The effect of spatial frequency on chromatic and achromatic steady-state visual evoked potentials. *Clin Neurophysiol* 1999; 110:1959–1964.

3. Aristotle quoted from Jaeger W: *Fundamentals of his Development.* Oxford, 1934.

4. Arden GB, Berninger TA, Hogg CR, Perry S: A survey of color discrimination in German ophthalmologists: Changes associated with the use of lasers and operating microscopes. *Ophthalmology* 1991; 98:565–566.

5. Arden GB, Gunduz K, Perry S: Color vision testing with a computer-graphics system: Preliminary results. *Doc Ophthalmol* 1988; 69:167–174.

6. Arden GB, Gunduz K, Perry S: Colour vision testing with a computer graphics system. *Clin Vis Sci* 1988; 2:303–320.

7. Arden GB, Hall MJ: Does occupational exposure to argon laser radiation decrease colour contrast sensitivity in UK ophthalmologists? *Eye* 1995; 9:686–696.

8. Arden GB, Wolf JE: Differential effects of light and alcohol on the electro-oculogragraphic responses of patients with age-related macular disease. *Invest Ophthalmol Vis Sci* 2003; 44:3226–3232.

9. Arden GB, Wolf JE: Colour vision testing as an aid to diagnosis management and treatment of ARM. *Br J Ophthalmol* 2004; 88:1180–1185.

10. Arden G, Wolf J, Berninger T, Hogg CR, Tzekov R, Holder GE: S-cone ERGs elicited by a simple technique in normals and in tritanopes. *Vision Res* 1999; 39:641–650.

11. Arden GB, Wrobleski J, Bhattacharya S, Fitzke F, Hogg CJ, Eckstein A, Bird AC: Peripheral colour contrast sensitivity in patients with inherited retinal degenerations. In Drum B (ed): *Colour Vision Deficiencies,* Vol. 12. Dordrecht, Kluwer, 1994.

12. Barbato L, Rinalduzzi S, Laurenti M, Ruggieri S, Accornero N: Color VEPs in Parkinson's disease. *Electroenceph Clin Physiol* 1994; 92:169–172.

13. Barbur JL, Harlow AJ, Plant GT: Insights into the different exploits of colour in the visual cortex. *Proc Roy Soc B* 1994; 258:327–334.

14. Barnes CS, Alexander KR, Fishman GA: A distinctive form of congenital stationary night blindness with cone ON-pathway dysfunction. *Ophthalmology* 2002; 109:575–583.

15. Berninger TA, Arden GB, Hogg CR, Frumkes TE: Separable evoked retinal and cortical potentials from each major visual pathway: Preliminary results. *Br J Ophthalmol* 1989; 73:502–512.

16. Berninger TA, Canning CR, Gunduz K, Strong N, Arden GB: Using argon laser blue light reduces ophthalmologists' color contrast sensitivity: Argon blue and surgeons' vision. *Arch Ophthalmol* 1989; 107:1453–1458.

17. Berninger TA, Canning C, Strong N, Gündüz K, Arden GB: Farbsinnstörungen bei Laser-Operateuren: Ein Vergleich zwischen Argon- und Dye-Lazer. *Kln Mbl* 1989.

18. Berninger TA, Canning C, Strong N, Gündüz K, Arden GB: Using argon laser blue light reduces ophthalmolgists' color contrast sensitivity. *Arch Ophthalmol* 1989; 107:1453–1458.

19. Berninger TA, Drobner B, Hogg C, Rudolph G, Arden GB, Kampik A: Farbensehen in Abhängigkeit vom Alter: Eine Normwertstudie. *Klin Monatsbl Augenheiligkd* 1999; 215:37–42.

20. Boyle R: *Some Uncommon Observations on Vitiated Sight.* London, J. Taylor, 1688.

21. Buchner H, Weyen U, Frackowiak RS, Romaya J, Zeki S: The timing of visual evoked potential activity in human area V4. *Proc R Soc Lond B* 1994; 257:99–104.

22. Castelo-Branco M, Faria P, Forjaz V, Kozak LR, Azevedo H: Simultaneous comparison of relative damage to chromatic pathways in ocular hypertension and glaucoma: Correlation with clinical measures. *Invest Ophthalmol Vis Sci* 2004; 45: 499–505.

23. Chiti Z, North RV, Mortlock KE, Drasdo N: The S-cone electroretinogram: A comparison of techniques, normative data and age-related variation. *Ophthalmic Physiol Opt* 2003; 23:370–376.

24. Crognale MA: Development, maturation, and aging of chromatic visual pathways: VEP results. *J Vis* 2002; 2(6):438–450.

25. Dalton J: *Memoir to Manchester Lit. and Phil. Soc.* London, 1781.

26. Dean FM, Arden GB, Dornhorst A: Partial reversal of protan and tritan colour defects with inhaled oxygen in insulin dependent diabetic subjects. *Br J Ophthalmol* 1997; 81:27–30.

27. Devos M, Devos H, Spileers W, Arden GB: Quadrant analysis of peripheral colour contrast thresholds can be of significant value in the interpretation of minor visual field alterations in glaucoma suspects. *Eye* 1995; 9:751–756.

28. Devos M, Spileers W, Arden GB: Colour contrast thresholds in congenital colour defectives. *Vision Res* 1996; 36:1055–1065.

29. Estevez O, Spekreijse H: The "silent substitution" method in visual research. *Vision Res* 1982; 22:681–691.

30. Ezra E, Arden GB, Riordan-Eva P, Aylward GW, Gregor ZJ: Visual field loss following vitrectomy for stage 2 and 3 macular holes. *Br J Ophthalmol* 1996; 80:519–525.

31. Falcao-Reis F, Spileers W, Hogg C, Arden GB: A new Ganzfeld electroretinographic stimulator powered by red and green light emitting diodes. *Acta Oftalmol* 1992; 3:36–49.

32. Felius J, van den Berg TJ, Spekreijse H: Peripheral cone contrast sensitivity in glaucoma. *Vision Res* 1995; 35:1791–1797.

33. Fletcher R, Voke J: *Defective Color Vision.* Bristol, Adam Hilger, 1985, pp 135–146.

34. Flitcroft DI: The interactions between chromatic aberration, defocus and stimulus chromaticity: Implications for visual physiology and colorimetry. *Vision Res* 1989; 29:349–360.

35. Frennesson IC: Prophylactic laser treatment in early age-related maculopathy: An 8-year follow up in a randomised pilot study shows a reduced incidence of exudative complications. *Acta Ophthalmol Scand* 2003; 81:449–454.

36. Frennesson C, Bergen J: Retinal function in Swedish ophthalmologists using argon lasers as reflected in colour contrast sensitivity: Normal thresholds in the great majority of the cases. *Acta Ophthalmol Scand* 1998; 76:610–612.

37. Frennesson IC, Nilsson SE: Colour contrast sensitivity in patients with soft drusen, an early stage of ARM. *Doc Ophthalmol* 1995; 90:377–386.

38. Frennesson IC, Nilsson SE: Effects of argon (green) laser treatment of soft drusen in early age-related maculopathy: A 6 month prospective study. *Br J Ophthalmol* 1995; 79:905–909.

39. Frennesson IC, Nilsson SE: Laser photocoagulation of soft drusen in early age-related maculopathy (ARM): The one

year results of a prospective randomised trial. *Eur J Ophthalmol* 1996; 6:307–314.

40. Gerth C, Delahunt PB, Crognale MA, Werner JS: Topography of the chromatic pattern-onset VEP. *J Vis* 2003; 3:171–182.

41. Goethe JW: Farbenlehre. In Sepper DL (ed): *Goethe Contra Newton: Polemics and the Project for a New Science of Color.* Cambridge, UK, Cambridge University Press, 1988.

42. Gouras P, MacKay CJ, Yamamoto S: The human S-cone electroretinogram and its variation among subjects with and without L and M-cone function. *Invest Ophthalmol Vis Sci* 1993; 34:2437–2442.

43. Grassmann H: Zur Theorie der Farbmischung. *Ann Phys Lpz* 1853; 89:60–84.

44. Greenstein VC, Zaidi Q, Hood DC, Spehar B, Cideciyan AV, Jacobson SG: The enhanced S cone syndrome: An analysis of receptoral and post-receptoral changes. *Vision Res* 1996; 36:3711–3722.

45. Gunduz K, Arden GB: Changes in colour contrast sensitivity associated with operating argon lasers. *Br J Ophthalmol* 1989; 73:241–246.

46. Gunduz K, Arden GB, Perry S, Weinstein GW, Hitchings RA: Colour vision defects in ocular hypertension and glaucoma: Quantification with a computer driven colour television system. *Arch Ophthalmol* 1988; 106:929–936.

47. Haider NB, Naggert JK, Nishina PM: Excess cone cell proliferation due to lack of a functional NR2E3 causes retinal dysplasia and degeneration in rd7/rd7 mice. *Hum Mol Genet* 2001; 16:19–26.

48. Haider NB, Jacobson SG, Cideciyan AV, Swiderski R, Streb LM, Searby C, Beck G, Hockey R, Hanna DB, Gorman S, Duhl D, Carmi R, Bennett J, Weleber RG, Fishman GA, Wright AF, Stone EM, Sheffield VC: Mutation of a nuclear receptor gene, NR2E3, causes enhanced S cone syndrome, a disorder of retinal cell fate. *Nat Genet* 2000; 24:127–131.

49. Helmholtz H: *Handbuch der Physiol Optik* 3. Auflage II. Band. Die Lehre von den Gesichtsempfindungen Hamburg-Leipzig, 1911.

50. Hood DC, Cideciyan AV, Roman AJ, Jacobson SG: Enhanced S cone syndrome: Evidence for an abnormally large number of S cones. *Vision Res* 1995; 35:1473–1481.

51. Horn FK, Jonas JB, Budde WM, Junemann AM, Mardin CY, Korth M: Monitoring glaucoma progression with visual evoked potentials of the blue-sensitive pathway. *Invest Ophthalmol Vis Sci* 2002; 43:1828–1834.

52. Huddart J: An account of persons who could not distinguish colours: A letter to the Rev. Joseph Priestley. *Phil Trans Roy Soc* 1777; 67(1):260–265.

53. Jacobson SG, Roman AJ, Roman MI, Gass JD, Parker JA: Relatively enhanced S cone function in the Goldmann-Favre syndrome. *Am J Ophthalmol* 1991; 111:446–453.

54. Jaeger W, Berninger TA, Krastel H: Pathophysiological consideration in dominant optic atrophy based upon spectral sensitivity, tritanomoloscopy, blue perimetry and visual electrophysiology. *Doc Ophthalmol Proc Ser 46* 1987; 397–411.

55. Juraske J: *Farbensehen untersucht mit dem VEP*, MD thesis. LMU, München, 1998.

56. Jurklies B, Weismann M, Kellner U, Zrenner E, Bornfeld N: Clinical findings in autosomal recessive syndrome of blue cone hypersensitivity. *Ophthalmologe* 2001; 98:285–293.

57. Kamiyama M, Yamamoto S, Nitta K, Hayasaka S: Undetectable S cone electroretinogram b-wave in complete congenital stationary night blindness. *Br J Ophthalmol* 1996; 80:637–639.

58. Kellner U, Foerster MH: Colored light stimuli in ERG for differential diagnosis of cone dystrophies. *Klin Monatsbl Augenheilkd* 1992; 201:102–106.

59. Kelly JP, Crognale MA, Weiss AH: ERGs, cone-isolating VEPs and analytical techniques in children with cone dysfunction syndromes. *Doc Ophthalmol* 2003; 106:289–304.

60. Kinnear PR, Sahraie A: New Farnsworth-Munsell 100 hue test norms of normal observers for each year of age 5–22 and for age decades 30–70. *Br J Ophthalmol* 2002; 86:1408–1411.

61. Knoblauch K, Vital-Durand F, Barbur JL: Variation of chromatic sensitivity across the life span. *Vision Res* 2001; 41:23–36.

62. Koelbing HM: Zur Geschichte der Farbenlehre. *Klin Mbl Augenheilkd* 1988; 192:186–192.

63. Korth M, Horn F: Luminance contrast and color contrast evoked pattern electroretinogram in normal eyes and in eyes with glaucoma. *Fortschr Ophthalmol* 1990; 87:403–408.

64. Kretschmann U, Stilling R, Ruther K, Zrenner E: Familial macular cone dystrophy: Diagnostic value of multifocal ERG and two-color threshold perimetry. *Graefes Arch Clin Exp Ophthalmol* 1999; 237:429–432.

65. Kries J von Zusätze zur 3. Auflage des Handb. Physiol Optik von v. Helmholtz Bd. II Hamburg-Leipzig, 1911, pp 333–378.

66. Kulikowski JJ, McKeefry DJ, Robson AG: Selective stimulation of colour mechanisms: An empirical perspective. *Spat Vis* 1997; 10:379–402.

67. Kulikowski JJ, Robson AG, McKeefry DJ: Specificity and selectivity of chromatic visual evoked potentials. *Vision Res* 1996; 36:3403–3405.

68. Kulikowski JJ, Robson AG, Murray IJ: Scalp VEPs and intra-cortical responses to chromatic and achromatic stimuli in primates. *Doc Ophthalmol* 2002; 105:243–279.

69. Landers JA, Goldberg I, Graham SL: Detection of early visual field loss in glaucoma using frequency-doubling perimetry and short-wavelength automated perimetry. *Arch Ophthalmol* 2003; 131:1705–1710.

70. Laties A, Zrenner E: Viagra (sildenafil citrate) and ophthalmology. *Prog Retin Eye Res* 2002; 21:485–506.

71. Livingstone MS, Hubel DH: Segregation of form, color, movement and depth: Anatomy, physiology and perception. *Science* 1988; 240:740–749.

72. Lois N, Holder GE, Bunce C, Fitzke FW, Bird AC: Phenotypic subtypes of Stargardt macular dystrophy-fundus flavimaculatus. *Arch Ophthalmol* 2001; 119:359–369.

73. Maar N, Tittl M, Stur M, Zajic B, Reitner A: A new colour vision arrangement test to detect functional changes in diabetic macular oedema. *Br J Ophthalmol* 2001; 85:47–51.

74. MacAdam DL: Visual sensitivities to color difference in daylight. *J Opt Soc Am* 1942; 32:247–263.

75. Maeda H, Nakamura M, Negi A: Selective reduction of the S-cone component of the electroretinogram in Posner-Schlossman syndrome. *Eye* 2001; 15:163–167.

76. Mantyvjarvi M, Maaranen T: Colour vision in central serous chorioretinopathy. In Mollon JD, Pokorny J, Knoblauch K (eds): *Normal and Defective Colour Vision*. Oxford, UK, Oxford University Press, 2003, pp 389–395.

77. Marmor MF, Jacobson SG, Foerster MH, Kellner U, Weleber RG: Diagnostic clinical findings of a new syndrome with night blindness, maculopathy, and enhanced S cone sensitivity. *Am J Ophthalmol* 1990; 110:124–134.

78. Marmor MF, Tan F, Sutter EE, Bearse MA Jr: Topography of cone electrophysiology in the enhanced S cone syndrome. *Invest Ophthalmol Vis Sci* 1999; 40:1866–1873.

79. McKeefry DJ, Murray IJ, Kulikowski JJ: Pattern ERGs from isoluminant gratings: Poor selectivity compared with VEPs. *Ophthalmic Physiol Opt* 1997; 17:499–508.

80. McKeefry DJ, Russell MH, Murray IJ, Kulikowski JJ: Amplitude and phase variations of harmonic components in human achromatic and chromatic visual evoked potentials. *Vis Neurosci* 1996; 13:639–653.

81. Mollon JD: "Tho' she kneele'd in that place where they grew." *J Exp Biol* 1989; 146:21–38.

82. Mollon JD, Pokorny J, Knoblauch K (eds): *Normal and Defective Colour Vision*, Oxford, UK, Oxford University Press, 2003, pp 422–438.

83. Mollon JD, Reffin JP: A computer controlled colour vision test that combines the principles of Chibret and Stilling. *J Physiol Lond* 1989; 414:5P.

84. Morrone MC, Burr DC, Fiorentini A: Development of contrast sensitivity and acuity of the infant colour system. *Proc R Soc Lond B* 1990; 242:134–139.

85. Nagel W: Zwei Aspekte für die augenärztliche Funktionsprüfung: Adaptometer und kleines Spektralphotometer (Anomaloskop). *Z Augenheilkd* 1907; 17:201–205.

86. Nakamura M, Hotta Y, Piao CH, Kondo M, Terasaki H, Miyake Y: Enhanced S-cone syndrome with subfoveal neovascularization. *Am J Ophthalmol* 2002; 133:575–577.

87. Nathans J, Piantandia TP, Eddy RL, Shows TB, Hogness DS: Molecular genetics of inherited variation in human color vision. *Science* 1986; 223:203–210.

88. Neitz M, Kraft TW, Neitz J: Expression of L-cone pigment gene subtypes in females. *Vision Res* 1998; 38:3321–3225.

89. Neitz M, Neitz J: Molecular genetics of color vision and color vision defects. *Arch Ophthalmol* 2000; 118:691–700.

90. Neubauer AS, Sameri-Kermani K, Schaller U, Welge-Lüssen U, Rudolph G, Berninger T: Detecting chloroquine retinopathy: Electro-oculogram versus colour vision. *Br J Ophthalmol* 2003; 87(7):902–908.

91. Newton I: *Opticks*. New ed., New York, Prometheus, 2003.

92. Ong GL, Ripley LG, Newsom RS, Casswell AG: Assessment of colour vision as a screening test for sight threatening diabetic retinopathy before loss of vision. *Br J Ophthalmol* 2003; 87:747–752.

93. Parry NRA, Kulikowski JJ, Murray JJ, Kranda K, Ort H: Visual evoked potentials and reaction times to chromatic and achromatic stimulation. In Hindmarch I, Aufdembrinke B, Ort H (eds): *Psychopharmacology and Reaction Time*. New York, Wiley, 1988.

94. Pieh S, Hanselmayer G, Lackner B, Marvan P, Grechenig A, Weghaupt H, Vass C, Skorpik C: Tritan colour contrast sensitivity function in refractive multifocal intraocular lenses. *Br J Ophthalmol* 2001; 85:811–815.

95. Plato: *Timaeus and Critias*, Lee, HDP (trans). London, Penguin, 1971.

96. Porciatti V, Di Bartolo E, Nardi N, Fiorentini A: Responses to chromatic and luminance contrast in glaucoma: A psychophysical and electrophysiological study. *Vision Res* 1997; 37:1975–1987.

97. Porciatti V, Sartucci F: The effect of spatial frequency on chromatic and achromatic steady-state visual evoked potentials. *Clin Neurophysiol* 1999; 110:1959–1964.

98. Porciatti V, Sartucci F: Normative data for onset VEPs to red-green and blue-yellow chromatic contrast. *Clin Neurophysiol* 1999; 110:772–781.

99. Potts MJ, Fells P, Falcao-Reis F, Buceti R, Arden GB: Colour contrast sensitivity, pattern ERGs and cortical evoked potentials in dysthyroid optic neuropathy. *Invest Ophthalmol Vis Sci* 1990; 31 (suppl):189.

100. Rabin J, Switkes E, Crognale M, Schneck ME, Adams AJ: Visual evoked potentials in three-dimensional color space: Correlates of spatio-chromatic processing. *Vision Res* 1994; 34:2657–2671.

101. Rayleigh: Experiments on colour (read Sept 2 1881). *Nature* 1881/1882; 25:64–68.

102. Regan D: Evoked potentials to changes in the chromatic contrast and to changes in the luminance contrast of checkerboard stimulus patterns. *Vision Res* 1971; 11:1203.

103. Regan D: Evoked potentials to changes in the chromatic contrast and luminance contrast of checkboard stimulus patterns. *Adv Exp Med Biol* 1972; 24:171–187.

104. Regan D: An evoked potential correlate of colour: Evoked potential findings and single cell speculations. *Vision Res* 1973; 13:1933–1941.

105. Regan D: Evoked potentials specific to spatial patterns of luminance and colour. *Vision Res* 1973; 13:2381–2402.

106. Regan D, Spekreijse H: Evoked potential indications of colour blindness. *Vision Res* 1974; 14:89–95.

107. Regan D: Electrophysiological evidence for colour channels in human pattern vision. *Nature* 1974; 250:437–439.

108. Regan D: Colour coding of pattern responses in man investigated by evoked potential feedback and direct plot techniques. *Vision Res* 1975; 15:175–183.

109. Regan D: Investigations of normal and defective colour vision by evoked potential recording. *Mod Probl Ophthalmol* 1978; 19:19–28.

110. Regan D, Tyler CW: Some dynamic features of colour vision. *Vision Res* 1971; 11:1307–1324.

111. Ruben ST, Arden GB, O'Sullivan F, Hitchings RA: Pattern electroretinogram and peripheral colour contrast thresholds in ocular hypertension and glaucoma: Comparison and correlation of results. *Br J Ophthalmol* 1995; 79:326–331.

112. Ruddock GA, Harding GF: Visual electrophysiology to achromatic and chromatic stimuli in premature and full term infants. *J Psychophysiol* 1994; 16:209–218.

113. Rudolph G: Genetische und klinische Aspekte des Farbensehens. *Orthoptik/Pleoptik* 2003; 27:63–72.

114. Sadun AA, Martone JF, Muci-Mendoza R, Reyes L, DuBois L, Silva JC, Roman G, Caballero B: Epidemic optic neuropathy in Cuba: Eye findings. *Arch Ophthalmol* 1994; 112:691–699.

115. Scholl HP, Kremers J, Vonthein R, White K, Weber BH: L- and M-cone-driven electroretinograms in Stargardt's macular dystrophy-fundus flavimaculatus. *Invest Ophthalmol Vis Sci* 2001; 42:1380–1389.

116. Schroeder A, Erb C, Falk S, Schwartze G: Colour vision disturbance in patients with arterial hypertension. In Mollon JD, Pokorny J, Knoblauch K (eds): *Normal and Defective Colour Vision*. Oxford, UK, Oxford University Press, 2003, pp 404–408.

117. Seebeck A: Über den bei manchen Personen vorkommenden Mangel an Farbensinn. *Ann Physik Chem* 1837; 42:177–233.

118. Sepper DI: *Goethe Contra Newton: Polemics and the Project for a New Science of Color.* Cambridge, UK, Cambridge University Press, 1988.

119. Silviera LCI, Damin ETB, Pinheiro MCN, Rodrigues AR, Moura ALA, Cortes MIT, Mello GA: Visual dysfunction following mercury exposure by breathing mercury vapour or by eating mercury-contaminated food. In Mollon JD, Pokorny J,

Knoblauch K (eds): *Normal and Defective Colour Vision*. Oxford, UK, Oxford University Press, 2003, pp 409–417.

120. Sjoberg SA, Neitz M, Balding SD, Neitz J: L-cone pigment genes suppressed in normal color vision. *Vision Res* 1998; 38:3359–3364.

121. Smith VC, Pokorny J, Davis M, Yeh T: Mechanisms subserving temporal modulation sensitivity in silent-cone substitution. *J Opt Soc Am A Opt Image Sci Vis* 1995; 12:241–249.

122. Spileers W, Falcao-Reis F, Arden GB: Evidence from human ERG a- and off-responses that colour processing occurs in the cones. *Invest Ophthalmol Vis Sci* 1993; 34:2079–2091.

123. Spileers W, Falcao-Reis F, Hogg C, Arden GB: A new Ganzfeld electroretinographic stimulator powered by red and green LEDs. *Clin Vis Sci* 1993; 8:21–39.

124. Stilling J: Die Prüfung des Farbensinnes beim Eisenbahn—und Marine personal. Cassel, Theodor Fischer, 1877.

125. Tak-Yu V, Falcao-Reis F, Spileers W, Arden GB, et al: Peripheral colour contrast: A new screening test for preglaucomatous visual loss. *Invest Ophthalmol Vis Sci* 1991; 32:2779–2789.

126. Terasaki H, Miyake Y, Nomura R, Horiguchi M, Suzuki S, Kondo M: Blue-on-yellow perimetry in the complete type of congenital stationary night blindness. *Invest Ophthalmol Vis Sci* 1999; 40:2761–2764.

127. Till C, Rovet JF, Koren G, Westall CA: Assessment of visual functions following prenatal exposure to organic solvents. *Neurotoxicology* 2003; 24:725–731.

128. Tobimatsu S, Tomoda H, Kato M: Human VEPs to isoluminant chromatic and achromatic sinusoidal gratings: Separation of parvocellular components. *Brain Topogr* 1996; 8:241–243.

129. Tzekov RT, Sohocki MM, Daiger SP, Birch DG: Visual phenotype in patients with Arg41Gln and Ala196+1 bp mutations in the CRX gene. *Ophthalmic Genet* 2000; 21:89–99.

130. Uji Y, Yokoyama M: Monochromatic electroretinogram of deutan defect in the presence of intense red adaptation. *Doc Ophthalmol* 1986; 63:173–178.

131. Ulbig MRW, Arden GB, Hamilton AMP: Colour contrast sensitivity and pattern electroretinographic findings after diode and argon laser photocoagulation in diabetic retinopathy. *Am J Ophthalmol* 1994; 117:583–588.

132. Ventura DF, Costa MF, Gualtieri M, Nishi M, Bernick M: Early vision loss in diabetic patients assessed by the Cambridge Colour Test. In Mollon JD, Pokorny J, Knoblauch K (eds): *Normal and Defective Colour Vision*. Oxford, UK, Oxford University Press, 2003, pp 395–403.

133. Ventura DF, Silviera GL, Rodrigues AR, deSouza JM, Gualtieri M, Ronci D, Costa MF: Preliminary norms for the Cambridge Colour Test. In Mollon JD, Pokorny J, Knoblauch K (eds): *Normal and Defective Colour Vision*. Oxford, UK, Oxford University Press, 2003.

134. Verriest G, Van Laethem J, Uvijls A: A new assessment of the normal ranges of the Farnsworth-Munsell 100-hue test scores. *Am J Ophthalmol* 1982; 93:635–642.

135. Weleber RG: Infantile and childhood retinal blindness: A molecular perspective (The Franceschetti Lecture). *Ophthalmic Genet* 2002; 23:71–97.

136. Windrickx J, Lindsey DT, Sanocki E, et al: Polymorphism in red photopigment underlies variation in colour matching. *Nature* 1992; 56:431–433.

137. Wissinger B, et al: CNGA3 Mutations in hereditary cone photoreceptors disorders. *Am J Hum Genet* 2001; 69:722–737.

138. Wolf J, Arden GB: The separation of parallel visual systems by disease processes. *Doc Ophthalmol* 1998–99; 95:271–281.

139. Woung LC, Jou JR, Liaw SL: Visual function in recovered ethambutol optic neuropathy. *J Ocul Pharmacol Ther* 1995; 11:411–419.

140. Wyszecki G, Stiles WS: *Colour Science*, ed 2. New York, Wiley, 1982, pp 525–549.

141. Yamamoto S, Hayashi M, Takeuchi S: Cone electroretinograms in response to color stimuli after successful retinal detachment surgery. *Jpn J Ophthalmol* 1998; 42:314–317.

142. Yamamoto S, Hayashi M, Takeuchi S: S-cone electroretinogram to Ganzfeld stimuli in patients with retinitis pigmentosa. *Doc Ophthalmol* 1999; 99:183–189.

143. Yamamoto S, Hayashi M, Takeuchi S: Electroretinograms and visual evoked potentials elicited by spectral stimuli in a patient with enhanced S-cone syndrome. *Jpn J Ophthalmol* 1999; 43:433–437.

144. Yamamoto S, Hayashi M, Takeuchi S, Shirao Y, Kita K, Kawasaki K: Normal S cone electroretinogram b-wave in Oguchi's disease. *Br J Ophthalmol* 1997; 81:1027.

145. Yamamoto S, Hayashi M, Tsuruoka M, Ogata K, Tsukahara I, Yamamoto T, Takeuchi S: Selective reduction of S-cone response and on-response in the cone electroretinograms of patients with X-linked retinoschisis. *Graefes Arch Clin Exp Ophthalmol* 2002; 240:457–460.

146. Yamamoto S, Hayashi M, Tsuruoka M, Yamamoto T, Tsukahara I, Takeuchi S: S-cone electroretinograms in multiple evanescent white dot syndrome. *Doc Ophthalmol* 2003; 106:117–120.

147. Yamamoto S, Nitta K, Kamiyama M: Cone electroretinogram to chromatic stimuli in myopic eyes. *Vision Res* 1997; 37:2157–2159.

148. Yamamoto S, Takeuchi S, Kamiyama M. The short wavelength-sensitive cone electroretinogram in diabetes: Relationship to systemic factors. *Doc Ophthalmol* 1997–98; 94:193–200.

48 Causes and Cures of Artifacts

GEOFFREY B. ARDEN

DIFFERENT ARTIFACTS occur in different situations, and it is convenient to consider these in turn.

Artifacts occurring in a new clinic

In a new clinic the user will have to purchase equipment. It should not be assumed too readily that the equipment actually works! If at all possible, one should use similar equipment, in a department where it is known to be functioning well, before making any purchase. If the equipment has not been used before, it should be installed by the makers, who should give demonstrations that the equipment works and describe how it works. Many manuals are so poorly written that they are only useful when you already know more or less what to do! Some tests for proper functioning are described below. Remember, computer-driven equipment may have some bugs in the program, and program updates may produce bugs in a previously well behaved program or may even introduce viruses.

While software faults can produce artifacts that may be irregular and difficult to analyze, the most common reasons for recording artifacts are due to poor techniques. An important part of the clinic is the rooms in which the equipment is housed and the tests performed. In general it is not necessary to have screened rooms that electrically isolate the equipment and patient from other sources, but it is wise to take precautions in a clinic that is being newly furbished. If a coaxial lead is attached to the input of a cathode ray oscilloscope (CRO) and the other end terminated with a few centimeters of wire attached to the braid of the shield, this will act as a "hum tracer." The wire can be carried round the clinic and any localized source of electrical interference detected. Other building faults that may escape attention and lead to anomalous results are sources of light present in rooms that should be dark: residual glow or light leakage around fittings in false ceilings can cause small elevations of the dark-adapted threshold, and if equipment is placed inside the patient cubicle, indicator lamps and light from the display screens can have the same effect. Such light leaks may make it impossible to elicit the threshold scotopic response.

However, the most common troublesome artifact is mains interference. A simplified description of the cause of this interference is given below. One should ensure that electrical power outlets do not form a source of mains inter-ference. They should be checked to see that they are properly grounded, and the supply should be totally enclosed by metallic conduit or trunking that has also been properly grounded. Ideally, the electrical supply of the clinic should be separate from other sources and taken from the main service panel of the building. A separate and heavy grounding cable that leads out of the building is also helpful. If separate circuits are not available and the power supply is contaminated by other users' equipment, a large and heavy isolation transformer may be required to act as a filter.

Any equipment near the patient can be a source of mains interference. If an apparatus is turned off and yet remains connected to the power outlet, it can introduce electrical interference. Equipment that uses considerable current, for example, motors used in elevators and commercial kitchens, can cause mains interference, even when placed a floor above or below the clinic. In many test situations, it is desirable to have the room lights turned on. Fluorescent tubes are arcs that produce pulses at double the mains frequency, and this may be a troublesome source of artifact. New varieties that operate at 40 K Hz are now readily available. The high-frequency pulses are more easily filtered from records. Interference of still higher frequency and intensity can be generated by medical pagers and similar sources: they produce broadcast signals that are designed to pass through walls and be picked up under adverse circumstances. The broadcast frequency is high, and the type of recording equipment in common use picks up and rectifies the envelope of the pulses. Fortunately, they are intermittent, for little can be done to remove the interference. Another source of interference that may be neglected is the power supply of a personal computer. These are almost always of the "switching" type and produce fast radiated spikes. These can cause noise on visual displays.

When an old disused facility is reinstalled, all of the above applies. In addition, remember that equipment that has not been used deteriorates, and "well it *was* working" is a statement to be treated with suspicion. Most commonly, records suddenly start to contain artifacts after periods of satisfactory use. The most frequent consists of mains interference, but slow drifts of voltage or higher-frequency noise may be encountered. If a sudden loss of all displays occurs, that does not count as recording an artifact and is beyond the scope of this chapter.

Theory of mains interference

The cause of mains interference is diagrammed in figure 48.1. When current flows through a device, electromagnetic radiation is radiated at right angles to the direction of current, according to well-known rules, and spreads to the recording site, in this case a patient's head. Within these tissues flows a small induced current. In another mode, the electrostatic voltage of the patient is altered because he forms one plate of a condenser, with the electrical equipment acting as the other plate and the intervening air as the dielectric. If metal plates are interposed between the source and the patient, he can be isolated from both electrostatic and electromagnetic radiation, although the latter is much more penetrating. Evidently, it is pointless to use shielding if a new source is placed between it and the patient, but in most screened rooms, one finds electrical cables and equipment inside the shield! With good equipment, such shielding is not often necessary. If it is, then the shield must be grounded so that induced currents and voltages in the shield are taken to ground. Often shielding need not be complete. A heavy metal couch, properly grounded, diverts radiated current away from the patient. Sheets of fine copper mesh in the form of roller blinds can be used and are effective, although not opaque. Various types of conductive glass are available, and these also act as shields. They are particularly useful in reducing emissions from monitor screens. The glass is often coated with a fine layer of tin alloy that is transparent and conductive; such sheets are expensive.

It is important that screening and other equipment be grounded in a proper manner. In figure 48.2, the patient is connected to a piece of equipment that injects a weak current into him. This is not a fanciful situation—all "real" amplifiers do just this—and current sources may be produced in a variety of other ways. The current return path is through the ground to the patient and then back through the ground of the equipment. This forms a *ground loop*, a most frequent cause of interference.

The causes of such loops may not be obvious. For example, a patient's moist hand touching a ground point may cause one. Frequently, the power supply of an apparently grounded item is a cause of a loop. In environments with many different pieces of equipment such as operating theaters, loops are more difficult to eradicate. Since current (usually at mains frequency or a multiple of it) continuously flows through the loop and the patient, electrodes placed along the current path record interference. Providing all precautions are taken and safety rules followed, the following general temporary procedure will localize loops and assist in their removal: make a new ground connection to all equipment. Use thick, flexible, insulated wire to make a very low resistance connection to each metallic portion of chairs, equipment racks, and all separate items of equipment. Check that the resistance between each of these grounds and all the other is very high (i.e., only one ground for each item). Connect all the separate wires to a common point, the

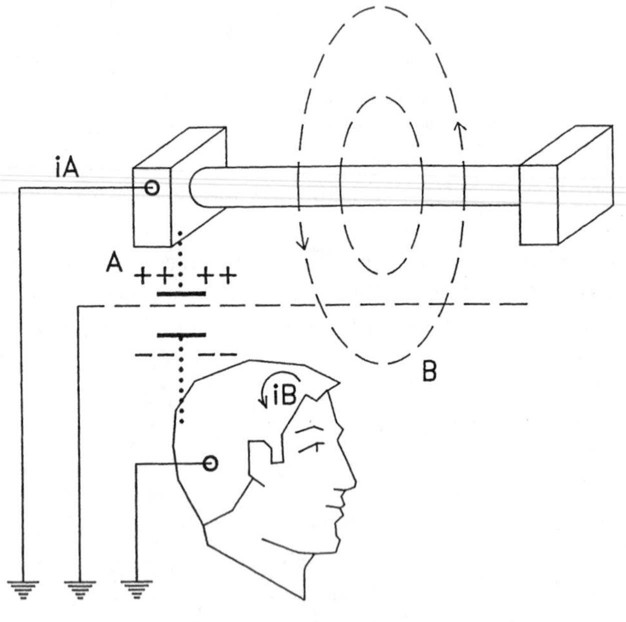

FIGURE 48.1   How mains interference enters the recording situation. A, Electrostatic interference. B, Electromagnetic. The shield (dotted line connected to the central ground) will prevent electrostatic interference but only reduce electromagnetic radiation.

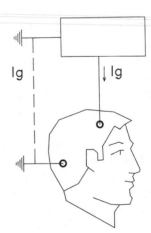

FIGURE 48.2   A ground loop. Current injected into the patient from any source flows through the tissues and sets up voltage gradients.

ground terminal of the lowest-level (input) amplifier. Then remove all other grounds, including all those in power cables, except for the main amplifier. If a loop is the source of the problem, the mains pickup will vanish or be much reduced. By replacing the old grounds one at a time the fault can be localized. Modern equipment is rarely dangerous if run without grounds (double insulation). A word of warning is required. If mains cables are modified in this way and the instruments used routinely in such a manner, there is a high probability that sooner or later someone will remove the new ground attached to the amplifier's front end, and then the equipment would be totally ungrounded. This is illegal in many countries and might be dangerous, so once the fault has been found, it should be corrected and a standard system installed.

Double-sided amplifiers and mains hum reduction

Figure 48.3 illustrates the principle of the double-sided or differential amplifier. The biological signal is developed down a resistance R_1 and little biological current flows down the resistance R_2 in series. The voltage across $R_1 + R_2$ is measured because the ground is connected to the far end of R_2. For example, R_2 and the ground electrode may correspond to placing a clip on the ear. If electrostatic or electromagnetic pickup produces a current that flows through *both* R_1 and R_2 and if $R_2 > R_1$, the mains voltage artifact may be

quite large. To minimize the interference, it is usual to differentially record across R_1. In the diagram, the one side of the amplifier measures $_AV_E$ and the other, $_BV_E$: the quantity amplified is $_AV_E - _BV_E = _AV_B$. This will reduce the mains interference by $R_1/(R_1 + R_2)$. An amplifier that does this is called a differential amplifier, and all modern equipment uses such amplifiers. While this may seem evident, errors in electrode placing are in fact quite frequent[1,4] and can lead to artifactual results.

The ability of a differential amplifier to reject signals that are presented to both its A and B inputs is called the common-mode rejection ratio (CMRR). Manufacturers are prone to quote very high figures for the CMRR. Such figures are often meaningless since the measurements are made under unreal conditions. Figure 48.3 shows the input of a "real" amplifier. The electrodes are connected to the source by resistances R_e, which represent the resistance of the electrodes and tissues. Since amplifiers are not perfect, some current flows into or out of the amplifier. This can be represented by a resistance to ground R_g, the input impedance of the amplifier. R_g is made as high as possible because otherwise the signal current produces a voltage that is divided between the two resistors; if R_e and R_g are equal, the signal amplitude will be halved. Normally, there is a limit on R_g because if it is made very high, the amplifier will be noisy: values between 1 and $10\,M\Omega$ are encountered. Now suppose that one electrode resistance becomes very high (R_{ea}); this

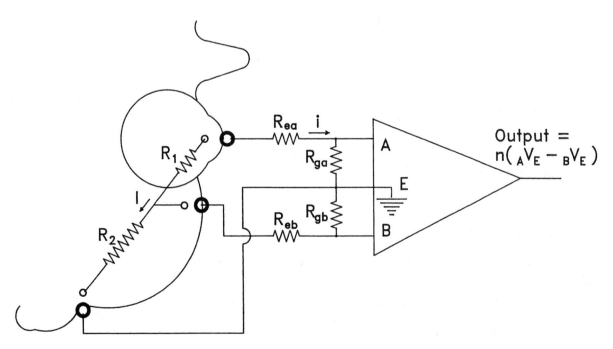

FIGURE 48.3 The principle of double-sided amplification, common-mode rejection, and its degradation in practice. For further explanation, see the text.

will unbalance the input circuit, and the signal seen by that side of the amplifier, the voltage across R_{g1}, will decrease. Therefore, the measured CMRR will decrease abruptly. In recording from the eye this imbalance almost always occurs. One electrode is a silver-silver chloride plate placed on abraded skin; the other may be a stainless steel wire placed on the cornea. If the latter polarizes, its effective resistance may be tenfold that of the skin electrode.

R_g may also change abruptly. The first stage in modern amplifiers is often a field effect transistor, and the gate of this device consists of a very thin layer of doped silicon. If an electrostatic charge is connected to the gate, e.g., by handling the electrode when its connector is inserted into the amplifier, the voltage gradient across the gate may damage it and reduce R_g. Nevertheless, if the electrodes are of low impedance, the amplifier may seem to work, after a fashion, but will be unbalanced, pick up more mains interference than previously, and will also be less stable.

When all else fails, mains interference can be removed by using a very narrow band–reject filter tuned to the mains frequency or in the main amplifier or by using a software equivalent. This is not good practice, and the filtering may itself distort the signal, especially in older equipment. The user should record the amplifier output to a series of square waves with different fundamental frequencies, with and without the "mains rejection filter" operational, to see whether the distortion is acceptable.

Electrode problems

Far and away the most common reason for encountering artifacts is poor electrode technique. For a detailed discussion of electrodes, see chapter 23. If electrodes are nominally nonpolarizable Ag-AgCl, the coating must be renewed, or else polarization will occur, and the input will be unbalanced. If exposed solder surfaces (i.e., the junction between the electrode proper and the connecting wires) come in contact with tears or saline, electrolysis will occur, and spurious slow voltage changes will be encountered.[2] Composite corneal electrodes like gold foil ones can break and develop hairline cracks that are difficult to detect but cause a high resistance. Common silver or gold skin electrodes have fewer problems but may also break at the junction with the lead. Placement of electrodes is important. The skin should be abraded with one of the proprietary abrasives to ensure an electrode resistance of $<3\,k\Omega$. The contact between skin and electrode is made with one of the proprietary contact gels and the electrode held by tape or some other adhesive medium. On the scalp the use of a modified bentonite paste is often helpful. This conducting paste is a water-soluble adhesive and holds the electrode onto hairy scalp, to which it is difficult to stick tape.

Checking for electrode problems

Many modern systems have built-in electrode checking devices, but these work by passing current through the electrodes. Sometimes this current may be high enough to cause some damage to corneal epithelium. It is useful to have a series of "dummy patients." These consist (figure 48.4) of three similar input wires connected together symmetrically. The simplest consists of the wire alone. When the three plugs are inserted into the amplifier sockets, the amplifier is shorted out, and the noise should disappear. If not, the

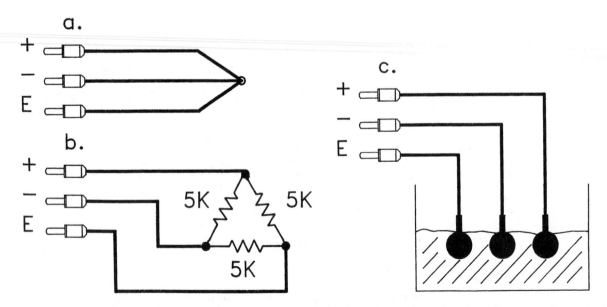

FIGURE 48.4 Diagrams of "dummy patients" are useful in fault detection to short the amplifier (A) and to see whether noise is present when the electrodes are truly symmetrical (B and C).

amplifier is very sick! A second dummy consists of three 5-kΩ resistors joined together as shown. It is useful to have another set with 100-kΩ resistors. If these introduce hum, the CMRR has decreased. In a further variant, the three input sockets may be connected to three similar non-polarizible electrodes that are placed in a small container of saline. If these produce the artifact, then the input stage is probably damaged. If these dummies produce a normal baseline value, the electrodes are at fault. Damaged input stages can cause slow fluctuations (drifts) of output voltage as well as higher-frequency noise and increased mains interference.

Stroboscopes require special mention. They operate at high voltages (typically 500 to 1,500 V) and discharge a high current for a very brief period. Thus electromagnetic radiations are intense and of high frequency. These penetrate shielding and are a common source of artifact that occurs at the moment of stimulation. If the artifactual voltage is small, this may be an advantage, e.g., in determining the time to peak of flicker wavelets, but frequently this is not the case. In an attempt to reduce the spikes, it is common practice to reduce the frequency response of the recording amplifier. This certainly reduces the peak height of the offending spike but also has the unfortunate effect of prolonging the declining phase of the artifact. In published records, the initial few milliseconds of the trace are sometimes removed (only for esthetic reasons, of course), but the telltail displacement of the initial portion can still be seen and the quality of the original records judged.

Eye movements and other muscle artifacts

Some of the artifacts in recording are produced by the patient. The most common are due to movement. This can affect the electrode wires (triboelectric effect), but it is also common to pick up electrical activity from muscles. The patient should be discouraged from chewing gum! A more serious problem is concerned with eye movements and blinking. Most corneal electrodes are displaced by these movements, the only exceptions being well-fitting contact lenses made to special order. Therefore the electrooculographic (EOG) potential at the corneal electrode changes, and this is often much larger than the response that is to be recorded. Patients with congenital nystagmus (rod monochromats, nyctalopes) therefore present a considerable problem in recording, as do those with some uncontrolled forms of midbrain degeneration. Often with patience, "quiet periods" occur when recordings can be made. A more common problem is eye movement linked in time to the flashing stimulus of the electroretinogram (ERG) or visual evoked response (VER): the flash causes the reflex blink. The delay is about 120 ms, and a large deflection distorts the b-wave. This commonly occurs in persons with photophobia, e.g., rod monochromats. Various tricks may be used to prevent blinking. If very weak flashes are used that only evoke the scotopic threshold response and minimal b-waves, blinking is less of a problem. With a light-adapted patient stimuli may be superimposed on a background and, in particular, with flicker, blinking is less evident. The provision of an adequate fixation spot may help, or the patient can be asked to make voluntary blinks before the flash is delivered. A variant of this problem occurs if the patient's eye converges or diverges after the flash. In such a case, the electrical sign of the artifact is opposite in the two eyes. The problem occurs in patients with phorias and partially compensated tropias. Again, adequate fixation may reduce these problems, but they may not vanish until there is considerable detail in the visual field, and this is not possible when the patient has to be in a completely dark-adapted state. Many of these eye movement problems are reduced if a contact lens-plus-speculum combination is used, as in the Burian-Allen lens. However, smaller movements of the lids and globe still occur, and small artifacts are often more of a problem than large ones are. They may be misinterpreted and will not be rejected by any software. In addition, patients who blink and whose eyes rove are those who are most likely to show corneal problems from the Burian-Allen lens.

A further artifact has been described by Johnson and Massof[3]—a very rapid reflex response of the neck muscles to the light flash. This has a delay of about 50 ms and could be confused with the pattern ERG (PERG). Since the PERG is a very small response, such contamination is serious. The artifact is seen when the patient is uncomfortable: it occurs when the neck is extended by placing the patient in a chin rest.

Another problem when the PERG is recorded is the involuntary pendular eye movements associated with a rapidly reversing pattern that appears to "stream." The movements need not be symmetrical about the fixation spot, and therefore the PERG may be superimposed on the sloping baseline caused by the eye movement. Unless the recording contains two or more cycles of response, the measurement of extreme positive-to-negative excursions is invalidated.

Recording the VER from scalp electrodes is often easier than recording a PERG since the electrical artifacts associated with eye movements are very small for occipital electrodes. One problem that may not be evident to those without experience of the electroencephalogram (EEG) is the phenomenon of alpha-entrainment. In children especially, the alpha rhythm can become temporarily phase locked to the stimulus, and in blind eyes this is often aided by the noise made by most xenon discharge lamps when they fire. Thus a large slow wave that appears to be a flash VER can develop. The waveform very rarely resembles a VER.

Averaging small signals: artifacts associated with amplifier saturation

All amplifiers in common use are ac-coupled, and the frequency response is determined by low- and high-pass filters. In most amplifiers, there are several stages of amplification, and the time constants of the intermediate stages are set to be longer than those of the initial and final stages so that further signal modification is not introduced. However, this can cause problems. If a very large and rapid potential change is amplified by the first amplifier stage, the input to an intermediate stage may be so large that its output voltage swings to the extreme value permitted by the power supply. The recovery of the intermediate stage is set by its own time constant. If the output stage has, as is usual, a smaller time constant, the output of the entire amplifier will return to zero while the intermediate stage of the amplifier is still saturated. Then the display will consist of a flat trace that appears to be noiseless. This is of consequence when very small signals are to be averaged and there are large artifacts caused, for example, by eye movements.

Most averagers reject signals that are too large, but few averagers reject signals that are too small; consequently, after a blink, the averager will continue to accept the flat trace that results from a saturated amplifier, and the final averaged signal will appear to be too small. If this artifact is known, it can be guarded against, but short of changing software and/or hardware, there is little that can be done except manual intervention.

REFERENCES

1. Arden GB, Hogg CH, Carter RM: Uniocular recording of the pattern ERG. *Vision Res* 1986; 26:281–286.
2. Arden GB, Siegel IM, Margolis S, Carter RM, Hogg CH: A gold foil electrode: Extending the horizons for clinical electroretinography. *Invest Ophthalmol Vis Sci* 1979; 14:421–426.
3. Johnson MA, Massof RW: The photomyoclonic reflex: An artifact in the clinical electroretinogram. *Br J Ophthalmol* 1982; 66:368–378.
4. Siepel WH, Siegel IM: Recording the pattern electroretinogram: A cautionary note. *Invest Ophthalmol Vis Sci* 1983; 24: 796–798.

IX PRINCIPLES OF CLINICAL TESTING AND EVALUATION OF VISUAL DYSFUNCTION FROM DEVELOPMENTAL, TOXIC, AND ACQUIRED CAUSES

49 Testing Levels of the Visual System

JOHN R. HECKENLIVELY, RICHARD G. WELEBER, AND GEOFFREY B. ARDEN

NONINVASIVE CLINICAL electrophysiological and psychophysical measurements allow an assessment of the health of every segment of the visual system from retinal pigment epithelium (RPE) to the visual cortex. An understanding of each test and their interrelationships assists the diagnosis of a number of diseases.[19] This is facilitated by the layered nature of the visual system and the assignment of electrical potentials from specific tests to particular cell layers.

Because most evoked responses stimulate the entire retina, regional loss of function might not be noticeable in the test results. By adjusting stimulus conditions and techniques of recording, a representation of the sequence of events along the visual pathway can be recognized, and the cone and rod systems can be measured separately. If the stimulus has an abrupt onset (as is usual), the delay between stimulus and response indicates additional signs of dysfunction that are not elicitable by other methods (e.g., psychophysics).

An understanding of the neuronal response order (from photoreceptor to visual cortex) and the interrelationships of the responses is important, since an abnormality at a lower level will usually give an abnormal response farther along the sequence chain, and misleading interpretations can be made if abnormal test results are inappropriately taken out of context. For instance, an abnormal visual evoked cortical potential (VECP) might be found in a number of retinal dystrophies and could be misinterpreted if an electroretinogram (ERG) is not performed to confirm that the defect is retinal, not in the optic pathway. Therefore, after taking an initial history from the patient, the tests to be performed on the patient should be ordered in such a manner as to maximize the success in diagnosing the level of dysfunction. For instance, if the patient has an abnormal ERG, then a VECP is seldom necessary. In practice, this approach must also be modified to maximize patient flow; in some clinics, tests are scheduled on different days, and patients who require further tests are recalled. In other cases, a VECP will be done before the ERG because the latter requires pupillary dilation and the patient cannot be recalled.

While the retina is composed of a complex neuronal matrix with both vertical and horizontal components, it is possible to detect abnormalities of the rods and cones, the photoreceptor layer generally, the middle retina, and the ganglion cell layer (table 49.1). If the central retina is reasonably healthy, then the VECP can detect abnormalities in the conduction of retina-generated signals to the visual cortex.

A directed approach to visual system evaluation is especially important for disorders that either have specific sites that have been shown to be abnormal on histopathology of the suspected disease or are believed to be abnormal on the basis of clinical appearance or other tests. For example, the ERG is well suited to evaluate generalized photoreceptor disease such as retinitis pigmentosa (RP) because the response is a mass one that is initiated by photoreceptors. Widespread photoreceptor dysfunction and loss are early features of RP. Best's macular dystrophy, on the other hand, presumably has a diffusely abnormal RPE, with inclusions of lipofuscin on histopathology but normal photoreceptors (except in regions of RPE loss or scarring). Therefore, it is not surprising that the ERG is normal in Best's dystrophy but the electro-oculogram (EOG), which tests potentials generated by the RPE, is abnormal.

While table 49.1 is helpful in forming a perspective on how the various tests can be used to evaluate cellular layers or "minisystems" in the visual system, it is useful, despite the risk of redundancy, to tabulate each test with the information that can be expected from doing it. These are presented in table 49.2.

The retinal pigment epithelium

The two main tests for evaluating the RPE are the EOG and the c-wave of the direct-coupled electroretinogram (DC-ERG) (see chapter 42). The EOG electrodes, placed on the inner and outer canthi of each eye, measure the standing potential of the pigment epithelium as the pigment fixates regularly between two points 30 degrees apart. This standing potential normally fluctuates but decreases with dark adaptation; subsequent light adaptation causes a large slow oscillation increase. The maximum value measured during light adaptation divided by the smallest dark-adapted value represents the Arden light peak/dark trough ratio, which is widely used to assess RPE function.

In certain disorders, the slow oscillations of the EOG can be abnormal to varying degrees, while the ERG is invariably

Table 49.1

Localization of lesions by electrophysiological testing*

Location	Test
Retinal pigment epithelium	Electro-oculogram
	DC ERG c-wave
	C-wave of the ERG (if the amplifier bandwidth is sufficient)
Outer segments	Early receptor potential
	Densitometry
Receptor layer	ERG a-wave (in general)
Cone system	Photopic ERG
	Color vision testing
	Flicker ERG
Rod system	Rod-isolated ERG
	Dim blue stimulus or white stimulus below the cone threshold
	Dark adaptation testing
Middle retinal layers/Müller cells	ERG b-wave
Amacrine/bipolar cells	Oscillatory potentials
	Pattern ERG (P50)
	Threshold negative response
Ganglion cell layer	Pattern ERG
Macula†	Focal ERG (specialized test)
Optic tract‡	Visual evoked cortical potential

*Details of each test can be found in the respective chapters.

†The flash ERG results in a panretinal response, and the macula contributes only 10% to 15% to the b-wave amplitude.[17] If a patient with a macular lesion has a poor photopic response, then the patient has a problem affecting the entire cone system.

‡If visual acuity is reduced, the VECP is reduced in amplitude and delayed no matter what the cause, such as refractive errors or retinal disease; thus, an abnormal VECP under these circumstances can be confused with a neuropathy unless a clinical examination is made.

normal or near normal. Examples of such diseases would include Best's vitelliform macular dystrophy, Stargardt's disease or fundus flavimaculatus, dominant drusen, and pattern dystrophy of the RPE. Of interest, the fast oscillations of the EOG are preserved in Best's macular dystrophy, even at a time when the slow oscillation is markedly abnormal.[18]

In other disorders, such as cone dystrophy, the EOG is normal, but the ERG is abnormal. In some forms of cone dysfunction, the standing potential of the eye may be subnormal even though the light-induced slow rise of this potential is of a normal absolute value. This results in a light-to-dark ratio for the slow oscillation that is greater than normal. Supernormal EOG light-to-dark ratios have been reported in X-linked cone dystrophy and cone dysfunction secondary to digoxin retinal toxicity.[19,21]

In certain subtypes of RP, the slow oscillations of the EOG may be relatively preserved. For example, type I RP, which is associated with early diffuse severe rod dysfunction, is usually associated with an abnormal EOG slow oscillation early in the disease.[18] On the other hand, type II RP, which is associated with regional loss of rod and cone function (often a cone-rod loss pattern) is more likely to have preservation of the EOG slow oscillation. Of importance with

regard to the site of pathology, the fast oscillations of the EOG appear abnormal earlier than do the slow oscillations of the EOG in some forms of RP.[18]

The large c-wave that is found with d.c. ERG testing correlates highly with the EOG Arden ratio when measured concurrently in patients in a number of different diseases.[16] Current techniques for measuring the c-wave are difficult to employ in the clinical setting, so the test is not widely used, even though it is a good measure of RPE function.

The early receptor potential

The early receptor potential (ERP) is evoked by an intense stimulus flash. It occurs with no detectable latency and precedes the a-wave. The initial corneal positive R1 has been correlated with the conversion of lumirhodopsin to metarhodopsin I.[15] The following negative R2 corresponds with the conversion of metarhodopsin I to metarhodopsin II.[6] The corneal voltage results from charge displacement across the outer limb membrane due to changes in the conformation of visual pigment. Capacitative current then flows from (or to) the inner limb. Cones contribute disproportionately to the ERP, since more of their pigment is present in the true surface membrane. In humans, Goldstein and

Test	Location/Information	Conditions Investigated
Visually evoked cortical response (using various types of stimuli)	Integrity of the primary and secondary visual cortex	Cortical blindness Malingering Assessment of visual acuity
	Proportion of crossed and uncrossed functional fibers in the chiasm (retinocortical projections)	Albinism[1,7] Prader-Willi syndrome[2] Septo-optic dysplasia Pituitary syndromes
	Continuity of optic nerve and tract radiations	Congenital defects Inflammation, injury Other optic atrophies Toxic neuropathy
	Demyelination	Multiple sclerosis Leukodystrophies
Pattern-evoked ERG	Amacrine and ganglion cell layer of the retina	Glaucoma Diabetic retinopathy Early maculopathies Traction on the macula
Components of the Flash ERG		
Oscillatory potentials	Amacrine cells, possibly horizontal, interplexiform cells	X-linked and autosomal recessive congenital stationary night blindness Defects of neurotransmission, Parkinson's disease, autism, drug toxicity
	Indicator of microvasculature status in the middle retinal layers	Diabetes mellitus Central vein occlusion
b-wave	Müller cells Bipolar cells	Disorders with negative ERG (CSNB, retinoschisis, quinine toxicity, etc.)
a-wave	Photoreceptors	Retinitis pigmentosa and other generalized retinal degenerations
c-wave	Hyperpolarization of apical membrane RPE	Diffuse RPE disease
Electro-oculogram[18]		
Fast oscillations	Hyperpolarization of basal membrane RPE after periodic light stimulation	Retinitis pigmentosa Diffuse RPE disease
Slow oscillations	Slow depolarization of the basal membrane of the RPE with light after dark adaptation	Best's macular dystrophy Stargardt's disease Dominant drusen Chloroquine toxicity Retinitis pigmentosa
Psychophysical Tests[8]		
Sustained spatial interaction (Westheimer sensitization-desensitization paradigm)	Inner and outer layer plexiform layers	Age-related macular degeneration
Transient spatial interaction (Werblin windmill paradigm)	Inner plexiform layer Dopaminergic amacrine	Parkinson's disease Effect of haloperidol on Tourette syndrome and schizophrenia
Rod-cone interactions	Rod-mediated inhibition of cone function	Some forms of CSNB Certain types of retinitis pigmentosa and related disorders
Cone-cone interactions	Cone-mediated inhibition of cone function (possible horizontal, interplexiform roles)	Currently unknown clinically
Dark adaptometry	Kinetics of dark adaptation and final sensitivity of rods and cones	Night blindness (occasionally due to cone dysfunction)

Berson found that of the total ERP amplitude, 60% to 80% was generated by cones and 20% to 40% by rods.[10] To record the ERP, investigators have used a lens filled with saline solution coupled to the electrode in a side arm that is covered with black tape to eliminate the photovoltaic artifact that occurs.[4] Because there is no neural amplification, flashes that elicit measurable ERPs bleach a considerable proportion of the pigment in the retina, and the interstimulus intervals should be at least several minutes. The ERP has been tested in a number of retinal dystrophies, and while delays have not been found, amplitude reduction has been observed that corresponds to a decrease in the quantity of visual pigment. Several types of RP have shown quicker regeneration time than normal.[3] The clinical usefulness of the ERP is limited, since the test has not been shown to be diagnostic of any particular disease and can be performed only in a limited number of research centers. A more extensive discussion of this topic can be found in chapter 40.

Electroretinogram

A number of studies[5] have been performed that correlate the mass ERG response to intracellular and intercellular retinal recordings, and there is general agreement that the a-wave is generated by the receptor layer and the b-wave is generated by Müller cells as a sequela to bipolar cell activity. While there is a temptation to think simplistically about origins of the ERG responses, various studies suggest complicated interactions involving inhibitory and excitatory cells affecting the receptor-bipolar-ganglion cell junctions and cell bodies.

Electroretinographic waveform changes characteristic of disease

There are several changes in waveform that, when present, greatly help in arriving at a diagnosis. These include a loss of oscillatory potentials, a negative response, that is, a large a-wave and reduced b-wave (table 49.3), the combination of a very abnormal photopic ERG with a normal rod ERG, and a highly abnormal cone and rod ERG. Specific loss of oscillatory potentials has been notably associated with X-linked and autosomal-recessive congenital stationary night blindness, vascular ischemia, and occasional cases of cone dysfunction and retinotoxicity, for example, to ethambutol. The negative waveform, seen under test conditions of dark adaptation when a bright flash stimulus is used, is a well-formed negative a-wave and a b-wave that may reach the isoelectric point. Negative a-waves are most commonly seen in cases of juvenile retinoschisis and congenital stationary night blindness, but other disorders are in the differential diagnosis and are presented in table 49.3. Historically, the term *negative waveform* has been applied to the scotopic bright-flash ERG, but many disorders can produce such a waveform in the photopic ERG as well.

Various degrees of negativity may be found. Thus, in some cases of retinoschisis and congenital night blindness, the b-wave is entirely absent, and the ERG consists of a PIII only. There is considerable amplification at the photoreceptor-bipolar synapse, so small photoreceptor responses produce large b-waves, and the latter "saturate" for flashes of intensity that are sufficient to evoke a measurable a-wave. The isolated PIII response is thus only seen with bright flashes under scotopic conditions.

Inferences about the site of pathological lesions can be made by considering at what level the dysfunction appears to occur and by comparing various tests of different levels. Thus, in juvenile retinoschisis, the patient typically has a large a-wave and a poor b-wave, which suggests that the dysfunction lies after the photoreceptor layer. Likewise, in congenital stationary night blindness, which also has a large negative wave (see tables 49.3 and 49.4), the rod ERG varies from very small to nonrecordable, while the dark-adapted bright-flash ERG has a large a-wave and a poor b-wave, again suggesting a problem in the rod system distal to the rod photoreceptor. Miyake covers the distinguishing features of the various forms of CSNB in chapter 74. A poor cone response (either flicker or photopic ERG) in the face of a full visual field and good response is typically seen in cone degenerations or dystrophies.

A comparison of tests is often useful in localizing the level of the visual system that is primarily affected. Table 49.4 lists multiple examples of this phenomena. An abnormal EOG and a normal ERG suggest RPE dysfunction, such as in Best's disease. A normal ERG with an abnormal VECP (assuming macular function is present) strongly suggests an optic neuropathy or retrochiasmal problem. An abnormal pattern ERG in the face of a normal VECP and flash ERG suggests ganglion cell dysfunction, as might be seen in early glaucoma, and also occurs in conditions such as Stargardt's disease before visual acuity is noticeably depressed.

Interpretation of the VECP and ERG may help to differentiate primary optic atrophy from optic atrophy secondary to retinal degeneration, but occasionally, this comparison can be difficult in situations such as long-standing advanced glaucoma, in which results of both tests may be abnormal. Also, some disorders, such as dominantly inherited optic atrophy, may have mildly abnormal ERGs as well as abnormal VECPs. Nevertheless, the combination of VECP and ERG is very useful to determine the site of pathology, especially in blond fundi in the face of subnormal visual acuity.

For a limited number of indications, the combination of VECP and pattern ERG (PERG) is extremely helpful. Disorders that produce dysfunction of ganglion cells but good acuity, such as early glaucoma, are most likely to produce

TABLE 49.3
Disorders with "negative" ERG waveforms

Disorder	Scotopic ERG		Photopic ERG	
	a-Wave	b-Wave	a-Wave	b-Wave
Stationary defects				
Autosomal recessive CSNB†	N‡	↓↓↓	N	±↓
X-linked recessive complete CSNB	N	↓↓↓	N	±↓
X-linked recessive incomplete CSNB (Miyake)	N	↓↓	N	±↓↓
Åland disease (Forsius-Eriksson ocular albinism)	N	↓↓	N	±↓↓
Oguchi's disease	N	±↓↓	N	±↓
Retinal dystrophies				
Early or transitional forms of RP	±↓	↓↓	±↓	±↓
Infantile Refsum's disease	↓↓	↓↓↓	↓↓	↓↓↓
Goldmann-Favre vitreoretinopathy	↓↓	↓↓↓	±↓	↓↓
X-linked recessive retinoschisis	N–↓↓	±↓–↓↓↓	±↓	±↓–↓↓
Congenital blindness				
Leber's congenital amaurosis	↓↓	↓↓↓	±↓↓	↓↓↓
Vascular disorders				
Ischemic central vein occlusion	±↓	±↓↓	NI	NI
Central retinal artery occlusion	±↓	±↓↓	±↓	±↓↓
Retinal Toxicity				
Quinine	±↓	↓↓	±↓	±↓↓
Vincristine	N	↓↓↓	N	N
Paraneoplastic melanoma	±↓	↓↓↓	NI	NI§
Optic Atrophy	N	±↓↓	N	±↓
Degenerative myopia	±↓	±↓↓	±↓	±↓↓

† CSNB = congenital stationary night blindness.

‡ N signifies normal amplitudes. NI indicates no information. The "±" sign indicates amplitudes variably reduced. Down-pointing arrows indicate severity of the subnormality, with a single arrow signifying mildly to moderately decreased amplitudes, two arrows denoting markedly decreased amplitudes, and three arrows denoting severely decreased amplitudes.

§ Thirty-hertz flicker ERG responses were normal.

Adapted from Weleber RG, Pillers DM, Hanna CE, Magenis RE, Buist NRM: *Arch Ophthalmol* 1989; 107:1170–1179; Francois J: *Int Ophthalmol Clin* 1968; 8(4):929–947; and Black RK, Jay B, Kolb H: *Br J Ophthalmol* 1966; 50:629–641.

abnormalities of the PERG with lesser defects of normal VECPs. This results from the fact that relatively few intact macular fibers are needed to produce an intact VECP, whereas current studies suggest that ganglion cell responses to the PERG may be abnormal early in the course of the disease.

Additional information about the RPE/receptor disease can be obtained by performing both EOGs and ERGs on the same patient. In some disorders, both results will be abnormal. In advanced and late stages of RP, both the ERG and the slow oscillation of the EOG will be markedly abnormal. However, in very early RP, the fast oscillations of the EOG may be more abnormal than the slow oscillation.

A distinctive pattern of abnormality that stands alone in electrophysiology is the abnormal misrouting of temporal retinostriate projections as detected by the VECP in oculocutaneous and ocular forms of albinism.[1] Testing must include measurements of cortical potentials over both the right and left occipital regions to obtain the required information. For reasons that are at present unclear, temporal retinal fibers that should pass to the ipsilateral visual cortex decussate in the chiasm in albinos to project the opposite visual cortex. Thus, patients with albinism show a deficiency of ipsilateral or uncrossed responses. This pattern of abnormal retinocortical visual representation is so characteristic of all types of albinism that it is included in the operational definition as to which disorders should be called albinism and which represent only a variable hypopigmentation state from other causes.

The best stimulus to elicit VECR, for detecting asymmetry of retinocortical projections appears to be the onset/disappearance of large patterns against a homogeneous gray field of equal mean luminance rather than flashes or pattern reversal.[7] The best way of demonstrating the abnormal cortical projections is an examination for asymmetry of the left-minus-right occipital VECP signals as stimulated through the right and left eyes. This avoids problems with interpretation of hemispheric differences related to ocular dominance or individual differences in cortical topography.

TABLE 49.4
Examples of definitive electrophysiological testing*

Tests and Findings	Disease	Supporting Clinical Information
Normal ERG Abnormal PERG	Optic neuropathy	Optic pallor Characteristic visual field changes
VECP testing to localize laterality demonstrates increased chiasmal crossing of temporal fibers	Albinism (all types)	Iris transillumination Blond fundus/skin/hair (varies with form)
Nonrecordable to poor photopic ERG Normal to near normal rod ERG Normal visual field (except possible central scotomas) loss	Cone degeneration or dysfunction	Occasional temporal optic atrophy Macular atrophy, often concentric
Negative-wave, bright-flash, dark-adapted ERG Nonrecordable rod ERG Normal to subnormal photopic ERG Missing to subnormal oscillatory potentials Normal visual field	Congenital stationary night blindness, X-linked and autosomal recessive	No fundus findings Myopia Congenital night blindness
Negative-wave, bright-flash, dark-adapted ERG Subnormal rod and cone ERG Macular changes are characteristic Visual field is usually full	X-linked retinoschisis	Macular and peripheral schisis May present with vitreous hemorrhage
Abnormal/nonrecordable rod ERG (changes in b-wave sensitivity, V/V_{max}) Abnormal to borderline cone ERG Visual field loss (may be relative scotoma early)	Rod-cone degeneration	Pigmentary retinopathy Visual field loss Night blindness Family history
Abnormal/nonrecordable cone ERG Abnormal rod ERG (greater in amplitude than cone) Visual field loss will determine if in RP or cone degeneration category Final rod threshold elevation <2.2 log units	Cone-rod dysfunction[18,19]	Temporal optic atrophy, telangiectatic optic nerve and adjacent retina Frequently less pigment deposits Occasional bull's-eye maculae
Normal ERG Abnormal EOG Dominant family history	Possible Best's disease Fundus and family examination will clarify if pattern dystrophy	Egg yolk lesion macula or symmetrical disturbance Visual acuity better than expected

*Mendelian inheritance pattern, course of the disease process, and fundus pattern often have to be utilized in addition to electrophysiological testing to determine a final diagnosis.

Alternately, monocular VECP testing with bilateral occipital recording may demonstrate disproportionate uncrossed nerve fibers characteristic of all types of albinism.

Correlation of test results with clinical findings

There is often a misconception that individual electrophysiological tests are always diagnostic and can be interpreted in isolation without other tests and often without regard to the ocular findings. Where there are some characteristic electrophysiological tests for specific disease states, the vast majority of patients need a combination of tests selected to properly arrive at a diagnosis. A few patients will present who have extensive testing but for whom a diagnosis is not found. To better define these patients, serial testing needs to be performed, often over years, in a search for diagnostic changes or for progression or stability in the disease; this allows for sensible counseling as well as placing the patient in a diagnostic category. Most patients accept the necessity to do serial testing if the rationale for evaluating the possibility of progression is explained.

Table 49.4 gives examples of ERG patterns that, when correlated with the clinical findings, are diagnostic of specific diseases or disorders. It is also important to correlate the clinical findings with the electrophysiological and psychophysical data; otherwise, a patient's condition might be misinterpreted. More frequently, the opposite occurs; that is, incorrect diagnoses are made because electrophysiological testing is not employed and clinical signs or symptoms suggesting a dystrophic or visual pathway disease are misinterpreted or neglected. Classic examples of conditions that are difficult to detect clinically but easy to diagnose electrophysiologically are RP sine pigmento, cone dystrophies with or without macular involvement, congenital stationary night blindness, Best's macular dystrophy, optic neuropathies without disk pallor, and hysterical amblyopia.

Kinetic visual fields correlating with the ERG and retinal findings often give a definitive answer as to the type of problem that a patient has; this is particularly relevant in cases of cone-rod dysfunction (with or without a bull's-eye macular lesion) in which the photopic b-wave is proportionately more affected than the rod signal but both are abnormal.

Patients with the cone-rod ERG pattern dysfunction may have a variety of problems, including a progressive disorder similar to RP, a cone degeneration with a subnormal rod response, occasionally juvenile retinoschisis (although the negative wave is present), advanced fundus flavimaculatus with severe macular loss, and cone-rod dystrophy.[11,12]

A proportion of cone-rod dystrophies in which the cone ERG is disproportionately depressed follow a course similar to typical RP (rod-cone degeneration) and exhibit, at some stage, alterations of the peripheral visual field, often with a ring scotoma. Others progress clinically with a pattern of change like that in cone degeneration or dysfunction and have (until very late in the condition) full peripheral visual fields and no ring scotomas but may have central scotomas. One of the more useful aspects of serial visual field testing of many patients with retinal dystrophies, particularly RP, is to reassure the patient that the condition is not progressing rapidly. Anxiety levels are usually high in these patients, and annual fields showing little change reinforce the concept that the patient has a chronic disease and that sudden blindness is very unlikely. A patient who is demonstrating rapid change should be carefully evaluated for the possibility of cystoid macular edema, hyperthyroidism, uveitis, serious systemic disease, and drug (or, rarely, light) toxicity. Occasional patients with RP will demonstrate reversible visual loss during episodes of viral or bacterial systemic or respirator infections. A few patients will complain of visual loss during pregnancy, but in most patients, this appears to be temporary.[13]

Dark-adaptation testing has traditionally been performed by measuring the threshold of vision after a preadapting bleaching with bright light. This must be done to standardize the test. Most laboratories use the Goldmann-Weekers dark adaptometer and a nonstandarized technique to determine the white light threshold of perception to a small light presented 10 degrees eccentrically. In normals, the threshold-time relationship is biphasic. If the preadaptation bleaches more than 50% of the rhodopsin, the scotopic system will take 10 minutes or more to become more sensitive than the photopic system. Therefore, after a rapid initial dark adaptation of 1–3 minutes, "cone" thresholds determine sensitivity until the cone-rod break, after which rods develop around 3.5 log unit greater sensitivity. More sophisticated dark adaptometers are automated and test various points in the peripheral retina; they employ red and blue-green test objects so that the relative sensitivities of the scotopic and photopic systems can be determined at various times during dark adaptation.[9,14]

In a number of patients with various types of retinal dystrophy, patients will relate a history of night blindness such that there are expectations, when psychophysical testing is done to measure rod sensitivity, that it should be very abnormal. Frequently, there is little correlation between final rod thresholds after 40 minutes of dark adaptation and the subjective complaint. Many patients with RP feel that their night vision is "fine," since it has not changed from childhood. It is useful to take measurements from at least two or three different retinal areas and take care to avoid known scotomas found on visual field testing. Patients with type I RP will typically have at least 3.5 log units of elevation of the final rod threshold, while patients with type II RP often have 2.5 log units or less. Patients with type II can have more severe loss in more advanced stages in which the visual field is less than 10 degrees.

REFERENCES

1. Apkarian P, Reits D, Spekreijse H, van Dorp D: A decisive electrophysiological test for human albinism. *Electroencephalogr Clin Neurophysiol* 1983; 55:513–531.
2. Apkarian P, Spekreijse H, van Swaay E, van Schooneveld M: Visual evoked potentials in Prader-Willi syndrome. *Doc Ophthalmol* 1989; 71:355–368.
3. Berson EL: Electrical phenomena in the retina. In Moses RA, Hart WM (eds): *Adler's Physiology of the Eye.* St. Louis, CV Mosby, 1987, pp 541–542.
4. Berson EL, Goldstein EB: Recovery of the human early receptor potential in dominantly inherited retinitis pigmentosa. *Arch Ophthalmol* 1970; 83:412.
5. Brown KT: The electroretinogram: Its components and their origins. *Vision Res* 1968; 8:633–677.
6. Cone RA: Early receptor potential: Photoreversible charge displacement in rhodopsin. *Science* 1967; 155:1128.
7. Creel D, Spekreijse H, Reits D: Evoked potentials in albinos: Efficacy of pattern stimuli in detecting misrouted optic fibers. *Electroencephalogr Clin Neurophysiol* 1981; 52:595–603.
8. Enoch JM, Fitzgerald CR, Campos EC: *Quantitative Layer-by-Layer Perimetry: An Extended Analysis.* New York, Grune & Stratton, 1981.
9. Ernst W, Faulkner DJ, Hogg CR, Powell DJ, Arden GB, Vaegan: An automated static perimeter/adaptometer using light emitting diodes. *Br J Ophthalmol* 1983; 67:431–442.
10. Goldstein EG, Berson EL: Rod and cone contributions to the early human receptor potential. *Vision Res* 1970; 10:207.

11. Heckenlively JR: Cone-rod dystrophy. *Ophthalmology* 1986; 93: 1450–1451.

12. Heckenlively JR, Martin DA, Rosales TR: Telangiectasia and optic atrophy in cone-rod degenerations. *Arch Ophthalmol* 1981; 99:1983–1991.

13. Heckenlively JR, Yoser SL, Friedman LH, Oversier JJ: Clinical findings and common symptoms in retinitis pigmentosa. *Am J Ophthalmol* 1988; 105:504–511.

14. Jacobson SG, Voigt WJ, Parel JM, Ets-G I, Apáthy PP, Nghiem-Phu L, Myers SW, Patella VM: Automated light- and dark-adapted perimetry for evaluating retinitis pigmentosa. *Ophthalmology* 1986; 93:1604–1611.

15. Pak WL: Some properties of the early electrical response in the vertebrate retina. *Cold Spring Harbor Symp Quant Biol* 1965; 30:493.

16. Röver J, Bach M: C-wave versus electrooculogram in diseases of the retinal pigment epithelium. *Doc Ophthalmol* 1987; 65: 385–392.

17. van Lith GHM: The macular function in the ERG. *Doc Ophthalmol Proc Ser* 1976; 10:405–415.

18. Weleber RG: Fast and slow oscillations of the EOG in Best's macular dystrophy and retinitis pigmentosa. *Arch Ophthalmol* 1989; 107:530–537.

19. Weleber RG, Eisner A: Retinal function and physiological studies. In Newsome DA (ed): *Retinal Dystrophies and Degenerations.* New York, Raven Press, 1988, pp 21–69.

20. Weleber RG, Pillers DM, Hanna CE, Magenis RE, Buist NRM: Åland Island eye disease (Forsius-Ericksson syndrome) associated with contiguous deletion syndrome at Xp21. Similarity to incomplete congenital stationary night blindness. *Arch Ophthalmol* 1989; 107:1170–1179.

21. Weleber RG, Shults WT: Dioxin retinal toxicity: Clinical and electrophysiologic evaluation of cone dysfunction syndrome. *Arch Ophthalmol* 1981; 99:1568–1572.

50 Effects of High Myopia on the Electroretinogram

STEVEN NUSINOWITZ

THE AMPLITUDE OF the electroretinogram (ERG) has long been reported to be reduced in highly myopic eyes. The first report of ERG changes in myopia is usually attributed to Karpe,[8] who reported abnormal ERGs in four eyes with high myopia. Several early reports on the ERG in myopia showed that ERG amplitudes were generally within normal limits up to 8 diopters of correction provided that there were no degenerative alterations in the retina but were abnormal with more severe myopia and associated retinopathy.[1,4,5,7] There was also some evidence in the early literature suggesting that photopic responses were affected earlier, and possibly to a greater degree, than scotopic responses,[1,2] although this observation has not been replicated in subsequent studies. With the development of more sophisticated and sensitive recording techniques, ERG abnormalities have been observed with less severe myopia.

Myopia is generally associated with change in eye shape resulting from elongation of the optic axis. Several studies have shown that ERG amplitudes are inversely proportional to axial length.[15,16,21] Pallin[15] demonstrated a significant negative correlation between ERG b-wave amplitude and the length of the optic axis, which was measured with ultrasonography. This study also demonstrated a high positive correlation between refractive error and the length of the optic axis (figure 50.1), with b-wave amplitudes higher in hyperopic and emmetropic eyes than in myopic eyes. Sex differences in ERG amplitudes have also been attributed to gender differences in average axial lengths.[15] The dependency of ERG amplitudes on axial length was confirmed in subsequent studies,[16,21] although the shape of the posterior segment, rather than the size and axial length alone, appeared to be the critical determinant of the saturated amplitude in a study reported by Chen et al.[3]

Some studies have reported selective losses in the b-wave of the electroretinogram in myopia, a finding that would imply differential effects on signal transmission from the photoreceptors to the proximal retina. However, deficits at the level of the b-wave seem to be more common in patients with high myopia who also have chorioretinal degeneration, atrophy, and thinning of the posterior sclera.[2,17] Perlman et al.[16] reported that all myopes demonstrate subnormal amplitudes but a normal waveform morphology, defined by a normal ratio between a- and b-wave amplitudes. However,

the characterization of ERG responses in hypermetropic eyes in the Perlman et al.[16] study was more complicated. While all myopic eyes had a- to b-wave amplitude ratios that were within normal limits despite generalized amplitude reductions, hypermetropic eyes had a- to b-wave amplitude ratios that were either subnormal, normal, or hypernormal. For example, the group of patients with subnormal a- to b-wave amplitude ratios was characterized by a relatively large a-wave and a subnormal b-wave, whereas the reverse applied to the group with hypernormal a- to b-wave amplitude ratios. These findings in the hypermetropic eyes were consistent with variable effects on the transmission of signals from the outer retina. However, no definite relationship was found between axial length of the eye and the a- to b-wave amplitude ratios, although there was an inverse relationship between axial length and the amplitude of the dark-adapted ERG evoked by a dim stimulus within each group. Westall et al.[21] did not show a selective loss of b-wave amplitude across a broad range of refractive error in patients who were carefully screened to exclude pathological defects.

Previous studies have reported a selective loss of short-wavelength cone (S-cone) spectral sensitivity and reduced cortical evoked potentials to short-wavelength light in myopia.[10,11] To investigate the retinal contribution to the S-cone deficits that had previously been documented, Yamamoto et al.[22] recorded cone-mediated ERGs to different chromatic stimuli in myopic and normal eyes to elicit short-wavelength-sensitive (S-), and mixed long- (L) and middle- (M) wavelength-sensitive responses. The S-cone and L,M-cone b-wave amplitudes decreased progressively with increasing myopia and were significantly lower in high myopia compared with emmetropic eyes. The S-cone and the L- and M-cone ERGs were almost equally affected in the myopic eye, with S-cone function decreasing at a slightly slower rate compared to L,M-cone ERGs as refractive error increased. These results suggest that the reduction of S-cone sensitivity may originate from inner retinal or higher-order changes that would not be reflected in the conventional ERG.

Westall et al.[21] performed an elegant study investigating the relationship between axial length, refractive error, and ERG responses. The extensive ERG protocol that was used included stimuli that conformed to the standards set forth by

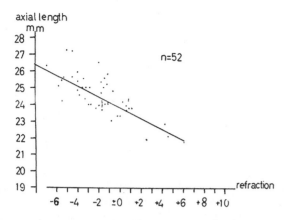

FIGURE 50.1 The relationship between refractive error (in diopters of correction) and the length of the optic axis measured with ultrasonography. (Data from Pallin O.[15])

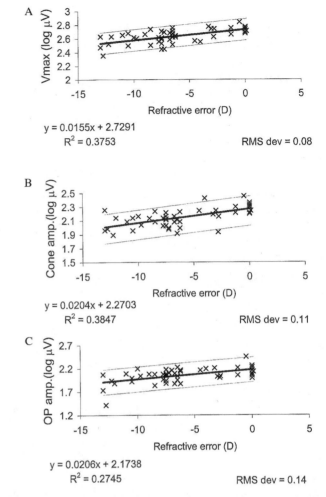

$$y = 0.0155x + 2.7291$$
$$R^2 = 0.3753 \qquad \text{RMS dev} = 0.08$$

$$y = 0.0204x + 2.2703$$
$$R^2 = 0.3847 \qquad \text{RMS dev} = 0.11$$

$$y = 0.0206x + 2.1738$$
$$R^2 = 0.2745 \qquad \text{RMS dev} = 0.14$$

FIGURE 50.2 ERG amplitude plotted against axial length. The *y*-axis shows the log ERG amplitude and the *x*-axis the axial length of the eye. Crosses represent individual data points. Regression lines (thick lines) and inner and outer ranges (thin lines) represent the expected value (from regression) plus and minus two standard deviations. Regression equations and R^2 values are shown for V_{max} (A), *b*-wave amplitude of the cone response (B), and the sum of the dark-adapted oscillatory amplitudes (C). (Data from Westall CA, Dhaliwal HS, Panton CM, et al.[21])

the International Society for Clinical Electrophysiology of Vision, which was the first study to have done this. ERGs from 60 subjects were recorded with varying degrees of myopia but without evidence of myopic retinopathy. The study revealed a significant difference between subjects with high myopia and subjects with small refractive error for V_{max}, the maximum saturated amplitude, the b-wave of the cone response, and the summed dark-adapted oscillatory potentials. A linear reduction in the logarithmic transform of the ERG amplitude with increasing axial length was demonstrated (figure 50.2). However, there were no differences in the implicit time of peak components, in the ratio of b- to a-wave amplitude derived from the maximal response, and in the semisaturation intensity estimated from the Naka-Rushton fit to the rod intensity series. In addition, they show relatively larger attenuation of later than earlier photopic oscillatory potentials, which suggests anomalies in pathways beyond the photoreceptors, possibly in the OFF-bipolar cell pathway in eyes with progressively greater myopia.

The finding of reduced ERG amplitudes in myopia using conventional full-field stimulation has also been reported when only the macula or adjacent regions are tested. Ishkawa et al.[6] examined the relationship between the amplitude of the photopic ERG recorded from the macula (focal ERG) and the degree of myopia. The amplitudes of the a- and b-waves of the focal ERG were significantly smaller than those of normal eyes, and the amplitudes were inversely proportional to the degree of myopia. The abnormal amplitude was interpreted by the authors to suggest a reduction in the number of macular cones that were contributing to the signal. More recently, Kawabata and Adachi-Usami[9] investigated local retinal function in patients with various degrees of myopia who had undergone multifocal electroretinography (mERG). In the mERG recording tech-

nique, small areas of the retina are stimulated simultaneously and local contributions to a massed electrical potential are extracted from a continuously recorded ERG (see chapter 17). The technique permits the mapping of the topography of local retinal function. Again, amplitudes were reduced as refractive error increased, the rate of change being slower for N1, the first negative peak of the mERG waveform, than for P1, the first positive peak. The latencies of N1 and P1 were also delayed, but the rates of change were more similar for each component in comparison to the amplitude parameter. What was particularly interesting about this study is the selective loss of function in more peripheral retinal regions in the myopic groups, as evidenced by the more rapid loss of local amplitudes in the parafoveal

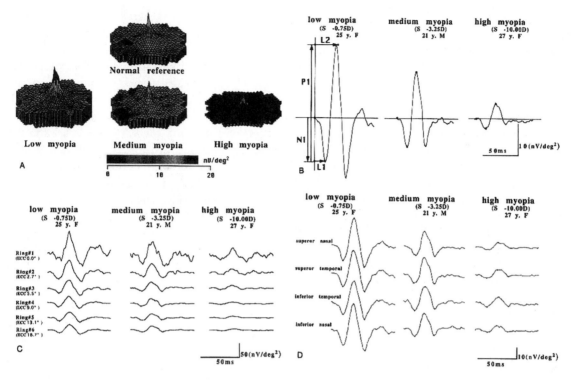

FIGURE 50.3 A, Multifocal electroretinographic topographies (three-dimensional view). The response densities (nV/degree^2) decreased in all measured retinal fields as the refractive errors increased. B, Summed responses from 103 individual hexagons. N1 and P1 amplitudes of the summed response decreased as the refractive error increased. Both L1 and L2 latencies for high myopia were significantly delayed in comparison to those of emmetropia/low myopia. C, Summed responses from six concentric rings centered on the macula. Response amplitudes were suppressed to a greater degree in the more peripheral rings in high myopia. D, Summed responses over four quadrants (superior-nasal, superior-temporal, inferior-nasal, and inferior-temporal regions). (Data from Kawabata H, Adachi-Usami E.[9])

areas (figure 50.3). This finding suggests that peripheral cones may be more sensitive to changes in eye shape produced by myopia, perhaps related to a more rapid change in the density of cones in these areas.

Implicit time of ERGs are generally within normal limits with high myopia. Perlman et al.[16] reported normal implicit times for both dark- and light-adapted responses. Lemagne et al.[13] also reported normal implicit times for rod-mediated responses to a single flash after 20 minutes of dark adaptation. Cone ERG implicit times to white flashes have been reported to be normal in patients with refractive errors ranging from −5.0 to −10 diopters,[12] and cone ERGs to chromatic stimuli have also been reported to be within normal limits.[22] In a group of patients with gyrate atrophy and high myopia, implicit times were normal or mildly elongated,[20] and in a complete form of congenital stationary night blindness, implicit times have been reported to be within normal limits in patients with a mean of −8.0 diopters of myopia.[14] Ishikawa et al.[6] also reported normal implicit time of macular focal ERGs in eyes showing only tigroid fundus, but those associated with posterior staphyloma involving the macula were significantly delayed. Kawabata and Adachi-Usami[9] reported mildly delayed latencies for the

mERG recordings in myopia. However, Westall et al.[21] reported no significant difference in implicit times for a broad range of ERG stimuli and refractive errors.

The cause of the changes in ERG amplitudes with refractive error is not well understood. Increased ocular resistance due to the elongated eyeball in myopia was thought to be the major cause of decreased ERG amplitudes.[15] Pallin[15] argued that the current passing from the retina to the surface of the eye passes through highly resistant conductors consisting of both intraocular and extraocular tissues and that the density of these conducting tissues increases with axial length. Lemagne et al.[13] designed a specially built system that allowed simultaneous recording of both the ERG and the resistance between the active and reference electrodes used for recording the ERG. The authors reported that ERG amplitudes were negatively correlated with the resistance measurements. However, there was broad variability in resistance measurements that was not correlated with refractive error, and the correlation between the resistance and amplitude measurements was relatively weak. Furthermore, resistance was measured between the electrode on the eye and a reference electrode on the midline of the forehead, which would not have allowed a specific test of resistance of ocular tissue. Whether the correlation between resistance and ERG amplitude holds when the active and reference electrodes are both positioned on the eye, and the relationship of the resistance measurements to axial length, has yet to be determined.

Chen et al.[3] dismiss the resistance argument as an explanation of reduced amplitudes because ocular current would be expected to increase with resistance, and according to these authors, a lower, not higher, resistance would be needed to explain the reduced ERG amplitudes in myopia. In contrast, Chen et al.[3] tested between two alternative hypotheses about the mechanism of reduced ERG amplitudes in myopia. One hypothesis, called the *stretched retina hypothesis*, predicted a reduced retinal sensitivity but a normal saturated amplitude because there would be fewer receptors per unit area of retina and more space between receptors as a result of the elongated eye. Thus, as a result of the reduced ability of photoreceptors to capture photons, higher intensities of light would be required to elicit a threshold response (sensitivity), but the saturated amplitude (responsivity) would be unaltered provided that sufficient light is provided. An alternative hypothesis in which function but not retinal spacing varies, predicted reduced saturated amplitudes and normal sensitivity. They reported significant reductions in the saturated amplitude with progressively higher degrees of myopia but normal retinal sensitivity. Thus, the data were consistent with the decreased cell responsivity hypothesis rather than the enlargement of the eye with wider spacing of retinal elements. In addition, the shape of the posterior segment, which was characterized with magnetic resonance images, rather than the size and axial length alone appeared to be the critical determinant of the saturated amplitude. It is not yet understood why retinal cells in myopia would have a lower responsivity. The finding of normal sensitivity and reduced saturated amplitudes has recently been confirmed.[21]

Optical factors have also been implicated as playing a role in the reduction of ERG amplitudes in myopia. Assuming a similar stimulus intensity and pupil size, retinal illuminance may be lower in the myopic eye compared to the normal eye. Retinal illuminance refers to the density of light falling on a unit area of retina, and with an elongated eye, light is spread over a wider area, thereby decreasing retinal illuminance. If the myopic eye functioned to shift the intensity-response curve so that a given light intensity is less effective, then retinal illuminance could be adjusted to equate amplitudes. The sensitivity but not the saturated amplitude of the myopic retina would be expected to be altered. However, several studies have demonstrated that saturated b-wave amplitudes are lower for the myopic eye,[3,9,21] ruling out the possibility that reduced retinal illuminance is the explanation for the reduced ERG amplitudes.

To summarize, ERG amplitudes are negatively correlated with refractive errors that are caused by elongation of the optic axis, with generally subnormal amplitudes for the highly myopic eye without pathological changes. This finding applies to both rod- and cone-mediated vision. Parafoveal and peripheral cone-mediated responses may be affected to a greater degree than more central regions, possibly related to the differences in the packing density of cones, and the deficits are slightly greater for the L- and M-cones compared to S-cones, possibly related to the greater number of L- and M-cones. Implicit timing of the peak components of the ERG are generally reported to be normal regardless of refractive state and with normal appearing fundi. The cause of the reduced amplitudes in myopia is not well understood. Differences in electrical and optical factors and loss of photoreceptor density have been implicated as the cause of the reduced ERG amplitudes in myopia.

REFERENCES

1. Aladjov S, Denev V, Penov G, Todorov S: The influence of galvanic current on the electroretinogram of the myopic eye. In Francois J (ed): *The Clinical Value of Electroretinography: XXth International Congress of Ophthalmology.* Basel/New York, Karger, 1966, pp 444–450.
2. Blach RK, Barrie J, Kolb H: Electrical activity of the eye in high myopia. *Br J Ophthal* 1966; 50:629–641.
3. Chen JF, Elsner AE, Burns SA, Hansen RM, Lou PL, Kwong KK, et al: The effect of eye shape on retinal responses. *Clin Vis Sci* 1992; 7:520–530.
4. Franceschetti A, Dieterle P, Schwartz A: Skotopisches elektroretinogram bei myopie mit und ohne vongenitaler hemeralopie: Symposium Luhacovice. *Acta Fac Med Univ Brunensis* 1960; 4:247–253.
5. Francois J, De Rouck A: L'electroretinographie dans la myopie et les decollements myopigenes de la retine. *Bull Soc Belge Ophthal* 1954; 107:323–331.
6. Ishikawa M, Miyake Y, Shiroyama N: Focal macular electroretinogram in high myopia. *Nippon Ganka Gakkai Zasshi* 1990; 94:1040–1047.
7. Jayle GE, Boyer RL: In *Electroretinographia*, 1960, pp 263–272.
8. Karpe G: Basis of clinical electroretinography. *Acta Ophthalmol* 1945; 24 (suppl):5–118.
9. Kawabata H, Adachi-Usami E: Multifocal electroretinogram in myopia. *Invest Ophthalmol Vis Sci* 1997; 38:2844–2851.
10. Kawabata H, Murayama K, Kakisu Y, Adachi-Usami E: Blue-cone spectral sensitivity in eyes with high myopia as estimated by the flash VECP. *Folia Ophthalmol Jpn* 1995; 46:535–539.
11. Koike A, Tokoro T: Spectral sensitivities in high myopic eyes. *J Jpn Ophthalmol Soc* 1986; 90:556–560.
12. Lachapelle P, Little JM, Polomeno RC: The photopic electroretinogram in congenital stationary night blindness with myopia. *Invest Ophthalmol Vis Sci* 1983; 24:442–450.
13. Lemagne JM, Gagne S, Cortin P: Resistance in clinical electroretinography: Its role in amplitude variability. *Can J Ophthalmol* 1982; 17:67–69.
14. Miyake Y, Yagasaki K, Horiguchi M, Kawase Y, Kanda T: Congenital stationary night blindness with negative electroretinogram: A new classification. *Arch Ophthalmol* 1986; 104:1013–1020.

15. Pallin O: The influence of the axial length of the eye on the size of the recorded b-wave potential in the clinical single-flash electroretinogram. *Acta Ophthalmol* 1969; 101 (suppl):1–57.

16. Perlman I, Meyer E, Haim T, Zonis S: Retinal function in high refractive error assessed electroretinographically. *Br J Ophthalmol* 1984; 68:79–84.

17. Ponte F: *Boll Oculist* 1962; 41:739–746.

18. Prijot E, Colmant I, Marechal-Courtois C: Electroretinography and myopia. In Francois J (ed): *The Clinical Value of Electroretinography: XXth International Congress of Ophthalmology.* Basel/New York, Karger, 1966, pp 440–443.

19. Uchida A: Studies of electrical activities of the eye in high myopia. *Nippon Ganka Gakkai Zasshi* 1977; 81(9):1328–1350.

20. Weleber RG, Kennaway NG: Gyrate atrophy of the choroid and retina. In Heckenlively JR (ed): *Retinitis Pigmentosa.* Lippincott, Philadelphia, 1988, pp 198–220.

21. Westall CA, Dhaliwal HS, Panton CM, Sigesmun D, Levin AV, Nischal KK, Heon E: Values of electroretinogram responses according to axial length. *Doc Ophthalmol* 2001; 102:115–130.

22. Yamamoto S, Nitta K, Kamiyama M: Cone electroretinogram to chromatic stimuli in myopic eyes. *Vision Res* 1997; 37:2157–2159.

51 Electrodiagnostic Testing in Malingering and Hysteria

GRAHAM E. HOLDER

SUSPECTED FUNCTIONAL visual loss is commonly encountered in routine clinical practice and often presents a challenge to the ophthalmologist. The main role of electrophysiology is to provide objective evidence of normal retinal and/or intracranial visual pathway function in the presence of subjective reports that suggest otherwise. In some patients, it is not possible to distinguish between malingering and hysteria; in others, there is little doubt. A clinical review of functional visual loss has addressed the diagnostic distinctions.[20] The term *nonorganic visual loss* is preferred, particularly if volitional aspects are uncertain.

It was commented in the first edition of this volume that although the clinical value of electrophysiology in the diagnosis of nonorganic visual loss was widely accepted, there were relatively few reports in the literature.[15] That remains the case. The first report appears to be that of Potts and Nagaya,[25] who reported that patients with hysterical amblyopia had normal foveal visual evoked potentials (VEP) to a 0.06-degree flashing red stimulus, whereas patients with strabismic amblyopia showed diminished or absent responses. The use of diffuse flash stimulation was also described by Arden's group,[1] and those authors cautioned against the unequivocal acceptance of electrophysiological criteria, citing one case of almost certain hysterical amblyopia in which scotopic flash VEP (FVEP) anomalies were observed. It is the case, however, that functional overlay superimposed on underlying organic dysfunction may be encountered. Subsequent reports, though mostly anecdotal, confirmed the finding of normal FVEPs in nonorganic visual loss.[2,3,11,22] The use of the FVEP in assisting disclose the nonorganic basis of suspect symptoms following trauma was also described.[21]

However, although the use of a luminance stimulus may be satisfactory in the evaluation of hysterical total blindness, which is not usually difficult to ascertain clinically, a contrast stimulus is necessary to evaluate less severe reported deficits. Halliday[19] first described the use of the pattern-reversal VEP (PVEP) in hysterical visual loss, reporting normal, symmetrical PVEPs in both eyes of patients despite markedly asymmetrical visual acuity. The technique was thought to be most useful in unilateral visual loss in which the good eye acts as a control. It was also stressed that a normal PVEP, although

strongly suggestive of nonorganic visual loss, does not preclude the existence of some organic disease.

The early studies using flashed-pattern VEPs[12,13,26] found that the maximum response amplitude occurred with check sizes of 10–30 minutes of arc. Later studies with pattern reversal came to similar conclusions for small fields but further suggested an interrelationship between check size and field size.[8,23,24] Small checks and fields are better for foveal stimulation, large checks and large fields for more peripheral retina.

The clinical management of patients with nonorganic visual loss would be facilitated if a simple relationship between VEP measurements and visual acuity existed that enabled an objective assessment of acuity. Unfortunately, most scaling methods that use pattern reversal perform relatively poorly as predictors of acuity,[7] although Halliday and McDonald[10] suggested that a well-formed pattern-reversal VEP is incompatible with a visual acuity of ~6/36 or worse. Despite the problems, attempts to assess acuity objectively in patients who are suspected of nonorganic visual loss have been made. Wildberger[32] reported the findings in two groups of patients: 17 "malingerers" (mostly schoolgirls) with no signs of an organic lesion and 10 patients (accident or disease) with signs but marked overlay. The findings in the patients were compared with those obtained in normal subjects to the same four check sizes in relation to insertion of graded orthoptic filters intended to reduce the acuity. The VEPs were easily able to detect malingering in the second group of patients, in whom acuities were usually claimed to be markedly reduced, but were not sensitive in the first group with milder claimed reductions. The VEP was assessed with the offset amplitude of the P100 component (P100–N135); in this author's laboratories, the onset amplitude of the pattern-reversal VEP (N75–P100) seems more sensitive. It is probably advisable routinely to measure both parameters. A recent publication[33] reported the use of pattern-reversal VEP in 72 patients with functional visual loss, suggesting that the discrepancy between acuity estimated by VEP and the best performed visual acuity was less than three lines on a Snellen chart in 88% of patients.

The use of pattern-onset stimulation, rather than pattern reversal, was previously described to yield improved results

(G. B. Arden, personal communication; see also Holder[15]). This has been confirmed in the authors' laboratories (V. McBain, et al., unpublished data). It is recognized that the pattern-onset or appearance VEP (PaVEP) is more susceptible to blur than is the pattern-reversal VEP. This enables a more direct relationship to be established between visual acuity and the presence or absence of a response to small check sizes of varying contrast. In addition, the spatiotemporal tuning function of the PaVEP is simpler and correlates closely with contrast sensitivity,[17,19,24] and the responses are often of larger amplitude than in reversal VEPs.[24] Furthermore, if a short (e.g., 40 ms) appearance time is used, it is difficult for the patient to defocus the pattern voluntarily.[18] PaVEP results are generally superior to those obtained with reversal when the patient is deliberately trying to influence the results.

Technical factors in the recording of patients who are suspected of hysteria or malingering are of paramount importance but receive little attention. The patient may fail to fixate, may attempt to defocus, may attempt prolonged eye closure during blinking, and so on. PVEP changes have been reported under such conditions.[5,28,29] Direct observation of the patient, with the patient aware of such monitoring, will often result in improved compliance (figure 51.1). Careful observation of both the raw electroencephalographic (EEG) input and the developing average is advisable; the appearance of an alpha rhythm in the ongoing EEG may indicate a failure in concentration. Equally, a tendency for the P100 component to broaden or increase in latency in the acquired average suggests that accommodation or fixation is unsatisfactory. Verbal commands to the patient to concentrate and attend to the fixation mark (or the center of the screen if perception of the fixation mark is denied) may be beneficial. If all perception is denied with one eye, fixation can be obtained by using the better eye, and an instruction to "try to keep your eyes still" will surprisingly often produce good results following occlusion of this eye and prompt commencement of stimulation. It may be necessary to stop averaging after fewer sweeps than usual to prevent waveform deterioration. A tendency for the P100 component to sharpen and remain of stable or slightly reducing latency during acquisition of the average only occurs with good patient compliance; observation of a broadening of the peak and/or increase in P100 latency suggests poor patient compliance and demands intervention by the recordist. A subjective report of stimulus perception should be obtained from the patient in all cases. Marked discrepancies between the subjective reports and the objective electrophysiological findings can be useful in alerting the examiner to nonorganic visual loss, particularly if marked interocular perceptual asymmetries are unaccompanied by VEP asymmetries.

It is advisable to record the PERG. The PERG P50 component is very susceptible to deterioration with poor compliance, and a normal PERG can only be obtained with

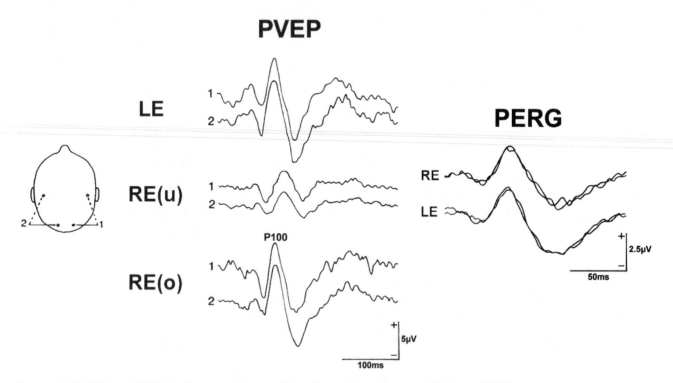

FIGURE 51.1 VEP and PERG findings in a 32-year-old female with reduced right visual acuity following trauma. Litigation was pending. Left eye findings (6/5) are normal. Ophthalmic examination was normal. Right eye PVEP was normal when the patient was aware that she was under direct observation [RE(o)] but delayed when she thought that she was unobserved [RE(u)].

satisfactory fixation, accommodation, and so on. Factors that affect the PERG are described elsewhere in this volume (see chapter 22). Equally, cases of mild maculopathy, with an unequivocally abnormal PERG, may sometimes have a PVEP within the normal range (Holder, unpublished observations); a normal PVEP should not therefore be presumed to preclude mild macular dysfunction. Rover and Bach[27] report the use of simultaneous recording of the PERG and PVEP to reveal malingering. Their patients complained of marked acuity loss, but only a few representative cases were discussed, and no quantitative patient data were presented. In particular, no mention was made as to whether their cases were bilateral or unilateral. A normal PERG and PVEP indicated malingering; a normal PERG and an abnormal PVEP indicated a "lesion of the visual pathway"; and an abnormal PERG and an abnormal PVEP indicated blurred image, poor cooperation, or retinal dysfunction.

Simultaneous PERG and PVEP can be particularly useful in unilateral cases; PVEP interpretation in a patient who is deliberately attempting to influence the results can be substantially improved by knowledge of the retinal response simultaneously recorded to the same stimulus. Binocular registration of the PERG, with the "good" eye enabling fixation, will usually reveal whether the PERG from the "bad" eye is abnormal or not (see figure 51.1). Significant macular dysfunction is excluded if the PERG from the bad eye is normal with binocular stimulation. If there is a unilateral PERG abnormality in the bad eye, the nature of the abnormality will indicate either ganglion cell/optic nerve or more distal dysfunction depending on whether the N95 or P50 component of the PERG is affected[16] (see chapter 22).

Routine ERG should also be performed; ERGs can be markedly abnormal in retinal dysfunction with no or minimal fundus abnormality but constricted visual fields, and field loss is often a feature of nonorganic visual loss. PERG and PVEP findings may be normal in such conditions if the maculae are spared. However, because normal PVEPs may be found in patients with cortical blindness, particular care should be taken before making the diagnosis of nonorganic visual loss if the symptoms suggest possible cortical dysfunction. Celesia's group[6] studied a 72-year-old woman with bilateral destruction of area 17 and attributed the

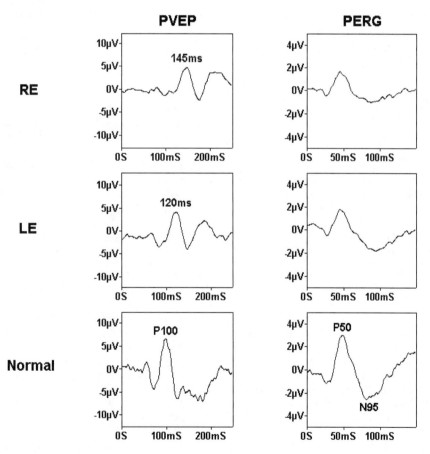

FIGURE 51.2 Electrophysiological findings in a 43-year-old female with a one-month history of sudden painless visual loss in the right eye. Ophthalmic examination was normal. The patient had a mother and sister who had previously had optic neuritis as part of multiple sclerosis, and it was suspected that the visual loss was nonorganic. The PVEPs from both right and left eyes are delayed; the lack of relative afferent pupillary defect presumably relating to the subclinical demyelination in the asymptomatic left optic nerve. Note the mild relative N95 reduction in the PERG from the right eye compared with the left.

presence of normal VEPs to conduction in extrageniculo-calcarine pathways. Bodis-Wollner et al.[4] reported normal VEPs in a 6-year-old boy with destruction of areas 18 and 19 but preservation of area 17. Similarly, retrochiasmal lesions may not give a PVEP abnormality even with a demonstrable field defect (see chapter 78). Evaluation of the P300 component may circumvent such problems.[30]

To conclude, electrodiagnostic testing is invaluable in the detection or confirmation of nonorganic visual loss, particularly if it is unilateral, so one eye can be judged against the other. Although the reader is reminded of the warning of Halliday[9] that normal electrophysiology does not preclude the presence of some underlying organic disease, the demonstration of normal electrophysiology can be reassuring, both for the clinician and, if the patient is a child, for concerned parents. Particular caution must be exercised if there is a possibility of cortical dysfunction. The most challenging patients are probably those with functional overlay superimposed on genuine underlying organic dysfunction. It is essential that an accurate history is taken and comprehensive ophthalmic and neurological examination performed; particular techniques for revealing functional deficit have been described in full elsewhere.[31] Electrophysiological examination is always advisable if there is any doubt. The objective nature of electrodiagnostic testing may not only demonstrate normal visual pathway function in patients whose symptoms suggest otherwise, but also reveal the presence of organic dysfunction in a patient with a presumed diagnosis of nonorganic visual loss (figure 51.2).

REFERENCES

1. Adams WL, Arden GB, Behrman J: Responses of human visual cortex following excitation of peripheral rods: Some applications in the clinical diagnosis of functional and organic visual defects. *Br J Ophthalmol* 1969; 53:439–452.
2. Beck EC, Dustman RE, Lewis EG: The use of the averaged evoked potential in the evaluation of central nervous system disorders. *Int J Neurol* 1975; 9:211–232.
3. Berman MS, Levi DM: Hysterical amblyopia: Electrodiagnostic and clinical evaluation. *Am J Optom Physiol Opt* 1975; 52:267–274.
4. Bodis-Wollner I, Atkin A, Raab E, et al: Visual association cortex and vision in man: Pattern evoked occipital potentials in a blind boy. *Science* 1977; 198:629–631.
5. Bumgarten J, Epstein CM: Voluntary alteration of visual evoked potentials. *Ann Neurol* 1982; 12:475–478.
6. Celesia GG, Archer CR, Kuroiwa Y, et al: Visual function of the extrageniculocalcarine system in man: Relationship to cortical blindness. *Arch Neurol* 1980; 37:704–706.
7. Chan H, Odom TV, Coldren L, et al: Acuity estimates by visually evoked potentials is affected by scaling. *Doc Ophthalmol* 1986; 62:107–117.
8. Erwin CW: Pattern reversal evoked potentials. *Am J Electroencephalogr Technol* 1981; 20:161–184.
9. Halliday AM: Evoked responses in organic and functional sensory loss. In Fessard A, LeLord G (eds): *Activities Evoquees et Leur Conditionnement Chez L'Homme Normal et en Pathologie Mentale.* Paris, Institut National de la Sante et de la Recherche Medicale, 1973, pp 189–212.
10. Halliday AM, McDonald WI: Visual evoked potentials. In Stalberg E, Young RR (eds): *Neurology 1: Clinical Neurophysiology.* London, Butterworths, 1981, pp 228–258.
11. Harding GFA: The visual evoked response. *Adv Ophthalmol* 1974; 28:2–28.
12. Harter MR, White CT: Effects of contour sharpness and check size on visually evoked cortical potentials. *Vision Res* 1968; 8:701–711.
13. Harter MR, White CT: Evoked cortical responses to checkerboard patterns: Effect of check size as a function of visual acuity. *Electroencephalogr Clin Neurophysiol* 1970; 28:48–53.
14. Holder GE: Significance of abnormal pattern electroretinography in anterior visual pathway dysfunction. *Br J Ophthalmol* 1987; 71:166–171.
15. Holder GE: Electrodiagnostic testing in malingering and hysteria. In Heckenlively JR, Arden GB (eds): *Principles and Practice of Clinical Electrophysiology of Vision.* St. Louis, Mosby Year Book, 1991, pp 573–577.
16. Holder GE: The pattern electroretinogram and an integrated approach to visual pathway diagnosis. *Prog Ret Eye Res* 2001; 20:531–561.
17. Howe JW, Mitchell KW: The objective assessment of contrast sensitivity by electrophysiological means. *Br J Ophthalmol* 1984; 68:626–638.
18. Howe JW, Mitchell KW, Robson C: Electrophysiological assessment of visual acuity. *Trans Ophthalmol Soc UK* 1981; 101:105–108.
19. Jetzel J, Parry N: Minimising the effects of spatial non-linearities on VEP estimation of resolution limit. *ARVO Abstracts* 2001; 42:4584.
20. Kathol RG, Cox TA, Corbett JJ, et al: Functional visual loss: 1. A true psychiatric disorder? *Psychol Med* 1983; 13:307–314.
21. Kooi KA, Yamada T, Marshall RE: Binocular and monocular visual evoked potential in the differential diagnosis of psychogenic and disease related disorders. *Int J Neurol* 1975; 9:272–286.
22. Lazurus GM: A clinical application of the visual evoked potential in the diagnosis of ophthalmic and neuroophthalmic pathology: Organic and functional lesions. *Am Optom Assoc* 1974; 45:1056–1063.
23. Meredith JT, Celesia GG: Pattern reversal visual evoked potentials and retinal eccentricity. *Electroencephalogr Clin Neurophysiol* 1982; 53:243–253.
24. Parry NRA, Murray IJ, Hadjzenonous C: Spatio-temporal tuning of VEPs: Effect of mode of stimulation. *Vision Res* 1999; 39:3491–3497.
25. Potts AM, Nagaya T: Studies on the visual evoked response: III. Strabismus amblyopia and hysterical amblyopia. *Doc Ophthalmol* 1969; 26:394–402.
26. Rietveld WJ, Tordoir WEM, Hagenouw JR, et al: Visual evoked responses to blank and to checkerboard patterned flashes. *Acta Physiol Pharmacol Neerl* 1967; 14:259–285.
27. Rover J, Bach M: Pattern electroretinogram plus visual evoked potential: A decisive test in patients suspected of malingering. *Doc Ophthalmol* 1987; 66:245–251.
28. Sokol S, Moskowitz A: Effect of retinal blur on the peak latency of the pattern evoked potential. *Vision Res* 1981; 21:1279–1286.

29. Tan CT, Murray NMF, Sawyers D, et al.: Deliberate alteration of the visual evoked potential. *J Neurol Neurosurg Psych* 1984; 47:518–523.

30. Towle VL, Sutcliffe E, Sokol S: Diagnosing functional visual deficits with the P300 component of the visual evoked potential. *Arch Ophthalmol* 1985; 103:47–50.

31. Walsh FB, Hoyt WF: The ocular signs of neurasthenia, hysteria, malingering, and the psychoses. In Walsh FB, Hoyt WF (eds): *Clinical Neuroophthalmology*. Baltimore, Williams & Wilkins, 1969, pp 2519–2537.

32. Wildberger H: Contrast evoked notentials in the evaluation of suspected malingering. *Doc Ophthalmol Proc Ser* 1981; 27:425–430.

33. Xu S, Meyer D, Yoser S, Mathews D, Elfervig JL. Pattern visual evoked potential in the diagnosis of functional visual loss. *Ophthalmology* 2001; 108:76–80.

34. Yiannakis C, Walsh JC: The variation of the pattern shift visual evoked response with the size of the stimulus field. In Chiappa KH (ed): *Evoked Potentials in Clinical Medicine*. New York, Raven Press, 1983, p 51.

52 Developmental Amblyopia

DOROTHY THOMPSON

AMBLYOPES CAN demonstrate many and various visual deficits, involving loss of spatial range, contrast and positional deficits (reviewed by Hess[46]), but the most widely accepted clinical definition of amblyopia is based on visual acuity. This suggests that amblyopia is a unilateral or bilateral decrease of visual acuity caused by a deprivation of form vision and/or an abnormal binocular interaction (usually early in life) for which no organic causes can be detected by physical examination of the eye and which, in appropriate cases, is reversible by therapeutic measures.[117]

Estimates of the prevalence of amblyopia are wide-ranging; it is said to affect between 1.6% and 3.5% of the population. This variation reflects the nature of the population studies from which the data are derived[88] and the arbitrary defining of amblyopia as two or more lines interocular difference on a recognition chart or more than one octave interocular difference, and the difficulty of clinically untangling subcategories of amblyopia. Subcategories, which relate to the etiology of amblyopia,[22] were introduced in an attempt to explain the varying degrees of success in amblyopia therapy.

The subcategories of functional amblyopia in which no organic lesion exists are broadly as follows:

1. Stimulus deprivation amblyopia, for example, due to media opacity (and occlusion amblyopia, the iatrogenic visual loss of the good eye after patching)
2. Strabismus amblyopia
3. Anisometropic amblyopia
4. Refractive or isometropia amblyopia with bilateral high refractive error (this includes meridional amblyopia)
5. Psychogenic amblyopia, a visual conversion reaction (treated separately in chapter 51)

Organic amblyopias, such as those due to nutritional or toxic effects, are dealt with separately in chapters 54 and 55.

Screening

In a population under 20 years of age, amblyopia is ten times more common a cause of visual loss than all other causes taken together.[40] Yet there is an absence of any rigorous clinical trials to demonstrate the worth of treatment or the impact on the quality of life of no treatment.[113] This has triggered a vigorous debate about the effectiveness of screening for amblyopia (e.g., at the Novartis meeting in the United Kingdom in 1999),[11] and has driven different international responses, governed, it seems, by public health resource and private insurance issues.[74] The outcome of these studies should begin to become available in the next few years and, it is hoped, will allow evidence-based decisions about screening to be reached.[16,49]

Within this general discussion, there is consensus that earlier detection has a better chance of remedy.[120] Of importance, only a minority of patients (10% of 253 patients) who lose their fellow eye after 11 years of age will subsequently show any improvement in the amblyopic eye.[86] Indeed, the projected lifetime risk of visual loss to an individual with amblyopia less than 6/12, or driving standard vision, is 1.2%, higher than was previously thought.[87] The outcome of therapy appears to be stable at least for anisometropia,[33,83] which prognostically has a better visual outcome and shows less sensitivity to the patient's age at presentation. Recent recommendations have suggested treatment for anisometropic amblyopia whatever the age.[28]

There continues to be some despair at both the lack of methods robust enough to reliably detect amblyopia in restless toddlers and the lack of coherence between centers using different test procedures.[58] Attempts are now being made to standardize ways in which individual tests are administered in different centers (e.g., Holmes et al.[48] and the HOTV test), but the range of behavioral tests for children is suboptimal for the detection of strabismic amblyopia,[35,91] for which crowded recognition acuity tests are best.[72] Testing visual acuity in young children is inherently noisy[59] and is all the more difficult because any measurements are taken on a moving staircase of visual maturation.[31] Some methods have reported interocular differences as little as 1/4 octave (e.g., Hamer et al.[41] reporting on sweep VEPs), and others recount difficulties in securing a reliable measure of interocular difference less than one octave.[10]

The site of amblyopia

The neurophysiological basis of amblyopia is still not fully understood. Amblyopia manifests as loss of spatial properties of neurons in the primary visual cortex, but there are almost certainly additional deficits at higher levels of the visual pathways.[2,45,54,60,65] There have been some discrepant reports that V1 might not be involved, such as early PET[30] and fMRI studies,[98] but other imaging studies provide evidence of deficits in V1, fMRI,[1,15] and MEG data.[2] These authors suggest that the discrepancies have arisen largely because of differences in the chosen stimuli, the temporal resolution of the techniques, and selecting patients with differing depths of amblyopia.

Evidence for a primary retinal involvement in amblyopia, suggested by animal work,[52] has not been substantiated (reviewed by Hess[45] and Simons[97]), and the flash electroretinogram (ERG) is normal in amblyopia.[56,75,123] Recently, Williams and Papkostopoulos[121] described a reduced electro-oculogram from amblyopic eyes (12 adults), implicating retinal pigment epithelial involvement in amblyopia. The authors speculate that this might reflect a deficiency in retinal dopaminergic function. Following levodopa (L-dopa) therapy in adult amblyopes and controls, there have been changes in spatial sensitivity related to both retinal and cortical changes.[37,38] Regression of visual acuity is similar in children who are given L-dopa and occlusion or occlusion alone, but Leguire et al.[64] suggest that the initial acuity gain after L-dopa therapy may beneficially reset the acuity baseline and produce a longer-term advantage. Pattern ERGs (PERGs) have been reported to be diminished in amblyopia,[8,9,84,107] but in other studies, when stimulus contrast and the retina area stimulated were compensated to provide good-sized PERGs, there was no difference between the amblyopic eye and the fellow eye.[39,45,47,48]

For the purposes of clinical detection, amblyopia is regarded as a predominantly cortical effect, and pattern visual evoked potentials (VEPs) are the electrophysiological test of choice. The amplitude attenuation and latency changes that are seen in association with amblyopia lend electrophysiological support to involvement of V1.[93]

Visual evoked potentials in amblyopia

There are three amblyopia challenges in clinical visual electrodiagnostic practice: whether VEPs can identify amblyopia and distinguish it from other causes of visual loss, whether VEPs can predict if the amblyopia is likely to respond to treatment, and whether VEPs can monitor the effect of patching treatment. Because amblyopia is frequently defined by the "bottom line," that is, the best recognition acuity at high contrast and luminance, many VEP studies have been directed toward making rapid assessment of the VEP acuity of each eye.[116] An alternative strategy is to assess the disruption to binocularity caused by reduced uniocular vision, but accounting for anomalous retinal correspondence can make this a complex task.

Interocular VEP differences

In amblyopia, pattern VEPs tend to be of reduced amplitude,[13,62,70,106,108] with increased latency to smaller check sizes,[6,118] akin to the effect of uncorrected refractive error.[73] Levi and Harwerth[66] showed that slopes of the regression of VEP amplitude versus stimulus contrast (below saturation) had a lower slope in the amblyopic eye than the fellow eye and suggest that this can demonstrate how amblyopia differs from optical blurring.[90]

Illiakis et al.[53] have suggested that the presence of pVEPs of normal latency, just smaller in amplitude, prior to occlusion has a better prognosis for eventual visual outcome (see also Hoyt[51]). This was related to central fixation. Others have found limited prognostic value in pattern-reversal VEPs.[34,43] However, Good et al.[36] have cautioned that pattern-reversal VEP grating acuity is superior to pattern ON/OFF grating acuity in detecting amblyopia. Pattern ON/OFF VEPs in amblyopia are found to be similar to those recorded when the central 3 degrees of visual field are occluded.[108] Shawkat et al.[95] further demonstrated that amblyopia can be detected with increased sensitivity if components of known macula predominance are measured, such as the n80 and p100 of the reversal VEP and, to a lesser extent, the onset contralateral p105 and CIII.

Recently, Davies et al.[29] have distinguished early- from late-onset strabismic amblyopes on the basis of the latency of the pattern onset VEP CII in adults. Those with earlier-onset amblyopia tended to have pVEP CII components of earlier latency and smaller amplitude in both eyes compared with normals. Late-onset strabismic amblyopes had attenuated pVEPs of markedly increased latency from the amblyopic eye, while the fellow eye was within normal range. Davies et al.[29] suggest that this could reflect an enhancement of magnocellular contribution relative to parvocellular contribution. (CII shows almost complete interocular transfer thought to relate to a prestriate origin and greater proportion of binocularly driven cells, in contrast to CI.[103]) Others have reported motion-onset VEPs are relatively robust compared to pattern-reversal VEPs in amblyopia,[61] and there is a report of an isolated reduction of P-stimuli steady-state responses in anisometropic amblyopia.[94] Alternatively, it is possible that an alteration in a preceding component of a composite waveform, such as the pattern-onset VEP, could also result in a shorter CII latency peak.

Vision measures using pattern VEPs

It is unrealistic to expect pattern VEP acuity assessment to correlate directly to behavioral measures. Resolution and recognition acuity demand different levels of processing and are influenced by different factors. The pattern-reversal VEP is a direct reflection of neural activation, or the extent of neural network stimulated per eye by the afferent impulses in V1, rather than an assessment of how these visual data are then processed by other areas. The distinction between the pathways tested by each acuity method is exceptionally important. There can be striking clinical discrepancies; for example, it is possible in optic atrophy to obtain fairly good 6/9–6/12 acuity yet for the pattern VEP to be very small and degraded. This may be explained if the few remaining functioning fibers are clustered sufficiently well centrally to give 6/9 at high contrast and good luminance but the overall volume of activation of the brain and the reduced VEP spatial frequency profile; normally the relation between VEP amplitude and pattern size has a "bandpass" function that causes considerable deficits in VEP. This indicates a significant deficit of cortical innervation that suggests that the patient will experience visual difficulties under less than optimal conditions. VEP abnormalities in amblyopia can persist despite normal acuity.[119] The spatial profile of the pattern VEP tends to be flattened in the amblyopic eye and the fellow eye if occlusion therapy has been carried out.[82]

Interocular differences in VEP amplitude and latency in normals are on the order of 10%.[3,104] Interocular differences in amplitude identify amblyopes with sensitivity between 46% and 85%. This is improved if amplitude is used in conjunction with latency.[105] Weiss and Kelly[119] noted a better prediction of final visual acuity if they made a linear combination of latencies of pattern-onset VEPs across three spatial frequencies. Occasionally, the amplitude of the amblyopic eye exceeds that of the fellow eye,[35,110] and a history of occlusion therapy and pressure of eccentric fixation then becomes very important in the analysis. Certainly, one measure is inadequate to detect amblyopia, and it is essential to assess a range of stimulus sizes.[80]

Effects of latent nystagmus and patching on pattern VEP

If there has been disruption to binocularity early on in life, monocular pattern VEP testing can be confounded by latent nystagmus (figure 52.1). This can in part be overcome by head positioning, by placing the eye that is being tested in adduction, and by using pattern-onset stimuli, but occasionally, the nystagmus will be too coarse for these strategies to compensate, and pattern VEPs will be confounded.

Similarly, when the effect of occlusion therapy is being monitored, a child will often attend wearing the patch. A few hours of patching will increase the response of the unoccluded eye in normals[116] and diminish the response of the patched eye.[6,7,81] It is possible that an interocular pattern VEP difference may decrease because the fellow eye response is diminished by patching rather than the amblyopic eye being improved. With prolonged occlusion, such as the extensive early occlusion used for unilateral cataract

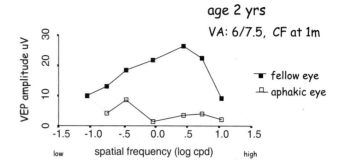

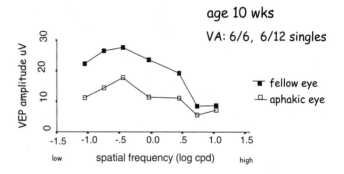

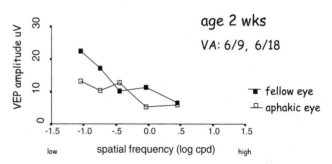

FIGURE 52.1 These three graphs are pattern-reversal VEP spatial tuning profiles for three patients operated on at 2 years, 10 weeks, and 2 weeks of age, respectively, for congenital cataract. The two patients operated on at 10 weeks and 2 weeks followed a patching regime of at least 50% of waking hours in the first year of life. Of note, the fellow eye acuities are similar, yet the spatial profiles of the fellow eye pattern VEP tuning are very different, changing from a bandpass function in the top trace to a broader bandpass with a lower spatial frequency peak in the second trace (patient operated on at 10 weeks) and becomes a low-pass function in the patient operated on at 2 weeks. This demonstrates the possible iatrogenic amblyogenic effect of early patching on the fellow eye and illustrates the importance of testing several spatial frequencies to uncover the extent of amblyopic loss rather than relying on the threshold measurement.

treatment, the changes to the fellow eye can be profound and in our experience sometimes irreversible.[115] It becomes important to compare the profile of spatial responses for both eyes across visits, noting the hours of pretest occlusion.

Threshold measurements of VEP acuity

To gain a threshold measurement, i.e., a VEP "acuity" measure, an extrapolation of the spatial profile of small check responses to baseline or noise level is necessary (e.g., Chan et al.[23]). In a group that was treated for congenital cataract, threshold check size was the only VEP parameter that correlated with single-letter visual acuity. This led to a suggestion that threshold check size may have greater clinical use than measures of pattern VEPs based on latency, amplitude, or waveform.[71]

Transient pattern-reversal and pattern-onset VEPs need 20–40 s of fixation per stimulus size, and a spatial profile may take 5–10 minutes per eye to acquire. Attempts have been made to speed things up with presentation rates approaching 8 Hz or 16 reversals per second with sweep techniques running through a series of different pattern sizes every second.[77,89,116] There are theoretical advantages that suggest that the regression to a threshold, either noise level or baseline, should be amplitude independent. Yet it is very difficult to regress low-amplitude signals, as might be recorded in amblyopia, with confidence. Also, sweep VEP stimulation rates are fast, and as the temporal frequency increases, the correlation with recognition acuity diminishes.[36,44] The spatiotemporal tuning profile that the sweep techniques tap into will not be at the high-recognition, static acuity range of older children. This is one of the reasons why the correlation of behavioral visual acuity matures with electrophysiological or sweep measures is higher in the first year, after which behavioral measures exceed the sweep VEP. The net result is an underestimate of high acuity and an overestimate of low acuity—the converse of the optimum that is required to detect mild amblyopia.

Vernier acuity

Vernier acuity is a hyperacuity measure that can take until 10 years of age to mature. As a positional acuity, it is considered the most sensitive measure of amblyopic deficit because it usually produces the greatest magnitude of deficit in comparison to other spatial measures (reviewed by Simmers et al.[96]). Transient vernier-offset VEPs are confounded by simultaneous motion stimulus. Levi et al.[67] noted that breaking collinearity elicited a greater response than the transition from noncollinearity to collinearity. This asymmetry uniquely manifests as odd harmonic components in the steady-state VEP. Skoczenski and Norcia[100] have reported steady-state recording of vernier-offset VEPs, distinct from the motion response, elicited by horizontal disparity of a vertical square wave grating in normal infants, but this has not yet been applied in amblyopia. Stereoscopic VEPs are also possible by using these techniques but are of small amplitude.[24,78]

As an alternative approach to measuring interocular differences in VEPs, there have been attempts to study the binocular consequences of amblyopia, i.e., suppression, lack of stereopsis, and fusion. This has been done indirectly with motion VEPs that show a nasotemporal asymmetry in normal infants of 2–3 months old that diminishes by 6–8 months. This shows a strong concordance with fusion.[19] Other, more direct studies are described below, but as yet, none of these techniques have proved to be a robust clinical screening method.

Binocular VEPs

There is a hierarchy of tests to assess binocular interaction that relies on (1) comparing monocular with binocular elicited VEPs, (2) using dichoptic stimulation to independently control the input of each eye and look at the resultant combination, and (3) cyclopean stimuli with, for example, random dot stereograms.

Binocular Summation and Facilitation   Binocular and monocular preferential looking (PL) acuity are comparable during the first 4–6 months; after this, binocular acuity is superior (reviewed by Birch[17]). VEPs to binocular stimulation (both eyes viewing the same stimulus) are greater, usually by the order of 1.4 (square root 2), than monocular responses, but there has been a large variation in findings owing to differences in stimuli, the VEP component measured, and electrode position.[4,5,63,70,90] If pattern VEPs are elicited by high-contrast patterns alone, the presence of summation cannot identify amblyopes. In general, summation is best seen to low-contrast (less than 40%), low-mean luminance, spatial frequencies less than 5 cycles per degree (cpd) and temporal frequencies less than 8 Hz.[11,26] Summation will be present with abnormal retinal correspondence but not with suppression.[25,79] At less than 6 months of age, binocular VEP acuity superiority is only 0.2 octaves; after this, monocular and binocular growth functions are almost identical.[41] When noted, even in subjects with normal vision, binocular summation has been termed *ephemeral*,[80] and an unreliable clinical index of normal binocularity.[67] Alternatively, the binocular response may be greater than the sum of the two monocular responses. This is called *binocular facilitation*.[12]

A reduction in binocular enhancement (1.6–1.2) of the pattern-reversal VEP during development has been reported to accompany increasing stereoacuity.[102] Others have suggested that the binocular advantage remains the same regardless of age.[114]

Dichoptic Stimulation   When two different stimuli are presented to each eye, the perception may be summation, suppression, or rivalry. Suppression is most easily observed if the same spatial frequency is presented to each eye at high contrast and luminance. Size-specific suppression of the VEP is abnormal in amblyopes. It is a more robust phenomenon than summation, but it is still inadequate to reliably detect in individual patients.[27,42,55,122]

Dichoptically presented stimuli may also test a hierarchy of binocular function:[99]

1. *Binocular fusion/dichoptic luminance or checkerboard stimuli.* Dichoptic checkerboard stimuli are regular checkerboard patterns that reverse at different rates or frequencies for each eye. Fourier analysis reveals beat VEPs generated at a nonlinear difference frequency that can come only from an interaction of monocular inputs; that is, this frequency is not present in the stimulation frequencies.[13,57,113] Stevens et al.[111] looked at dichoptic luminance beat VEPs and found that stereo-blind children had significantly lower dichoptic signal-to-noise ratios than did stereo-normal children. Sato et al.[92] have used pseudo-binary sequences dichoptically to record speedier simultaneous monocular VEPs and to remove any ambiguity induced by temporal correlation between eyes that may arise from analysis in the frequency domain.

2. *Dynamic random dot correlograms.* Correlograms are generated when moving random dot patterns that are presented to each eye alternate between two phases: correlated and anticorrelated.

3. *Dynamic random dot stereograms.* With the stereograms, portions of random dot patterns that are presented to each eye are shifted horizontally relative to each other at a fixed rate, alternately producing crossed and uncrossed binocular disparities. Subjectively, these patterns appear to shift in depth.

Data suggest that sensory fusion, when measured by VEP responses to dynamic random dot correlograms, is more robust than is stereopsis to abnormal binocular experience and support the notion that pathways processing correlated/anticorrelated stimuli might not completely overlap with pathways processing disparity information.[32] Skrandies[101] demonstrated with topographic techniques that higher visual processing areas are most likely involved in stereoscopic vision, for example, V2. Rivalry appears to become more prominent as the extrastriate regions are ascended, but it has not yet been resolved where in the brain rivalry occurs.[20]

In the human visual cortex, rivalry is undetectable by fMRI in Brodman's areas 17 and 18, is weak in area 19, and becomes increasingly prominent in frontoparietal cortex,[69] but in another study using stimuli of different contrast, area V1 was as active as other higher areas.[85] Lumer[68] suggests that a relative asynchrony in the timing of firing in V1 distinguishes conflicting from congruent stimuli.

It has been noted that binocular rivalry in human infants seems to develop rapidly over the same developmental period as do horizontal disparity and interocular correlation: age 3–5 months.[18] However, Brown et al.[21] have recently shown electrophysiologically that infants between 5 and 15 months of age do not demonstrate a VEP marker of physiological rivalry to dichoptically presented phase-reversing gratings despite the presence of binocular interactions. These electrophysiological data suggest that unlike stereopsis, rivalry does not require separate eye-of-origin information and appears to be a competition between percepts, that is, beyond binocular convergence, a higher-level mechanism compared to the interocular comparisons that are required for stereopsis. It is not yet clear how useful this higher-level test will be clinically.

Summary

Interocular assessment of pattern VEPs to assess the spatial profile of each eye before patching can indicate poor vision levels consistent with amblyopia.

Monitoring patching therapy demands a critical appraisal of amount and timing of pretest patching to account for the possible iatrogenic effects of patching.

Distinguishing amblyopia from other causes of postretinal dysfunctions depends on the relative effect and combination with other clinical data. This can be especially difficult when amblyopia is gross, for example, if it is of early onset and untreated.

REFERENCES

1. Algaze A, Roberts C, Leguire L, Schmalbrock P, Rogers G: Functional magnetic resonance imaging as a tool for investigating amblyopia in the human visual cortex: A pilot study. *J Am Assoc Pediatr Ophthalmol Strabismus* 2002; 6(5):300–308.
2. Anderson SJ: Functional neuroimaging in amblyopia. In Moseley M, Fielder A (eds): *Amblyopia: A Multidisciplinary Approach.* Oxford, UK, Butterworth Heineman, 2002, pp 43–67.
3. Amigo G, Fiorentini A, Pirchio M, Spinelli D: Binocular vision tested with visual evoked potentials in children and infants. *Invest Ophthalmol Vis Sci* 1978; 17:910–915.
4. Apkarian P, Levi D, Tyler CW: Binocular facilitation in the visual-evoked potential of strabismic amblyopes. *Am J Optom Physiol Opt* 1981; 58:820–830.
5. Apkarian PA, Nakayama K, Tyler CW: Binocularity in the human evoked potential: Facilitation, summation and suppression. *Electroencephalogr Clin Neurophysiol* 1981; 51:32–48.
6. Arden GB, Barnard WM: Effect of occlusion on the visual evoked response in amblyopia. *Trans Ophthalmol Soc U K* 1979; 99:419–426.
7. Arden GB, Barnard WM, Mushin AS: Visually evoked responses in amblyopia. *Br J Ophthalmol* 1974; 58:183–192.
8. Arden GB, Vaegan, Hogg CR, Powell D, Carter RM: Pattern ERGs are abnormal in most amblyopes. *Trans Ophthalmol Soc* 1980; 308:82–83.
9. Arden GB, Wooding SL: Pattern ERG in amblyopia. *Invest Ophthalmol Vis Sci* 1985; 26:88–96.

10. Atkinson J: Discussion. In Moseley M, Fielder A (eds): *Amblyopia: A Multidisciplinary Approach*. Oxford, UK, Butterworth Heineman, 2002, p 138.

11. Bagolini B, Porciatti V, Falsini B: Binocular interaction and steady-state visual evoked potentials: I. A study in normal subjects and in subjects with defective binocular vision. *Graefes Arch Clin Exp Ophthalmol* 1988; 226:401–406.

12. Bagolini B, Falsini B, Cermola S, Porciatti V: Binocular interactions and steady-state VEPs. A study in normal and defective binocular vision (Part II). *Graefes Arch Clin Exp Ophthalmol* 1994; 232(12):737–744.

13. Baitch LW, Levi DM: Evidence for nonlinear binocular interactions in human visual cortex. *Vision Res* 1988; 28(10):1139–1143.

14. Barris MD, Dawson WW, Trick LR: LASCER Bode plots for normal, amblyopic, and stereoanomalous observers. *Doc Ophthalmol* 1981; 51:347–363.

15. Barnes GR, Hess RF, Dumoulin SO, Achtman RL, Pike GB: The cortical deficit in humans with strabismic amblyopia. *J Physiol* 2001; 533:281–297.

16. Beck RW: Clinical research in pediatric ophthalmology: The Pediatric Eye Disease Investigator Group. *Curr Opin Ophthalmol* 2002; 13(5):337–340.

17. Birch E: Stereopsis in infants and its developmental relation to visual acuity. In Simons K (ed): *Early Visual Development, Normal and Abnormal*. New York, Oxford University Press, 1993, pp 224–236.

18. Birch E, Petrig B: FPL and VEP measures of fusion, stereopsis and stereoacuity in normal infants. *Vision Res* 1996; 36(9):1321–1327.

19. Birch EE, Fawcett S, Stager D: Co-development of VEP motion response and binocular vision in normal infants and infantile esotropes. *Invest Ophthalmol Vis Sci* 2000; 41:1719–1723.

20. Blake R, Logothetis NK: Visual competition. *Nat Rev Neurosci* 2002; 3(1):13–21.

21. Brown RJ, Candy TR, Norcia AM: Development of rivalry and dichoptic masking in human infants. *Invest Ophthalmol Vis Sci* 1999; 40(13):3324–3333.

22. Campos EC, Prampolini ML, Gulli R: Contrast sensitivity differences between strabismic and anisometropic amblyopia: Objective correlate by means of visual evoked responses. *Doc Ophthalmol* 1984; 58:45–50.

23. Chan H, Odom JV, Coldren J, Dove C, Chao GM: Acuity estimated by visually evoked potentials is affected by scaling. *Doc Ophthalmol* 1986; 62:107–117.

24. Chao GM, Odom JV, Karr D: Dynamic stereoacuity: Comparison of normal and stereoblind observers' electrophysiological and psychophysical responses. *Doc Ophthalmol* 1988; 70:45–58.

25. Chiesi C, Sargentini AD, Bokani R: Binocular visual perception in strabismics studied by means of visual evoked responses. *Doc Ophthalmol* 1984; 58:51–56.

26. Ciganek L: Binocular addition of the visually evoked response with different stimulus intensities in man. *Vision Res* 1970; 10:479–487.

27. Ciganek L: Binocular addition of the visual response evoked by dichoptic patterned stimuli. *Vision Res* 1971; 11:1289–1297.

28. Cobb CJ, Russell K, Cox A, MacEwen CJ: Factors influencing visual outcome in anisometropic amblyopes. *Br J Ophthalmol* 2002; 86(11):1278–1281.

29. Davis AR, Sloper JJ, Neveu MM, Hogg CR, Morgan MJ, Holder GE: Electrophysiological and psychophysical differences between early- and late-onset strabismic amblyopia. *Invest Ophthalmol Vis Sci* 2003; 44(2):610–617.

30. Demer JL, Noorden GK, Volkow ND, Gould KL: Imaging of cerebral blood flow and metabolism in amblyopia by positron emission tomography. *Am J Ophthalmol* 1988; 105:337–347.

31. Dobson V: Visual acuity testing in infants from laboratory to clinic. In Simons K (ed): *Early Visual Development, Normal and Abnormal*. New York, Oxford University Press, 1993, pp 318–334.

32. Eizenman M, Westall CA, Geer I, Smith K, Chatterjee S, Panton CM, Kraft SP, Skarf B: Electrophysiological evidence of cortical fusion in children with early-onset esotropia. *Invest Ophthalmol Vis Sci* 1999; 40(2):354–362.

33. FitzGerald DE, Krumholtz I: Maintenance of improvement gains in refractive amblyopia: A comparison of treatment modalities. *Optometry* 2002; 73(3):153–159.

34. Furuskog P, Persson HE, Wanger P: Subnormal visual acuity in children: Prognosis and visual evoked cortical potential findings. *Acta Ophthalmol* 1987; 65:648–652.

35. Geer I, Westall CA: A comparison of tests to determine acuity deficits in children with amblyopia. *Ophthalmic Physiol Opt* 1996; 16(5):367–374.

36. Good WV, Hou C, Norcia AM: Sweep VEP pattern reversal grating acuity is superior to on/off grating acuity for the detection of amblyopia. *Invest Ophthalmol Vis Sci* 2002; 43:2938.

37. Gottlob I, Charlier J, Reinecke RD: Visual acuities and scotomas after one week levodopa administration in human amblyopia. *Invest Ophthalmol Vis Sci* 1992; 33:2722–2728.

38. Gottlob I, Weghaupt H, Vass C, Auff E: Effect of levodopa on the human pattern electroretinogram and pattern visual evoked potentials. *Graefes Arch Clin Exp Ophthalmol* 1989; 227(5):421–427.

39. Gottlob I, Welge-Luessen L: Normal pattern electroretinograms in amblyopia. *Invest Ophthalmol Vis Sci* 1987; 28:187–191.

40. Grounds A: Amblyopia. In Barnard S, Edgar D (eds): *Pediatric Eye Care*. Oxford, Blackwell Science, 1998, pp 75–101.

41. Hamer RD, Norcia AM, Tyler CW, Hsu-Winges C: The development of monocular and binocular VEP acuity. *Vision Res* 1989; 29(4):397–408.

42. Harter MR: Binocular interaction: Evoked potentials to dichoptic stimulation. In Desmedt JM (ed): *Visual Evoked Potentials in Man: New Developments*. Oxford, UK, Clarendon Press, 1977.

43. Henc-Petrinovic L, Deban N, Gabric N, Petrinovic J: Prognostic value of visual evoked responses in childhood amblyopia. *Eur J Ophthalmol* 1993; 3(3):114–120.

44. Heravian SJ, Douthwaite WA, Jenkins TC: Acuity predictions from visually evoked potential to checkerboard pattern reversal stimuli: The effect of reversal rate. *Clin Exp Optom* 1999; 82(6):244–249.

45. Hess RF: Amblyopia: Site unseen. *Clin Exp Optom* 2001; 84:321–336.

46. Hess RF: Sensory processing in human amblyopia. In Moseley M, Fielder A (eds): *Amblyopia: A Multidisciplinary Approach*. Oxford, UK, Butterworth Heineman, 2002, pp 19–42.

47. Hess RF, Baker CL: Assessment of retinal function in severely amblyopic individuals. *Vision Res* 1984; 24:1367–1376.

48. Hess RF, Baker CL, Verhoeve JN, Keesey UT, France TD: The pattern evoked electroretinogram: Its variability in

normals and its relationship to amblyopia. *Invest Ophthalmol Vis Sci* 1985; 26:1610–1623.

49. Holmes JM, Beck RW, Repka MX: Amblyopia: Current clinical studies. *Ophthalmol Clin North Am* 2001; 14(3):393–398.

50. Holmes JM, Beck RW, Repka MX, Leske DA, Kraker RT, Blair RC, Moke PS, Birch EE, Saunders RA, Hertle RW, Quinn GE, Simons KA, Miller JM: Pediatric Eye Disease Investigator Group. The amblyopia treatment study visual acuity testing protocol. *Arch Ophthalmol* 2001; 119(9): 1345–1353.

51. Hoyt CS, Jastrzebski GB, Marg E: Amblyopia and congenital esotropia. *Arch Ophthalmol* 1984; 102:58–61.

52. Ikeda H, Tremain KE: Amblyopia occurs in retinal ganglion cells in cats reared with convergent squint without alternating fixation. *Exp Brain Res* 1979; 35:559–582.

53. Iliakis E, Moschos M, Hontos N, Tsalouki JK, Chimonidou E: The prognostic value of visual evoked response latency in the treatment of amblyopia caused by strabismus. *Doc Ophthalmol* 1996–97; 92(3):223–228.

54. Imamura K, Richter H, Fischer H, Lennerstrand G, Franzen O, Rydberg A, Andersson J, Schneider H, Onoe H, Watanabe Y, Langstrom B: Reduced activity in the extrastriate visual cortex of individuals with strabismic amblyopia. *Neurosci Lett* 1997; 225(3):173–176.

55. Jacobson SG, Sandberg MA, Effron MH, Berson EL: Foveal cone electroretinograms in strabismic amblyopia: Comparison with juvenile macular degeneration, macular scars, and optic atrophy. *Trans Ophthalmol Soc U K* 1979; 99:353–356.

56. Jacobsson P, Lennerstrand G: A comparison of different VEP methods for the assessment of binocular vision. *Doc Ophthalmol Proc Ser* 1981; 27:337–344.

57. Katsumi O, Peli E, Oguchi Y, Kawaras T: Effect of contrast on fusional visual evoked potential (VEP): Model and experimental results. *Am J Optom Physiol Opt* 1985; 62:233–239.

58. Kemper AR, Margolis PA, Downs SM, Bordley WC: A systematic review of vision screening tests for the detection of amblyopia. *Pediatrics* 1999; 104(5, Pt 2):1220–1222. Comment in *Pediatrics* 2001; 107(4):809.

59. Kheterpal S, Jones HS, Auld R, Moseley MJ: Reliability of visual acuity in children with reduced vision. *Ophthalmic Physiol Opt* 1996; 16(5):447–449.

60. Kiorpes L, McNee SP: Neural mechanisms underlying amblyopia. *Curr Opin Neurobiol* 1999; 9:480–486.

61. Kubova Z, Kuba M, Juran J, Blakemore C: Is the motion system relatively spared in amblyopia?: Evidence from cortical evoked responses. *Vision Res* 1996; 36(1):181–190.

62. Lawwill T: Electrophysiologic aspects of amblyopia. *Ophthalmology* 1978; 85:451–463.

63. Leguire LE, Fellows RR, Rogers GL, Burian HM: Binocular summation and facilitation of latency in flash and pattern VERs in 6 to 30 month old children. *Binoc Vis* 1987; 2:15–23.

64. Leguire LE, Komaromy KL, Nairus TM, Rogers GL: Long-term follow-up of L-dopa treatment in children with amblyopia. *J Pediatr Ophthalmol Strabismus* 2002; 39(6):326–330.

65. Levi DM: Pathophysiology of binocular vision and amblyopia. *Curr Opin Ophthalmol* 1994; 5(5):3–10.

66. Levi D, Harwerth R: Contrast evoked potentials in strabismic and anisometropic amblyopia. *Invest Ophthalmol Vis Sci* 1978; 17:571–575.

67. Levi DM, Manny RE, Klein S, Steinman SB: Electrophysiological correlates of hyperacuity in the human visual cortex. *Nature* 1983; 306:468–470.

68. Lumer ED: A neural model of binocular integration and rivalry based on the coordination of action potential timing in primary visual cortex. *Cereb Cortex* 1998; 8(6):553–561.

69. Lumer ED, Friston KJ, Rees G: Neural correlate of perceptual rivalry in the human brain. *Science* 1998; 280:1930–1934.

70. Manny RE, Levi DM: The visually evoked potential in humans with amblyopia: Pseudorandom modulation of uniform field and sine-wave gratings. *Exp Brain Res* 1982; 47:15–27.

71. McCulloch DL, Skarf B: Pattern reversal visual evoked potentials following early treatment of unilateral, congenital cataract. *Arch Ophthalmol* 1994; 112(4):510–518.

72. McGraw PV, Winn B, Gray LS, Elliott DB: Improving the reliability of visual acuity measures in young children. *Ophthalmic Physiol Opt* 2000; 20(3):173–184.

73. McKerral M, Lachapelle P, Tremblay F, Polomeno RC, Roy MS, Beneish R, Lepore F: Monocular contribution to the peak time of the binocular pattern visual evoked potential. *Doc Ophthalmol* 1995–96; 91(2):181–193.

74. Membreno JH, Brown MM, Brown GC, Sharma S, Beauchamp GR: A cost-utility analysis of therapy for amblyopia. *Ophthalmology* 2002; 109(12):2265–2271.

75. Miyake Y, Awaya S: Stimulus deprivation amblyopia: Simultaneous recording of local macular electroretinogram and visual evoked response. *Arch Ophthalmol* 1984; 102:998–1003.

76. Moseley M, Fielder A (eds): *Amblyopia: A Multidisciplinary Approach.* Oxford, Butterworth Heineman, 2001.

77. Moskowitz A, Sokol S, Hansen V: Rapid assessment of visual function in pediatric patients using pattern VEPs and acuity cards. *Clin Vis Sci* 1987; 2:11–20.

78. Norcia A: Improving infant evoked response measurement. In Simons K (ed): *Early Visual Development, Normal and Abnormal.* New York, Oxford University Press, 1993, pp 536–552.

79. Nuzzi G, Franchi A: Binocular interaction in visual evoked responses: Summation, facilitation and inhibition in a clinical study of binocular vision. *Ophthalmic Res* 1983; 15:261–264.

80. Odom JV: Amblyopia. In Arden G, Heckenliveley J (eds): *Clinical Electrophysiology,* St. Louis, Mosby Year Book, 1991, pp 589–593.

81. Odom JV, Hoyt CS, Marg E: Eye patching and visual evoked potential acuity in children four months to eight years old. *Am J Optom Physiol Opt* 1982; 59:706–717.

82. Ohn YH, Katsumi O, Matsui Y, Tetsuka H, Hirose T: Snellen visual acuity versus pattern reversal visual-evoked response acuity in clinical applications. *Ophthalmic Res* 1994; 26(4): 240–252.

83. Ohlsson J, Baumann M, Sjostrand J, Abrahamsson M: Long term visual outcome in amblyopia treatment. *Br J Ophthalmol* 2002; 86(10):1148–1151.

84. Persson HE, Wanger P: Pattern-reversal electroretinograms in squint amblyopia, artificial anisometropia, and simulated eccentric fixation. *Acta Ophthalmol* 1982; 60:123–132.

85. Polonsky A, Blake R, Braun J, Heeger DJ: Neuronal activity in human primary visual cortex correlates with perception during binocular rivalry. *Nat Neurosci* 2002; 3(11):1153–1159.

86. Rahi JS, Logan S, Borja MC, Timms C, Russell-Eggitt I, Taylor D: Prediction of improved vision in the amblyopic eye after visual loss in the non-amblyopic eye. *Lancet* 2002; 360(9333):621–622.

87. Rahi J, Logan S, Timms C, Russell-Eggitt I, Taylor D: Risk, causes, and outcomes of visual impairment after loss of vision in the non-amblyopic eye: A population-based study. *Lancet* 2002; 360(9333):597–602.

88. Reeves BC: Taxonomy and epidemiology of amblyopia. In Moseley M, Fielder A (eds): *Amblyopia: A Multidisciplinary Approach*. Oxford, UK, Butterworth Heineman, 2002, pp 68–80.

89. Regan D: Speedy assessment of visual acuity in amblyopia by the evoked potential method. *Ophthalmologica* 1977; 175: 159–164.

90. Regan D: *Human Brain Electrophysiology: Evoked Potentials and Evoked Magnetic Fields in Science and Medicine*. New York, Elsevier, 1989.

91. Rydberg A, Ericson B, Lennerstrand G, Jacobson L, Lindstedt E: Assessment of visual acuity in children aged 1 1/2–6 years, with normal and subnormal vision. *Strabismus* 1999; 7(1):1–24.

92. Sato E, Taniai M, Mizota A, Adachi-Usami E: Binocular interaction reflected in visually evoked cortical potentials as studied with pseudorandom stimuli. *Invest Ophthalmol Vis Sci* 2002; 43:3355–3358.

93. Schroeder CE, Tenke CE, Givre SJ, Arezzo JC, Vaughan HG Jr: Striate cortical contribution to the surface-recorded pattern-reversal VEP in the alert monkey. *Vision Res* 1991; 31(7–8):1143–1157. Erratum in *Vision Res* 1991; 31(11):1.

94. Shan Y, Moster ML, Roemer RA, Siegfried JB: Abnormal function of the parvocellular visual system in anisometropic amblyopia. *J Pediatr Ophthalmol Strabismus* 2000; 37(2):73–78.

95. Shawkat FS, Kriss A, Timms C, Taylor DS: Comparison of pattern-onset, -reversal and -offset VEPs in treated amblyopia. *Eye* 1998; 12(5):863–869.

96. Simmers AJ, Gray LS, McGraw PV, Winn B: Functional visual loss in amblyopia and the effect of occlusion therapy. *Invest Ophthalmol Vis Sci* 1999; 40:2859–2871.

97. Simons K: Stereoscopic neurontropy and the orginis of amblyopia and strabismus. In Simons K (ed): *Early Visual Development, Normal and Abnormal*. New York, Oxford University Press, 1993, pp 409–453.

98. Sireteanu R, Tonhausen N, Muckli L, et al: Cortical site of the amblyopia deficit in strabismic and anisometropic subjects investigated with fMRI. *Invest Ophthalmol Vis Sci* 1998; S909.

99. Skarf B, Eizenman M, Katz LM, Bachynski B, Klein R: A new VEP system for studying binocular single vision in human infants. *J Pediatr Ophthalmol Strabismus* 1993; 30(4): 237–242.

100. Skoczenski AM, Norcia AM: Development of VEP vernier acuity and grating acuity in human infants. *Invest Ophthalmol Vis Sci* 1999; 40(10):2411–2417.

101. Skrandies W: The processing of stereoscopic information in human visual cortex: Psychophysical and electrophysiological evidence. *Clin Electroencephalogr* 2001; 32(3):152–159.

102. Sloper JJ, Collins AD: Reduction in binocular enhancement of the visual-evoked potential during development accompanies increasing stereoacuity. *J Pediatr Ophthalmol Strabismus* 1998; 35(3):154–158.

103. Smith AT, Jeffreys DA: Evoked potential evidence for differences in binocularity between striate and prestriate regions of human visual cortex. *Exp Brain Res* 1979; 36:375–380.

104. Sokol S: Pattern visual evoked potentials: Their use in pediatric ophthalmology. *Int Ophthalmol Clin* 1980; 20:251–268.

105. Sokol S: Abnormal evoked potential latencies in amblyopia. *Br J Ophthalmol* 1983; 67:310–314.

106. Sokol S, Bloom B: Pattern reversal visually evoked potentials in infants. *Invest Ophthalmol Vis Sci* 1973; 12:936–939.

107. Sokol S, Nadler D: Simultaneous electroretinograms and visually evoked potentials from adult amblyopes in response to a patterned stimulus. *Invest Ophthalmol Vis Sci* 1979; 18: 848–855.

108. Spekreijse H, Khoe LH, van der Tweel LH: A case of amblyopia: Electrophysiology and psychophysics of luminance and contrast. In Arden GB (ed): *The Visual System*. New York, Plenum, 1972, pp 141–156.

109. Spekreijse H, van der Tweel LH, Regan UM: Interocular sustained suppression: Correlations with evoked potential amplitude and distribution. *Vision Res* 1972; 12:521–526.

110. Srebro R: Visually evoked potentials in eccentrically and centrally fixing amblyopes. *Br J Ophthalmol* 1984; 68:468–471.

111. Stevens JL, Berman JL, Schmeisser ET, Baker RS: Dichoptic luminance beat visual evoked potentials in the assessment of binocularity in children. *J Pediatr Ophthalmol Strabismus* 1994; 31(6):368–373.

112. Stewart Brown S, Snowdon SK: Evidence based dilemmas in pre-school vision screening. *Arch Dis Child* 1998; 78:406–407.

113. Suter S, Suter PS, Perrier DT, Parker KL, Fox JA, Roessler JS: Differentiation of VEP intermodulation and second harmonic components by dichoptic, monocular, and binocular stimulation. *Vis Neurosci* 1996; 13(6):1157–1166.

114. Sutija VG, Ficarra AP, Paley RT, Zhang H, Solan HA, Wurst SA: Age and binocular advantage: A VEP assessment. *Optom Vis Sci* 1990; 67(2):111–116. Erratum in *Optom Vis Sci* 1990; 67(4):290.

115. Thompson DA, Moller H, Russell-Eggitt I, Kriss A: Visual acuity in unilateral cataract. *Br J Ophthalmol* 1996; 80(9): 794–798.

116. Tyler CW, Apkarian PA, Nakayama K, Levi DM: Rapid assessment of visual function: An electronic sweep technique for the pattern VEP. *Invest Ophthalmol Vis Sci* 1979; 18: 703–713.

117. van Noorden GK: *Binocular Vision and Ocular Motility: Theory and Management of Strabismus*, 3 ed. St Louis, Mosby, 1985.

118. Watts PO, Neveu MM, Holder GE, Sloper JJ: Visual evoked potentials in successfully treated strabismic amblyopes and normal subjects. *J Am Assoc Pediatr Ophthalmol Strabismus* 2002; 6(6):389–392.

119. Weiss A, Kelly JP: VEP correlations with anisometropic and strabismic amblyopia in children before and after patching. *Invest Ophthalmol Vis Sci* 2002; 43:4699.

120. Williams C, Northstone K, Harrad RA, Sparrow JM, Harvey I: ALSPAC Study Team. Amblyopia treatment outcomes after screening before or at age 3 years: Follow up from randomised trial. *BMJ* 2002; 324(7353):1549.

121. Williams C, Papakostopoulos D: Electro-oculographic abnormalities in amblyopia. *Br J Ophthalmol* 1995; 79(3):218–224.

122. Wright KW, Ary JP, Shors TJ, Eriksen KJ: Suppression and the pattern visual evoked potential. *J Pediatr Ophthalmol Strabismus* 1986; 23(5):252–257.

123. Yinjon U, Auerbach E: The electroretinogram of children deprived of pattern vision. *Invest Ophthalmol* 1974; 17: 538–543.

53 Visual Evoked Potentials in Cortical Blindness

EMIKO ADACHI-USAMI

"CORTICAL BLINDNESS" is bilateral visual loss due to dysfunction of both occipital lobes. It is diagnosed on the basis of behavioral observations that reflect problems in seeing, even though the patients can hardly describe their visual loss. Therefore, laboratory tests such as computed tomography, magnetic resonance imaging, electroencephalography, and visual evoked cortical potentials (VECP) must be relied on to provide the diagnosis of cortical blindness.

Among such objective tests, the VECP has raised the hope that it could be used to quantify functional visual loss because correspondences between subjective visual functions such as visual acuity, color vision, and central visual field defects and the VECP have been reported to occur. However, the results appearing in the literature are still in conflict. In the present chapter, the VECP and cortical blindness will be described.

General clinical visual signs

In textbooks, visual acuity loss in cortical blindness is described as being total in both eyes. However, when we carefully read published case reports, descriptions of visual acuity even during the recovery stage do not sufficiently clarify whether the patients are still totally blind or not because expressions are used such as "light perception" and "counting fingers," which depend on the patients' behavior. Nonetheless, visual agnosia is a characteristic sign of cortical blindness. As a result, the definitive patterns of visual dysfunction such as color sense, binocularity, spatial sense, and macular sparing are obscure. On the other hand, pupillary light reflexes and ocular movements generally remain normal.

Causes of cortical blindness

The most common cause of cortical blindness is generalized cerebral hypoxia at the striate, parietal, and premotor regions, as well as vascular lesions of the striate cortex. Cerebral hypoxia can be caused by intoxication with carbon monoxide or nitrogen oxide and by inflammation such as meningitis, encephalitis, vascular occlusion, trauma, and so on. It occurs secondarily to transtentorial herniation, hemodialysis, hypoglycemia, and congenital malformations.

In any case, hypoxia is the final result. Recently, single-photon emission tomography (SPECT) and positron emission tomography (PET) have been used to demonstrate changes in cerebral blood flow.[18] These methods may develop more widely in the future.

Visual evoked potentials in cortical blindness

The VECP is generally considered to originate from central retinogeniculocalcarine pathways. However, the involvement of extrageniculate pathways cannot be completely ruled out. Therefore, VECPs in cortical blindness have received considerable attention. However, there is still no agreement about the VECP findings.

In the majority of published papers, VECP studies were done with flash stimulation. With the recent advances of technique in recording VECPs, it is generally said that the evaluation of flash VECPs is not as reliable as that of pattern VECPs. For example, Hess et al.[11] found in four patients with acute occipital blindness that no pattern VECP could be obtained, but a flash VECP was recorded. They concluded that the flash method was not appropriate for differentiating occipital blindness from psychogenic visual disorders.

Nevertheless, flash VECP is still being used effectively for patients who cannot fixate on the stimulus field such as in cortical blindness, infants, mentally retarded children, and unconscious patients.

The studies described below are concerned mainly with flash VECPs; their results are classified simply as normal, abnormal, and recovering.

WORKS REPORTING NORMAL VISUAL EVOKED CORTICAL POTENTIALS Spehlmann et al.[19] reported a 66-year-old patient with cortical blindness caused by numerous bilateral cerebral infarcts; no light perception was reported, but the patient showed flash VECPs of normal amplitude on repeated examinations.

Frank and Torres[10] recorded flash VECPs in 30 children with cortical blindness and found no significant differences between the patients and age-matched children with central nervous system diseases but without blindness. Only 1 patient with encephalopathy and increased intracranial pressure showed no response. As described above, Hess et al.[11] found normal flash VECPs and an absence of pattern VECPs. Normal flash *and* pattern VECPs were reported by Celesia et al.[6] in a 72-year-old patient who had infarction in bilateral areas 17 and part of area 18. They concluded that VECPs are mediated by extrageniculocalcarine pathways.

Newton et al.[16] reported a 16-month-old child with cortical blindness following *Haemophilus influenzae* meningitis. The flash VECP was normal, as were the fundi. Using both flash and pattern stimuli, Celesia et al.[7] found that VECPs were preserved, and positron-emission tomography showed a functioning island of occipital cortex that most likely represented the generator of the VECP.

These reports may support the evidence that extrageniculate pathways are also involved in the generation of flash VECPs. However, as Hoyt[12] pointed out, although the second visual system may be capable of mediating VECPs in some cases, it does not seem to be capable of sustaining any kind of cognitive vision.

WORKS REPORTING ABNORMAL VISUAL EVOKED CORTICAL POTENTIALS   Because of interindividual variations of flash VECP waves and poor cooperation or fixation of the patient, it is hard to make a definite diagnosis of an abnormal response. Careful studies that demonstrate the abnormality of VECPs have been reported by a number of authors.

Kooi and Sharbrough[13] reported a case with posttraumatic cortical blindness whose flash VECPs were abnormal, with none of the normal initial five waves being identifiable, while the vertex potential was recordable.

Regan et al.[17] followed an infant for 15 months whose cortical blindness had presumably begun at the age of 3.5 months. VECPs recorded at 4 months were monophasic, and the latency was prolonged; the VECP waves grew progressively more complex with age. However, recovery could be anticipated from the VECP development.

Chisholm[8] reported a case of cortical blindness due to bilateral occipital infarction and found VECPs to be absent.

Aldrich et al.[2] found that flash or pattern VECPs recorded during blindness were abnormal in 15 of 19 patients but were not correlated with visual loss.

WORKS REPORTING THE RECOVERY OF VISUAL EVOKED CORTICAL POTENTIALS IN ACCORDANCE WITH VISUAL IMPROVEMENTS   Several authors reported that VECP improvement paralleled vision recovery. Barnet et al.,[3] in six clinically blind patients, observed that flash VECPs were depressed in three of them and that in two others the VECPs were preserved several days before visual improvement

became evident. Duchowny et al.[9] reported that changes in short-latency VECP components were correlated with visual ability. However, up to the present, there is no irrefutable evidence that short-latency components are related to the striate cortex.

A work by Makino et al.[14] described in a follow-up study that the flash VECP configuration became normal with the passage of time. Miyata et al.[15] studied a case of transient cortical blindness caused by recurrent hepatic encephalopathy and found prolonged latency and a reduced amplitude of the second wave when the patient lost vision completely but a return to normal values after treatment.

Two other papers[1,4] pointed out that either flash or pattern VECPs were present in normal configurations when the patient could see well and that they were nonrecordable when the patient claimed no vision. The configuration of the VECPs might be a criterion for evaluating the abnormality of VECPs, even though it is nonspecific.

Bodis-Wollner and Mylin,[5] using VECPs of monocular and dynamic random-dot pattern stimuli, found that the recovery of binocular vision was delayed in comparison to the recovery of monocular vision. They concluded that it was not due to simple acuity impairment or convergence deficiency and thus provided evidence for the vulnerability of postsynaptic cortical mechanisms of human binocular vision.

Conclusion

As mentioned above, the VECP findings in cortical blindness are still controversial. There are two reasons for this. One is that the patient's visual loss cannot be quantitatively determined by subjective testing of visual acuity, binocular vision, color sense, and spatial vision because of the uncertainty of the patient's responses. It is therefore hard to make a comparison between the VECP results and the subjective and clinical visual signs.

Another reason is that the pathological lesions that cause cortical blindness are not often localized in the striate cortex or extrastriate cortex but spread widely throughout the parietal and temporal regions.

In any case, the theme of the relationship between cortical blindness and VECPs is fascinating, at least from the point of view of study of the origin of VECPs and the hope of differentiating cortical blindness from psychogenic visual disturbances.

REFERENCES

1. Abraham FA, Melamed E, Lavy S: Prognostic value of visual evoked potentials in cotical blindness following basilar artery occlusion. *Appl Neurophysiol* 1975; 38:126–135.
2. Aldrich MS, Alessi AG, Beck RW, Gilman S: Cortical blindness: Etiology, diagnosis and prognosis. *Ann Neurol* 1987; 21:149–158.

3. Barnet AB, Manson JI, Wilner E: Acute cerebral blindness in childhood. *Neurology* 1970; 20:1147–1156.
4. Bodis-Wollner I: Recovery from cerebral blindness: Evoked potentials and psychophysical measurements. *Electroencephalogr Clin Neurophysiol* 1977; 42:178–184.
5. Bodis-Wollner I, Mylin L: Plasticity of monocular and binocular vision following cerebral blindness: Evoked potential evidence. *Electroencephalogr Clin Neurophysiol* 1987; 68:70–74.
6. Celesia GG, Archer CR, Kuroiwa Y, Goldfader PR: Visual function of the extrageniculo-calcarine system in man. Relationship to cortical blindness. *Arch Neurol* 1980; 37:704–706.
7. Celesia GG, Polcyn RD, Holden JE, Nickles RJ, Gatley JS, Koeppe RA: Visual evoked potentials and positron emission tomographic mapping of regional cerebral blood flow and cerebral metabolism: Can the neuronal potential generators be visualized? *Electroencephalogr Clin Neurophysiol* 1982; 54:243–256.
8. Chisholm IH: Cortical blindness in cranial arteritis. *Br J Ophthalmol* 1975; 59:323–333.
9. Duchowny MS, Weiss I, Majlessi H, Barnet AB: Visual evoked responses in childhood cortical blindness after head trauma and meningitis. *Neurology* 1974; 24:933–940.
10. Frank Y, Torres F: Visual evoked potentials in the evaluation of "cortical blindness" in children. *Ann Neurol* 1979; 6:126–129.
11. Hess ChW, Meienberg O, Ludin HP: Visual evoked potentials in acute occipital blindness. Diagnostic and prognostic value. *J Neurol* 1982; 227:193–200.
12. Hoyt CG: Cortical blindness in infancy. In Crawford et al (eds): *Pediatric Ophthalmology and Strabismus: Trans New Orleans Acad Ophthalmal.* New York, Raven Press, 1986, pp 235–243.
13. Kooi KA, Sharbrough FW III: Electrophysiological findings in cortical blindness. Report of a case. *Electroencephalogr Clin Neurophysiol* 1966; 20:260–263.
14. Makino A, Soga T, Obayashi M, Seo Y, Ebisutani D, Horie S, Ueda S, Matsumoto K: Cortical blindness caused by acute general cerebral swelling. *Surg Neurol* 1988; 29:393–400.
15. Miyata Y, Motomura S, Tsuji Y, Koga S: Hepatic encephalopathy and reversible cortical blindness. *Am J Gastroenterol* 1988; 83:780–782.
16. Newton NL Jr, Reynolds JD, Woody RC: Cortical blindness following *Hemophilus influenzae* meningitis. *Ann Ophthalmol* 1985; 17:193–194.
17. Regan D, Regal DM, Tibbles JAR: Evoked potentials during recovery from blindness recorded serially from an infant and his normally sighted twin. *Electroencephalogr Clin Neurophysiol* 1982; 54:465–468.
18. Silverman IE, Galetta SL, Gray LG, Moster M, Atlas SW, Maurer AH, Alavi A: SPECT in patients with cortical visual loss. *J Nucl Med* 1993; 34:1447–1451.
19. Spehlmann R, Gross RA, Ho SU, Leestma JE, Norcross KA: Visual evoked potentials and postmortem findings in a case of cortical blindness. *Ann Neurol* 1977; 2:531–534.

54 Drug Side Effects and Toxicology of the Visual System

EBERHARDT ZRENNER

ACCORDING TO AN estimate by Crofton and Sheets,[16] almost half of all neurotoxic chemicals affect some aspect of sensory function, the visual system being most frequently affected. Grant and Schuhman,[36] in their encyclopedic *Toxicology of the Eye*, list approximately 3000 substances that produce unwanted side effects in the visual system. Quite often, alterations in visual function are the first symptoms following chemical exposure,[26] occurring in absence of any clinical signs of toxicity.[4] This not only suggests that the sensory systems, in particular the retina and the central visual system, are especially vulnerable to toxic insults, but also requires highly sensitive tests to be applied at a stage at which neither subjective function nor biomicroscopic morphology indicates such side effects. On the other hand, many of these effects are not necessarily toxic but may indicate undesired (though quite physiological) side effects on metabolic processes in one or several of the various stages of transforming the optical image of an object into the perceived neuronal image. Numerous proteins, such as transmitters or enzymes, and their metabolic processes are involved in processing information in photoreceptors and in the many connected neurons transmitting visual information to perceptual centers (table 54.1), whose function can be affected by neurotropic agents, drugs, food, and environmental agents. Additionally, there are numerous non-neuronal cells whose function is important for the integrity of the information processing, such as pigment epithelial cells, glial cells, and vascular structures, that are easily affected by immunological processes, for example. Considering the incredibly large number of substances that potentially affect visual function, this chapter can only discuss principal considerations and procedures recommended in cases of suspected adverse reactions of the more common potentially toxic compounds in the visual system.

Of further general concern are the factors that determine whether a particular chemical can reach a particular ocular site: concentration and duration of exposure, mode of application, and interaction with the various ocular structures as well as integrity of natural barriers. The blood-retinal barrier formed by the continuous type of capillaries is largely impermeable under normal physiological conditions to such chemicals as glucose and amino acids.[3] However, in certain areas of the retina, e.g., around the optic disk, the continuous type of capillaries is lacking, and hydrophylic molecules can enter the optic nerve head by diffusion from the extravascular space.

The outer retina is supplied by the choriocapillaris, and these capillaries have loose epithelial junctions and multiple fenestrae and are highly permeable to large proteins. During systemic exposure to chemicals and drugs by inhalation, transdermally, or parenterally, compounds can be distributed to all parts of the eye via the bloodstream.

The chapter aims at mediating a basic understanding of toxic mechanisms by pointing out cell-specific functional changes and typical symptoms in unwanted, toxic side effects. In an individual case, I strongly recommend consulting referenced publications such as Grant and Schuhman[36] and Fraunfelder,[32] where references on the primary literature on the various substances can be found. Additionally, there are very interesting general chapters and books that concern ocular toxicology that can often be of help.[5,15,26,47,73]

Cell-specific functional alterations

THE RETINAL PIGMENT EPITHELIUM   The retinal pigment epithelium (RPE) has four major functions: phagocytosis, vitamin A transport and storage, potassium metabolism, and protection from light damage. Accordingly, RPE functions can be altered, for example, by inhibitors of phagocytosis, modulation of potassium metabolism, metabolic alterations in the visual cycle, and the action of melanin-binding substances. Additionally, melanin is found in several different locations, such as the pigmented cells of the iris, the ciliary body, and the uveal tract. Melanin has a high binding affinity for polycyclic, aromatic carbons; calcium; and toxic heavy metals such as aluminum, iron, lead, and mercury.[24,63,74,86] This may result in excessive accumulation and slow release of numerous drugs and chemicals that bind to melanin granula, such as phenothiazines, glycosides, and chloroquine.

Chloroquine   Two of the most extensively studied retinotoxic drugs are chloroquine diphosphate (Aralen, Resochin) and hydroxychloroquine sulfate (Plaquenil), which shows a lower

TABLE 54.1

Examples of neurotransmitters and neuromodulatory active substances and their cellular sources in the vertebrate retina

Neuroactive Substance	Cell Type
Glutamate	Photoreceptors (cones and rods), bipolar cells, ganglion cells
Gamma aminobutyric acid (GABA)	Horizontal cells, amacrine cells
Glycine	Amacrine cells, bipolar cells, ganglion cells
Taurine	Photoreceptors, amacrine cells, bipolar cells
Dopamine	Amacrine cells (including interplexiform cells)
Melatonin	Photoreceptors
Serotonin	Amacrine cells, bipolar cells (in nonmammalian vertebrates)
Acetylcholine	Amacrine cells (in the INL and displaced in the GCL)
Substance P	Amacrine cells, ganglion cells
Vasoactive intestinal polypeptide	Amacrine cells
Somatostatin	Amacrine cells, ganglion cells
Angiotensin II	Amacrine cells
Nitric oxide	Amacrine cells
ATP	Amacrine cells, ganglion cells
Adenosine	Amacrine cells, ganglion cells
Brain-derived neurotrophic factor (BDNF)	Amacrine cells, ganglion cells
Kynurenic acid	Amacrine cells

incidence of retinopathy; Primaquine, Daraprim, and Quensyl also belong to this group. In retinal pigment epithelial cells, chloroquine phosphate is bound for a half-lifetime of five years in an eightyfold higher concentration in the retina relative to the liver.[63] The drug is used not only for malaria prevention, but also as basic therapy in chronic rheumatic diseases. With a typical dosage of 4–6 mg per kilogram body weight, a critical total dose can be achieved after 3–6 months.[38]

The typical signs of chloroquine retinopathy are as follows:

- Relative ring scotomata or paracentral scotomata
- Bilateral, increasing errors in color vision testing
- Increased pigmentation of the RPE
- Loss of RPE cells, initially often as a ring around the macula
- Electro-oculogram (EOG): reduced light/dark ratio
- Electroretinogram (ERG): reduced b-wave amplitude and prolonged latency in advanced cases
- Bull's-eye (incidence of 0.04–40%, depending on the study)

To avoid ocular damage by chloroquine, the dose has to be strictly related to body weight. Patients with low body weight or reduced renal excretion ability are at particular risk. A dose of less than 250 mg chloroquine or 400 mg hydroxychloroquine per day appears to produce little or no retinopathy, even after prolonged therapy.[49,69] From a 6-year cohort study in more than 400 patients, Mavrikakis et al.[62] conclude that patients with normal renal function may receive hydroxychloroquine at a maximal daily dose of 6.5 mg/kg and continue safely for 6 years. Annual screening is recommended, with central visual field screening, color testing, monitoring best corrected visual acuity, and careful funduscopy with dilated pupils to keep the incidence of retinal toxicity below 1% of patients treated.

Before starting long-term therapy with chloroquine, every patient should have an initial ophthalmic checkup, including fundus photography, visual fields, and color vision. In cases of reduced renal excretion or very low body weight or in elderly patients, an initial EOG and a biannual follow-up reexamination of visual field and color vision are recommended. In cases of suspected incipient retinopathy, the EOG should be done. Although the value of the EOG was questioned in some studies, individual cases clearly show the initial signs in the EOG. In advanced cases, standardized electroretinography helps in monitoring the function of rods and cones.

Cytostatica It should be mentioned that some cytostatic drugs have a retinotoxic potential that is closely related to that of chloroquine, such as sparsomycin, triaziquone, vincristine, and vinblastine, acting primarily through a biochemical inhibition of protein synthesis.[10]

Phenothiazine Phenothiazine-derivative drugs, such as chlorpromazine, piperidylchlorophenothiazine, and thioridazine, are quite commonly used for the treatment of schizophrenia and other psychoses. Some drugs of this group are known to cause night blindness and pigmentations in the pigment epithelium as well as changes in the EOG.[2,44]

Indomethacin Indomethacin is a nonsteroidal, anti-inflammatory drug that inhibits prostaglandin synthesis by inhibiting cyclooxygenase.[47] Long-term intake of indomethacin can produce discrete pigment scattering of the RPE perifoveally, followed by decreases in visual acuity, altered visual fields, increased thresholds for dark adaptation, blue-yellow discrimination problems, and decreases in ERG amplitudes as well as in the EOG dark/light ratio.[13,45,70] ERG responses after the cessation of drug treatment as well as color vision almost return to normal; pigmentary changes, however, are irreversible. The exact mechanisms of retinotoxicity are unknown.

FUNCTIONAL ALTERATIONS IN PHOTORECEPTORS Numerous substances can alter visual function by acting on the visual transduction process and/or the visual cycle. Besides the more commonly used antibiotic chloramphenicol these include also glycosides such as digoxin and digitoxin. Digitalis (or foxglove)-induced visual abnormalities were reported already over two centuries ago by Withering.[90] Most frequently, the complaints are hazy or blurred vision, flickering lights, colored spots surrounded by halos, and increased glare sensitivity. Color vision problems have been confirmed,[20,42,75,81] probably acting through the inhibition of the retinal sodium/potassium ATPase. ERG analysis reveals typically a depressed critical flicker fusion frequency, reduced rod and cone amplitudes, and increased implicit times as well as elevated rod and cone thresholds.[60,76] Also phosphodiesterase (PDE) inhibitors, such as sildenafil (Viagra), can affect the photoreceptor transduction process, acting on the retinal PDE. In therapeutic doses, sildenafil can lead to reversible color discrimination problems, blurred vision, glare sensitivity, blue-tinged borders between bright and dark areas, and ERG changes at higher doses.[57,95]

Mild effects of this kind were also reported with other phosphodiesterase inhibitors, such as theophylline and even caffeine.[53,82] Apparently, phosphodiesterase inhibitors affect the spectrally different cones in the retina in a slightly different manner, and even minor imbalances in the excitation of short-, middle-, and long-wavelength-sensitive cones can produce color vision disturbances.[58,59,92,97] Alterations of color perception do therefore belong among early signs of drug-induced functional alterations of the visual system.

FUNCTIONAL ALTERATIONS IN CELLS OF THE INNER RETINA (OUTER PLEXIFORM TO INNER PLEXIFORM LAYER) In the outer and inner plexiform layers, numerous transmitters and modulators are known (figure 54.1; see table 54.1).[23,56] Actions of drugs and toxic agents on transmitter function can easily alter visual function, especially if GABA, glycine, glutamate, dopamine, and acetylcholine functions are involved.

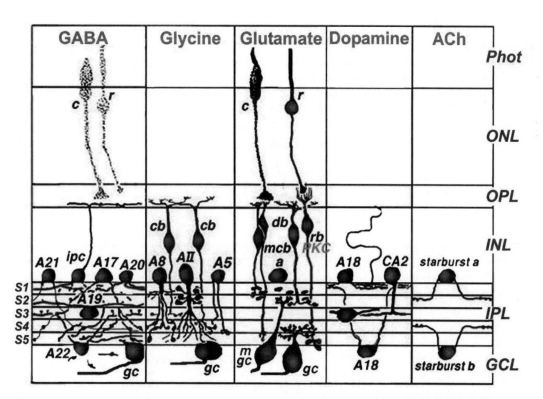

FIGURE 54.1 The various transmitters that are present in the retina are found in particular layers. A multitude of transmitters and neuromodulators is found in the more than 20 different types of amacrine cells in the inner plexiform layer (IPL). Compounds that affect the function of such transmitters thereby act specifically on the function and electrophysiological characteristics of these target cells. This specificity often allows correlation of functional alterations in electrophysiological parameters to action and adverse reactions of neurotropic compounds. (Source: Konrad Kohler, personal communication.)

GABA Antiepileptic drugs that act on the GABA metabolism quite commonly alter visual function.[11,21,41] Such antiepileptics are carbamazepine (Tegretal), phenytoin (Phenhydan), and vigabatrin (Sabril). While these drugs can cause color vision disturbances, vigabatrin can also produce irreversible concentric visual field defects. Vigabatrin raises GABA levels by irreversibly binding to GABA transaminase, thus preventing the metabolism of GABA. Incidences of reported visual field changes vary between 0.1% and 30%.[65,80] The earliest report of retinal electrophysiological changes in humans associated with vigabatrin treatment is that of Bayer et al.[8] All patients with visual field defects revealed altered oscillatory potential waveforms in the ERG, especially patients with marked visual field defects,[11] also visible in multifocal ERGs,[77] that are usually irreversible.[79] In about half of the patients, a delayed cone single-flash response was found in the Ganzfeld ERG, and a reduced Arden ratio was found in the electro-oculogram. Harding developed a special VEP stimulus with a high sensitivity and specificity in identifying visual field defects.[41] At high doses, vigabatrin in animal studies had revealed microvacuolation in the myelin sheath.

Agents that modulate GABA can be expected to alter the GABA-ergic functions of horizontal cells and thereby can alter contrast vision and presumably functions of adaptation as well.

Dopamine A number of drugs, such as fluphenazine, haloperidol, and sulpiride, can affect the dopamine metabolism and thereby modify retinal function.[83] In animal experiments, all three dopamine antagonists increased the rod b-wave, while b-wave latency and implicit time showed no drug-induced changes. On the other hand, the D1 antagonist fluphenazine increases the fast transient ON-component while simultaneously strongly decreasing the OFF-component. In contrast, concentrations of the D2 antagonist sulpiride that had a comparable effect on the fast transient ON-component of the ONR (optic nerve response) did not influence the OFF-component. These findings indicate that D1 and D2 receptors play different roles in the transmission of rod signals at the border of middle and inner retina. As reported in patch clamp investigations by Guenther et al.,[39] application of the receptor antagonists haloperidole, spiperone, and SCH23390 reduce calcium influx between 8% and 77%, while an effect of dopamine itself was not observed. The study of Dawis and Niemeyer[19] in arterially perfused cat eyes suggests that dopamine itself has an inhibitory effect on the rod visual pathway, since the rod b-wave amplitude is reduced after dopamine application. The functional roles of dopamine were lined out very nicely by Witkovsky and Dearry.[91] The action of these drugs may be based on a particular cell population of dopaminergic neurons, the density of which ranges from 10 to 80 cells/mm^2. They surround other amacrine pericaria, probably amacrine cells of the AII type that transmit rod pathway information onto cone bipolar cells.

Inorganic lead Lead intoxication can also reduce the activity of dopamine synthesis. Since dopamine is used by the rod-specific AII amacrine cells, lead can induce special changes in rod signals in the ERG,[29] accompanied by histological alterations.[28,54] Rhesus monkeys that were exposed prenatally and postnatally to moderate or high levels of lead for 9 years had decreased tyrosine hydroxylase immunoreactivity in the dopaminergic amacrine cells.[54] Fox et al.[27] reported selective apoptotic cell death in rod and bipolar cells after 3 weeks of low or moderate levels of lead exposure in neonatal rats. In vivo and in vitro data suggest that lead can also inhibit the rod cGMP phosphodiesterase, thereby producing an elevation of the rod Ca^{2+} concentration[30] with changes in the scotopic ERG. Even nanomolar or micromolar concentrations of lead can selectively depress the amplitude and absolute sensitivity of rod (not cone) photoreceptor potentials,[31,85] similar to changes that are observed in ERG studies in occupationally lead-exposed workers.[14,84] Clearly, lead has multisite actions in the nervous system, depending on concentration, duration of exposure, and other external functions such as corticosteroid treatment that may release stored lead from bones (personal observations).

Studies in occupationally endangered workers have revealed that the sensitivity and amplitude of the a- and b-waves of the dark-adapted ERG are decreased.[37,40]

In addition to retinal deficits, oculomotor deficits can occur in chronically lead-exposed workers,[35] as well as optic atrophy after chronic lead exposure or acute high-level exposures.[52]

Other retinal transmitters and modulators More than 20 different transmitter substances are used in the various types of amacrine cells as shown in table 54.1. Consequently, numerous drugs can affect the function of amacrine cells, and individual wavelets of the oscillatory potentials that have their origins in amacrine cells can even be affected differently. As an example of drug-induced functional changes in the inner retina, angiotensinergic amacrine cells may be mentioned.[18,50,55,89] Angiotensin II antagonists can considerably alter retinal function, as shown in ERGs and optic nerve responses of the arterially perfused cat eye[17,96] and by electroretinography in cats.[48]

FUNCTIONAL CHANGES IN RETINAL GANGLION CELLS Retinal ganglion cells have quite different tasks: The parvocellular system is mainly responsible for coding of fine spatial resolution and color, while the magnocellular system codes primarily movement and contrast. Drugs that affect ganglion cell function therefore can show different effects on the parvocellular and magnocellular systems.

Ethambutol Ethambutol is widely used for the treatment of tuberculosis. It causes the following:

- Color vision disturbances as early symptoms
- Contrast vision changes
- Visual field defects, especially central scotomata with loss of visual acuity
- Changes in visual evoked cortical potentials

These alterations can occur within a few weeks after starting the treatment. Also, ethambutol may act at different sites. While initially, horizontal cell function and thereby color discrimination is altered as seen in VEPs[98] as well as in fish retina single-cell recordings,[87] advanced forms may lead to loss of ganglion cells and degeneration of the optic nerve. After cessation of drug intake, the functions improve, as can easily be seen by anomaloscopy.[67]

Methanol and ethanol Methanol is readily absorbed from all routes of exposure, easily crosses all membranes, and is oxidized by alcohol dehydrogenase to formaldehyde, excreted as formic acid in the urine. Humans are highly sensitive to methanol-induced neurotoxicity owing to our limited capacity to oxidized formic acid. Acute methanol poisoning in humans and experimental animals leads to profound and permanent structural alterations in the retina and the optic nerve. Symptoms range from blurred vision to decreased visual acuity and blindness due to optic nerve degeneration.[6] The ERG b-wave amplitude in humans starts to decrease significantly when the blood format concentration exceeds 7 millimolar.[66,72] At higher doses, the a-wave amplitudes also decrease. Interestingly, besides the effect on ganglion cells, methanol may have a direct toxic effect on Müller glial cells[33,34] and thereby indirectly affect particularly the depolarizing rod bipolar cells or the synaptic transmission between photoreceptors and bipolar cells.

Other compounds Other substances that typically modify ganglion cell functions are chloramphenicol, quinine, thallium, and ergotamine derivatives. It should be mentioned that ethanol even in modest concentrations can affect the EOG and color vision.[99]

GLIAL CELLS The retina contains several groups of glial cells, Müller cells, oligodentrocytes, and astrocytes. Müller cells are important not only for the metabolism of glutamate and other neurotransmitters, but also for buffering of the potassium released after illumination. Since the b-wave of the electroretinogram is intricately connected with the function of Müller cells, any drug action on Müller cells can strongly affect b-wave amplitude and implicit time. Direct toxic effects on glial cells are known, for example, in ammonia intoxication occurring in the alcohol syndrome[22] and methanol poisoning (see above) or in poisoning with methyl mercury (see below).

THE OPTIC NERVE There is a series of drugs that particularly affects axonal fibers of ganglion cells. For example, exposure to acrylamide produces a particular damage of the axons of the parvocellular system while sparing axons of the magnocellular system, leading to specific visual deficits such as increased in threshold for visual acuity and flicker fusion as well as prolonged latency of pattern evoked cortical potentials.[64]

Carbon disulfide Carbon disulfide (CS₂) has a marked effect on vision (for a survey, see Beauchamp et al.[9]). The changes in the visual function are central scotoma, depressed visual sensitivity in the periphery, optic atrophy, pupillary disturbances, disorders of color perception, and blurred vision. Vasculopathies including some in the retina were reported as well, but histology in animals points primarily to an optic neuropathy,[25] and alterations in the VEP are expected in such conditions.

Tamoxifen Widespread axonal degeneration induced by tamoxifen in the macular and perimacular area was reported by Kaiser-Kupfer et al.,[51] accompanied by retinopathy as well. Clinical symptoms include a permanent decrease in visual acuity and abnormal visual fields.[1] Following cessation of low-dose tamoxifen therapy, most of the keratopathy accompanying tamoxifen intake and some of the retinal alterations were seen to be reversible.[68]

Nutritional deficiencies Optic neuropathies can also occur in an epidemic fashion, as happened in 1992 and 1993 in Cuba, with over 50,000 people suffering from optic neuropathy, sensory and autonomic peripheral neuropathy, with high-frequency neural hearing loss and myelopathy. In addition to low food intake, habits such as frequent smoking and high cassava consumption may contribute to such optic neuropathies. Nutritional deficiencies are what primarily contribute to such epidemic outbreaks, but it is not clear whether some people have a genetically determined higher susceptibility to nutritional deficiencies or viral exposures that otherwise would have been tolerated.[78]

Other toxic optic neuropathies Other, more common drugs that can produce alterations of optic nerve function with concomitant VEP changes are ethambutol (see above), isoniazid (INH), streptomycin, and chloramphenicol.

CENTRAL NERVOUS SYSTEM Direct effects of drugs, such as those described in the retina and optic nerve, can of course also affect peripheral nerves and cortical neurons directly. Besides the direct action of a compound, increased cerebrospinal pressure can cause secondary alterations of the optic nerve with papilledema, for example, that observed after the treatment with ergotamines that may produce prolonged latency in the pattern VEP.[43] Since many cortical areas are involved in processing visual information, alteration of vision can also be caused by direct drug action on neurons in higher cortical areas and can produce visual hallucinations and neurological deficits. This is true not only for lead, as described above, but also for methyl mercury, which can accumulate in the food chain and reach toxic concentration after consumption of fish and shellfish. Methyl mercury poisoning leads to constriction of visual field caused by destruction of cortical, neural, and glial cells, as observed during an epidemic methyl mercury poisoning in Minamata Bay in Japan ("Minamata disease"). Methyl mercury–poisoned individuals also experience poor night vision with scotopic visual deficits.[46] Interestingly, mercury also accumulates in the retina of animals exposed to methyl mercury and produces rod-selective electrophysiological and morphological alterations.[12,31]

From symptom to diagnosis

Although electrophysiological results certainly are an important part of the diagnostic puzzle,[92] they should always be judged in conjunction with a complete workup of a case.

Since the toxic origin of visual symptoms is usually difficult to establish, some more general aspects of an ophthalmological damage are discussed in the following section.

HISTORY   It is very important to carefully record history in case of suspected intoxication, changes in digestion, metabolic alterations, and diseases of the kidney or liver that may lead to reduced excretion and thereby to high toxic serum levels. Resection of parts of the stomach can lead to nutritional deficiencies and cause nutritive optic atrophy. It is also very important to properly record the amount and duration of medication. Additionally, the amount of tobacco and alcohol as well as possible exposure to solvents or metals in industrial production should be recorded.

Usually, symptoms are equally present in both eyes, and uniocular symptoms may occur only in case of increased risk of thrombosis or other local vascular changes induced by chemical agents. The typical key symptoms of many drug-induced functional alterations of the visual system should be asked for:

- Increased glare sensitivity
- Chromatopsias
- Changes of light and dark adaptation, difficulties in mesopic vision
- Phosphenes

Common additional symptoms in case of toxic visual disturbances may be related to other sensory organs or to the central nervous system, leading, for example, to the following:

- Vertigo
- Headache
- Loss of hearing
- Paresthesias

SPECIAL CONSIDERATIONS FOR TESTING PROCEDURES IN TOXIC VISUAL DISTURBANCES   The ophthalmologic basic investigation should carefully consider changes in visual acuity, color vision disturbances, visual field alterations, changes in the oculomotor system, pupillary function and accommodation, and possible deposits on cornea, iris, and lens, along with a careful investigation of the retina and the pigment epithelium as well as the optic disk. Depending on symptoms reported in the patient's history, tests should be performed concerning glare sensitivity, dark adaptation, and changes in ERG, EOG, and/or VEP and to test contrast vision.

Visual acuity and visual fields   In testing visual acuity and visual fields, it should be kept in mind that substances that affect the papillomacular bundle and thereby produce central scotomata and decreased visual acuity often can be barbiturates, benzenes, tobacco and/or alcohol, ethambutol, lead, and methanol. Substances that produce typically peripheral concentric visual field defects that are not necessarily accompanied by visual acuity loss include vigabatrin, phenothiazines, nalidixic acid, chloramphenicol, nitrofurantoin, and salicylates.

Typically, ring and arcuate scotomata are found in cases of intoxication with chloroquine, INH, or streptomycin.

Color vision disturbances   There are numerous substances that typically produce color vision disturbances.[71] Such color vision disturbances are often caused by imbalances between the short-, middle-, and long-wavelength cones, which are differently affected by individual drugs.

The desaturated version of the Panel D 15 test or the Roth 28 hue test, the FM 100 hue test, and the anomaloscope are well suited to monitor color vision disturbances and their variation during the course of an intoxication. There is a particular color vision table for acquired color vision disturbances by Ishikawa (SPP2) that respects the varying ranges of cone spectral sensitivity occurring in such disturbances, while most other isochromatic tables are designed for congenital color vision deficiencies. The widening of the matching range and/or a shift toward the achromatic axis in the anomaloscope is of particular value in tracking down acquired color vision disturbances.[71,93]

Contrast vision and dark adaptation   Contrast and glare sensitivity can be tested by the nyctometer or other contrast and glare sensitivity testers, such as the Oculus mesoptometer. Quite commonly, drugs (e.g., vincristine or phenothiazines) can change the threshold and the time course of the dark adaptation function, especially if the pigment epithelium or the rhodopsin metabolism is affected.

Intraocular and extraocular muscles   Several drugs, such as direct adrenergics (adrenaline or neosynephrine) as well as indirectly acting forms (thyramine and cocaine) can lead to increased pupillary diameters, while cholinergica (carbachol, physostigmine, etc.) lead to a narrowing of the pupils. Mydriasis is reported in drugs for treatment of Parkinson's, as well as in antihistamines, tranquilizers, neuroleptic agents, and antidepressive agents, while miosis occurs in cholinesterase inhibitors, antihypertensive drugs, and opium derivatives.

Drug-induced changes of accommodation are quite common. Acute transitory myopization without spasm of accommodation and without miosis occurs with administration of aminophenazones, acetylsalicylic acid, sulfonamides, tetracycline, certain diuretics, and carboanhydrase inhibitors as well as in neuroleptic drug application.

Ptosis can be a side effect of barbiturates and other hypnotics and sedatives, such as chloral hydrate and carbromal. It also occurs in metal poisoning drugs with muscle relaxant action and during treatment with sympatholytica.

Overshooting saccades are observed with MAO inhibitors. Slowed oculomotor action has been seen also after intravenous application of diazepam.

Final comments

All these tests should be employed, not as a strict complete sequence of tests but step by step according to hints in the patient's history and the ophthalmological basic investigation, depending on the possibility of functional changes the particular test is assessing.

As far as the application of electrophysiological tests is concerned, the reader is referred to the particular chapters in this book.

Again, actions of drugs happen quite frequently at multiple sites. They may vary depending on the genetic background of individuals, and I recommend consulting the standard references mentioned in the introduction.

ACKNOWLEDGMENT   I wish to thank Mrs. Regina Nicolaidis, M.A., for checking and proofreading the manuscript.

REFERENCES

1. Ah-Song R, Sasco AJ: Tamoxifen and ocular toxicity. *Cancer Detect Prev* 1997; 21:522–533.
2. Alkemade PPH: Phenothiazine-retinopathy. *Ophthalmologica* 1968; 155:70–76.
3. Alm A: Ocular circulation. In Hart WM (ed): *Adler's Physiology of the Eye*, 9 ed. St. Louis, Mosby Year Book, 1992, pp 198–227.
4. Anger WK, Johnson BL: Chemicals affecting behaviour. In O'Donoghue JL (ed): *Neurotoxicity of Industrial and Commercial Chemicals*. Boca Raton, CRC Press, 1985, pp 51–148.
5. Ballantyne B: Toxicology related to the eye. In Ballantyne B, Marrs TC, Syversen T (eds): *General and Applied Toxicology*. New York, McGraw Hill, 1999, pp 737–774.
6. Baumbach GL, Cancilla PA, Martin-Amat G, Tephly TR, McMartin KE, Makar AB, Hayreh MS, Hayreh SS: Methyl alcohol poisoning: IV. Alterations of the morphological findings of the retina and optic nerve. *Arch Ophthalmol* 1977; 95:1859–1865.
7. Bayer AU, Thiel H-J, Zrenner E, Dichgans J, Kuehn M, Paulus W, Schmidt D: Colour vision tests for early detection of antiepileptic drug toxicity. *Neurology* 1997; 48:1394–1397.
8. Bayer A, Zrenner E, Ried S, Schmidt D: Effects of anticonvulsant drugs on retinal function: Psychophysical and electrophysiological findings in patients with epilepsy. *Invest Ophthalmol Vis Sci* 1990; 31(4):417.
9. Beauchamp RO Jr, Bus JS, Popp JA, Boreiko CJ, Goldberg L: A critical review of the literature on carbon disulfide toxicity. *CRC Crit Rev Toxicol* 1983; 11:168–277.
10. Bernstein HN: Chloroquine ocular toxicity. *Surv Ophthalmol* 1967; 12:415–477.
11. Besch D, Kurtenbach A, Apfelstedt-Sylla E, Sadowski B, Dennig D, Asenbauer C, Zrenner E, Schiefer U: Visual field constriction and electrophysiological changes associated with vigabatrin. *Doc Ophthalmol* 2002; 104:151–170.
12. Braekevelt CR: Morphological changes in rat retinal photoreceptors with acute methyl mercury intoxication. In Hollyfield JG (ed): *The Structure of the Eye*. New York, Elsevier, 1982, pp 123–131.
13. Burns CA: Ocular effects of indomethacin: Slit lamp and electroretinographic ERG study. *Invest Ophthalmol* 1966; 5:325–331.
14. Cavelleri A, Trimarchi F, Gelmi C, Baruffini A, Minoia C, Biscaldi G, Gallo G: Effects of lead on the visual system of occupationally exposed subjects. *Scand J Work Environ Health* 1982; 8 (suppl 1):148–151.
15. Chiou GCY: *Ophthalmic Toxicology*. New York, Raven Press, 1992.
16. Crofton KM, Sheets LP: Evaluation of sensory system function using reflex modification of the startle response. *J Am Coll Toxicol* 1989; 8:199–211.
17. Dahlheim P, Schneider T, Reiter W, Zrenner E: Das Angiotensin-I Converting enzyme (ACE): Aktivitätsverteilung im Auge und neurophysiologische Funktion auf die Netzhautfunktion. *Fortschr Ophthalmol* 1988; 85:709–715.
18. Datum KH, Zrenner E: Angiotensin-like immunoreactive cells in the chicken retina. *Exp Eye Res* 1991; 53:157–165.
19. Dawis S, Niemeyer G: Dopamine influences the light peak in the perfused mammalian eye. *Invest Ophthalmol Vis Sci* 1986; 27:330–335.
20. Duncker G, Krastel H: Ocular digitalis effects in normal subjects. *Lens Eye Tox Res* 1990; 7:281–303.
21. Dyer RS: The use of sensory evoked potentials in toxicology. *Fundam Appl Toxicol* 1985; 5:24–40.
22. Eckstein A, Reichenbach A, Jacobi P, Weber P, Gregor M, Zrenner E: Hepatic retinopathia: Changes in retinal function. *Vision Res* 1997; 37(12):1699–1706.
23. Ehinger B: Connexions between retinal neurons with identified neurotransmitters. *Vision Res* 1983; 23:1281–1291.
24. Eichenbaum JW, Zheng W: Distribution of lead and transthyretin in human eyes. *Clin Toxicol* 2000; 38:371–381.

25. Eskin TA, Merigan WH, Wood RW: Carbon disulfide effects on the visual system: II. Retinogeniculate degeneration. *Invest Ophthalmol Vis Sci* 1988; 29:519–527.

26. Fox DA, Boyes W: Toxic responses of the ocular and visual system. In Klaassen CD (ed): *Casarett & Doull's Toxicology: The Basic Science of Poisons.* 6 ed. New York, McGraw-Hill, 2001.

27. Fox DA, Campbell ML, Blockers YS: Functional alterations and apoptotic cell death in the retina following developmental or adult lead exposure. *Neurotoxicology* 1997; 18:645–665.

28. Fox DA, Chu LWF: Rods are selectively altered by lead: II. Ultrastructure and quantitative histology. *Exp Eye Res* 1988; 46:613–625.

29. Fox DA, Farber DB: Rods are selectively altered by lead: I. Electrophysiology and biochemistry. *Exp Eye Res* 1988; 46:579–611.

30. Fox DA, Katz LM: Developmental lead exposure selectively alters the scotopic ERG component of dark and light adaptation and increases rod calcium content. *Vision Res* 1992; 32:249–252.

31. Fox DA, Sillman AJ: Heavy metals affect rod, but not cone photoreceptors. *Science* 1979; 206:78–80.

32. Fraunfelder FT: *Drug-Induced Ocular Side Effects,* 5 ed. Oxford, UK, Butterworth-Heinemann, 2000.

33. Garner CD, Lee EW, Louis-Ferdinand RT: Müller cell involvement in methanol-induced retinal toxicity. *Toxicol Appl Pharmacol* 1995; 130:101–107.

34. Garner CD, Lee EW, Terzo TS, Louis-Ferdinand RT: Role of retinal metabolism in methanol-induced retinal toxicity. *J Toxicol Environ Health* 1995; 44:43–56.

35. Glickman L, Valciukas JA, Lilis R, Weisman I: Occupational lead exposure: Effects on saccadic eye movements. *Int Arch Occup Environ Health* 1984; 54:115–125.

36. Grant WM, Schuhman JS: *Toxicology of the Eye,* 4 ed. Springfield, Ill, Charles C Thomas, 1993.

37. Guguchkova PT: Electroretinographic and electrooculographic examinations of persons occupationally exposed to lead. *Vestnik Oftalmolog* 1972; 85:60–65.

38. Guldenschuh I, Niemeyer G: Zur Früherfassung von Netzhautschäden durch Chloroquin und Hydroxychloroquin als Antirheumatika. *Hausarzt* 1987; 38:313.

39. Günther E, Wilsch V, Zrenner E: Inhibitory action of haloperidol, spiperone and SCH23390 on calcium currents in rat retinal ganglion cells. *Neuroreport* 1994; 5(11):1373–1376.

40. Hajek A, Goldmann A, Zrenner E: Hat die Bleibelastung durch die Umwelt einen Effekt auf den Verlauf tapetoretinaler Degenerationen? *Klin Mbl Augenheilk* 1989; 195:49.

41. Harding GFA, Robertson EL, Spencer EL, Holliday I: Vigabatrin: Its effect on the electrophysiology of vision. *Doc Ophthalmol* 2002; 104:213–299.

42. Haustein KO, Schmidt C: Differences in colour discrimination between three cardioactive glycosides. *Int J Pharmacol Ther Toxicol* 1988; 26:517–520.

43. Heider W, Berninger T, Brunk G: Electroophthalmological and clinical findings in a case of chronic abuse of ergotamine. *Fortschr Ophthalmol* 1986; 83:539–541.

44. Henkes HE: Electro-oculography as a diagnostic aid in phenothiazine retinopathy. *Trans Ophthalmol Soc Uk* 1967; 87:285–287.

45. Henkes HE, van Lith GHM, Canta LR: Indomethacin retinopathy. *Am J Ophthalmol* 1972; 73:846–856.

46. Iwata K: Neuro-ophthalmological findings and a follow-up study in the Agano area. In Tsubari T, Irukayama K (eds): *Minimata Disease: Methylmercury Poisoning in Minimata and Niigata, Tokyo.* Tokyo, Kodansha, 1977, pp 166–185.

47. Jaanus SD, Bartlett JD, Hiett JA: Ocular effects of systemic drugs. In Bartlett JD, Jaanus SD (eds): *Clinical Ocular Pharmacology,* 3 ed. Boston, Butterworth-Heinemann, 1995, pp 957–1006.

48. Jacobi P, Oswald H, Jurklies B, Zrenner E: Neuromodulatory effects of the renin-angiotensin system on the cat electroretinogram. *Invest Ophthalmol Vis Sci* 1994; 35(3):973–980.

49. Johnson MW, Vine AK: Hydroxychloroquine therapy in massive total doses without retinal toxicity. *Am J Ophthalmol* 1987; 104:139–144.

50. Jurklies B, Eckstein A, Jacobi P, Kohler K, Risler T, Zrenner E: The reinin-angiotensin system: A possible neuromodulator in the human retina? *German J Ophthalmol* 1995; 4:144–150.

51. Kaiser-Kupfer MI, Kupfer C, Rodrigues MM: Tamoxifen retinopathy: A clinocopathologic report. *Ophthalmology* 1981; 88:89–93.

52. Karai I, Horiguchi SH, Nishikawa N: Optic atrophy with visual vield defect in workers occupationally exposed to lead for 30 years. *J Toxicol Clin Toxicol* 1982; 19:409–418.

53. Kohen L, Zrenner E, Schneider T: Der Einfluß von Theophyllin und Coffein auf die sensorische Netzhautfunktion des Menschen. *Fortsch Opthalmol* 1986; 83:338–344.

54. Kohler K, Lilienthal H, Guenther E, Winneke G, Zrenner E: Persistent decrease of the dopamine-synthesizing enzyme tyrosine hydroxylase in the rhesus monkey retina after chronic lead exposure. *Neurotoxicology* 1997; 18:623–632.

55. Kohler K, Wheeler-Schilling T, Jurklies B, Guenther E, Zrenner E: Angiotensin II in the rabbit retina. *Vis Neurosci* 1997; 14:63–71.

56. Kolb H, Fernandez E, Nelson R: The organization of the vertebrate retina. Available at: www.webvision.med.utah.edu.

57. Laties AM, Zrenner E: Viagra (sildenafil citrate) and ophthalmology. *Prog Retin Eye Res* 2002; 21:485–506.

58. Lyle WM: Drugs and conditions which may affect colour vision: I. Drugs and chemicals. *J Am Optom Assoc* 1974; 45:47.

59. Lyle WM: Drugs and conditions which may affect colour vision: II. Diseases and conditions. *J Am Optom Assoc* 1974; 45:173.

60. Madreperla SA, Johnson MA, Nakatani K: Electrophysiological and electroretinographic evidence for photoreceptor dysfunction as a toxic effect of digoxin. *Arch Ophthalmol* 1994; 112:807–812.

61. Marmor MF, Zrenner E. Standard for clinical electroretinography (1999 update). *Doc Ophthalmol* 1999; 97:143–156.

62. Mavrikakis I, Sfikakis PP, Mavrikakis E, Rougas K, Nikolaou A, Kostopoulos C, Mavrikakis M: The incidence of irreversible retinal toxicity in patients treated with hydroxychloroquine. *Ophthalmology* 2003; 110(7):1321–1326.

63. Meier-Ruge W: Drug induced retinopathy. *CRC Toxicol* 1972; 1:325–360.

64. Merigan WH, Barkdoll E, et al: Acrylamide effects on the macaque visual system: I. Pychophysics and electrophysiology. *Invest Ophthalmol Vis Sci* 1985; 26:309–316.

65. Miller NR, Johnson MA, Paul SR, Girkin CA, Perry JD, Endres M, Krauss GL: Visual dysfunction in patients receiving vigabatrin: Clinical and electrophysiological findings. *Neurology* 1999; 53(9):2082–2087.

66. Murray TG, Burton TC, Rajani C, Lewandowski MF, Burke JM, Eells JT: Methanol poisoning: A rodent model with structural and functional evidence for retinal involvement. *Arch Ophthalmol* 1991; 109:1012–1016.

67. Nasemann J, Zrenner E, Riedel KG: Recovery after severe ethambutol intoxication: Psychophysical and electrophysiological correlations. *Doc Ophthalmol* 1989; 71:279–292.

68. Noureddin BN, Seoud M, Bashshur Z, Salem Z, Shamseddin A, Khalil A: Ocular toxicity in low-dose tamoxifen: A prospective study. *Eye* 1999; 13:729–733.

69. Ochsendorf FR, Runne U, Goerz G, Zrenner E: Chloroquin-Retinopathie: Durch individuelle Tagesdosis vermeidbar. *Dtsch Med Wschr* 1983; 118:1895–1898.

70. Palimeris G, Koliopoulos J, Velissaropoulos P: Ocular side effects of indomethacin. *Ophthalmologica* 1972; 164:339–353.

71. Pokorny J, Smith VS, Verriest G, Pinckers A: *Congenital and Acquired Color Vision Defects.* New York, Grune and Stratton, 1979.

72. Potts AM: The visual toxicity of methanol: VI. The clinical aspects of experimental methanol poisoning treated with base. *Am J Ophthalmol* 1955; 39:76–82.

73. Potts AM: Toxic responses of the eye. In Klaassen CD (ed): *Casarett's and Doull's Toxicology: The Basic Science of Poisons,* 5 ed. New York, McGraw-Hill, 1996, pp 583–615.

74. Potts AM, Au PC: The affinity of melanin for inorganic ions. *Exp Eye Res* 1976; 22:487–491.

75. Rietbrock N, Alken RG: Colour vision deficiencies: A common sign of intoxication in chronically digoxin-treated patients. *J Cardiovasc Pharmacol* 1980; 2:93–99.

76. Robertson DM, Hollenhorst RW, Callahan JA: Ocular manifestations of digitalis toxicity. *Arch Ophthalmol* 1966; 76:640–645.

77. Ruether K, Pung T, Kellner U, Schmitz B, Hartmann C, Seeliger M: Electrophysiologic evaluation of a patient with peripheral visual field contraction associated with vigabatrin. *Arch Ophthalmol* 1998; 116:817–819.

78. Sadun AA: Acquired mitochondrial impairment as a cause of optic nerve disease. *Trans Am Ophthalmol Soc* 1998; 96:881–923.

79. Schmidt T, Ruther K, Jokiel B, Pfeiffer S, Tiel-Wilck K, Schmitz B: Is visual field constriction in epilepsy patients treated with vigabatrin reversible? *J Neurol* 2002; 249:1066–1071.

80. Schmitz B, Schmidt T, Jokiel B, Pfeiffer S, Tiel-Wilck K, Ruther K: Visual field constricition in epilepsy patients treated with vigabatrin and other antiepileptic drugs: A prospective study. *J Neurol* 2002; 249(4):469–475.

81. Schneider T, Dahlheim P, Zrenner E: Tierexperimentelle Untersuchungen zur okulären Toxizität von Herzglykosiden. *Fortschr Ophthalmol* 1989; 86:751–755.

82. Schneider T, Zrenner E: The influence of phosphodiesterase inhibitors on ERG and optic nerve response of the cat. *Invest Ophthal Vis Sci* 1986; 27:1395–1403.

83. Schneider T, Zrenner E: Effects of D1- and D2-dopamine antagonists on ERG and optic nerve response of the cat. *Exp Eye Res* 1991; 52:425–430.

84. Signorino M, Scarpino O, Provincialli L, Marchesi GF, Valentino M, Governa M: Modifications of the electroretinogram and of different components of the visual evoked potentials in workers exposed to lead. *Ital Electroenceph J* 1983; 10:51P.

85. Tessier-Lavigne M, Mobbs P, Attwell D: Lead and mercury toxicity and the rod light response. *Invest Ophthalmol Vis Sci* 1985; 26:1117–1123.

86. Ulshafer RJ, Allen CB, Rubin ML: Distributions of elements in the human retinal pigment epithelium. *Arch Ophthalmol* 1990; 108:113–117.

87. van Dijk BW, Spekreijse H: Ethambutol changes the colour coding of carp retinal ganglion cells reversibly. *Invest Ophthalmol Vis Sci* 1983; 24:128–133.

88. Vaney DI: The mosaic of amacrine cells in the mammalian retina. *Progr Retin Res* 1990; 9:49–100.

89. Wheeler-Schilling TH, Sautter E, Guenther E, Kohler K: Expression of angiotensin-converting enzyme (ACE) in the developing chicken retina. *Exp Eye Res* 2001; 72:173–182.

90. Withering W: *An Account of the Foxglove and Some of Its Medicinal Uses: With Practical Remarks on Dropsy and Other Diseases.* London, Broomsleigh Press, 1785.

91. Witkovsky P, Dearry A: Functional roles of dopamine. *Prog Retin Res* 1991; 11:247–292.

92. Zrenner E: Electrophysiological characteristics of the blue sensitive mechanism: Test of a model of cone interaction under physiological and pathological conditions. *Doc Ophthalmol Proc Ser* 1982; 33:103–125.

93. Zrenner E: Farbsinnprüfungen: Grundlagen, Meßverfahren und Anwendungen bei angeborenen und erworbenen Farbsinnstörungen. In *Bücherei des Augenarztes, Vol. 106.* Stuttgart, Enke Verlag, 1985, pp 263–286.

94. Zrenner E: Tests of retinal function in drug toxicity. In Hockwin O, Green K, Rubin LF (eds): *Manual of Oculotoxicity Testing Drugs.* Stuttgart, Fischer Verlag, 1992, pp 331–361.

95. Zrenner E: No cause for alarm over retinal side-effects of sildenafil. *Lancet* 1999; 353:340–341.

96. Zrenner E, Dahlheim P, Datum KH: A role of the angiotensin-renin system for retinal neurotransmission?. In Weiler R, Osborne NN (eds): *Neurobiology of the Inner Retina,* Berlin, Springer-Verlag, 1989, pp 375–387.

97. Zrenner E, Kramer W, Bittner C, Bopp M, Schlepper M: Rapid effects on colour vision, following intravenous injection of a new, non glycoside positive inotropic substance (AR-L 115 BS). *Doc Ophthalmol Proc Seri* 1982; 33:493–507.

98. Zrenner E, Krüger CJ: Ethambutol mainly affects the function of red/green opponent neurons. *Doc Ophthalmol Proc Ser* 1981; 27:13–25.

99. Zrenner E, Riedel KG, Adamczyk R, Gilg T, Liebhardt E: Effects of ethyl alcohol on the electrooculogram and colour vision. *Doc Ophthalmol* 1986; 63:305–312.

55 Mitochondrial Diseases

ALVIN B. H. SEAH AND NANCY J. NEWMAN

THE MITOCHONDRIAL disorders are a heterogenous group of disorders in which biochemical or genetic analysis, inheritance pattern, histopathology, or clinical presentation suggests a primary dysfunction of the mitochondria.[5,8,20,28] Mitochondria are tiny intracellular organelles that are essential for oxidative phosphorylation and play a role in other metabolic processes. They are responsible for generating much of the energy needed by the cell, in the form of adenosine triphosphate (ATP). The central nervous system, including the ocular tissues such as retina and optic nerve, are particularly reliant on mitochondrial energy production.

Every human cell contains hundreds of mitochondria. Each mitochondrion contains its own DNA and all the elements necessary for local transcription, translation, and replication. Like nuclear DNA, mitochondrial DNA (mtDNA) is read onto messenger RNAs that are then translated into proteins. These processes take place within the mitochondrion. Unlike nuclear DNA, which is organized in chromosomes, mtDNA exists in the form of circular molecules that are similar to the DNA found in bacteria. Each circle of mtDNA consists of a pair of complementary chains of DNA, totaling approximately 16,500 base pairs. Each mitochondrion contains between two and ten such circles of mtDNA. Mitochondrial DNA replicates at random within the mitochondria, and the mitochondria themselves divide by a budding process, unlike the elaborate cell cycle and mitosis of eukaryotic cells. During cellular mitosis, intracytoplasmic organelles, including mitochondria, are randomly partitioned into each daughter cell. If a new mutation in mtDNA occurs, intracellular populations of both mutant and normal mtDNA coexist, a condition known as heteroplasmy.

However, not all of the proteins found within the mitochondria are encoded by mtDNA. In fact, most of the proteins found in mitochondria are encoded by nuclear genes, synthesized in the usual way in the cytoplasm on cytoplasmic ribosomes, and subsequently transported into the mitochondria. Hence, primary mitochondrial dysfunction can result from different origins, with different inheritance patterns. Mutations can arise involving mtDNA, including single-nucleotide substitutions, such as in Leber's hereditary optic neuropathy (see chapter 76), which will be inherited maternally. Other mutations resulting in disease include segmental deletions and rearrangements involving entire regions of mtDNA.[14] Other mutations can arise involving nuclear genes that participate in mitochondrial function. These genes may code for mitochondrial proteins or may otherwise be involved in the normal functioning of mitochondria and even mtDNA. Diseases resulting from abnormalities in these genes will be transmitted in classic Mendelian fashion.

The criteria required to label a disease as *mitochondrial* has evolved over time. Initially, diseases were considered *mitochondrial myopathies* if somatic muscle biopsy showed morphological evidence of abnormalities involving the mitochondria, usually by using the modified Gomori trichrome stain to produce the so-called ragged red appearance.[30] Later, abnormalities of muscle mtDNA were found in such patients.[14,15,26,51] Therefore, the label of *mitochondrial disease* was expanded to include diseases that had genetic evidence to suggest mitochondrial abnormalities, even if the muscle fibers were morphologically normal. Several clinical syndromes were designated as mitochondrial diseases, include Leber's hereditary optic neuropathy,[49] MELAS (mitochondrial myopathy, encephalopathy, lactic acidosis, and strokelike episodes),[33] MERRF (myoclonic epilepsy with ragged red fibers),[10] and KSS (Kearns-Sayre syndrome).[21]

Clinically, the mitochondrial diseases manifest with a surprising amount of heterogeneity. There is poor correlation among the genetic defect, the biochemical abnormality, and the clinical presentation.[5,28] Thus, a single genetic defect can give rise to a range of clinical presentations. Similarly, a single clinical syndrome can arise from a number of different genetic defects. In general, however, the most common ophthalmologic manifestations of mitochondrial disease can be grouped into syndromes of bilateral optic neuropathy, progressive external ophthalmoplegia (PEO), pigmentary retinopathy, and retrochiasmal visual loss, although there is frequently overlap among these categories.[5] For example, KSS encompasses both ophthalmoplegia and pigmentary retinopathy and may rarely include optic atrophy.[26,51]

The literature on electrophysiological studies of the visual pathways in mitochondrial diseases is difficult to interpret, both because of the evolving definition of mitochondrial disease and because of the use of different electrophysiological techniques in the various reports. Older articles, prior to modern molecular genetic diagnosis, include information collected on patients with "mitochondrial myopathy," a diagnosis that was usually established by the presence of ragged red fibers on muscle biopsy. These studies typically included patients with varying clinical presentations but with common histopathological findings. Newer articles focus primarily on patients or pedigrees with either a defined clinical presentation or, more frequently, a specific genetic defect. Because of the range of presentation, some of the patients who were reported, although genetically carriers, were clinically unaffected. In addition, many of these reports focus on other issues, and information on the electrophysiological findings may be sparse.

The electrophysiological investigations described in both the earlier and more recent studies include primarily various forms of the electroretinogram (ERG) and the visual evoked potential (VEP). Data from the electro-oculogram (EOG) are reported in a few studies. Results are variably reported as either normal or subnormal, without further details or, less commonly, with more detailed descriptions of photopic or scotopic abnormalities. Studies in the English-language literature that provide electrophysiological data are summarized in the tables and detailed below.

Electrophysiological studies in patients without genetic diagnosis

FULL-FIELD (FLASH) ERG   A review of the literature found a total of 101 patients with ragged red fibers who were investigated with full-field ERGs (table 55.1).[1,3,4,13,27,37] Two studies were in children;[13,37] the others were in adult patients. Only two studies[3,4] gave details on individual eyes; the patients reported by the other authors presumably had comparable results in both eyes. There were 42 (42%) patients who had normal ERGs. Another patient had a normal ERG in one eye and scotopic abnormalities in the other. Of the patients with abnormal results, 16 patients had subnormal ERGs in both eyes with no further details, and another patient had a subnormal ERG in one eye and no response in the other.[3] Twenty-three patients had both scotopic and photopic abnormalities in both eyes, and one other patient had both scotopic and photopic abnormalities in one eye and only scotopic abnormalities in the other eye.[4] Three patients had only photopic abnormalities in both eyes, and two more had only scotopic abnormalities in both eyes. Ten patients had absent responses in both eyes. Interestingly, in the study by Riguardiere and coworkers,[37] all eight pediatric patients had normal ERGs. Because half of the patients in this study were younger than 6 years old, this supports the impression that clinical and electrophysiological evidence of retinal involvement in these diseases increases with age.[27]

ROD PHOTORECEPTOR RESPONSES   Cooper and coworkers[7] studied 22 pediatric patients (median age 5 years) with presumed mitochondrial disease, 20 defined by biochemical enzyme complex deficiencies, one by a large mitochondrial deletion, and one by a mtDNA mutation at nucleotide posi-

TABLE 55.1

Full-field ERG results in patients without specific genetic diagnosis but presumed mitochondrial disease

Authors	Year	Number	Normal	Abnormal (Unspecified)	Abnormal (Scotopic and Photopic)	Abnormal (Photopic Only)	Abnormal (Scotopic Only)	Abnormal 30-Hz Flicker	Absent
Bastiaensen[3]*	1978	45	12	14.5	7	1	3	NR	7.5
Harden et al.[13]	1982	12	7	2	—	—	—	NR	3
Mullie et al.[27]†	1985	7	0	—	5	2	—	7	0
Berdjis et al.[4]‡	1985	11	6 OU, 1 w/scotopic 1 w/amblyopia	—	2 OU, 1 w/scotopic	—	2 eyes	NR	—
Rigaudiere et al.[37]	1993	9	8	—	—	—	—	NR	—
Ambrosio et al.[1]	1995	17	8	—	9	—	—	9	—

*Bastiaensen[3] reported four patients and reviewed the literature for ERG results in 41 other patients.

†Mullie et al.[27] reported ERG results in 11 patients. Mitochondrial DNA analysis results on a number of his patients were reported subsequently by Smith and Harding.[44] Three patients had mtDNA deletions, and another had the 3243 mutation. These patients are included in tables 55.2 and 55.3, respectively.

‡Berdgis et al.[4] reported results for separate eyes. One of their patients had an amblyopic eye that was not tested, and the other eye proved normal. A patient had one normal eye with scotopic abnormalities in the other eye, and another patient had scotopic abnormalities in one eye and both scotopic and photopic abnormalities in the other eye.

NR = not reported.

OU = both eyes.

tion 8993. They used the Hood and Birch[17] formulation of the Lamb and Pugh[23,36] model of rod phototransduction to study photoreceptor response parameters, specifically S and R_{mp3} derived from the scotopic a-wave and $\log \sigma$ and V_{max} derived from the b-wave. Results were obtainable in 19 patients. These parameters showed some abnormality in most of the patients, being completely normal in only five patients, of whom three were among the youngest patients studied.

PATTERN ERG Sartucci and coworkers[39] described 17 patients with histologically defined mitochondrial myopathy. Of these, ten patients had PEO, and the remaining seven had symptoms including ptosis, bulbar weakness, and cerebellar signs. None of these patients fulfilled the exact diagnostic criteria for KSS, MELAS, or MERRF syndromes. Fourteen patients underwent pattern ERG (PERG). The PERGs showed abnormal responses in 11 patients. Of these, 13 eyes showed no response, and the P50 was delayed in four eyes. The same group also performed VEPs (see below) and calculated the retinocortical time (RCT). The RCT was prolonged unilaterally in four eyes and not evaluable in 15 other eyes.

VISUAL EVOKED POTENTIAL Techniques for recording the VEP were varied. Harden and coworkers[13] recorded flash VEPs (fVEP) with both eyes open in 12 patients. The potentials were present with well-defined early components in six of 12 patients; five others had either absent or ill-defined early components; in the last case, the VEP was of "unusual configuration with enlarged components." Rigaudiere and coworkers[37] reported fVEPs in eight pediatric patients, four with mitochondrial myopathy and the remainder with mitochondrial encephalopathy. The fVEPs were normal in four patients and showed hyperamplitudes in two patients with mitochondrial myopathy, associated with normal latencies. Another two patients, both with mitochondrial encephalopathy, had decreased amplitudes and increased latencies. The abnormal VEPs were seen in the older patients; the mitochondrial myopathy patients were aged 6 and 9 years compared to 5 months and 2 years, while the encephalopathy patients were both aged 15 years, compared to 21 months and 5 years.

Using a mixture of both flash and pattern-reversal VEPs, Smith and Harding[44] reported VEP results in 20 patients, some of whom had genetic abnormalities, including one patient with MERRF and three patients with MELAS (see below). Of the remaining 16 patients, six patients had normal results, and ten had abnormal results. Berdgis and coworkers[4] obtained normal fVEP results in 21 eyes.

Pattern-shift VEP (PSVEP) was reported in a total of 83 other patients, some of whom were known to have mitochondrial deletions.[1,4,39,40,42,48] Five studies[1,4,39,40,42] gave PSVEP results in a total of 77 patients. Six patients[40] had mitochondrial deletions, but details were not reported. Of 153 eyes, 80 (52%) were normal, 45 eyes had prolonged latencies, four eyes had side-to-side latency differences, and 24 more eyes showed absent responses.

Versino and coworkers[48] investigated the effect of check size in 13 patients with PEO and histopathologically proven mitochondrial disease, using both 15' and 30' check sizes. Seven of these patients had mitochondrial deletions. The P100 latency was delayed bilaterally in eight patients, regardless of check size. In three patients, the P100 latency was normal for the 30' check size but delayed for the 15' check size, and in the last two patients the VEP was normal for both the 15' and 30' check sizes.

ELECTRO-OCULOGRAM EOGs were not commonly reported. Bastiaensen[3] obtained EOGs in four patients and reviewed the literature for PEO patients. The EOGs were normal in three of his patients and at the lower limit of normal for the other patient. He found in the previous literature another two patients with normal EOG and four patients with subnormal EOG. However, he commented that the EOGs often could not be recorded because of abnormal ocular motility. Mullie and coworkers[27] performed EOGs in 11 patients and reported their results as the EOG light rise, instead of the Arden index. Six patients had subnormal results, while two more had supernormal results. The remaining three patients had such poor eye motility that EOG proved impossible to perform.

Electrophysiological studies in patients genetically defined

With the advent of molecular genetics, mitochondrial diseases became better characterized genetically. Given the rapid advances in this field, earlier papers in the molecular era reported abnormalities in restriction splice sites, while later studies used the polymerase chain reaction and DNA sequencing techniques to better define and specify the genetic abnormalities. Many patients with morphologically abnormal muscle fibers were found to have abnormalities involving the mtDNA. Partial deletions, usually with some degree of heteroplasmy, were found in many patients with the CPEO/KSS phenotype. Single-nucleotide substitutions were found in other disorders, the common mutations being the 3243A-G mutation in MELAS[11,12] and the 8344A-G mutation in MERRF.[41]

In addition to these syndromes, which typically have ragged red fibers on biopsy, other syndromes without such histological findings are now known to be the result of mtDNA defects. One such syndrome of particular interest to the ophthalmologist is the syndrome of neurogenic muscle weakness, ataxia, and retinitis pigmentosa (NARP), a maternally inherited disorder resulting from a point mutation at position 8993 in the ATPase 6 gene of the mtDNA.[16] This condition has a heterogenous clinical presentation, ranging from isolated retinal changes to Leigh's syndrome with psychomotor regression, seizures, and death in early childhood.[6,25,31,47,50] The NARP mutation has been associated with pigmentary degeneration of the retina in a salt-and-pepper pattern as well as a bone spicule pattern.[31] Indeed, a salt-and-pepper appearance in childhood may progress to a full-blown retinitis pigmentosa pattern over the years.[22]

Another syndrome associated with a mtDNA point mutation is the syndrome of maternally inherited diabetes and deafness (MIDD) resulting from a point mutation at position 3243, the mutation that is most commonly found in association with the MELAS phenotype.[2] Leber's hereditary optic neuropathy, associated primarily with mtDNA mutations[28] at positions 3468, 11778, and 14484, is described in chapter 76. Although the above diseases are very well described clinically, biochemically, and genetically, electrophysiological information is sparse, with the exception of the NARP syndrome.

mtDNA DELETIONS AND REARRANGEMENTS Nine patients with the CPEO/KSS phenotype who were confirmed to have mitochondrial deletions had ERGs performed[19,27,32] (table 55.2). Two patients had normal ERGs, while seven others had abnormal results. In one of the patients reported by Mullie and coworkers,[27] who was later determined to have mtDNA deletions,[44] serial ERGs were performed three years apart. Deterioration was apparent in all ERG variables over time, although visual function remained clinically normal.

MELAS AND MIDD (3243 MUTATION) Most patients with the MELAS and MIDD syndromes have the same common mtDNA mutation at position 3243.[5,28] Case series include patients with either clinical presentation. Flash ERGs on patients with the 3243 mutation were reported in a total of 16 patients[18,19,24,27,43,46] (table 55.3), of which nine were

TABLE 55.2

Results of electrophysiological testing in patients with confirmed mtDNA deletions

Authors	Year	No. of Patients	ERG	EOG
Mullie et al.[27]*	1985	3	Cone: all 3 abnormal Rod: 2 abnormal, 1 normal	NR
Ota et al.[32]	1994	1	Normal photopic and scotopic	Normal Arden ratio
Isashiki et al.[19]	1998	5	1 normal, 4 abnormal	NR

*Mullie et al.[27] reported ERG results in 11 patients, and three of his patients were reported subsequently by Smith and Harding[44] to have mitochondrial deletions.

NR = not reported.

TABLE 55.3

Results of electrophysiological testing in patients with the 3243 (MELAS and MIDD) mtDNA mutation

Authors	Year	No. of patients	ERG	VEP	EOG Results
Mullie et al.[27]*	1985	1	Abnormal rod Abnormal cone	NR	NR
Smith and Harding[44]*	1993	3	NR	2 normal, 1 abnormal	NR
Hwang et al.[18]	1997	2	NR	2 abnormal	NR
Sue et al.[46]	1997	11	11 normal (PERG)	7 normal OU, 2 abnormal one eye 2 abnormal OU	NR
Isashiki et al.[19]	1998	1	Abnormal	NR	NR
Latkany et al.[24]	1999	1	Abnormal photopic and scotopic	NR	NR
Smith et al.[43]	1999	12	Scotopic: 6 abnormal eyes, 18 normal eyes Photopic: 5 abnormal eyes, 19 normal eyes	NR	4 normal, 8 abnormal

*Mullie et al.[27] reported ERG results in 11 patients, and one of his patients was reported subsequently by Smith and Harding[44] to have the 3243 mutation.

NR = not reported.

OU = both eyes.

TABLE 55.4

Full-field ERG results in patients with the 8993 (NARP) mtDNA mutation

Authors	Year	No. of Patients	Retinal Pigmentation	CPEO	Ragged Red Fibers	Leigh's Disease	ERG
Holt et al.[16]	1990	4	4/4	0/4	0/4	0/4	1/4 "small responses," 3/4 NR
Fryer et al.[9]	1993	9	4/9	0	NR	2/9	1 "low amplitude, poorly defined," others not done
Puddu et al.[35]	1993	3	2/3 "RP," 1/3 normal	0/4	0/4	0/4	1/3 "normal," 2/3 dec phot a, b, inc b implicit time
Ortiz et al.[31]	1993	13	1/13 "RP," 6/13 "SP," 1/13 "BS"	0/13	0/13	4/13	1/13 "normal," 3/13 "rod-cone dysfunction," 4/13 not done
Chowers et al.[6]	1999	7	2/3 pigmentation	0/3	0/3	0/3	1/3 "normal," 1/3 "cone," 1/3 "rod-cone"
Porto et al.[34]	2001	4	3/4 "BS"	0	NR	1/4	1/3 "cone-rod," 1/4 "no response," 2/4 NR

RP = retinitis pigmentosa, BS = bone spicules, SP = salt-and-pepper changes, NR = not reported, CPEO = chronic progressive external ophthalmoplegia.

normal and seven were abnormal. Sue and coworkers[46] reported PERG data on 11 patients in four 3243-positive pedigrees, all of which were normal. Because of the association with diabetes, a number of patients may also have diabetic retinopathy and laser treatment, potentially confounding the ERG results. EOGs were reported in 12 patients by Smith and coworkers,[43] four of which were normal and eight of which were abnormal.

MERRF There are only a few reports of visual electrophysiological investigations in MERRF patients with the 8344 mutation. Seventeen patients had VEPs.[29,38,44,45] Of these, seven patients were normal, four had delayed P100 latencies, one had absent responses, and five had high amplitudes. The patients with high amplitudes were all from the study by Rosing and coworkers,[38] and the authors postulated that this finding was also found in other myoclonic and photosensitive epilepsies. A similar finding of increased amplitudes was seen in the somatosensory evoked potentials of these patients. This may reflect a general hyperexcitability to all stimuli as part of startle myoclonus. ERG and EOG data have not been reported in MERRF patients.

THE T8993G (NARP) SYNDROME The NARP syndrome may present clinically with a wide range of findings, including retinal pigmentation. The range of electrophysiological findings is equally variable (table 55.4) and may reflect the age at which these patients were tested (figures 55.1 and 55.2). Details are summarized in table 55.4.[6,9,16,31,34,35] Of 14 patients studied with flash ERG, only three had normal ERGs, ten had various abnormalities, and one had an unrecordable ERG.

Conclusions

Electrophysiological studies of the visual pathways are not uncommonly abnormal among patients with mitochondrial disease. ERG abnormalities are frequently present in patients with overt retinal pigmentation as well as in patients with apparently normal funduscopy. Abnormalities have been found with various techniques, including full-field ERG and pattern ERG. Although longtitudinal studies have not been reported, children with mitochondrial diseases may have normal ERGs initially and later progress to manifest abnormalities, a process that is often mirrored by the retinal appearance. Use of more sophisticated indices of photoreceptor transduction might provide a more sensitive indicator of photoreceptor stress.[7]

VEP abnormalities are also frequently present in patients with mitochondrial disease, even if there is no apparent optic nerve or brain involvement. Hyperamplitudes may be present in MERRF syndrome as part of a generalized sensitivity to stimuli.

The advent of molecular genetics has led to more precise characterization of the mitochondrial disorders. However, a particular clinical presentation can frequently result from different genetic abnormalities, and each genetic defect may produce a wide range of clinical presentations. The electrophysiological findings in patients with mitochondrial disease are equally variable.

ACKNOWLEDGMENTS This study was supported in part by a departmental grant (Department of Ophthalmology) from Research to Prevent Blindness, Inc., New York, New York, and by core grant P30-EY06360 (Department of Ophthalmology) from the National Institutes of Health, Bethesda, Maryland. Dr. Newman is a recipient of a Research to Prevent Blindness Lew R. Wasserman Merit Award.

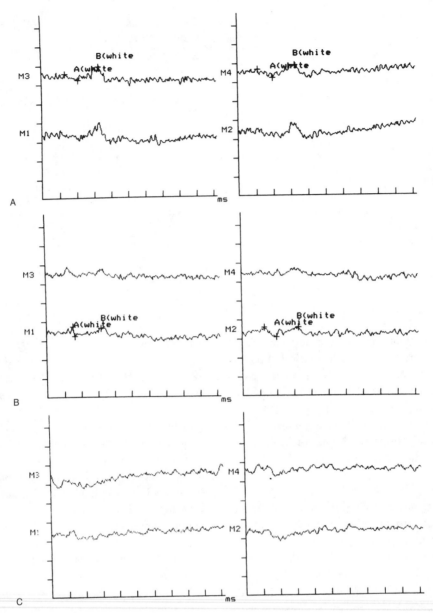

A

B

C

FIGURE 55.1   Serial ERGs of a patient with the 8993 (NARP) mutation performed in 1994 (A), 1996 (B), and 1998 (C), showing progressing loss of responses to a full-field white flash stimulus.

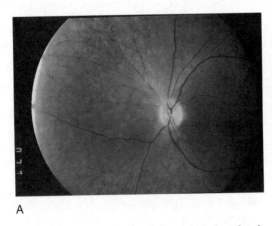

A

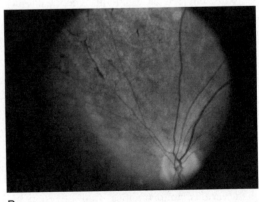

B

FIGURE 55.2   Serial fundus photographs of the same patient dated 1986 (A) and 1994 (B) showing increased retinal pigmentation from salt-and-pepper retinopathy to frank bone spiculing. Note that the magnification in part B is higher, showing more central encroachment of the pigmentary changes. Both images demonstrate substantial arterial attenuation. (See also color plate 22.)

REFERENCES

1. Ambrosio G, de Marco R, Loffredo L, et al: Visual dysfunction in patients with mitochondrial myopathies. *Doc Ophthalmol* 1995; 89:211–218.

2. Ballinger SW, Shoffner JM, Hedaya EV, et al: Maternally transmitted diabetes and deafness associated with a 10.4 kb mitochondrial DNA deletion. *Nat Genet* 1992; 1:11–15.

3. Bastiaensen LAK: Pigment changes of the retina in chronic progressive ophthalmoplegia (CPEO). *Acta Ophthalmol* 1978; 56 (suppl 138):5–36.

4. Berdjis H, Heider Y, Demisch K: ERG and VEP in chronic progressive external ophthalmoplegia (CPEO). *Doc Ophthalmol* 1985; 60:427–434.

5. Biousse V, Newman NJ: Neuro-ophthalmology of mitochondrial diseases. *Semin Neurol* 2001; 21:275–291.

6. Chowers I, Lerman-Sagie T, Elpeleg ON, et al: Cone and rod dysfunction in the NARP syndrome. *Br J Ophthalmol* 1999; 83:190–193.

7. Cooper LL, Hansen RM, Darras BT, et al: Rod photoreceptor function in children with mitochondrial disorders. *Arch Ophthalmol* 2002; 120:1055–1062.

8. DiMauro S, Bonilla E, Zeviani M, et al: Mitochondrial myopathies. *Ann Neurol* 1985; 17:521–538.

9. Fryer A, Appleton R, Sweeney MG, Rosenbloom L, Harding AE: Mitochondrial DNA 8993 (NARP) mutation presenting with a heterogeneous phenotype including 'cerebral palsy.' *Arch Dis Child* 1994; 71:419–422.

10. Fukuhara N, Tokiguchi S, Shirakawa K, et al: Myoclonus epilepsy associated with ragged red fibers (mitochondrial abnormalities): Disease entity or syndrome? Light and electron microscopic studies of two cases and review of the literature. *J Neurol Sci* 1980; 47:117–133.

11. Goto Y, Nonaka I, Honai S: A mutation in the tRNA Leu (UUR) gene associated with the MELAS subgroup of mitochondrial encephalomyopathies. *Nature* 1990; 348:651–653.

12. Goto Y, Nonaka I, Haroi S: A new mtDNA mutation associated with mitochondrial myopathy, encephalomyopathy, lactic acidosis and stroke-like episodes. *Biochim Biophys Acta* 1991; 1097:238–240.

13. Harden A, Pampiglione G, Battaglia A: "Mitochondrial myopathy" or mitochondrial disease? EEG, ERG, VEP studies in 13 children. *J Neurol Neurosurg Psychiatry* 1982; 45:627–632.

14. Holt IJ, Harding AE, Cooper JM, et al: Mitochondrial myopathies: Clinical and biochemical features of 30 patients with major deletions of muscle mitochondrial DNA. *Ann Neurol* 1989; 26:699–798.

15. Holt IJ, Harding AE, Morgan-Hughes JA: Deletions of mitochondrial DNA in patients with mitochondrial myopathies. *Nature* 1988; 331:717–719.

16. Holt IJ, Harding AE, Petty RKH, et al: A new mitochondrial disease associated with mitochondrial DNA heteroplasmy. *Am J Hum Genet* 1990; 46:428–433.

17. Hood DC, Birch DG: Rod phototransduction in retinitis pigmentosa: Estimation and interpretation of parameters derived from the rod a-wave. *Invest Ophthalmol Vis Sci* 1994; 35:2948–2961.

18. Hwang JM, Park HW, Kim SJ: Optic neuropathy associated with mitochondrial tRNA[Leu(UUR)] A3243G mutation. *Ophthalmic Genet* 1997; 18:101–105.

19. Isashiki Y, Nakagawa M, Ohba N, et al: Retinal manifestations in mitochondrial diseases associated with mitochondrial DNA mutation. *Acta Ophthalmol Scand* 1998; 76:6–13.

20. Johns DR: Mitochondrial DNA and disease. *N Engl J Med* 1995; 333:638–644.

21. Kearns TP, Sayre GP: Retinitis pigmentosa, external ophthalmoplegia and complete heartblock: Unusual syndrome with histologic study in one of two cases. *Arch Ophthalmol* 1958; 60:280–289.

22. Kerrison JB, Biousse V, Newman NJ: Retinopathy of NARP syndrome. *Arch Ophthalmol* 2000; 118:298–299.

23. Lamb TD, Pugh EN: A quantitative account of the activation steps involved in phototransduction in amphibian photoreceptors. *J Physiol* 1992; 449:719–758.

24. Latkany P, Ciulla TA, Cucchillo P, et al: Mitochondrial maculopathy: Geographic atrophy of the macula in the MELAS associated A to G 3243 mitochondrial DNA point mutation. *Am J Ophthalmol* 1999; 128:112–114.

25. Makela-Bengs P, Suomalainen A, Majander, et al: Correlation between the clinical symptomatology and the proportion of mitochondrial DNA carrying the 8993 point mutation in the NARP syndrome. *Pediatr Res* 1995; (37):634–639.

26. Moraes CT, DiMauro S, Zeviani M, et al: Mitochondrial DNA deletions in progressive ophthalmoplegia and Kearns-Sayre syndrome. *N Engl J Med* 1989; 320:1293–1299.

27. Mullie MA, Harding AE, Petty RKH, et al: The retinal manifestations of mitochondrial myopathy: A study of 22 cases. *Arch Ophthalmol* 1985; 103:1825–1830.

28. Newman NJ: Mitochondrial disease and the eye. *Ophthalmol Clin N Am* 1992; 5:405–424.

29. Ohtsuka Y, Amano R, Oka E, et al: Myoclonus epilepsy with ragged red fibers: A clinical and electrophysiologic follow-up study on two sibling cases. *J Child Neurol* 1993; 8:366–371.

30. Olson W, Engel WK, Walsh GP, et al: Oculocraniosomatic neuromuscular disease with 'ragged red' fibers: Histochemical and ultrastructural changes in limb muscles in a group of patients with idiopathic progressive external ophthalmoplegia. *Arch Neurol* 1972; 26:193–211.

31. Ortiz RG, Newman NJ, Shoffner JM, et al: Variable retinal and neurologic manifestations in patients harboring the mitochondrial DNA 8993 mutation. *Arch Ophthalmol* 1993; 111:1525–1530.

32. Ota Y, Miyake Y, Awaya S, et al: Early retinal involvement in mitochondrial myopathy with mitochondrial DNA deletion. *Retina* 1994; 14:270–276.

33. Pavlakis SG, Phillips PC, DiMauro S, et al: Mitochondrial myopathy, encephalopathy, lactic acidosis and stroke-like episodes: A distinctive clinical syndrome. *Ann Neurol* 1984; 3:455–458.

34. Porto FBO, Mack G, Sterboul MJ, et al: Isolated late-onset cone-rod dystrophy revealing a familial neurogenic muscle weakness, ataxia and retinitis pigmentosa syndrome with the T8993 mitochondrial mutation. *Am J Ophthalmol* 2001; 132:935–937.

35. Puddu P, Barboni P, Mantovani V, et al: Retinitis pigmentosa, ataxia, and mental retardation associated with mitochondrial DNA mutation in an Italian family. *Br J Ophthalmol* 1993; 77:84–88.

36. Pugh EN, Lamb TD: Amplification and kinetics of the activation steps in phototransduction. *Biochem Biophys Acta* 1993; 1141:111–149.

37. Rigaudiere F, Manderieux N, Le Gargasson JF, et al: Electrophysiological exploration of visual function in mitochondrial diseases. *Electroencephalogr Clin Neurophysiol* 1995; 96:495–501.

38. Rosing HS, Hopkins LC, Wallace DC, et al: Maternally inherited mitochondrial myopathy and myoclonic epilepsy. *Ann Neurol* 1985; 17:228–237.

39. Sartucci F, Rossi B, Tognoni G, et al: Evoked potentials in the evaluation of patients with mitochondrial myopathy. *Eur Neurol* 1993; 33:428–435.

40. Schubert M, Zierz S, Dengler R: Central and peripheral nervous system conduction in mitochondrial myopathy with chronic progressive external ophthalmoplegia. *Electroencephalogr Clin Neurophysiol* 1994; 90:304–412.

41. Shoffner JM, Lott MT, Lezza AM, et al: Myoclonic epilepsy and ragged red fiber disease (MERRF) is associated with a mitochondrial DNA tRNA (Lys) mutation. *Cell* 1990; 61:931–937.

42. Sjo O, Trojaborg W: A multimodality electrophysiological study of patients with progressive ophthalmoplegia, pigmentary retinopathy and mitochondrial myopathy. In Gallai V (ed): *Maturation of Central Nervous System.* Amsterdam, Elsevier, 1986, pp 297–306.

43. Smith PR, Bain SC, Good PA, et al: Pigmentary retinal dystrophy and the syndrome of maternally inherited diabetes and deafness caused by the mitochondrial DNA 3243 tRNA(Leu) A to G mutation. *Ophthalmology* 1999; 106:1101–1108.

44. Smith SJ, Harding AE: EEG and evoked potential findings in mitochondrial myopathies. *J Neurol* 1993; 240:367–372.

45. So N, Berkovic S, Andermann F, et al: Myoclonus epilepsy and ragged red fibers (MERRF). *Brain* 1989; 112:1261–1276.

46. Sue CM, Mitchell P, Crimmins DS, et al: Pigmentary retinopathy associated with the mitochondrial DNA 3243 point mutation. *Neurology* 1997; 49:1013–1017.

47. Tatuch Y, Cristodoulou J, Feigenbaum A, et al: Heteroplasmic mtDNA mutation (T → G) at 8993 can cause Leigh disease when the percentage of abnormal mtDNA is high. *Am J Hum Genet* 1992; 50:852–858.

48. Versino M, Piccolo G, Callieco R, et al: Multimodal evoked potentials in progressive external ophthalmoplegia with mitochondrial myopathy. *Acta Neurol Scand* 1991; 84:107–110.

49. Wallace DC, Singh G, Lott MT, et al: Mitochondrial DNA mutation associated with Leber's hereditary optic neuropathy. *Science* 1998; 242:1427–1430.

50. White SL, Shanske S, Biros I, Warwick L, Dahl HM, Thorburn DR, Di Mauro S: Two cases of prenatal analysis for the pathogenic T to G substitution at nucleotide 8993 in mitochondrial DNA. *Prenat Diagn* 1999; 19:1165–1168.

51. Zeviani M, Moraes CT, DiMauro S, et al: Deletions of mitochondrial DNA in Kearns-Sayre syndrome. *Neurology* 1988; 38:1339–1346.

X   EVALUATION OF VASCULAR DISEASES, INFLAMMATORY STATES, AND TUMORS

56 Diseases of the Middle Retina: Venous and Arterial Occlusions

MARY A. JOHNSON

BRANCH AND CENTRAL retinal vein occlusion are common retinal vascular disorders, second only to diabetic retinopathy in frequency of occurrence. They are both easy disorders to diagnose using clinical techniques. For this reason, investigations into the value of the electroretinogram (ERG) in these disorders have focused on prognosis, not diagnosis.

Central retinal vein occlusion

It is estimated that about 20% of eyes with central retinal vein occlusion (CRVO) are ischemic and are therefore at risk for developing neovascularization of the iris (NVI).[5,15] The determination of ischemia in this disorder, however, is problematic; fluorescein angiograms (FA) often do not capture peripheral capillary nonperfusion, they might be difficult to read because of intraretinal hemorrhage or other factors, the FA changes associated with ischemia in CRVO might not be completely understood,[19] and CRVO eyes that have no apparent capillary dropout occasionally develop NVI.[2,9,14]

The ERG has been shown to be a sensitive and specific test for identifying CRVO eyes that are at risk for the development of NVI. It has the advantages over angiography of providing an evaluation of the entire retina, including far peripheral areas, and of quantifying the amount of ischemia with regard to the retinal area that is affected, the extent of the damage within the area affected, and the amount of functional loss in perfused but still ischemic eyes. In a prospective study involving 140 eyes of 128 patients, Hayreh and colleagues[2] found that the ERG as well as other measures of visual function proved far superior to the morphological tests of fluorescein angiography and fundoscopic appearance in differentiating ischemic from nonischemic CRVO during the early acute phase. Their most sensitive test in uniocular CRVO was the RAPD, followed closely by the ERG, then visual field and visual acuity. The combination of RAPD and ERG differentiated 97% of ischemic from nonischemic cases. The authors stated that ophthalmoscopic appearance was the "least reliable, most misleading" parameter.

Researchers have categorized the ERG changes that occur in CRVO in a number of ways. Eyes with CRVO often have reduced ERG b/a amplitude ratios, reduced b-wave amplitudes, reduced or enhanced a-wave amplitudes, delays in the implicit times of the a- and b-waves and the multifocal ERG, reductions in oscillatory potential amplitudes, and changes in the Naka-Rushton R_{max} and log K parameters derived from intensity-response analysis. ERGs recorded from most cases of CRVO will show significant changes in some of these parameters, even if the eye is perfused and has a good prognosis. However, eyes with CRVO that develop NVI demonstrate large ERG changes, and it is generally not difficult to identify eyes that are at risk for NVI even when the ERG is recorded only once, at the patient's initial visit.[1,10,13,19,20]

ERG amplitudes

The work of Sabates and colleagues[20] has focused attention on the dramatic reductions that are often seen in the b/a ratio in ischemic eyes with CRVO. The b/a ratio is the amplitude of the b-wave, measured from a-wave trough to b-wave peak, to the amplitude of the a-wave, measured from the baseline to the trough of the a-wave. Sabates et al.[20] reported that five out of eight eyes in his study that had b-wave reductions that were so large that the b-wave did not extend beyond the prestimulus baseline (the b/a ratio measured less than 1; see figure 56.1) developed NVI, whereas only one eye that did not have this characteristic developed the complication. Kaye and Harding recently obtained similar results,[14] and Breton et al.[1] confirmed findings that date to Karpe's original monograph, published in 1945.[12] Johnson and McPhee[10] found the b/a ratio to be specific but not sensitive for NVI in a prospective study of 93 eyes with CRVO. They attributed some of the differences between studies to the different stimulus luminances that were used; the b/a ratio is not an invariant characteristic of the ERG but rather depends strongly on stimulus intensity, as illustrated in figures 56.2A and 56.2B.

Much of the reduction in b/a ratios can be attributed to preferential reductions in the b-wave amplitude. In a prospective study of 30 CRVO eyes, seven that later developed NVI and 23 that did not, Kaye and Harding[14] reported that b-wave amplitudes were decreased on average by $102\,\mu V$ in eyes that developed NVI when compared to the

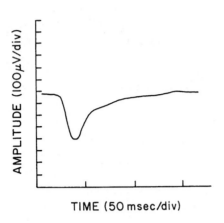

FIGURE 56.1 An ERG recorded from an eye with CRVO and NVI. The b/a amplitude ratio measures <1.

normal fellow eyes and by 63 μV when compared to affected eyes that did not develop NVI. Mean a-wave amplitudes were not significantly different for any of the comparisons. This latter result may be due to the fact that in CRVO, the a-wave may either increase or decrease with disease severity. Curiously, the b/a ratio was found to be a better predictor of NVI development than was b-wave amplitude. This paradox might be explained by two factors: the large variability on ERG amplitude and the fact that the a-wave amplitude may be either abnormally large or abnormally small in CRVO. Abnormally small a-waves, of course, suggest that more than the middle retina is involved in the disorder.

Other investigators have also demonstrated substantial b-wave reductions in CRVO.[1,9,10] These studies will be discussed more fully in the section dealing with intensity-response functions.

Oscillatory potential (OP) amplitudes are reduced in CRVO, but while there is a significant difference between the means of distributions of OPs recorded from eyes that develop NVI when compared to eyes that do not develop this complication, there is a substantial overlap between these distributions. This overlap results from the fact that CRVO eyes not at risk for NVI have substantial OP reductions.[11]

Temporal factors

Large delays in ERG implicit times are found in CRVO eyes that develop NVI. Values for the scotopic single-flash a- and b-waves, the photopic b-wave, and the peak of the 30-Hz flicker response have been reported.[1,2,9,10,14] In a prospective study of 62 CRVO patients, Johnson and McPhee[10] showed

that both the scotopic b-wave and the 30-Hz response recorded from patients at their first visit identified patients who had or would later develop NVI, with high sensitivity and specificity. Their data for scotopic b-wave implicit time, measured from stimulus onset to peak of the b-wave, are illustrated in figure 56.3A. While ERGs from most of the CRVO eyes showed delays in b-wave timing, eyes that had or that would develop NVI showed much larger changes than the eyes that did not develop NVI. A risk factor criterion of 58 ms, which was 8 ms longer than the upper limit of the range of normal values for b-wave implicit time, yielded a sensitivity of 94% and a specificity of 64% for this data set. Figure 56.3B, which pictures the affected and normal eyes of a patient with CRVO and NVI, illustrates the size of the effect that is often seen.

B-wave implicit time delays were the most discriminant feature of the CRVO ERGs recorded by Kaye and Harding.[14] In agreement with Johnson and McPhee's data, they found that the difference between the means of the ERGs recorded from eyes that developed NVI versus the eyes that did not develop NVI was 7.4 ms, a difference that was significant at the $p < .001$ level. Furthermore, there was no overlap between these two distributions at the 99% confidence level. They also found significant intereye differences for both groups. These differences measured 9.6 ms for the NVI group and 2 ms for the comparison between the ERGs recorded from the nonproliferative CRVO eyes and their fellow eyes.

A similar picture is seen for the 30-Hz flicker ERG.[1,9,10,17] McPhee et al.[17] showed that, by using a criterion of 40 ms, a value that is 7 ms greater than the upper limit of the normal range, the 30-Hz flicker ERG shows performance equivalent to that of the scotopic b-wave in identifying eyes that had or that would develop NVI (figure 56.4A). At this criterion value, the sensitivity for this data set was 100%, and the specificity was 68%. Figure 56.4B illustrates a 30-Hz flicker ERG recorded from the normal and affected eyes of a patient with CRVO. McPhee et al.[17] measured implicit time as the phase of a 30-Hz sine wave fit to the data and not to the amplitude peak of the waveform because high-frequency components, which usually occur in healthy eyes at the leading edge of the flicker ERG, often disappear in eyes with CRVO. In these cases, measuring implicit time as the time to peak will accentuate the actual shift in time in waveforms recorded in normal eyes and in affected but non-proliferative eyes, thus reducing the ability to identify the individuals who have real time shifts and who are at risk for NVI.[22]

The NIH-sponsored ERG ancillary study to the Central Vein Occlusion Study (CVOS) confirmed the discriminability of the ERG implicit time delay in CRVO. Investigators from eight centers participated in the ERG-CVOS, testing a total of 333 patients, or about half of the patients enrolled

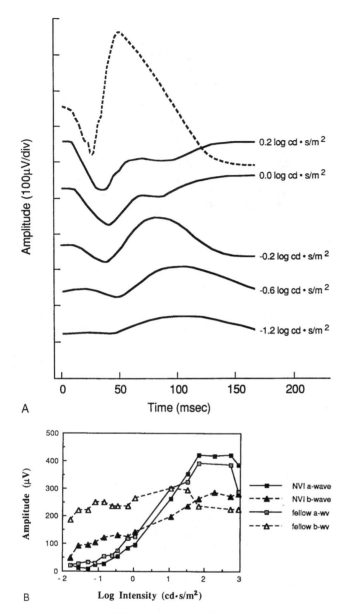

FIGURE 56.2 A, ERGs recorded as a function of stimulus luminance for an eye with CRVO and NVI (solid lines). For comparison, the dotted line is a normal ERG recorded at 0.2 log cd s/m². Note that the b/a ratio is less than 1 here only for the two brightest stimuli. B, a- and b-wave amplitudes plotted as a function of stimulus luminance. Note that as stimulus luminance increases, the a-wave amplitude grows at a faster rate than does the b-wave amplitude, and this results in smaller b/a ratios. This figure shows ERG amplitudes for the normal and affected eyes of a patient with central retinal vein occlusion and iris neovascularization. For this patient, the greatest recorded difference between eyes occurs at the 0.03 log cd s/m² intensity. Here, the difference in b/a ratio between eyes of 2.13 (fellow eye) versus 1.50 (affected eye) is due largely to a reduction in b-wave amplitude.

in the CVOS. They were able to compare the performance of the ERG to visual acuity, fundus photography, and fluorescein angiography, collected in a prescribed fashion and analyzed in reading centers. Not only was the ERG the most discriminant measure, it also was able to identify at-risk eyes in which a fluorescein angiogram could not be performed.[2]

The recent development of the multifocal ERG has illustrated that ERG timing delays occur throughout the retina in CRVO. Dolan et al.[3] reported that implicit times of the wide-field multifocal ERG (mfERG) were delayed in 98% of the central responses and 91% of the peripheral responses of the CRVO eyes that were examined. Furthermore, almost 60% of the fellow eyes showed implicit time delays, suggesting either predisposing factors for development of a CRVO in the fellow eye or that other vascular pathology is contributing to ocular ischemia in these patients. Thus, mfERG implicit times, like OP amplitudes, are very sensitive to retinal functions changes secondary to CRVO. However, it is not yet known how specific the mfERG can be in identifying eyes that later develop iris neovascularization.

Intensity-response analysis

ERG b-wave amplitude increases with stimulus intensity up to moderately high levels of luminance. These intensity-response data are typically analyzed by fitting them to a saturating, nonlinear function of a form first used by Naka and Rushton in 1966 in their work on the S-potential in fish.[18] This so-called Naka-Rushton function has the following form:

$$R = \frac{R_{max}I^n}{I^n + K^n} \tag{1}$$

where R and I are intensity-response ordered pairs, R_{max} is the asymptotic amplitude, K is the semisaturation constant, that is, the intensity at which R_{max} reaches half of its asymptotic value, and n is related to the slope at $I = K$. The value of performing this analysis is that the parameters derived from equation (1) can be evaluated in terms of putative pathophysiological mechanisms of disease. A number of studies have examined how the Naka-Rushton parameters change in CRVO and whether these changes can be used to predict neovascularization.

Eyes with CRVO usually show reductions in R_{max} and n and elevations in K. An elevation in K indicates that more light is required to produce normal amplitude ERGs, i.e., retinal sensitivity is reduced. Retinal heterogeneity is reflected in the slope parameter. Using Monte Carlo simulations, it has been formally demonstrated that heterogeneity in either R_{max} or K will decrease n.[16]

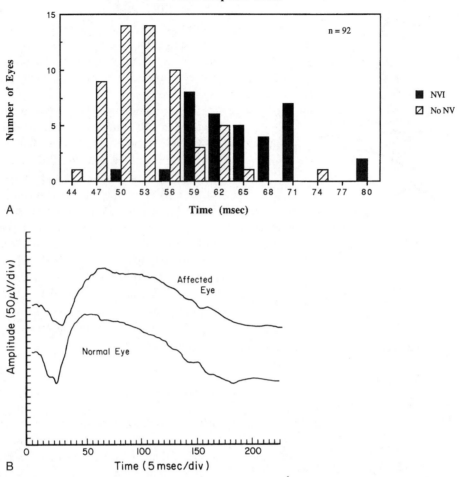

FIGURE 56.3 A, B-wave implicit time for CRVO eyes with NVI (solid bars) and without NVI (hatched bars). B, ERGs recorded from the affected and normal eyes of a patient with CRVO and NVI. The ERG recorded from the affected eye shows reduced a- and b-wave amplitudes and delays in implicit times when compared with the normal, fellow eye.

As with the other ERG parameters that have been examined, eyes that develop NVI have large elevations in K and often have large reductions in R_{max}. Using ROC analysis, which is a method of comparing entire distributions of data and which reflects the amount of overlap between distributions, Johnson and McPhee[10] have shown that the probability of detection (P_d) for K is 0.83, and P_d for R_{max} is 0.65. These numbers indicate the probability of detecting an eye that will progress to NVI using only the parameter and no additional patient information. A linear discriminant analysis performed on the data showed that virtually all of the information contained in the Naka-Rushton parameters was contained in K.

Breton and colleagues[1] have also shown that R_{max} and K are highly predictive of NVI in eyes with CRVO, but in their study, R_{max} was more discriminant than K. These conflicting results are likely due to differences in the algorithms used for fitting the data.[10]

CRVO eyes with elevations in K act as though they are seeing less light, and this is a major reason that delays in ERG timing occur in this disease. Examination of the scotopic b-wave implicit time versus stimulus luminance functions pictured in figure 56.5 (parts c and d) for the normal and affected eyes of a CRVO patient with NVI illustrates two facts: that a dimmer stimulus produces a response occurring later in time and that, for this patient, the implicit time versus luminance function recorded from the normal eye requires at least some horizontal translation (i.e., along the log intensity axis) to fit the data recorded from the affected eye. In CRVO, these implicit time delays reflect losses in sensitivity;[8,10] the highly significant correlation between the logarithm of K and the scotopic b-wave implicit time is 0.81, and the correlation between log K and the 30-Hz flicker response implicit time is 0.74.[10]

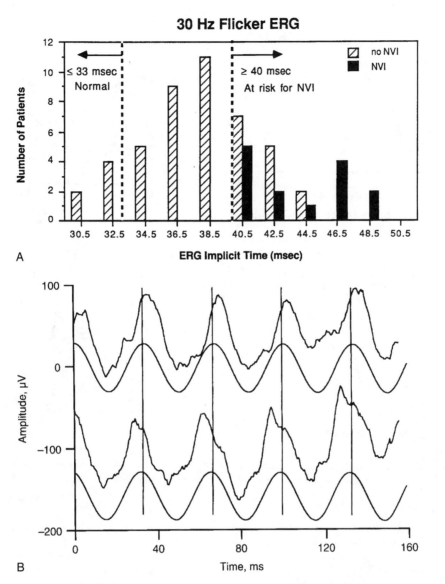

FIGURE 56.4 A, 30-Hz ERG implicit time for CRVO eyes with NVI (solid bars) and without NVI (hatched bars). B, ERGs recorded from the affected (top trace) and fellow eyes (third trace) of a patient with CRVO. While the peaks of the waveforms occur at considerably different points in time, the fundamental frequencies of these waveforms (traces 2 and 4, respectively) differ by only 2.3 ms. (Reprinted courtesy of the Archives of Ophthalmology.)

Photoreceptor function in CRVO

Johnson and Hood[8] used the Hood and Birch[6] model of the a-wave to determine that a change in the gain of the photoreceptor response occurs in CRVO patients that develop NVI. In their study of 52 patients, they found that reduction in photoreceptor sensitivity (S) accounted for about one third of the elevation in K and in the b-wave implicit time delay (figure 56.5). This was an unusual finding in a disorder that is thought to involve only the inner retina. Johnson and McPhee[10] hypothesized that photoreceptor sensitivity loss in CRVO may be due to a proximal shift in the retinal O_2 gradient due to reduced inner nuclear layer perfusion. Alternatively, reduced choroidal perfusion could account for reduced photoreceptor activation, particularly in individuals with minimal disruption in circulation to the inner retina. A global reduction in perfusion may also explain the functional abnormalities that are seen in so many of the fellow eyes of patients with vein occlusion.[10,21]

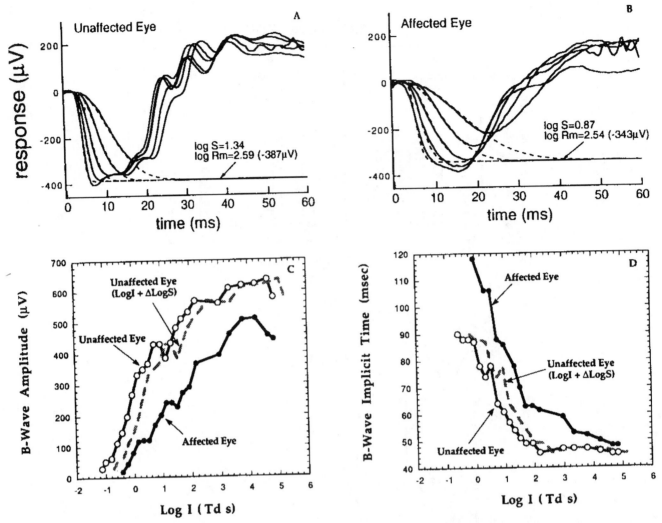

FIGURE 56.5 ERGs recorded from a patient with unilateral CRVO and NVI. Solid curves are the data, and dashed curves are the model's fit to the leading edge of the a-wave. Photoreceptor gain (log S) was reduced by 0.53 log unit in the affected eye (B) compared with the unaffected eye (A), but the a-wave amplitude (R_m) was about the same in both eyes. The reduction in log S was not sufficient to account for either the shift in the b-wave intensity response function (C) or the shift in the implicit time function (D). Dashed curves (C, D) represent the responses from the normal eye shifted by the difference in log S between eyes. (Reprinted courtesy of the Optical Society of America.)

Branch retinal vein occlusion

The same types of effects observed in CRVO also occur in branch retinal vein occlusion (BRVO) but on a much smaller scale. In fact, for the most part, the changes observed cannot be used to manage patients on an individual basis, undoubtedly because a much smaller area of the retina is affected.[12] Johnson et al.[7] showed that ERGs recorded from eyes with BRVO and retinal NV showed reductions in R_{max}, elevations in K, and delays in the scotopic b-wave and 30-Hz flicker implicit times, but the overlap in the distributions of these parameters for the proliferative and affected but nonproliferative eyes was substantial. Thus, while this result is scientifically interesting, it is not clinically useful.

Retinal artery occlusion

In cases of complete and long-standing central retinal artery occlusion (CRAO), the ERG consists of a supernormal a-wave and a very reduced if not absent b-wave. The highly negative ERG is present soon after the onset of the occlusion. The reduced b-wave and supernormal a-wave are presumably due to damage to ON-bipolar cells. Less severe artery occlusions, or situations in which the cilioretinal artery provides circulation, produce the intermediate ERG findings of partially increased a-wave and decreased b-wave amplitudes. The ERG is useful in diagnosing acute CRAO because fundus changes are not apparent immediately following an occlusion. The ERG can also be useful in diagnosing CRAO in the presence of other pathology, because only CRAO and CRVO produce large unilateral reductions in the b/a ratio.

Karpe and Uchermann[13] described ERG findings in a study of 16 CRAO eyes (13 patients). Fifteen of these eyes had large reductions in the b/a ratio, in which the b-wave potential did not approach the potential of the prestimulus baseline. The other eye had an extinguished ERG but also had concomitant diabetic retinopathy that could not be evaluated because of cataract. The visual acuities in the group were very poor, except in one case in which the cilioretinal artery provided blood flow to the macula. In one instance, administration of a vasodilator increased the b-wave from 0 or less (measured from prestimulus baseline) to $120\,\mu V$. Similar attempts to reoxygenate the retina using hyperbaric oxygen also increased b-wave amplitudes in CRAO patients who had a favorable visual outcome.[23] Occlusion of a branch of the retinal artery, described by the authors in seven cases, resulted in a subnormal ERG b-wave, presumably because of the smaller retinal area that was affected.[12]

Complete occlusions of the ophthalmic artery result in an extinguished ERG. The ophthalmic artery provides circulation to both the central retinal artery and the choroid plexus; therefore, the lack of recordable retinal potentials is presumed to be due to infarction of both outer and inner retinal layers.

ACKNOWLEDGMENT Supported by an unrestricted grant to the University of Maryland Department of Ophthalmology from Research to Prevent Blindness.

REFERENCES

1. Breton ME, Quinn GE, Keene SS, Dahmen JC, Brucker AJ: Electroretinogram parameters at presentation as predictors of rubeosis in central retinal vein occlusion patients. *Ophthalmology* 1989; 96:1343–1352.

2. Brigell M, the CVOS-ERG Study Group: The role of the baseline ERG in prediction of subsequent neovascular changes following central retinal vein occlusion. Presented at the 1996 annual meeting of the International Society for Clinical Electrophysiology of Vision, July 20–24, 1996, Tubingen, Germany.

3. Dolan FM, Parks S, Keating D, Dutton GN, Evans AL: Multifocal electroretinographic features of central retinal vein occlusion. *Invest Ophthalmol Vis Sci* 2003; 44:4954–4959.

4. Hayreh SS, Klugman MR, Beri M, Kimura AE, Podhajsky P: Differentiation of ischemic from non-ischemic central retinal vein occlusion during the early acute phase. *Graefes Arch Clin Exp Ophthalmol* 1990; 228:201–217.

5. Hayreh SS, Rojas P, Podhajsky P, Montague P, Woolson RF: Ocular neovascularization with retinal vascular occlusion: III. Incidence of ocular neovascularization with retinal vein occlusion. *Ophthalmology* 1983; 90:488–506.

6. Hood DC, Birch DG: The a-wave of the human ERG and rod receptor function. *Invest Ophthalmol Vis Sci* 1990; 31:2070–2081.

7. Johnson MA, Finkelstein D, Massof RW: Retinal function in branch vein occlusion. *Invest Ophthalmol Vis Sci* 1983; 24 (suppl):296.

8. Johnson MA, Hood DC: Rod photoreceptor transduction is affected in central retinal vein occlusion associated with iris neovascularization. *J Opt Soc Am A Opt Image Sci Vis* 1996; 13:572–576.

9. Johnson MA, Marcus S, Elman MJ, McPhee TJ: Neovascularization in central retinal vein occlusion: Electroretinographic findings. *Arch Ophthalmol* 1988; 106:348–352.

10. Johnson MA, McPhee TJ: Electroretinographic findings in iris neovascularization due to acute central retinal vein occlusion. *Arch Ophthalmol* 1993; 111:806–814.

11. Johnson MA, Procope J, Quinlan PM: Electroretinographic oscillatory potentials and their role in predicting treatable complications in patients with central retinal vein occlusion. *Opt Soc Am Techn Dig* 1990; 3:62–65.

12. Karpe G: The basis of clinical electroretinography. *Acta Ophthalmol Suppl* 1945; 24:1–118.

13. Karpe G, Uchermann A: The clinical electroretinogram: IV. The electroretinogram in circulatory disturbances of the retina. *Acta Ophthalmol* 1955; 33:493–516.

14. Kaye SB, Harding SP: Early electroretinography in unilateral central retinal vein occlusion as a predictor of rubeosis iridis. *Arch Ophthalmol* 1988; 106:353–356.

15. Magargal LE, Donoso LA, Sanborn GE: Retinal ischemia and risk of neovascularization following central retinal vein obstruction. *Ophthalmology* 1982; 89:1241–1245.

16. Massof RW, Marcus S, Dagnelie G, Choy D, Sunness JS, Albert M: Theoretical interpretation and derivation of flash-on-flash threshold parameters in visual system diseases. *Appl Optics* 1988; 27:1014–1029.

17. McPhee TJ, Johnson MA, Elman MJ: Electroretinography findings in iris neovascularization due to acute central retinal vein occlusion. *Invest Ophthal Vis Sci Suppl* 1988; 29:67.

18. Naka KI, Rushton WAH: S-potentials from colour units in the retina of fish (Cyprinidae). *J Physiol* 1966; 185:536–555.

19. Quinlan PM, Johnson MA, Hiner CJ, Elman MJ: Fluorescein angiography and electroretinography as predictors of neovascularization in central retinal vein occlusion. *Invest Ophthalmol Vis Sci* 1989; 30 (suppl):392.

20. Sabates R, Hirose T, McMeel JW: Electroretinography in the prognosis and classification of central retinal vein occlusion. *Arch Ophthalmol* 1983; 101:232–235.

21. Sakaue H, Katsumi O, Hirose T: Electroretinographic findings in fellow eyes of patients with central retinal vein occlusion. *Arch Ophthalmol* 1989; 107:1459–1462.

22. Severns ML, Johnson MA, Merritt SA: Automated estimation of latency and amplitude from the flicker electroretinogram. *Appl Optics* 1991; 30:2106–2112.

23. Yotsukura J, Adachi-Usami E: Correlation of electroretinographic changes with visual prognosis in central retinal artery occlusion. *Ophthalmologica* 1993; 207:13–18.

57 Acute Disorders of the Outer Retina, Pigment Epithelium, and Choroid

SCOTT E. BRODIE

IN THE LAST SEVERAL decades, several acute and subacute disorders of the outer retina, pigment epithelium, and choroid have been described, primarily on the basis of their clinical features. These include central serous chorioretinopathy (CSC),[10] birdshot chorioretinitis,[31] multifocal evanescent white dot syndrome (MEWDS),[22] acute zonal occult outer retinopathy (AZOOR),[13] punctate inner choroidopathy (PIC),[36] multifocal choroiditis with panuveitis (MCP),[8] serpiginous choroiditis,[32] and acute multifocal posterior placoid pigment epitheliopathy (AMPPPE).[11] In many cases, these disorders exhibit features suggestive of an inflammatory or autoimmune etiology. As awareness of these disease entities has emerged from the clinical descriptions, with little understanding of their underlying causes, it has seldom been possible to differentiate between them with confidence.[16] In some cases, there may also be overlap with syndromes that are defined in terms of retinal disturbances (e.g., acute macular neuroretinopathy) or in terms of the resulting visual disturbance (e.g., acute idiopathic blind spot enlargement syndrome).[17] While it is not feasible here to fully reconcile the nosology of these overlapping conditions, this chapter will summarize the clinical and electrophysiological features of several of those conditions (central serous chorioretinopathy, birdshot chorioretinitis, multifocal evanescent white dot syndrome, and acute zonal occult outer retinopathy) in which electrophysiological studies may play a useful role.

Central serous chorioretinopathy

Central serous chorioretinopathy is an acute or subacute disorder characterized by the development of a localized serous retinal detachment in the posterior pole.[18] The initial disturbance appears to be at the level of the retinal pigment epithelium (RPE), which often develops one or more small detachments or loci of angiographic leakage. In the most characteristic cases, leakage from underneath the pigment epithelium into the subretinal space can be dramatically visualized by fluorescein angiography as a plume of fluorescent fluid, which is seen to emerge from a hot spot in the RPE and ascend through the cooler subretinal fluid as a "smokestack" or "mushroom cloud" (figure 57.1). Indocyanine green angiography frequently demonstrates additional choroidal hot spots elsewhere in the fundus. Symptoms depend on the location of the detachment: If the macula is elevated, decreased acuity (with a hyperopic shift) is likely, along with micropsia and metamorphopsia. With prolonged detachment, dark adaptation becomes impaired, and vision may be permanently reduced.

In chronic cases, the affected sectors of the retinal pigment epithelium become mottled and atrophic, often in a dependent pattern that suggests lengthy tracks of subretinal fluid emanating from the optic nerve or the central serous lesion. The pigmentary changes may mimic those of retinitis pigmentosa.

CSC frequently heals spontaneously, often with good recovery of vision. Unfortunately, recurrences are common, often leading to RPE degeneration and more permanent visual loss. Recovery is often accompanied by formation of a pigment epithelial scar, generally corresponding to the site of the RPE leak noted acutely. Some authors have suggested that light laser treatment to the site of leakage may hasten recovery, though the ultimate visual outcome appears to be unchanged.[35]

The etiology of CSC remains unclear. The condition is most frequently seen in young males, though the predominance of this group appears to be less than was previously thought.[18] CSC has been associated with the "Type A" personality (prone to increased stress),[37] as well as pregnancy. In some cases, systemic steroid medication or increases in levels of endogenous steroids, as seen in Cushing's disease, appear to precipitate CSC.[4]

The diagnosis of CSC is made on clinical grounds, primarily based on history, ophthalmoscopic appearance, and angiography with fluorescein or indocyanine green. Focal

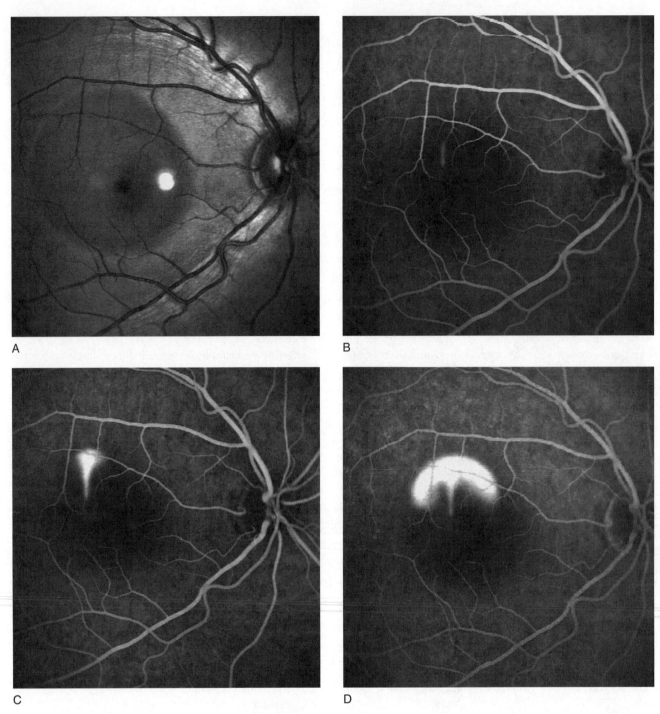

FIGURE 57.1 Central serous chorioretinopathy. A, Red-free image. The serous detachment of the macular region appears as a darker gray zone in the posterior pole. Distortion of the retinal blood vessels is evident. B–D, Fluorescein angiogram. A thin plume of fluorescent fluid is seen emanating from a point source in the retinal pigment epithelium. In subsequent frames, it grows larger ("smoke-stack") and starts to fill the subretinal space ("mushroom cloud"). (Courtesy of Mr. Ken Boyd.)

electroretinography shows a moderate reduction of the a-wave and b-wave, with marked reduction of the oscillatory potentials, in the detached retinal sector.[25,26] This stands in contrast to a rhegmatogenous detachment, which is electrically silent owing to short-circuiting of the retinal currents through the retinal hole.

Multifocal electroretinogram (ERG) technique similarly demonstrates disturbance of retinal function in the area of the serous retinal detachment[24,34] (figure 57.2). There is controversy as to whether the retinal dysfunction is confined to the detached retinal sector or extends beyond the detachment into clinically normal areas. Some investigators also report electroretinographic abnormalities in the clinically normal fellow eye. Localized abnormalities of the multifocal ERG show substantial recovery after resolution of the serous detachments but do not return completely to normal.[6,33]

Birdshot chorioretinitis

Birdshot chorioretinitis is the term given to a group of diseases of the retina and choroid characterized by a peculiar pattern of oval depigmented lesions underlying the sensory retina. The term was chosen "because of the multiple, small, white spots that frequently have the pattern seen with birdshot in the scatter from a shotgun"[31] (figure 57.3). The cause is unknown, though an autoimmune mechanism appears likely. Clinical features include a quiet eye, minimal anterior segment inflammation, chronic vitritis, retinal vascular leakage, and frequent cystoid macular edema.[9] Indications of compromised retinal physiology include abnormalities of dark adaptation and abnormalities of the ERG and electro-oculogram (EOG). Late complications include subretinal neovascularization, rhegmatogenous retinal detachment, rubeosis iridis, posterior subcapsular cataract, glaucoma, and anterior ischemic optic neuropathy.

Most patients with birdshot chorioretinitis present initially with reduced visual acuity, floaters, or occasionally photopsia. Patients may also report night blindness as an initial or subsequent symptom. Later in the course of the disease, abnormal color vision is frequently noted. Visual acuity fluctuates throughout the course of the disease.

Fluorescein angiography reveals findings that are suggestive of retinal inflammation, including vascular leakage, with cystoid macular edema seen in severe cases. The retinal blood vessels, which may appear attenuated clinically, are often hypofluorescent throughout the angiogram. The birdshot lesions are frequently inert angiographically, at least early in the study.[15] On indocyanine green angiography, the birdshot lesions appear as hypofluorescent spots at the level of the choroid and are typically more numerous than the pale spots that are seen opthalmoscopically.[5]

The ERG in birdshot chorioretinitis may vary from supernormal to extinguished. Often, the ERG waveforms are uniformly reduced in amplitude.[12,23] The electronegative waveform, with smaller b-wave than a-wave, is also commonly observed.[19] Variations in the ERG amplitudes, particularly the response to 30-Hz flicker and the scotopic response to the International Society for Clinical Electrophysiology of Vision (ISCEV) standard flash, have been found helpful in the monitoring of the course of the disease and in guiding the adjustment of immunosuppressive therapy.[38] The Arden ratio of the EOG is typically reduced.[29]

The specific mechanism of cellular dysfunction in birdshot chorioretinopathy is not known, although a significant inflammatory component is clearly present. Reports of a strong association between this disease and the HLA-A29 antigen (as many as 90% of patients may be HLA-A29-positive) would seem to implicate an autoimmune etiology, possibly with a genetic component.[2,27] This is said to be the closest linkage between any human disease and a specific HLA type.[9]

Multiple evanescent white dot syndrome

Multiple evanescent white dot syndrome (MEWDS) is an acute disorder of the deep retina and choroid that is characterized by central or paracentral scotomas associated with numerous pale fundus lesions at the level of the deep retina or pigment epithelium (figure 57.4). As the name implies, these fundus lesions are transient, typically fading from view several weeks after the onset of symptoms. An antecedent flulike illness is frequently reported.[22]

In many cases, formal perimetry reveals enlargement of the physiologic blind spot or other visual field defects. In this regard, patients with MEWDS appear similar to many of those described in the neuro-ophthalmologic literature with an "enlarged blind spot syndrome," and a considerable overlap between these syndromes is probable.[16] Most cases recover spontaneously, though pigmentary abnormalities in the fundus may persist indefinitely. Visual field abnormalities may seem disproportionate to the extent of the fundus lesions and may outlast the loss of visual acuity. Field loss is occasionally permanent.

Angiographically, the retinal circulation appears normal. With fluorescein angiography, the white dots seen clinically appear as hyperfluorescent lesions. Late staining of the optic nerve is typical.[14] With indocyanine green angiography, the lesions appear as hypofluorescent spots, more numerous and much more clearly evident than the ophthalmoscopic lesions.[20]

During the acute phase of the illness, the Ganzfeld ERG often shows variable reductions in amplitude, with attenuation of a-waves and early receptor potentials.[22] EOG

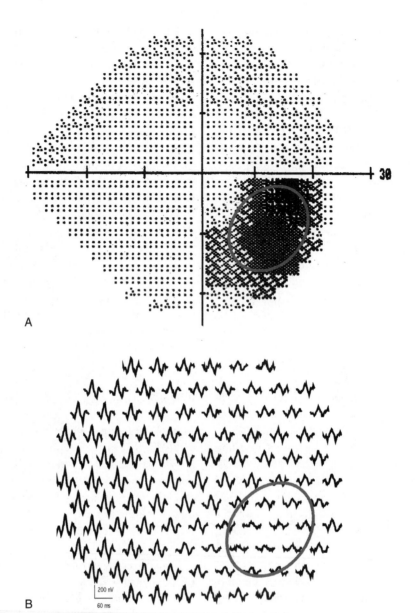

A

B

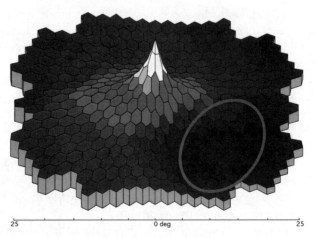

C

FIGURE 57.2 Central serous chorioretinopathy. A, An eccentric serous detachment superior to the optic disk causes a localized visual field defect inferior to the physiologic blind spot. B,C: Atten-uation of the multifocal ERG is seen in the region corresponding to the visual field defect. (Courtesy of Donald Hood, Ph.D.) (See also color plate 23.)

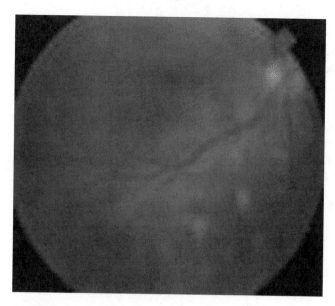

FIGURE 57.3 Birdshot chorioretinitis. Pale fundus lesions are neither raised nor depressed relative to the surrounding retina. (Courtesy of Alan Friedman, M.D.) (See also color plate 24.)

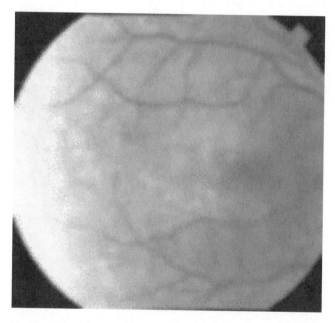

FIGURE 57.4 Multiple evanescent white dot syndrome (MEWDS). Pale white dots are seen early in the course of the disorder. (Courtesy of Wayne Fuchs, M.D.) (See also color plate 25.)

recordings are also abnormal. Recovery of the ERG parallels normalization of the clinical findings.[7] Focal and multifocal ERG technique typically reveals the inhomogeneous, patchy nature of the disorder.[3]

The diagnosis of MEWDS requires that it be differentiated from numerous other inflammatory disorders of the

retina, pigment epithelium and choroid, also characterized by pale fundus lesions with a multifocal distribution. In comparison with MEWDS, AMPPPE causes a much more dramatic disruption of the choriocapillaris, with sharply demarcated patches of choroidal hypofluoresence. In retinal pigment epitheliitis, the typical fundus lesions are dark spots surrounded by a yellow-white halo. The lesions of multifocal choroiditis and punctate inner choroidopathy are pale, punched-out lacunae of the choriocapillaris, typically larger and more numerous in the former than the latter condition. In contrast with MEWDS, ERG abnormalities and some degree of visual loss are much more often permanent in multifocal choroiditis and PIC.[28]

Acute zonal occult outer retinopathy

More subtle in initial presentation than the preceding entities, acute zonal occult outer retinopathy (AZOOR) is characterized by acute development of localized visual field abnormalities and visual disturbances and ERG changes that are suggestive of disturbance of outer retinal function, with little or no alteration in the ophthalmoscopic appearance of the fundus.[13] The condition is typically monocular, with a strong preponderance of females. The course is frequently protracted, and permanent visual field changes, often accompanied by late onset of pigmentary changes in the retina, akin to those of retinitis pigmentosa, are common. Indeed, the resemblance of these eyes after the acute phase of the illness to RP has led to the suggestion that many cases of so-called unilateral RP may in fact be previously unrecognized cases of AZOOR.[17]

Angiographically, the findings are subtle, but deep hypofluorescent rings with hyperfluorescent haloes have been reported with both fluorescein and indocyanine green angiography.[30]

In the absence of overt ophthalmoscopic abnormalities, the electroretinographic abnormalities are important elements of the diagnosis of AZOOR.[21] The disease is commonly monocular, so interocular differences in the ERG may be at least as important as overt abnormalities in individual ERG parameters. Abnormalities are reported in nearly all aspects of the Ganzfeld ERG, including photopic amplitude for single-flash and flicker stimuli, scotopic rod b-wave amplitudes, and scotopic mixed rod-cone responses (a-wave and b-wave amplitude) to the ISCEV standard flash stimulus (figure 57.5). Multifocal ERG recordings correlate closely with the visual fields that are obtained clinically.[1]

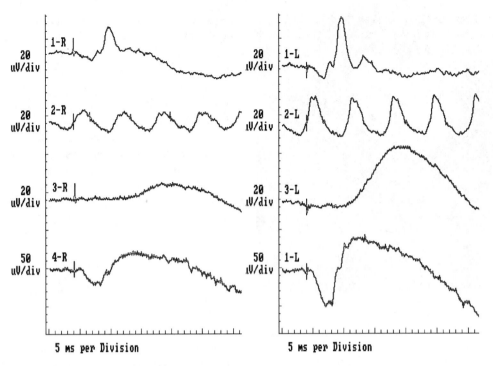

FIGURE 57.5 ERG abnormalities in acute zonal occult outer retinopathy (AZOOR). ISCEV standard Ganzfeld ERGs recorded from the right eye (reduced amplitudes) and left eye (normal responses) of a patient with AZOOR.

REFERENCES

1. Arai M, et al: Multifocal electroretinogram indicates visual field loss in acute zonal occult outer retinopathy. *Am J Ophthalmol* 1998; 126:466–469.

2. Baarsma GS, Kijlstra A, Oosterhuis JA, Kruit PJ, Rothova A: Association of birdshot retinochoroidopathy and HLA-A29 antigen. *Doc Ophthalmol* 1986; 61:267–269.

3. Bultman S, Marin M, Rohrschneider K: Aussagekraft von Fundus-perimetrie und multfokalem ERG mittels SLO bei MEWDS. *Ophthalmologe* 2002; 99:719–723.

4. Carvalho-Recchia CA, et al: Corticosteroids and central serous chorioretinopathy. *Ophthalmology* 2002; 109:1834–1837.

5. Chang B, et al: Birdshot chorioretinopathy. In Yannuzzi LA, Flower RW, Slakter JS (eds): *Indocyanine Green Angiography*. St. Louis, Mosby, 1997, pp 231–238.

6. Chappelow AV, Marmor MF: Multifocal electroretinogram abnormalities persist following resolution of central serous chorioretinopathy. *Arch Ophthalmol* 2000; 118:1211–1215.

7. Chen D, Martidis A, Baumal CR: Transient multifocal electroretinogram dysfunction in multiple evanescent white dot syndrome. *Ophthalmic Surg Lasers* 2002; 33:246–249.

8. Dreyer RF, Gass DJ: Multifocal choroiditis and panuveitis: A syndrome that mimics ocular histoplasmosis. *Arch Ophthalmol* 1984; 102:1776–1784.

9. Duker JS: Birdshot retinochoroidopathy. In Guyer DR, et al (eds): *Retina, Vitreous, Macula*. Philadelphia, WB Saunders, 1999, pp 565–568.

10. Gass JDM: Pathogenesis of disciform detachment of the neuroepithelium: II. Idiopathic central serous choroidopathy. *Am J Ophthalmol* 1960; 63:587–615.

11. Gass JDM: Acute posterior multifocal placoid pigment epitheliopathy. *Arch Ophthalmol* 1968; 80:177–185.

12. Gass JDM: Vitiliginous chorioretinitis. *Arch Ophthalmol* 1981; 99:1778–1787.

13. Gass JDM: Acute zonal occult outer retinopathy. *J Clin Neurol Ophthalmol* 1993; 13:79–97.

14. Gass JDM: *Stereoscopic Atlas of Macular Diseases: Diagnosis and Treatment, ed 4*. St. Louis, Mosby, 1997, pp 678–681.

15. Gass JDM: *Stereoscopic Atlas of Macular Diseases: Diagnosis and Treatment, ed 4*. St. Louis, Mosby, 1997, pp 710–713.

16. Gass JDM: Overlap among acute idiopathic blind spot enlargements syndrome and other conditions. *Arch Ophthalmol* 2001; 119:1729–1730.

17. Gass JDM, Agarwal A, Scott IU: Acute zonal occult outer retinopathy: A long-term follow-up study. *Am J Ophthalmol* 2002; 134:329–339.

18. Hall LS, Guyer DR, Yannuzzi LA: Central serous chorioretinopathy. In Guyer DR, et al (eds): *Retina, Vitreous, Macula*. Philadelphia, WB Saunders, 1999, pp 206–216.

19. Hirose T, et al: Retinal function in birdshot retinochoroidopathy. *Acta Ophthalmol* 1991; 69:327–337.

20. Ie D, Yannuzzi LA, Slakter JS: Multiple evanescent white dot syndrome. In Yannuzzi LA, Flower RW, Slakter JS (eds): *Indocyanine Green Angiography*. St. Louis, Mosby, 1997, pp 231–238.

21. Jacobson SG, et al: Pattern of retinal dysfunction in acute zonal occult outer retinopathy. *Ophthalmology* 1995; 102:1187–1198.

22. Jampol LM, Sieving PA, Pugh D, Fishman GA, Gilbert H: Multiple evanescent white dot syndrome: I. Clinical findings. *Arch Ophthalmol* 1984; 102:671–674.

23. Kaplan HJ, Aaberg TM: Birdshot retinochoroidopathy. *Am J Ophthalmol* 1980; 90:773–782.

24. Marmor MF, Tan F: Central serous chorioretinopathy: Bilateral multifocal electroretinographic abnormalities. *Arch Ophthalmol* 1999; 117:184–188.

25. Miyake Y: Macular oscillatory potentials in humans: Macular OPs. *Doc Ophthalmol* 1990; 75:111–124.

26. Miyake Y, et al: Local macular electroretinographic responses in idiopathic central serous chorioretinopathy. *Am J Ophthalmol* 1988; 106:546–550.

27. Nussenblatt RB, Mittal KK, Ryan S, Green WR, Maumenee AE: Birdshot retinochoroidopathy associated with HLA-A29 antigen and immune responsiveness to retinal S-antigen. *Am J Ophthalmol* 1982; 94:147–158.

28. Oh KT, et al: Multifocal electroretinography in multifocal choroiditis and the multiple evanescent white dot syndrome. *Retina* 2001; 21:581–589.

29. Priem HA, et al: Electrophysiologic studies in birdshot chorioretinopathy. *Am J Ophthalmol* 1988; 106:430–436.

30. Rodriguez-Coleman H, et al: Zonal occult outer retinopathy. *Retina* 2002; 22:665–669.

31. Ryan SJ, Maumenee AE: Birdshot retinochoroidopathy. *Am J Ophthalmol* 1980; 89:31–45.

32. Schatz H, Maumenee AE, Patz A: Geographic helicoids peripapillary choroidopathy: Clinical presentation and fluorescein angiographic findings. *Trans Am Acad Ophthalmol Otolaryngol* 1974; 78:747–761.

33. Suzuki K, et al: Multifocal electroretinogram in patients with central serous chorioretinopathy. *Jpn J Ophthalmol* 2002; 46:308–314.

34. Vajaranant TS, et al: Localized retinal dysfunction in central serous chorioretinopathy as measured using the multifocal electroretinogram. *Ophthalmology* 2002; 109:1243–1250.

35. Watzke RC, Burton TC, Leverton PE: Ruby laser photocoagulation therapy of central serous retinopathy: I. A controlled clinical trial: 11. Factors affecting prognosis. *Trans Am Acad Ophthalmol Otolaryngol* 1974; 78:205–211.

36. Watzke RC, Packer AJ, Folk JC, et al: Punctate inner choroidopathy. *Am J Ophthalmol* 1984; 98:572–584.

37. Yannuzzi LA: Type A behavior and central serous chorioretinopathy. *Trans Am Ophthalmol Soc* 1986; 84:799–845.

38. Zacks DN, et al: Electroretinograms as an indicator of disease activity in birdshot retinochoroidopathy. *Graefes Arch Clin Exp Ophthalmol* 2002; 240:601–607.

58 Autoimmune Retinopathy, CAR and MAR Syndromes

JOHN R. HECKENLIVELY, NATALIA APTSIAURI, AND GRAHAM E. HOLDER

THE ELECTRORETINOGRAM can play a central role in diagnosing cases with autoimmune retinopathy (AIR). Patients with AIR frequently present with photopsias, night blindness, decreased central vision, and narrowed or scotomatous visual fields and may be mistaken as having retinitis pigmentosa.[4,14] Making the situation more complicated, a few retinitis pigmentosa (RP) patients may develop AIR as a complication of their underlying disease (see below). Very often, the patient swears that his or her vision was normal a year before but now has noticeable changes. On examination, patients frequently have minimal retinal changes, and many are referred to neuro-ophthalmology clinic for evaluation. Most AIR patients develop a diffuse panretinal atrophy, which on viewing manifests as a blond fundus with mild to severe retinal vessel attenuation, and often a fine pigmentation or granularity to the subretinal space. A large majority of AIR patients have blond fundi with diffuse atrophy, and they do not have bone spicule–like dark pigment deposits. The signs and findings in AIR are often subtle and confusing, but an electoretinographic study *will demonstrate severe retinal dysfunction* in the face of often minimal changes in the fundus (figures 58.1A and 58.1B). Many patients have negative or greatly reduced waveforms in the dark-adapted bright-flash electroretinogram (ERG). The above findings alone do not give a diagnosis of AIR, but is the first step in establishing a more firm diagnosis.

Autoimmune retinopathy is a complex subject because there are many variations on the theme. Rare patients have cancer-associated retinopathy (CAR syndrome), and even rarer is melanoma-associated retinopathy (MAR syndrome). There has even been a report of AIR associated with a teratoma.[28] Because different combinations of antiretinal antibodies have different levels of pathogenicity and because of other factors such as blood-retinal barrier integrity and family history of autoimmune diseases, can influence the severity. Most AIR patients present without cancer, but an associated carcinoma needs to be ruled out if the patient has newly diagnosed autoimmune retinopathy. If a patient has a carcinoma or melanoma and then presents with visual dysfunction, the diagnosis is much easier but still needs to be confirmed with a thorough evaluation, including ERG. Because many of these cases are treatable with immunosuppression, which can have significant side effects, it is important to be as certain as possible of the diagnosis.

Autoimmune complications also can occur in patients with RP, and the most typical form shows up as severe cystoid edema of the posterior pole or macula. Some patients will have severe striae (wrinkles) of the macular area (not cellophane retinopathy, which has more of a mild shimmer effect). These patients typically complain of having noticeable loss of visual field over a short period of time, and if their kinetic visual fields are followed over a year, there is noticeable contraction of their isopters every 3–4 months. This subgroup of RP patients has been termed "*CAR-like syndrome*," since they have the same findings as CAR patients but do not have carcinomas. Most patients fall into the category of simplex RP, but have the additional findings of cystoid edema, retinal striae, diffuse retinal atrophy with minimal to no pigment deposits, and faster progression than occurs in typical RP (figure 58.2).

To better understand the role of antiretinal antibodies in RP, we evaluated a group of 521 RP patients by doing Western blots on their serum. Fifty-one patients had antibody immunoreactivity in the range of 23 to 26 kDa, and those in turn had dot-blot antirecoverin testing. Eight of 51 patients had immunoreactivity to recoverin.[10] Since antirecoverin antibodies have been shown to be associated with CAR syndrome and cytotoxicity has been demonstrated in cell retinal cell cultures, these antibodies in RP patients are likely to be contributing to the patients' pathology.

Family histories

There is seldom a family history of RP in patients who present with AIR. Occasionally, a patient with familial RP will develop cystoid edema and will be found to have antiretinal antibodies on Western blots. Some of these patients also may exhibit faster than usual visual field loss.[9] A majority of the time, a history will be found that first-degree relatives of the patient will have autoimmune diseases such as lupus erythematosis, scleroderma, severe asthma, thyroid disease, diabetes, rheumatoid arthritis, fibromyalgia, or multiple sclerosis, and there is usually a mix of different

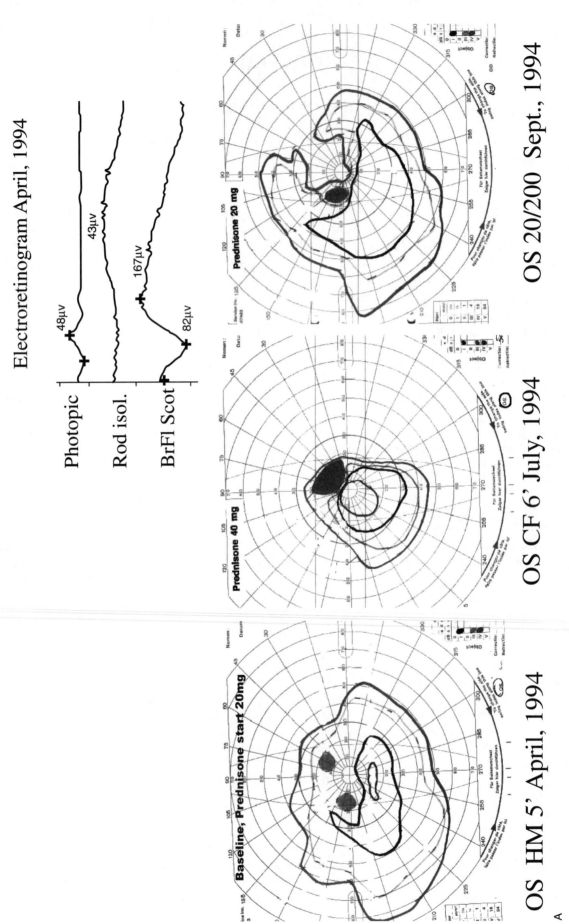

Electroretinogram April, 1994

Photopic — 48μv

Rod isol. — 43μv

BrFl Scot — 167μv / 82μv

Baseline; Prednisone start 20mg

OS HM 5' April, 1994

Prednisone 40 mg

OS CF 6' July, 1994

Prednisone 20 mg

OS 20/200 Sept., 1994

A

FIGURE 58.1   Cases of CAR syndrome. A, Case 1. Eighty-four-year-old man who was found to have colon carcinoma in October 1994. No vision in OD from advanced glaucoma. Found to have CAR in April 1994. Relatively low doses of prednisone gave good visual recovery. Larger doses would be used today. (See also color plate 26.)

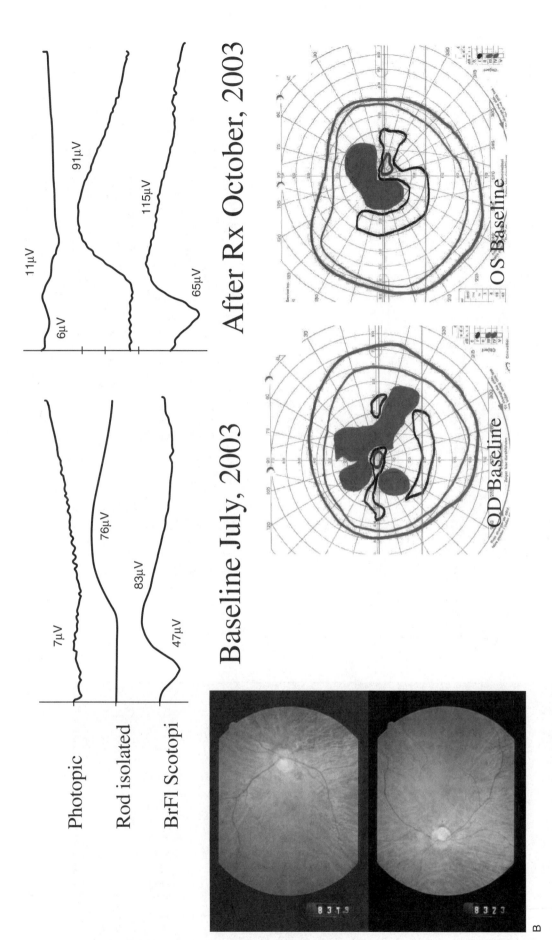

After Rx October, 2003

Baseline July, 2003

11μV
91μV
115μV
6μV
65μV

OS Baseline

7μV
76μV
83μV
47μV

OD Baseline

Photopic

Rod isolated

BrFl Scotopi

B

FIGURE 58.1   (continued) B, Case 2. Seventy-one-year-old woman with ovarian carcinoma found in October 2002. Vision was severely diminished six months later. She was placed on 60 mg prednisone, 100 mg Immuran, and 100 mg cyclosporine. ERG values increased, while Goldmann visual fields remained the same on follow-up visit. Fundus showed diffuse atrophy without pigment deposits. (See also color plate 27.)

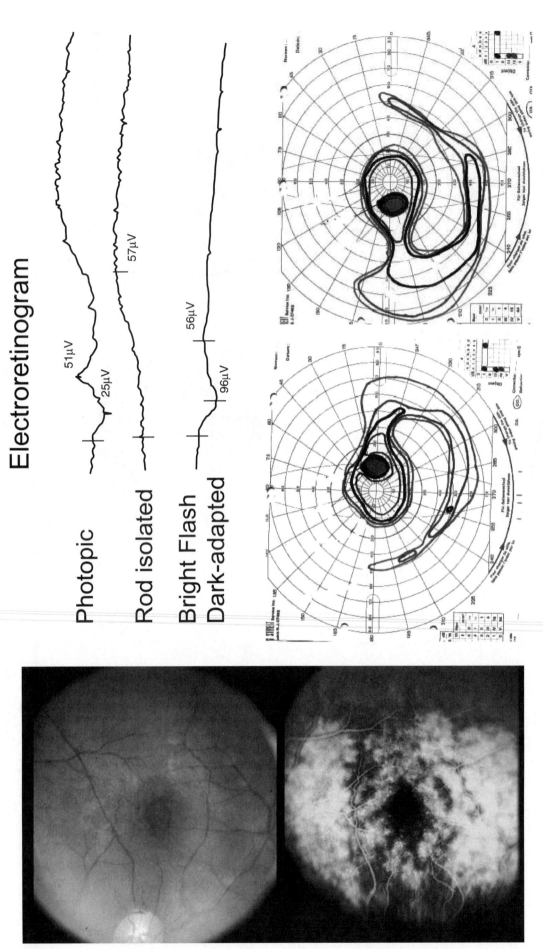

FIGURE 58.2 Forty-two-year-old woman with CAR-like syndrome and severe cystic edema of the posterior pole and no pigment deposits in the periphery. This patient had antirecoverin antibodies with bands of activity to seven other retinal proteins. There was no history of cancer. (See also color plate 28.)

autoimmune diseases in the first-degree relatives of the patient.

The diagnosis of AIR is often based on putting a number of different factors together, which may include the following:

1. Rapid loss of vision over a 1- to 6-month period. The patient is usually insistent that there is a problem even though the examination might not show much.

2. Frequently, a lack of findings on ophthalmoscopy. The atrophy is diffuse, the retinal pigment epithelium becomes depigmented, and pigment deposits are uncommon. Retinal vascular attenuation and cystoid edema may be present.

3. Kinetic visual fields demonstrated contraction of isopters, often with ring scotomata. There may be asymmetry in the amount of involvement between eyes. Over 3–6 months, the loss of field may be dramatic and not typical of RP. Often, the ERG will be more severely affected, while there may be a large amount of visual field on kinetic testing. Some cases that have milder loss of visual field also have macular edema.

4. Involvement of the posterior pole with a cystic edematous process correlates well with a strong presence of autoimmune antibodies. RP patients with cystoid macular edema also have a positive correlation with the presence of antiretinal antibodies on Western blotting.[11]

5. Western blots of the patients' serum against normal retinal protein extracts will typically show antiretinal IgG and sometimes IgM bands of activity (see figure 58.1). Demonstrated activity against recoverin is pathognomic for AIR and, when it is against α-enolase, arrestin, carbonic anhydrase, and photoreceptor-specific nuclear receptor (PNR), strongly support the diagnosis if other features are present. Most cases have a minimum of three different antiretinal antibodies on Western blot. It should be noted that just having random antiretinal antibodies does not mean that AIR is present. Antibodies against recoverin, arrestin, enolase, and PNR are likely to have significance.

6. The definitive test for MAR syndrome is checking for reactivity against donor normal retina bipolar cells on immunohistology. Some of these patients are showing anti-PNR reactivity. Many patients with positive Western blots will also light up specific cell types on immunohistology examinations of normal retina, but it is not known yet how this correlates with pathogenicity. Cytotoxic studies have been done that suggest toxicity by various antiretinal antibodies.[1,9,27]

7. The patient has a family history of autoimmune diseases in first-degree relatives as noted previously.

Summary of electroretinographic findings

Many AIR patients undergo electroretinographic testing because the ophthalmologist is not sure what they really have, and a retina-based problem needs to be ruled out. The retinal changes can be subtle and nonspecific, and it is often a surprise when the ERG results are so abnormal. The changes on the ERG are dependent on the stage of disease at which the patient is tested and what combinations of antibodies are affecting the retina. At least half the time, the patient will have a negative waveform, but it should be remembered that this finding is not pathognomonic for AIR but that there is a large differential for conditions associated with this disease (see chapter 72). Various patterns of dysfunction can be found in these patients depending on what damage the antibodies are doing in the retina, from cone-rod or rod-cone patterns, or from nonspecific loss.

Cancer-associated retinopathy

Paraneoplastic retinopathies associated with carcinomas have been most commonly associated with small cell carcinoma of the lung, but cases have been reported from a variety of other carcinomas, including breast, endometrial, and colon cancers, and even from lymphomas. Presumably, the tumor is producing retinal proteins that are antigenic and stimulate antibody production. In many cases, the presence of autoimmune genes makes some patients more susceptible to developing the retinopathy. Paraneoplastic autoimmune optic neuritis also has been reported numerous times.[5,29]

Many patients who develop CAR syndrome attribute their visual symptoms to the chemotherapy or just having cancer. In some cases, the visual symptoms precede the discovery of the malignancy. Various immunosuppressive therapies have been tried in patients, including prednisone, stronger immunosuppression with immuran and cyclosporine, intravenous immunoglobulin administered monthly, and plasmaphoresis administered monthly, with varying degrees of success. The first author had one patient with ovarian carcinoma and antirecoverin antibodies who recovered peripheral visual fields on monthly subtenons injections of depomedrol, as her internist did not want her to be on systemic immunosuppression.

A variety of antiretinal antibodies have been identified in these patients, and different combinations can be seen. The ones that have been identified to date are listed in table 58.1. It should be noted that a number of unknown proteins have been seen in Western blots, and these inciting proteins have yet to be identified and proven to be pathogenic. Jankowska and colleagues did an assay against known retinal proteins using sera from patients with lung cancer and sarcoidosis. They found high levels of antiretinal antibody acitivity in the lung cancer and sarcoid groups compared to controls, and the lung cancer sera had high levels of antibodies to recoverin and α-enolase.[16]

Table 58.1

Proteins which have been associated with autoimmune retinopathy[1,12,13,14]

Name	Weight
Recoverin	23 kD
Carbonic anhydrase	30 kD
Transducin β	35 kD
α-enolase	46 kD
Arrestin	48 kD
TULP1	78 kD
PNR photoreceptor cell-specific nuclear receptor	41 kD
Heat shock protein HSC 70	65 kD

Melanoma-associated retinopathy

The electrophysiological findings in melanoma-associated retinopathy (MAR) were first described by Berson and Lessell in a patient with shimmering of vision and nyctalopia following cutaneous malignant melanoma (MM).[3] The principal observation was a negative ERG with a bright white flash delivered under scotopic conditions, in keeping with dysfunction postphototransduction. Fishman's group reported a second case in which ON- and OFF-response recording using long-duration stimulation was also performed.[2] This showed reduction in the ON b-wave but sparing of the OFF-response and the ON-response a-wave. A recent report from Sieving's group showed that intravitreal injection into a primate eye of IgG from an affected patient produced the characteristic ERG changes approximately 1 hour after injection.[22] Milam and coworkers first reported the presence of autoantibodies against bipolar cells, and this was endorsed by histopathological findings of reduced bipolar cell density in the inner nuclear layer.[7,23] Jacobson reported a patient with colon adenocarcinoma and antibipolar antibodies with attenuated ERG signals.[15]

Of great interest, a recent report describes asymptomatic retinopathy in three of 28 patients with cutaneous MM; four patients had symptoms and ERG findings suggestive of MAR.[25] A large summary article on MAR syndrome patients that included a review of the literature and 11 new patients was published by Keltner in 2001.[18] They noted that immunohistological staining of bipolar cells is typical, but other staining can also be seen. They cited several patients who reported improvement with immunosuppression therapies.

The clinical presentation is typically shimmering photopsias and nyctalopia with normal ophthalmological examination, but vitritis has been described in one patient, and an absence of nyctalopia has been described in another.[17,20] The clinical features have recently been reviewed.[4]

At Moorfields Eye Hospital, we have examined seven cases of clinically ascertained MAR.[12] Shimmering photopsias and nyctalopia dominated the clinical picture in all

patients. Two patients had mild vitritis. Investigations were usually negative, but in one patient, white dots that were visible on ophthalmoscopy were hyperfluorescent on fundus autofluorescence imaging. The significance of this is unknown. Electrophysiologically, the rod-specific ERG was undetectable in six cases and almost so in the seventh. The maximal response showed a profoundly negative waveform in all patients. These data reflect profound dysfunction postphototransduction and are in keeping with dysfunction of the rod ON or depolarizing bipolar cells (DBCs). Superficially, the full-field ERG cone responses appeared much less affected, with minimal if any abnormality of cone flicker response implicit time. However, close inspection reveals subtle but highly significant changes. In particular, the single-flash photopic response shows a distinctive broadened a-wave and a sharply rising b-wave with a reduced b/a ratio and lack of photopic oscillatory potentials. It is suggested that this appearance is pathognomonic of marked dysfunction of cone DBCs, with preservation of cone OFF or hyperpolarizing bipolar cells. The profoundly negative ON response, with preservation of the ON a-wave and loss of the ON b-wave, accompanied by a normal OFF response supports this proposal. The somewhat broadened trough of the 30-Hz flicker ERG with a sharply rising peak is thought to be a manifestation of the same phenomenon. The PERG was severely reduced in all patients in whom it was recorded. S-cone-specific ERGs, when recorded, were always reduced. No significant interocular electrophysiological asymmetry was present in any patient. Color contrast sensitivity testing, when performed, showed no elevation of protan and tritan axis thresholds but significant elevation in the tritan axis.[8]

It is widely accepted that S-cones have only an ON bipolar cell pathway, unlike L- and M-cones that have both ON and OFF pathways.[6] The loss of S-cone ERGs and the elevated tritan axis on color contrast sensitivity testing are thus in keeping with additional ON pathway involvement in relation to the S-cone pathway. The profoundly abnormal PERGs, in keeping with the observations of Kim et al. in a study of four patients before the introduction of International Society for Clinical Electrophysiology of Vision standard ERGs,[19] are notable given the often-normal visual acuity and fundus appearance. However, it has recently been suggested that the PERG has a particular dependence on ON bipolar cell function.[13] Overall, the electrophysiological data are in keeping with global ON-pathway dysfunction affecting rods and all cone types.

Some authors have commented on the similarity between the ERG findings in their cases of MAR and those in complete X-linked congenital stationary night blindness with myopia.[21,24,26] To facilitate this comparison, a full set of electrophysiological data from a typical patient with cCSNB with myopia is also shown in figure 58.3. The undetectable rod-specific ERG, the profoundly negative maximal

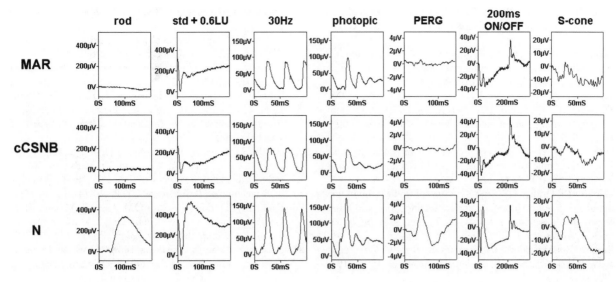

FIGURE 58.3 ERG and PERG findings from a patient with melanoma-associated retinopathy and a patient with complete X-linked congenital stationary night blindness. Note the identical findings. See text for full details.

response, the photopic single-flash ERG with a broadened a-wave and sharply rising b-wave, the markedly subnormal PERG, the negative ON response with sparing of the OFF response, and the reduced S-cone ERG are all indistinguishable from the findings in a patient with MAR. These data extend those described in the case report of Alexander and colleagues.[2]

The identical pattern of electrophysiological abnormalities in MAR and cCSNB exemplify the need always to interpret electrophysiological data in clinical context. Patients with MAR have an acquired nyctalopia with shimmering photopsias, they can be of either gender, they need not be myopic, and they almost invariably have had cutaneous MM. Patients will not always be aware of the diagnosis of malignant melanoma, and a history of removal of a "pigmented mole" or similar cutaneous lesion might be revealed only by direct questioning.

Future diagnostic techniques in AIR

It is likely that more definitive laboratory tests will be forthcoming to better make the diagnosis of AIR, likely based on the exciting antigens (and their antibodies) and specific inflammatory products such as specific cytokines that are involved in the pathologic process. The ERG will play a major role in identifying affected patients and possibly in monitoring treatment.

REFERENCES

1. Adamus G, Amundson D, Seigel GM, Machnicki M: Anti-enolase-α autoantibodies in cancer-associated retinopathy: Epitope mapping and cytotosicity on retinal cells. *J Autoimmun* 1998; 11:671–677.

2. Alexander KR, Fishman GA, Peachey NS, Marchese AL, Tso MO: "On" response defect in paraneoplastic night blindness with cutaneous malignant melanoma. *Invest Ophthalmol Vis Sci* 1992; 33:477–483.

3. Berson EL, Lessell S: Paraneoplastic night blindness with malignant melanoma. *Am J Ophthalmol* 1988; 106:307–311.

4. Chan JW: Paraneoplastic retinopathies and optic neuropathies: Survey of *Ophthalmology* 2003; 48:12–38.

5. Cross S, Salomao DR, Parisi JE, Kryzer TJ, Bradley EA, Mines JA, Lam BL, Lennon VA: Paraneoplastic autoimmune optic neuritis with retinitis defined by CRMP-5-IgG. *Ann Neurol* 2003; 54:38–50.

6. Evers HU, Gouras P: Three cone mechanisms in the primate electroretinogram: Two with, one without OFF-center bipolar responses. *Vision Res* 1986; 26:245–254.

7. Gittinger JW Jr, Smith TW: Cutaneous melanoma-associated paraneoplastic retinopathy: Histopathologic observations. *Am J Ophthalmol* 1999; 127:612–614.

8. Gunduz K, Arden GB: Changes in colour contrast sensitivity associated with operating argon lasers. *Br J Ophthalmol* 1989; 73:241–246.

9. Heckenlively JR, Aptsiauri N, Nusinowitz S, Peng C, Hargrave P: Investigations of antiretinal antibodies in pigmentary retinopathy and other retinal degenerations. *Trans Am Ophthalmol Soc* 1996; 94:179–206.

10. Heckenlively JR, Fawzi AA, Oversier J, Jordan BL, Aptsiauri N: Autoimmune retinopathy: Patients with antirecoverin immunoreactivity and panretinal degeneration. *Arch Ophthalmol* 2000; 118:1525–1533.

11. Heckenlively J, Jordan B, Aptsiauri N: An association of antiretinal antibodies and cystoid macular edema in retinitis pigmentosa patients. *Am J Ophthalmol* 1999; 127:565–578.

12. Holder GE: Electrophysiological features of melanoma associated retinopathy (MAR). *Invest Ophthalmol Vis Sci* 2000; 41:S568.

13. Holder GE: The pattern electroretinogram and an integrated approach to visual pathway diagnosis. *Prog Ret Eye Res* 2001; 20:531–561.

14. Hooks JJ, Tso MOM, Detrick B: Retinopathies associated with antiretinal antibodies. *Clin Diagn Lab Immunol* 2001; 8:853–858.

15. Jacobson DM, Adamus G: Retinal anti-biolar cell antibodies in a patient with paraneoplastic retinopathy and colon carcinoma. *Am J Ophthalmol* 2001; 131:806–808.

16. Jankowska R, Witkowska D, Porębska I, Kuropatwa M, Kurowska E, Gorczyca WA: Serum antibodies to retinal antigens in lung cancer and sarcoidosis. *Pathobiology* 2004; 71:323–328.

17. Kellner U, Bornfeld N, Foerster MH: Severe course of cutaneous melanoma associated paraneoplastic retinopathy. *Br J Ophthalmol* 1995; 79:746–752.

18. Keltner JL, Thirkill CE, Yip PT: Clinical and immunologic characteristics of melanoma-associated retinopathy syndrome: Eleven new cases and a review of 51 previously published cases. *J Neuroophthalmol* 2001; 21(3):173–187.

19. Kim RY, Retsas S, Fitzke FW, Arden GB, Bird AC: Cutaneous melanoma-associated retinopathy. *Ophthalmology* 1994; 101:1837–1843.

20. Kiratli H, Thirkill CE, Bilgic S, Eldem B, Kececi A: Paraneoplastic retinopathy associated with metastatic cutaneous melanoma of unknown primary site. *Eye* 1997; 11:889–892.

21. Klopfer M, Schmidt T, Leipert KP, Ugi I, Boeck K, Hofmann S: Melanoma-associated retinopathy with night blindness: Case report. *Ophthalmologe* 1997; 94:563–567.

22. Lei B, Bush RA, Milam AH, Sieving PA: Human melanoma-associated retinopathy (MAR) antibodies alter the retinal ON-response of the monkey ERG in vivo. *Invest Ophthalmol Vis Sci* 2000; 41:262–266.

23. Milam AH, Saari JC, Jacobson SG, Lubinski WP, Feun LG, Alexander KR: Autoantibodies against retinal bipolar cells in cutaneous melanoma-associated retinopathy. *Invest Ophthalmol Vis Sci* 1993; 34:91–100.

24. Miyake Y, Yagasaki K, Horiguchi M, Kawase Y, Kanda T: Congenital stationary night blindness with negative electroretinogram: A new classification. *Arch Ophthalmol* 1986; 104:1013–1020.

25. Pfohler C, Haus A, Palmowski A, Ugurel S, Ruprecht KW, Thirkill CE, Tilgen W, Reinhold U: Melanoma-associated retinopathy: High frequency of subclinical findings in patients with melanoma. *Br J Dermatol* 2003; 149:74–78.

26. Potter MJ, Thirkill CE, Dam OM, Lee AS, Milam AH: Clinical and immunocytochemical findings in a case of melanoma-associated retinopathy. *Ophthalmology* 1999; 106:2121–2125.

27. Shiraga S, Adamus G: Mechanism of CAR syndrome: Anti-recoverin antibodies are the inducers of retinal cell apoptotic death via the caspase 9- and caspase 3-dependent pathway. *J Neuroimmunol* 2002; 132:72–82.

28. Suhler EB, Chan CC, Caruso RC, Schrump DS, Thirkill C, Smith JA, Nussenblatt RB, Buggage RR: Presumed teratoma-associated paraneoplastic retinopathy. *Arch Ophthalmol* 2003; 121:133–136.

29. Thirkill CE, FitzGerald P, Sergott RC, Roth Am, Tyler NK, Keltner JL: Cancer-associated retinopathy (CAR syndrome) with antibodies reacting with retinal, optic nerve, and cancer cells. *N Engl J Med* 1989; 321:1589–1594.

59 Ischemic Optic Neuropathy

GRAHAM E. HOLDER

ANTERIOR ISCHEMIC optic neuropathy usually presents in the older patient with painless, often severe visual loss of sudden onset that can be irreversible. Ophthalmoscopy reveals pallid swelling of the optic disc that may be accompanied by superficial peripapillary hemorrhages. The findings probably relate to acute ischemia of the anterior portion of the optic nerve.[6,13,17] The initial report of severe visual loss in association with giant cell arteritis appears to be that of Jennings,[27] but the term *ischemic optic neuritis* was first used by Wagener.[46] It is now usually known as *ischemic optic neuropathy* (ION).[35] Clinical reviews have identified two groups of patients: those with giant cell arteritis (arteritic, AAION) and those without (nonarteritic, NAION).[3,17,34,39] Many nonarteritic cases are idiopathic, but systemic hypertension, ischemic heart disease, hypercholesterolaemia, and diabetes mellitus are risk factors.[17,39,41] There are reports of ION in association with hypotension,[44] migraine,[4,33,47] acute hypotension and anemia consequent on gunshot wound or lipsuction,[36,43] following internal carotid artery dissection,[2] and following cataract surgery.[30,38]

Clinically, patients with NAION present with visual loss in one eye, possibly with previous involvement of the other eye. The optic disc is swollen, and the more extensive the disc swelling, the greater is the degree of visual impairment.[3] Flame hemorrhages are usually present. The majority of patients have inferior altitudinal field defects, but approximately 20% have a central scotoma.[7] The field defect may correlate poorly with the fundus appearance, but some patients have clear superior or inferior swelling with corresponding altitudinal field loss. In one large series,[17] more than 35% of the NAION patients had a visual acuity of 6/36 or worse, but 30% had normal (6/9 or better) acuity.

Patients with AAION often have symptoms associated with temporal arteritis: malaise, muscle pain, scalp tenderness, etc., whereas the nonarteritic patients do not feel unwell. There is often generalized field constriction in the affected eye. Visual acuity may be severely reduced, with 60% having an acuity of counting fingers or worse,[17] but also may be unimpaired. A percentage of both groups may have had previous transient visual dysfunction. The blood erythrocyte sedimentation rate (ESR) is usually raised in temporal arteritis, but a low ESR does not exclude the diagnosis,[17,34] and a positive temporal artery biopsy is necessary for confirmation. It is important to distinguish the cases due to temporal arteritis from idiopathic cases because high-dose steroids are the treatment of choice in arteritic ION.[9,18,34] The addition of methotrexate may be effective.[28] There have been reports of improvement following steroid administration in nonarteritic patients,[17] but as yet there is no satisfactory treatment. Optic nerve sheath decompression initially seemed to improve outcome in some patients with progressive NAION,[42] but the results from the Ischemic Optic Neuropathy Decompression Trial not only failed to confirm significant therapeutic benefit, but also suggested that nerve sheath decompression may actually be potentially harmful in NAION.[24–26]

The histological changes in AAION were reviewed by Henkind et al.[19] The orbital vessels, including the posterior ciliary arteries, the ophthalmic artery, and the intraneural central retinal artery, may be involved in the arteritic process, but involvement of the intraocular retinal or choroidal vessels is unusual. Hayreh and Baines[16] suggested that the posterior ciliary arteries feed fairly well delineated areas of the choroid and nerve head and that posterior ciliary artery occlusions may infarct the optic disc and adjacent retrolaminar optic nerve. The reader is referred elsewhere for a comprehensive discussion of the blood supply to the optic nerve head.[14,15] A case report, without clinical details, of the histopathological findings in nonarteritic ION showed focal infarction 3 mm behind the lamina cribrosa that was caused by thromboembolism in three discrete pial and pial-derived arterioles.[32] The temporal aspect of the macula showed ischemic necrosis. A recent large series further defined the histopathology of ischemic optic neuropathy in relation to localized ischemic edema, cavernous degeneration, or an area of atrophy located superior or inferior in the optic nerve.[29]

The first detailed report of the electrophysiological findings in NAION was that of Wilson,[49] although "delays" in the pattern visual evoked potential (PVEP) had previously been mentioned.[20] Wilson[49] examined both PVEP and flash VEPs (FVEPs) in a mixed group of 15 arteritic and nonarteritic patients. Both PVEPs and FVEPs showed reduced amplitude, but only four patients showed minimal (<10 ms) latency changes. The clinically uninvolved eye invariably had normal visual evoked potentials (VEPs). Those findings were contrasted with those in optic nerve demyelination, in which latency delays in excess of 10 ms are common and there is often subclinical involvement of the fellow eye. Other authors[5,8,10,21,48] confirmed the high incidence of reduced amplitude, normal latency VEPs, but Glaser and Laflamme[8] found a predominance of P100 component delays in acute cases. Harding's group[10] noted that all affected eyes showed a reduced VEP and that those with a delayed or triphasic response to flash had temporal arteritis. The FVEP delay in association with temporal arteritis was confirmed by this author,[21] who further reported that the PVEP was more sensitive than the FVEP in nonarteritic patients. Amplitude reductions were usually relative to the uninvolved eye. Typical findings are shown in figure 59.1. Cox et al.[5] compared the PVEPs from 24 eyes with NAION with 22 eyes with optic nerve demyelination. The mean latency difference between the involved and the uninvolved eyes was 3 ms for NAION but 21 ms in demyelination. Wildberger[48] found amplitude changes but also reported that patients with an inferior altitudinal defect touching the horizontal meridian showed apparent latency delays that were attributed to preservation of the normal longer latency response from the superior field.[31]

Definite latency delays have been reported,[37] but stimulus and recording parameters were not given. A later study[45] emphasized the difficulties in accurate component identification with a single midline recording channel. (See also chapter 15 for a discussion of normal PVEP components and their distribution.) Those authors, using a 15 degree radius, 50 minute check stimulus, found "delays" in some cases that could be explained by complete or partial substitution of the paramacular P135 subcomponent for the usually dominant, macular-derived P100 component. It should be remembered that this interpretation only applies with a large field. Most of their patients had single-channel recordings with central field stimulation. PVEPs were often extinguished, but delays were observed. Follow-up studies suggested that the abnormalities remained essentially unchanged.

Posterior ischemic optic neuropathy may also occur but is much less common[12,40] and has not been satisfactorily characterized electrophysiologically.

This author reported PERG abnormalities in seven cases of NAION, five with involvement of the P50 component and two with an abnormality confined to N95.[22] As P50 component reduction is usually associated with dysfunction anterior to the retinal ganglion cells in the visual pathway,[23] the histopathological observations of macular necrosis in ION[32] may be relevant.

To conclude, the finding of a normal latency, reduced amplitude PVEP suggests NAION in a patient with sudden, painless loss of vision and a swollen optic disc. If there has been a previous episode in the fellow eye with resultant disc pallor, the appearances may be mistaken for the Foster-Kennedy syndrome (see figure 59.2). An abnormal VEP is not a feature of papilloedema per se, and electrophysiology should help to resolve any diagnostic difficulties in such cases. The findings from clinically uninvolved eyes are normal. PVEP delays can occasionally be observed but are less marked than in optic nerve demyelination. There are

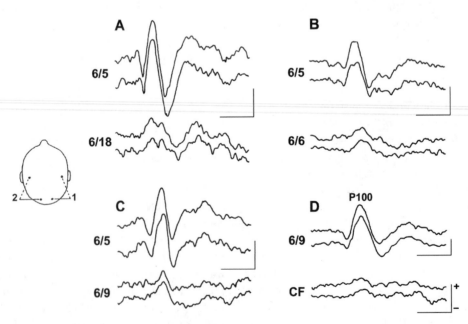

FIGURE 59.1 VEP findings in four patients with nonarteritic ischemic optic neuropathy. The affected eye in each patient is shown as the lower of the two pairs of traces for each patient. Patient A shows a broadening of the major positive P100 component with increased N135 component latency, but the dominant feature is amplitude reduction; patient B shows marked P100 amplitude reduction with mild latency increase; patient C shows amplitude reduction with no latency change; patient D shows a questionable P100, of normal latency if present. Calibration: 5 μV, 80 ms.

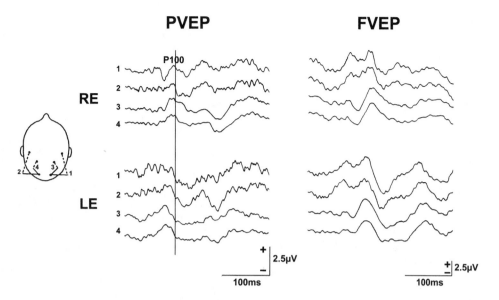

PVEP　　　　　**FVEP**

P100

RE

LE

＋ 2.5μV
－
100ms

＋ 2.5μV
－
100ms

FIGURE 59.2　Pattern and flash VEPs in a 62-year-old patient with pseudo Foster-Kennedy syndrome due to acute anterior ischemic optic neuropathy with disc swelling in the right eye and old anterior ischemic optic neuropathy with disk pallor in the left eye. Visual acuities were 6/12 right, 6/36 left. Pattern VEPs from both eyes fall within the normal latency range (vertical line = upper limit of normal for age) but show mild increase in P100 latency from the right eye relative to the left. Flash VEPs show mild interocular asymmetry in later components from the right eye but show no definite abnormality.

usually associated systemic symptoms and elevation of the blood ESR with AAION.

REFERENCES

1. Asselman P, Chadwick DW, Marsden CD: Visual evoked responses in the diagnosis and management of patients suspected of multiple sclerosis. *Brain* 1975; 98:261–282.
2. Biousse V, Schaison M, Touboul PJ, D'Anglejan-Chattillon J, Bousser MG: Ischemic optic neuropathy associated with internal carotid artery dissection. *Arch Neurol* 1998; 55:715–719.
3. Boghen DR, Glaser JS: Ischaemic optic neuropathy. *Brain* 1975; 98:689–708.
4. Cowan CL, Knox DL: Migraine optic neuropathy. *Ann Ophthalmol* 1982; 14:164–166.
5. Cox TA, Thompson HS, Hayreh SS, et al: Visual evoked potential and pupillary signs. *Arch Ophthalmol* 1982; 100:1603–1607.
6. Feldon SE: Anterior ischemic optic neuropathy: Trouble waiting to happen. *Ophthalmology* 1999; 106:651–652.
7. Gerling J, Meyer JH, Kommerell G: Visual field defects in optic neuritis and anterior ischemic optic neuropathy: Distinctive features. *Graefes Arch Clin Exp Ophthalmol* 1998; 236:188–192.
8. Glaser JS, Laflamme P: The visual evoked response: Methodology and application in optic nerve disease. In Thompson HS (ed): *Topics in Neuro-ophthalmology.* Baltimore, Williams & Wilkins, 1979, pp 199–218.
9. Hamilton CR, Shelley WM, Tumulty PA: Giant cell arteritis: Including temporal arteritis and polymyalgia rheumatica. *Medicine (Baltimore)* 1971; 50:1–27.
10. Harding GFA, Crews SJ, Good PA: VEP in neuroophthalmic disease. In Barber C (ed): *Evoked Potentials.* Lancaster, UK, MTP Press, 1980, pp 235–241.
11. Hayreh SS: Pathogenesis of visual field defects: Role of the ciliary circulation. *Br J Ophthalmol* 1970; 54:289–311.
12. Hayreh SS: Posterior ischemic optic neuropathy. *Ophthalmologica* 1981:29–41.
13. Hayreh SS: Anterior ischemic optic neuropathy. *Clin Neurosci* 1997; 4:251–263.
14. Hayreh SS: The blood supply of the optic nerve head and the evaluation of it: Myth and reality. *Prog Ret Eye Res* 2001; 20:563–593.
15. Hayreh SS: Blood flow in the optic nerve head and factors that may influence it. *Prog Ret Eye Res* 2001; 20:565–624.
16. Hayreh SS, Baines JAB: Occlusion of the posterior ciliary artery, I, II, III. *Br J Ophthalmol* 1972; 56:719–764.
17. Hayreh SS, Podhajsky P: Visual field defects in anterior ischaemic optic neuropathy. *Doc Ophthalmol Proc Ser* 1979; 19:53–71.
18. Hayreh SS, Zimmerman B, Kardon RH: Visual improvement with corticosteroid therapy in giant cell arteritis: Report of a large study and review of literature. *Acta Ophthalmol Scand* 2002; 80:355–367.
19. Henkind P, Charles NC, Pearson J: Histopathology of ischaemic optic neuropathy. *Am J Ophthalmol* 1970; 6:78–90.
20. Hennerici M, Wenzel D, Freund HJ: The comparison of small size rectangle and checkerboard stimulation for the evaluation of delayed visual evoked responses in patients suspected of multiple sclerosis. *Brain* 1977; 100:119–136.
21. Holder GE: The visual evoked potential in ischaemic optic neuropathy. *Doc Ophthalmol Proc Ser* 1981; 27:123–129.
22. Holder GE: Abnormalities of the pattern electroretinogram in optic nerve lesions: Changes specific for proximal retinal dysfunction. In Barber C, Blum T (eds): *Evoked Potentials III.* London, Butterworths, 1987, pp 221–224.

23. Holder GE: The pattern electroretinogram and an integrated approach to visual pathway diagnosis. *Prog Ret Eye Res* 2001; 20:531–561.

24. Ischemic Optic Neuropathy Decompression Trial Research Group: Optic nerve decompression surgery for non-arteritic ischemic optic neuropathy (NAION) is not effective and may be harmful. *JAMA* 1995; 273:625–632.

25. Ischemic Optic Neuropathy Decompression Trial Study Group: Characteristics of patients with non-arteritic ischemic optic neuropathy eligible for the Ischemic Optic Neuropathy Decompression Trial. *Arch Ophthalmol* 1996; 114:1366–1374.

26. Ischemic Optic Neuropathy Decompression Trial Research Group: Ischemic optic neuropathy decompression trial: Twenty-four-month update. *Arch Ophthalmol* 2000; 118:793–798.

27. Jennings GH: Arteritis of temporal arteries. *Lancet* 1938; 1:424–428.

28. Jover JA, Hernandez-Garcia C, Morado IC, et al: Combined treatment of giant-cell arteritis with methotrexate and prednisone: A randomised, double-blind, placebo controlled trial. *Ann Intern Med* 2001; 134:106–114.

29. Knox DL, Kerrison JB, Green WR: Histopathologic studies of ischemic optic neuropathy. *Trans Am Ophthalmol Soc* 2000; 98:203–220.

30. Lavy S, Neumann E: Changes of the optic nerve after cataract extraction simulating the Foster-Kennedy syndrome. *Confin Neurol* 1959; 19:383–389.

31. Lehmann D, Skrandies W: Visually evoked scalp potential fields in hemiretinal stimulation. *Doc Ophthalmol Proc Ser* 1980; 23:237–243.

32. Lieberman MF, Shahi A, Green WR: Embolic ischaemic optic neuropathy. *Am J Ophthalmol* 1978; 86:206–210.

33. McDonald WL, Sanders MD: Migraine complicated by ischaemic papillopathy. *Lancet* 1971; 1:521–523.

34. McFadzean RM: Ischemic optic neuropathy and giant cell arteritis. *Curr Opin Ophthalmol* 1998; 9:10–17.

35. Miller GR, Smith JL: Ischaemic optic neuropathy. *Am J Ophthalmol* 1966; 62:103–115.

36. Minagar A, Schatz NJ, Glaser JS: Liposuction and ischemic optic neuropathy: Case report and review of literature. *J Neurol Sci* 2000; 181:132–136.

37. Moschos M: Visual evoked potential findings in ischaemic optic neuropathy. *Doc Ophthalmol Proc Ser* 1984; 40:227–230.

38. Oliver M: Posterior pole changes after cataract extraction in elderly subject. *Am J Ophthalmol* 1966; 62:1145–1148.

39. Repka MX, Savino PJ, Schatz NJ, et al: Clinical profile and long term implications of anterior ischemic optic neuropathy. *Am J Ophthalmol* 1983; 96:478–483.

40. Sadda SR, Nee M, Miller NR, Biousse V, Newman NJ, Kouzis A: Clinical spectrum of posterior ischemic optic neuropathy. *Am J Ophthalmol* 2001; 132:743–750.

41. Salomon O, Huna-Baron R, Kurtz S, et al: Analysis of prothrombotic and vascular risk factors in patients with nonarteritic anterior ischemic optic neuropathy. *Ophthalmology* 1999; 106:739–742.

42. Sergott RC, Cohen MS, Bosley TM, et al: Optic nerve decompression may improve the progressive form of non-arteritic ischemic optic neuropathy. *Arch Ophthalmol* 1989; 107:1743–1754.

43. Shaked G, Gavriel A, Roy-Shapira A: Anterior ischemic optic neuropathy after haemorrhagic shock. *J Trauma* 1998; 44:923–925.

44. Sweeney PJ, Breuer AC, Selhorst JB, et al: Ischaemic optic neuropathy: A complication of cardiopulmonary bypass surgery. *Neurology* 1982; 32:560–562.

45. Thompson PD, Mastaglia FL, Carroll WM: Anterior ischaemic optic neuropathy: A correlative clinical and visual evoked potential study of 18 patients. *J Neurol Neurosurg Psychiatry* 1986; 49:128–135.

46. Wagener HP: Temporal arteritis and loss of vision. *Am J Med Sci* 1946; 212:225–228.

47. Weinstein JM, Feman SS: Ischaemic optic neuropathy in migraine. *Arch Ophthalmol* 1982; 100:1097–1100.

48. Wildberger H: Pattern-evoked potentials and visual field defects in ischaemic optic neuropathy. *Doc Ophthalmol Proc Ser* 1984; 40:193–201.

49. Wilson WB: Visual evoked response differentiation of ischaemic optic neuritis from the optic neuritis of multiple sclerosis. *Am J Ophthalmol* 1978; 86:530–535.

XI CLINICAL DESCRIPTIONS: RETINAL PIGMENT EPITHELIUM DISEASES

60 Gyrate Atrophy of the Choroid and Retina

RICHARD G. WELEBER

History of the disease

Gyrate atrophy of the choroid and retina is one of scores of genetic dystrophies allied to retinitis pigmentosa. Although it was first described by Cutler in 1895[8] and Fuchs in 1896,[11] interest in gyrate atrophy was sparked by the reports by Simmel and Takki in 1973[49] and Takki in 1974[54] of hyperornithinemia associated with this condition. Since then, the enzyme defect (ornithine aminotransferase, or OAT) has been detected,[46] the abnormal gene product has been characterized biochemically and enzymatically,[25,27] the gene for the missing enzyme has been cloned,[19] and studies have been performed on a molecular level to uncover the mechanism of the loss of functional gene product.[1,6,14–18,28–31,34,35,41] OAT is a pyridoxal phosphate–dependent enzyme, and pyridoxine-responsive and -nonresponsive forms of the condition have been described. Over 100 cases of gyrate atrophy have been reported worldwide. Considerable allelic heterogeneity exists for OAT-deficient gyrate atrophy for both pyridoxine-responsive and -nonresponsive cases. Interestingly, the largest group of patients with gyrate atrophy is Finnish, the great majority of whom are homozygous or compound heterozygous for one of two common founder mutations (L402P and R180T), neither of which is pyridoxine-responsive.[35] For more extensive coverage of the clinical, biochemical, and molecular genetic aspects of gyrate atrophy, the reader is referred to reviews.[56,61]

The electroretinogram (ERG) is severely abnormal in most patients with gyrate atrophy, even in childhood (figures 60.1 and 60.2).[5,29,30,54] Stoppoloni et al.[53] reported an allegedly normal ERG in a 3-year, 9-month-old girl, but the technique was inadequately described, and the amplitudes for the patient and the normal ranges were not presented. Rinaldi et al.[44] reported that the ERG for this same patient at 4 years of age was normal for the left eye (photopic a-wave: 40 μV, b-wave: 80 μV; scotopic a-wave: 40 μV, b-wave: 200 μV) but that for the right eye was now subnormal (photopic a- and b-waves: 40 μV; scotopic a-wave: 40 μV, b-wave: 125 μV). However, again the range of normal responses for the technique employed were not given. Most reports, especially those of older patients, describe the ERG as undetectable, but averaging was usually not performed, and the

lower limits of detectability were not given for the system used. Patients with pyridoxine-responsive gyrate atrophy have had some of the largest reported ERG amplitudes, with maximal bright white stimulus scotopic and photopic b-wave amplitudes in the 100- to 200-μV and 50- to 65-μV range, respectively (see figures 60.1 and 60.2). For those patients with sizable ERGs, although both rod- and cone-mediated responses are subnormal, the rod responses appear more subnormal than do those from the cone system.[5,23,60] The oscillatory potentials range from moderately to severely subnormal but are often still clearly discernible and, in rare instances, relatively well preserved in comparison with the loss of b-wave amplitude. The implicit times are usually normal, although mild prolongation of cone b-wave implicit can occur (see figures 60.1 and 60.2).[63]

To assess the course of change of visual function outcome variables in patients who might become candidates for gene replacement therapy, Caruso et al.[7] have studied the rate of decline of static perimetry, kinetic perimetry, and ERG b-wave amplitudes for the ISCEV standard maximum scotopic bright-flash and the 30-Hz flicker responses for patients with pyridoxine-nonresponsive gyrate atrophy. They found that in the 4 to 6 years of follow-up, the visual field half-lives were variable, but the median was 17.0 years for static perimetry and 11.4 years for kinetic perimetry. ERG amplitudes likewise had variable half-lives, but the median was 16 years for the scotopic bright-flash responses and 10.7 years for the flicker responses. Thus, the rates of change of visual function outcome measures in these subjects were slow, indicating that a long-term clinical trial would be needed to assess the efficacy of therapeutic intervention that is intended to preserve existing visual function. The rate of change of visual function outcome measures appears even slower for those rare individuals with pyridoxine-responsive gyrate atrophy (R. G. Weleber, unpublished data, 2003).

The electro-oculogram (EOG) can range from low normal to severely subnormal.[23,54,64] Fast oscillations of the EOG were subnormal for three pyridoxine responders (Weleber and Kennaway[61] and R. G. Weleber, unpublished observations, 1983–1987) (figure 60.3).

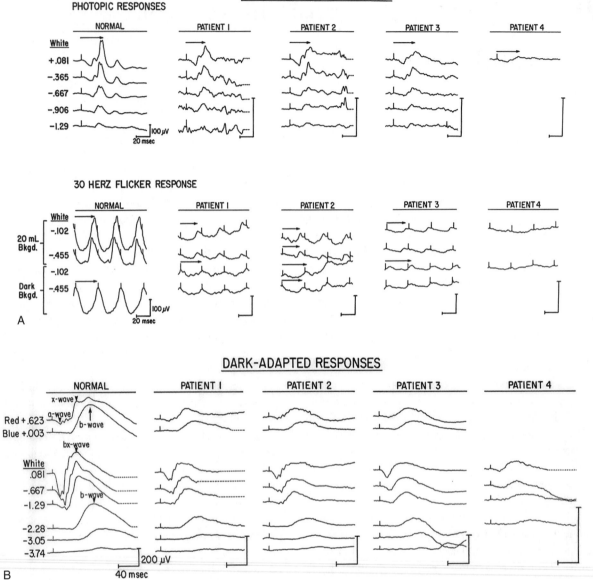

FIGURE 60.1 ERGs from patients with pyridoxine-responsive (patients 1–3) and pyridoxine-nonresponsive (patient 4) gyrate atrophy. Note that the calibration scale is different in height for the patients compared with the normal ERG. A, Photopic cone and 30-Hz flicker. Note the prolonged implicit time for some of the 30-Hz flicker responses for patients 2 and 3. The calibration scale indicates 100 μV vertically and 20 ms horizontally for all tracings. The numbers to the left of the normal tracing indicate the intensity of the stimulus in log foot-lambert-seconds. B, Scotopic ERG responses. The calibration scale indicates 200 μV vertically and 40 ms horizontally for all tracings. The numbers to the left of the normal tracing indicate the intensity in log foot-lambert-seconds for the white light stimuli and in log μJ/cm² steradian for the red and blue light stimuli. (From Weleber RG, Kennaway NG: Clinical trial of vitamin B6 for gyrate atrophy of the choroid and retina. *Ophthalmology* 1981; 88:316–324. Used by permission.)

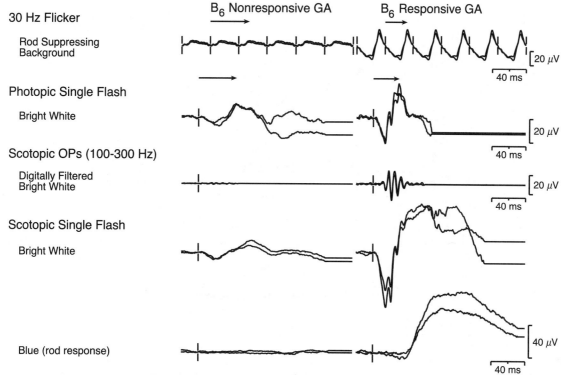

30 Hz Flicker
Rod Suppressing Background

Photopic Single Flash
Bright White

Scotopic OPs (100–300 Hz)
Digitally Filtered Bright White

Scotopic Single Flash
Bright White

Blue (rod response)

B6 Nonresponsive GA

B6 Responsive GA

20 μV
40 ms

20 μV
40 ms

20 μV
40 ms

40 μV
40 ms

FIGURE 60.2   International Society for Clinical Electrophysiology of Vision standard ERGs of a 12-year-old girl with pyridoxine-nonresponsive gyrate atrophy (same patient as in figures 60.4A and 60.5) (left column) and a 38-year-old woman with pyridoxine-responsive gyrate atrophy (patient 2 in figure 60.1) (right column). The responses for the right and left eyes are superimposed. Note that for the patient with pyridoxine-nonresponsive gyrate atrophy, the flicker timing and single-flash cone b-wave implicit times (arrows) are prolonged, the scotopic OPs are profoundly subnormal, and the rod response is indiscernible from noise.

Clinical description and natural history

Gyrate atrophy begins in the first decade of life as circular areas of total vascular atrophy of the choroid and retina in the midperiphery and far periphery (figure 60.4). As the patient ages, these lesions enlarge, coalesce, and eventually form the characteristic scalloped border between the atrophic peripheral choroid and retina and the more intact posterior fundus that led to the term *gyrate atrophy*. In some patients who are not responsive to pyridoxine, atrophy also develops around the optic nerve and in a ring around the macula.[39] The earliest symptoms are loss of peripheral visual fields (figure 60.5) and night blindness (figure 60.6). Eventually, progressive extension of the lesions toward the posterior pole produces constriction of visual fields and, in most patients, legal blindness from tunnel vision by the fourth to fifth decade. Loss of central vision can occur from cataracts, macular edema, or involvement of the atrophic process in the macula itself. All patients are myopic, the degree of myopia ranging from mild to severe.

Dark adaptometry curves range from normal[54] to an elevation of both cone and rod segments (see figure 60.6).[54,61,64]

Color vision is usually good until visual acuity falls below 20/40; tritan defects can occur.[54]

Careful funduscopy and fluorescein angiography usually show a zone of disturbed retinal pigment epithelium (RPE) between the atrophic and more intact areas of the retina (figure 60.7). This zone of disturbed RPE is the area into which the atrophic lesions will extend with time. Enoch et al.,[10] using detailed perimetry, have shown that the disruption of retinal function occurs abruptly in this zone but that some function persists within islands of more peripheral remaining retina.

Although intelligence is normal in the vast majority of cases, several patients have had abnormal electroencephalography results, seizures, or abnormal MRIs.[57] Although this is of no discernible clinical significance, all but one[23] (Case 2) of the patients who have been investigated have had abnormal inclusions within type 2 muscle fibers on muscle biopsy (figure 60.8).[27,32,52] Abnormalities on electrocardiography have also been noted in several patients.[52]

Inheritance is clearly autosomal-recessive. Carriers, who are clinically normal, can be distinguished from normal by assay of enzyme activity in cultured fibroblasts.[27,48]

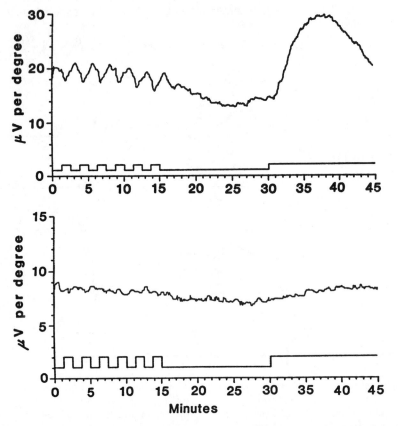

FIGURE 60.3 EOG from a normal subject (light to dark ratio 2.26) (top) and a 38-year-old woman with pyridoxine-responsive gyrate atrophy (patient 3) (light-to-dark ratio: 1.25, normal: >1.85) (bottom).

(From Weleber RG, Kennaway NG: Gyrate atrophy of the choroid and retina. In Heckenlively JR (ed): *Retinitis pigmentosa*. Philadelphia, JB Lippincott, 1988, pp 198–220. Used by permission.)

Known histopathology/pathophysiology of gyrate atrophy

HISTOPATHOLOGY In only one case of gyrate atrophy have the eyes been studied histopathologically.[65] This 97-year-old woman (patient 6 in previous reports) had pyridoxine-responsive gyrate atrophy,[64,66] and the kinetics of her mutant enzyme have been studied.[25] In the regions of atrophy, there was total loss of all retinal and choroidal elements, but the retina posterior to the scalloped abrupt border was essentially intact.

The abnormalities on muscle biopsy appear as subsarcolemmal inclusions that on electron microscopy represent accumulations of tubular inclusions (see figure 60.8). These defects within muscle are believed to be secondary to a localized deficiency of creatine phosphate, created by end-product inhibition of arginine glycine transamidinase by the high levels of ornithine in patients with gyrate atrophy.[50] However, since arginine glycine transamidinase activity has not been detected in the retina, such a mechanism cannot explain the pathophysiology in this tissue.[43]

Abnormal, swollen mitochondria have been observed in liver[2] and iridectomy specimens[59] and are believed to result from the toxicity of high ornithine levels within mitochondria.

PHYSIOLOGY Although much is known about the enzyme defect and more recently about the molecular defects in gyrate atrophy, little is known about how the enzyme deficiency actually produces the atrophy. Proposed theories have centered on the possibility of direct toxic effects of elevated ornithine levels within mitochondria and a localized deficiency of either creatine or proline within the retina. Evidence does exist that ornithine concentrations similar to those seen in patients are toxic to RPE cells in vitro.[9] Whereas creatine phosphate is a known major source of energy for muscle, its role as an energy store for the eye is unknown. The most tenable theory for the ocular pathology is localized deficient proline synthesis within the retina. This results from the inhibitory effects of ornithine, through glutamic γ-semialdehyde, on the enzyme Δ^1-pyrroline 5-carboxylate (P5C) synthase, which is necessary for the formation of P5C, and hence proline, from glutamate (figure 60.9).[45]

BIOCHEMISTRY Although in her original report, Takki alluded to the finding of deficient OAT, Sengers et al. were the first to demonstrate conclusively that OAT was the defective enzyme in gyrate atrophy.[46] Others confirmed this deficiency in lymphocytes[55] and cultured fibroblasts.[26,37,47] OAT is a pyridoxal phosphate–dependent enzyme (see

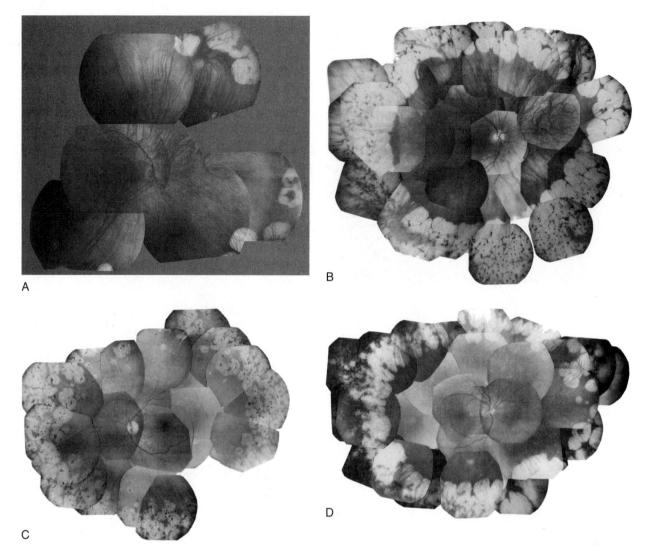

FIGURE 60.4   Fundus appearance of right eye of a 12-year-old girl with early pyridoxine-nonresponsive gyrate atrophy (A) (same patient as in figure 12.1 in Weleber and Kennaway), a 28-year-old woman with pyridoxine-responsive gyrate atrophy (B) (patient 1), a 37-year-old woman with pyridoxine-responsive gyrate atrophy (C) (patient 3), and a 40-year-old man with pyridoxine-nonresponsive gyrate atrophy (D) (patient 4). (From Weleber RG, Kennaway NG: Gyrate atrophy of the choroid and retina. In Heckenlively JR (ed): *Retinitis Pigmentosa*. Philadelphia, JB Lippincott, 1988, pp 198–220. Used by permission.) (See also color plate 29.)

Figure 60.9) that catalyzes the interconversion of ornithine and glutamic-γ-semialdehyde, the latter being metabolized to either glutamate or proline. The vast majority of patients with gyrate atrophy are not responsive to pyridoxine. However, six patients,[5,12,27,47,62,64,66] none of Finnish extraction, have been found to respond to pyridoxine, either in vivo, with approximately a 50% reduction of serum ornithine levels, or in vitro, with elevation of residual OAT activity and increased concentrations of pyridoxal phosphate. The residual OAT activity is greater in patients who respond to pyridoxine. Characterization of the mutant enzyme in pyridoxine-responsive and -nonresponsive patients has provided interesting correlations with the

clinical and biochemical features in these patients.[25] In pyridoxine-responsive gyrate atrophy, the K_m for pyridoxal phosphate is elevated, and the enzyme shows increased heat lability in some cases. Surprisingly, although her enzyme showed the greatest heat stability of the mutant enzymes studied, the pyridoxine-responsive patient with the mildest disease had the highest K_m for pyridoxal phosphate. Western blot analysis of mitochondrial proteins by using antiserum to human OAT demonstrated reduced but easily detectable protein in four pyridoxine-responsive patients and normal protein in two of five patients who did not respond to pyridoxine. Three other nonresponsive patients showed very low to undetectable OAT protein. Low residual enzyme activity

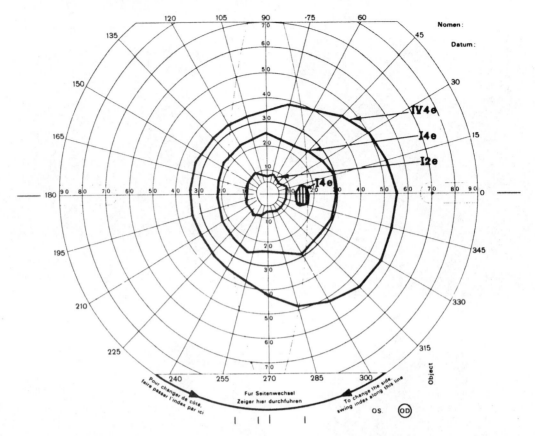

FIGURE 60.5   Visual field by Goldmann perimetry for a 12-year-old girl with pyridoxine-nonresponsive gyrate atrophy (same patient as figure 60.4A). Note that the visual field is more contracted than would be anticipated from the appearance of the retina. (Same patient as in figure 12.1 in Weleber and Kennaway.)

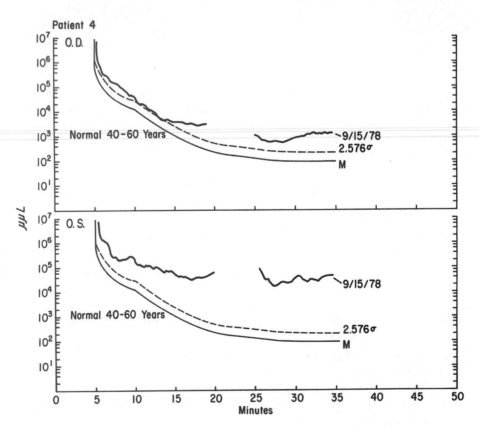

FIGURE 60.6   Full dark-adaptation curves for a 40-year-old man with pyridoxine-nonresponsive gyrate atrophy (patient 4). Note that the cone and rod segments of the curve are only mildly elevated for the right eye but markedly elevated for the left eye. (From Weleber RG, Kennaway NG. Gyrate atrophy of the choroid and retina, in Heckenlively JR (ed): *Retinitis Pigmentosa*. Philadelphia, JB Lippincott, 1988, pp 198–220. Used by permission.)

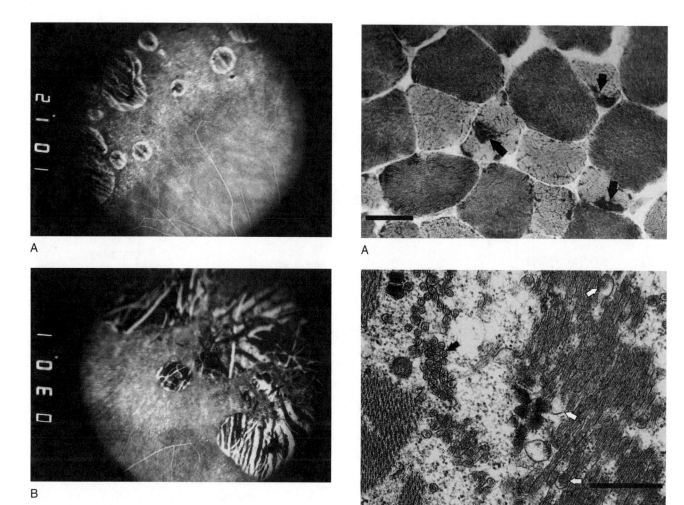

FIGURE 60.7 Fluorescein angiograms of zone between areas of atrophy and more intact retina in left eye of a 37-year-old woman with pyridoxine-responsive gyrate atrophy (A and B) (patient 3, same patient as in figure 60.4C). Note the diffuse RPE transmission defects in the zone just posterior to areas of atrophy. (From Weleber RG, Kennaway NG: Gyrate atrophy of the choroid and retina. In Heckenlively JR (ed): *Retinitis Pigmentosa*. Philadelphia, JB Lippincott, 1988, pp 198–220. Used by permission.)

FIGURE 60.8 Muscle biopsy material from patient with pyridoxine-responsive gyrate atrophy (patient 2), demonstrates subsarcolemmal inclusions (solid arrows) in type 2 muscle fibers on light microscopy (NADH-tetrazolium reductase stain) (A) and tubular aggregates (solid arrows) and dilated saccules (open arrows) on electron microscopy (B). Calibration bars indicate 20 μm for light micrography and 0.5 μm for electron micrograph. (From Kennaway NG, Weleber RG, Buist NRM: Gyrate atrophy of the choroid and retina with hyperornithinemia: Biochemical and histologic studies and response to vitamin B6. *Am J Hum Genet* 1980; 32:529–541. Used by permission.)

in mitochondrial preparations from patients who are not responsive to pyridoxine has made enzyme kinetic studies difficult, but the K_m for ornithine and pyridoxal phosphate appear normal. These studies reflect mutation heterogeneity within, as well as between, pyridoxine-responsive and -nonresponsive patients with OAT-deficient gyrate atrophy.[25]

Therapeutic trials for patients with gyrate atrophy have involved a reduction of plasma ornithine levels by supplementation with vitamin B-6 for the uncommon pyridoxine-responsive patients or by reduction of protein, and hence arginine, in the diet. Arginine restriction has lowered ornithine levels to within the normal range, and this has been associated with apparent mild short-term improvement of visual function.[22,33] Mild short-term improvement was

also noted in pyridoxine-responsive patients who were given supplemental vitamin B-6.[60] Others have reported either no improvement or worsening of fundus lesions while receiving diet or pyridoxine supplementation.[4] Vannas-Sulonen et al.[58] have reported continued progression despite normal or near-normal plasma ornithine concentrations achieved with dietary arginine restriction. Long-term follow-up on patients who were able to maintain rigorous arginine restriction have shown evidence that the rate of disease progression appears to be slowed by dietary therapy.[20,21] Proline supplementation has been tried as a means of therapy,[13] but

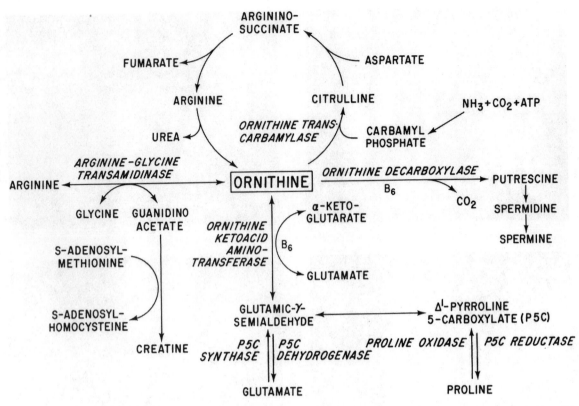

FIGURE 60.9 Biochemical pathways involved in the metabolism of ornithine. (From Weleber RG, Kennaway NG, Buist NRM: Gyrate atrophy of the choroid and retina: Approaches to therapy. *Int Ophthalmol* 1981; 4:122–132. Used by permission.)

no conclusive evidence of its benefit on a long-term basis has been shown. Creatine supplementation reversed some of the abnormalities on muscle biopsy but had no effect on the eye.[51,59]

MOLECULAR GENETICS O'Donnell et al. in 1985 demonstrated that the gene for OAT resides on chromosome 10.[36] The mRNA for human OAT was cloned and the sequence for human cDNA determined in 1986 by Inana et al.,[19] Barrett et al.,[3] and Ramesh et al.[40] in 1987 localized OAT gene sequences to the long arm of chromosome 10 and the short arm of the X-chromosome, the latter probably representing nonfunctional pseudogenes. O'Donnell et al. showed that only the gene sequence on chromosome 10 transcribes OAT activity.[38] Most patients with gyrate atrophy have apparently normal OAT mRNA,[16,24] and a variable amount of immunoreactive OAT protein.[16,25] These findings suggest that the underlying molecular defect can be subtle, such as a point mutation that results in poor translation of mRNA, a labile gene product, defective transport to the mitochondria, or a gene product that is inactive. A variety of defects have been characterized at the molecular level,[1,6,14–18,28–31,34,35,41] including several instances of single base changes, possibly affecting the pyridoxal phosphate–binding site,[41] the recognition signal for mitochondrial

uptake,[41] or in one case the initiator codon,[34] which results in a loss of the entire mitochondrial leader frame and 113 amino acids of the mature protein. For one patient, OAT gene expression was completely lacking owing to deletion of part of the gene.[14,16] These studies attest to the heterogeneity of gyrate atrophy at the molecular level.

Relevant testing and differential diagnosis

The differential diagnosis of gyrate atrophy includes choroideremia, especially in later stages, paving-stone peripheral retinal degeneration, which can be seen in high myopia, and an uncommon form of peripheral atrophy of the choroid and retina that begins in middle age or older patients with fundus features that closely mimic gyrate atrophy but are milder.[24,61] These latter patients and indeed all patients with other disorders that might be confused with gyrate atrophy have failed to show hyperornithinemia and have shown normal OAT activity in cultured fibroblasts or lymphocytes. Choroideremia can usually be easily distinguished from gyrate atrophy, especially in the early stages, by the characteristic fundus appearance and fluorescein angiogram. The fundus in choroideremia shows a somewhat patchy but more generalized loss of RPE and choriocapillaris.

The best means of establishing the diagnosis of gyrate atrophy is by measurement of serum or plasma ornithine levels. Additional testing is indicated for determining pyridoxine responsiveness. This can be achieved by measuring ornithine levels before and after oral supplementation with vitamin B-6 (100–200 mg/day). Pyridoxine responsiveness can also be demonstrated by assay of OAT activity in cultured fibroblasts with and without increased levels of pyridoxal phosphate. Chronic supplementation of the diet with vitamin B-6 is not recommended unless pyridoxine responsiveness is shown by in vitro or in vivo methods. Because of the risks involved in the severe protein restriction that is required to significantly reduce plasma ornithine levels, dietary restriction of arginine is not recommended unless adequate metabolic monitoring is done. There are no studies that have studied whether more modest, long-term reductions of arginine (protein) intake may be beneficial.

Perimetric visual field testing is indicated for periodic assessment of level of visual impairment and is the most practical means of functionally monitoring the disease for progression. ERG and EOG are valuable for establishing the severity of retinal dysfunction and are useful for following patients who have measurable responses.

ACKNOWLEDGMENTS Supported by the Foundation Fighting Blindness and by Research to Prevent Blindness.

REFERENCES

1. Akaki Y, Hotta Y, Mashima Y, et al: A deletion in the ornithine aminotransferase gene in gyrate atrophy. *J Biol Chem* 1992; 267:12950–12955.
2. Arshinoff SA, McCulloch JC, Matuk Y, Phillips MJ, Gordon BA, Marliss EB: Amino-acid metabolism and liver ultrastructure in hyperornithinemia with gyrate atrophy of the choroid and retina. *Metabolism* 1979; 28:979–988.
3. Barrett DJ, Bateman JB, Sparkes RS, Mohandas T, Klisak I, Inana G: Chromosomal localization of human ornithine aminotransferase gene sequences to 10q26 and Xp11.2. *Invest Ophthalmol Vis Sci* 1987; 28:1037–1042.
4. Berson EL, Hanson AH, Rosner B, Shih VE: A two year trial of low protein, low arginine diets or vitamin B$_6$ for patients with gyrate atrophy. *Birth Defects* 1982; 18:209–218.
5. Berson EL, Schmidt SY, Shih VE: Ocular and biochemical abnormalities in gyrate atrophy of the choroid and retina. *Ophthalmology* 1978; 85:1018–1027.
6. Brody LC, Mitchell GA, Obie C, et al: Ornithine-d-aminotransferase mutations causing gyrate atrophy: Allelic heterogeneity and functional consequences. *J Biol Chem* 1992; 267:3302–3307.
7. Caruso RC, Nussenblatt RB, Csaky KG, Valle D, Kaiser-Kupfer MI: Assessment of visual function in patients with gyrate atrophy who are considered candidates for gene replacement. *Arch Ophthalmol* 2001; 119:667–669.
8. Cutler CW: Drei ungewöhnliche Fälle von Retino-Choroideal-Degeneration. *Arch Augenheilkd* 1895; 30:117–122.
9. Del Monte MA, Hu DN, Maumenee IH, Valle D, Simell O: Selective ornithine toxicity to cultured human retinal pigment epithelium (abstract). *Invest Ophthalmol Vis Sci* 1982; 22: 173.
10. Enoch JM, O'Donnell J, Williams RA, Essock EA: Retinal boundaries and visual function in gyrate atrophy. *Arch Ophthalmol* 1984; 102:1314–1316.
11. Fuchs E: Ueber zwer der Retinitis pigmentosa verwante Krankheiten. [Retinitis punctata albescens und atrophia gyrata choroideae et retinae.] *Arch Augenheilkd* 1896; 32:111–116.
12. Hayasaka S, Saito T, Nakajima H, et al: Gyrate atrophy with hyperornithinaemia: Different types of responsiveness to vitamin B6. *Br J Ophthalmol* 1981; 65:478–483.
13. Hayasaka S, Saito T, Nakajima H, Takahashi O, Mizuno K, Tada K: Clinical trials of vitamin B6 and proline supplementation for gyrate atrophy of the choroid and retina. *Br J Ophthalmol* 1985; 69:283–290.
14. Hotta Y, Kennaway NG, Weleber RG, Inana G: Inheritance of ornithine aminotransferase gene, mRNA, and enzyme defect in a family with gyrate atrophy of the choroid and retina. *Am J Hum Genet* 1989; 44:353–357.
15. Inana G, Chambers C, Hotta Y, et al: Point mutation affecting processing of the ornithine aminotransferase precursor protein in gyrate atrophy. *J Biol Chem* 1989; 264:17432–17436.
16. Inana G, Hotta Y, Zintz C, et al: Expression defect of ornithine aminotransferase gene in gyrate atrophy. *Invest Ophthalmol Vis Sci* 1988; 29:1001–1005.
17. Inana G, Hotta Y, Zintz C, et al: Molecular genetics of ornithine aminotransferase defect in gyrate atrophy. *Prog Clin Biol Res* 1989; 314:99–111.
18. Inana G, Hotta Y, Zintz C, et al: Molecular basis of ornithine aminotransferase defect in gyrate atrophy. *Prog Clin Biol Res* 1991; 362:191–219.
19. Inana G, Totsuka S, Redmond M, et al: Molecular cloning of human ornithine aminotransferase mRNA. *Proc Natl Acad Sci U S A* 1986; 83:1203–1207.
20. Kaiser-Kupfer MI, Caruso RC, Valle D: Gyrate atrophy of the choroid and retina: Long-term reduction of ornithine slows retinal degeneration. *Arch Ophthalmol* 1991; 109:1539–1548.
21. Kaiser-Kupfer MI, Caruso RC, Valle D: Gyrate atrophy of the choroid and retina: Further experience with long-term reduction of ornithine levels in children. *Arch Ophthalmol* 2002; 120:146–153.
22. Kaiser-Kupfer MI, de Monasterio FM, Valle D, Walser M, Brusilow S: Gyrate atrophy of the choroid and retina: Improved visual function following reduction of plasma ornithine by diet. *Science* 1980; 210:1128–1131.
23. Kaiser-Kupfer MI, Ludwig IH, de Monasterio FM, Valle D, Krieger I: Gyrate atrophy of the choroid and retina: Early findings. *Ophthalmology* 1985; 92:394–401.
24. Kellner U, Weleber RG, Kennaway NG, Fishman GA, Foerster MH: Gyrate atrophy-like phenotype with normal plasma ornithine. *Retina* 1997; 17:403–413.
25. Kennaway NG, Stankova L, Wirtz MK, Weleber RG: Gyrate atrophy of the choroid and retina: Characterization of mutant ornithine aminotransferase and mechanism of response to vitamin B6. *Am J Hum Genet* 1989; 44:344–352.
26. Kennaway NG, Weleber RG, Buist NR: Gyrate atrophy of choroid and retina: Deficient activity of ornithine ketoacid aminotransferase in cultured skin fibroblasts. *N Engl J Med* 1977; 297:1180.

27. Kennaway NG, Weleber RG, Buist NR: Gyrate atrophy of the choroid and retina with hyperornithinemia: Biochemical and histologic studies and response to vitamin B6. *Am J Hum Genet* 1980; 32:529–541.

28. Mashima Y, Murakami A, Weleber RG, et al: Nonsense-codon mutations of the ornithine aminotransferase gene with decreased levels of mutant mRNA in gyrate atrophy. *Am J Hum Genet* 1992; 51:81–91.

29. Mashima Y, Shiono T, Tamai M, Inana G: Heterogeneity and uniqueness of ornithine aminotransferase mutations found in Japanese gyrate atrophy patients. *Curr Eye Res* 1996; 15:792–796.

30. Mashima Y, Weleber RG, Kennaway NG, Inana G: A single-base change at a splice acceptor site in the ornithine aminotransferase gene causes abnormal RNA splicing in gyrate atrophy. *Hum Genet* 1992; 90:305–307.

31. Mashima YG, Weleber RG, Kennaway NG, Inana G: Genotype-phenotype correlation of a pyridoxine-responsive form of gyrate atrophy. *Ophthalmic Genet* 1999; 20:219–224.

32. McCulloch C, Marliss EB: Gyrate atrophy of the choroid and retina with hyperornithinemia. *Am J Ophthalmol* 1975; 80:1047–1057.

33. McInnes RR, Arshinoff SA, Bell L, Marliss EB, McCulloch JC: Hyperornithinaemia and gyrate atrophy of the retina: Improvement of vision during treatment with a low-arginine diet. *Lancet* 1981; 1:513–516.

34. Mitchell GA, Brody LC, Looney J, et al: An initiator codon mutation in ornithine-delta-aminotransferase causing gyrate atrophy of the choroid and retina. *J Clin Invest* 1988; 81:630–633.

35. Mitchell GA, Brody LC, Sipila I, et al: At least two mutant alleles of ornithine delta-aminotransferase cause gyrate atrophy of the choroid and retina in Finns. *Proc Natl Acad Sci U S A* 1989; 86:197–201.

36. O'Donnell J, Cox D, Shows T: The ornithine aminotransferase gene is on human chromosome 10 (abstract). *Invest Ophthalmol Vis Sci* 1985; 26:128.

37. O'Donnell JJ, Sandman RP, Martin SR: Deficient L-ornithine: 2-oxoacid aminotransferase activity in cultured fibroblasts from a patient with gyrate atrophy of the retina. *Biochem Biophys Res Commun* 1977; 79:396–399.

38. O'Donnell JJ, Vannas-Sulonen K, Shows TB, Cox DR: Gyrate atrophy of the choroid and retina: Assignment of the ornithine aminotransferase structural gene to human chromosome 10 and mouse chromosome 7. *Am J Hum Genet* 1988; 43:922–928.

39. Peltola KE, Nänto-Salonen K, Heinonen OJ, et al: Ophthalmologic heterogeneity in subjects with gyrate atrophy of choroid and retina harboring the L402P mutation of ornithine aminotransferase. *Ophthalmology* 2001; 108:721–729.

40. Ramesh V, Eddy R, Bruns GA, Shih VE, Shows TB, Gusella JF: Localization of the ornithine aminotransferase gene and related sequences on two human chromosomes. *Hum Genet* 1987; 76:121–126.

41. Ramesh V, McClatchey AI, Ramesh N, et al: Molecular basis of ornithine aminotransferase deficiency in B-6-responsive and -nonresponsive forms of gyrate atrophy. *Proc Natl Acad Sci U S A* 1988; 85:3777–3780.

42. Ramesh V, Shaffer MM, Allaire JM, Shih VE, Gusella JF: Investigation of gyrate atrophy using a cDNA clone for human ornithine aminotransferase. *DNA* 1986; 5:493–501.

43. Rao GN, Cotlier E: Ornithine delta-aminotransferase activity in retina and other tissues. *Neurochem Res* 1984; 9:555–562.

44. Rinaldi E, Stoppoloni GP, Savastano S, Russo S, Cotticelli L: Gyrate atrophy of choroid associated with hyperornithinaemia: Report of the first case in Italy. *J Pediatr Ophthalmol Strabismus* 1979; 16:133–135.

45. Saito T, Omura K, Hayasaka S, Nakajima H, Mizuno K, Tada K: Hyperornithinemia with gyrate atrophy of the choroid and retina: A disturbance in de novo formation of proline. *Tohoku J Exp Med* 1981; 135:395–402.

46. Sengers RCA, Trijbels JMG, Brussaart JH, et al: Gyrate atrophy of the choroid and retina and ornithine-ketoacid aminotransferase deficiency (abstract). *Pediatr Res* 1976; 10:894.

47. Shih VE, Berson EL, Mandell R, Schmidt SY: Ornithine ketoacid transaminase deficiency in gyrate atrophy of the choroid and retina. *Am J Hum Genet* 1978; 30:174–179.

48. Shih VE, Mandell R, Berson EL: Pyridoxine effects on ornithine ketoacid transaminase activity in fibroblasts from carriers of two forms of gyrate atrophy of the choroid and retina. *Am J Hum Genet* 1988; 43:929–933.

49. Simell O, Takki K: Raised plasma-ornithine and gyrate atrophy of the choroid and retina. *Lancet* 1973; 1:1031–1033.

50. Sipilä I: Inhibition of arginine-glycine amidinotransferase by ornithine: A possible mechanism for the muscular and chorioretinal atrophies in gyrate atrophy of the choroid and retina with hyperornithinemia. *Biochim Biophys Acta* 1980; 613:79–84.

51. Sipilä I, Rapola J, Simell O, Vannas A: Supplemental creatine as a treatment for gyrate atrophy of the choroid and retina. *N Engl J Med* 1981; 304:867–870.

52. Sipilä I, Simell O, Rapola J, Sainio K, Tuuteri L: Gyrate atrophy of the choroid and retina with hyperornithinemia: Tubular aggregates and type 2 fiber atrophy in muscle. *Neurology* 1979; 29:996–1005.

53. Stoppoloni G, Prisco F, Santinelli R, Tolone C: Hyperornithinemia and gyrate atrophy of choroid and retina: Report of a case. *Helv Paediatr Acta* 1978; 33:429–433.

54. Takki K: Gyrate atrophy of the choroid and retina associated with hyperornithinemia. *Br J Ophthalmol* 1974; 58:3–23.

55. Valle D, Kaiser-Kupfer MI, Del Valle LA: Gyrate atrophy of the choroid and retina: Deficiency of ornithine aminotransferase in transformed lymphocytes. *Proc Natl Acad Sci U S A* 1977; 74:5159–5161.

56. Valle D, Simell O: The hyperornithinemias. In Scriver CR, Beaudet AL, Sly WS, Valle D (eds): *The Metabolic and Molecular Bases of Inherited Disease*, ed 8. New York, McGraw-Hill, 2001, pp 1857–1895.

57. Valtonen M, Nanto-Salonen K, Jaaskelainen S, et al: Central nervous system involvement in gyrate atrophy of the choroid and retina with hyperornithinaemia. *J Inherit Metab Dis* 1999; 22:855–866.

58. Vannas-Sulonen K, Simell O, Sipilä I: Gyrate atrophy of the choroid and retina: The ocular disease progresses in juvenile patients despite normal or near normal plasma ornithine concentration. *Ophthalmology* 1987; 94:1428–1433.

59. Vannas-Sulonen K, Sipilä I, Vannas A, Simell O, Rapola A: Gyrate atrophy of the choroid and retina: A five year follow-up of creatine supplementation. *Ophthalmology* 1985; 92:1719–1727.

60. Weleber RG, Kennaway NG: Clinical trial of vitamin B6 for gyrate atrophy of the choroid and retina. *Ophthalmology* 1981; 88:316–324.

61. Weleber RG, Kennaway NG: Gyrate atrophy of the choroid and retina. In Heckenlively JR (ed): *Retinitis Pigmentosa*. Philadelphia, JB Lippincott, 1988, pp 198–220.

62. Weleber RG, Kennaway NG, Buist NRM: Vitamin B$_6$ in management of gyrate atrophy of choroid and retina. *Lancet* 1978; 2:1213.

63. Weleber RG, Kennaway NG, Buist NR: Gyrate atrophy of the choroid and retina: Approaches to therapy. *Int Ophthalmol* 1981; 4:23–32.

64. Weleber RG, Wirtz MK, Kennaway NG: Gyrate atrophy of the choroid and retina: Clinical and biochemical heterogene-ity and response to vitamin B$_6$. *Birth Defects: Orig Article Series* 1982; 18:219–230.

65. Wilson DJ, Weleber RG, Green WR: Ocular clinicopathologic study of gyrate atrophy. *Am J Ophthalmol* 1991; 111:24–33.

66. Wirtz MK, Kennaway NG, Weleber RG: Heterogeneity and complementation analysis of fibroblasts from vitamin B$_6$ responsive and non-responsive patients with gyrate atrophy of the choroid and retina. *J Inher Metab Dis* 1985; 8:71–74.

61 Dominant Drusen

ELISE HÉON, FRANCIS MUNIER, AND COLIN WILLOUGHBY

DRUSEN ARE SMALL, extracellular deposits that accumulate below the retinal pigment epithelium on Bruch's membrane.[7] "Hard" drusen, including basal laminar drusen and cuticular drusen, represent focal thickening of Bruch's membrane or the basal membrane underlying the retinal pigment epithelium (RPE). "Soft" drusen are usually larger (small RPE detachments) and carry a higher risk of degenerative changes.[37] Although drusen are located in the posterior pole, they are biomarkers of a more diffuse disease process that is complex and at least partly genetically determined. Drusen are usually a hallmark of a progressive macular degeneration process, and their formation parallels changes in Bruch's membrane and the RPE. The deposits seen in dominant drusen are distinguished from those seen in Stargardt's disease, Best disease, or other "flecked" retinopathies. These pathologies can be characterized on the basis of clinical and pathophysiological findings. These conditions will not be discussed in this chapter, nor will optic nerve drusen, also a distinct entity. Drusen are usually seen in the aging eye but can be seen as early as the first decade, especially when a hereditary pattern is documented. These changes are usually not associated with any systemic findings, although drusen can be documented in conditions such as mesangiocapillary glomerulonephritis type II.[11]

The nature of drusen

Although drusen are widely accepted as the hallmark of age-related macular degeneration,[52] their composition and the mechanism of their formation are not understood.[7] The nature of drusen appears to be partly environmentally determined and partly genetically determined. Histochemical and immunocytochemical studies have shown that drusen contain a variety of lipids, polysaccharides, and glycoaminoglyans, and over 20 drusen-related proteins have been identified.[1,2,7,22,31,35,38,41] The nature of drusen is being further elucidated through various approaches.[7]

Dominant drusen

The term *dominant drusen* refers to a genetically heterogeneous group of disorders of autosomal-dominant inheritance. Individuals affected with this genetically determined type of deposits are at 50% risk of transmitting the related genetic defect. The penetrance of dominant drusen is not always complete, which implies that despite carrying a causal genetic defect, the retina may look normal even late in life. This often challenges the recognition of the inheritance or heritability pattern.[8] The appearance and distribution of the drusen can be variable within and between families.[8,46] The deposits are usually located in the posterior pole. In dominant drusen, they are also often seen nasal to and/or very close to the optic nerve (figure 61.1). Inherited drusen are usually bilateral and symmetric and tend to appear earlier in life than age-related sporadic drusen. They may appear decades before any symptoms. Other than these observations, there is no specific clinical or pathological clue to distinguish the heritable drusen from the sporadic nonhereditary variant.[18,51]

In some instances, a specific pattern of distribution may be recognized, leading to the diagnosis of Sorsby's fundus dystrophy,[27,48,59–61] Doyne's honeycomb dystrophy,[9,45] malattia Leventinese,[17] or Hutchinson-Tay choroiditis.[28] When no specific pattern is recognized, the pathology is simply referred to as *dominant drusen* (figure 61.2).

Dominantly inherited drusen models have been studied genetically in an attempt to elucidate the basis of the more commonly observed sporadic cases. Although dominant drusen were long thought to constitute one entity,[8] this was disproved by recent molecular studies showing the genetic heterogeneity of these deposits. At least four disease gene loci have been identified,[26,34,47,73] and three genes have been characterized: peripherin/RDS (*RDS*), tissue inhibitor of metalloproteinase 3 (*TIMP-3*), and EGF-containing fibulin-like extracellular matrix protein 1 (*EFEMP1*).[47,63,73] The genetic heterogeneity of drusen implies that the pathophysiological mechanisms that lead to their formation are also varied. This may explain the range of psychophysical and electrophysiological findings that have been documented. Further molecular characterization of drusen should assist in understanding the electrophysiological changes observed. The study of dominant drusen is useful to define the changes that are related to drusen per se, as in those cases, changes related to the aging of the retina are less of a confounding factor.

Functional changes associated with dominant drusen

Functional changes of the retina associated with drusen, although somewhat controversial, are usually minimal

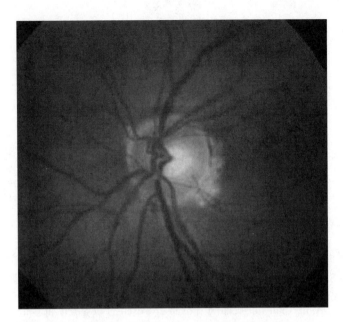

FIGURE 61.1 Fundus photography of peripapillary drusen in a case of "aborted" malattia Leventinese.

except for decrease in central visual acuity, contrast sensitivity, and color vision. Progression of the disease is usually associated with the development of central scotoma and changes in dark adaptation. The variability in the psychophysical and electrophysiological abnormalities that have been documented in the literature may reflect not only the various pathophysiological events that are involved, but also the evolving sophistication of the testing techniques available. Full-field electroretinograms (ERGs) are typically normal in drusen, although subnormal recordings have been documented.[37] No electrophysiological criteria can currently differentiate patients with familial drusen from those with nonfamilial drusen.[18] The standardization of testing procedures (http://www.iscev.org/standards) and the use of newer recent techniques such as the multifocal ERG should provide useful information in the near future.[2]

ELECTRO-OCULOGRAPHY Electro-oculography of small cohorts of patients who are affected with dominant drusen shows normal value in all cases.[16,65] This suggests that dominant drusen are primarily not a diffuse disease of the RPE. This contrasts with previously documented abnormal electro-oculogram (EOG) reports from patients with fundus flavimaculatus and supports the hypothesis that drusen are functionally and pathophysiologically distinct from flecks.[37] Studies of patients affected with nonexudative age-related macular degeneration (AMD) provide different results, 20% of patients having abnormal EOG recording, especially in soft drusen.[18,72] The size of the area of retina that is involved at the time of testing as well as the recording technique used may be confounding factors.

ELECTRORETINOGRAPHY Subnormal ERG recordings have been documented in several patients with dominant drusen and nonexudative AMD, in which decreases of both rod and cone function have been documented.[18,43,72] Changes in amplitudes can precede changes in implicit times.[72] Recent studies showed that the cone b-wave implicit time was prolonged in at least two subtypes of hereditary drusen: malattia Leventinese and codon 172-RDS–related maculopathy.[21] This variability in results partly reflects differences in recording technique and the control populations that were used. When drusen of the elderly are assessed, a decrease in dark-adapted retinal sensitivity is measured in the central retina in the area of drusen as well as the nondrusen area.[54,65] This sensitivity loss appears to reflect a diffuse retinal disease process and disruption of rod-mediated kinetic parameters of dark adaptation in early nonexudative AMD.[44] These observations support the hypothesis that the presence of drusen in the posterior pole reflects a diffuse retinal disease process.

In AMD patients with a variable amount of soft drusen, retinal cone-mediated flicker sensitivity losses can be detected with the focal ERG as a function of flicker modulation depth. Early lesions have been associated with reduced response gain and phase delays, with normal thresholds.[15,54] In patients with early nonexudative AMD, the focal ERG changes parallel the extent and severity of fundus lesions. However, a functional impairment of outer macular layers detected by focal ERG losses could precede morphological changes that are typical of more advanced disease.[14] In more recent evaluations of AMD populations, it was found that the amplitude of the oscillatory potential OP2 was significantly reduced in addition to the abnormal photopic responses compared with an age-matched control group.[72]

Significant abnormalities in the foveal amplitude and the foveal latency of multifocal ERG (MERG) can also be detected in pre-AMD or early AMD eyes as well as in the asymptomatic controlateral eyes, suggesting MERG as a sensitive tool in detecting early foveal abnormalities in AMD. By using the concentric configuration, the foveal amplitude of pre-AMD or early AMD eyes was significantly suppressed when compared with the age-matched control group, and their average latency was longer in the fovea than in outer rings and significantly prolonged when compared with the normal control group. Similar changes in amplitude and latency were also observed in the asymptomatic fellow eyes.[36]

Genetic influences

Several studies have shown that the genetic predisposition of drusen is now accepted to be a major risk factor for the development of macular degeneration.[25,33,40,55,57,58] This is especially true when there is a large number (>20) of small hard drusen and large (≥125 micron) soft drusen[24] or when drusen are seen nasal to the disc.[8] These findings should

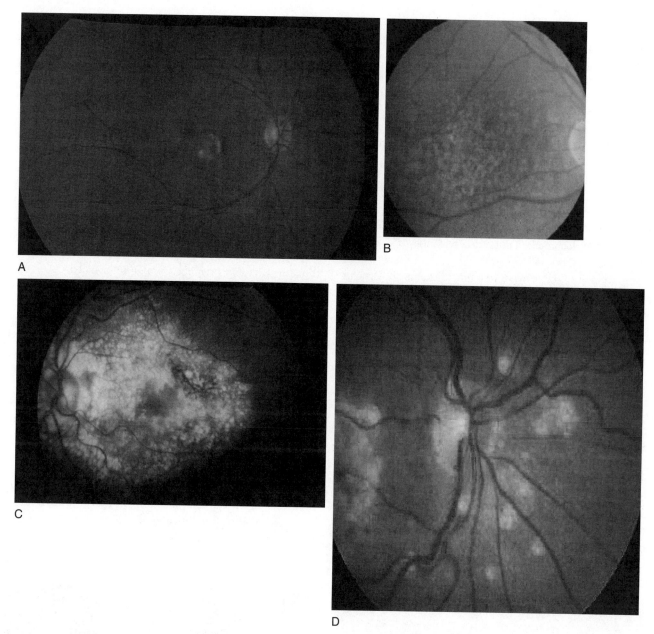

FIGURE 61.2 *Clinical range of dominant drusen. Fundus photography of a 37-year-old female with Sorsby's fundus dystrophy (A), a 40-year-old with dominant macular drusen with no pattern (B) (courtesy of Dr. J. Hopkins), a 43-year-old male affected with fine* radial drusen (malattia Leventinese) (C), and a 39-year-old male affected with Doyne's honeycomb dystrophy (D). Note the coarse macular and peripapillary deposits. (Courtesy of Dr. William Pearce.)

prompt the examination of family members, as the diagnosis of dominant drusen may influence counseling and management. Three specific genetic models of dominant drusen for which the gene has been identified are discussed below.

Specific genetic models

TIMP-3–RELATED DRUSEN More than 50 years ago, Sorsby et al.[60] described a dominantly inherited fundus dystrophy

with onset of central visual loss between the fifth and sixth decades, leading eventually to the loss of ambulatory vision in the mid-seventies. Early ophthalmoscopic changes can be seen during the third decade (see figure 61.2A) and may take the form of either discrete drusenlike deposits or a confluent yellow deposit at the level of the retinal pigment epithelium.[27,48] Confluent thickening of Bruch's membrane may be difficult to identify by ophthalmoscopy alone but was suggested as a possible barrier to diffusion of nutrients to the photoreceptors.[61] The first sign of the disease can be the delay in choriocapillaris filling on fluorescein angiography, usually confined to the posterior pole in the young individuals. The most obvious clinical change is the drusenlike deposits seen along the arcades and nasal to the optic disk rather than at the central macula. These deposits are associated with the subsequent development of geographic atrophy or neovascularization.[27,48,61] Drusen are very infrequently centered over the fovea, making the distinction between Sorsby's fundus dystrophy (SFD) and other forms of age-related and genetically determined drusen relatively straightforward. Night blindness is an early symptom that is usually not correlated with an abnormal full-field ERG.[56] Photoreceptor dysfunction has been documented in some severe cases,[4,30,54] but the EOG is usually normal. Steinmetz et al.[61] and Jacobson et al.[29] proposed a testable hypothesis that thickening of Bruch's membrane caused night blindness by blocking the passage of vitamin A from the choriocapillaris to the photoreceptors. This was confirmed by the reversal of psychophysical and electrophysiological abnormalities following high-dose vitamin A supplementation (50,000 IU/d).[29]

Sorsby's fundus dystrophy was mapped to chromosome 22q,[74] and point mutations in the *TIMP-3* gene were subsequently identified in affected members of unrelated SFD pedigrees.[73] These mutations are found to disrupt the functional properties of the mature protein; they are not seen in the normal population and most probably are disease causing. The role of *TIMP-3* is being elucidated, and it is thought to play a role in the degradation process of Bruch's membrane[78] and as an inhibitor of angiogenesis.[49] The recent development of the Sorsby mouse model should contribute to a better understanding of the mechanisms that underlie this disease.[75]

CODON 172 RDS–RELATED DRUSEN A very wide range of phenotype, including that of drusen, result from mutations in the *RDS/peripherin* gene.[3,42,47,50,62,76] For example, mutations in codon 172, especially the Arg172Trp mutation, cause a highly penetrant, progressive form of macular degeneration with subtle dominant drusen[47,77] (figures 61.3, 61.4B, and 61.4D). Even though the disease can be detected early by ophthalmoscopy in the asymptomatic adolescent, severe visual loss does not occur before the fifth decade. The early stage is characterized by the presence of bilateral and symmetric macular drusen with no specific pattern of distribution (see figures 61.4B and 61.4D). In later stages, it resembles atrophic AMD except when the chorioretinal atrophy extends to the optic nerve head. In most affected cases, the macular changes are bilateral and symmetric, and the optic disk and periphery remain uninvolved.

Although the product of the *RDS/peripherin* gene is a photoreceptor-specific glycoprotein detected exclusively in the outer segment of rods and cones,[6,67–69] these individuals do not complain of nyctalopia and do not have constricted visual fields. The primary symptoms include early-onset photophobia and difficulty in dark adaptation as early as the second decade. This has been reflected in abnormal color-contrast sensitivity and reduced pattern and cone ERG in some cases.[77] Visual acuity and retinal function changes are first noted around the third decade, when the cone and in some cases rod amplitudes were mildly altered before the b-wave implicit time. Overall, the full-field retinal function remains remarkably preserved until the late stages of the disease. In general, cone and rod thresholds are elevated, and color-contrast sensitivities are absent in the central visual field.[77] Cone ERGs are usually diminished in amplitudes and delayed. Peripherally, the scotopic sensitivities

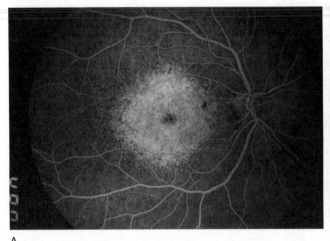

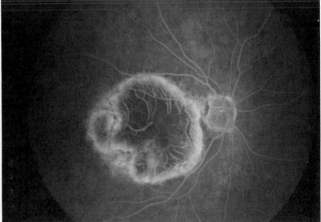

A

B

FIGURE 61.3 Fluorescein angiography of early and late stage of codon 172 RDS–related maculopathy. A, Intravenous fluorescein angiography (IVFA) of a 31-year-old male affected with a Arg172Trp-related maculopathy, B, IVFA of a 60-year-old male relative with the same Arg172Trp mutations. Their respective fundus photography and electrophysiology are shown in figures 61.4B and 61.4D.

remain normal until late, as does the recovery to bleach.[77] Rod ERGs also usually remain normal until very late in the disease, around the sixth or seventh decade. At that time, some ERG recordings have showed subnormal function of both the cone and rod systems, resembling cone-rod degeneration.[21,26] Codon 172-RDS–related maculopathy is characterized by a relatively continuous decrease of central vision starting during the third decade of life, in contrast with *EFEMP1*-related maculopathy (see below), in which visual acuity is retained until the fifth decade.[21] EOGs were shown to be normal with Arden ratios ranging between 170% and 220%.

On evaluation by static perimetry, the areas of elevated threshold and absolute scotomas corresponded closely to the extension of the macular changes. Static and dynamic perimetry would not show peripheral field constriction.[47]

EFEMP1-RELATED DRUSEN   The first convincing evidence of dominantly inherited drusen was provided by Doyne in 1899.[9] Histopathological examination of one of Doyne's patients[5,70] revealed the abnormalities to be hyaline thickenings of Bruch's membrane. Klainguti, Wagner, and Forni later fully characterized this condition and demonstrated its autosomal-dominant inheritance.[17,32,71] This disorder has been referred to as *malattia Leventinese*, after the origin of the Swiss affected individuals. Malattia Leventinese shows clinical overlap and a shared molecular background with Doyne's honeycomb dystrophy and the radial drusen maculopathy of Gass.[19] Although it was originally recognized in Switzerland, families affected with autosomal-dominant radial drusen have been identified throughout the world, including Czechoslovakia,[10,64] Australia, Japan, and the United States.[10,20]

As suspected by Deutman, Doyne's honeycomb dystrophy and mallatia Leventinese are allelic variants due to a mutation in *EFEMP1*.[8] Families that are affected with malattia Leventinese and radial drusen maculopathy were mapped to chromosome 2p16-21,[26] and the disease-causing gene (*EFEMP1*) was identified through the analysis of additional families, including some affected with the Doyne's honeycomb dystrophy phenotype.[63] The same mutation, Arg345Trp, was seen in all families that were studied, producing the malattia Leventinese, radial drusen, and Doyne's honeycomb dystrophy phenotypes.[39] Drusen are genetically heterogeneous, as *EFEMP1* is not associated with sporadic drusen,[53] and there appears to be a radial drusen family without a EFEMP1 mutation.[66] No *EFEMP1* mutations have been identified in patients affected with AMD.[63]

EFEMP1 is predicted to be an extracellular matrix protein but is otherwise completely uncharacterized. Mutant EFEMP1 is misfolded and secreted inefficiently and is retained within cells. In normal eyes, EFEMP1 is not present at the site of drusen formation. In eyes that are affected with malattia Leventinese, EFEMP1 accumulated within the retinal pigment epithelial cells and between the RPE and drusen, not being a major component of drusen. In AMD eyes, EFEMP1 is found to accumulate beneath the RPE overlaying the drusen.[38]

The malattia Leventinese phenotype is characterized by an early-onset radial distribution of basal laminar type of drusen in the macular and peripapillary area (see figure 61.4A). The nasal retina is also frequently involved. The disease is progressive, the drusen increasing in size and number with age and some developing dense pigmentation. In the early and end stages of the disease, the radial pattern of distribution of the drusen may be difficult to detect without fluorescein angiography (see figure 61.4C). When drusen are larger and coarser with virtually no radial pattern of distribution of the drusen, we refer to Doyne's honeycomb dystrophy (DHRD) (see figure 61.2D). The severity of radial distribution of drusen (basal laminar) that are seen clinically is the main feature that can be used to differentiate between the DHRD and malattia Leventinese phenotypes. In either case, the deposits are characterized by abnormal autofluorescence patterns and an *EFEMP1* mutation. Radial drusen maculopathy, like many autosomal-dominant conditions, is characterized by an intrafamilial and interfamilial phenotypic variability that remains unexplained.[12] This variability involves the severity, pattern, and progression of the disease. Some molecularly affected patients carry only subtle clinical signs of the disease and fail to show progression. This clinical subtype was identified by Forni in the 1960s as the "aborted form"[17] (see figure 61.1). Similarly, the highly variable phenotype suggests that the influence of the *EFEMP1* gene may be modulated by other genetic and/or environmental factors.[13]

Patients usually remain asymptomatic until the fourth decade, when they notice some difficulty in adapting from a brightly lit to a dim lit environment. Some may also develop a variable degree of metamorphopsia, photophobia, and reading difficulty in part owing to the developing paracentral scotomas. The condition relentlessly progresses to a variable degree of visual loss by the fifth decade, which becomes more severe in the sixties and seventies. By the age of 75, most affected individuals are legally blind from the disease. Although considered a rare complication, choroidal neovascularization may be encountered.

Symptomatic visual dysfunction may well precede the stage of retinal atrophy. Patients may complain of reduced central vision, difficulty in adapting to a dimly lit environment, and decreased contrast vision.[23] However, most patients with *EFEMP1* mutations retain good visual function (0.8–1.0) until the fifth decade, followed by a rapid decrease in the fifth or sixth decade. This contrasts with the RDS-related maculopathy described earlier, in which the natural history is characterized by a relatively continuous decrease

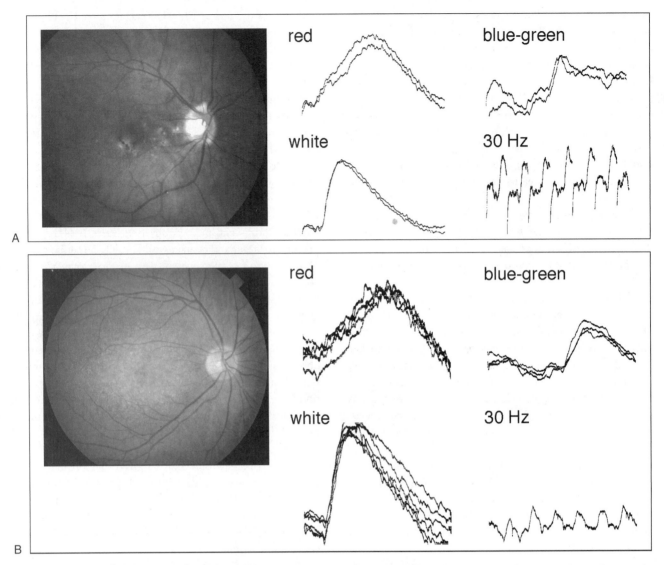

FIGURE 61.4   Clinical-electrophysiological correlation of different stages of the *EFEMP1*-related and codon 172 RDS–related maculopathies. A, Fundus photography of a 29-year-old male (early stage) affected with an *EFEMP1* maculopathy (left) and the corre-sponding full-field ERG recording (right). B, Fundus photography of a 31-year-old male affected with an Arg172Trp-related maculopathy (left) and the corresponding full-field ERG recording (right).

in visual acuity with increasing age. Rod-driven and cone-driven ERG b-wave amplitudes decrease nearly linearly in both conditions in accord with the normal loss of amplitude with increasing age. Implicit times of cone b-waves for *EFEMP1*-related disease increased more markedly with age when compared to RDS-related disease, in which the values were always prolonged beyond the normal range with a slight increase with age (see figures 61.4A and 61.4C).[21,23] The documented change of the rod and cone ERG ampli-tudes is not different from that related to age.[21] Color-contrast thresholds and both pattern and foveal ERGs show abnormal recordings when tested in adulthood.[23] Dark adaptation kinetics can be markedly prolonged when meas-ured in a central location over the confluent deposits, unlike the case when they are measured peripherally to these

deposits.[23] This work highlights the geographic importance of dark adaptation kinetics measurements. In a study of six patients (age range: 34–51 years), a variety of modest ERG changes were observed, which include reduced oscillatory potential and a marginally delayed 30-Hz response cone b-wave. The pattern and focal ERGs were variably reduced in most patients.[23]

Distinguishing between the different types of dominant drusen based on electrophysiological testing alone is diffi-cult.[21] The conflicting reports regarding the functional attributes of various dominantly inherited drusen may reflect the various ages that were tested with respect to the progressive nature of the condition in addition to the genetic heterogeneity of this group of conditions and the different methodologies used through time.

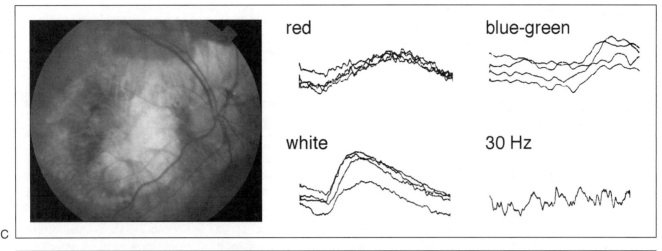

C

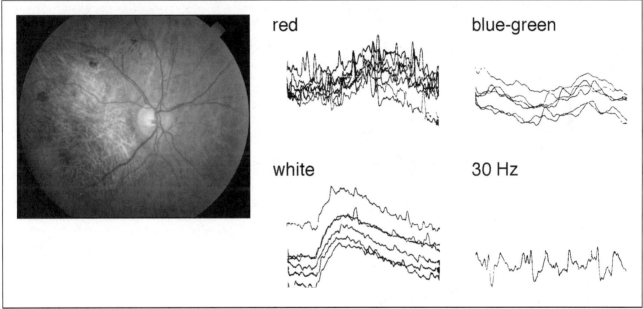

D

FIGURE 61.4   (continued) C, Fundus photography of a 60-year-old male (late stage) affected with an *EFEMP1* maculopathy (left) and the corresponding full-field ERG recording (right). D, Fundus pho-tography of a 60-year-old male affected with an Arg172Trp-related maculopathy (left) and the corresponding full-field ERG recording (right).

Summary

The clinical distinction between hereditary and nonheredi-tary drusen is challenging. Newer electrophysiological tech-niques that are now available may document retinal dysfunction related to drusen but are not diagnostic of drusen.

The known pathological changes associated with drusen do not significantly alter the electrical properties of the RPE cells.[37] Hereditary drusen usually show an early abnormal autofluorescence pattern and correlated abnormal contrast sensitivity, color vision, and cone ERG responses.

At least three early-onset dominant drusen models have led to the identification of a macular degeneration gene. Although these genes are not AMD genes, they are helping the investigation of the pathways involved in age-related macular degeneration. This allowed us to start learning about what AMD genes could look like, where they are expressed, and what they can do. For example, we know that genes that lead to drusen may involve various mechanisms, such as photoreceptors, Bruch's membrane stability, vitamin A transport, and angiogenesis.

The generation of animal models will facilitate the explo-ration of the mechanisms underlying phenotype variability. For example, TIMP-3 is present in drusen, and early animal work suggest that TIMP-3 may play a role in the modula-tion of neovascularization. The knock-in mice display early features of age-related changes in Bruch's membrane and the RPE that may represent the primary clinical manifesta-tions of SFD. The fact that the night blindness associated with Sorsby fundus dystrophy can be reversed over the short term with high-dose vitamin A supports the ideas of nutritional manipulation in some cases. Accumulation of EFEMP1 in RPE suggest that misfolding and aberrant accumulation may lead to drusen formation and cellular degeneration. These biological findings combined with the more sophisticated electrophysiological approaches to macular degeneration should provide critical information relating to drusen-related vision loss.

ACKNOWLEDGMENTS The authors are grateful to Professor Günter Niemeyer, Zurich, for the electrophysiological expertise provided.

REFERENCES

1. Abdelsalam A, Del Priore L, Zarbin MA: Drusen in age-related macular degeneration: Pathogenesis, natural course, and laser photocoagulation-induced regression. *Surv Ophthalmol* 1999; 44:1–29.

2. Anderson DH, et al: Local cellular sources of apolipoprotein E in the human retina and retinal pigmented epithelium: Implications for the process of drusen formation. *Am J Ophthalmol* 2001; 131:767–781.

3. Apfelstedt-Sylla E, et al: Extensive intrafamilial phenotypic variation among patients with autosomal dominant retinal dystrophy and mutations in the human RDS/peripherin gene. *Br J Ophthalmol* 1995; 79:28–34.

4. Clarke M, et al: Clinical features of a novel TIMP-3 mutation causing Sorsby's fundus dystrophy: Implications for disease mechanism. *Br J Ophthalmol* 2001; 85:1429–1431.

5. Collins T: A pathological report upon a case of Doyne's choroiditis ("honeycomb" or "familial choroiditis"). *Ophthalmoscope* 1913; 11:537–538.

6. Connell G, et al: Photoreceptor peripherin is the normal product of the gene responsible for retinal degeneration in the rds mouse. *Proc Natl Acad Sci U S A* 1991; 88:723–726.

7. Crabb JW, et al: Drusen proteome analysis: An approach to the etiology of age-related macular degeneration. *Proc Natl Acad Sci U S A* 2002; 99:14682–14687.

8. Deutman AF, Jansen LM: Dominantly inherited drusen of Bruch's membrane. *Br J Ophthalmol* 1970; 54:373–382.

9. Doyne RW: Peculiar condition of choroiditis occurring in several members of the same family. *Trans Ophthalmol Soc UK* 1899; 19:71.

10. Dusek J, Streicher T, Schmidt K: Hereditäre drusen der bruchschen membran: I. Klinische und lichtmikroskopische beobachtungen. *Klin Monatsbl Augenheilkd* 1982; 181:27–31.

11. Duvall-Young J, MacDonald MK, McKechnie NM: Fundus changes in (type II) mesangiocapillary glomerulonephritis simulating drusen: A histopathological report. *Br J Ophthalmol* 1989; 73:297–302.

12. Edwards AO, et al: Malattia leventinese: Refinement of the genetic locus and phenotypic variability in autosomal dominant macular drusen. *Am J Ophthalmol* 1998; 126:417–424.

13. Evans K, et al: Assessment of the phenotypic range seen in Doyne honeycomb retinal dystrophy. *Arch Ophthalmol* 1997; 115:904–910.

14. Falsini B, et al: Focal electroretinograms and fundus appearance in nonexudative age-related macular degeneration: Quantitative relationship between retinal morphology and function. *Graefes Arch Clin Exp Ophthalmol* 1999; 237:193–200.

15. Falsini B, et al: Retinal sensitivity to flicker modulation: Reduced by early age-related maculopathy. *Invest Ophthalmol Vis Sci* 2000; 41:1498–1506.

16. Fishman GA, Carrasco C, Fishman M: The electro-oculogram in diffuse (familial) drusen. *Arch Ophthalmol* 1976; 94:231–233.

17. Forni S, Babel J: Etude clinique et histologique de la malattia Levantinese. *Ophthalmologica* 1962; 143:313–322.

18. Gass JD: Drusen and disciform macular detachment and degeneration. *Arch Ophthalmol* 1973; 90:206–217.

19. Gass JDM: *Stereoscopic Atlas of Macular Diseases: Diagnosis and Treatment.* St. Louis, Mosby, 1977.

20. Gass J: In Klein E (ed): *Stereoscopic Atlas of Macular Diseases.* St. Louis, Mosby, 1987, pp 92–97.

21. Gerber DM, Munier FL, Niemeyer G: Cross-sectional study of visual acuity and electroretinogram in two types of dominant drusen. *Invest Ophthalmol Vis Sci* 2003; 44:493–496.

22. Hageman GS, Mullins RF, Russell SR, Johnson LV, Anderson DH: Vitronectin is a constituent of ocular drusen and the vitronectin gene is expressed in human retinal pigmented epithelial cells. *Faseb J* 1999; 13:477–484.

23. Haimovici R, et al: Symptomatic abnormalities of dark adaptation in patients with EFEMP1 retinal dystrophy (malattia Leventinese/Doyne honeycomb retinal dystrophy). *Eye* 2002; 16:7–15.

24. Hammond CJ, et al: Genetic influence on early age-related maculopathy: A twin study. *Ophthalmology* 2002; 109:730–736.

25. Heiba IM, Elston RC, Klein BE, Klein R: Sibling correlations and segregation analysis of age-related maculopathy: The Beaver Dam Eye Study. *Genet Epidemiol* 1994; 11:51–67.

26. Heon E, et al: Linkage of autosomal dominant radial drusen (malattia leventinese) to chromosome 2p16-21. *Arch Ophthalmol* 1996; 114:193–198.

27. Hoskin A, Sehmi K, Bird AC: Sorsby's pseudoinflammatory macular dystrophy. *Br J Ophthalmol* 1981; 65:859–865.

28. Hutchinson J, Tay W: Symmetrical central choroidoretinal disease occuring in senile persons. *R London Ophthalmol Hosp Rep* 1875; 8:231–244.

29. Jacobson SG, et al: Night blindness in Sorsby's fundus dystrophy reversed by vitamin A. *Nat Genet* 1995; 11:27–32.

30. Jacobson SG, et al: Novel mutation in the TIMP3 gene causes Sorsby fundus dystrophy. *Arch Ophthalmol* 2002; 120:376–379.

31. Kamei M, Hollyfield JG: TIMP-3 in Bruch's membrane: Changes during aging and in age-related macular degeneration. *Invest Ophthalmol Vis Sci* 1989; 40:2367–2375.

32. Klainguti R: Die tapeto-retinal degenration im Kanton Tessin. *Klin Monatsbl Augenheilkd* 1932; 89:253–254.

33. Klaver CC, et al: Genetic association of apolipoprotein E with age-related macular degeneration. *Am J Hum Genet* 1998; 63:200–206.

34. Klein ML, et al: Age-related macular degeneration: Clinical features in a large family and linkage to chromosome 1q. *Arch Ophthalmol* 1998; 116:1082–1088.

35. Kliffen M, et al: The APO(*)E3-Leiden mouse as an animal model for basal laminar deposit. *Br J Ophthalmol* 2000; 84:1415–1419.

36. Li J, Tso MO, Lam TT: Reduced amplitude and delayed latency in foveal response of multifocal electroretinogram in early age related macular degeneration. *Br J Ophthalmol* 2001; 85:287–290.

37. Marmor MF: Pattern dystrophy. In Heckenlively JR, Arden GB (eds): *Principles and Practice of Clinical Electrophysiology of Vision.* St. Louis, Mosby Year-Book, 1991, pp 664–668.

38. Marmorstein LY, et al: Aberrant accumulation of EFEMP1 underlies drusen formation in Malattia Leventinese and age-related macular degeneration. *Proc Natl Acad Sci U S A* 2002; 99:13067–13072.

39. Matsumoto M, Traboulsi EI: Dominant radial drusen and Arg345Trp EFEMP1 mutation. *Am J Ophthalmol* 2001; 131:810–812.

40. Meyers SM: A twin study on age-related macular degeneration. *Trans Am Ophthalmol Soc* 1994; 92:775–843.

41. Mullins RF, Russell SR, Anderson DH, Hageman GS: Drusen associated with aging and age-related macular degeneration contain proteins common to extracellular deposits associated with atherosclerosis, elastosis, amyloidosis, and dense deposit disease. *Faseb J* 2000; 14:835–846.

42. Nakazawa M, et al: Ocular findings in patients with autosomal dominant retinitis pigmantosa and transversion mutation in codon 244 (Asn244Lys) of the peripherin/RDS gene. *Arch Ophthalmol* 1994; 112:1567–1573.

43. Niemeyer G, Demant E: Cone and rod ERGs in degenerations of central retina. *Graefes Arch Clin Exp Ophthalmol* 1983; 220:201–208.

44. Owsley C, Jackson GR, White M, Feist R, Edwards D: Delays in rod-mediated dark adaptation in early age-related maculopathy. *Ophthalmology* 2001; 108:1196–1202.

45. Pearce WG: Doyne's honeycomb retinal degeneration: Clinical and genetic features. *Br J Ophthalmol* 1968; 52:73–78.

46. Piguet B, Haimovici R, Bird AC: Dominantly inherited drusen represent more than one disorder: A historical review. *Eye* 1995; 9(1):34–41.

47. Piguet B, et al: Full characterization of the maculopathy associated with an Arg-172-Trp mutation in the RDS/peripherin gene. *Ophthalmic Genet* 1996; 17:175–186.

48. Polkinghorne PJ, et al: Sorsby's fundus dystrophy: A clinical study. *Ophthalmology* 1989; 96(12):1763–1768.

49. Qi JH, et al: A novel function for tissue inhibitor of metalloproteinases-3 (TIMP3): Inhibition of angiogenesis by blockage of VEGF binding to VEGF receptor-2. *Nat Med* 2003; 9:407–415.

50. Richards S, Creel D: Pattern dystrophy and retinitis pigmentosa caused by a peripherin/RDS mutation. *Retina* 1995; 15:68–72.

51. Russell SR, Mullins RF, Schneider BL, Hageman GS: Location, substructure, and composition of basal laminar drusen compared with drusen associated with aging and age-related macular degeneration. *Am J Ophthalmol* 2000; 129:205–214.

52. Sarks SH: Council lecture: Drusen and their relationship to senile macular degeneration. *Aust J Ophthalmol* 1980; 8:117–130.

53. Sauer CG, et al: EFEMP1 is not associated with sporadic early onset drusen. *Ophthalmic Genet* 2001; 22:27–34.

54. Scullica L, Falsini B: Diagnosis and classification of macular degenerations: An approach based on retinal function testing. *Doc Ophthalmol* 2001; 102:237–250.

55. Seddon JM, Ajani UA, Mitchell BD: Familial aggregation of age-related maculopathy. *Am J Ophthalmol* 1997; 123:199–206.

56. Sieving PA, Boskovich S, Bingham E, Pawar H: Sorsby's fundus dystrophy in a family with a Ser-181-CVS mutation in the TIMP-3 gene: Poor outcome after laser photocoagulation. *Trans Am Ophthalmol Soc* 1996; 94:275–294; discussion, 295–297.

57. Silvestri G, Johnston PB, Hughes AE: Is genetic predisposition an important risk factor in age-related macular degeneration? *Eye* 1994; 8(5):564–568.

58. Smith W, et al: Risk factors for age-related macular degeneration: Pooled findings from three continents. *Ophthalmology* 2001; 108:697–704.

59. Sorsby A: Choroidal angio-sclerosis with special reference to its hereditary character. *Br J Ophthalmol* 1939; 23:433–444.

60. Sorsby A, Mason MEJ, Gardener N: A fundus dystrophy with unusual features. *Br J Ophthalmol* 1949; 33:67–97.

61. Steinmetz R, Polkinghorne P, Fitze F, Kemp C, Bird A: Abnormal dark adaptation and rhodopsin kinetics in Sorsby's fundus dystrophy. *Invest Ophthalmol Vis Sci* 1992; 33:1633–1636.

62. Stone EM, et al: Novel mutations in the peripherin (RDS) and rhodopsin genes associated with autosomal dominant retinitis pigmentosa (ADRP). *Invest Ophthalmol Vis Sci* 1993; 34:1149.

63. Stone EM, et al: A single EFEMP1 mutation associated with both malattia Leventinese and Doyne honeycomb retinal dystrophy. *Nat Genet* 1999; 22:199–202.

64. Streicher T, Schmidt K, Dusek J: [Hereditary drusen of Bruch's membrane: I. Clinical and light microscopical study.] *Klin Monatsbl Augenheilkd* 1982; 181:27–31.

65. Sunness JS, Johnson MA, Massof RW, Marcus S: Retinal sensitivity over drusen and nondrusen areas: A study using fundus perimetry. *Arch Ophthalmol* 1988; 106:1081–1084.

66. Toto L, et al: Genetic heterogeneity in malattia Leventinese. *Clin Genet* 2002; 62:399–403.

67. Travis GH, Brennan MB, Danielson PE, Kozak CA, Sutcliffe JG: Identification of a photoreceptor-specific mRNA encoded by the gene responsible for retinal degeneration slow (rds). *Nature* 1989; 338:70–73.

68. Travis G, Sutcliffe J, Bok D: The retinal degeneration slow (rds) gene product is a photoreceptor disc membrane-associated glycoprotein. *Neuron* 1991; 6:61–70.

69. Travis GH, et al: The human retinal degeneration slow (RDS) gene: Chromosome assignment and structure of the mRNA. *Genomics* 1991; 10:733–739.

70. Treacher C: A pathological report upon a case of Doyne's choroiditis ("honeycomb" or "family" choroiditis). *Ophthalmoscope* 1913; 11:537–538.

71. Wagner H, Klainguti R: Weitere Untersuchungen über die Malattia leventinese. *Ophthalmologica (Basel)* 1943; 105:225–228.

72. Walter P, Widder RA, Luke C, Konigsfeld P, Brunner R: Electrophysiological abnormalities in age-related macular degeneration. *Graefes Arch Clin Exp Ophthalmol* 1999; 237:962–968.

73. Weber B, Vogt G, Pruett R, Stöhr H, Felbor U: Mutations in the tissue inhibitor of metalloproteinases-3 (TIMP3) in patients with Sorsby's fundus dystrophy. *Nat Genet* 1994; 8:352–356.

74. Weber BHF, Vogt G, Wolz W, Ives EJ, Ewing CC: Sorsby's fundus dystrophy is genetically linked to chromosome 22q13-qter. *Nature Genet* 1994; 7:158–161.

75. Weber BH, et al: A mouse model for Sorsby fundus dystrophy. *Invest Ophthalmol Vis Sci* 2002; 43:2732–2740.

76. Weleber RG, Carr RE, Murphey WH, Sheffield VC, Stone EM: Phenotypic variation including retinitis pigmentosa, pattern dystrophy, and fundus flavimaculatus in a single family with a deletion of codon 153 or 154 of the peripherin/RDS gene. *Arch Ophthalmol* 1993; 111:1531–1542.

77. Wrobleski J, et al: Macular dystrophy associated with mutations at codon 172 in the human retinal degeneration slow gene. *Ophthalmology* 1994; 101:12–22.

78. Yeow KM, et al: Sorsby's fundus dystrophy tissue inhibitor of metalloproteinases-3 (TIMP-3) mutants have unimpaired matrix metalloproteinase inhibitory activities, but affect cell adhesion to the extracellular matrix. *Matrix Biol* 2002; 21:75–88.

62 Stargardt Disease

DAVID BIRCH

STARGARDT DISEASE (STGD), first described in 1909 by Karl Stargardt,[35] is by far the most common form of juvenile macular degeneration. Although the incidence of one in 10,000 is frequently cited, precise estimates of prevalence are not available. STGD is characterized by discrete yellowish deposits within the posterior pole. One variant of STGD, fundus flavimaculatus, was described by Franceschetti and Francois in 1963.[19] The term was used to describe patients who had white pisciform flecks throughout the fundus but who typically retained good visual acuity until later in life. Molecular studies have more recently shown that autosomal recessive forms of fundus flavimaculatus, STGD, and some more widespread forms of cone-rod dystrophy (CRD) and retinitis pigmentosa (RP) are all associated with mutations in the ABCA4 (formerly ABCR) gene. A rare dominant form of macular disease with phenotypic similarity to STGD has been related to mutations in ELOVA4, a gene that is believed to be related to long-chain fatty acid metabolism.[40]

STGD typically begins in the first or second decade of life. Presenting symptoms include visual acuity that cannot be corrected to 20/20. Typically, there is a fairly rapid decline in acuity during the teenage years, with final acuity of 20/200 to 20/400 by adulthood.[17] The full-field ERG is useful for ruling out more widespread forms of retinal degeneration.[4] As shown in figure 62.1, responses are usually within the normal range in children with the disease. The cone electroretinogram (ERG) to 31-Hz flicker typically lies toward the lower limit of normal, and the cone b-wave implicit time is usually longer than mean normal but still within the normal range.[22] Older patients with extensive macular generation may show subnormal cone and rod amplitudes (see figure 62.1), but the magnitude of loss is roughly predictable from the extent of macular degeneration. An important characteristic of STGD is that cone b-wave implicit time remains borderline normal despite advanced disease. This is an important prognostic indicator, since patients who retaining normal or near normal b-wave implicit times are likely to retain useful peripheral function throughout life.[6] As we shall see, this discriminates patients with STGD from those with CRD, who, despite having similar gene mutations, nevertheless have a distinctly different visual prognosis.

While the full-field ERG is useful for discriminating the more localized pathology of STGD from widespread forms of retinal degeneration, it is of little value in the early detection of macular disease and for following patients in longitudinal studies and clinical trials. In evaluating the possible retinal basis for reduced acuity in a child, it is necessary to obtain a focal or multifocal ERG. The focal ERG should be conducted with direct visualization of the fundus to ensure that the response originates from the area of interest.[34] Typically, in evaluating an acuity loss, the region of interest is the fovea. With the stimulus as small as 4 degrees, the stimulus is flickered at a frequency that is higher than the rod fusion frequency. The Maculoscope™, for example, based on the work of Sandberg et al.,[34] employs a spot flickering at 42 Hz within a more intense, steady surround. The sensitivity and utility of this test for documenting the retinal basis of acuity loss have been reviewed previously.[7] It is generally thought that the foveal response drops below the lower normal amplitude limit when visual acuity is 20/50 or less owing to macular degeneration.[15] In STGD, the amplitude may be below the lower limit of normal before substantial loss of acuity, making this an important prognostic test.[11,15,26]

The multifocal ERG (mfERG) adds the capability for simultaneously measuring retinal function at dozens of locations throughout the macula.[38] With the recent development of the fundus camera-based stimulus delivery system, it is now possible to monitor fundus position while testing. This is particularly important for patients with STGD, who may use a preferred eccentric locus of fixation whenever possible. In practice, it is useful to assess the fixation behavior of the patient through a fundus camera prior to mfERG testing. It is then possible to correct for eccentric fixation during testing. Maintaining the position of the optic disk helps to ensure that the stimulus pattern is centered on the fovea. Figure 62.2A shows the fundus of the left eye of a 20-year-old female with STGD. Characteristic flecks (lipofuscin) are scattered throughout the posterior pole but are not present in the macula, which has an atrophic appearance (more evident on fluorescein angiography). The mfERG from the same eye is characteristic of responses in a patient with recently diagnosed STGD (figure 62.2B). Despite only a modest reduction in acuity, responses from the central 10 degrees are severely reduced in amplitude, while responses from outside the macula are normal. The pattern of loss in the mfERG corresponds to that seen in the visual field (figure 62.2C).

Mutations in the ABCA4 gene were identified as a cause of STGD in 1997.[2,3] It is now thought that all cases of

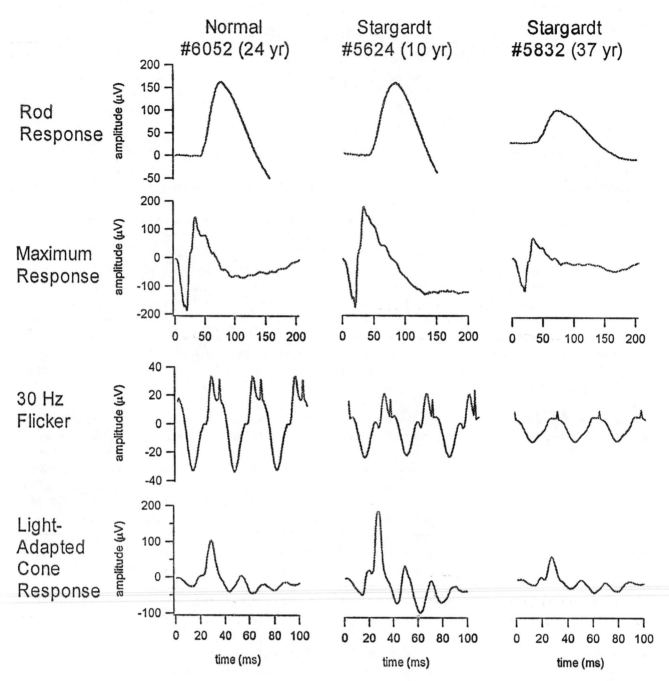

FIGURE 62.1 Representative full-field ERGs from a normal subject (left column) and two patients with STGD at different stages of disease (middle and right column). Response amplitudes are bor- derline reduced in the older patient, but b-wave implicit times are at the upper end of normal.

autosomal recessive STGD are due to ABCA4 mutations.[20] The protein encoded by the ABCA4 gene is called rim protein (RmP) because it was initially described in frog rod outer segment rims.[30] RmP is a member of the adenosine triphosphate–binding cassette (ABC) transporter superfamily.[3] Because it produces increased ATPase activity from RmP in vivo, a likely substrate of RmP is all-*trans*-retinal.[36] On the basis of findings in the *abcr*−/− mouse model, in which RmP is completely absent, Travis and colleagues have proposed a model for RmP (figure 62.3A).[39] According to the model, RmP participates in the metabolism of vitamin A in the photoreceptors after exposure to light. After exposure of rhodopsin to light (*hv*), all-*trans*-retinal is released within the outer segment disk. All-*trans*-retinal combines with phosphatidylethanolamine (PE) normally present in the disk membranes. The all-*trans* retinal-PE complex is called N-retinylidine-PE (N-ret-PE). The RmP protein normally transports the N-ret-PE out of the disk, where all-*trans*-retinal is reduced to all-*trans* retinol (a*t*ROL) and eventually reconverted back to 11-*cis*-retinal within the RPE.

With missing or defective RmP, N-ret-PE accumulates within the intradiskal space (figure 62.3B). The consequences of this are far reaching. One consequence is that "naked" opsin may be activated by the excess levels of free all-*trans*-retinal within the intradiskal space (ops/a*t*RAL). This activation is believed to produce a noisy receptor in the dark, leading to an equivalent background and consequently, to delays in dark adaptation. These delays have been reported in patients with STGD after exposure to adapting light that bleaches a substantial fraction of the visual pigment.[16] This delay in dark adaptation parallels that found in both homozygote[39] and heterozygote[24] *abcr* knock-out mice.

A second consequence of the buildup of N-ret-PE is the combining of a second molecule of all-*trans*-retinal with N-ret-PE to produce N-retinylidene-N-retinyl-PE (A2PE-H$_2$). A2PE-H$_2$ is ultimately hydrolyzed to form N-retinylidene-N-retinyl-ethanolamine (A2E). Many of these reactions occur in the RPE after disks containing the excessive trapped A2PE-H$_2$ are shed as part of the normal phagocytotic process. The A2E accumulates as lipofuscin in the RPE and may ultimately damage intracellular membranes and destroy the overburdened RPE cells within the macula.[14]

Also associated with ABCA4 mutations and therefore part of the spectrum of STGD is a subset of cone-rod dystrophy, a progressive retinal degeneration that is typically inherited as an autosomal-recessive disease. A common early symptom is decreased visual acuity due to macular degeneration. In fact, young patients with CRD form may be thought to have STGD because of the similarity in appearance, but with time, it develops into a more progressive disorder. The severe visual loss manifests as a posterior pole cellophane maculopathy and expanding central scotoma or widespread posterior pole flecks, which then degenerate, leaving an atrophic macular scar. Both forms show the dark choroid effect outside the macular areas that may show hyperfluorescence due to the central degeneration. Patients with CRD have characteristic changes in the full-field ERG that include delayed cone b-wave implicit times.[5] A subset of patients with CRD shows a prolonged time course of dark adaptation following a bleach.[18] CRD is distinguished from RP on the basis of visual acuity, fundus appearance, ERG findings, and the absence of night blindness as a presenting symptom. In a large prospective study of 100 patients with either CRD or RP, it was shown that the rate of rod ERG loss was significantly lower in CRD than in RP.[9] Moreover, the rate of rod loss in CRD was similar to the rate of cone loss. This is quite different from RP, in which rod ERG function is lost approximately three times faster than cone function.[9] In addition, the patterns of visual field loss[8] and ERG loss[10] are different in CRD and RP. Thus, when ABCA4 mutations take the CRD pathway, it is a clinically distinct retinal disorder from STGD and RP that has widespread involvement of both cone and rod photoreceptors.

Despite the distinctive characteristics of each phenotype, mutations in the human ABCA4 gene that cause STGD have been implicated in a subset of patients with recessive RP and recessive CRD.[13,23,27,37] As in STGD, one consequence of the defect in RmP is the accumulation of all-*trans*-retinaldehyde within the rod outer segment disks and the production of a persistent "equivalent background" due to transient accumulation of the "noisy" photoproduct. This equivalent background is believed to be a major factor causing the slowed time course of adaptation in patients with ABCA4 mutations. The time course of dark adaptation following a photobleach is shown in figure 62.4 for a patient with CRD. Also shown is the average time course (±1 standard deviation) based on the 15 control subjects. Compared to normal, the time course of recovery in the patient with CRD is remarkably slow. Whereas the average control subject returns to within 0.2 log unit of the prebleach (fully dark-adapted) threshold by 25.4 minutes, it took 59 minutes for this patient with CRD to return to within 0.2 log unit of the preexposure value. The median recovery time for 11 patients with CRD associated with ABCA4 mutations of 41.6 minutes was significantly longer ($t = −4.38$, $p < .001$) than the 25.4 minutes required for the average control subject.[12] Similar delays in the time course of dark adaptation have been reported previously in a subset of patients with CRD.[18] Also similar to this phenotype in CRD patients is the delayed recovery of rod sensitivity following light exposure in mice homozygous[39] and heterozygous[24] for a null mutation in the *abcr* gene.

After 30 minutes of dark adaptation following a photobleach, thresholds for normal subjects were at their prebleach values, while thresholds for the majority of patients

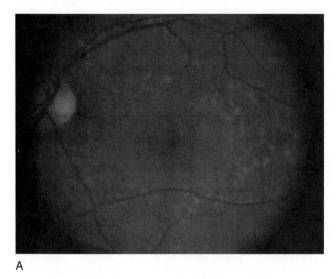

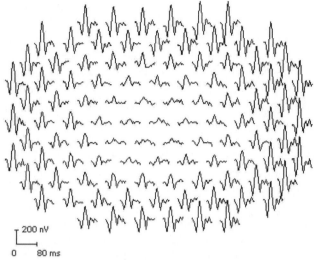

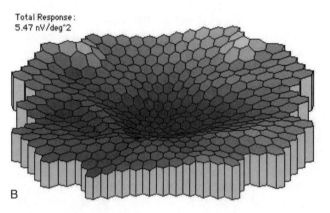

FIGURE 62.2   A, Fundus photo from left eye showing lipofuscin accumulation within the posterior pole. B, mfERG from same patient showing selective loss of responses from the central 10 degrees. (See also color plate 30.)

with CRD remained elevated. To determine whether the persistent elevation was associated with an equivalent or noisy background, pupil size was measured after 30 minutes in the dark.[30] Patients with CRD and associated ABCA4 mutations had significantly smaller pupil diameters than did normal subjects 30 minutes following a bleach, and the test eye pupil diameter (OS) was consistently smaller than the chemically dilated pupil diameter (OD). This phenotype is apparently due to the accumulation of all-*trans*-retinaldehyde, which interacts with opsin apoprotein to form a "noisy" photoproduct.[21,23,37] Loss of this transport activity also results in the accumulation of toxic bis-retinoids in the retinal pigment epithelium,[24,25] which may predispose to photoreceptor degeneration.

Research with patients and with animal models of STGD and CRD may also shed light on the mechanisms involved in age-related macular degeneration (AMD). In analyzing data from over 1700 patients with AMD at several centers, Allikmets found that particular ABCA4 alleles raise the risk of AMD.[1] The two most commonly associated variants were

G1961E and D2177N. The increase in risk is between three-fold and fivefold. Consistent with a role for ABCA4 mutations in heterozygote carriers of ABCA4 are the findings from of transgenic mice. *Abcr*+/− (*abca4*+/−) heterozygous mice accumulate A2E in the RPE at a rate approximately intermediate between wild-type and homozygeous mice.[24] Delays in recovery from a bleach are also present but are less severe than those in the *abcr*−/− mice. Interestly, delayed dark adaptation has also been reported in AMD.[28,29]

It is interesting that a single gene, ABCA4, can be associated with STG, CRD, RP, and, to some extent, AMD. It has been proposed that the severity of disease is related to the amount of residual RmP activity in a given patient.[13] Thus, a heterozygote carrying one mutant ABCA4 allele may be at risk for AMD, the degree of risk being related to the severity of the allele. A patient with two mild to moderate mutant alleles would have SRGD. CRD or RP would be the result of inheriting two severe mutant alleles. Although of heuristic value, this model is clearly an oversimplification, and exceptions to this scheme have been documented.[12] Patients with CRD may

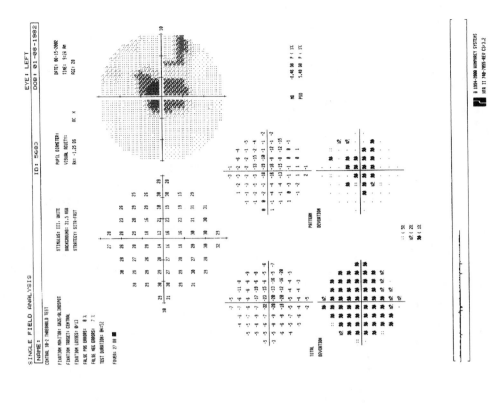

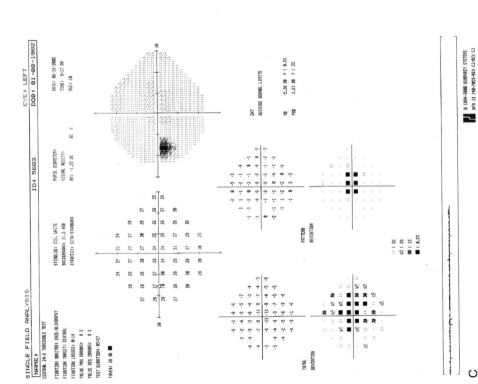

C, Humphrey static perimetric fields from central 24 degrees (left) and 10 degrees (right) showing loss of sensitivity corresponding to mfERG regional loss.

FIGURE 62.2 (continued)

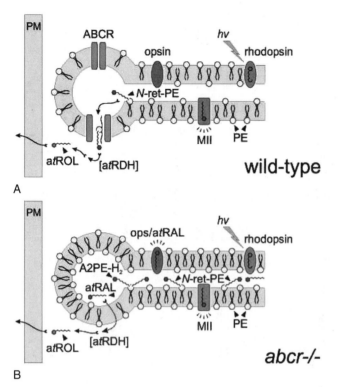

A

B

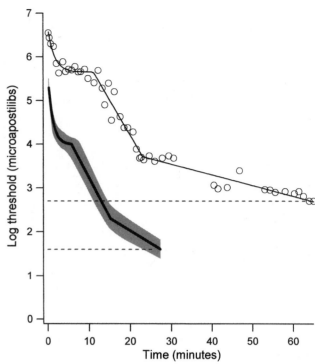

FIGURE 62.3 Model for the function of RmP (ABCR) protein in disk membranes. A, Wild-type, in which ABCT is a transporter (flippase) for N-ret-PE. B, *abcr*−/− mouse (and patients with reduced flippase activity). N-ret-PE trapped in the disk combines with a second molecule of all-*trans*-retinal to produce A2PE-H$_2$. A2PE-H$_2$ is ultimately hydrolyzed to form A2E. Many of these reactions occur in the RPE after disks containing the excessive trapped A2PE-H$_2$ are shed as part of the normal phagocytotic process. The A2E accumulates as lipofuscin in the RPE and may ultimately damage intracellular membranes and destroy the over-burdened RPE cells within the macula. A2E: N-retinylidene-N-retinyl-ethanolamine; A2PE-H$_2$: N-retinylidene-N-retinyl-PE; a*t*RAL: all-*trans*-retinal; a*t*RDH: all-*trans*-retinal dehydrogenase; a*t*ROL: all-*trans*-retinol; ops: opsin; PE: phosphatidylethanolamine; PM: plasma membrane. (From Weng J, Mata NL, Azarian SM, Tzekov RT, Birch DG, Travis GH: Insights into the function of Rim protein in photoreceptors and etiology of Stargardt's disease from the phenotype in abcr knockout mice. *Cell* 1999; 98:13–23.) (See also color plate 31.)

have the same allele as patients with STGD, even within the same family, and there is no obvious difference in predicted RmP activity that would explain whether a patient has CRD or RP. At the present time, molecular biology appears to have a limited diagnostic role in ABCA4 mutations. Electrophysiology continues to be the technique of choice for determining whether a patient with an ABCA4 mutation has STGD, CRD, or RP. Clearly, the implications of these phenotypic distinctions are enormous for visual prognosis.

Our rapidly evolving understanding of the etiology of STGD is already leading to suggestions for clinical trials to arrest visual loss. On the basis of work in *abcr*−/− mice, which show less A2E buildup when kept in the dark,[39] it

FIGURE 62.4 Time course of dark-adaptation in patient with CRD. Open circles are measured thresholds, solid line is best fit of linear component dark adaptation model. Also shown is the best-fit function for values from 15 normal subjects. The gray area shows ±1 standard deviation. Thresholds were followed until they returned to within 0.2 log unit of the patient's prebleach threshold (dashed lines).

seems prudent to recommend that patients with STGD minimize light exposure to the greatest extent practical. Drugs may be available or under development that could inhibit the accumulation of A2E in RPE cells. In this regard, isotretinoin was recently reported to be effective in limiting A2E accumulation in *abcr*−/− mice.[31] Finally, drugs and gene therapy have the potential to stimulate under active RmP activity.

ACKNOWLEDGMENTS Supported by EY05235, EY09076, and the Foundation Fighting Blindness.

REFERENCES

1. Allikmets R: Further evidence for an association of ABCR alleles with age-related macular degeneration. *Am J Hum Genet* 2000; 67:487–491.
2. Allikmets R, Singh N, Sun H, Shroyer NF, Hutchinson A, Chidambaram A, Gerrard B, Baird L, Stauffer D, Peiffer A, Rattner A, Smallwood P, Li Y, Anderson KL, Lewis RL, Nathans J, Leppert M, Dean M, Lupski JR: A photoreceptor cell-specific ATP-binding transporter gene (*ABCR*) is mutated in recessive Stargardt macular dystrophy. *Nat Genet* 1997; 15:236–246.
3. Azarian SM, Travis GH: The photoreceptor rim protein is an ABC transporter encoded by the gene for recessive Stargardt's disease (ABCR). *FEBS Lett* 1997; 409:247–252.

4. Berson EL: Retinitis pigmentosa. *Invest Ophthalmol Vis Sci* 1993; 34:1659–1676.

5. Berson EL, Gouras P, Gunkel RD: Progressive cone-rod degeneration. *Arch Ophthalmol* 1968; 80:68–76.

6. Berson EL, Gouras P, Hoff M: Temporal aspects of the electroretinogram. *Arch Ophthalmol* 1969; 81:207–214.

7. Birch DG: Focal and multifocal electroretinography. In Fishman GA, Birch DG, Harding GE, Brignell MG (eds): *Electrophysiologic Testing*. San Francisco, American Academy of Ophthalmology, 2001, pp 177–195.

8. Birch DG, Anderson JL: Rod visual fields in cone-rod degeneration: Comparisons to retinitis pigmentosa. *Invest Ophthalmol Vis Sci* 1990; 31:2288–2299.

9. Birch DG, Anderson JL, Fish GE: Yearly rates of rod and cone functional loss in retinitis pigmentosa and cone-rod dystrophy. *Ophthalmology* 1999; 106:258–268.

10. Birch DG, Fish GE: Rod ERGs in retinitis pigmentosa and cone-rod degeneration. *Invest Ophthalmol Vis Sci* 1987; 28:140–150.

11. Birch DG, Fish GE: Focal cone electroretinograms: Aging and macular disease. *Doc Ophthalmol* 1988; 69:211–220.

12. Birch DG, Peters AY, Locke KL, Megarity CF, Travis GH: Visual function in patients with cone-rod dystrophy (CRD) associated with ABCR mutations. *Vision Sci Appl* 2000; 1:53–56.

13. Cremers FP, van de Pol DJ, van Driel M, den Hollander AI, van Haren FJ, Knoers NV, Tijmes N, Bergen AA, Rohrschneider K, Blankenagel A, Pinckers AJ, Deutman AF, Hoyng CB: Autosomal recessive retinitis pigmentosa and cone-rod dystrophy caused by splice site mutations in the Stargardt's disease gene ABCR. *Hum Mol Genet* 1998; 7:355–362.

14. Eldred GE, Laskey MR: Retinal age pigments generated by self-assembling lysosomotrophic detergents. *Nature* 1993; 361:724–726.

15. Fish GE, Birch DG: The focal electroretinogram in the clinical assessment of macular disease. *Ophthalmology* 1989; 96:109–114.

16. Fishman GA, Farbman JS, Alexander KR: Delayed rod dark adaptation in patients with Stargardt's disease. *Ophthalmology* 1991; 98:957–962.

17. Fishman GA, Farber M, Patel BS, Derlacki DJ: Visual acuity loss in patients with Stargardt's macular dystrophy. *Ophthalmology* 1987; 94:809–814.

18. Fishman GA, Pullura P, Alexander KR, Derlacki DJ, Gilbert LD: Prolonged rod dark adaptation in patients with cone-rod dystrophy. *Am J Ophthalmol* 1994; 118:362–367.

19. Franceschetti A, Francois J: Fundus flavimaculatus. *Arch D'Ophthal* 1965; 25:505–530.

20. Glazer LC, Dryja TP: Understanding the etiology of Stargardt's disease. *Ophthalmol Clin N Am* 2002; 15:93–100.

21. Jager S, Palczewski K, Hofmann KP: Opsin/all-trans-retinal complex activates transducin by different mechanisms than photolyzed rhodopsin. *Biochemistry* 1996; 35:2901–2908.

22. Lachapelle P, Little JM, Roy MS: The electroretinogram in Stargardt's disease and fundus flavimaculatus. *Doc Ophthalmol* 1990; 73:395–404.

23. Martinez-Mir A, Paloma E, Allikmets R, Ayuso C, del Rio T, Dean M, Vilageliu L, Gonzalez-Duarte R, Balcells S: Retinitis pigmentosa caused by a homozygous mutation in the Stargardt disease gene ABCR [letter, comment]. *Nat Genet* 1998; 18:11–12.

24. Mata NL, Tzekov RT, Liu X, Weng J, Birch DG, Travis GH: Delayed dark-adaptation and lipofuscin accumulation in abcr+/− mice: Implications for involvement of ABCR in age-related macular degeneration. *Invest Ophthalmol Vis Sci* 2001; 42:1685–1690.

25. Mata NL, Weng J, Travis GH: Biosynthesis of a major lipofuscin fluorophore in mice and humans with ABCR-mediated retinal and macular degeneration. *Proc Natl Acad Sci U S A* 2000; 97:7154–7159.

26. Matthews GP, Sandberg MA, Berson MA: Foveal cone electroretinograms in patients with central visual loss of unexplained etiology. *Arch Ophthalmol* 1992; 110:1568–1570.

27. Maugeri A, Klevering BJ, Rohrschneider K, Blankenagel A, Brunner HG, Deutman AF, Hoyng CB, Cremers FP: Mutations in the ABCA4 (ABCR) gene are the major cause of autosomal recessive cone-rod dystrophy. *Am J Hum Genet* 2000; 67:960–966.

28. Owsley C, Jackson GR, Cideciyan AV, Huang Y, Fine SL, Ho AC, Maguire MG, Lolley V, Jacobson SG: Psychophysical evidence for rod vulnerability in age-related macular degeneration. *Invest Ophthalmol Vis Sci* 2000; 41:267–273.

29. Owsley C, Jackson GR, White M, Feist R, Edwards D: Delays in rod-mediated dark adaptation in early age-related maculopathy. *Ophthalmology* 2001; 108:1196–1202.

30. Papermaster DS, Schneider BG, Zorn M, Kraehenbuhl JP: Immunocytochemical localization of a large intrinsic membrane protein to the incisures and margins of frog rod outer segment disks. *J Cell Biol* 1978; 78:415–425.

31. Radu RA, Mata NL, Nusinowitz S, Liu X, Sieving PA, Travis GH: Treatment with isotretinoin inhibits lipoduscin accumulation in a mouse model of recessive Stargardt's macular degeneration. *Proc Nat Acad Sci U S A* 2003; 100:4742–4747.

32. Rozet JM, Gerber S, Ghazi I, Perrault I, Ducroq D, Souied E, Cabot A, Dufier JL, Munnich A, Kaplan J: Mutations of the retinal specific ATP binding transporter gene (ABCR) in a single family segregating both autosomal recessive retinitis pigmentosa RP19 and Stargardt disease: Evidence of clinical heterogeneity at this locus. *J Med Genet* 1999; 36:447–451.

33. Sachs K, Maretzki D, Meyer CK, Hofman KP: Diffusible ligand all-trans-retinal activates opsin via a palmitoylation-dependent mechanism. *J Biol Chem* 2000; 2754:6189–6619.

34. Sandberg MA, Jacobson SG, Berson EL: Foveal cone electroretinograms in retinitis pigmentosa and juvenile maular degeneration. *Am J Ophthalmol* 1979; 88:702–707.

35. Stargardt K: Uber familiare, progressive degeneationin der makulagegend des auges. *Graefes Arch Clin Exp Ophthalmol* 1909; 71:534–550.

36. Sun H, Nathans J: Stargardt's ABCR is localized to the disc membrane of retinal rod outer segments. *Nature Genet* 1997; 17:15–16.

37. Surya A, Foster KW, Knox BE: Transducin activation by the bovine opsin apoprotein. *J Biol Chem* 1995; 270:5024–5031.

38. Sutter EE, Tran D: The field topography of ERG components in man: I. The photopic luminance response. *Vision Res* 1992; 32:433–446.

39. Weng J, Mata NL, Azarian SM, Tzekov RT, Birch DG, Travis GH: Insights into the function of Rim protein in photoreceptors and etiology of Stargardt's disease from the phenotype in abcr knockout mice. *Cell* 1999; 98:13–23.

40. Zhang K, Kniazeva M, Han M, Li W, Yu Z, Yang Z, Li Y, Metzker ML, Allikmets R, Zack DJ, Kakuk LE, Lagali PS, Wong PW, MacDonald IM, Sieving PA, Figueroa DJ, Austin CP, Gould RJ, Ayyagari R, Petrukhin K: A 5-bp deletion in ELOVL4 is associated with two related forms of autosomal dominant macular dystrophy. *Nat Genet* 2001; 27:89–93.

63 Bietti's Crystalline Dystrophy of Cornea and Retina

RICHARD G. WELEBER AND DAVID J. WILSON

History of the disease

In 1937, Bietti[4,5] described three patients with retinal degeneration beginning in the third decade of life. All were characterized by glittering crystals in the posterior pole and in the superficial paralimbal cornea. Welch, in 1977, first used the term *crystalline retinopathy*, which so aptly describes the most characteristic feature of this disease.[37] Over 90 cases have been reported worldwide. The disease appears to be more frequent among Asians.[16,21] Although most accepted cases have crystals in both the cornea and the retina, some patients, who are otherwise typical, lack crystals in the cornea.[10,14,28,33] Other patients will show only retinal crystals for years before corneal crystals become evident.[19] As the disease progresses to later stages, the crystals in the retina become less apparent and eventually disappear.[3,35] Heterogeneity probably exists for Bietti's crystalline dystrophy (BCD). Wilson et al.[38] have suggested that the electrophysiological findings can differentiate two subtypes of BCD: a diffuse type (figures 63.1 to 63.3), with a profoundly abnormal electroretinogram (ERG),[2,4,38,39] and a regional or localized type (figures 63.4 to 63.6), with a more intact ERG that may be either normal or only mildly abnormal (figure 63.7).[14,34,38,39] Reports have detailed the progressive nature of BCD and have provided long-term follow-up information for 11,[38] 16,[21] 20,[2] 26,[21] and 30 years.[19,20] Some reports suggest that patients can progress from the regional to the diffuse phenotype.[3,19,20] Whether these two types represent allelic or genetic homogeneity remains unclear. Interestingly, the patient reported by Jurlies et al.[19] demonstrated at 34 years of age an electronegative scotopic ERG, a feature that was not reported by others with regional expression of the disease, even at age 58 years.[38]

Clinical description and natural history

Little information has been assembled on the natural history of BCD, especially with regard to consideration of the two possible subtypes. Patients report onset of symptoms anywhere from the second to the sixth decade of life, with the great majority in the third decade of life.[35] When patients are first examined, their Snellen visual acuity may be rela-

tively good, but as paracentral scotomas develop, deepen, and enlarge, near visual tasks such as reading become progressively more difficult. Symptoms related to paracentral scotomas may exist early but often are difficult for patients to verbalize other than noting that their central vision is blurred or that reading is difficult. With the diffuse type of BCD, early symptoms of night blindness and peripheral field loss are prominent and indicate diffuse photoreceptor abnormalities. With the localized or regional type, patients become symptomatic from scotomas close to fixation, which are generally perceived as central or pericentral vision loss. With both types, the scotomas correspond to the areas of retinal pigment epithelium (RPE) and choriocapillaris abnormalities. With the diffuse type, progression is more rapid, and the final visual impairment and subsequent disability are much greater (see figure 63.3). Color vision can be abnormal in both diffuse and regional disease and is usually of the tritan type.[38–40]

The two types differ in fundus appearance. In the diffuse type, tiny yellow crystals are present at various levels in the retina. RPE defects with pigment mottling and deposition can be seen diffusely throughout the fundus. In the localized or regional type, the disease begins in the posterior pole in the form of RPE defects. Subsequent atrophy of the choriocapillaris leads to prominence of medium-sized and larger choroidal vessels. With fluorescein angiography, a zone of hyperfluorescence will often separate the involved retina from the more normal-appearing peripheral retina (see figures 63.4 and 63.6). This type of BCD progresses by slow extension of the areas of RPE hyperfluorescence with further atrophy of the RPE and choroid in these regions.

The concept of subtypes of Bietti's dystrophy is not universally accepted, and many researchers have previously explained the wide range of clinical manifestations by different stages of the same disease. For example, Yuzawa et al. describe three stages of evolution to explain the disparity of clinical involvement seen with Bietti's crystalline dystrophy.[39] Stage 1 involved primarily RPE disease, stage 2 involved subsequent localized atrophy of the choriocapillaris, and stage 3 involved diffuse atrophy of the choriocapillaris. Presumably, all patients progress from stage 1 to stage 2, but to our

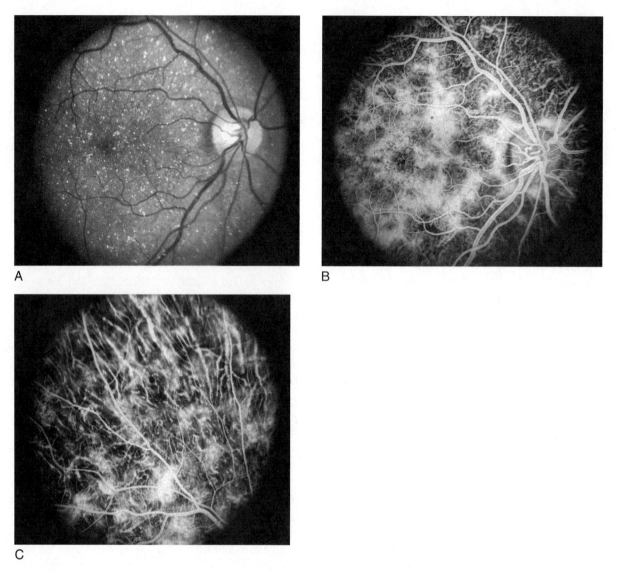

A

B

C

FIGURE 63.1 Fundus appearance (A) and fluorescein angiogram (B and C) of the right eye of a Japanese woman (patient of Wilson et al.[38]) with the diffuse form of Bietti's crystalline dystro-phy of cornea and retina at 36 years of age. (From Wilson DJ, Weleber RG, Klein ML, Welch RB, Green WR.[38] Used by permission.)

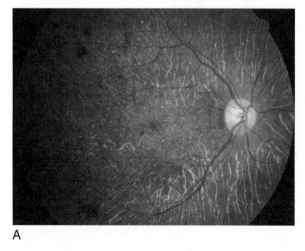

A

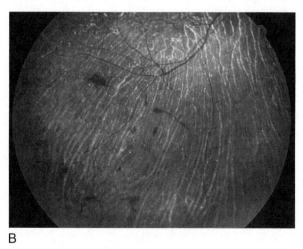

B

FIGURE 63.2 Same patient as in figure 63.1 at 45 years of age (A and B). Note the further loss of pigment epithelium and choriocapillaris over the nine-year interval. (From Wilson DJ, Weleber RG, Klein ML, Welch RB, Green WR.[38] Used by permission.) (See also color plate 32.)

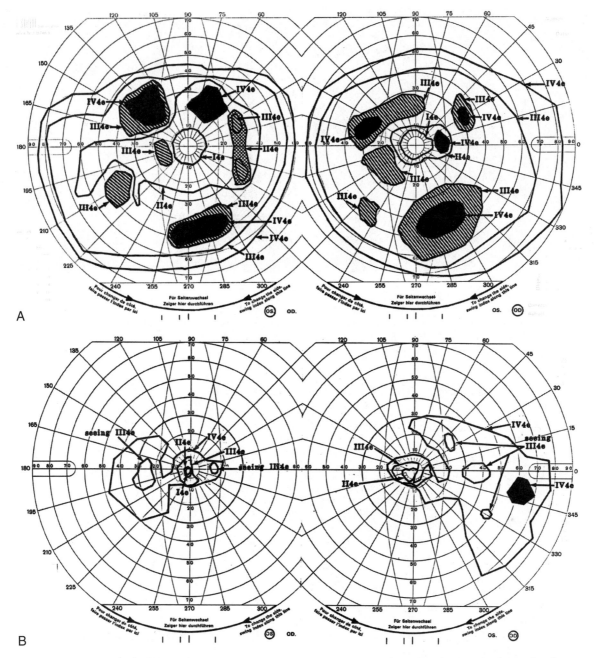

FIGURE 63.3   Goldmann perimetric visual fields for patient shown in figure 63.1 with the diffuse form of Bietti's dystrophy at 36 (A) and 45 (B) years of age. Her visual acuity decreased from 20/30 J1 OU at 36 years of age to 20/50 J1 OU at 47 years of age. From 47 to 48 years of age, her visual acuity dropped to finger counting at 4 feet OD and at 7 feet OS; she was unable to read any Jaeger type at near distance. (From Wilson DJ, Weleber RG, Klein ML, Welch RB, Green WR.[38] Used by permission.)

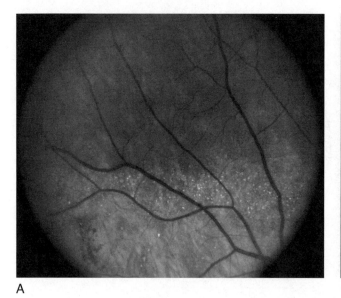
A

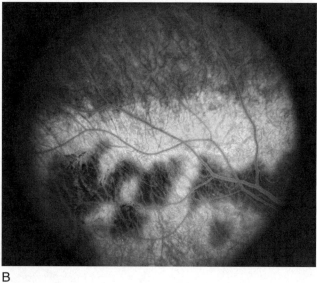
B

FIGURE 63.4 Fundus appearance (A) and fluorescein angiogram (B) of the superior border of atrophic lesions in the posterior pole of the right eye of a 52-year-old man with the regional form of Bietti's crystalline dystrophy (patient 2 in Wilson DJ, Weleber RG, Klein ML, Welch RB, Green WR.[38]). Note that crystals are prominent in the transition zone of disturbed RPE between atrophic retina and normal peripheral retina.

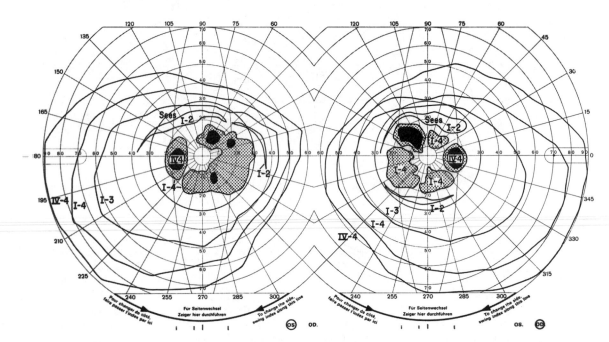

FIGURE 63.5 Goldmann perimetric visual fields of a 49-year-old man with the regional form of Bietti's crystalline dystrophy (patient 2 in Wilson DJ, Weleber RG, Klein ML, Welch RB, Green WR.[38]). Same patient as shown in figure 63.4. Although his visual acuity was 20/25 in each eye, the patient was greatly bothered by pericentral scotomas.

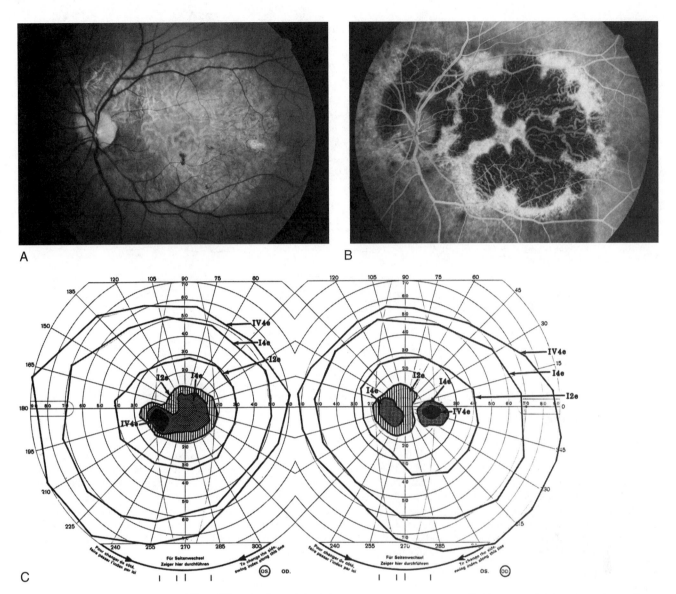

FIGURE 63.6   Fundus appearance (A) and fluorescein angiogram (B) of the left eye and Goldmann perimetric visual fields (C) of a 61-year-old man with the regional form of Bietti's crystalline dystrophy (patient 3 in Wilson et al.[38]). The visual fields had not changed over those determined nine years previously, but the visual acuity had decreased from 20/30 J1 to 20/40 J2. (See also color plate 33.)

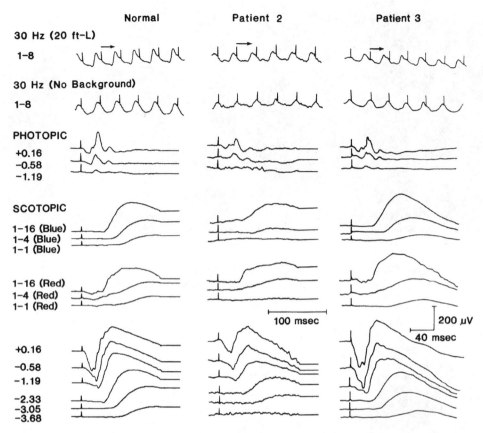

| Normal | Patient 2 | Patient 3 |

30 Hz (20 ft-L)

1–8

30 Hz (No Background)

1–8

PHOTOPIC

+0.16
−0.58
−1.19

SCOTOPIC

1–16 (Blue)
1–4 (Blue)
1–1 (Blue)

1–16 (Red)
1–4 (Red)
1–1 (Red)

100 msec

200 µV
40 msec

+0.16

−0.58

−1.19

−2.33
−3.05
−3.68

FIGURE 63.7 Ganzfeld ERGs of two patients with the regional form of Bietti's crystalline dystrophy (patients 2 and 3 in Wilson et al.[38]) as compared with a normal ERG on the left. ERGs from the right and left eyes were averaged to produce the tracings shown for the normal individual and patient 2. The stimulus spikes for the 30-Hz flicker and the photopic and scotopic responses for the normal ERG and patient 2 were set at 50, 50, and 75 µV and 75, 75, and 100 µV, respectively, to provide a vertical calibration scale. For these tracings, the 100-ms horizontal scale applies. For patient 3, the calibration scale is noted for 40 ms and 200 µV. The numbers to the left of the normal waveforms preceded by a plus or minus sign indicate the intensity of the white light stimulus in log foot-lambert-seconds. For the red and blue light responses, the numbers indicate the photostimulator intensity settings. (From Wilson DJ, Weleber RG, Klein ML, Welch RB, Green WR.[38] Used by permission.)

knowledge, no case has ever been reported to progress from purely regional disease with preservation of normal peripheral retina to diffuse disease of the entire fundus. This observation has led us to propose that two subtypes of the disease exist.

The corneal lesions, which have been reported in approximately one fourth of cases,[21] are very fine, whitish-yellow crystals that appear just inside the limbus in superficial stroma and often require high magnification for detection (figure 63.8). With time, the crystals become less apparent. Unlike those seen with nephropathic infantile cystinosis, the crystals are not visible within the more central cornea or the conjunctiva on biomicroscopy.

Reports of affected siblings, both males and females being affected, and the high frequency of consanguinity among otherwise normal parents,[2,9,10,14–16,33,39] strongly argue for autosomal-recessive inheritance. Two reports, however, suggest autosomal-dominant inheritance.[30,31]

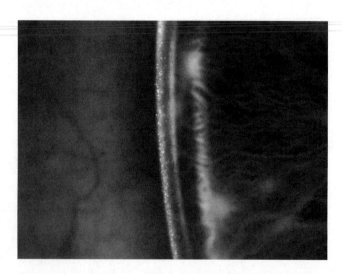

FIGURE 63.8 Corneal crystals in peripheral corneal stroma of the right eye of a 54-year-old man with regional retinal involvement (patient 2 in Wilson et al.[38]). (From Wilson DJ, Weleber RG, Klein ML, Welch RB, Green WR.[38] Used by permission.)

Known histopathology/pathophysiology of the disease

HISTOPATHOLOGY   On biopsy, crystals that have the appearance of cholesterol or cholesterol ester are present within corneal and conjunctival fibroblasts (figure 63.9).[38] Complex lipid inclusions are also present. Wilson et al.[38] have demonstrated inclusions in circulating lymphocytes similar to those seen in the cornea (figure 63.10), which suggests that this disorder may represent a systemic abnormality of lipid metabolism.

Kaiser-Kupfer et al.[21] reported studies on crystalline lysosomal material in lymphocytes and fibroblasts from three members of a Chinese family with BCD and the ocular pathology of eyes from the 88-year-old grandmother of the proband. Biochemistry failed to show that the deposits were cholesterol or cholesterol ester, and the true nature of the stored compounds remains uncertain.[21] The ocular pathology showed panretinal degeneration with complex lipid deposition within choroidal fibroblasts.[21]

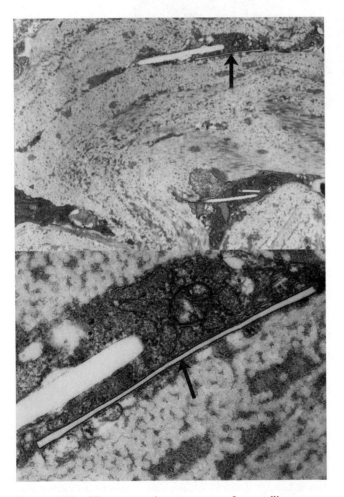

FIGURE 63.9   Ultrastructural appearance of crystalline spaces (arrows) seen on a corneal biopsy specimen from a patient previously reported by Welch[37] (Top, 13,000×; bottom, 64,000×). (From Wilson DJ, Weleber RG, Klein ML, Welch RB, Green WR.[38] Used by permission.)

PHYSIOLOGY   Although the finding of inclusions in circulating lymphocytes suggests a systemic defect of lipid metabolism, no consistent abnormalities have been found with routine laboratory evaluations, including plasma and urine levels of amino acids, plasma lipoproteins and steroid determination, serum protein electrophoresis and immunoelectrophoresis, and leukocyte cellular cystine assay. Mild elevations of serum cholesterol have been reported in some but not all patients, and the significance of such a finding in older patients is unclear.[2,14,34,38]

At present, nothing definitive is known about the pathophysiology of this disease. Lee et al.[25] have found a 32-kDa fatty acid–binding protein missing from lymphocytes in Bietti crystalline dystrophy. Biochemistry studies found that BCD is characterized by a lower than normal conversion of FA precursors into n-3 polyunsaturated fatty acids and suggest that BCD is the result of deficient lipid binding, elongation, or desaturation.[26] Linkage studies have found a localization to chromosome 4q35.[18] There is no consensus as to whether the diffuse and regional phenotypes are truly different genetic diseases or different stages of one disease. Although some suggest that the variable phenotypes of BCD reflect different stages of progression, we believe that locus or allelic heterogeneity or the effects of modifying genes could easily account for the variable phenotypes and natural history.*

Relevant testing and findings

Since the diagnosis is easily made by clinical examination, reports on affected individuals are often incomplete with regard to other studies. Few investigators have reported the results of extensive retinal function tests on patients with Bietti's dystrophy. Patients tend to fall into two groups: those with regional disease, in whom the retinal function tests appear as one would predict considering a localized process, and those with diffuse disease, in whom the retinal function tests indicate widespread abnormalities. The ERG reflects the degree of involvement of the fundus. The ERG is normal to moderately abnormal in the regional type[14,21,33,34,38,39] and severely subnormal to nonrecordable in the diffuse type.[2,38,39] Negative ERGs have been reported.[2,10] The a-wave analyses of three cases of BCD have shown

*The gene for Bietti's crystalline dystrophy has been found to be a novel gene, CYP4V2, the product of which has homology to other proteins of the CYP540 family, suggesting a role of the gene product in fatty acid and steroid metabolism. (Li A, Jiao X, Munier FL, Schorderet DF, Yao W, Iwata F, Hayakawa M, Kanai A, Chen MS, Lewis RA, Heckenlively J, Weleber RG, Traboulsi EI, Zhang Q, Xiao X, Kaiser-Kupfer M, Sergeev Y, Hejtmancik JF: Bietti crystalline corneoretinal dystrophy is caused by mutations in the novel gene CYP4V2. Am J Hum Genet 2004; 78:817–826.)

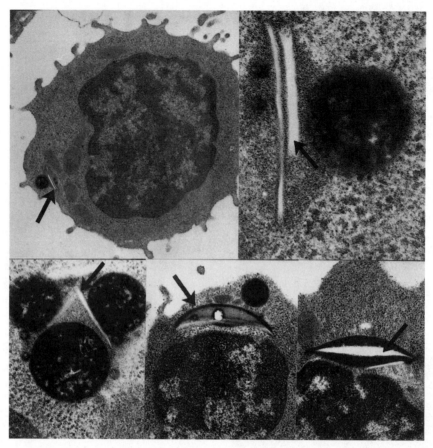

FIGURE 63.10   Ultrastructural appearance of crystals seen in circulating lymphocytes (top left, 13,000×; top right, 110,000×; bottom left, 44,000×; bottom center, 20,000×; bottom right, 22,000×). (From Wilson DJ, Weleber RG, Klein ML, Welch RB, Green WR.[38] Used by permission.).

variable findings with normal to decreased Rm_{p3} for rod and cone responses and reduced rod S (sensitivity). However, for all three subjects, the cone S was normal, suggesting that cones may be less involved than rods in this disease.[33] No eyes were found to have normal Rm_{p3} and decreased S in rods and cones, suggesting that in the early stage of the disease, photoreceptor loss and/or outer segment shortening may be present with normal phototransduction. Although two-color static perimetry has not yet been reported on these patients, the finding of diffuse and regional forms of Bietti's dystrophy is similar to the reported classification of autosomal-dominant retinitis pigmentosa (RP) into type I (diffuse) and type II (regional) disease.[24,27]

The electro-oculogram (EOG) appears abnormal in diffuse disease or advanced disease[38] but can be normal or only mildly abnormal in early disease of the regional type.[21,38] In one patient with late regional disease, the EOG was abnormal, and the fast oscillations of the EOG were found to be absent.[38] Dark adaptometry showed an elevation of both the cone and rod portions of the curve, with minimal if any discernible cone-rod break. Further dark adaptation occurred in one patient with moderately advanced diffuse disease after patching for 14 hours, but the retinal threshold was still elevated 1.3 log units above that normally seen after 30 minutes.[38]

Differential diagnosis

The differential diagnosis of Bietti's crystalline dystrophy includes retinal oxalosis secondary to prolonged anesthesia with methoxyflurane,[7] cystinosis,[11,32] canthaxanthine retinopathy,[6,8] talc emboli,[1,12] tamoxifen retinopathy,[22,23,29] and Sjögren-Larsson syndrome.[13,17] X-linked retinoschisis has also been reported with retinal crystals.[36] The diagnosis of Bietti's dystrophy is almost always made or suspected on clinical grounds. Perimetry is performed to assess the extent of visual field loss and to allow correlation of fundus appearance with visual field defects. The ERG appears to play a major role in defining diffuse from regional disease. EOG, dark adaptometry, and color vision tests are ancillary tests that help to establish the level and extent of retinal dysfunction and are useful in providing vocational and prognostic counseling and in following patients for rate of progression.

ACKNOWLEDGMENTS Supported by The Foundation Fighting Blindness and by Research to Prevent Blindness.

REFERENCES

1. Atlee WE Jr: Talc and cornstarch emboli in eyes of drug abusers. *JAMA* 1972; 219:49–51.

2. Bagolini B, Ioli-Spada G: Bietti's tapetoretinal degeneration with marginal corneal dystrophy. *Am J Ophthalmol* 1968; 65:53–60.

3. Bernauer W, Daicker B: Bietti's corneal-retinal dystrophy: A 16-year progression. *Retina* 1992; 12:18–20.

4. Bietti G: Su alcune forme atipiche o rare di degenerazione retinica (degenerazioni tappeto-retiniche e quadri morbosi similari). *Boll Oculist* 1937; 16:1159–1244.

5. Bietti GB: Ueber familiäres Vorkommen von retinitis punctata albescense (verbunden mit'dystrophia marginalis cristallinea cornea'): Glitzern des Glaskörpers und anderen degenerativen Augenveränderungen. *Klin Monatsbl Augenheilkd* 1937; 99:737–756.

6. Boudreault G, Cortin P, Corriveau LA, Rousseau AP, Tardif Y, Malenfant M: La rétinopathie à la canthaxanthine: 1. Étude clinique de 51 consommateurs. [Canthaxanthine retinopathy: 1. Clinical study in 51 consumers.] *Can J Ophthalmol* 1983; 18:325–328.

7. Bullock JD, Albert DM: Flecked retina: Appearance secondary to oxalate crystals from methoxyflurane anesthesia. *Arch Ophthalmol* 1975; 93:26–31.

8. Cortin P, Boudreault G, Rousseau AP, Tardif Y, Malenfant M: La rétinopathie à la canthaxanthine: 2. Facteurs prédisposants. [Retinopathy due to canthazanthine: 2. Predisposing factors.] *Can J Ophthalmol* 1984; 19:215–219.

9. François J: Discussion of Bietti's tapetoretinal degeneration with marginal corneal dystrophy: Crystalline retinopathy. *Trans Am Ophthalmol Soc* 1977; 75:179.

10. François J, De Laey JJ: Bietti's crystalline fundus dystrophy. *Ann Ophthalmol* 1978; 10:709–716.

11. François J, Hanssens M, Coppieters R, Evens L: Cystinosis: A clinical and histopathologic study. *Am J Ophthalmol* 1972; 73:643–650.

12. Friberg TR, Gragoudas ES, Regan CD: Talc emboli and macular ischemia in intravenous drug abuse. *Arch Ophthalmol* 1979; 97:1089–1091.

13. Gilbert WR Jr, Smith JL, Nyhan WL: The Sjogren-Larsson syndrome. *Arch Ophthalmol* 1968; 80:308–316.

14. Grizzard WS, Deutman AF, Nijhuis F, de Kerk AA: Crystalline retinopathy. *Am J Ophthalmol* 1978; 86:81–88.

15. Hayasaka S, Okuyama S: Crystalline retinopathy. *Retina* 1984; 4:177–181.

16. Hu D: Ophthalmic genetics in China. *Ophthalmic Pediatr Genet* 1983; 21:39–45.

17. Jagell S, Polland W, Sandgren O: Specific changes in the fundus typical for the Sjogren-Larsson syndrome: An ophthalmological study of 35 patients. *Acta Ophthalmol (Copenh)* 1980; 58:321–330.

18. Jiao X, Munier FL, Iwata F, et al: Genetic linkage of Bietti crystalline corneoretinal dystrophy to chromosome 4q35. *Am J Hum Genet* 2000; 67:1309–1313.

19. Jurklies B, Jurklies C, Schmidt U, Wessing A: Bietti's crystalline dystrophy of the retina and cornea. *Retina* 1999; 19:168–171.

20. Jurklies B, Jurklies C, Schmidt U, Wessing A, Bornfeld N: [Corneoretinal dystrophy (Bietti): Long-term course of one patient over a period of 30 years, and interindividual variability of clinical and electrophysiological findings in two patients.] *Klin Monatsbl Augenheilkd* 2001; 218:562–569.

21. Kaiser-Kupfer MI, Chan C-C, Markello TC, et al: Clinical, biochemical and pathologic correlations in Bietti's crystalline dystrophy. *Am J Ophthalmol* 1994; 118:569–582.

22. Kaiser-Kupfer MI, Kupfer C, Rodrigues MM: Tamoxifen retinopathy: A clinicopathologic report. *Ophthalmology* 1981; 88:89–93.

23. Kaiser-Kupfer MI, Lippman ME: Tamoxifen retinopathy. *Cancer Treat Rep* 1978; 62:315–320.

24. Kemp CM, Jacobson SG, Faulkner DJ: Two types of visual dysfunction in autosomal dominant retinitis pigmentosa. *Invest Ophthalmol Vis Sci* 1988; 29:1235–1241.

25. Lee J, Jiao X, Hejtmancik JF, Kaiser-Kupfer M, Chader GJ: Identification, isolation, and characterization of a 32-kDa fatty acid-binding protein missing from lymphocytes in humans with Bietti crystalline dystrophy (BCD). *Mol Genet Metab* 1998; 65:143–154.

26. Lee J, Jiao X, Hejtmancik JF, et al: The metabolism of fatty acids in human Bietti crystalline dystrophy. *Invest Ophthalmol Vis Sci* 2001; 42:1707–1714.

27. Massof RW, Finkelstein D: Two forms of autosomal dominant retinitis pigmentosa. *Doc Ophthalmol Proc Series* 1981; 51:289–346.

28. Mauldin WM, O'Connor PS: Crystalline retinopathy (Bietti's tapetoretinal degeneration without marginal corneal dystrophy). *Am J Ophthalmol* 1981; 92:640–646.

29. McKeown CA, Swartz M, Blom J, Maggiano JM: Tamoxifen retinopathy. *Br J Ophthalmol* 1981; 65:177–179.

30. Miyauchi O, Murayama K, Adachi-Usami E: A family with crystalline retinopathy demonstrating an autosomal dominant inheritance pattern. *Retina* 1999; 19:573–574.

31. Richards BW, Brodstein DE, Nussbaum JJ, Ferencz JR, Maeda K, Weiss L: Autosomal dominant crystalline dystrophy. *Ophthalmology* 1991; 98:658–665.

32. Sanderson PO, Kuwabara T, Stark WJ, Wong VG, Collins EM: Cystinosis: A clinical, histopathologic, and ultrastructural study. *Arch Ophthalmol* 1974; 91:270–274.

33. Usui T, Tanimoto N, Takagi M, Hasegawa S, Abe H: Rod and cone a-waves in three cases of Bietti crystalline chorioretinal dystrophy. *Am J Ophthalmol* 2001; 132:395–402.

34. Weber U, Adler K, Hennekes R: Kristalline Chorioretinopathie mit marginaler kornealer Beteiligung. [Crystalline chorioretinopathy with marginal corneal involvement.] *Klin Monatsbl Augenheilkd* 1984; 185:268–271.

35. Weber U, Owczarek J, Kluxen G, Bernsmeier H: [Clinical course in Bietti crystalline tapetoretinal degeneration.] *Klin Monatsbl Augenheilkd* 1983; 183:259–261.

36. Weinberg DV, Sieving PA, Bingham EL, Jampol LM, Mets MB: Bietti crystalline retinopathy and juvenile retinoschisis in a family with a novel RS1 mutation. *Arch Ophthalmol* 2001; 119:1719–1721.

37. Welch RB: Bietti's tapetoretinal degeneration with marginal corneal dystrophy crystalline retinopathy. *Trans Am Ophthalmol Soc* 1977; 75:164–179.

38. Wilson DJ, Weleber RG, Klein ML, Welch RB, Green WR: Bietti's crystalline dystrophy: A clinicopathologic correlative study. *Arch Ophthalmol* 1989; 107:213–221.

39. Yuzawa M, Mae Y, Matsui M: Bietti's crystalline retinopathy. *Ophthalmic Paediatr Genet* 1986; 7:9–20.

40. Yoshida A, Nara Y, Takahashi M: Crystalline retinopathy: Evaluation of blood-retinal barrier by vitreous fluorophotometry. *Jpn J Ophthalmol* 1985; 29:290–300.

64 Leber Congenital Amaurosis

ROBERT K. KOENEKOOP

LEBER CONGENITAL amaurosis (LCA, MIM 204000) represents a group of congenital retinal diseases that lead to blindness, with a worldwide prevalence of three in 100,000.[3] Although rare, it accounts for at least 5% of all inherited retinopathies and approximately 20% of children attending schools for the blind.[3] We estimate that 180,000 patients are affected worldwide.

In 1869, Leber defined LCA as a congenital form of retinitis pigmentosa, with severe visual loss at or near birth, wandering nystagmus, amaurotic pupils, a pigmentary retinopathy, and autosomal-recessive inheritance.[3,54] In 1956, Franceschetti and Dieterli reported a nondetectable electroretinogram (ERG) in the early course of LCA as essential in the diagnosis.[25] Dominant inheritance has also been reported, but this is thought to be rare.[26,46,74,81,82] LCA is genetically heterogeneous, and since 1996, eight genes[12,15,20,29,59,61,67,79,83] (six of which have been cloned) with disparate retinal functions have been implicated. Five of the LCA genes (tables 64.1, 64.2, and 64.3) are expressed in the photoreceptors, namely, retinal guanylate cyclase (*GUCY2D*), cone-rod homeobox (*CRX*), Aryl hydrocarbon receptor–interacting protein-like 1 (*AIPL-1*), retinitis pigmentosa (RP) GTPase interacting protein 1 (*RPGRIP-1*), and crumbs-like protein 1 (*CRB-1*), while one is predominantly expressed in the retinal pigment epithelium (RPE), the *RPE65* gene.

The study of LCA is proving central to our understanding of normal retinal development and physiology and also improves our understanding of other retinal degenerations. In the near future, LCA may be treatable by pharmacological intervention and/or gene replacement therapy, as both mouse[90] and dog[1] LCA models showed dramatic short-term improvements in rod and cone physiology and restoration of vision, by ERG, pupillometry, and behavioral testing.[1] These future therapies for human LCA will likely be gene-specific, giving major significance to gene identification and genotype-phenotype studies.

The clinical variability of LCA is striking. We find variability in visual acuities (20/200 to no light perception), visual evolution (stable, deteriorating, or rarely improving),[7,30,40,52,75] refractions (from high hyperopia to high myopia), retinal appearance (from near normal to severe pigmentary retinopathy), associated ocular features (keratoconus, cataracts), associated systemic features, and retinal histopathology (from essentially normal[43] to extensive degeneration.[5,23,51,55,66,74,92,95] Some patients have an essen-

tially normal retinal aspect; others may have yellow flecks, salt-and-pepper changes, a marbled pattern, atrophic changes, nummular pigment clumps, a "macular coloboma," white dots, or preserved para-arteriolar RPE. Keratoconus and cataracts may develop in the course of the disease in some patients. LCA may rarely be associated with systemic disease, and this adds additional variability to the disease spectrum. Mental retardation, deafness, polycystic kidney disease (also known as Senior Loken disease), skeletal anomalies (also known as Saldino Mainzer disease), or osteopetrosis may be found in addition to the ocular disease.

In approximately 40% of LCA cases it is now possible to identify the causative mutations in one of the seven LCA genes. Several strategies are now available to provide a molecular diagnosis for a child affected with LCA. The most rapid and comprehensive is the new LCA genotyping array (LCA disease chip), which includes all 300 currently documented LCA mutations. In a period of four hours per sample it is possible to determine the genotype in ~35% of the new cases.[97] Conventional SSCP, dHPLC combined with automated sequencing also allows identification of mutations but is much more cumbersome. Genotyping LCA patients is extremely helpful for providing 1) a more accurate clinical diagnosis, 2) a more accurate visual prognosis, 3) a molecular classification of disease, 4) a prenatal diagnosis in selected cases, and 5) a way of separating LCA patients who may be treatable in the near future and those that may be treatable later.

The clinical understanding of the diagnostic findings in LCA has been evolving as more patients have molecular diagnoses and it becomes possible to go back and correlate test and phenotype to a confirmed known type of early onset retinal degeneration. Because LCA represents a group of diseases with at least seven and potentially as many as 20 genes, it can be expected that there will be variation in severity at onset and in the severity of the disability. For many years, with the lack of availability of the electroretinogram (ERG) and a reluctance to test infants and young children, many patients did not have an ERG until they were older. By then the patients were frequently blind and had a nondetectable ERG signal. Foxman et al.[24] suggested ERG testing in blind infants before the age of 1 year to separate LCA from early onset RP. ERG testing is also crucial to differentiate albinism, complete and incomplete achromatopsia, and complete and incomplete congenital stationary night blindness from LCA.[50] Infants can now easily have

TABLE 64.1

LCA genes to date, protein and chromosomal locations

LCA Gene	Discovered	LCA Protein	Chromosome
GUCY2D	1996	Retinal guanylate cyclase	17p13.3
RPE65	1997	Retinal pigment epithelial protein 65	1p31
CRX	1998	Cone-rod homeobox	19q13
AIPL-1	2000	Aryl hydrocarbon receptor–interacting protein-like 1	17p13.1
CRB-1	2001	Crumbs homolog 1	1q31
RPGRIP-1	2001	Retinitis pigmentosa GTPase regulator interacting protein 1	14q11

TABLE 64.2

LCA genes, their retinal expression, and functional pathways

LCA Gene	Retinal Location	Functional Pathway
GUCY2D	Photoreceptor	Phototransduction cascade
RPE65	RPE	Retinoid cycle
CRX	Photoreceptor	Photoreceptor development/expression phototransduction proteins
AIPL-1	Photoreceptor	Biosynthesis of phosphodiesterase
CRB-1	Photoreceptor	Apical-basal polarity determination of the PR
RPGRIP-1	Photoreceptor	Structural component of ciliary axoneme in connecting cilium

TABLE 64.3

LCA genes, a proposal of their detailed defects, and proposed type of defect

LCA Gene	Detail of the Proposed Defect	Proposed Type of Defect
GUCY2D	Inability to replenish cGMP and restore the phototransduction cascade	Metabolic/biochemical
RPE65	Inability to resynthesize 11-*cis*-retinal and rhodopsin	Metabolic/biochemical
CRX	Inability to form PR outer segments, and express key phototransduction proteins	Structural
AIPL-1	Unable to synthesize PDE	Metabolic/biochemical
CRB-1	Unable to form zonula adherence during PR morphogenesis	Structural
RPGRIP-1	Unable to form ciliary axoneme and connecting cilium	Structural

standardized ERGs in a visual physiology laboratory, a site which is accustomed to managing infants.

Because the infant ERG is not equivalent to that of older children, caution is needed in interpreting these infantile ERGs. Fulton et al. have published standardized first-year values to assist in the interpretation of waveforms from this age group.[30] If it is necessary to perform ERG testing under anesthesia, then great care must be given to interpreting the resulting waveforms. Operating room conditions are seldom standardized, and more importantly some anesthetics may suppress or alter ERG waveforms. We recommend that a child suspected of having LCA or any other retinal dystrophy have an ERG at around age 6 months and then a repeat ERG at 1 year.

Repeat ERGs are important because infantile testing is so difficult—children frequently cry and the electrodes fall out, or the tears may interfere with the signals and the ERG signals still mature in the first year of life.[30] It is possible to have a small ERG signal early in the LCA disease process, and this certainly does not preclude the diagnosis of LCA. Also, a small number of children with early visual impairment have developmental delay and with repeat testing may have more robust or normal ERG signals on repeat testing.

The aim of this chapter is to discuss in detail, the seven types of LCA associated with the seven currently known LCA genes. Furthermore, we will summarize the management of the blind infant.

LCA caused by RPE65 defects

LCA caused by mutations in the *RPE65* gene result in a block in the retinoid cycle and an inability to restore levels of 11-*cis*-retinal (table 64.3). *RPE65* is abundantly expressed in the retinal pigment epithelium (RPE),[37] which plays an important role in the vitamin A cycle. Recently, *RPE65* expression has been documented in mammalian cone but not rod photoreceptors.[99] The *RPE65* gene is located on chromosome 1p22 and was cloned by Hamel et al. in 1993.[36] It is highly conserved in all vertebrates. The genomic structure of *RPE65* was elucidated by Nicoletti et al.[65] and is composed of 14 exons; the protein consists of 533 amino acids. *RPE65* mutations have been found both in juvenile RP patients[35] and in LCA patients.[61] In some populations, *RPE65* mutations can account for up to 16% of LCA.[64] Other large-scale studies found the relative burden of *RPE65* in LCA to be 3%,[16] 6%,[60] and 11.4%.[86] The new

LCA disease microarray revealed that 2.4% of LCA patients had *RPE65* mutations (N = 205).[97]

The phenotype of LCA patients resulting from *RPE65* defect appears to be distinct, as LCA patients with the *RPE65* genotype appear to have measurable visual function, unlike LCA patients with *GUCY2D* mutations.[70] In a longitudinal study of four LCA patients with *RPE65* mutations, Lorenz et al.[58] found that a typical LCA child with *RPE65* mutations would present at 3 or 4 months old with suspected blindness. In bright light, a visual reaction was noted, there was nystagmus, and the pupillary light response was dimished. On retinoscopy, mild hyperopia (+4.00 D) was found, while on fundoscopy at age 3–4 months, mild retinal changes were seen, with increased granularity of the RPE and retinal arteriolar thinning. At age 1 year, measurable visual acuities were present when measured by Teller Acuity Cards, and the ERG showed a measurable cone response and a nondetectable rod response. At age 3 years, the acuity was found to be 20/200. At age 5 years, both cone and rod ERG responses were nondetectable, and the retina revealed optic disk pallor, a bull's-eye maculopathy, thinned retinal arterioles, and RPE granularity. Acuities remained at 20/200, and the Goldmann visual fields were recordable and showed a well-preserved response.

In summary, the clinical phenotype of LCA patients with *RPE65* mutations may consist of severe visual impairment in infancy, with gradual visual improvement in the first few years of life, unlike the visual performance that is usually seen in LCA. Gradually, visual function may then decline and is associated with nondetectable ERG responses, and retinal findings indicating a diffuse retinal degeneration. This suggests that *RPE65* type LCA represents a rod-cone dystrophy. We also found that *RPE65* type LCA patients have measurable visual acuities (20/200), Goldmann visual fields, and small ERG amplitudes followed by slow deterioration of their visual function when measured over 20 years.[15]

In an important study by Porto et al.,[72] the retinal phenotype of a fetus with LCA and mutations in the *RPE65* gene was assessed by histopathological and immunocytochemical analysis. They obtained retinal tissue from a voluntarily aborted 33-week-old fetus with a homozygous C330Y *RPE65* mutation and studied the histopathological changes compared to an age-matched fetus. They found 55% fewer cell nuclei in the outer nuclear layer (ONL) in the central retina, while the midperiphery and far periphery counts were similar to those of the control. The cell counts of the inner nuclear layer (INL) (i.e., bipolar, horizontal, and amacrine cells) were also less in the *RPE65* fetus, while the ganglion cell layer (GCL) was normal. Specific immunolabeling revealed both rod and cone photoreceptor outer segment abnormalities. No apoptosis or gliosis was detected, and there was no neurite sprouting or Muller cell activation,

as is seen in some RP retinal specimens. The RPE showed abnormal inclusions, while the Bruch's membrane was thickened, and the choriocapillaris was engorged.

These are the first histopathological retinal changes documented in a human LCA baby with a known gene defect, in this case *RPE65*, and therefore are very important. The results are also unexpected, as the animal models and their responses to treatments indicate essentially normal retinal architecture and viable photoreceptors. Not all human LCA retinas with *RPE65* mutations are necessarily abnormal, however; in Van Hooser et al.,[90] a relatively normal retinal architecture was noted by optical coherence tomography in vivo in an LCA patient with *RPE65* defects. Also, the question remains whether the changes found in the Porto et al.[72] study represent retinal degeneration or a failure to develop normal retinal cell numbers. Finally, it remains to be determined whether abnormal retinal histology can still support gene therapy.

The clinical phenotype and ERG phenotype of carriers (parents with LCA offsprings) of heterozygous mutations of LCA genes may have distinct features, which may give insight into the pathophysiology of the causative gene and point to the defective gene in the offspring.[47] The phenotype of carrier parents who harbor heterozygous *RPE65* mutations has not yet been extensively studied but is predicted to reveal a rod-cone-type dysfunction. Felius et al.[22] found extensive dark-adapted visual field defects (1–2 log units above normal) and delayed 30-Hz flicker ERG in one carrier parent of a *RPE65* mutation (but not in the other) of a child with juvenile RP.

In the *RPE65* mouse model of LCA[66] (knock-out of the *RPE65* gene, *RPE65*[−/−]), rods and cones are present at birth and appear normal with intact outer segments until 15 weeks, when the outer nuclear layer declines from 10–11 layers to 8–9 layers and then down to 7 layers at 28 weeks. The rod ERG is absent from the beginning, but the cone ERG is intact. Furthermore, although opsin levels are normal, the rhodopsin molecule is absent. In conclusion, the RPE[−/−] mouse model likely represents a rod-cone degeneration and therefore provides a model of human LCA.

The *RPE65* dog model[4] of LCA is found in the Swedish Briard dog and represents a natural knock-out of the *RPE65* gene.[91] A 4-bp deletion is present in the *RPE65* gene in homozygous state in exon 5 and results in a frameshift and a premature stop codon, with two thirds of the polypeptide missing, making this likely a null allele.[91] The dogs develop an autosomal-recessive early-onset, slowly progressive retinal dystrophy. Histopathology of the dog shows a relatively well-preserved retina, with relative minor photoreceptor changes but with prominent inclusions in the RPE layer and slowly progressive degeneration.[3] The rod and cone ERG are essentially nondetectable.

Therapeutic studies

Acland et al.[1] studied the effects of *RPE65* gene replacement in the Briard dog. Subretinal injections in one eye of three dogs containing the AAV virus with cDNA of dog *RPE65*, with a CMV promotor, B-actin enhancer, and internal ribosome entry sequence were performed at age 4 months. Rod-mediated and cone-mediated ERGs, visual evoked potential, pupillometry, and behavioral testing all showed dramatic improvements in visual function at about 8 months of age. In eyes that were treated with subretinal AAV-RPE65, a rod and cone ERG response was found that represents approximately 16% of normal, which was significantly different from untreated or intravitreally injected eyes. These results were obtained in three eyes, which were injected subretinally in only one of the four retinal quadrants. Genomic PCR and RT PCR demonstrated expression of the wild-type message in the retina and RPE, while immunoblots showed persistant RPE65 protein in RPE cells. This is the first study to demonstrate restoration of visual function in a large-eyed animal model with LCA due to an *RPE* gene defect. It is currently not known whether the retinas of human LCA patients with *RPE65* defects are intact and whether the photoreceptor layer is present. The time window before the retina undergoes cell death is also not known. Also, whether LCA photoreceptor gene replacements have similar dramatic effects will now have to be evaluated. A human clinical trial involving well-characterized LCA gene defects in babies with LCA is likely not far off.

Van Hooser et al.,[90] using recent knowledge that *RPE65* mutations in mice lead to an inability to form 11-*cis*-retinal (which binds to rod opsin to form the light-sensitive photopigment rhodopsin), supplemented the mouse diet with the oral vitamin A derivative 9-*cis*-retinal, and consequently showed short-term improvements in rod photopigment production and rod physiology. The long-term consequences of this intervention are not yet known.

LCA caused by GUCY2D defects

LCA caused by mutations in the retinal guanylate cyclase gene, *GUCY2D*, is the result of a block in the recovery of the phototransduction cascade (table 64.3). The phototransduction gene retinal guanylate cyclase, *GUCY2D*, was cloned by Shyjan et al. in 1992 and mapped to 17p13.1.[77] Camuzat et al.[8] mapped a LCA gene by homozygosity mapping to the same 17p13.1 interval. In 1996, Perrault et al.[67] reported mutations in *GUCY2D* in four unrelated LCA probands. The human gene contains 20 exons (figure 64.1) and has thus far been implicated in autosomal-recessive (AR) LCA[67] and autosomal-dominant (AD) cone-rod dystrophy[45,69] (also known as CORD6). *GUCY2D* is expressed in the photoreceptor outer segments but at higher levels in cones than in rods.[18,56]

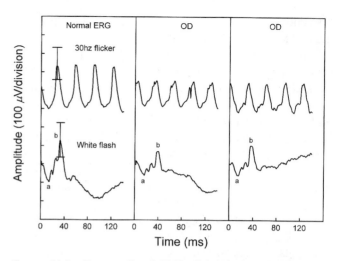

FIGURE 64.1   Cone-mediated 30-Hz flicker (top) and white-flash ERG (bottom) of the right eye (OD) of a normal 45-year-old; the father (middle); and mother (right) of a LCA patient with compound heterozygous *GUCY2D* mutations. The father carries a 1-bp deletion (bp 2843 del G) in exon 15 of *GUCY2D*, and the mother carries a L954P mutation in *GUCY2D*, also in exon 15. Both the 30-Hz flicker and white-flash cone mediated amplitudes are clearly decreased in comparison to normal.

Functional studies have revealed that mutations in the kinase homology domain of the retinal guanylate cyclase severely compromise the ability to produce cGMP.[21] We found LCA mutations in the extracellular, kinase homology, and catalytic domains and performed expression experiments to compare their impact on enzyme activity. We found that LCA mutations from the extracellular domain (C105Y and L325P) cause a mild decrease in the catalytic ability of the enzyme,[48] while catalytic domain mutations (L954P and P858S) severely compromise the ability of GCAP to stimulate cGMP production and cause dominant negative effects on the wild-type allele.[49] As we added more of the mutant allele, we noted a progressive decrease in the ability of the enzyme to produce cGMP.[49] Dominant negative effects are seen with dominant mutations, we were therefore surprised to find dominant negative behavior with autosomal-recessive mutations.[88] Classical teaching about recessive mutations dictates that in the heterozygous state, the wild-type allele provides enough protein product to have a normal phenotype. Membrane guanylyl cyclases are thought to exist in a dimeric state,[10,87] and our results showing a significant decrease in wild-type RetGCf-1 activity when L954P or P858S are coexpressed with wild-type suggest that any heterodimers that are formed are inactive or poorly active.[88]

These in vitro findings prompted us to test the hypothesis of in vivo dominant negative effects, by ERG of parents of LCA children with *GUCY2D* mutations.[47] We found normal rod ERGs (see figure 64.1) but significant (see figure 64.1) and repeatable cone ERG abnormalities in parents of LCA patients.[47] Our findings are most consistent with a mild cone dysfunction in the carrier state, and this correlates well with the expression profile of *GUCY2D*, which is much higher in cones than in rods,[18,56] and with the *GUCY2D* knock-out mouse, which develops a cone dystrophy.[96] We then studied a second LCA family with a *GUCY2D* mutation, and we found very similar results[47] (not shown). These findings have prompted us to make the following two hypotheses:

1. Heterozygous parents of LCA patients have an ERG phenotype and that this ERG phenotype is LCA gene-specific, and these changes may point to the causal gene or pathway. A simple ERG of the parents at the time of the initial visit of the LCA child may therefore direct the subsequent genotyping strategy.

2. Because the ERG of the LCA child is nondetectable by definition, it has no information content in terms of pathophysiology. We propose that the ERG phenotypes of carriers of LCA genes give insights into the pathophysiology of LCA itself.

In some populations, *GUCY2D* may be the most commonly mutated LCA gene, with 20% of LCA patients carrying *GUCY2D* mutations.[68] Other studies found the relative burden to be 6%.[16,60] The phenotype of *GUCY2D* type LCA patients may be distinct, as most authors have noted a severe phenotype (with vision in the light perception or count finger range) with high hyperopia and photoaversion,[70] while others found a severe but stable phenotype over a period of 20 years, with an essentially normal retinal appearance.[16]

In the *GUCY2D* mouse model of LCA[96] (knock-out of the *GUCY2D* gene, *GUCY2D*[-/-]), rods and cones are present at birth with normal OS. By 5 weeks, there is a dramatic decrease in the number of cones only. By age 1 month, the cone ERG was not detectable, and despite their normal number and morphology, the rod ERG was markedly decreased. This model represents a severe cone-rod degeneration with much more cone than rod disease and therefore again only partially mimics human LCA.

In the *GUCY2D* chicken model of LCA[76] (naturally occurring deletions in both copies of the *GUCY2D* gene, *GUCY2D*[-/-]), a different pathological response occurs. At hatching, photoreceptors are normal in number and morphology, but on day 7, their numbers start to decline from the center to the periphery, and by 6–8 months, the entire photoreceptor layer is gone. The RPE layer then undergoes atrophy.[76] While the number of photoreceptors is still normal, it is of interest that the ERG is nondetectable. Semple-Rowland et al.[76] propose the following set of events to explain the LCA type disease in this rd chicken: A deletion and insertion of the *GUCY2D* gene representing a null allele results in an absent cGMP and permanent closure of the cGMP-gated cation channels. This would lead to chronic hyperpolarization of the cells, as in constant light exposure.

Glutamate levels would be chronically elevated, and phototransduction would not be able to take place, which explains the nondetectable ERG. Evidently, these circumstances do not impair normal rod and cone development but do cause a rapid cone rod degeneration. This excellent model of human LCA may represent an *early biochemical dysfunction with a superimposed cone rod degeneration.*

LCA caused by CRX defects

LCA caused by mutations in the *CRX* gene result in a block in photoreceptor outer segment development and inability to express several key retinal genes (table 64.3). The cone-rod homeobox gene *CRX* was cloned by Freund et al. by screening a human retinal cDNA library with a fragment of a homologous gene.[27] *CRX* resides on chromosome 19q13.3, has three exons, and encodes a protein with 299 amino acids. *CRX* is highly conserved in the animal kingdom, is specifically expressed in developing photoreceptors and the pineal gland, and plays an important role in regulating important photoreceptor genes, including rhodopsin, and is necessary for the formation of rod and cone outer segments.[31,32] *CRX* is implicated in a variety of severe retinal diseases, including autosomal-dominant LCA,[29] autosomal-recessive LCA,[85] autosomal-dominant cone rod dystrophy (CORD2),[28] and autosomal-dominant RP.[81] *CRX* mutations are probably a rare cause of LCA. We estimate that *CRX* mutations are responsible for approximately 2–3% of LCA,[16] which is in agreement with others.[60] Three regions of the predicted CRX protein are highly conserved and include the homeobox, the WSP domain, and the OTX tail domain. According to Rivolta et al.,[74] *CRX* mutations fall into two groups. Group 1 are missense mutations and one short in-frame deletion that preferentially affect the homeobox domain. In the second group are nine frameshift mutations, which are all found in the terminal exon 3. Most frameshift mutations are assumed to create null alleles because they lead to premature termination of translation. This is not the case for the exon 3 *CRX* mutations, according to Rivolta et al.,[74] because of new emerging information about mRNA decay mechanisms that lead to rapid mRNA degradation and no translated protein when the mutations occur upstream of an intron. As the *CRX* frameshift mutations occur in a terminal exon, they escape detection, and the mRNA molecule is predicted to be stable and translated. Therefore, *CRX* mutations are dominant, fully penetrant, and likely act through a dominant negative mechanism to cause the disease phenotype.[74]

Most authors report a severe phenotype for patients with mutations in *CRX*,[16,79] while we have reported one LCA patient with a heterozygous *CRX* mutation (A177 1 bp del) and a marked improvement in acuity, visual field, and cone ERG when measured over a period of 11 years.[46] We found a dramatic improvement in Snellen visual acuity from

20/900 at age 6 to 20/150 at age 11, with a rapid change at age 10, at the same time that we found measurable cone ERG activity and visual fields. Furukawa et al.[32] found that both rod and cone photoreceptor outer segments were not developed in the *CRX* knock-out mouse ($CRX^{-/-}$) and also found that in the heterozygous knock-out mouse ($CRX^{+/-}$), the cone photoreceptor outer segments were initially shorter than the wild-type mouse. They noted the absence of a cone ERG in their heterozygous ($CRX^{+/-}$) four-week old mice, a time when the wild-type cone ERG is already present. At two months, the cone ERG of the heterozygotes ($CRX^{+/-}$) increased but was still slightly decreased in comparison to wild-type. After a delay of six months, the heterozygous mice ($CRX^{+/-}$) developed normal cone ERGs and normal-length cone outer segments. The delay in cone ERG and cone photoreceptor outer segment formation in the heterozygous knock-out mouse ($CRX^{+/-}$) is initially similar to the delay in the cone ERG development of our LCA patient with the A177 1bp del *CRX* mutation and may correspond to delayed expression of cone opsin genes and/or cone outer segment formation in our patient.

We have not yet examined the ERGs of a carrier parent with a *CRX* mutation, but Swaroop et al.[85] found mild rod and cone ERG abnormalities in both parents of a LCA child with a homozygous *CRX* mutation.

LCA caused by AIPL-1 defects

LCA caused by *AIPL-1* mutations potentially result in a defect in the biosynthesis of the phototransduction enzyme phosphodiesterase (table 64.3). The gene for aryl hydrocarbon receptor–interacting protein like-1, *AIPL-1*, was discovered and cloned by Sohocki et al. in 1999,[79] by screening a human cDNA library containing retinal and pineal gland sequences. It is located on chromosome 17p13.1 and contains eight exons. It is expressed in the retina and pineal gland, but its exact function is not yet known. *AIPL-1* interacts with NUB-1, which is thought to control cell cycle progression.[2] Immunocytochemistry studies with an *AIPL-1* antibody revealed that *AIPL-1* is exclusively expressed in rod and not cone photoreceptors.[89]

The original pedigree for linkage analysis was of Pakistani origin, and many LCA patients developed keratoconus. We also found *AIPL-1* mutations in four Pakistani pedigrees with LCA from remote mountain villages who exhibited a severe phenotype, with count finger to light perception vision, severe retinal degeneration, a maculopathy, and keratoconus.[11] We estimate that mutations in *AIPL-1* are found in up to 7% of patients with LCA.[80]

ERGs of carrier parents of *AIPL-1* mutations may provide insight into the pathophysiology of LCA caused by *AIPL-1*. We found significant rod isolated ERG abnormalities and normal cone mediated ERGs in an *AIPL-1* carrier parents

with a single copy of W88X (figure 64.2), suggesting that *AIPL-1* type LCA represents a rod-cone disease (Dharmaraj et al., 2003, personal communication).

LCA caused by CRB-1 defects

LCA caused by mutations in the crumbs gene, *CRB-1* result in a defect in the molecular scaffold that controls zonula adherens assembly and in elongation of the photoreceptor outer segment (table 64.3). The crumbs homolog 1 gene, *CRB1*, was cloned by den Hollander et al.,[13,14] and mutations were found in 10 of 15 patients with RP12,[13] a specific form of ARRP with preservation of the para-arteriolar RPE (PPRPE type of RP). The gene resides on 1q31, has 12 exons, and encodes a protein of 1376 amino acids. The CRB1 protein shows conspicuous structural similarity to drosophila crumbs, a protein essential in establishing and maintaining epithelial cell polarity of ectodermally derived cells. Because of the severity of the PPRPE type RP, *CRB1* was postulated also to cause LCA. Den Hollander et al.[12] and Lotery et al.[59] recently found that 13% of cases with LCA can be explained by mutations in the *CRB1* gene, making it a common and important gene for LCA. In addition, *CRB1* mutations were identified in five of nine patients with RP and Coats'-like exudative vasculopathy, a severe complication of RP.[12] LCA patients with *CRB1* mutations in three of seven cases also show the PPRPE picture. Although the number of patients with LCA and *CRB1* mutations is still relatively small, it is noted that three of seven LCA patients and at most one of 15 patients with RP12 or ARRP carry two CRB1 protein truncating mutations, suggesting that combinations of severe *CRB1* mutations cause LCA and that combinations of severe and moderately severe mutations cause RP12 or ARRP. Further details of the *CRB1* phenotype of LCA and the carrier phenotype are still lacking.

LCA caused by RPGRIP-1 defects

LCA caused by mutations in the gene *RPGRIP-1*, result in defects in the connecting cilium, which connects the inner and outer segment of photoreceptors (table 64.3) and disk morphogenesis.[98] The *RPGRIP-1* defects may result in problems with vesicular trafficking of proteins. The *RPGRIP-1* gene, encoding the retinitis pigmentosa GTPase regulator interacting protein-1, was discovered by Boyle and Wright[6] by performing protein-protein interaction studies using RPGR as bait in yeast-two hybrid screening of retinal cDNA libraries. Mutations in the *RPGR* gene are the major cause of X-linked RP3. *RPGRIP1* resides on 14q11 and has 25 exons. It is expressed in rods and cones and localizes to the connecting cilium, which connects the inner to the outer segment.[42] The RPGRIP1 protein may be a structural component of the ciliary axoneme.[42] Dryja et al.[20] found that 6%

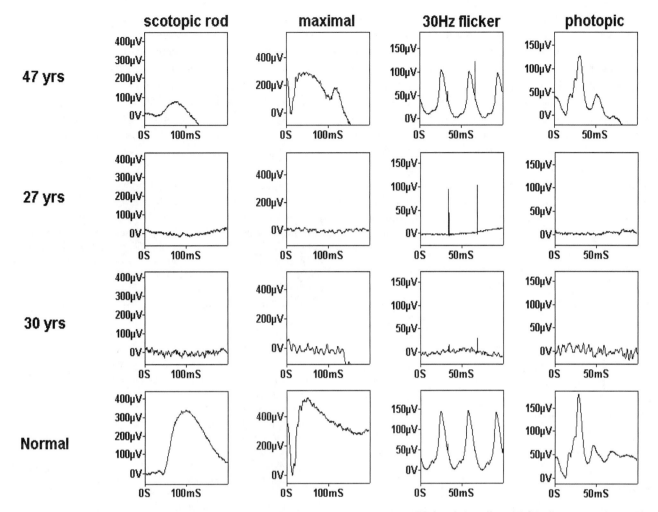

FIGURE 64.2 Scotopic rod-mediated ERGs, maximal ERGs, 30-Hz flicker, and photopic ERGs of normal (bottom), two LCA sibs (middle, ages 30 and 27 years), and carrier mother of the sibs (top, age 47 years). The sibs are both homozygous for the W88X mutation in *AIPL-1*, while the mother is a heterozygous carrier of this mutation. The ERGs of the affected LCA sibs are nondetectable, consistent with LCA. The mother's ERG clearly shows an abnormality in the rod-mediated signals, where the rod amplitudes are markedly decreased compared to normal. Cone-mediated signals appear normal.

of LCA harbor mutations in this gene. The LCA phenotype has not yet been delineated; nor has the carrier phenotype.

LCA caused by RDH12 defects

The relatively new LCA gene *RDH12* maps to 14q23.3 consists of 7 exons and encodes a retinol dehydrogenase expressed in photoreceptors, which participates in the vitamin A cycle, as does *RPE65*.[44] The retinol dehydrogenase encoded by *RDH12* is involved in the conversion of all *trans* retinal to all *trans* retinol. The exact biochemical consequences of *RDH12* defects are not yet known. Clinically, the LCA and/or juvenile RP patients harboring *RDH12* mutations thus far were found to have a severe and progressive rod-cone dystrophy with severe macular atrophy but no or mild hyperopia.[44,71]

Management of the blind infant

The role of the primary ophthalmologist making the initial diagnosis of LCA is difficult, complex, and consists of at least six aspects.

First and foremost it is essential that the *proper diagnosis* is made, and both overlapping ocular and systemic diseases must be ruled out. The main ocular diseases are albinism, achromatopsia, congenital stationary night blindness, optic nerve hypoplasia, delayed visual maturation, and cortical visual impairment. The main systemic diseases are all peroxisomal disorders, neuronal lipoid fuscinosis, abetalipoproteinemia, Bardet-Biedl syndrome, Alstrom syndrome, Senior Loken syndrome, Joubert syndrome, and Saldino-Mainzer syndrome.[50]

Second, the recessive *inheritance* must be communicated and counseled. If not possible, a genetic counselor must be consulted. Third, the *visual prognosis* must be given. Most patients with LCA will have significant lifelong visual handicaps and need extra help at home, school, and work. Most LCA patients have stable visual function, while a subgroup may decline, and rare improvements have been documented. Fourth, a *molecular diagnosis* is now a must as it is relatively easy to do and provides essential information to the family (carrier status, prenatal screening), the eye-care giver, and the scientist (prognosis, definitive diagnosis, treatment trials). Fifth, it is essential to provide the family with *information* such as family support groups, websites, and other information (www.FFB.ca; www.FFB.org; www.cafamily.org.uk; American Council of the Blind www.acb.org). Finally, it is imperative that the family is put in touch with a local *blindness institute* for social, psychological, and low-vision support. A good example is the Los Angeles Blind Children's Center (see Toni Marcy in Heckenlively 1988[39]). Many issues relating to a mother's and father's feelings of guilt and the affected child's issues of self-stimulation (mannerisms of "blindisms") if he or she is not stimulated to explore the outside world are addressed at this type of institution. Their program consists of six goals, including 1) acceptance of the blindness, 2) promotion of parent-child attachment, 3) furthering gross motor development (motility training), 4) stimulating object handling, 5) stimulating language development, and 6) prevention of deviant behavior (autism and self-stimulatory behavior).

Summary

In summary, there are currently seven genes responsible for LCA, and mutations in these genes can explain approximately 40% of the cases. Genotype-phenotype correlations of both the LCA and the carrier phenotype suggest that although highly variable, there are clinical features that are specific for the gene defect. These studies are still in progress, but initial results show that *GUCY2D* defects can lead to a severe cone-rod type LCA, with poor but stable visual function, an essentially normal retinal appearance, and a cone dysfunction in the obligate carriers. *RPE65* defects lead to a different phenotype, with an initially milder form of LCA than *GUCY2D*, with signs of retinal degeneration and slowly progressive visual loss later in life. *AIPL-1* defects lead to a very severe form of LCA, often with cataracts, keratoconus and a maculopathy, while some carriers have a striking rod dysfunction on ERG. *CRX* defects lead to a variable LCA phenotype, with most LCA patients showing a severe retinal degeneration and visual loss, but may rarely be associated with an improving phenotype. The carrier signs seem to be a rod and cone dysfunction on ERG. *CRB-1* defects can lead to a unique LCA phenotype, with preservation of the para-arteriolar RPE. The complete phenotype and the carrier phenotype of *CRB-1* are still unknown. The *RPGRIP-1*

phenotype has not yet been fully delineated but appears to consist of a severe pigmentary retinopathy. Similarly, the *RDH12* phenotype has not been fully delineated but appears to consist of a severe rod-cone degeneration with a prominent maculopathy.

At least seven retinal and/or RPE genes are responsible for LCA, but five of the seven genes (*GUCY2D, RPE65, CRX, AIPL-1,* and *CRB-1*) are also associated with adult or later onset retinal diseases such as cone-rod or rod-cone degenerations. Future therapies for LCA may be gene specific, making genotype-phenotype correlations very useful in reclassifying LCA at the molecular level.

ACKNOWLEDGMENTS Support for the author's LCA studies comes from both the Foundation Fighting Blindness Canada and the FRSQ. The author is much indebted to colleagues Drs. Rando Allikmets, Frans Cremers, Gerry Fishman, Pierre Lachapelle, Irma Lopez, Irene Maumenee, and Melanie Sohocki for their thoughtful discussions.

REFERENCES

1. Acland GM, Aguire GD, Ray J, Zang Q, et al: Gene therapy restores vision in a canine model of childhood blindness. *Nat Genet* 2001; 28:92–95.
2. Akey DT, Zhu X, Dyer M, Li A, Sorensen A, Blackshaw S, et al: The inherited blindness associated protein AIPL1 interacts with the cell cycle regulator protein NUB1. *Hum Mol Genet* 2002; 11(22):2723–2733.
3. Alstrom CH, Olson O: Heredo-retinopathia congenitalis monohybrida recessiva autosomalis. *Hereditas* 1957; 43:1–178.
4. Aquire G, Balswin V, Pearce-Kelling S, Narfstrom K, Ray K, Acland GM: Congenital stationary nightblindness in the dog: Common mutation in the *RPE65* gene indicates founder effect. *Mol Vis* 1998; 4:23.
5. Aubineau M: Retinite pigmentaire congenitale familiale: Examen anatomique. *Ann Oculistique* 1903; 129:432–439.
6. Boylan JP, Wright AF: Identification of a novel protein interacting with *RPGR. Hum Mol Genet* 2000; 9:2085–2093.
7. Brecelj J, Stirn-Kranjc B: ERG and VEP follow up study in children with Leber congenital amaurosis. *Eye* 1999; 13:47–54.
8. Camuzat A, Dollfus H, Rozet JM, et al: A gene for Leber's congenital amaurosis maps to chromosome 17p. *Hum Mol Genet* 1995; 4:1447–1452.
9. Camuzat A, Rozet JM, Dollfus H, et al: Evidence of genetic heterogeneity of Leber's congenital amaurosis (LCA) and mapping of LCA1 to chromosome 17p13. *Hum Genet* 1996; 97:798–801.
10. Chinkers M, Wilson EM: Ligand-independent oligomerization of natriuretic peptide receptors: Identification of heteromeric receptors and a dominant negative mutant. *J Biol Chem* 1992; 267:18589–18597.
11. Damji KF, Sohocki MM, Khan R, Bulman D, Gupta SK, Rahim M, Loyer M, Hussein N, Ladak S, Jamal A, Koenekoop RK: Leber congenital amaurosis with anterior keratoconus in Pakistani families is caused by the Trp278X mutation in the *AIPL1* gene on 17p. *Can J Ophthalmol* 2001; 36:252–259.
12. den Hollander AI, Heckenlively JR, van den Born LI, de Kok YJM, van der Velde-Visser SD, Kellner U, Jurklies B, van Schooneveld MJ, Blankenagel A, Rohrschneider K, et al:

Leber congenital amaurosis and retinitis pigmentosa with Coats-like exudative vasculopathy are associated with mutations in the crumbs homologue 1 (*CRB1*) gene. *Am J Hum Genet* 2001; 69:198–203.

13. den Hollander AI, ten Brink JB, de Kok YJM, van Soest S, van den Born LI, van Driel MA, van de Pol DJR, Payne AM, Bhattacharya SS, Kellner U, Hoyng CB, Westerveld A, Brunner HG, Bleeker-Wagemakers EM, Deutman AF, Heckenlively JR, Cremers FPM, Bergen AAB: Mutations in a human homologue of drosophila crumbs cause retinitis pigmentosa (RP12). *Nat Genet* 1999; 23:217–221.

14. den Hollander AI, van Driel MA, de Kok YJM, van de Pol DJR, Hoyng CB, Brunner HG, Deutman AF, Cremers FPM: Isolation and mapping of novel candidate genes for retinal disorders using suppression subtractive hybridization. *Genomics* 1999; 58:240–249.

15. Dharmaraj S, Li Y, Robitaille J, et al: A novel locus for Leber congenital amaurosis maps on chromosome 6q. *Am J Hum Genet* 2000; 66:319–326.

16. Dharmaraj S, Silva E, Pina A-L, Li Y, Yang J, Carter RC, Loyer M, El-Hilali H, Traboulsi E, Sundin O, Zhu D, Koenekoop RK, Maumenee I: Mutational analysis and clinical correlation in LCA. *Ophthalmic Genet* 2000; 21(3):135–150.

17. Dizhoor AM, Lowe DG, Olshevskaya EV, et al: The human photoreceptor membrane guanylyl cyclase, RetGC, is present in outer segments and is regulated by calcium and a soluble activator. *Neuron* 1994; 12:1345–1352.

18. Dizhoor AM, Lowe DG, Olshevskaya EV, et al: Expression patterns of *RetGC-1* in rod and cone photoreceptors. *Neuron* 1994; 12:1345–1352.

19. Dizhoor AM, Olshevskaya EV, Henzel WJ, et al: Cloning, sequencing, and expression of a 24-kDa Ca(2+)-binding protein activating photoreceptor guanylyl cyclase. *J Biol Chem* 1995; 270:25200–25206.

20. Dryja TP, Adams SM, Grimsby JL, McGee TL, Hong DH, et al: Null *RPGRIP1* alleles in patients with Leber congenital amaurosis. *Am J Hum Genet* 2001; 68:1295–1298.

21. Duda T, Venkataraman V, Goraczniak R, Lange C, Koch K-W, Sharma RK: Functional consequences of a rod outer segment membrane guanylate cyclase (ROS-GC1) gene mutation linked with Leber's congenital amaurosis. *Biochemistry* 1999; 38:509–515.

22. Felius J, Bingham EL, Kemp JA, Khan NW, Thompson DA, Sieving PA: Clinical course and visual function in a family with mutations in the *RPE65*. *Arch Ophthalmol* 2002; 120:55–61.

23. Flanders M, Lapointe ML, Brownstein S, et al: Keratoconus and Leber's congenital amaurosis: A clinicopathological correlation. *Can J Ophthalmol* 1984; 19:310–314.

24. Foxman SG, Heckenlively JR, Bateman JB, et al: A classification of congenital and early-onset retinitis pigmentosa. *Arch Ophthalm* 1985; 108:1502–1506.

25. Franceschetti A, Dieterlé P: Die Differentaldiagnostische Bedeutung des ERG's bei tapeto-retinalen Degenerationen: Elektroretinographie. *Bibl Ophth* 1956; 48:161.

26. François J: Leber's tapetoretinal reflex. *Int Ophthalmol Clin* 1968; 8:929–947.

27. François J, Hanssens M: Étude histo-pathologique de deux cas de dégénérescence tapéto-rétinienne congénitale de Leber. *Ann Oculistique* 1969; 202:127–155.

28. Freund CL, Gregory-Evans CY, Furukawa T, Papaioannou M, Looser J, Ploder L, Bellingham J, Ng D, Herbrick JA, Duncan A, Scherer SW, Tsui LC, Loutradis-Anagnostou A, Jacobson SG, Cepko CL, Bhattacharya SS, McInnes RR: Cone-rod dystrophy due to mutations in a novel photoreceptor-specific homeobox gene (*CRX*) essential for maintenance of the photoreceptor. *Cell* 1997; 91:543–553.

29. Freund CL, Wang Q-L, Chen S, Muskat BL, Wiles CD, Sheffield VC, Jacobson SG, McInnes RR, Zack DJ, Stone EM: De novo mutations in the *CRX* homeobox gene associated with Leber congenital amaurosis (letter). *Nat Genet* 1998; 18:311–312.

30. Fulton AB, Hansen RM, Mayer DL: Vision in Leber congenital amaurosis. *Arch Ophthalmol* 1996; 114:698–703.

31. Furukawa T, Morrow EM, Cepko CL: *Crx*, a novel otx-like homeobox gene, shows photoreceptor-specific expression and regulates photoreceptor differentiation. *Cell* 1997; 91:531–541.

32. Furukawa T, Morrow EM, Li T, et al: Retinopathy and attenuated circadian entrainment in Crx-deficient mice. *Nat Genet* 1999; 23:466–470.

33. Gerber S, Perrault I, Hanein S, Barbet F, Ducroq D, Ghazi I, Martin-Coignard D, Leowski C, Homfray T, Dufier JL, Munnich A, Kaplan J, Rozet JM: Complete exon-intron structure of the RPGR-interacting protein (*RPGRIP1*) gene allows the identification of mutations underlying Leber congenital amaurosis. *Eur J Hum Genet* 2001; 9:561–571.

34. Gillespie FD: Congenital amaurosis of Leber. *Am J Ophthalmol* 1966; 61:874–880.

35. Gu S, Thompson DA, Srikumari CRS, Lorenz B, Finckh U, Nicoletti A, Murthy KR, Rathmann M, Kumaramanickavel G, Denton MJ, Gal A: Mutations in *RPE65* cause autosomal recessive childhood-onset severe retinal dystrophy. *Nature Genet* 1997; 17:194–197.

36. Hamel CP, Jenkins NA, Gilbert DJ, Copeland NG, Redmond TM: The gene for the retinal pigment epithelium-specific protein *RPE65* is localized to human 1p31 and mouse 3. *Genomics* 1994; 20:509–512.

37. Hamel CP, Tsilou E, Pfeffer BA, Hooks JJ, Detrick B, Redmond TM: Molecular cloning and expression of *RPE65*, a novel retinal pigment epithelium-specific microsomal protein that is post-transcriptionally regulated in vitro. *J Biol Chem* 1993; 268:15751–15757.

38. Hanein S, Perrault I, Gerber S, Tanguy G, Barbet F, Ducroq D, Calvas P, Dollfus H, Hamel C, Lopponen T, Munier F, Santos L, Shalev S, Zafeiriou D, Dufier JL, Munnich A, Rozet JM, Kaplan J: Leber congenital amaurosis: Comprehensive survey of the genetic heterogeneity, refinement of the clinical definition, and genotype-phenotype correlations as a strategy for molecular diagnosis. *Hum Mutat* 2004; 23:306–317.

39. Heckenlively JR: *Retinitis Pigmentosa*. Philadelphia, JB Lippincott Company, 1988.

40. Heher KL, Traboulsi EI, Maumenee IH: The natural history of Leber's congenital amaurosis. *Ophthalmology* 1992; 99:241–245.

41. Henkes HE, Verduin PC: Dysgenesis or abiotrophy?: A differentiation with the help of the electro-retinogram (ERG) and electro-oculogram (EOG) in Leber's congenital amaurosis. *Ophthalmologica* 1963; 145:144–160.

42. Hong D-H, Yue G, Adamian M, Li T: Retinitis pigmentosa GTPase regulator (*RPGR*)-interacting protein is stably associated with the photoreceptor ciliary axoneme and anchors RPGR to the connecting cilium. *J Biol Chem* 2001; 276:12091–12099.

43. Horsten GP: Development of the retina of man and animals. *Arch Ophthalmol* 1960; 63:232–242.

44. Janecke AR, Thompson DA, Utermann G, Becker C, Hubner CA, Schmid E, McHenry CL, Nair AR, Ruschendorf

F, Heckenlively J, Wissinger B, Nurnberg P, Gal A: Mutations in RDH12 encoding a photoreceptor cell retinol dehydrogenase cause childhood-onset severe retinal dystrophy. *Nat Genet* 2004; 36:850–854.

45. Kelsell RE, Gregory-Evans K, Payne AM, Perrault I, Kaplan J, Yang R-B, Garbers DL, Bird AC, Moore AT, Hunt DM: Mutations in the retinal guanylate cyclase (RETGC-1) gene in dominant cone-rod dystrophy. *Hum Molec Genet* 1998; 7: 1179–1184.

46. Koenekoop RK, Loyer M, Dembinska O, Beneish R: Improvement in visual function in Leber congenital amaurosis and the *CRX* genotype. *Ophthalmic Genet* 2002; 23(1):49–59.

47. Koenekoop RK, Fishman GA, Ianacconne A, Loyer M, Sunness JS, Ezzeldin H, Ciccarelli ML, Baldi A, Lotery AJ, Jablonski MM, Pittler SJ, Maumenee I: Electroretinographic (ERG) abnormalities in parents of patients with Leber congenital amaurosis who have heterozygous *GUCY2D* mutations. *Arch Ophthalmol* 2002; 120(10):1325–1330.

48. Koenekoop RK, Ramamurthy V, Pina AL, Loyer M, Dharmaraj S, Elhilali H, Maumenee I, Hurley J: Biochemical consequences of *RetGC-1* mutations found in children with Leber congenital amaurosis. *Invest Ophthalmol Vis Sci* 2000; 41(4):S200 (abstract 1050).

49. Koenekoop RK, Tucker C, Pina AL, Loyer M, Maumenee IH, Hurley J: Expression studies of retinal guanylate cyclase mutations in children with Leber's congenital amaurosis. *Invest Ophthalmol Vis Sci* 1999; 40(4):S930 (abstract 4905).

50. Koenekoop RK: Major Review: An overview of recent developments in Leber congenital amaurosis: A model to understand human retinal development. *Surv Ophthalmol* 2004; 49(4):379–398.

51. Kroll AJ, Kuwabara T: Electron microscopy of a retinal abiotrophy. *Arch Ophthalmol* 1964; 71:683–690.

52. Lambert SR, Kriss A, Taylor D, et al: Follow-up and diagnostic reappraisal of 75 patients with Leber's congenital amaurosis. *Am J Ophthalmol* 1989; 107:624–631.

53. Laura RP, Dizhoor AM, Hurley JB: The membrane guanylyl cyclase, retinal guanylyl cyclase-1, is activated through its intracellular domain. *J Biol Chem* 1996; 271:11646–11651.

54. Leber T: Uber retinitis pigmentosa und angeborene amaurose. *Graefes Arch Klin Ophthalmol* 1869; 15:1–25.

55. Li Z, Kljavin I, Milam A: Rod photoreceptor sprouting in retinitis pigmentosa. *J Neurosci* 1995; 15(8):5429–5438.

56. Liu X, Seno K, Nishizawa Y, et al: Ultrastructural localization of retinal guanylate cyclase in human and monkey retinas. *Exp Eye Res* 1994; 59:761–768.

57. Liu X, Bulgakov OV, Wen XH, Woodruff ML, Pawlyk B, Yang J, Fain GL, Sandberg MA, Makino CL, Li T: AIPL1, the protein that is defective in Leber congenital amaurosis, is essential for the biosynthesis of retinal rod cGMP phosphodiesterase. *Proc Natl Acad Sci U S A* 2004; 101:13903–13908.

58. Lorenz B, Gyurus P, Preising M, et al: Early-onset severe rod cone dystrophy in young children with *RPE 65* mutations. *Invest Ophthalmol Vis Sci* 2000; 41(9):2735–2742.

59. Lotery AJ, Jacobson SG, Fishman GA, Weleber RG, et al: Mutations in the *CRB1* gene cause Leber congenital amaurosis. *Arch Ophthalmol* 2001; 119:415–420.

60. Lotery AJ, Namperumalsamy P, Jacobson SG, et al: Mutation analysis of three genes in patients with Leber congenital amaurosis. *Arch Ophthalmol* 2000; 118:538–543.

61. Marlhens F, Bareil C, Griffoin J-M, Zrenner E, Amalric P, Eliaou C, Liu S-Y, Harris E, Redmond TM, Arnaud B, Claustres M, Hamel CP: Mutations in *RPE65* cause Leber's congenital amaurosis (letter). *Nature Genet* 1997; 17:139–141.

62. Marmor MF, Arden GB, Nilsson SEG, Zrenner E, for the Standardization Committee of the International Society for Clinical Electrophysiology of Vision (ISCEV): Standard for clinical electrophysiology. *Arch Ophthalmol* 1989; 107:816–819.

63. Milam A, Li Z, Fariss R: Histopathology of the human retina in retinitis pigmentosa. *Prog Retin Eye Res* 1998; 17(2):175–205.

64. Morimura H, Fishman GA, Grover SA, Fulton AB, Berson EL, Dryja TP: Mutations in the *RPE65* gene in patients with autosomal recessive retinitis pigmentosa or Leber congenital amaurosis. *Proc Natl Acad Sci U S A* 1998; 95:3088–3093.

65. Nicolletti A, Wong DJ, Kawase K, et al: Molecular characterization of the human gene encoding an abundant 61 kDA protein specific to the retinal pigment epithelium. *Hum Mol Genet* 1995; 4:641–649.

66. Noble KG, Carr RE: Leber's congenital amaurosis. *Arch Ophthalmol* 1978; 96:818–821.

67. Perrault I, Rozet JM, Calvas P, et al: Retinal-specific guanylate cyclase gene mutations in Leber's congenital amaurosis. *Nat Genet* 1996; 14:461–464.

68. Perrault I, Rozet J, Gerber S, Ghazi I, et al: Spectrum of RetGC1 mutations in Leber congenital amaurosis. *Eur J Hum Genet* 2000; 8:578–582.

69. Perrault I, Rozet JM, Gerber S, et al: A RetGC-1 mutation in autosomal dominant cone-rod dystrophy. *J Hum Genet* 1998; 63:651–654.

70. Perrault I, Rozet JM, Ghazi I, Leowski C, Bonnemaison M, et al: Different outcome of *RetGC1* and *RPE65* gene mutations in Leber congenital amaurosis. *Am J Hum Genet* 1999; 64:1225–1228.

71. Perrault I, Hanein S, Gerber S, Barbet F, Ducroq D, Dollfus H, Hamel C, Dufier JL, Munnich A, Kaplan J, Rozet JM: Retinal dehydrogenase 12 (RDH12) mutations in leber congenital amaurosis. *Am J Hum Genet* 2004; 75:639–646.

72. Porto FB, Perrault I, Hicks D, Rozet JM, Manoteau N, Hanein S, Kaplan J, Sahel AJ: Prenatal human ocular degeneration occurs in Leber congenital amaurosis (LCA2). *J Gene Med* 2002; 4(4):390–396.

73. Redmond TM, Yu S, Lee E, Bok D, Hamasaki D, Chen N, Goletz P, Ma J-X, Crouch RK, Pfeifer K: Rpe65 is necessary for production of 11-cis-vitamin A in the retinal visual cycle. *Nature Genet* 1998; 20:344–351.

74. Rivolta C, Berson E, Dryja TP: Dominant Leber congenital amaurosis, cone-rod degeneration, and retinitis pigmentosa caused by mutant versions of the transcription factor *CRX*. *Hum Mutat* 2001; 18:488–498.

75. Schappert-Kimmijser J, Henkes HE, Bosch J: Amaurosis congenita (Leber). *AMA Arch Ophthal* 1959; 61:218.

76. Semple-Rowland S, Lee NR, Van Hooser JP, et al: A null mutation in the photoreceptor guanylate cyclase gene causes the retinal degeneration chicken phenotype. *Proc Natl Acad Sci U S A* 1998; 95:1271–1276.

77. Shyjan AW, de Sauvage FJ, Gillett NA, Goeddel DV, Lowe DG: Molecular cloning of a retina-specific membrane guanylyl cyclase. *Neuron* 1992; 9:727–737.

78. Silva E, Yang JM, Li Y, et al: A *CRX* null mutation is associated with both Leber congenital amaurosis and a normal ocular phenotype. *Invest Ophthalmol Vis Sci* 2000; 41:2076–2079.

79. Sohocki MM, Bowne SJ, Sullivan LS, Blackshaw S, Cepko CL, Payne AM, Bhattacharya SS, Khaliq S, Mehdi SQ, Birch DG, Harrison WR, Elder FFB, Heckenlively JR, Daiger SP: Muta-

tions in a new photoreceptor-pineal gene on 17p cause Leber congenital amaurosis. *Nature Genet* 2000; 24:79–83.

80. Sohocki MM, Perrault I, Leroy BP, Payne AM, Dharmaraj S, Bhattacharya SS, Kaplan J, Maumenee IH, Koenekoop R, Meire FM, Birch DG, Heckenlively JR, Daiger SP: Prevalence of *AIPL1* mutations in inherited retinal degenerative disease. *Mol Genet Metab* 2000; 70:142–150.

81. Sohocki MM, Sullivan LS, Mintz-Hittner HA, Birch D, Heckenlively JR, Freund CL, McInnes RR, Daiger SP: A range of clinical phenotypes associated with mutations in *CRX*, a photoreceptor transcription-factor gene. *Am J Hum Genet* 1998; 63:1307–1315.

82. Sorsby A, Williams CE: Retinal aplasia as a clinical entity. *Br Med J* 1960; 1:293–297.

83. Stockton DW, Lewis RA, Abboud EB, et al: A novel locus for Leber congenital amaurosis on chromosome 14q24. *Hum Genet* 1998; 103:328–333.

84. Sullivan TJ, Heathcote JG, Brazel SM, Musarella MA: The ocular pathology in Leber's congenital amaurosis. *Aust N Z J Ophthalmol* 1994; 22:25–31.

85. Swaroop A, Wang QL, Wu W, et al: Leber congenital amaurosis caused by a homozygous mutation (R90W) in the homeodomain of the retinal transcription factor CRX: Direct evidence for the involvement of CRX in the development of photoreceptor function. *Hum Mol Genet* 1999; 8:299–305.

86. Thompson DA, Gyurus P, Fleischer LL, Bingham EL, McHenry CL, et al: Genetics and phenotypes of *RPE65* mutations in inherited retinal degeneration. *Invest Ophthalmol Vis Sci* 2000; 41:4293–4299.

87. Thompson DK, Garbers DL: Dominant negative mutations of the guanylyl cyclase-A receptor: Extracellular domain deletion and catalytic domain point mutations. *J Biol Chem* 1995; 270:425–430.

88. Tucker C, Pina AL, Loyer M, Maumenee IH, Hurley J, Koenekoop RK: Dominant negative effects of retinal guanylate cyclase (*GUCY2D*) mutations in children with Leber congenital amaurosis: Genotype-phenotype correlations. *Exp Eye Res* 2003 (submitted).

89. van der Spuy J, Chapple JP, Clark BJ, Luthbert PJ, et al: The Leber congenital amaurosis gene product AIPL-1 is localized exclusively in rod photoreceptors of the adult human retina. *Hum Mol Genet* 2002; 11(7):823–831.

90. Van Hooser JP, Aleman TS, He YG, Cideciyan AV, et al: Rapid restoration of visual pigment and function with oral retinoid in a mouse model of childhood blindness. *Proc Natl Acad Sci U S A* 2000; 97(15):8623–8628.

91. Veske A, Nilson SD, Narfstrom K, Gal A: Retinal dystrophy of Swedish briard/briard beagle dogs is due to a 4 bp deletion in *RPE65. Genomics* 1999; 57:57–61.

92. Vrabec F: Un cas de degenerance pigmentaire congenitale de la retine examinee histoloquement. *Ophthalmologica* 1951; 122:65–75.

93. Waardenburg PJ: Does agenesis or dysgenesis neuroepithelialis retinae, whether or not related to keratoglobus, exist? *Ophthalmologica* 1957; 133:454–461.

94. Waardenburg PJ, Schappert-Kimmijser J: On various recessive biotypes of Leber's congenital amaurosis. *Acta Ophthalmol* 1963; 41:317–320.

95. Winkelman JE, Horsten GPM: Congenital blindness in the presence of a normal fundus. *Ophthalmologica* 1959; 137:423–425.

96. Yang RB, Robinson SW, Xiong WH, et al: Disruption of a retinal guanylyl cyclase gene leads to cone-specific dystrophy and paradoxical rod behavior. *J Neurosci* 1999; 19:5889–5897.

97. Zernant J, Kulm M, Dharmaraj S, den Hollander AI, Perrault I, Preising MN, Lorenz B, Kaplan J, Cremers FP, Maumenee I, Koenekoop RK, Allikmets R: Genotyping microarray (disease chip) for leber congenital amaurosis: Detection of modifier alleles. *Invest Ophthalmol Vis Sci* 2005; 46:3052–3059.

98. Zhao Y, Hong DH, Pawlyk B, Yue G, Adamian M, Grynberg M, Godzik A, Li T: The retinitis pigmentosa GTPase regulator (RPGR)-interacting protein: Subserving RPGR function and participating in disk morphogenesis. *Proc Natl Acad Sci U S A* 2003; 100:3965–3970.

99. Znoiko SL, Crouch RK, Moiseyev G, Ma JX: Identification of the RPE65 protein in mammalian cone photoreceptors. *Invest Ophthalmol Vis Sci* 2002; 43:1604–1609.

65 Pattern Dystrophies

MICHAEL F. MARMOR

THE TERM *PATTERN dystrophy* was suggested by the author[12] and Hsieh et al. in 1977[7] to describe a group of related dystrophies of the retinal pigment epithelium (RPF) that are characterized by granular or reticular pigmentation patterns and a relatively benign clinical course. Earlier literature had described a variety of RPE dystrophies with unusual pigmentary patterns such as reticular dystrophy,[18] butterfly dystrophy,[5] fundus pulverulentus,[19] dystrophia macroreticularis,[15] and others. Some families with dominant pattern dystrophy, often with a butterfly pattern, have now been found to have mutations of the peripherin/RDS gene (a gene that can also cause retinitis pigmentosa).[9,16,17] And a pattern dystrophy has been described in families with a mitochondrial DNA mutation that also causes maternal diabetes and deafness.[2,14] However, many families lack any known mutation,[13,22] and inheritance can be recessive as well as dominant. Thus, the designation "pattern dystrophy" provides a way of describing and categorizing a variety of genetic disorders that behave in a similar fashion with respect to RPE involvement and limited functional changes.[11]

Clinical findings

The pattern dystrophies represent inherited disorders in which there is a primary granular or reticular disturbance of the RPE without any predisposing factor such as age-related macular degeneration, pigment epithelial detachment, vitelliform macular lesions, juvenile macular dystrophy, or other secondary causes of pigmentary dispersion in the fundus. The pigmentary patterns can vary widely, and some families have extensive peripheral changes as in reticular dystrophy[18] (figure 65.1), whereas in other families, the pigmentation is limited to the macula (figure 65.2). Families have been described in which there are individual differences among the members in their pattern of pigmentation[1,4,7,12] (compare figures 65.2 and 65.3).

The pattern dystrophies typically cause few symptoms during youth or the early adult years.[1,4,10,11,21] Visual acuity may be mildly subnormal, but severe visual loss as often characterizes pigment epithelial detachment, Stargardt's disease, or vitelliform dystrophy would be unusual and would in general argue against the diagnosis. Older individuals can develop more extensive RPE thinning or atrophic changes in the macula (figures 65.3 and 65.4), however, and

sometimes have significant visual loss (see figure 65.4).[13,22] It is unclear whether pattern dystrophy increases the risk of age-related decompensation of whether these late atrophic changes are specific to the dystrophy.

Fluorescein angiography is extremely important in the evaluation of pattern dystrophies, since the RPE changes are often difficult to see on ophthalmoscopic examination (see figures 65.1 through 65.3). A fundus that shows only mild nonspecific pigment epithelial changes on direct examination may display striking granular or pigmentary patterns on angiography that extend more peripherally than expected. The pigmentary patterns that are visible on angiography are not associated with leakage of dye through the pigment epithelium or with secondary changes such as choroidal neovascularization (except in elderly patients[12] or isolated cases[3] in which pattern dystrophy might not be the only cause).

Physiological findings

By definition, the pattern dystrophies are associated with relatively little functional deficit until (possibly) old age. We have already noted that visual acuity may be mildly reduced, depending on the degree of foveal involvement, and there may be a mild degree of contrast sensitivity loss or color vision disturbance.[6] The visual fields and dark adaptation have been normal in the vast majority of reported cases, although individual pedigrees with central sensitivity loss[4] and subnormal dark adaptation[10] have been described. Severe loss of acuity should make one think of other disorders such as Stargardt's disease, vitelliform dystrophy, or age-related macular degeneration.

In young and middle-aged patients with pattern dystrophy, multifocal electroretinogram (mfERG) abnormalities may be present in areas of macular damage,[8] but diffuse electrophysiological findings are essentially limited to the electro-oculogram (EOG) in youth and middle age. The electroretinogram (ERG) has universally been reported as normal (figure 65.5) in these eyes, while the EOG (which might be expected to reflect pigment epithelial abnormality) is either normal or only modestly subnormal.[1,5,7,8,21] Individual cases with very low light/dark ratios have been noted, but most commonly, the ratio is in the 1.5–1.8 range if suppressed at all (see figure 65.6). The EOG findings are quite distinct and distinguishable from those in vitelliform

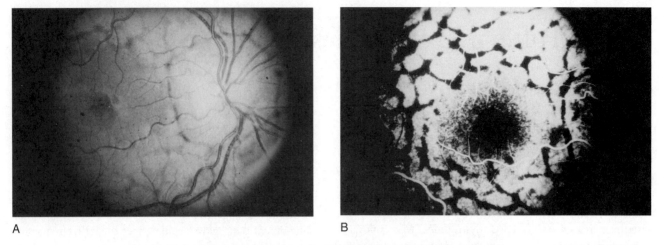

A

B

FIGURE 65.1   Reticular dystrophy. A, Fundus photograph. B, Fluorescein angiogram.

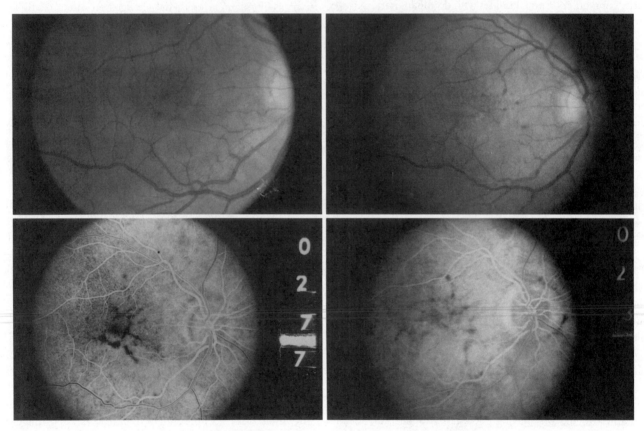

FIGURE 65.2   Macular changes in a patient with pattern dystrophy. Top, Fundus photographs at ages 19 and 38. Bottom, Fluorescein angiograms at ages 19 and 38. The pigmentary changes were more visible by angiography than photography. With aging, there was more diffuse thinning of the RPE.

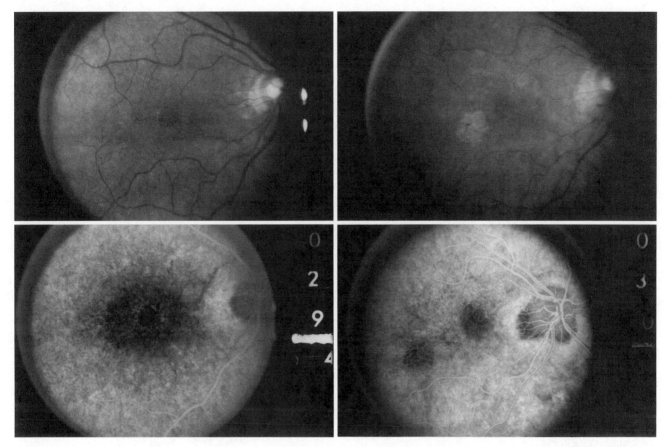

FIGURE 65.3 Mother of the patient in figure 65.2. She shows more granular than reticular pigmentary patterns and developed increasing RPE atrophy with age. Top, Fundus photographs at ages 43 and 62. Bottom, Fluorescein angiograms at ages 43 and 62. Note the parafoveal patches of atrophy at age 62. She also showed a significant diminution of her ERG (see figure 65.5).

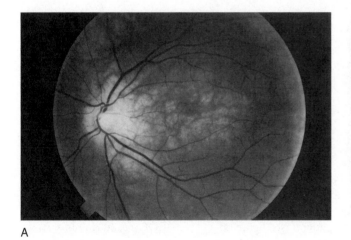

A

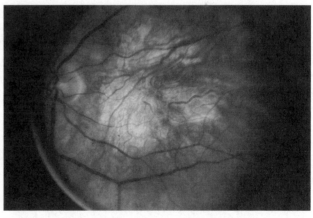

B

FIGURE 65.4 Two older cousins of the patients in figures 65.2 and 65.3, showing atrophic loss of RPE. A, Fundus photograph at age 69 (visual acuity 20/50). B, Fundus photograph of the mother of the patient on the left at age 80 (visual acuity 20/200).

ELECTRORETINOGRAMS IN PATTERN DYSTROPHY

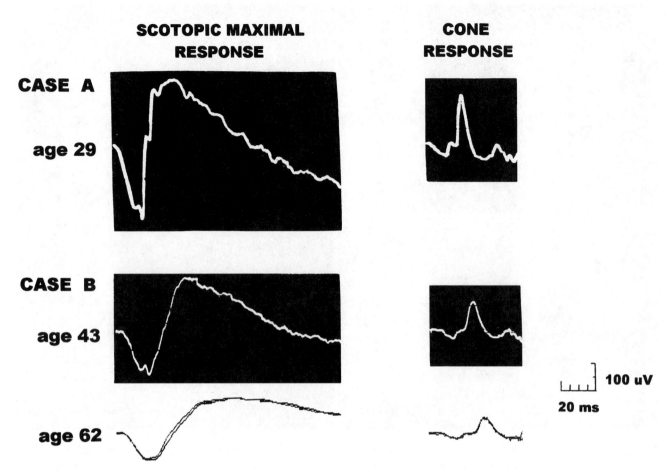

SCOTOPIC MAXIMAL RESPONSE

CONE RESPONSE

CASE A

age 29

CASE B

age 43

age 62

100 uV

20 ms

FIGURE 65.5 Electroretinograms in pattern dystrophy. Case A: A 29-year-old patient with a normal ERG. Case B: Patient from figure 65.3. The ERG was low-normal at age 43 and fell to subnormal levels by age 62.

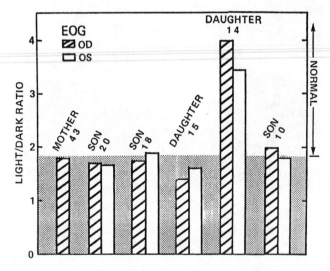

FIGURE 65.6 EOG light/dark ratios in a family with pattern dystrophy (including the patients in figures 65.2 and 65.3). The affected members all had borderline values; the daughter with a high ratio had a normal-appearing fundus and did not have the disease.

dystrophy, in which every affected family member (regardless of fundus lesions) has an extremely reduced light/dark ratio. The hyperosmolarity response has also been found to be abnormal in one patient with pattern dystrophy who had a normal EOG.[20] In older individuals, as the RPE atrophic changes become more extensive, there can be corresponding functional abnormalities, including mfERG losses. Paracentral scotomas may be found, as well as blue-yellow (tritan) color confusions and a mild rise in dark adaptation threshold. The full-field ERG drifts toward borderline levels and may be moderately (though not severely) reduced in some patients (see figure 65.5).[13] The EOG results do not seem to change much with age.

Summary

The pattern dystrophies represent a group of inherited pigment epithelial disorders in which there is pigment clumping and rearrangement at the level of the RPE in the macula and/or periphery, with little or no loss of acuity or retinal sensitivity until late in life. This includes disorders such as butterfly dystrophy, reticular dystrophy, and fundus pulverulentus along with patients whose familial pattern of fundus pigmentation may be less dramatic or more variable. The pattern dystrophies are clinically quite distinct from drusen, vitelliform dystrophy, and fundus flavimaculatus. Young to middle-aged individuals may show mild mfERG changes in the affected areas of the macula and may show a borderline or mildly subnormal EOG. Older individuals can develop more extensive macular atrophy and may show some modest reduction of the full-field ERG.

REFERENCES

1. Ayazi S, Fagan R: Pattern dystrophy of the pigment epithelium. *Retina* 1981; 1:287–289.
2. Bonte CA, Matthijs GL, Cassiman JJ, Leys AM: Macular pattern dystrophy in patients with deafness and diabetes. *Retina* 1997; 17:216–221.
3. Burgess D: Subretinal neovascularization in a pattern dystrophy of the retinal pigment epithelium. *Retina* 1981; 1:151–155.
4. deJong PTVM, Delleman JW: Pigment epithelial pattern dystrophy. *Arch Ophthalmol* 1982; 100:1416–1421.
5. Deutman AF, van Blommestein DA, Henkes HE, Waardenburg PJ, Sollevand-van Dreist E: Butterfly-shaped pigment dystrophy of the fovea. *Arch Ophthalmol* 1970; 83:558–569.
6. Duinkerke-Eerola KU, Pinckers A, Cruysberg JRM: Pattern dystrophy of the retinal pigment epithelium. *Int Ophthalmol* 1987; 11:65–72.
7. Hsieh RC, Fine BS, Lyons JS: Patterned dystrophies of the retinal pigment epithelium. *Arch Ophthalmol* 1977; 95:429–435.
8. Kellner U, Jandeck C, Kraus H, Foerster MH: Hereditäre makula dystrophien. *Ophthalmologe* 1998; 95:597–601.
9. Kim RY, Dollfus H, Keen TJ, Fitzke FW, Arden GB, Bhattacharya SS, Bird AC: Autosomal dominant pattern dystrophy of the retina associated with a 4-base pair insertion at Codon 140 in the peripherin/RDS gene. *Arch Ophthalmol* 1995; 224:451–455.
10. Kingham JD, Fenzl RE, Willerson D, Aaberg TM: Reticular dystrophy of the retinal pigment epithelium. *Arch Ophthalmol* 1978; 96:1177–1184.
11. Marmor MF: Dystrophies of the retinal pigment epithelium. In Zinn KM, Marmor MF (eds): *The Retinal Pigment Epithelium.* Cambridge, Mass, Harvard University Press, 1979, pp 424–453.
12. Marmor MF, Byers B: Pattern dystrophy of the pigment epithelium. *Am J Ophthalmol* 1977; 84:32–44.
13. Marmor MF, McNamara JA: Pattern dystrophy of the retinal pigment epithelium and geographic atrophy of the macula. *Am J Ophthalmol* 1996; 122:382–392.
14. Massin P, Virally-Monod M, Vialettes B, Paques M, Gin H, Porokhov B, Caillat-Zucman S, Froguel P, Paquis-Fluckinger V, Gaudric A, Guillausseau P-J (on behalf of the GEDIAM Group): Prevalence of macular pattern dystrophy in maternally inherited diabetes and deafness. *Ophthalmol* 1999; 106:1821–1827.
15. Mesker RP, Oosterhuis JA, Delleman JW: A retinal lesion resembling Sjögren's dystrophia reticularis laminae pigmentosae retinae. In *Perspectives in Ophthalmology, vol 26.* Princeton, NJ, Excerpta Medica, 1970, pp 40–45.
16. Richards SC, Creel DJ: Pattern dystrophy and retinitis pigmentosa caused by a peripherin/RDS mutation. *Retina* 1995; 15:68–72.
17. Sears JE, Aaberg TA, Daiger SP, Moshfeghi DM: Splice site mutation in the peripherin/RDS gene associated with pattern dystrophy of the retina. *Am J Ophthalmol* 2001; 132:693–699.
18. Sjögren H: Dystrophia reticularis laminae pigmentosae retinae. *Acta Ophthalmol* 1950;28:279–295.
19. Slezak H, Hommer K: Fundus pulverulentus. *Graefes Arch Clin Exp Ophthalmol* 1969; 178:177–182.
20. Wakabayashi K, Yonemura D, Kawasaki K: Electrophysiological analysis of Best's macular dystrophy and retinal pigment epithelial pattern dystrophy. *Ophthalmic Paediatr Genet* 1983; 3:13–17.
21. Watzke RC, Folk JC, Lang RM: Pattern dystrophy of the retinal pigment epithelium. *Ophthalmology* 1982; 89:1400–1406.
22. Weigell-Weber M, Kryenbühl C, Büchi ER, Spiegel R: Genetic heterogeneity in autosomal dominant pattern dystrophy of the retina. *Mol Vis* 1996; 20:2–6.

66 Best Vitelliform Macular Dystrophy

GERALD A. FISHMAN

BEST VITELLIFORM macular dystrophy is an autosomal-dominantly inherited disorder whose familial occurrence was first described in 1905 by Friedrich Best in a family of German ancestry.[6] Previously, in 1883, Adams had described a single patient with this disease.[1] In 1950, the Belgian ophthalmologists Zanen and Rausin[53] first used the description *vitelliform* when referring to the macular lesion that they observed in patients with this disease. The term *vitelliform* ("egg-yolk-like") has its origin from the Latin word *vitellus* meaning "egg-yolk."

The fundus findings include a spectrum of phenotypic expressions. The most distinctive macular lesion, which is most often initially discovered between the ages of 3 and 15 years, demonstrates a sharply circumscribed, bilateral, yellow, "egg-yolk-like" sunny-side-up appearance (figure 66.1). This clinical phenotype has been observed as early as 1 week and 3 weeks of age[3,13] and as late as age 74 years.[11] It is generally between 1 and 2 disk diameters in size, although its size may vary from as small as approximately one half to as large as three or four times the diameter of the optic disk.[29] The presence of this macular lesion is still consistent with visual acuity that is most frequently 20/25 or better. Although only a single isolated foveal lesion is usually present, multiple nonfoveal foci of yellow, egg-yolk-like lesions may also be seen, and patients with unilateral lesions have also been described.[11,25,29,34] A vitelliform lesion can develop in a previously normal-appearing macula.[4,11] Of historical interest, none of the eight patients described by Best showed the classic vitelliform macular lesion.[6]

The initial and primary pathogenetic changes in this disease involve the retinal pigment epithelial (RPE) cells. Consistent with this, Weingeist et al.[52] histologically observed an abnormal accumulation of a lipofuscinlike material in all RPE cells of a patient with Best macular dystrophy, a finding also noted by O'Gorman et al.[39] in another patient.

Progressive impairment of visual acuity tends to parallel a subsequent course in which the yellow egg-yolk-like material appears to rupture or become fragmented into a "scrambled-egg" appearance, the so-called vitelliruptive stage.[30] Eventually, in turn, this lesion can be replaced by a fibrotic (gliotic) hypertrophic-appearing scar.[16,36] In some patients, the yellow material may resorb and subsequently be resecreted. Infrequently, in other patients, subretinal hemorrhage with identifiable or unidentified choroidal neovascular membranes may develop.[3,5,7,35,38] Variability in phenotypic expression of the macular lesion can occur between different families and within the same family.[25,32] Approaches to classifying the various stages of macular changes observed in patients with Best dystrophy have been published.[11,16,29,36]

Most patients are visually asymptomatic or show only slight-to-moderate visual loss bilaterally until between 40 and 50 years of age.[11,29] In one study of 47 patients, 30 of 39 (76%) younger than 30 years of age had a visual acuity of 20/40 or better in at least one eye.[16] Peripheral visual field remains normal. Patients are characteristically hypermetropic and esotropia is commonly observed.[11,27] Astigmatism and amblyopia are also often found.[11,27] ERG cone and rod a- and b-wave amplitudes are typically normal, as is the dark adaptation recovery time, in patients with Best vitelliform macular dystrophy.[2,10,11,30] However, Nilsson and Skoog[37] as well as Rover et al.[43] reported either absent or small ERG c-wave amplitudes in patients with this disorder (indicative of diffuse RPE cell dysfunction). Using a Siles-Crawford test to determine the directional sensitivity of the fovea in a patient with a vitelliform macular lesion and 20/20 vision, Benson et al.[5] showed the foveal receptor orientation to be normal. This finding is most consistent with the conclusion that the egg-yolk-like changes reside within, and also probably below, the RPE cells.

The definitive diagnostic test in this disease is the electrooculogram (EOG), which is markedly abnormal in affected patients. Appreciably reduced EOG light-peak to dark-trough ratios are observed at all stages of clinically evident disease,[9,20,21,25,30,45,49] as well as in those who inherit the gene yet show no clinically apparent fundus changes.[10,11,19,49] In instances when only one eye manifests a clinically apparent retinal lesion, both eyes show reduced EOG ratios.[11,20,21] Since the EOG is regarded as a functional test of the entire retina, an abnormal EOG recording implies overall retinal dysfunction. The large interindividual variation of the EOG standing potential limits it diagnostic usefulness. However, the mean baseline values of the EOG standing potential in patients with Best disease for both those expressing and those

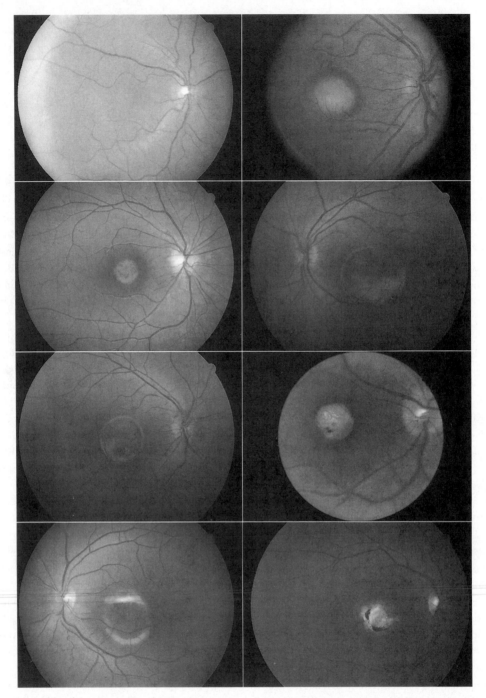

FIGURE 66.1 Fundus photographs representing various stages of macular lesions that can be observed in patients with Best macular dystrophy. Top left, Stage I: mild degree of foveal pigment mottling and nonspecific hypopigmentation. Top right, Stage II: typical vitelliform or egg-yolk-like lesion. Second row left, Stage IIIa: scrambled or "fried egg" phase as the vitelliform lesion becomes diffusely more amorphous and diluted in appearance. Second row right, Stage IIIb: pseudohypopyon phase in which the yellow substance in the vitelliform cyst develops a layered appearance as a consequence of partial resorption. Third row left, Stage IIIc: only a sparse amount of yellowish substance remains as resorption of the vitelliform lesion is almost complete. Third row right, Stage IIId shows atrophic changes of both the retinal pigment epithelium and choriocapillaris vessels. Bottom, Stage IV: both less and more extensive examples are depicted. Characteristic feature is a fibrotic-gliotic-appearing scar in addition resorption of the vitelliform material. (See also color plate 34.)

not expressing clinically apparent retinal changes have been reported as below the mean of a control population.[49] Weleber[51] found that not only was the EOG slow-oscillation light peak subnormal, but also it was delayed in reaching its peak in patients with Best dystrophy. He additionally observed that the EOG fast oscillations were preserved in patients with this disease.

On occasion, a patient with Best macular dystrophy can have bilateral atrophic-appearing foveal lesions that may show some phenotypic similarities to other hereditary macular lesions, such as those seen in Stargardt macular dystrophy or cone dystrophy. However, the absence of fundus flecks in Best disease, the presence of a dark choroid in Stargardt macular dystrophy, and a markedly abnormal EOG in patients with Best dystrophy help to distinguish patients with Best disease from those with Stargardt disease. The normal ERG and abnormal EOG in patients with Best macular dystrophy differentiate these patients who show an atrophic foveal lesion from patients with cone dystrophy. Additionally, with few exceptions, patients with cone dystrophy manifest abnormal cone ERG a- and b-wave amplitudes but a normal EOG response.[14,15] Unlike a number of patients with cone dystrophy, those with Best disease, as a rule, do not complain of photoaversion or impairment of color vision. In addition to Stargardt disease and cone dystrophy, some patients with Best macular dystrophy with an atrophic-appearing foveal lesion may present with a phenotype having certain clinical similarities to lesions that are observed in patients with North Carolina macular dystrophy. Normal EOG ratios in this disorder are distinct from the EOG abnormality found in Best disease.[17]

There are a group of macular disorders other than Best vitelliform macular dystrophy that may present with a vitelliform lesion. They include (1) those described as either a peculiar foveomacular dystrophy,[22] adult foveomacular vitelliform dystrophy,[8,40] dominant slowly progressive macular dystrophy,[47] or adult-onset foveomacular pigment epithelial dystrophy;[50] (2) those associated with leakage from retinal perifoveal capillaries;[18] (3) those observed as a spectrum of age-related macular degeneration associated with an elevation of the retinal pigment epithelium;[23,33,48] (4) those unassociated with any of the above descriptions or clinical findings;[12,28,33,44] and (5) a variant expression of pattern dystrophy.[24,26] The macular lesions within the first four categories can collectively be considered forms of adult-onset foveomacular vitelliform dystrophies/degenerations (AOFVD). Table 66.1 summarizes the differential diagnosis of vitelliform macular lesions. In general, a normal EOG light-peak to dark-trough ratio helps to distinguish these disorders from Best dystrophy. However, there are reports of both slightly subnormal and even more substantially subnormal EOG findings in some patients with vitelliform lesions unassociated with Best disease. The use of optical

TABLE 66.1

Differential diagnosis of vitelliform macular lesions

A. Classic Best vitelliform macular dystrophy
B. Adult-onset foveomacular vitelliform dystrophies/ degenerations
  Group I:
  1. A peculiar foveomacular dystrophy
  2. Adult foveomacular vitelliform dystrophy
  3. Dominant slowly progressive macular dystrophy
  4. Adult-onset foveomacular pigment epithelial dystrophy
  Group II: Leakage from perifoveal retinal capillaries
  Group III: A spectrum of age-related macular degeneration associated with an elevation of the retinal pigment epithelium
  Group IV: Unassociated with any of the above descriptive terms or clinical findings
C. Variant expression of pattern dystrophy
  At least some patients subcategorized (1–4) within Group I likely have the same genetic disease. Autosomal-dominant transmission with variable expressivity should always be considered in Group I patients.
  Some patients within either Group I or Group IV may harbor a mutation in the peripherin/RDS gene similar to that observed in a segment of patients with pattern dystrophy (C).

coherence tomography has been reported to be of possible value in differentiating at least some patients with AOFVD from those with Best vitelliform macular dystrophy.[42]

In addition to the aforementioned hereditary, or likely hereditary, disorders with either a vitelliform phenotype or atrophic-appearing macular changes with phenotypic similarity to some patients with Best dystrophy, certain acquired disorders may also show changes that might resemble atypical presentations of Best dystrophy. These include inflammatory macular lesions associated with chorioretinitis or central serous choroidopathy. Normal EOG light-peak to dark-trough ratios in these latter disorders can resolve any lingering diagnostic uncertainty.

Mutations in a novel retina-specific gene on the long arm of chromosome 11 (11q13) have been identified in patients affected with Best macular dystrophy.[31,41] This gene encodes a 585-amino-acid protein known as bestrophin, which is selectively expressed in the RPE cells of the retina.[41]

REFERENCES

1. Adams JE: Case showing peculiar changes in the macula. *Trans Ophthal Soc U K* 1883; 3:113.
2. Baca W, Fishman GA, Alexander KR, Glenn AM: Dark adaptation in patients with Best vitelliform macular dystrophy. *Br J Ophthalmol* 1994; 78:430–432.
3. Barkman Y: A clinical study of central tapetoretinal degeneration. *Acta Ophthalmol* 1961; 39:663–671.
4. Barricks ME: Vitelliform lesions developing in normal fundi. *Am J Ophthalmol* 1977; 83:324–327.

5. Benson WE, Kolker AE, Enoch JM, Van Loo JA, Honda Y: Best's vitelliform macular dystrophy. *Am J Ophthalmol* 1975; 79:59–66.

6. Best F: Über eine hereditäre maculaaffektion. *Beiträge Zur Vererbungslehre Zschr Augenheilk* 1905; 13:199–212.

7. Braley AE: Dystrophy of the macula. *Am J Ophthalmol* 1966; 61:1–24.

8. Burgess DB, Olk J, Uniat LM: Macular disease resembling adult foveomacular vitelliform dystrophy in older adults. *Ophthalmology* 1987; 94:362–366.

9. Cross HE, Bard L: Electro-oculography in Best's macular dystrophy. *Am J Ophthalmol* 1974; 77:46–50.

10. Deutman AF: Electro-oculography in families with vitelliform dystrophy of the fovea. *Arch Ophthalmol* 1969; 81:305–316.

11. Deutman AF: *The Hereditary Dystrophies of the Posterior Pole of the Eye*. Springfield, Ill, Charles C. Thomas, 1971, pp 198–299.

12. Epstein GA, Rabb MF: Adult vitelliform macular degeneration: Diagnosis and natural history. *Br J Ophthalmol* 1980; 64:733–740.

13. Falls H: The polymorphous manifestations of Best's disease (vitelliform eruptive disease of the retina). *Trans Am Ophthalmol Soc* 1969; 67:265–279.

14. Fishman GA: Hereditary progressive macular dystrophies. In Smith JL (ed): *Neuro-ophthalmology Update*. New York, Masson, 1977, pp 73–89.

15. Fishman GA: Electroretinography and inherited macular dystrophies. *Retina* 1985; 60:107–119.

16. Fishman GA, Baca W, Alexander KR, Derlacki DJ, Glenn AM, Viana M: Visual acuity in patients with Best vitelliform macular dystrophy. *Ophthalmology* 1993; 100:1665–1670.

17. Fishman GA, Birch DG, Holder GE, Brigell MG: *Electrophysiologic Testing in Disorders of the Retina, Optic Nerve, and Visual Pathway*. San Francisco, The Foundation of the American Academy of Ophthalmology, 2001, p 59.

18. Fishman GA, Trimble S, Rabb MF, Fishman M: Pseudovitelliform macular degeneration. *Arch Ophthalmol* 1977; 95:73–76.

19. François J: Vitelliform macular degeneration. *Ophthalmologica* 1971; 163:312–324.

20. François J, De Rouck A, Fernandez-Sasso D: Electro-oculography in vitelliform degeneration of the macula. *Arch Ophthalmol* 1967; 77:726–733.

21. François J, de Rouck A, Fernandez-Sasso D: Electroretinography and electro-oculography in diseases of the posterior pole of the eye. *Bibl Ophthalmol* 1969; 80:132–163.

22. Gass JDM: A clinicopathologic study of a peculiar foveomacular dystrophy. *Trans Am Ophthalmol Soc* 1974; 72:139–156.

23. Gass JDM, Jallow S, Davia B: Adult vitelliform macular detachment occurring in patients with basal laminar drusen. *Am J Ophthalmol* 1985; 99:445–459.

24. Giuffre G, Lodato G: Vitelliform dystrophy and pattern dystrophy of the retinal pigment epithelium: Concomitant presence in a family. *Br J Ophthalmol* 1986; 70:526–532.

25. Godel V, Chaine G, Regenbogen L, Coscas G: Best's vitelliform macular dystrophy. *Acta Ophthalmol* 1986; 175:5–31.

26. Gutman I, Walsh JB, Henkind P: Vitelliform macular dystrophy and butterfly-shaped epithelial dystrophy: A continuum? *Br J Ophthalmol* 1981; 66:170–173.

27. Huysmans J: Exudative central detachment of the retina in a family (macular pseudo-cysts). *Ophthalmologica* 1940; 99:449–455.

28. Kingham JD, Lochen GP: Vitelliform macular degeneration. *Am J Ophthalmol* 1977; 84:526–531.

29. Krill AE: *Hereditary Retinal and Choroidal Diseases, vol 2*. New York, Harper & Row, 1972, pp 665–704.

30. Krill AE, Morse PA, Potts AM, Klien BA: Hereditary vitrelliruptive macular degeneration. *Am J Ophthalmol* 1966; 61:1405–1415.

31. Lotery AJ, Munier FL, Fishman GA, Weleber RG, Jacobson SG, Affatigato LM, Nichols BE, Schorderet DF, Sheffield VC, Stone EM: Allelic variation in the VMD2 gene in Best disease and age-related macular degeneration. *Invest Ophthalmol Vis Sci* 2000; 41:1291–1296.

32. Maloney WF, Robertson DM, Duboff SM: Hereditary vitelliform macular degeneration: Variable fundus findings within a single pedigree. *Arch Ophthalmol* 1977; 95:979–983.

33. Marmor MF: Vitelliform lesions in adults. *Ann Ophthalmol* 1979; 11:1705–1712.

34. Miller SA: Multifocal Best's vitelliform dystrophy. *Arch Ophthalmol* 1977; 95:984–990.

35. Miller SA, Bresnick GH, Chandra SR: Choroidal neovascular membrane in Best's vitelliform macular dystrophy. *Am J Ophthalmol* 1976; 82:252–255.

36. Mohler CW, Fine SL: Long-term evaluation of patients with Best's vitelliform dystrophy. *Ophthalmology* 1981; 88:688–692.

37. Nilsson SE, Skoog KO: The ERG c-wave in vitelliform macular degeneration (VMD). *Acta Ophthalmol* 1980; 58:659–666.

38. Noble KG, Scher BM, Carr RE: Polymorphous presentations in vitelliform macular dystrophy: Subretinal neovascularization and central choroidal atrophy. *Br J Ophthalmol* 1978; 62:561–570.

39. O'Gorman S, Flaherty WA, Fishman GA, Berson EL: Histopathologic findings in Best's vitelliform macular dystrophy. *Arch Ophthalmol* 1988; 106:1261–1268.

40. Patrinely JR, Lewis RA, Font RI: Foveomacular vitelliform dystrophy, adult type: A clinicopathologic study including electron microscopic observations. *Ophthalmology* 1985; 92:1712–1718.

41. Petrukhin K, Koisti MJ, Bakall B, Li W, Xie G, Marknell T, Sandgren O, Forsman K, Holmgren G, Andréasson S, Vujic M, Bergen AAB, McGarty-Dugan V, Figueroa D, Austin CP, Metzker ML, Caskey CT, Wadelius C: Identification of the gene responsible for Best macular dystrophy. *Nat Genet* 1998; 19:241–247.

42. Pierro L, Tremolada G, Intronini U, Calori G, Brancato R: Optical coherence tomography findings in adult-onset foveomacular vitelliform dystrophy. *Am J Ophthalmol* 2002; 134:675–680.

43. Rover J, Huttel M, Shaubele G: The DC-ERG: Technical problems in recording from patient. *Doc Ophthalmol Proc Ser* 1982; 31:73–79.

44. Sabates R, Pruett RC, Hirose T: Pseudovitelliform macular degeneration. *Retina* 1982; 2:197–205.

45. Sabates R, Pruett RC, Hirose T: The electror-oculogram in "vitelliform" macular lesions. *Doc Ophthalmol Proc Ser* 1983; 37:93–103.

46. Schwartz LJ, Metz HS, Woodward F: Electrophysiologic and fluorescein studies in vitelliform macular degeneration. *Arch Ophthalmol* 1972; 87:636–641.

47. Singerman LJ, Berkow JW, Patz A: Dominant slowly progressive macular dystrophy. *Am J Ophthalmol* 1977; 83:680–693.

48. Snyder DA, Fishman GA, Witteman G, Fishman M: Vitelliform lesions associated with retinal pigment epithelial detachment. *Ann Ophthalmol* 1978; 10:1711–1715.

49. Thorburn W, Norstrom S: EOG in a large family with hereditary macular degeneration (Best's vitelliform macular dystrophy): Identification of gene carriers. *Acta Ophthalmol* 1978; 56:455–464.

50. Vine AK, Schatz H: Adult-onset foveomacular pigment epithelial dystrophy. *Am J Ophthalmol* 1980; 89:680–691.

51. Weleber RG: Fast and slow oscillations of the electro-oculogram in Best's macular dystrophy and retinitis pigmentosa. *Arch Ophthalmol* 1989; 107:530–537.

52. Weingeist TA, Kobrin JL, Watzke RC: Histopathology of Best's macular dystrophy. *Arch Ophthalmol* 1982; 100: 1108–1114.

53. Zanen J, Rausin G: Kyste vitelliform congénital de la macula. *Bull Soc Belge Ophtal* 1950; 96:544–549.

67 Sorsby's Fundus Dystrophy

MICHAEL P. CLARKE AND KEITH W. MITCHELL

In 1949, SORSBY and Mason described five families with a dominantly inherited central retinal dystrophy leading to visual loss in the fifth decade.[34] Visual loss occurred either because of subretinal neovascular membranes leading to disciform scarring or because of chorioretinal atrophy at the macula. There was gradual progression of the condition to involve the retinal periphery, such that ambulatory vision was lost up to 35 years later.[34] The condition has become known as Sorsby's fundus dystrophy (SFD). For general and electrophysiological reviews, see Berninger,[5] Iannaccone,[22] and Scullica and Falsini.[32]

Clinical features

Family members who have been studied before the onset of the macular lesion demonstrate drusen, pigment epithelial atrophy,[21] and a yellow subretinal deposit throughout the fundus.[7] Night blindness is a feature in some patients.[17,22]

The onset of central visual loss has subsequently been noted from the third[17] to the seventh[23] decades. Distortion and sudden loss of vision occur in the presence of a subretinal neovascular membrane (figure 67.1), but gradual visual failure due to macular atrophy is equally common[31] (figure 67.2).

Densely packed drusen and angioid streaks are noted in some patients.[21] The disciform scars are always large (see figure 67.1) and become pigmented in late stages.[7] As the scar flattens, atrophy occurs, leading to choroidal sclerosis. One fortunate patient has been reported with a small island of preserved central vision.[28] Subsequent gradual loss of peripheral vision is the rule. There are no associated systemic health problems.[11]

Histopathology

The few eyes that have been studied histopathologically have had end-stage pathology. There is a widespread eosinophilic deposit at the level of Bruch's membrane, atrophy of the choriocapillaris, and, at the macula, either photoreceptor and pigment epithelial atrophy or disciform scarring associated with breaks in Bruch's membrane.[3]

Electrophysiology

Capon et al. found normal electroretinograms (ERGs) in eyes with normal vision.[7] There was no abnormality of a- or b-wave amplitudes, latencies, or waveforms under scotopic or photopic conditions. Electro-oculograms (EOGs) showed a reduced light rise in all cases, with a range from 120% to 165%. Hoskin et al. found normal ERGs and EOGs in eight patients, all under the age of 45, at 50% risk of having SFD.[21] Felbor et al. found the ERG to be normal initially in one patient but subnormal four years after presentation with visual loss in one eye.[16] The same authors reported early-onset disease associated with subbnormal ERGs and EOGs. Also reported, albeit in a single-case study, is the finding that the EOG may be affected before the onset of symptoms.[28]

Other studies of patients with central visual loss have demonstrated attenuated ERGs, more marked under scotopic than photopic conditions[24,39] (see figures 67.3 through 67.5). No effect was observed on response implicit time. Clarke et al.[12] have also shown that pattern ERGs (PERGs) are markedly abnormal in most patients with central visual loss (see figures 67.6 and 67.7), but even in the case in which a small central island of vision is preserved, the PERG is significantly reduced.[28] A mouse model of SFD has so far shown normal ERGs throughout life.[39]

Color vision

Both deuteranomaly[18] and tritanomaly[6,7] have been described in different members of British families who are now known to have the same causative mutation. Other families have had normal color vision.[21]

Psychophysics

Dark adaptation is usually abnormal from an early stage in SFD, and the abnormality worsens with age. The rod-cone break is delayed, as is the return to prebleach rod sensitivity.[7,10,16,25,36] The abnormality is worse centrally than peripherally before the onset of central vision loss.[25] A member of one of the original families described by Sorsby, however, showed abnormal but nonprogressive dark adaptation.[28]

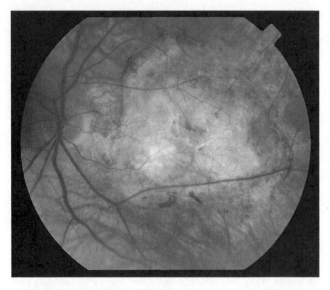

FIGURE 67.1   Left fundus of a patient with SFD showing large disciform scar. (See also color plate 35.)

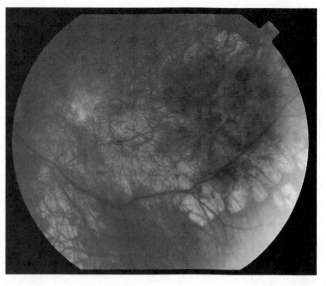

FIGURE 67.2   Left fundus of a patient with SFD showing atrophy of the retinal pigment epithelium and choriocapillaris at the posterior pole. (See also color plate 36.)

Representative Flash ERG's

Male Control, Age 46, LE ERG

Sorsby's Patient DP, Age 52, LE ERG

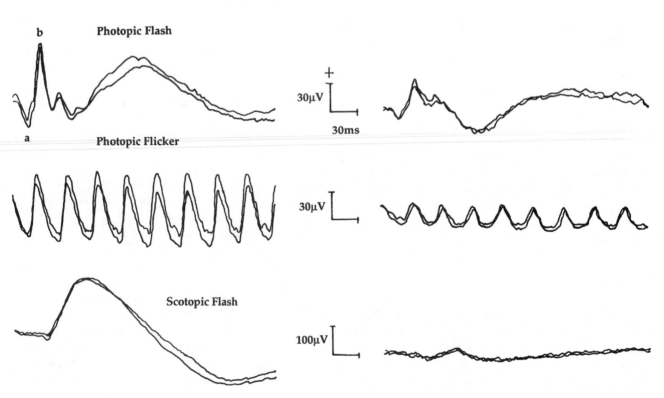

FIGURE 67.3   Representative flash ERGs (elicited to ISCEV ERG Standard 1999) from a male control subject (left) and a similarly aged patient with SFD (right).

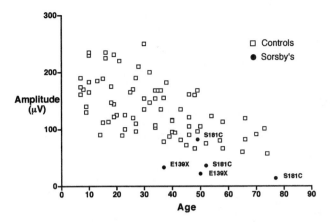

FIGURE 67.4   Scattergram of age versus photopic b-wave amplitude for control subjects and patients with SFD. Each data point for the SFD cases is labeled with the specific gene mutation for that patient.

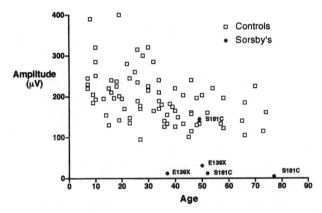

FIGURE 67.5   Scattergram of age versus scotopic b-wave amplitude for control subjects and patients with SFD.

Visual fields

Central and paracentral scotomas have been reported,[19,28] although a tiny central island has been shown to be preserved in one case.[28] These latter authors have also commented that the underreporting of field losses in the literature may misrepresent the nature and extent of such loss in the condition.

Genetics

Inheritance is autosomal-dominant with high penetrance, and males and females are affected equally. The discovery of mutations in the tissue inhibitor of metalloproteinase-3 (TIMP-3) gene in some families labeled as SFD indicated that it was truly a separate disorder[40] and not just the severe end of the spectrum of dominant drusen (also known as Doyne's honeycomb degeneration or malattia Leventinese). Seven mutations have been described in the TIMP-3 gene. All of these mutations are in exon 5, apart from one that is in the intron/exon junction and may cause abnormal splicing of TIMP-3 mRNA.[37] This mutation has been found in a Japanese family and is associated with a later onset of central visual loss.[23] All but one of the mutations in exon 5 cause a cysteine substitution, which is thought to lead to aberrant disulphide bonding that causes oligomerization of the TIMP-3 protein. The exception is the E139X mutation described in a British family, which causes truncation of the TIMP-3 protein.[11]

The TIMP-3 protein is part of a family of metalloproteinase enzyme inhibitors that are involved in the turnover of the extracellular matrix. There are four very similar tissue inhibitors of metalloproteinases (TIMPs)[2] composing a gene family with 12 highly conserved cysteine residues that form six disulphide bridges essential for correct protein folding and function. TIMPs consist of two domains, each stabilized by three disulphide bonds, an amino terminal inhibitory domain through which they bind to an active matrix metalloproteinase, and a carboxy terminal domain that is involved in interactions with proform matrix metalloproteinases and with binding to the extracellular matrix.[26]

Immunohistochemistry of human eyes shows TIMP-3-specific staining in Bruch's membrane, particularly in the basement membranes of retinal pigment epithelial and endothelial cells.[14] The eosinophilic deposit that is seen histologically in eyes with SFD stains for TIMP-3.[13] The mechanism by which mutations in TIMP-3 give rise to retinal disease is not known but is unlikely to be due to loss of TIMP-3 function, as expression studies have shown all known disease causing mutants to be functional metalloproteinase inhibitors.[27] TIMP-3 has antiangiogenic properties in vitro,[1] and overexpression of TIMP-3 in transfected rat retinal pigment epithelium inhibits experimental choroidal neovascularization.[38] TIMP-3 is expressed in subretinal neovascular membranes.[35] TIMP-3 is known to express apoptotic properties when overexpressed in vitro,[4,29] and an alternative mechanism, particularly for the patients with atrophic maculopathy, could be apoptosis of photoreceptor and retinal pigment epithelial cells induced by accumulation of dimerized TIMP-3. The TIMP-3 deposit seen in SFD may represent an insoluble dimerized form of the inhibitor produced by abnormal disulphide bond formation by the mutated protein, which may be associated with elastin.[9] Dimerization of the protein product of S181C, S156C, G166C, and E139X has been demonstrated.[27] One possible mechanism for retinal disease may therefore be impairment of the nutrition and metabolism of the outer retina because of abnormal deposition of dimerized TIMP-3 in Bruch's membrane.

Treatment

Laser treatment has generally been ineffective in controlling subretinal neovascularization in SFD,[20,33] although one study

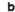

a

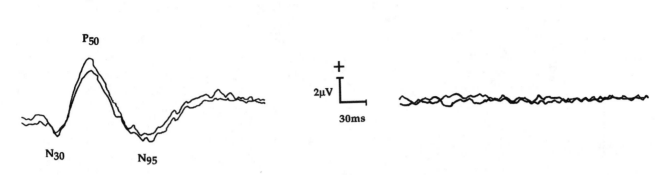

b

FIGURE 67.6 Representative transient PERGs (elicited to ISCEV PERG Standard 2000) to 25′ check size, four reversals per second stimulation. The responses from the left eye of a 48-year-old male control subject (A) and a 52-year-old patient with SFD (B) are shown.

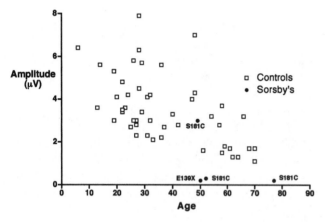

FIGURE 67.7 Scattergram of age versus PERG P50/N95 amplitude for control subjects and patients with SFD.

reported benefit.[8] Jacobson et al. demonstrated reversal of night blindness in SFD by treatment with high-dose vitamin A.[25] Peripheral rod sensitivity returned to normal or near normal, and rod ERGs improved in one patient. The doses that are used, however, are associated with significant side effects, including liver damage and teratogenicity, and the regime is not generally employed in the treatment of SFD.

Relationship to age-related macular degeneration

SFD is of particular interest because the macular lesions closely resemble those seen in age-related macular degeneration (ARMD). Mutations in TIMP-3 have been excluded as causative in ARMD.[15,30] However, the possibility exists that the accumulation of TIMP-3 protein that occurs in Bruch's membrane as part of normal aging may be important in the etiology of ARMD.

Conclusion

It appears that the SFD phenotype arises following a gradual accumulation of TIMP-3 protein over many years. For unknown reasons, presumably related to the biochemistry of the mutant protein, the S156C mutation has an earlier onset of central visual loss, and the splice site mutation seen at the intron4/exon5 junction has a later onset. The EOG seems to be affected early in the course of the disease, which may be expected, as the site of deposition of TIMP-3 is in Bruch's membrane. Dark adaptation appears to be next affected in the time course of the condition, with accompanying and progressive effects on the ERG being observed. The latter seems to be a function of the duration of the disease, indicating a gradual deterioration of photoreceptor function, with rods being affected first.

Color vision and central/paracentral field abnormalities may also be noted in some patients. As macular function becomes compromised, allied effects on the PERG are also to be expected. Further studies of SFD are likely to develop our understanding of the pathogenesis of ARMD.

REFERENCES

1. Anand-Apte B, Pepper M, Voest E, et al: Inhibition of angiogenesis by tissue inhibitor of metalloproteinase-3. *Invest Ophthalmol Vis Sci* 1997; 38(12):2433–2434.
2. Apte S, Olsen B, Murphy G: The gene structure of tissue inhibitor of metalloproteinases (TIMP)-3 and its inhibitory activities define the distinct TIMP gene family. *J Biol Chem* 1995; 270:14313–14318.
3. Ashton N, Sorsby A: Fundus dystrophy with unusual features: A histological study. *Br J Ophthalmol* 1951; 35:751–764.
4. Baker A, Zaltsman A, George S, et al: Divergent effects of tissue inhibitor of metalloproteinase-1, -2, or -3 overexpression on rat vascular smooth muscle cell invasion, proliferation, and death in vitro. *J Clin Invest* 1998; 101(6):1478–1487.

5. Berninger T: Sorsby's fundus syndrome. In Heckenlively JD, Arden GB (eds): *Principles and Practice of Clinical Electrophysiology of Vision.* St. Louis, Mosby Year Book, 1991, pp 705–706.

6. Berninger T, Polkinghorne P, Capon M, Arden G, Bird A: Color vision defect: An early sign of Sorsby retinal dystrophy? [in German]. *Ophthalmologe* 1993; 90(5):515–518.

7. Capon M, Polkinghorne P, Fitzke F, Bird A: Sorsby's pseudoinflammatory macular dystrophy: Sorsby's fundus dystrophies. *Eye* 1988; 2(1):114–122.

8. Carr R, Noble K, Nasaduke I: Hereditary hemorrhagic macular dystrophy. *Am J Ophthalmol* 1978; 85:318.

9. Chong N, Alexander R, Gin T, Bird A, Luthert P: TIMP-3, collagen and elastin immunohistochemistry and histopathology of Sorsby's fundus dystrophy. *Invest Ophthalmol Vis Sci* 2000; 41(3):898–902.

10. Cideciyan A, Pugh EJ, Lamb T, Huang Y, Jacobson S: Rod plateaux during dark adaptation in Sorsby's fundus dystrophy and vitamin A deficiency. *Invest Ophthalmol Vis Sci* 1997; 38(9):1786–1794.

11. Clarke M, Mitchell K, Goodship J, et al: Clinical features of a novel TIMP-3 mutation causing Sorsby's fundus dystrophy: Implications for disease mechanism. *Br J Ophthalmol* 2001; 85:1429–1431.

12. Clarke M, Mitchell K, McDonnell S: Electroretinographic findings in macular dystrophy. *Doc Ophthalmol* 1997; 92:325–339.

13. Fariss R, Apte S, Luthert P, Bird A, Milam A: Accumulation of tissue inhibitor of metalloproteinases-3 in human eyes with Sorsby's fundus dystrophy or retinitis pigmentosa. *Br J Ophthalmol* 1998; 82(11):1329–1334.

14. Fariss R, Apte S, Olsen B, Iwata K, Milam A: Tissue inhibitor of metalloproteinases-3 is a component of Bruch's membrane of the eye. *Am J Pathol* 1997; 150:323–328.

15. Felbor U, Doepner D, Schneider U, Zrenner E, Weber B: Evaluation of the gene encoding the tissue inhibitor of metalloproteinases-3 in various maculopathies. *Invest Ophthalmol Vis Sci* 1997; 38(6):1054–1059.

16. Felbor U, Stohr H, Amann T, Schoherr U, Apfelstedt-Sylla E, Weber B: A second independent Tyr168Cys mutation in the tissue inhibitor of metalloproteinases-3 (TIMP3) in Sorsby's fundus dystrophy. *J Med Genet* 1996; 33:233–236.

17. Felbor U, Stohr H, Amann T, Schoherr U, Weber B: A novel Ser156Cys mutation in the tissue inhibitor of metalloproteinases-3 (TIMP3) in Sorsby's fundus dystrophy with unusual clinical features. *Hum Mol Genet* 1995; 4:2415–2416.

18. Fraser H, Wallace D: To get Sorsby's familial pseudoinflammatory macular dystrophy. *Am J Ophthalmol* 1971; 71:1216–1220.

19. Hamilton W, Ewing C, Elizabeth J, Carruthers J: Sorsby's fundus dystrophy. *Ophthalmology* 1989; 96:1755–1762.

20. Holz F, Haimovici R, Wagner D, Bird A: Recurrent choroidal neovascularisation after laser photocoagulation in Sorsby's fundus dystrophy. *Retina* 1994; 14(4):329–334.

21. Hoskin A, Sehmi K, Bird A: Sorsby's pseudoinflammatory macular dystrophy. *Br J Ophthalmol* 1981; 65:859–865.

22. Iannaccone A: Genotype-phenotype correlations and differential diagnosis in autosomal dominant macular disease. *Doc Ophthalmol* 2001; 102:197–236.

23. Isashiki Y, Tabata Y, Kamimura K, Ohba N: Sorsby's fundus dystrophy in two Japanese families with unusual clinical features. *Jpn J Ophthalmol* 1999; 43(6):472–480.

24. Jacobson S, Cideciyan A, Bennett J, Kingsley R, Sheffield V, Stone E: Novel mutation in the TIMP3 gene causes Sorsby fundus dystrophy. *Arch Ophthalmol* 2002; 120(3):376–379.

25. Jacobson S, Cideciyan A, Regunath G, et al: Night blindness in Sorsby's fundus dystrophy reversed by vitamin A. *Nat Genet* 1995; 11:27–32.

26. Langton K, Barker M, McKie N: Localization of the functional domains of human tissue inhibitor of metalloproteinases-3 and the effect of a Sorsby's fundus dystrophy mutation. *J Biol Chem* 1998; 273(27):16778–16781.

27. Langton K, McKie N, Curtis A, et al: A novel TIMP-3 mutation reveals a common molecular phenotype in Sorsby's fundus dystrophy. *J Biol Chem* 2000; 275(35):27027–27031.

28. Lip P, Good P, Gibson J: Sorsby's fundus dystrophy: A case report of 24 years follow up with electrodiagnostic tests and indocyanine green angiography. *Eye* 1999; 13(1):16–25.

29. Majid M, Smith V, Easty D, Baker A, Newby A: Adenovirus mediated gene delivery of tissue inhibitor of metalloproteinases-3 induces death in retinal pigment epithelial cells. *Br J Ophthalmol* 2002; 86(1):97–101.

30. Paz MDL, Pericak-Vance M, Lennon F, Haines J, Seddon J: Exclusion of TIMP3 as a candidate locus in age-related macular degeneration. *Invest Ophthalmol Vis Sci* 1997; 38(6):1060–1065.

31. Polkinghorne P, Capon M, Berninger T, Lyness A, Sehmi K, Bird A: Sorsby's fundus dystrophy: A clinical study. *Ophthalmology* 1989; 96(12):1763–1768.

32. Scullica L, Falsini B: Diagnosis and classification of macular degenerations: An approach based on retinal function testing. *Doc Ophthalmol* 2001; 102(3):237–250.

33. Seiving P, Boskovich S, Bingham E, Pawar H: Sorsby's fundus dystrophy in a family with a Ser181Cys mutation in the TIMP-3 gene: Poor outcome after laser photocoagulation. *Trans Am Ophthalmol Soc* 1996; 94:275–294.

34. Sorsby A, Mason M: A fundus dystrophy with unusual features. *Br J Ophthalmol* 1949; 33:67–97.

35. Steen B, Sejersen S, Berglin L, Seregard S, Kvanta A: Matrix metalloproteinases and metalloproteinase inhibitors in choroidal neovascular membranes. *Invest Ophthalmol Vis Sci* 1998; 39(11):2194–2200.

36. Steinmetz R, Polkinghorne P, Fitzke F, Kemp C, Bird A: Abnormal dark adaptation and rhodopsin kinetics in Sorsby's fundus dystrophy. *Invest Ophthalmol Vis Sci* 1992; 33(5):1633–1636.

37. Tabata Y, Isashiki Y, Kamimura K, Ohba N: A novel splice site mutation in the tissue inhibitor of metalloproteinases-3 in Sorsby's fundus dystrophy with unusual clinical features. *Hum Genet* 1998; 103:179–182.

38. Takahashi T, Nakamura T, Hayashi A, et al: Inhibition of experimental choroidal neovascularisation by overexpression of tissue inhibitor of metalloproteinases-3 in retinal pigment epithelial cells. *Am J Ophthalmol* 2000; 130:774–781.

39. Weber B, Lin B, White K, et al: A mouse model for Sorsby fundus dystrophy. *Invest Ophthalmol Vis Sci* 2002; 43(8):2732–2740.

40. Weber B, Vogt G, Pruett R, Stohr H, Felbor U: Mutations in the tissue inhibitor of metalloproteinases-3 (TIMP3) in patients with Sorsby's fundus dystrophy. *Nat Genet* 1994; 8:352–356.

XII DISEASES OF THE
OUTER RETINA

68 Choroideremia

IAN M. MACDONALD AND MIGUEL C. SEABRA

CHOROIDEREMIA (CHM, OMIM 303100) is a distinct diagnosis that can be clinically distinguished from other retinal degenerations, such as other forms of retinitis pigmentosa (RP). CHM represents 6% of cases in one practice that focused on RP-related conditions.[10] Mauthner first used the term to indicate that the choroid was missing while the retinal vessels were preserved and no optic atrophy was noted.[14] These characteristics set CHM apart from RP, which has significant pigment dispersion in the retina, retinal vessel narrowing, and optic nerve gliosis. In some cases, patients with CHM have posterior subcapsular cataracts that are also commonly seen in RP. CHM is an ocular disorder with no systemic manifestations. The extensive study of a large Canadian family with CHM by McCulloch and McCulloch in 1948 indisputably showed CHM to be X-linked.[15]

Clinical characteristics

Boys affected by choroideremia begin to recognize difficulty seeing at night during grade school years. The fundus will show signs of retinal pigment epithelial (RPE) mottling throughout the fundus, most marked in the equatorial region. These changes have been identified in boys as young as 3–10 months of age.[12] The findings evolve with progressive loss of choriocapillaris, RPE, and retina in a scalloped fashion with coincident loss in visual field. The chorioretinal atrophy spans the entire peripheral retina, while the anatomy of the central macula remains relatively intact (figure 68.1). In some cases, remnants of normal retina remain near the optic nerve, which shows no gliosis or pallor. Deep choroidal vessels of normal diameter may be seen beyond the areas of chorioretinal atrophy, and the retinal vessels do not show narrowing that marks cases of RP. In a study of 115 patients with CHM from three centers, most patients retained central visual acuity and macular fields until their late sixties.[18] Two cases of subretinal neovascularization have been reported in a CHM male and a carrier.[5]

Female carriers tend to be asymptomatic in their youth and middle years. Testing will demonstrate poor dark adaptation and in some cases defects in the visual field.[12] Many older females will complain of trouble seeing at night. The fundus findings of patchy chorioretinal degeneration in the female begin predominantly in the midperiphery of the fundus (figure 68.2). An intravenous fluorescein angiogram may occasionally be helpful in defining the extent of changes in the female carrier (figure 68.3), demonstrating pigment dispersion and atrophy of the choriocapillaris and RPE beyond what may be seen clinically.[23] In our experience and that of others, these findings are slowly progressive and are not limited to the midperipheral fundus but may be seen with careful examination around the disk and in the macula.[6] Occasionally, young female carriers may demonstrate a disorder as severe as the affected male, presumably as a result of lyonization.[7,9]

Electrophysiology

The electroretinogram (ERG) of an affected male may be nonrecordable but, early in the disorder, will mimic that of a patient with RP and is not specifically diagnostic. A certain amount of variability is seen in the ERG within families and between families affected by CHM. The ERG is frequently normal in a carrier of CHM despite a disproportionate degree of RPE mottling. By comparison, the ERG of a carrier of X-linked RP is frequently abnormal and minimal changes are seen with fundus examination.[1] Sieving and colleagues showed that of the ERG responses to three stimuli—a dim blue flash, a dark-adapted white flash, or a flickering stimulus—not one response consistently predicted carrier status of CHM.[22] Over a 10-year interval, they recorded a decrease in the ERG amplitudes in two CHM carriers, suggesting progressive loss of function. The electro-oculogram is not usually helpful to assess patients with CHM. Female carriers show a decrease in the Arden ratio with age, perhaps again consistent with the slow but progressive nature of the disorder.[17] The visual field is a more practical clinical parameter than the ERG to monitor the function of a CHM patient over time.

Differential diagnosis

The end stage of CHM should not be confused with X-linked RP. In general, CHM does not show the degree of pigment migration into the retina that is seen in RP. Signs in a carrier female within the family that are consistent with CHM will help to differentiate the two diagnoses. Cystoid macular edema that is found occasionally in patients with X-linked RP has not been identified in patients with CHM.[10]

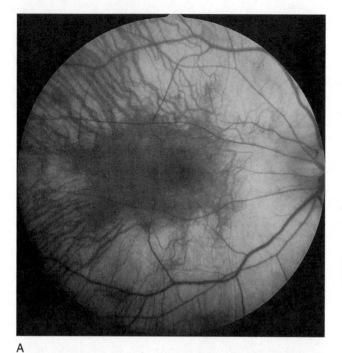

A

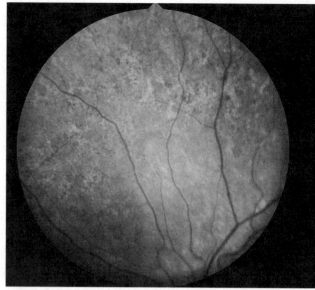

FIGURE 68.2   Fundus photograph (nasal midperiphery) of a 29-year-old female carrier with patchy RPE changes. Vision: 20/20 OS. (See also color plate 38.)

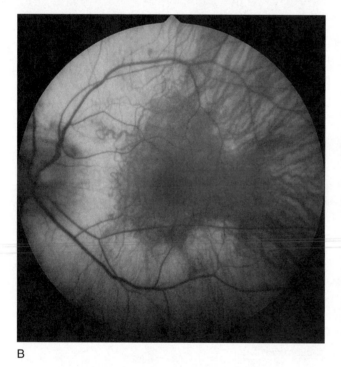

B

FIGURE 68.1   Fundus photographs of a 17-year-old CHM affected male showing preserved deep choroidal vessels and central macula, normal-appearing retinal vessels and optic nerve, and no pigment dispersion. A, OD. B, OS. Vision: 20/20 OU. (See also color plate 37.)

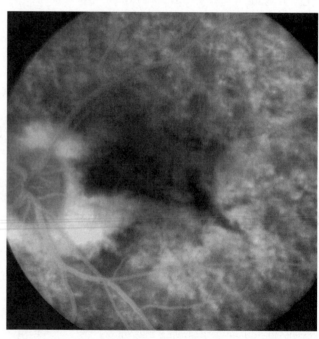

FIGURE 68.3   Intravenous fluorescein angiogram in a 34-year-old female carrier with areas of RPE and pigment disruption. Vision: 20/30 OS.

An association between CHM and deafness is rare and is due to a contiguous gene syndrome that results from the deletion of both the CHM gene and a gene for deafness, DFN3.[16] Some cases of CHM and deafness could be confused with Usher syndrome. Usher syndrome is an autosomal-recessively inherited RP-related disorder with varying degrees of hearing impairment. The fundus of Usher syndrome does not show the distinct pattern of retinal degeneration that is typical of CHM.

Gyrate atrophy is often referenced as one of the disorders that might be confused with CHM. Gyrate atrophy is an autosomal-recessive metabolic disorder in which mutations in the gene for ornithine aminotransferase result in hyperornithinemia. The fundus of patients with gyrate atrophy and the progressive nature of the associated retinal degeneration could suggest CHM, but in general, the RPE in gyrate atrophy tends to be more hyperpigmental than that in CHM. The fundus of a patient with gyrate atrophy has bilateral midperipheral and peripheral areas of scalloped coalescent loss of retina, RPE, and choriocapillaris.[11]

Gene function

The CHM gene was identified by Cremers and colleagues, using a positional cloning strategy.[3] The function of the gene was later revealed by Seabra and colleagues, who showed that the gene was homologous to component A of Rab geranylgeranyl transferase, now termed Rab escort protein-1 (REP-1).[20] REP-1 functions in the prenylation of Rab GTPases by the covalent addition of 20-carbon geranylgeranyl units. Lymphocytes from patients with CHM show a marked inability to prenylate Rab proteins, in particular Rab27a.[19,21] Rab proteins play a role in organelle formation and the trafficking of vesicles in exocytic and endocytic pathways. To date, all mutations and deletions of the CHM gene result in truncation of the gene product, resulting in its functional loss or absence. This fact allows the confirmation of the clinical diagnosis by noting the absence of REP-1 with immunoblot analysis of protein from peripheral white blood cells of affected males.[13] As all mutations create the same effect, helpful genotype-phenotype correlations cannot be found in our experience and that of others.[8]

The absence of REP-1 in CHM and its relationship to the pathophysiology of the disorder remain to be determined. Another protein, REP-2, encoded by the CHM-like gene, may not function sufficiently in the eye to compensate for the lack of REP-1.[2] No effective treatment has been found for choroideremia. Nutritional approaches may have some benefit as, for example, dietary supplementation with lutein to protect residual macular function.[4]

ACKNOWLEDGMENTS The authors thank Bernd Schwanke, Holly Ridyard, and Dr. Deborah Carper for their technical and editorial assistance.

REFERENCES

1. Berson EL, Rosen JB, Simonoff EA: Electroretinographic testing as an aid in detection of carriers of X-chromosome-linked retinitis pigmentosa. *Am J Ophthalmol* 1979; 87:460–468.

2. Cremers FP, Molloy CM, van de Pol DJ, van den Hurk JA, Bach I, Geurts van Kessel AH, Ropers HH: An autosomal homologue of the choroideremia gene colocalizes with the Usher syndrome type II locus on the distal part of chromosome 1q. *Hum Mol Genet* 1992; 1:71–75.

3. Cremers FP, van de Pol DJ, van Kerkhoff LP, Wieringa B, Ropers HH: Cloning of a gene that is rearranged in patients with choroideraemia. *Nature* 1990; 347:674–677.

4. Duncan JL, Aleman TS, Gardner LM, De Castro E, Marks DA, Emmons JM, Bieber ML, Steinberg JD, Bennett J, Stone EM, MacDonald IM, Cideciyan AV, Maguire MG, Jacobson SG: Macular pigment and lutein supplementation in choroideremia. *Exp Eye Res* 2002; 74:371–381.

5. Endo K, Yuzawa M, Ohba N: Choroideremia associated with subretinal neovascular membrane. *Acta Ophthalmol Scand* 2000; 78:483–486.

6. Forsius H, Hyvärinen L, Nieminen H, Flower R: Fluorescein and indocyanine green fluorescence angiography in study of affected males and in female carriers with choroidermia: A preliminary report. *Acta Ophthalmol (Copenh)* 1977; 55:459–470.

7. Fraser GR, Friedmann AI: Choroideremia in a female. *Brit Med J* 1968; 2:732–734.

8. Fujiki K, Hotta Y, Hayakawa M, Saito A, Mashima Y, Mori M, Yoshii M, Murakami A, Matsumoto M, Hayasaka S, Tagami N, Isashiki Y, Ohba N, Kanai A: REP-1 gene mutations in Japanese patients with choroideremia. *Graefes Arch Clin Exp Ophthalmol* 1999; 237:735–740.

9. Harris GS, Miller JR: Choroideremia: Visual defects in a heterozygote. *Arch Ophthalmol* 1968; 80:423–429.

10. Heckenlively JR: Choroideremia. In Heckenlively JR, Arden GB (eds): *Principles and Practice of Electrophysiology of Vision*. St. Louis, Mosby, 1991, pp 659–663.

11. Kaiser-Kupfer MI, Ludwig IH, de Monasterio FM, Valle D, Krieger I: Gyrate atrophy of the choroid and retina: Early findings. *Ophthalmology* 1985; 92:394–401.

12. Karna J: Choroideremia: A clinical and genetic study of 84 Finnish patients and 126 female carriers. *Acta Ophthalmol Suppl* 1986; 176:1–68.

13. MacDonald IM, Mah DY, Ho YK, Lewis RA, Seabra MC: A practical diagnostic test for choroideremia. *Ophthalmology* 1998; 105:1637–1640.

14. Mauthner L: Ein Fall von Choideremia. *Berd Naturw Med Ver Innsbruck* 1871; 2:191.

15. McCulloch C, McCulloch RPJ: A hereditary and clinical study of choroideremia. *Trans Am Acad Ophthalmol Otolaryngol* 1948; 542:160–190.

16. Merry DE, Lesko JG, Sosnoski DM, Lewis RA, Lubinsky M, Trask B, van den Engh G, Collins FS, Nussbaum RL: Choroideremia and deafness with stapes fixation: A contiguous gene deletion syndrome in Xq21. *Am J Hum Genet* 1989; 45:530–540.

17. Pinckers A, van Aarem A, Brink H: The electrooculogram in heterozygote carriers of Usher syndrome, retinitis pigmentosa, neuronal ceroid lipofuscinosis, Senior syndrome and choroideremia. *Ophthalmic Genet* 1994; 15:25–30.

18. Roberts MF, Fishman GA, Roberts DK, Heckenlively JR, Weleber RG, Anderson RJ, Grover S: Retrospective,

longitudinal, and cross sectional study of visual acuity impairment in choroideraemia. *Br J Ophthalmol* 2002; 86:658–662.

19. Seabra MC, Brown MS, Goldstein JL: Retinal degeneration in choroideremia: Deficiency of rab geranylgeranyl transferase. *Science* 1993; 259:377–381.

20. Seabra MC, Brown MS, Slaughter CA, Südhof TC, Goldstein JL: Purification of component A of Rab geranylgeranyl transferase: Possible identity with the choroideremia gene product. *Cell* 1992; 70:1049–1057.

21. Seabra MC, Ho YK, Anant JS: Deficient geranylgeranylation of Ram/Rab27 in choroideremia. *J Biol Chem* 1995; 270:24420–24427.

22. Sieving PA, Niffenegger JH, Berson EL: Electroretinographic findings in selected pedigrees with choroideremia. *Am J Ophthalmol* 1986; 101:361–367.

23. van Dorp DB, van Balen AT: Fluorescein angiography in potential carriers for choroideremia: An additional aid for final diagnosis, when funduscopy shows equivocal symptoms. *Ophthalmic Paediatr Genet* 1985; 5:25–30.

69 Retinitis Pigmentosa

DAVID G. BIRCH

PIGMENTARY RETINAL degeneration, as seen through the ophthalmoscope, was first described by van Trigt in 1853 and named retinitis pigmentosa by Donders in the Netherlands.[40] The term *retinitis pigmentosa (RP)* has traditionally included a group of hereditary retinal degenerations with characteristic features. These features include night blindness, progressive field constriction with relative preservation of macular function, and pigmentary disturbances within the posterior pole (figure 69.1). The prevalence of RP in different countries varies from one in 3000 to one in 4000 individuals.[100] The number of affected individuals in the United States is estimated to be between 50,000 and 100,000. Approximately 20% of these cases are autosomal-dominant, 10% are X-linked, 20% are autosomal-recessive, and the remainder are isolated (simplex RP; no known family history).[30] Most patients with RP are nonsyndromic; that is, they do not have any other associated systemic disease. The most common exception is Usher syndrome, which accounts for approximately 10–15% of RP and is associated with either profound (Type I), partial (Type II), or, extremely rarely, progressive (Type III) hearing loss. Other syndromic conditions with associated RP include Bassen-Kornzweig syndrome (abetalipoproteinemia), Refsum disease, Laurence-Moon-Bardet-Biedl syndrome, neuronal ceroid lipofuscinosis (Batten disease), Alström disease, and Kearns-Sayre syndrome.

The term *retinitis pigmentosa* has been retained for historical reasons even though it is merely descriptive and inappropriate, since it implies an inflammatory condition. In fact, this descriptive term for the entire category of diseases will gradually be replaced by specific mechanistic disease names reflecting the disease-causing mutation. At the present time, we have a transitional situation, in which we are still trying to force patients into descriptive categories such as retinitis pigmentosa, cone-rod dystrophy, and pattern dystrophy. In many cases, the fits do not work, and even within a single family with a RDS-peripherin mutation, for example, we may find individuals with different "diagnoses."[64,112] As knowledge evolves, it will become increasingly more informative to describe patients with names related to their mutations, such as RP1 or RDS/peripherin, than just RP. When the specific mutation is known, the patient can be counseled more accurately with respect to rate of progression. The number of known locations and specific cloned genes is constantly growing (see http://www.sph.uth.tmc.edu/retnet). In the summary that follows, the current state of knowledge with regard to genes that cause retinitis pigmentosa will be presented. In the second part of the chapter, a summary will be given of some of the ERG protocols that are available for characterizing phenotype. It should become clear that one current challenge is to broaden the scope of the ERG and ancillary functional techniques to enrich the description of phenotype.

Genetic analysis of retinitis pigmentosa

Because the eye is readily accessible, retinal disorders have played an important role in the development of mammalian genetics.[12] The first autosomal-dominant pedigree in human genetics to be fully documented involved the descendents of Jean Nougaret (1637–1719), a French butcher who had congenital stationary night blindness (CSNB). The first mammalian genetic linkage, by Haldane in 1915, was between the mouse pink-eye dilute and albino loci.[12]

The first mapped gene for RP was RP2, a gene for X-linked retinitis pigmentosa (XlRP) that maps to Xp11.[13] Subsequently, one form of adRP was mapped to 3q.[79] Shortly thereafter, the 3q form of adRP was shown to be caused by mutations in rhodopsin.[41,44] Since then, additional genes causing adRP have been mapped to 6p, 7p, 8q, 17p, and 18q. Of these, the gene on 6p has been identified as the gene for peripherin; RP1 on 8q has been identified as a photoreceptor-specific protein of unknown function but with similarity over a short region to doublecortin.[26] AdRP can also result from mutations in developmental regulatory genes such as *NRL*, a neural lucine zipper.[115] Autosomal-dominant cone-rod dystrophy (CORD2) results from mutations in *CRX*, a cone-rod otx-like photoreceptor transcription factor.[46,47,102,107] Linkage analysis suggests that there are at least four additional genes for XlRP.[48,53,83,88] The RP GTPase regulator (*RPGR*) gene maps to Xp21.1[80] and is responsible for RP3, the most common form of XlRP. A rare form of XlRP (RP24) maps to Xq26–27.[48] Autosomal-recessive RP may be caused by mutations in any of a number of genes, including rhodopsin;[99] *PDE6B*, which maps to 4p;[77] the rod cGMP-gated channel (*CNGA1*), which also maps to 4p;[76] *PDE6A*, which maps to 5q;[42] *TULP1*, which maps to 6p;[52] and *RLBP1*, cellular retinaldehyde–binding protein, which maps to 15q.[81] Table 69.1, modified from a table in

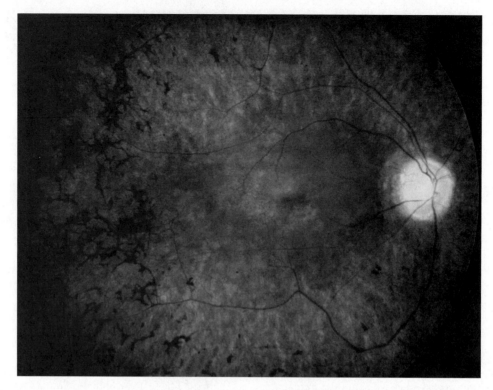

FIGURE 69.1   Fundus photograph showing the posterior pole of a 42-year-old patient with XlRP. Note the "waxy disk," the attenuated retinal vessels, and the bone spicule–like pigmentary deposits throughout the midperiphery. (See also color plate 39.)

TABLE 69.1

Genes and loci for retinitis pigmentosa

Protein	Gene	Locus	Inheritance
RPE65	*RPE65*	1p31	AR
RP18		1q13–q23	AD
Crumbs homolog	*CRB1*	1q31–q32.1	AR
RP23		2p11–p16	AR
c-mer receptor tyrosine kinase	*MERTK*	2q14.1	AR
RP26		2q31–q33	AR
Rhodopsin	*RHO*	3q21–q24	AD
Prominin (mouse)–like-1	*PROML1*	4p	AR
cGMP phosphodiesterase-β	*PDEβ*	4p16.3	AR
cGMP gated channel protein	*CNGCa*	4p14–q13	AR
cGMP phosphodiesterase-α	*PDEa*	5q31.2–qter	AR
RP29		4q32–q34	AR
Peripherin-RDS	*RDS*	6p21.1	AD digenic
Tubby-like protein	*TULP1*	6p21.3	AR
RP25		6cen–q15	AR
RP9		7p15–p13	AD
RP10		7q31.3	AD
RP1 protein	*RP1*	8p11–q21	AD
Rod outer membrane protein-1	*ROM1*	11q13	Digenic
Neural retina leucine zipper	*NRL*	14q11.1–12.1	AD
Retinaldehyde-binding protein	*RLBP1*	15q26	AR
RP22		16p12.1–p12.3	AR
RP13		17p13.3	AD
RP17		17q22	AD
RP11		19q13.4	AD
RP23		Xp22	XL
RP6		Xp21.3–p21.2	XL
RP GTPase regulator	*RGPR (RP3)*	Xp21	XL
RP2 protein	*RP2*	Xp11.3–p11.2	XL
RP24		Xq26–q27	XL

AD, autosomal-dominant; *AR*, autosomal-recessive; *cGMP*, cyclic guanine monophosphat; *XL*, X-linked.

Bessant et al.,[12] provides a list of genes and chromosomal loci known to cause retinitis pigmentosa.

Considerable progress has been made recently in determining the phenotype and mechanisms of functional loss for mutations that are primarily structural. Approximately 30–40% of all adRP cases are caused by rhodopsin mutations. Rhodopsin plays both a structural role as the most abundant outer segment protein and a functional role as the chromophore and initiator of the phototransduction cascade. Consequently, rhodopsin mutations produce a spectrum of clinical phenotypes, including type 1 adRP, type 2 adRP, sector adRP, and autosomal-dominant congenital stationary night blindness. In addition, rhodopsin mutations have been shown to be the cause of approximately 2% of recessive cases of RP.[99] The second most common gene known to cause adRP is peripherin/*RDS*, the human homolog of the gene that was first identified and isolated as the cause of mouse "retinal degeneration slow" (rds).[36,110] The *rds* gene encodes an integral membrane glycoprotein located in outer segment discs.[3] Rod outer segment protein 1 (*ROM1*) has a similar predicted secondary structure and the same outer segment distribution as peripherin/*RDS*.[5] Although the function of peripherin/*RDS* and *ROM1* have not been firmly established, there is indirect evidence that they may be members of a new class of adhesion proteins that stabilize the rims of outer segment disks through homophilic and/or heterophilic interactions across the intradiscal space.[5,49,109] In particular, these interactions may involve residues within their highly conserved extracellular (intradiscal) D2 loops. The clinical phenotypes include adRP, dominant retinitis punctata albescens, dominant butterfly-shaped pigment dystrophy of the fovea, and autosomal-dominant macular degeneration. That peripherin/*RDS* mutation can cause either RP and/or macular degeneration is consistent with the observation that the protein is expressed in both rods and cones, though its exact functional role in each photoreceptor must be different. Arg-172-Trp mutations, for example, cause cone degeneration but appear to have no deleterious effects on rods.[114] Finally, there is digenic RP[66] that results from a combination of one mutation in peripherin/*RDS* and one in *ROM1*. Neither mutation alone in a heterozygote causes clinically significant degeneration.

Several approaches are available for studying mechanisms by which specific mutations lead to rod cell functional abnormalities and eventual death. Mutant opsins have been grouped on the basis of their behavior in tissue culture cells.[105] Class I mutants had characteristics similar to those of wild-type rhodopsin. For example, their absorbance spectrum was normal, and transport from the endoplasmic reticulum (ER) to the plasma membrane was apparently successful. Class II mutants differed substantially from the wild-type. Their absorbance was 1–5% of wild-type levels,

their glycosylation patterns were abnormal, and transport of the proteins to the plasma membrane was not successful. Some of these proteins failed to leave the ER at all (Class IIa), while others were found equally distributed between the ER and the plasma membrane (Class IIb). However, the behavior of mutations in model systems must be compared to their action in vivo and ultimately in human patients, in whom the consequences are not always predictable. Transgenic mouse technology offers one in vivo system for studying the action of mutant genes. Among the many transgenic lines available are those expressing P23H, Q344X, K296E, and P347S rhodopsin mutations; P216L and L185P peripherin/RDS mutations; rom1 knock-outs; and rhodopsin knock-outs. Differences in vitro and in vivo are seen, for example, with the Q344X rhodopsin mutation. In vivo studies show increased retention in the cell body,[106] whereas in culture, Q344X is a Class I mutant that is efficiently transported to the cell membrane. The P23H rhodopsin mutation is a Class II mutant in culture,[105] but the mutant protein is present in the outer segment of the transgenic mouse.[87] The mutant protein reduces the gain of transducin activation in patients[22] but apparently not early in degeneration for the VPP transgenic mouse expressing the P23H mutation.[50] The K296E mutant activates transducin independent of light in vitro[97] but is phosphorylated and stably bound to arrestin in the transgenic mouse.[73]

In both human RP and mouse models of RP due to mutations in genes specific to rods, it is nevertheless the case that the loss of rod photoreceptors is accompanied by the gradual degeneration of cones. Photoreceptor loss occurs primarily through programmed cell death (apoptosis).[96] It appears that degenerating photoreceptors induce apoptosis in initially healthy neighboring cells,[63] and there is an accumulating body of evidence that neuroprotective factors may be capable of rescuing photoreceptors from this fate.[72]

MUTATIONS AFFECTING THE PHOTOTRANSDUCTION CASCADE
Whereas many of the negative effects of dominantly inherited mutations appear to be due to the effect on structural proteins, it is clear that the mutations that cause recessive forms of RP tend to involve either phototransduction or the visual cycle. Processes underlying activation and recovery in vertebrate rods are now understood in great detail. During the excitation phase of the rod photoresponse, light stimulates an enzymatic cascade that culminates in the hydrolysis of cyclic GMP.[68,104] The interaction of excited rhodopsin (R*) with many G-protein molecules (transducin) causes each of them to release GDP and bind GTP. Transducin-GTP then activates cGMP phosphodiesterase (PDE), which hydrolyzes cGMP to 5'-GMP. The drop in cGMP caused by PDE activation causes closure of channels held open by cGMP in darkness, halting the continuous entry of Na^+ and Ca^{2+} ions, and results in a transient hyperpolarization of the cell. Several

processes contribute to the recovery phase of the photoresponse. First, photolyzed rhodopsin is phosphorylated by rhodopsin kinase, which decreases the ability of R* to stimulate transducin. It also stimulates the binding of arrestin to the photolyzed rhodopsin, further reducing its ability to activate transducin. Activated transducin α subunits (Tα) already formed by photolyzed rhodopsin deactivate when their bound GTP is hydrolyzed to GDP. GTP hydrolysis appears to be modulated by the RGS-9.[31,54] Tα-GDP then reassociates with Tβγ and releases the PDEγ subunit, which reinhibits PDE activity. Light-stimulated hydrolysis of cGMP within rod photoreceptors reduces the activity of cGMP-gated cation channels in the photoreceptor plasma membrane. Because these channels are the major route by which Ca^{2+} enters the photoreceptor, the intracellular concentration of Ca^{2+} falls. Lowered Ca^{2+} levels stimulate the activity of guanylate cyclase, which then accelerates cGMP resynthesis and the restoration of the dark conductance.

It is clear that rod photoreceptors in many warm-blooded animals, including rats, rabbits, cows, monkeys,[84,108] and humans,[59] show the same kind of background adaptation once thought to be characteristic of lower vertebrates. Flashes superimposed on a steady background become smaller and more rapid than in the dark, with a pronounced shortening in the time to peak photoresponse.[7,43,86] The flash sensitivity, defined as the change in current per photon absorbed, declines linearly with log increases in background intensity. During recovery in the dark following bright light exposure, sensitivity remains low (bleaching adaptation) as long as naked opsin is still present. Recent evidence suggests that the underlying mechanism may be similar to background adaptation.[35,37] At this time, it is not clear where in the photoreceptor enzymatic cascade adaptation occurs, but there is evidence that it may occur at almost any step. It probably does not occur in the initial kinetics of transducin activation[6,59,70,92] (but see Jones[65] and Lagnado and Baylor[69]). However, adaptation could influence the duration of transducin activation, the turnoff of activated PDE or channel sensitivity. A large body of evidence suggests that the drop in cytoplasmic Ca^{2+} caused by channel closing activates a negative feedback loop by stimulating guanylate cyclase and cGMP recovery.[104] Thus, the decrease in cytoplasmic calcium may be crucial in regulating the adaptation of the photoresponse.[78,93]

MUTATIONS AFFECTING THE VISUAL CYCLE   The first step in rod vision is the absorption of a photon by rhodopsin in the rod outer segment. This leads to the 11-*cis* to all-*trans* isomerization of the retinaldehyde chromophore. Before light sensitivity can be regained through the regeneration of rhodopsin, the all-*trans*-retinaldehyde must dissociate from the opsin apoprotein and reisomerize to 11-*cis*-retinaldehyde. This process, known as the visual cycle, is well under-stood in the rods.[25,39,94] Following photoisomerization and reduction by all-*trans*-retinal dehydrogenase, the resulting all-*trans*-retinol is translocated across the extracellular space from the rod outer segment to the RPE. It is reisomerized to 11-*cis*-retinol in a two-step process involving synthesis of a fatty-acyl ester by lecithin-retinol acyltransferase and ester hydrolysis coupled energetically to *trans*-to-*cis* isomerization by isomerohydrolase. Finally, 11-*cis*-retinol is oxidized to 11-*cis*-retinal by 11-*cis*-retinol dehydrogenase in RPE cells. The 11-*cis*-retinal moves back to the rod outer segments, where it combines with opsin to form rhodopsin.

Only recently has it become apparent that mutations in genes encoding components of the visual cycle can lead to retinal disease. Mutations in the gene for *RPE65*, which has been proposed as the isomerohydrolase in the RPE for the *trans*-to-*cis* isomerization,[95] lead to a form of Leber congenital amaurosis.[82] Mutations in *ABCR*, which encodes a rod disk rim transporter for retinal,[4,113] cause Stargardt disease,[1] and recessive CRD[23,38] and may be risk factors for age-related macular degeneration.[2] Mutations in *RDH5*, the gene that encodes NAD/NADP-dependent 11-*cis*-retinol dehydrogenase, are associated with fundus albipunctatus.[116]

ERG measures of retinal function in retinitis pigmentosa

The preceding brief review illustrates the dramatic progress that has been made in molecular biology relating to retinitis pigmentosa over the past 20 years. To adequately characterize phenotype, it is necessary to conduct tests that reflect properties of photoreceptor structure, phototransduction, the visual cycle, and adaptation. Many of the properties can be assesses by evolving ERG protocols. These protocols can be applied to patients with retinitis pigmentosa to reveal mechanisms of photoreceptor degeneration and guide the search for disease-causing mutations.

ISCEV STANDARD PROTOCOL   Representative ERGs from a normal subject are shown in figure 69.2. The responses shown are those of the ISCEV (International Society for Clinical Electrophysiology and Vision) standard protocol.[75] The ISCEV standard prescribes a standard stimulus of $1-3\,cd\,s/m^2$ and recording guidelines so that ERGs can be compared and interpreted across different clinics worldwide. The standard provides a core of key responses for comparison. The standard is not intended to be a comprehensive protocol; indeed, clinics are expected to expand the protocol as appropriate for the particular disease under consideration. Examples of expansions of the protocol for RP will be shown in subsequent sections.

Each ERG clinic needs to establish upper and lower limits of normal. Generally, this is done by recruiting and testing normal subjects of different ages. Although there is no

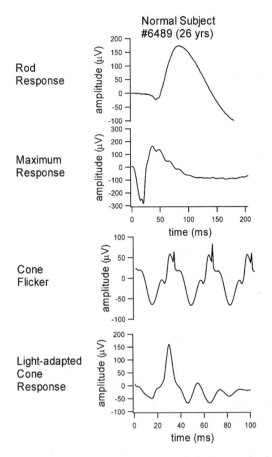

Rod
Response

Maximum
Response

Cone
Flicker

Light-adapted
Cone
Response

FIGURE 69.2 ISCEV standard responses from a normal subject. Spikes superimposed on the cone flicker (31 Hz) indicate the stimulus flash.

"right" number, 100 is probably a reasonable target number so that age trends can be identified. Generally, amplitudes are converted to log values because these more closely approximate a normal distribution.[11,15] It is then possible to determine the upper and limits of normal (typically with $p < .05$) from the mean and standard deviation of this distribution example. These normal limits can also be adjusted for age. Figure 69.3, for example, shows the age-related variation in rod amplitude (figure 69.3A) and in cone ERG amplitude to 30-Hz flicker (figure 69.3B). Much of the decline in sensitivity with age appears to originate at the photoreceptor level.[24]

Examples of ISCEV protocol responses from patients with different forms of RP are shown in figure 69.4. These examples are chosen to illustrate some very broad generalizations. One is that rod ERG responses are severely attenuated at an early age. An exception to this generalization can occur in some types of adRP mutation, where individuals can retain rod responses well into adulthood. XlRP tends to be the most severe form, with severe attenuation of both rod and cone responses by the teenage years. Patients with cone-rod dystrophy tend to have low acuity owing to macular involvement and cone ERG loss that is equal to or greater than rod ERG loss. Leber congenital amaurosis is characterized by severe loss of retinal function at or soon after birth. Note that a consistent finding in virtually all kinds of RP and allied retinal degenerations is the delay in cone b-wave implicit time.[9] The upper limit ($p < .05$) of cone b-wave implicit time to 30-Hz flicker is slightly less than 33.3 ms (one

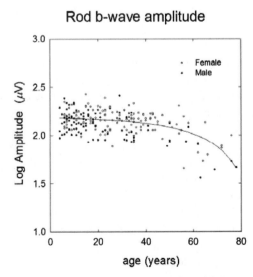

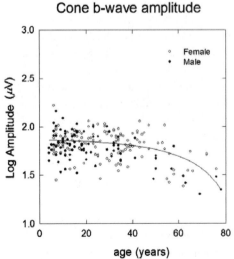

FIGURE 69.3 Variation in log amplitude with age. Left, Rod response. Solid curve is best-fit exponential with half amplitude at age 69 years. Right, Cone response to 31-Hz flicker. Solid curve is best-fit exponential with half-amplitude at age 70 years. Open circles indicate female; solid circles indicate male. (From Birch DG, Anderson JL.[15])

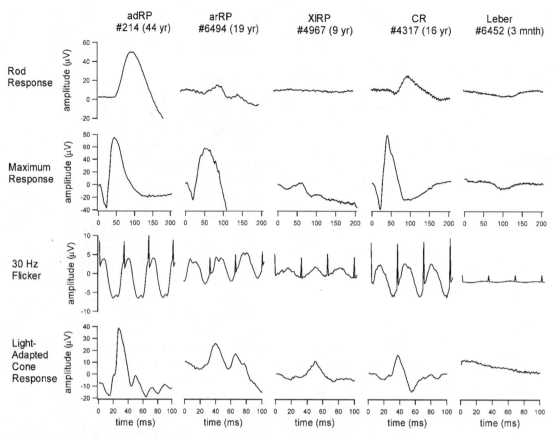

FIGURE 69.4 ISCEV standard ERG responses in selected patients with retinitis pigmentosa. All show reduced rod responses and reduced and delayed cone responses. (See text for details.)

cycle). The spikes superimposed on the flicker responses indicate each flash (cycle). Thus, responses that peak to the right of the spike are delayed well beyond the normal upper limit of cone b-wave implicit time. Despite considerable attention over the past 20 years, the cause of these delays is still not understood completely. A small portion of the delay originates in the cone photoreceptors, which typically have reduced sensitivity in their response to light.[61] This reduction in gain will be reflected in the b-wave as an increase in implicit time, but the magnitude should be on the order of 2–3 ms rather than the 10–15 ms that is often found. Abnormal rod-cone interactions have also been proposed as the source of the delay, since rods act to speed up cones in normal subjects.[21]

SENSITIVITY OF FULL-FIELD ERG   One of the key questions concerning the full-field ERG in diagnostic use involves the sensitivity of the test. How confident can we be, for example, that an individual with a normal ERG will never develop RP? Traditionally, it has been difficult to answer this question, since patients receiving ERGs tend to have prior clinical evidence of RP. In those rare reports of attempts to rule out disease in asymptomatic family members, there are few

reported assessments of accuracy from following the status of the individuals later in life. ERG testing of asymptomatic individuals is usually performed in XlRP or adRP pedigrees. In the case of XlRP, the ERG seems to be abnormal in virtually all infants and children. This is particularly important, since we can readily identify carriers of the XlRP gene through either clinical exam[45] or full-field ERG.[10] These women are often eager to have their sons tested at an early age. We tested and followed a group of 14 at-risk males with full-field pupillometric measures and ERGs. The nine who subsequently were diagnosed with XlRP had elevated pupil thresholds as infants, and all had reduced amplitudes and delayed b-wave implicit times when first tested with the ERG at age 5. Five of the infants with normal test results did not subsequently show any evidence of XlRP. Subsequently, we have tested 106 boys with a subsequently-confirmed diagnosis of XlRP. Only two (1.8%) showed full-field ERG amplitudes within the normal range and none had normal cone implicit time.

Our ability to determine the prognostic value of the full-field ERG has also been changed by the molecular revolution, which has provided a gold standard for evaluating the sensitivity of the ERG in families where the disease-

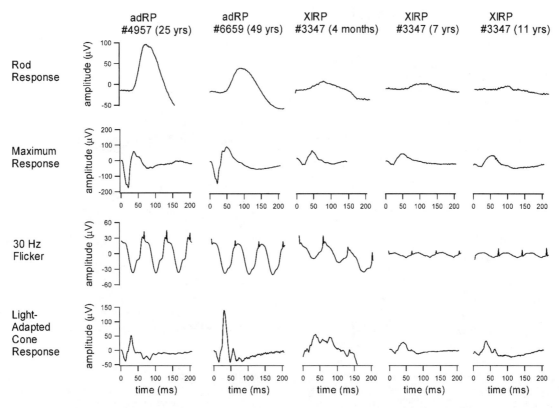

FIGURE 69.5   ISCEV standard ERG responses in selected patients with retinitis pigmentosa. The first two columns show responses from patients with adRP and known mutations retaining normal (#4957) or near-normal (#6659) responses. The final three columns are from a patient with XlRP followed over 11 years. Soon after birth, rod and cone responses were within the normal range for this age. By 7 years, rod and cone responses were small and delayed.

associated gene is known. Particularly in families with adRP, DNA samples can be obtained at the time of the ERG to determine the presence or absence of a mutation. The vast majority of affected infants show abnormal full-field ERG responses on their initial visit, but very occasionally, we encounter normal responses in a young patient with a mutation that is thought to be disease-causing. Examples of both normal and reduced ISCEV standard ERGs from select patients with RP are shown in figure 69.5. The examples of ERGs within the normal range should provide ample evidence of the caution that must be exercised in interpreting results, especially from young family members.

Extensions of the ISCEV ERG protocol

AMPLITUDE-RETINAL ILLUMINANCE FUNCTIONS   The ISCEV standard rod response is elicited by a retinal illuminance lying at the upper end of the linear range of the b-wave amplitude-retinal illuminance function. Either a change in effective light energy (neutral density effect) or a change in the response per unit energy (response compression) can produce a reduction in amplitude. These alternatives can be distinguished by recording responses to a range of retinal illuminances and plotting the amplitude-retinal illuminance relationship.

Responses to an extended range of retinal illuminances are shown in figure 69.6 for a normal subject and a patient with retinitis pigmentosa. At high retinal illuminances, responses to short-wavelength flashes include a small cone component. The amplitude of this cone component can be determined from the matched cone responses to long-wavelength stimuli and subtracted to obtain the actual rod amplitude. Corresponding rod peak-to-peak amplitudes are plotted as a function of retinal illuminance in figure 69.7. The solid curve is the best fit of the saturating exponential relationship attributed to Michaelis and Menton in chemistry and first used by Naka and Rushton[85] to describe intracellular responses to light. The curve plots

$$\frac{V}{V_{\max}} = \frac{I^n}{I^n + k^n}$$

where V = rod peak-to-peak amplitude, $V_{\max}$ = maximum rod amplitude, I = retinal illuminance, k = retinal illuminance at half-amplitude, and n is an exponent describing the slope of the function. In most normal subjects and patients, n is roughly equal to 1.0.[18] Therefore, an abnormality in rod

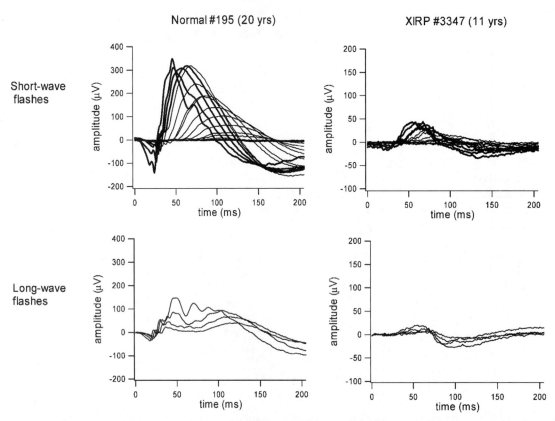

Normal #195 (20 yrs)

XlRP #3347 (11 yrs)

Short-wave flashes

Long-wave flashes

FIGURE 69.6   Full-field ERGs obtained over an extended series of retinal illuminances in a normal subject and a patient with XlRP. Upper panels show responses to short-wave stimuli; lower panels show responses to long-wave stimuli matched photometrically to the four most intense short-wave responses (darker traces in upper panels). By subtracting the cone components, rod-only amplitudes can be isolated.

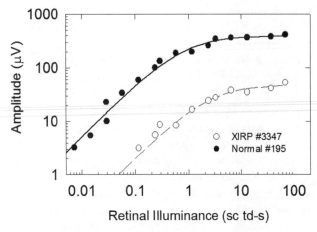

FIGURE 69.7   Plots of log rod-only amplitude as a function of log retinal illuminance in a normal subject (solid symbols) and a patient with XlRP (open symbols). Curves are best fit Naka-Rushton functions. Compared to mean normal, log k was elevated 0.5 log unit and log V_{max} was reduced by 0.9 log unit.

b-wave function in retinitis pigmentosa can be attributed to either a decrease in log V_{max} or an increase in log k. A change in log V_{max} in a given patient leads to a vertical shift, while a change in log k produces a horizontal shift. The vast major-

ity of patients show a decrease in log V_{max}.[18] V_{max} reflects the total activity of all rod bipolar cells. If all rod bipolars are functioning, even with reduced sensitivity, it follows that with enough stimulation it should be possible to elicit a normal maximum response. The fact that V_{max} is reduced in most patients implies that a substantial number of rod bipolars are nonfunctional, that is, have complete loss of their input due to photoreceptor degeneration. Log k reflects the sensitivity of the rod bipolar cells. Since each rod bipolar cell reflects the pooled input from many rods, it follows that either the complete loss of some of the rods from the receptive field or a shortening of the outer segments of all the rods in the receptive field will have roughly the same effect on log k.[62]

Extended amplitude-retinal illuminance functions are useful for following patients over time, either to determine the natural history of the disease[17] or to evaluate the efficacy of therapy. ISCEV standard ERGs, extended amplitude-retinal illuminance functions, and rod static perimetric fields (figure 69.8) were obtained annually in 67 patients with RP.[17] On the average, log V_{max} decreased by 0.06 log unit per year (12%), while log k increased by 0.08 log unit per year (16%). Since the exponent of the Michaelis-Menton function was set to 1, the variation in log rod threshold is the sum of the

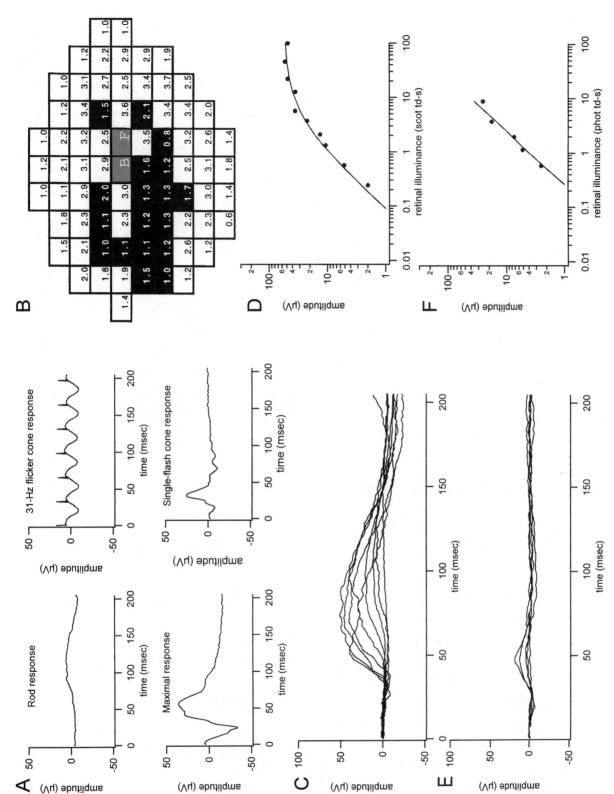

FIGURE 69.8 Full-field ERGs and rod visual fields in retinitis pigmentosa. A, ISCEV standard responses. B, Log rod perimetric sensitivity values (unshaded regions lie within 2.0 log units of normal). C, Rod-only ERG series. D, Rod ERG amplitude as a function of retinal illuminance. E, Dark-adapted cone ERG series. F, Cone ERG amplitude as a function of retinal illuminance. (From Birch DG, Anderson JL.[16])

Normal Subject #6051 Age: 65 yrs

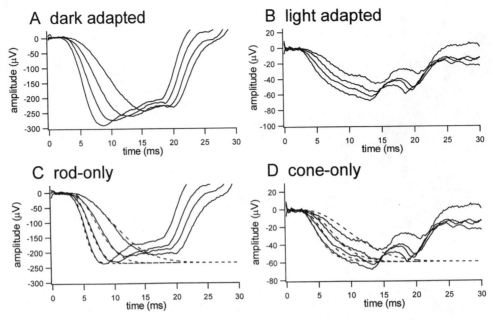

FIGURE 69.9   Representative a-wave responses from a 65-year-old control subject. A, Responses in dark to intensities ranging from 3.2 to 4.4 log scotopic troland-seconds (log sc td s). B, Same four intensities presented against a 3.2 log td background. C, Rod-isolated responses. Dashed lines show fit of the computational phototransduction model.[59] D, Cone responses and model fits (dashed curves). (From Birch DG et al.[24])

XIRP #5046 Age: 23 yrs

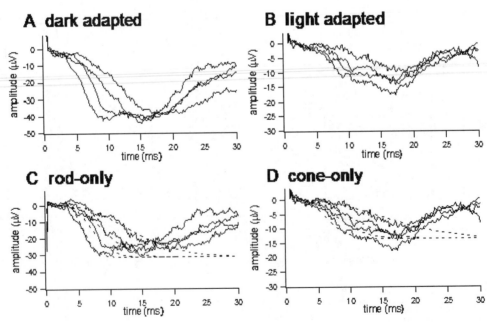

FIGURE 69.10   Representative a-wave responses from a 23-year-old man with XIRP. A, Responses in the dark to intensities ranging from 3.2 to 4.4 log sc td s. B, Same four intensities presented against a 3.2 log td background. C, Rod-isolated responses with best fit of model. D, Cone responses and model fits (dashed lines). (From Birch DG et al.[24])

changes in $\log k$ and $\log V_{max}$. In this particular sample of 67 patients with retinitis pigmentosa tested yearly in a prospective study, the annual increase in rod ERG threshold was 0.14 log unit (28%).

A-WAVE ANALYSIS The ERG generated by a brief flash includes an initial cornea-negative a-wave, the early portion of which reflects the massed transduction activity of rod and cone photoreceptors[29,55,89,101] and the later portion of which reflects inner retinal negative components.[98,103] Several new developments have vastly increased the value of the ERG as a research tool for studying abnormal rod function in inherited retinal degenerations. Lamb and Pugh recently provided a quantitative description of the activation stages of transduction.[71] We had previously concluded that the leading edge of the human a-wave provides a measure of human rod photoreceptor activity, since it could be fitted by traditional receptor models based on n-stage exponential filters.[56–58] More recently, we showed that the Lamb and Pugh model fits the leading edge in normal human subjects slightly better than does the n-stage model.[59] Since the Lamb and Pugh model is based on the actual biochemical steps in the G-protein activation cascade, it can be used to evaluate defects in the activation stages of phototransduction resulting from specific gene mutations in RP.

The leading edge of the a-wave recorded from the human eye spans approximately 5–20 ms (figure 69.9). The rod-mediated component of this initial segment of the ERG is essentially a linear monitor of the rod photocurrent response[27,56,57] and can be quantitatively analyzed in relation to the activation steps of phototransduction.[28,33,34,60] Virtually all patients with RP show a decrease in the maximum amplitude of the photoresponse, consistent with a reduced number of cyclic GMP-gated channels (figure 69.10). The leading edge reflects the gain of phototransduction and may or not be abnormal in a given patient, depending at least in part on the type of RP.[111] The b-wave and other postreceptor components begin to dominate the human ERG at approximately 10–20 ms and thus obscure the subsequent response of the rods. Photocurrent data obtained from mammalian rods in vitro[8,32,67,84,108] predict a time scale of several hundred milliseconds or more, depending on flash intensity, for the rod response in vivo. Thus, in the human ERG, the period of development of the leading edge of the rod a-wave represents only a tiny fraction of the duration of the rod flash response. However, techniques have recently been developed for deriving the entire rod photoresponse from the ERG in human patients. Properties of the derived response from the human ERG (time course, sensitivity, adaptation) are comparable to those of in vitro rod photocurrent responses obtained in previous studies.[90] The technique employs the paired-flash method used in recent studies of the human ERG[14,19,20,90,91] and in similar in vivo studies of the mouse

ERG[51,74] to analyze the recovery kinetics of the rod a-wave after a saturating test flash. In this method, the extent of recovery from rod saturation (i.e., from a condition of zero circulating current in the rods) at a given time after the test flash is determined from the a-wave response to a bright probe flash that rapidly reestablishes rod saturation (figure 69.11). It is anticipated that quantitative analysis of the full time course of the photoresponse will become an important component of phenotypic assessment in patients with RP and should provide insights into the mechanism of disease.

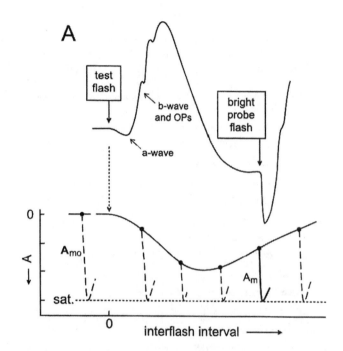

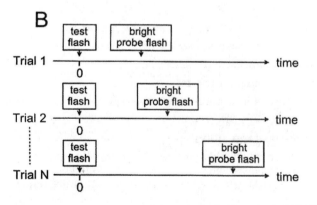

FIGURE 69.11 Paired-flash ERG method. A, Hypothetical ERG response to a test flash and a subsequently presented bright test flash. The lower part of the panel shows hypothetical responses to a group of probe flashes presented at differing times. Peaks of these responses are aligned to reflect the presumed fixed state of the rods at photocurrent saturation. B, Protocol for paired-flash trials to determine time course of the derived response to a fixed test flash. (From Pepperberg DR, Birch DG, Hood DC.[91])

Summary

The remarkable advances in molecular biology over the past 20 years have led to a wealth of information about disease-causing mutations. Our ability to genotype patients must be matched by a comprehensive set of tools for establishing the phenotype. More specific knowledge of genotype-phenotype relationships can provide insight into mechanism, help in patient counseling, and, perhaps most important, provide the foundation for future treatment trials as appropriate interventions become available.

REFERENCES

1. Allikmets R, et al: A photoreceptor cell-specific ATP-binding transporter gene (ABCR) is mutated in recessive Stargardt macular dystrophy. *Nature Genetics* 1997; 15:236–246.
2. Allikmets R, et al: Mutation of the Stargardt disease gene (ABCR) in age-related macular degeneration. *Science* 1997; 277:1805–1807.
3. Arikawa K, et al: Localization of peripherin/rds in the disk membranes of cone and rod photoreceptors: Relationship to disk membrane morphogenesis and retinal degeneration. *J Cell Biol* 1992; 116:659.
4. Azarian SM, Papermaster DS, Travis GH: Molecular characterization of the rim protein in bovine photoreceptors. *Invest Ophthalmol Vis Sci* 1996; 37 (suppl):S805.
5. Bascom RA, et al: Cloning of the cDNA for a novel photoreceptor membrane protein (rom-1) identifies a disk rim protein family implicated in human retinopathies. *Neuron* 1992; 8:1171–1184.
6. Baylor DA, Hodgkin AL: Changes in time scale and sensitivity in turtle photoreceptors. *J Physiol (Lond)* 1974; 242:729–758.
7. Baylor DA, Lamb TD, Yau K-W: Two components of electrical dark noise in toad retinal rod outer segments. *J Physiol (Lond)* 1980; 309:591–621.
8. Baylor DA, Nunn BJ, Schnapf JL: The photocurrent, noise and spectral sensitivity of rods of the monkey: *Macaca fascicularis. J Physiol* 1984; 357:575–607.
9. Berson EL, Gouras P, Hoff M: Temporal aspects of the electroretinogram. *Arch Ophthalmol* 1969; 81(2):207–214.
10. Berson EL, Rosen JB, Simonoff EA: Electroretinographic testing as an aid in detection of carriers of X-chromosome-linked retinitis pigmentosa. *Am J Ophthalmol* 1979; 87(4):460–468.
11. Berson EL, et al: Natural course of retinitis pigmentosa over a three-year interval. *Am J Ophthalmol* 1985; 99(3):240–251.
12. Bessant D, Kaushal S, Bhattacharya S: Genetics and biology of the inherited retinal dystrophies. In Kaufman PL, Alm A (eds): *Adler's Physiology of the Eye*, ed 10. St. Louis, Mosby, 2003, pp 358–381.
13. Bhattacharya SS, et al: Close genetic linkage between X-linked retinitis pigmentosa and a restriction fragment length polymorphism identified by recombinant DNA probe L1.28. *Nature* 1984; 309:253–255.
14. Birch DG: ERG measures of photoreceptor deactivation in retinitis pigmentosa. *Digital J Ophthalmol* 1999; 5:1–11.
15. Birch DG, Anderson JL: Standardized full-field electro-retinography: Normal values and their variation with age. *Arch Ophthalmol* 1992; 110(11):1571–1576.
16. Birch DG, Anderson JL: Yearly rates of rod and cone functional loss in retinitis pigmentosa ad cone-rod degeneration. *Vision Science and its Applications, OSA Technical Digest Series* 1993; 3:334–337.
17. Birch DG, Anderson JL, Fish GE: Yearly rates of rod and cone functional loss in retinitis pigmentosa and cone-rod dystrophy. *Ophthalmology* 1999; 106(2):258–268.
18. Birch DG, Fish GE: Rod ERGs in retinitis pigmentosa and cone-rod degeneration. *Invest Ophthalmol Vis Sci* 1987; 28(1):140–150.
19. Birch DG, Pepperberg DR, Hood DC: The effects of light adaptation on recovery kinetics of the human rod photoresponse. *Vision Science and Its Applications, OSA Technical Digest Series* 1996; 1:60–63.
20. Birch DG, Pepperberg DC, Hood DC: Recovery of dark- and light-adapted flash responses of human rods and cones. *Invest Ophthalmol Vis Sci* 1996; 37:3733.
21. Birch DG, Sandberg MA: Dependence of cone b-wave implicit time on rod amplitude in retinitis pigmentosa. *Vision Res* 1987; 27(7):1105–1112.
22. Birch DG, et al: Abnormal activation and inactivation mechanisms of rod transduction in patients with autosomal dominant retinitis pigmentosa and the pro-23-his mutation. *Invest Ophthalmol Vis Sci* 1995; 36(8):1603–1614.
23. Birch DG, et al: Homozygous and compound-heterozygous mutations in the ABCR gene associated with a distinct phenotype of cone-rod dystrophy. *Invest Ophthalmol Vis Sci* 1999; 40:S722.
24. Birch DG, et al: Quantitative electroretinogram measures of phototransduction in cone and rod photoreceptors: Normal aging, progression with disease, and test-retest variability. *Arch Ophthalmol* 2002; 120(8):1045–1051.
25. Bok D: Processing and transport of retinoids by the retinal pigment epithelium. *Eye* 1990; 4:326–332.
26. Bowne SJ, et al: Mutations in the RP1 gene causing autosomal dominant retinitis pigmentosa. *Hum Mol Genet* 1999; 8(11):2121–2128.
27. Breton ME, Montzka DP: Empiric limits of rod photocurrent component underlying a-wave response in the electroretinogram. *Doc Ophthalmol* 1992; 79:337–361.
28. Breton ME, et al: Analysis of ERG a-wave amplification and kinetics in terms of the G-protein cascade of phototransduction. *Invest Ophthalmol Vis Sci* 1994; 35(1):295–309.
29. Brown KT, Wiesel TN: Localization of origins of electroretinogram components by intraretinal recording in the intact cat eye. *J Physiol* 1961; 158:257–280.
30. Bunker CH, et al: Prevalence of retinitis pigmentosa in Maine. *Am J Ophthalmol* 1984; 97(3):357–365.
31. Chen CK, et al: Slowed recovery of rod photoresponse in mice lacking the GTPase accelerating protein RGS9-1. *Nature* 2000; 403:557–560.
32. Chen J, et al: Mechanisms of rhodopsin inactivation in vivo as revealed by a COOH-terminal truncation mutant. *Science* 1995; 267:374–377.
33. Cideciyan AV, Jacobson SG: Negative electroretinograms in retinitis pigmentosa. *Invest Ophthalmol Vis Sci* 1993; 34:3253–3263.
34. Cideciyan AV, Jacobson SG: An alternative phototransduction model for human rod and cone ERG a-waves: Normal parameters and variation with age. *Vision Res* 1996; 36(16):2609–2621.
35. Clack JW, Pepperberg DR: Desensitization of skate photoreceptor by bleaching and background light. *J Gen Physiol* 1982; 80:863–883.

36. Connell G, et al: Photoreceptor peripherin is the normal product of the gene responsible for retinal degeneration in the rds mouse. *Proc Nat Acad Sci U S A* 1991; 88: 723–726.

37. Cornwall MC, Fain GL: Bleaching of rhodopsin in isolated rods causes a sustained activation of PDE and cyclase which is reversed by pigment regeneration. *Invest Ophthalmol Vis Sci* 1992; 33:1103.

38. Cremers FP, et al: Autosomal recessive retinitis pigmentosa and cone-rod dystrophy caused by splice site mutations in the Stargardt's disease gene ABCR. *Hum Mol Genet* 1998; 7(3): 355–362.

39. Crouch RK, et al: Retinoids and the visual process. *Photochem Photobiol* 1996; 64(4):613–621.

40. Donders FC: Beitrage zur pathologischen anatomie des auges; 2) Pigmentbildung in der netzhaut. *Graefes Arch Ophthalmol* 1857; 3:139–150.

41. Dryja TP, et al: Mutations within the rhodopsin gene in patients with autosomal dominant retinitis pigmentosa. *N Engl J Med* 1990; 323:1302–1307.

42. Dryja TP, et al: Frequency of mutations in the gene encoding the alpha subunit of rod cGMP-phosphodiesterase in autosomal recessive retinitis pigmentosa. *Invest Ophthalmol Vis Sci* 1999; 40(8):1859–1865.

43. Fain GL: Sensitivity of toad rods: Dependence on wavelength and background illumination. *J Physiol (Lond)* 1976; 261: 71–101.

44. Farrar GJ, et al: Autosomal dominant retinitis pigmentosa: Linkage to rhodopsin and evidence for genetic heterogeneity. *Genomics* 1990; 8:35–40.

45. Fishman GA, Cunha-Vaz JE: Carriers of X-linked recessive retinitis pigmentosa: Investigation by vitreous fluorophotometry. *Int Ophthalmol* 1981; 4(1–2):37–44.

46. Freund CL, et al: Cone-rod dystrophy due to mutations in a novel photoreceptor-specific homeobox gene (CRX) essential for maintenance of the photoreceptor. *Cell* 1997; 91(4): 543–553.

47. Furukawa T, Morrow EM, Cepko CL: Crx, a novel otx-like homeobox gene, shows photoreceptor-specific expression and regulates photoreceptor differentiation. *Cell* 1997; 91(4): 531–541.

48. Gieser L, et al: A novel locus (RP24) for X-linked retinitis pigmentosa maps to Xq26–27. *Am J Hum Genet* 1998; 63(5): 1439–1447.

49. Goldberg AF, Moritz OL, Molday RS: Heterologous expression of photoreceptor peripherin/rds and Rom-1 in COS-1 cells: Assembly, interactions, and localization of multisubunit complexes. *Biochemistry* 1995; 34(43):14213–14219.

50. Goto Y, et al: Functional abnormalities in transgenic mice expressing a mutant rhodopsin gene. *Invest Ophthalmol Vis Sci* 1995; 36(1):62–71.

51. Goto Y, et al: Rod phototransduction in transgenic mice expressing a mutant opsin gene. *J Opt Soc Am A Opt Image Sci Vis* 1996; 13(3):577–585.

52. Hagstrom SA, et al: Recessive mutations in the gene encoding the tubby-like protein TULP1 in patients with retinitis pigmentosa. *Nat Genet* 1998; 18(2):174–176.

53. Hardcastle AJ, et al: Evidence for a new locus for X-linked retinitis pigmentosa (RP23). *Invest Ophthalmol Vis Sci* 2000; 41(8):2080–2086.

54. He W, et al: RSG9, a GTPase accelerator for phototransduction. *Neuron* 1998; 20:95–102.

55. Heynen H, van Norren D: Origin of the electroretinogram in the intact macaque eye: I. Principal component analysis. *Vision Res* 1985; 25:697–707.

56. Hood DC, Birch DG: The a-wave of the human electroretinogram and rod receptor function. *Invest Ophthalmol Vis Sci* 1990; 31:2070–2081.

57. Hood DC, Birch DG: A quantitative measure of the electrical activity of human rod photoreceptors using electroretinography. *Vis Neurosci* 1990; 5(4):379–387.

58. Hood DC, Birch DG: The relationship between models of receptor activity and the a-wave of the human ERG. *Clin Vis Sci* 1990; 5:293.

59. Hood DC, Birch DG: Light adaptation of human rod receptors: The leading edge of the human a-wave and models of rod receptor activity. *Vision Res* 1993; 33(12):1605–1618.

60. Hood DC, Birch DG: Rod phototransduction in retinitis pigmentosa: Estimation and interpretation of parameters derived from the rod a-wave. *Invest Ophthalmol Vis Sci* 1994; 35(7):2948–2961.

61. Hood DC, Birch DG: Abnormalities of the retinal cone system in retinitis pigmentosa. *Vision Res* 1996; 36(11): 1699–1709.

62. Hood DC, Shady S, Birch DG: Understanding changes in the b-wave of the ERG caused by heterogeneous receptor damage. *Invest Ophthalmol Vis Sci* 1994; 35(5):2477–2488.

63. Huang PC, et al: Cellular interactions implicated in the mechanism of photoreceptor degeneration in transgenic mice expressing a mutant rhodopsin gene. *Proc Natl Acad Sci U S A* 1993; 90:8484–8488.

64. Jacobson SG, et al: Photoreceptor function in heterozygotes with insertion or deletion mutations in the RDS gene. *Invest Ophthalmol Vis Sci* 1996; 37(8):1662–1674.

65. Jones GL: Light adaptation and the rising phase of the flash photocurrent of salamander retinal rods. *J Physiol* 1995; 487(2):441–451.

66. Kajiwara K, Berson EL, Dryja TP: Digenic retinitis pigmentosa due to mutations at the unlinked peripherin/RDS and ROM1 loci. *Science* 1994; 264(5165):1604–1608.

67. Kraft TW, Schneeweis DM, Schnapf JL: Visual transduction in human rod photoreceptors. *J Physiol* 1993; 464:747–765.

68. Lagnado L, Baylor D: Signal flow in visual transduction. *Neuron* 1992; 8:995–1002.

69. Lagnado L, Baylor D: Calcium controls light-triggered formation of catalytically active rhodopsin. *Nature* 1994; 367:273–277.

70. Lamb TD: Effects of temperature changes on toad rod photocurrents. *J Physiol (Lond)* 1984; 346:557–578.

71. Lamb TD, Pugh EN: A quantitative account of the activation steps involved in phototransduction in amphibian photoreceptors. *J Physiol* 1992; 499:719.

72. LaVail MM, et al: Multiple growth factors, cytokines and neurotrophins rescue photoreceptors from the damaging effects of constant light. *Proc Natl Acad Sci U S A* 1992; 89:11249–11253.

73. Li T, et al: Constitutive activation of phototransduction by K296E opsin is not a cause of photoreceptor degeneration. *Proc Natl Acad Sci U S A* 1995; 92(8):3551–3555.

74. Lyubarsky AL, Pugh EN: Recovery phase of the murine rod photoresponse reconstructed from electroretinographic recordings. *J Neurosci* 1996; 16(2):563–571.

75. Marmor MF, et al: Standard for clinical electroretinography. *Arch Ophthalmol* 1989; 107:816–819.

76. McGee TL, Berson EL, Dryja TP: Defects in the rod cGMP-gated gene in patients with retinitis pigmentosa. *Invest Ophthalmol Vis Sci* 1994; 35:1716.

77. McLaughlin ME, et al: Recessive mutations in the gene encoding the beta-subunit of rod phosphodiesterase in patients with retinitis pigmentosa. *Nat Genet* 1993; 4(2): 130–134.

78. McNaughton PA: Light response of vertebrate photoreceptors. *Physiol Rev* 1990; 70:847–884.

79. McWilliams P, et al: Autosomal dominant retinitis pigmentosa (ADRP): Localization of an ADRP gene to the long arm of chromosome 3. *Genomics* 1989; 5:619–622.

80. Meindl A, et al: A gene (RPGR) with homology to the RCC1 guanine nucleotide exchange factor is mutated in X-linked retinitis pigmentosa (RP3). *Nat Genet* 1996; 13: 35–42.

81. Morimura H, Berson EL, Dryja TP: Recessive mutations in the RLBP1 gene encoding cellular retinaldehyde-binding protein in a form of retinitis punctata albescens. *Invest Ophthalmol Vis Sci* 1999; 40(5):1000–1004.

82. Morimura H, et al: Mutations in the RPE65 gene in patients with autosomal recessive retinitis pigmentosa or leber congenital amaurosis. *Proc Natl Acad Sci U S A* 1998; 95(6): 3088–3093.

83. Musarella MA: Mapping of the X-linked recessive retinitis pigmentosa gene. A review. *Ophthalmic Paediatr Genet* 1990; 11(2):77–88.

84. Nakatani K, Tamura T, Yau K-W: Light adaptation in retinal rods of the rabbit and two other nonprimate mammals. *J Gen Physiol* 1991; 97:413–435.

85. Naka KI, Rushton WAH: S-potential colour units in the retina of the fish (cyprimidae). *J Physiol* 1966; 185:536.

86. Nicol GD, Bownds MD: Calcium regulates some, but not all, aspects of light adaptation in rod photoreceptors. *J Gen Physiol* 1989; 94:233–259.

87. Olsson JE, Gordon JW, Pawlyk BS: Transgenic mice with a rhodopsin mutation (Pro23His): A mouse model of autosomal dominant retinitis. *Neuron* 1992; 9:815–830.

88. Ott J, et al: Localizing multiple X chromosome-linked retinitis pigmentosa loci using multilocus homogeneity tests. *Proc Natl Acad Sci U S A* 1990; 87(2):701–704.

89. Penn RD, Hagins WA: Signal transmission along retinal rods and the origin of the electroretinographic a-wave. *Nature* 1969; 223:201–205.

90. Pepperberg DR, Birch DG, Hood DC: Photoresponses of human rods in vivo derived from paired-flash electroretinograms. *Vis Neurosci* 1997; 14:73–82.

91. Pepperberg DR, Birch DG, Hood DC: Electroretinographic determination of the human rod flash response in vivo. *Methods Enzymol* 2000; 316:202–223.

92. Pepperberg DR, et al: Light-dependent delay in the falling phase of the retinal rod response. *Vis Neurosci* 1992; 8:9–18.

93. Pugh EN Jr, Lamb TD: Cyclic GMP and calcium: The internal messengers of excitation and adaptation in vertebrate photoreceptors. *Vision Res* 1990; 30:1923–1948.

94. Rando RR: Molecular mechanisms in visual pigment regeneration. *Photochem Photobiol* 1992; 56:1145–1156.

95. Redmond TM, et al: Rpe65 is necessary for production of 11-cis-vitamin A in the retinal visual cycle. *Nat Genet* 1998; 20(4):344–351.

96. Reme CE: Apoptotic cell death in retinal degenerations. *Prog Retinal Eye Res* 1998; 17:443.

97. Robinson PR, et al: Constitutively active mutants of rhodopsin. *Neuron* 1992; 9:719–725.

98. Robson JG, Frishman LJ: Photoreceptor and bipolar cell contributions to the cat electroretinogram: A kinetic model of the early part of the flash response. *J Opt Soc Am A Opt Image Sci Vis* 1996; 13(3):613–622.

99. Rosenfeld PJ, et al: A null mutation in the rhodopsin gene causes rod photoreceptor dysfunction and autosomal recessive retinitis pigmentosa. *Nat Genet* 1992; 1:209–213.

100. Sharma RK, Ehinger B: Management of hereditary retinal degenerations: Present status and future directions. *Surv Ophthalmol* 1999; 43(5):427–444.

101. Sillman AJ, Ito H, Tomita T: Studies on the mass receptor potential of the isolated frog retina: I. General properties of the response. *Vision Res* 1969; 9:1435–1442.

102. Sohocki MM, et al: A range of clinical phenotypes associated with mutations in CRX, a photoreceptor transcription factor. *Am J Hum Genet* 1998; 63:1307–1315.

103. Steinberg RH, Frishman LJ, Sieving PA: Negative components of the electroretinogram from proximal retina and photoreceptor. In Osborne NN, Chader GJ (eds): *Progress in Retinal Research*. Oxford, UK, Pergamon, 1991, pp 121–160.

104. Stryer L: Cyclic GMP cascade of vision. *Ann Rev Neurosci* 1986; 9:87–119.

105. Sung C-H, et al: Functional heterogeneity of mutant rhodopsins responsible for autosomal dominant retinitis pigmentosa. *Proc Natl Acad Sci U S A* 1991; 88:8840–8844.

106. Sung CH, et al: A rhodopsin gene mutation responsible for autosomal dominant retinitis pigmentosa results in a protein that is defective in localization to the photoreceptor outer segment. *J Neurosci* 1994; 14(10):5818–5833.

107. Swain PK, et al: Mutations in the cone-rod homeobox gene are associated with the cone-rod dystrophy photoreceptor degeneration. *Neuron* 1997; 19(6):1329–1336.

108. Tamura T, Nakatani K, Yau K-W: Light adaptation in cat retinal rods. *Science* 1989; 245:755–758.

109. Travis GH, Sutcliffe JG, Bok D: The retinal degeneration slow (rds) gene product is a photoreceptor disc membrane-associated glycoprotein. *Neuron* 1991; 6:61–70.

110. Travis G, et al: The human retinal degeneration slow (RDS) gene: Chromosome assignment and structure of the mRNA. *Genomics* 1991; 10:733.

111. Tzekov RT, et al: Cone and rod ERG phototransduction parameters in retinitis pigmentosa. *Invest Ophthalmol Vis Sci* 2003; 44:3993–4000.

112. Weleber RG, et al: Phenotypic variation including retinitis pigmentosa, pattern dystrophy, and fundus flavimaculatus in a single family with a deletion of codon 153 or 154 of the peripherin/RDS gene. *Arch Ophthalmol* 1993; 111(11):1531–1542.

113. Weng J, et al: Insights into the function of Rim protein in photoreceptors and etiology of Stargardt's disease from the phenotype in abcr knockout mice. *Cell* 1999; 98(1):13–23.

114. Wroblewski JJ, et al: Macular dystrophy associated with mutations at codon 172 in the human retinal degeneration slow gene. *Ophthalmology* 1994; 101(1):12–22.

115. Yang-Feng TL, Swaroop A: Neural retina-specific leucine zipper gene NRL (D14S46E) maps to human chromosome 14q11.1–q11.2. *Genomics* 1992; 14(2):491–492.

116. Yamamoto H, et al: Mutations in the gene encoding 11-cis retinol dehydrogenase cause delayed dark adaptation and fundus albipunctatus. *Nat Genet* 1999; 22(2):188–191.

70 Cone Dystrophies and Degenerations

JOHN R. HECKENLIVELY

THE STANDARDIZED electroretinogram (ERG) is the main clinical test that will confirm a cone degeneration or dystrophy. Cone degeneration or dysfunction may be congenital or acquired, but the diagnosis is often difficult to make, since the early fundus changes can be subtle. A standardized protocol with carefully established normal values is essential for optimally recognizing a cone dysfunction pattern. The clinician may have minimal physical evidence to motivate asking for an ERG or even, if suspicious, might not realize that the ERG is the definitive diagnostic test. Traditionally, cone dystrophy refers to congenital or very early onset cases, usually called *achromatopsia*, and cases with family inheritance patterns. The term *cone degeneration* is often used in acquired cases in which there is no family history.

Depending on the stage of disease and genetic type of cone disorder, clinical signs and fundus changes provide strong diagnostic clues that a cone disorder may be present. Patients with cone dysfunction typically complain of light sensitivity and tend to see better at dusk or in the dark.[3] Most have uncorrectable subnormal vision, dark-to-light adaptation problems, and loss of hues or color blindness (variable finding). Frequently, patients do not volunteer these symptoms unless questioned directly for them. Some patients who are city dwellers will have "urban night blindness," since at night, their cones do not function well in semilighted city areas where it is not dark enough for rods to be effective.

Common fundus findings include a circumscribed granularity or atrophy of the macular area and temporal optic pallor or atrophy. Congenital or early-onset cases will typically have nystagmus, which is often the symptom that brings the child to the eye doctor. Some X-linked cone dystrophy patients have confluent retinal areas of tapetal-like sheen (figure 70.1A and 70.1B), and rare patients have crystalline deposits in the macular area (figure 70.2). Krill reported a group of patients who had abnormal retinal blood vessel formation with cone dystrophy, including cases in which the retinal vessels crossed the raphe in the macula (figure 70.3).[6,8]

A diagnosis of cone degeneration or dysfunction is easily confirmed by a standardized ERG. The International Society for Clinical Electrophysiology and Vision (ISCEV) standardized protocol calls for the cone and rod systems to be tested separately, as well as together in the dark-adapted bright-flash testing. Besides using a single or averaged bright flash under light-adapted conditions, another technique for isolating the cone response is to employ a flickering bright stimulus light with a frequency greater than 20–30 cycles per second (Hz), since the rod response under standard conditions will attenuate fairly severely after 8 Hz and is absent by 20 Hz.[4] The flicker stimulus, which maximally stimulates the cone system, is useful in bringing out subtle dysfunction or partial cone degenerations, which may not be as apparent by single flash techniques, as the response may be disportionately worse than the single-flash photopic response.[2]

Cone system dysfunction should be suspected in all patients who complain of photosensitivity, problems in light adaptation, and difficulties with color saturation or discrimination (table 70.1). Patients present with subnormal or abnormal visual acuity that is noncorrectable. A number of patients will have macular atrophy or degenerative changes, some of which start as bull's-eye macular lesions or demonstrated "cookie cutter"—shaped macular atrophy (figure 70.4A and 70.4B). Temporal optic nervehead pallor or atrophy is common in many cone dystrophies (figure 70.5). This change may be mistaken as a "tiled" disk. Abnormal color vision is not an exclusive finding in cone degeneration and may be seen in macular degeneration in macular dystrophies without panretinal cone degeneration. Unless there is a known family history of a cone disorder, an ERG is needed to confirm the diagnosis of cone dystrophy or degeneration, since this diagnosis implies a panretinal cone disorder.

An important fact to remember is the foveal centralis contributes at most only 10–15% to the photopic b-wave amplitude. This fact was confirmed many years ago by examining patients who had foveal scars but otherwise normal retinas. In the face of a macular lesion, a large reduction in the photopic ERG means that there is a cone system dysfunction.[12]

Traditionally, the hereditary cone degenerations and dysfunction disorders have been classified into congenital and later onset forms (table 70.2).[6,8] The two congenital cone dysfunction disorders, blue monocone monochromatism, which is X-linked, and rod monochromatism, which is

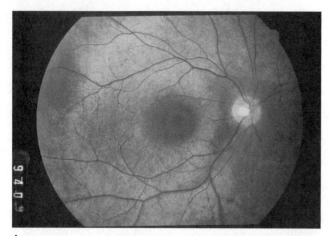

A

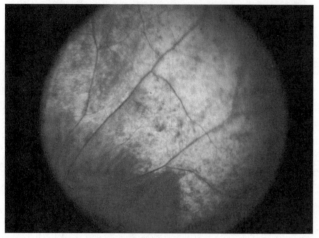

B

FIGURE 70.1 Symmetric, round atrophy of fovea centralis is typically seen in a number of types of cone dystrophy or degeneration. A, In this case of X-linked cone dystrophy with tapetal sheen, the atrophy of the foveal centralis is highlighted by the surrounding sheen. This 54-year-old man had photosensitivity OU and a history of retinal detachment in his right eye; his visual acuity was 20/200 OU. B, While the sheen is seen as patches in the periphery. These patients exhibit the Mizuo-Nakamura effect on dark adaptation. (See also color plate 40.)

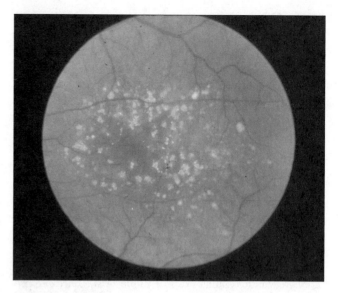

FIGURE 70.2 Cone dystrophy with foveal crystals. Right eye of a 58-year-old woman with urban night blindness with nonrecordable photopic ERG and normal scotopic ERGs. Visual acuity was OD 20/40, OS 20/60, and Goldmann visual fields were full. (See also color plate 41.)

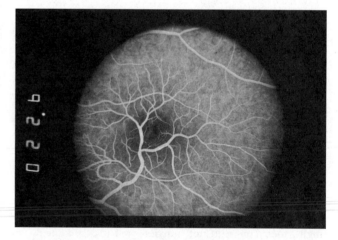

FIGURE 70.3 Fluorescein angiogram of a 13-year-old girl with a cone dystrophy. The left eye had a large retinal vessel crossing the macula with telangiectatic branches giving some late leakage and edema to the macula. The retinal vessels OD were normal.

autosomal-recessive, typically present with congenital nystagmus, and the diagnosis may be missed, or it may be misjudged as congenital nystagmus unless an ERG is performed. The term *dystrophy* has been broadly used in the ophthalmologic literature, so it is appropriate to use it in congenital-onset cone-loss cases.

Hereditary cone degenerations have been found in all three Mendelian modes of inheritance. A list of the ones currently known are listed in table 70.2. Genetic disease databases, such as RetNet or PubMed, can be used to update this information (see http://www.sph.uth.tmc.edu/retnet or http://www.ncbi.nlm.nih.gov/entrez/query.fcgi).

The electroretinographic pattern in all of these cone-loss disorders is generally the same pattern: The photopic ERG is severely abnormal to nonrecordable by single-flash or computer-averaged methods, while the rod ERG is normal to subnormal (figure 70.6). While the rod tracing might not have a normal amplitude, it is well formed and stable over time in cone dystrophy patients. Dark-adapted tracings frequently show a blink response near the peak of the b-wave, since most patients are photophobic (see figure 70.6). If a scotopic red flash stimulus is employed, the early cone response will be absent, and the later rod response will be present.

Conditions that can be confused initially with cone degeneration are early cases of cone-rod retinitis pigmentosa or cases of RP inversa, in which a cone-rod ERG pattern with dense progressive central scotoma may be found and could otherwise be mistaken for a cone degeneration with mild rod involvement.[5] Checking the peripheral visual field is an important adjunctive test in all these disorders, and the field is typically stable and full over time. Visual fields, often per-

formed serially, are an important confirmatory test for distinguishing cone disorders from progressive disorders with peripheral loss and may be diagnostic on the initial test. Some cone disorders will have central scotomata whose size is consistent with the level of visual acuity.

Clinical features of cone degeneration

The diagnosis of cone degeneration or dysfunction can be extraordinarily difficult to make in the clinical setting since, in many patients, the signs and symptoms are very subtle. However, there are diagnostic indicators that ordinarily might be ignored. These are presented below to aid in determining whether an ERG should be ordered to confirm the diagnosis (see table 70.1).

The most common presenting symptoms of cone dysfunction are subnormal visual acuity and complaints of photosensitivity, loss of color saturation, or problems in adapting from a darkened environment to a lighted one. Some patients state that they see better at dusk or in the dark. An unusual symptom that a few city-dwelling cone dystrophy patients may have is urban night blindness; in a city environment, there is usually enough light at night so that rods are unable to undergo full dark adaptation, while cones do not function well. These patients will give a history of night blindness and, from the symptoms, may be mistakenly

TABLE 70.1

Signs and symptoms commonly seen in cone degeneration patients

Presenting symptoms:
1. Decreased visual acuity without obvious reason
2. Complaints of photosensitivity or glare
3. Color vision (often hue) problems
4. Problems in light or dark adaptation, particularly dark to lighted conditions
5. Central scotomata

Ophthalmoscopic signs of cone degeneration:
1. Nerve fiber loss
2. Temporal optic nervehead atrophy or loss
3. Macular degeneration, early may appear granular, later occurs as symmetric or round atrophy of fovea centralis
4. X-linked later onset patients have tapetal-like retinal sheen

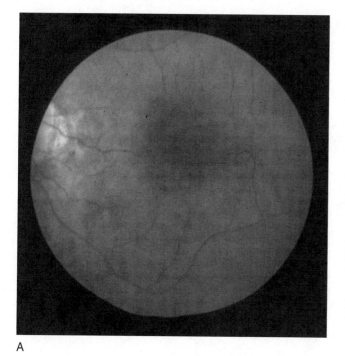

A

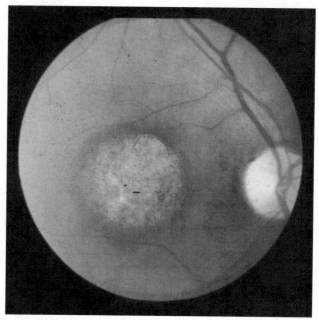

B

FIGURE 70.4   Fundus photographs of patients with inherited cone dystrophies; A, A 60-year-old man with blue-cone monochromatism who recently noted some mild decreases in his central vision from 20/60 to 20/200, presumably from aging. B, A 54-year-old woman with 20/400 vision OU from a large dominant pedigree with cone dystrophy from a GUCY2D gene mutation, with foveal centralis atrophy giving a "cookie cutter" appearance to macula. This pattern is characteristic of many cone dystrophies. (See also color plate 42.)

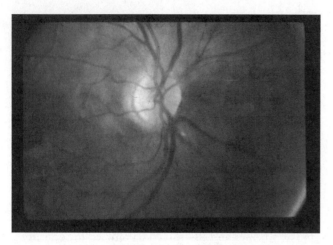

FIGURE 70.5 Temporal optic nerve head atrophy is commonly seen in many cone degenerations; illustrated here by a 9-year-old boy with rod monochromatism with temporal pallor. Sometimes the temporal edge of the nerve is flattened or missing. (See also color plate 43.)

thought to have some form of RP. Another poorly understood group of patients who have urban night blindness have rod-cone interaction dysfunction (Frumkes effect).

The most important sign to the clinician is that the patient's vision is not correctable to normal levels, and at times, there may be no obvious reason for the visual deficit. Many patients will have obvious macular changes such as bull's-eye lesions (see figure 70.4B), or macular atrophy, but there are other patterns to macular tissue loss that give clues that a panretinal cone degeneration is occurring. Some patients will demonstrate crystalline deposits in the fovea centralis region, sometimes associated with a geographic atrophy pattern.

One key to recognizing cone degeneration patterns of tissue loss is to note that in most patients, the atrophy is confined to the fovea centralis and usually is symmetric between eyes (see figures 70.2A through 70.2D); the tissue change itself may consist of diffuse atrophic loss, a confluent sheen

TABLE 70.2

Hereditary forms of cone degeneration or dysfunction

Congenital
Rod monochromatism (achromatopsia), autosomal-recessive
    GNAT2 gene on 1p13.3; cone-specific transducin alpha subunit, rare
    GNGA3 gene on 2q11.2; cone photoreceptor cGMP-gated cation channel
    Alpha subunit; accounts for 20–30% of cases
    GNGB3 gene on 8q21.3, cone cyclic nucleotide-gated cation channel
    Beta 3 subunit; accounts for 40–50% of achromatopsia cases

Cone monochromacy
    OPN1LW at Xq28; one to five copies of 3′ to red pigment gene
    OPN1MW at Xq28; green pigment gene alterations
    RCD1 at 6q25 autosomal-dominant
    Blue cone monochromatism, X-linked recessive, alterations in red and green visual pigment gene cluster

Later onset
Autosomal-dominant cone dystrophy
    GUCA1A gene on 6p21.1; guanylate cyclase–activating protein 1A
    RIMS1 gene on 6q13; regulating synaptic membrane exocytosis protein 1
    RCD1 linked to 6q25–q26

X-linked recessive cone dystrophy
    COD1 lined to Xp11.4 progressive cone dystrophy[1]
    COD2 linked to Xq27 progressive cone dystrophy[13]

X-linked recessive red cone dystrophy

Cone-rod dystrophy genes (see text for distinguishing features from cone dystrophy)
    CORD8 on 1q12–q24
    ALMS1 AR gene on 2p13.1; Alström's syndrome protein
    SCA7 AD gene, on 3p14.1 dominant spinocerebellar ataxia
    AIPL1 on 17p13.2 dominant cone-rod dystrophy (recessive homozygous mutations cause Lebers amaurosis)
    GUCY2D on 17p13.1 dominant cone-rod dystrophy (recessive homozygous mutations cause Lebers amaurosis)
    CORD4 on 17q
    UNC119 on 17q11.2 dominant cone-rod dystrophy
    CORD1 on 81q21.1 cone-rod dystrophy, de Grouchy syndrome
    CRX on 19q13.32 dominant cone-rod dystrophy, recessive mutations may give Lebers amaurosis or cone-rod dystrophy
    COD4 linked to Xp11.4
    RPGR on Xp11.4 associated with dominant and recessive RP, cone-rod dystrophy

Source: RetNet (http://www.sph.uth.tmc.edu/Retnet).

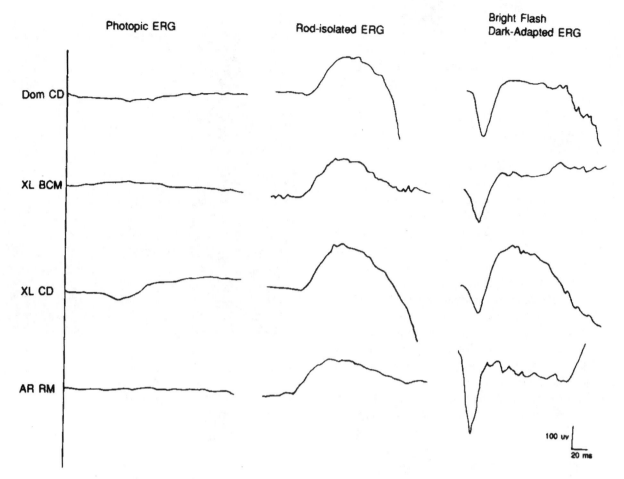

Photopic ERG	Rod-isolated ERG	Bright Flash Dark-Adapted ERG

Dom CD

XL BCM

XL CD

AR RM

100 uv
20 ms

FIGURE 70.6 ERG tracings of typical cases of cone dystrophy in which the photopic (cone) signal is nonrecordable to barely discernible (left tracings). In the rod-isolated signal (middle column), the ERG is well formed and is typically normal to subnormal. The bright-flash dark-adapted tracings are subnormal to abnormal in amplitude, and if interpreted alone without the other two tracings, would be misleading and not diagnostic of any condition. The cases illustrated here are a 54-year-old woman with dominant inherited cone dystrophy DOM CD (see figure 70.6B), whose vision was OD 20/200, OS 20/300; a 60-year-old man with X-linked blue cone monochromatism (XL BCM), who came from a large X-linked pedigree—his visual acuity as a young man was 20/60, but by 60 years of age it was 20/200 OU (see figure 70.6A); a 58-year-old man with X-linked cone dystrophy (XL CD) with tapetal-like sheen (see figures 70.3A and 70.3B), who presented with 20/200 vision; and a 20-year-old woman with autosomal-recessive rod monochromatism (AR RM), who presented with 20/200 vision.

with atrophy, a granular pigmentary reaction, or even crystals. Rare cone dystrophy patients will have peripheral pigmentary deposits. Concentric confluent loss is not pathognomonic of cone degeneration but is a strong indicator for performing a standardized ERG.

Patients with congenital onset and most hereditary forms of cone dystrophy will have temporal optic atrophy; since many of these patients are myopic, the atrophy may be confused or misinterpreted as a tilted disk, or the change may be a combined effect of myopic alterations in scleral canal development and atrophy of temporal disk tissue. Many of these patients, particularly those with a congenital-onset form, will demonstrate a flattened or squashed appearance to the temporal disc (see figure 70.3B). Other patients will have distinct pallor of the temporal portion of the disk

without obvious tissue loss (see figure 70.5), while adult-onset cone degeneration may have no disk changes.

Another pattern of disk atrophy that can be seen is a rim of white granular or sometimes crystalline-appearing material, often present in conjunction with disk pallor. Nerve fiber layer loss is a final clue that a panretinal degeneration is present but is a nonspecific finding in a number of hereditary retinal degenerations.

Known hereditary forms of cone dysfunction or dystrophy

Rod monochromatism, often called achromatopsia, is inherited in the autosomal-recessive fashion and the clinical condition has turned out to be due to a number of different gene mutations (see table 70.2). Patients may have full to partial expression of the cone loss, with visual acuity ranging from 20/60 to 20/200. There also may be varying amounts of nystagmus, which usually improves with age. Since many of these patients have blond fundi and minimal granularity of the macula, they may be thought to have ocular albinism, but an ERG will quickly distinguish the cone dysfunction. Another clinical diagnostic technique that may be helpful for distinguishing albinism from cone dystrophy is to transilluminate the iris looking for iris atrophy; electrophy-siological testing for albinism can be done by performing lateralizing visually evoked testing (see chapter 25).

Blue cone monochromatism is an X-linked recessive congenital cone dysfunction disorder that tends to be milder than rod monochromatism. An X-linked recessive pattern of inheritance in the face of a congenital absence of cone function is a reliable indicator of this disease (see table 70.2), but molecular testing is needed to confirm the diagnosis.

Blue cone monochromatism patients may have visual acuity as good as 20/30 and occasionally as poor as 20/200; the macula develops a granular atrophy, and there is frequently severe temporal disk atrophy (see figures 70.4A and 70.4B). Carriers for the disorder may show a loss of the cone portion (x-wave) of the red stimulus dark-adapted ERG; the amount of loss is dependent on the degree of lyonization.

A late-onset X-linked cone dystrophy has been reported that has a characteristic tapetal-like sheen (see figures 70.1A and 70.1B) and changes with dark adaptation (Mizuo-Nakamura effect). These patients in later stages often will show an inverselike macular atrophy in that their sheen highlights the macular atrophy (see figure 70.1A). As was noted above, there is a pattern of symmetric anatomic foveal tissue loss, and the sheen is missing from this area in this group of patients. Several of the affected family members have had round atrophic holes leading to retinal detachment, so these patients should be checked on a regular basis for hole formation, which will need laser prophylaxis if found. The gene for this disorder is currently unknown.

An X-linked red cone degeneration has been reported in a pedigree in which the DNA analysis with a cDNA probe found a 6.5-kb deletion in the red cone pigment gene. Clinically, patients have photosensitivity in childhood and a red color deficiency.[10] The 15-year-old propositus's maternal grandfather and great uncle had 20/200 vision with macular atrophy. The ERG showed loss of red cone function, and the 30-Hz flicker appeared to be the most affected.

Partial cone degeneration or dysfunction

A number of adult and senile patients will demonstrate partial cone loss on standardized full-field electroretinographic testing. Many of these cone degeneration patients

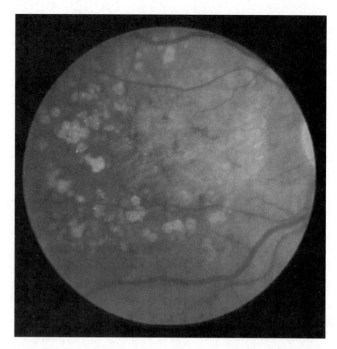

FIGURE 70.7 Senile cone degeneration in an 80-year-old woman with failing vision over ten years, who was found to have poor photopic ERGs with both eyes. Her right eye had a 45 uV b-wave amplitude while the left eye was barely recordable with count finger vision. Rod responses were abnormal. Visual fields were full with central scotomata. Many patients with senile cone degeneration have regional atrophy with crystallike drusen deposits. (See also color plate 44.)

have no family history and will show subnormal vision, photosensitivity, or complaints of light or dark adaptation and foveal atrophy. A few patients will have golden or yellow deposits in the macular area (figure 70.7). Some may have temporal disk atrophy. The cone ERG in some will be attenuated from 30% to 60% of normal often with increased implicit times up to 40 ms. There is a wide variety of presenting visual acuities in these patients, but they typically range from 20/40 to 20/200. Ladewig identified a group of senile cone degeneration patients, whom he did not find to be otherwise distinguishable from patients with age-related macular degeneration.[9]

Autosomal-dominant cone dystrophy

Autosomal-dominant cone dystrophy in most families has a distinctive appearance and clinical history. Frequently, subnormal vision will begin by the teenage years, and early macular atrophy will be seen.[7] At this stage, the disease is frequently thought to be Stargardt's disease, and some patients even have a few yellow deposits similar to flecks (see figure 70.5). In some families, patients aged 10–30 may show cone ERGs, which are barely recordable to extinguished, while in others, the cone ERGs will be only mildly affected. In all cases over time, however, the cone ERG progressively worsens and becomes nonrecordable by single-flash technique. In some cases, flicker function may be worse than single-flash cone testing. These patients universally develop round, symmetric macular atrophy (see figures 70.7A and 70.7B). To date, three genes associated with dominant cone dystrophy have been identified (see table 70.2). The number of types of dominant cone dystrophy is not known, but it is of interest that benign concentric annular dystrophy on a follow-up report was found to have a slow cone degeneration in a dominant family.[11]

Autosomal-recessive cone dystrophy

Autosomal-recessive forms of cone dystrophy clearly exist and have been reported in the literature, but this group of diseases is not well understood, in part because many cases appear as isolated occurrences, and family studies have not been productive.

Management of cone disorders

By the time cone dysfunction patients are examined, most have discovered that tinted lenses are beneficial to their vision, both indoors and outdoors, although a few patients will not have tried sunglasses at all. The clinician can play an important role, emphasizing that patients with cone dysfunction do better on average than patients with more progressive problems such as retinitis pigmentosa and can be given a more encouraging outlook. The ophthalmologist also can help by recommending to patients who are not doing so that they use multiple pairs of variably tinted lenses worn according to the lighting conditions. Particularly important is reassurance that wearing tinted glasses indoors is perfectly acceptable and necessary for their condition.

Once patients with a retinal dystrophy learn that they have a problem that is considered untreatable, they often fail to seek ophthalmological care, and refractive problems may be neglected. Since many cone dystrophy patients have myopia, a current refraction is always in order. Patients with central scotomas and subnormal central vision may benefit from low visual aids and eccentric viewing. Some patients report relief of glare with antioxidant vitamins such as beta-carotene and lutein.

Occasional patients will be seen who appear to have foveal structure on ophthalmoscopy yet have extinguished photopic ERGs (figure 70.8). This occurrence is in contrast to patients with bull's-eye or cookie cutter macular lesions. The ERG will give a clear answer to whether a panretinal degenerative process is occurring in the patient and should be done

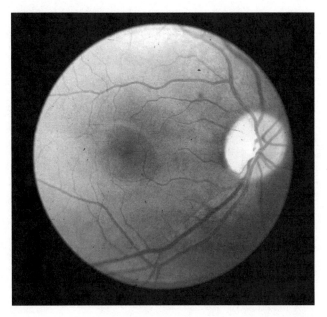

FIGURE 70.8   Cone dystrophy with apparent foveal structure. This 22-year-old woman presented with a history of color blindness and photosensitivity for at least ten years. The family history was negative. Her vision was 20/200 OU, and her photopic ERG was nonrecordable, while her scotopic waveforms were within normal limits. Her Goldmann visual field was full OU. On fundus examination, she appeared to have some foveal structure; but on close inspection, the fovea centralis showed atrophy and mild granularity. (See also color plate 45.)

when there is unexplained subnormal vision or symptoms of color desaturation and glare in patients who may have minimal fundus findings.

REFERENCES

1. Bergen AAB, Pinckers AJLG: Localization of a novel X-linked progressive cone dystrophy gene to Xq27: Evidence for genetic heterogeneity. *Am J Hum Genet* 1997; 60:1468–1473.
2. Carr RE, Siegel I: *Electrodiagnostic*. Philadelphia, FA Davis, 1990.
3. Goodman G, Ripps H, Siegel IM: Cone dysfunction syndromes. *Arch Ophthalmol* 1963; 70:214–231.
4. Hecht S, Schlaer S: Intermittent stimulation by light: V. The relation between intensity and critical frequency for different parts of the spectrum. *J Gen Physiol* 1936; 19:965.
5. Heckenlively JR: RP cone-rod degeneration. *Trans Am Ophthalmol Soc* 1987; 85:438–470.
6. Krill AE: Cone degenerations. In Krill AE, Deutman A (eds): *Hereditary Retinal and Choroidal Dystrophies*. Hagerstown, Md, Harper and Roy, 1977.
7. Krill AE, Deutman AF: Dominant macular degenerations: The cone dystrophies. *Am J Ophthalmol* 1972; 73:352–369.
8. Krill AE, Deutman AF, Fishman M: The cone degenerations. *Doc Ophthalmol* 1973; 35:1–80.

9. Ladewig M, Kraus H, Foerster MH, Kellner U: Cone dysfunction in patients with late-onset cone dystrophy and age-related macular degeneration. *Arch Ophthalmol* 2003; 121(11):1557–1561.

10. Reichel E, Bruce AM, Sandberg MA, et al: An electroretinographic and molecular genetic study of x-linked cone degeneration. *Am J Ophthalmol* 1989; 108:540–547.

11. van den Biesen P, Deutman A: Evolution of benign concentric annular macular dystrophy. *Am J Ophthalmol* 1985; 100:73–78.

12. van Lith, GHM: The macular function in the ERG. *Doc Ophthalmol Proc Ser* 1976; 10:405–415.

13. Yang Z, Peachey NS, Moshfeghi DM, Thirumalaichary S, Chorich L, Shugart YY, Fan K, Zhang K: Mutations in the *RPGR* gene cause X-linked cone dystrophy. *Hum Mol Genet* 2002; 11:605–611.

71 Vitamin A Deficiency

RONALD E. CARR

NIGHT BLINDNESS DUE to vitamin A deficiency has been recognized since ancient Egyptian times, and of the many systemic complications of vitamin A deficiency, the retinal reaction to low vitamin A levels is the best understood. A brief discussion of the metabolism of vitamin A follows to more clearly understand these problems. Vitamin A is transported across the intestinal mucosa and is bound to lipoprotein molecules and then transported and stored in the liver as vitamin A ester. As the body needs vitamin A, these esters are transported as vitamin A alcohol (retinol) to peripheral tissues, including the retina, in conjunction with retinol-binding protein, a transport protein manufactured by the endoplasmic reticulum of the liver. In the retina, vitamin A alcohol is stored in the retinal pigment epithelium and only can be utilized by the photoreceptors after conversion to the aldehyde (retinal). This conversion utilizes the zinc-dependant enzyme alcohol dehydrogenase. Retinal then combines with the protein opsin in darkness to form rhodopsin, and if the retina is bleached by light, this complex breaks down, and the aldehyde is again reduced to the alcohol.

With vitamin A deficiency, as shown in the rat, after the initial stores of vitamin A in the liver and blood have been exhausted, the level of rod visual pigment (rhodopsin) also falls, and reciprocally, the visual threshold rises, thus leading to night blindness.[4]

The classic fundus picture of vitamin A deficiency, first recognized in 1915, is that of scattered multiple white or gray-white spots in the retina, seen mainly in the periphery, with their diameter being that of a retinal vein (figure 71.1).[11] Such fundus changes are easily separable from other "white-dot" retinal lesions by the finding of a low vitamin A level and the clearing of these lesions with normalization of vitamin A levels.

In recent years small-bowel bypass surgery has been performed for morbid obesity and Crohn's disease, and several reports have been forthcoming that note the development of night blindness, usually several years after surgery.[3,13] In all cases parenteral vitamin A has alleviated the symptoms.

Electroretinographic (ERG) findings consist of reduced rod and cone responses with normal implicit times.[7] The abnormality of both photoreceptor systems is further borne out by the dark adaptation curves, which show elevation of both rod and cone segments. With psychophysical measurements of dark adaptation, the more peripheral rods respond more quickly than do the perifoveal rods.

Heckenlively (personal communication) has noted in two of his patients with vitamin A deficiency secondary to malabsorption that the photopic and dark-adapted bright-flash ERG waveforms are very similar in shape and timing, quite unlike the usual situation where the dark-adapted bright-flash ERG has larger a- and b-waves as compared with the photopic ERG. Perlman et al. found a similar change in his reported case (figure 71.2).[7]

Kemp et al.[6] studied visual function and rhodopsin levels in three subjects with vitamin A deficiency secondary to primary biliary cirrhosis and Crohn's diseases by using two-color adaptometry and fundus reflectometry. Employing green and red targets to test rod and cone dark adaptation thresholds before and after vitamin A supplementation, the authors were able to correlate serum vitamin A levels with cone and rod sensitivity (figure 71.3). Fundus reflectometry was used in one patient with liver disease to measure rhodopsin levels before and 3 and 9 days after starting vitamin A supplementation; there was complete recovery to normal of rhodopsin, which was correlated with the dark adaptation testing (figure 71.4).

Abnormalities in liver function have also been associated with vitamin A deficiency and night blindness, possibly due to either abnormal synthesis of retinol-binding protein, lowered serum zinc levels, or simply impaired storage areas for vitamin A esters. Diseases that illustrate these processes include biliary cirrhosis,[12] cystic fibrosis,[8] and chronic alcoholism,[9] the latter presumably with alcoholic cirrhosis. White dots are rarely seen in these conditions and, if present, tend to be more amorphous. Electrophysiological and psychophysical studies in such patients showed elevated rod and cone thresholds on dark adaptation testing as well as reduced or undetectable rod ERGs with reduced-amplitude cone ERGs and normal implicit times. Full recovery was obtained in virtually all patients following parenteral or oral vitamin A supplements.

The syndrome of abetalipoproteinemia (Bassen-Kornzweig syndrome) is associated with steatorrhea, acanthocytosis, a progressive neuromuscular degeneration, and a generalized degeneration of the retina.[1] In this disorder there is a low level of all fats including the fat-soluble vitamins. The associated absence or near-absence of

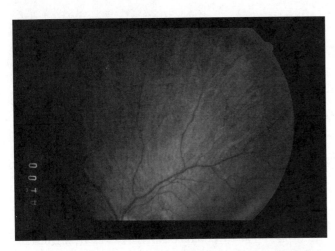

FIGURE 71.1 Fundus photograph of a 53-year-old woman with documented vitamin A deficiency from complications secondary to bowel resection in Crohn's disease. Her barely recordable ERG and night vision became normal after parenteral vitamin A and E therapy. (Courtesy of John Heckenlively, M.D.) (See also color plate 46.)

lipoproteins, among them the lipoproteins responsible for the transport of vitamin A in the blood, is the metabolic abnormality responsible for the concomitant low serum levels of this vitamin. Several studies have shown that some patients given vitamin A with subsequent normalization of their vitamin A levels will show an improvement in both dark adaptation as well as the ERG.[5,10] Bishara et al. suggested that vitamin E should also be administered comcomitantly.[2]

In summary, from a clinical perspective, vitamin A deficiency with subsequent night blindness can occur from a number of diseases affecting different metabolic sites; these include (1) reduced intake of vitamin A and/or carotenoids such as in malnutrition, (2) reduced intestinal absorption of vitamin A such as follows intestinal bypass or resection surgery, (3) defects in the transport of vitamin A as in Bassen-Kornzweig syndrome, and (4) liver disease that leads to abnormalities in the normal vitamin A pathway due to reduced production of retinol-binding protein, reduced amounts of zinc, or reduced storage areas for vitamin A esters.

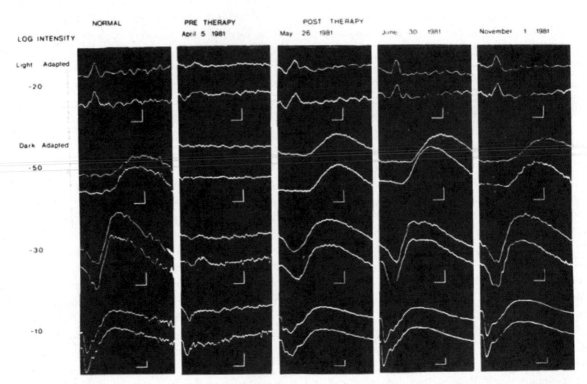

FIGURE 71.2 ERGs of a normal subject (first column) and a patient with vitamin A malabsorption. The patient's ERG responses were measured at different dates before (second column) and after (third to fifth columns) therapy. The ERG responses were evoked by single white flashes of different intensities during the light- (1st row) and dark-adapted states (second to fourth rows). The intensity of the test light is given as the density of the neutral filter interposed in the light path. The upper tracing is from the left eye and the lower from the right eye. The calibration mark equals 100 µV vertically and 25 ms horizontally. (From Perlman I, Barsilai D, Haim T, Schramek A.[7] Used by permission.)

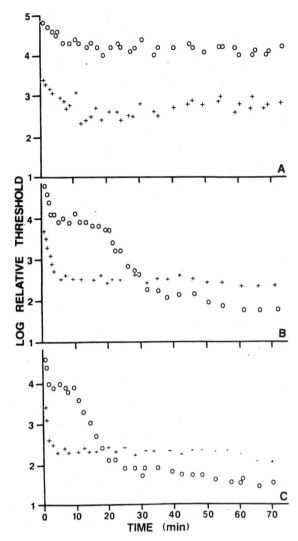

FIGURE 71.3 Two-color dark adaptometry of a subject with vitamin A deficiency: Relative thresholds to the green (*circles*) and red (*crosses*) stimuli. Measurements were made at a retinal eccentricity of 25 degrees along the horizontal meridian in the nasal field and followed a white bleaching exposure that removed virtually all visual pigment. A, results obtained on the first test; B, data obtained when vitamin A supplementation had led to partial recovery of visual function; C, data obtained when systemic vitamin A levels were normal. (From Kemp CM, Jacobson SG, Faulkner DJ, Walt RW.[6] Used by permission.)

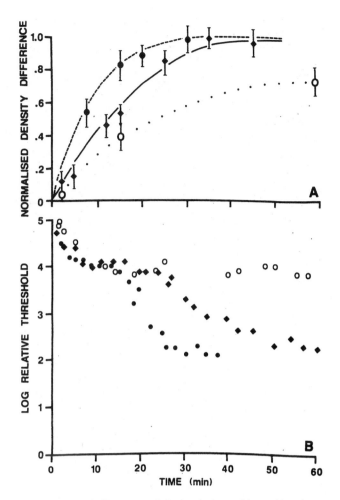

FIGURE 71.4 A, Recovery of rhodopsin in a subject with primary bilary cirrhosis and vitamin A deficiency following a full bleaching exposure on days when serum levels were normal (filled circle), mildly abnormal (diamond), and more severely abnormal (open circle). All double-density changes have been normalized to the value obtained at 30 minutes (0 to 0.12 density units) on the day when the serum vitamin A level was normal. Error bars are 1 SD. B, corresponding dark adaptometry data for a green stimulus. (From Kemp CM, Jacobson SG, Faulkner DJ, Walt RW.[6] Used by permission.)

REFERENCES

1. Bassen FA, Kornzweig AL: Malformation of erythrocytes in a case of atypical retinitis pigmentosa. *Blood* 1950; 5:381–387.

2. Bishara S, Merin S, Cooper M, Aziz E, Delpre G, Deckelbaum RJ: Combined vitamin A & E therapy prevents retinal electrophysiological deterioration in abetalipoproteinemia. *Br J Ophthalmol* 1982; 66:767–770.

3. Brown GC, Felton SM, Benson WE: Reversible night-blindness associated with intestinal bypass surgery. *Am J Ophthalmol* 1980; 89:776–779.

4. Dowling JE, Wald G: The biologic formation of vitamin A acid. *Proc Natl Acad Sci USA* 1960; 46:587–608.

5. Gouras P, Carr RE, Gunkel RD: Retinitis pigmentosa in abetalipoproteinemia: Effects of vitamin A. *Invest Ophthalmol* 1971; 10:784–793.

6. Kemp CM, Jacobson SG, Faulkner DJ, Walt RW: Visual function and rhodopsin levels in humans with vitamin A deficiency. *Exp Eye Res* 1988; 46:188.

7. Perlman I, Barsilai D, Haim T, Schramek A: Night vision in a case of vitamin A deficiency due to malabsorption. *Br J Ophthalmol* 1983; 67:37–42.

8. Petersen RA, Petersen VS, Robb RM: Vitamin A deficiency with xerophthalmia and night blindness in cystic fibrosis. *Am J Dis Child* 1968; 116:662–665.

9. Sandberg MA, Rosen JB, Berson EL: Cone and rod function in vitamin A deficiency with chronic alcoholism and retinitis pigmentosa. *Am J Ophthalmol* 1977; 84:658–665.

10. Sperling MA, Hiles DA, Kennerdel JS: ERG responses following vitamin A therapy in abetalipoproteinemia. *Am J Ophthalmol* 1972; 73:342–351.

11. Teng KH: Further contributions to the fundus xerophthalmicus. *Ophthalmologica* 1965; 150:219–238.

12. Walt RW, Kemp CM, Lyness L, Bird AC, Sherlock S: Vitamin A treatment for night blindness in primary biliary cirrhosis. *Br Med J* 1984; 288:1030–1031.

13. Wechsler HL: Vitamin A deficiency following small-bowel bypass surgery for obesity. *Arch Dermatol* 1979; 115:73–75.

XIII DISEASES OF THE MIDRETINA (INCLUDING NEGATIVE WAVEFORM DISEASES)

72 Differential Diagnosis of the Electronegative Electroretinogram

RICHARD G. WELEBER AND PETER J. FRANCIS

THE ELECTRONEGATIVE electroretinogram (ERG), also referred to as a *negative ERG*, is a very distinctive electrophysiological finding that has significant importance in not only establishing the correct diagnosis, but also localizing the source of the abnormality within the retina. An electronegative ERG has classically been defined as an ERG in which the a-wave amplitude is normal but the b-wave amplitude is severely subnormal, being smaller in amplitude than the a-wave. Within the past two decades, the term *electronegative ERG* has been expanded to include not only the classic definition, but also any ERG in which the b-wave is smaller than the a-wave, even when the a-wave itself is clearly subnormal. Moreover, although the term was initially applied only to the dark-adapted mixed rod-cone bright-flash ERG, the term has recently been used to describe a similar configuration for the light-adapted cone ERG.[34,72]

Origins of the negative ERG

The human maximal full-field electoretinogram presented to the dark-adapted eye is mainly rod-derived and has two predominant components: An initial negative a-wave followed rapidly by a supervening positive b-wave. The a-wave has been shown to be linked to the kinetics of rod phototransduction. It is now generally agreed that the b-wave arises from ON bipolar cell depolarisation,[26,40,67] though it is likely that rod inner segments, the synaptic layer between rod and bipolar cells[63] and third-order neurons also contribute.[83]

The basic underlying retinal pathology for all electronegative ERGs must thus be a disturbance at or proximal to the photoreceptor inner segments but that relatively spares photoreceptor outer segment function. This may include disturbance of neurotransmitter release from photoreceptor inner segments, defects of the postsynaptic receptors of bipolar cells where they synapse with the photoreceptors, or any disturbance of the microvasculature of the middle retinal neurons. Etiologies that should therefore be considered include inherited retinal dystrophies and acquired processes such as inflammatory, autoimmune, vascular, or neurotoxic retinopathies.

Disorders associated with an electronegative ERG

Many disorders have been described with electronegative ERGs. A complete listing is shown in table 72.1 together with references to chapters in this text in which more detailed descriptions may be found. Some show selective reduction in the b-wave, for example, congenital stationary night blindness (CSNB) and melanoma-associated retinopathy (MAR). Disorders in which the a-wave amplitude is typically also abnormal include diseases that affect multiple retinal cell types, such as ocular siderosis, quinine toxicity, methanol toxicity, and certain forms of retinitis pigmentosa, and vascular diseases that compromise or disrupt both choroidal and retinal circulation, such as birdshot choroidopathy and carotid insufficiency.

CONGENITAL STATIONARY NIGHT BLINDNESS Probably the most frequent and best-recognized cause of a negative ERG is X-linked CSNB (Schubert-Bornschein types; see also chapter 74). CSNB is a recessive, nonprogressive retinal disorder characterized by night blindness, decreased visual acuity, myopia, nystagmus, and strabismus. In 1986, Miyake et al. proposed the existence of two distinct subtypes of CSNB, termed *complete* and *incomplete*.[50] Patients with complete CSNB show moderate to severe myopia, profoundly subnormal rod function, abnormal scotopic and photopic oscillatory potentials, and a normal or near-normal photopic cone amplitude (figure 72.1). Patients with incomplete CSNB show moderate myopia to hyperopia, subnormal but measurable rod responses, subnormal but more intact oscilatory potentials, and subnormal cone function (see figure 72.1). Weleber and Tongue reported siblings with visual developmental delay and presumed autosomal-recessive CSNB with markedly subnormal ERG amplitudes during early infancy that increased at age 1 year to became consistent with the complete form of CSNB.[80] Typically, with both autosomal and X-linked CSNB, the maximal scotopic ERG b-wave amplitude is markedly reduced, but the a-wave is normal or only minimally subnormal.

Two genes have been discovered for the X-linked forms of CSNB (reviewed in Weleber[76]). Incomplete CSNB results from mutation of the gene *CACNA1F*, which encodes the

TABLE 72.1
Disorders associated with electronegative electroretinograms

Disorder	Reference
Inherited (common)	
Schubert-Bornschein type X-linked congenital stationary night blindness (CSNB)	Miyake et al.[50]
X-linked juvenile retinoschisis	Peachey et al.[54]
Inherited (rare associations)	
Retinitis pigmentosa	Cideciyan and Jacobson[16]
Inherited electronegative ERG without fundus abnormalities	Fishman et al.[17]
Fundus albipunctatus	Miyake et al.[49]
Bietti's crystalline dystrophy	Jurklies et al.[31]
Macular cell sheen dystrophy	Kellner et al.[35]
Hereditary optic atrophy	Weleber and Miyake[77]
Cone-rod dystrophy	GUCY2D mutation,[24] CRX mutation R41W,[72] autosomal-dominant[20]
Bull's eye macular dystrophy	Miyake et al.[24]
Åland Island eye disease (Fossius–Eriksson syndrome)	Weleber et al.[78]
Oregon eye disease	Pillers et al.[56]
Neural ceroid lipofuscinoses (NCL)	Marshman et al.,[43] Weleber[74]
Duchenne muscular dystrophy	Jensen et al.,[27] Pillers et al.,[55] Sigesmund et al.,[69] Weleber et al.[78]
Mucolipidosis IV	Pradhan et al.[59]
Infantile Refsum disease	Weleber,[75] Weleber et al.[79]
Autosomal-dominant neovascular inflammatory vitreoretinopathy (ADNIV)	Bennett et al.,[5] Stone et al.[70]
Acquired	
Melanoma-associated retinopathy (MAR)	Berson and Lessell[7]
Central retinal vascular occlusion (artery, vein)	Bresnick,[9] Karpe and Uchermann[32]
Birdshot chorioretinopathy	Priem et al.[60]
Ocular siderosis (from intraocular metallic foreign body)	Schechner et al.[66]
Quinine toxicity	Bacon et al.[2]
Vincristine-induced retinotoxicity	Ripps et al.[62]
Methanol toxicity	McKeller et al.[46]
MS-222 (fish anesthetic)	Bernstein et al.[6]

α-subunit of the L-type voltage-gated calcium channel present within retinal synapses.[3,71] Presumably, the mutations cause a decrease in neurotransmitter release from photoreceptor presynaptic terminals.[71] Complete CSNB results from a mutation of the gene *NYX*, which encodes nyctalopin, a small leucine-rich proteoglycan that is thought to be essential for the development of functional ON pathway retinal interconnections, including ON bipolar cells.[4,61]

Controversy exists as to whether Åland Island eye disease (AIED) (also called Forsius-Eriksson ocular albinism)[19] is a separate disorder or should be considered a subset of X-linked incomplete CSNB.[13,83] Family studies suggest that the two disorders have the same genetic interval,[1,23,66] and although mutations in *CACNA1F* have been found in rare AIED-like patients, no mutations have been identified in the *CACNA1F* gene in the original AIED patients.[84] Nonetheless, AIED and incomplete CSNB are electrophysiologically similar, if not indistinguishable.[78]

X-LINKED JUVENILE RETINOSCHISIS X-linked juvenile retinoschisis (XLRS) is probably the next most frequent and recognized genetic cause of an electronegative ERG (figure 72.2) (see chapter 73).[25,36,54,68] This progressive retinal dystrophy is the most common cause of juvenile macular degeneration in males.[52] The condition exhibits considerable variability at presentation. Classically, multiple peripheral retinoschises and vitreoretinal degeneration can be seen associated with a cystic, spoke-wheel maculopathy.[21]

Electrophysiological and psychophysiological studies of XLRS have been interpreted to suggest that oscillatory potentials (OPs) may be generated, at least in part, by interplexiform cells rather than entirely from amacrines or horizontal cells.[54] Furthermore, the negative ERG in association with normal psychophysical function is strongly supportive of Müller cell dysfunction. Müller cells are not the direct generators of the OPs but reflect the signal generated in other cells.[54] Abnormal a-wave responses are also seen and

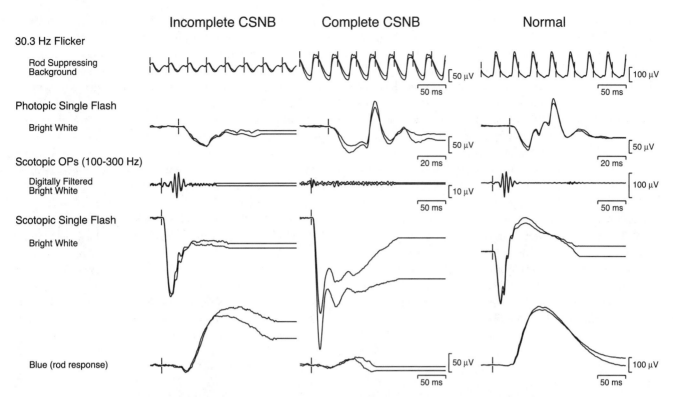

FIGURE 72.1   International Society for Clinical Electrophysiology of Vision (ISCEV) standard ERG for patient with incomplete CSNB, complete CSNB, and an age-similar normal for comparison. The right and left eyes are superimposed. Note that sizable rod responses, detectable oscillatory potentials, and severely subnormal photopic b-waves distinguish the incomplete from the complete form of CSNB. (Reproduced with permission from Weleber RG. Infantile and childhood retinal blindness: A molecular perspective (The Franceschetti Lecture). Ophthalmic Genet 2002; 23:71–97.)

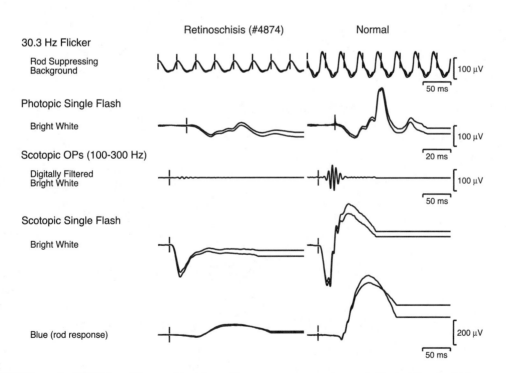

FIGURE 72.2   ISCEV standard ERG for a 36-year-old patient with X-linked retinoschisis, compared to a normal. The right and left eyes are superimposed. Typical foveal schisis was not evident, but the foveal umbo was absent.

indicate that photoreceptor as well as inner retinal layer function may be affected in XLRS, at least in some patients.[8]

XLRS results from mutations within the XLRS1 gene, which encodes retinoschisin. This protein acts as a cell adhesion protein to maintain cellular organization and the synaptic structure of the retina.[81] Disruption of this gene function presumably leads to the disruption of Müller cells, which results in the splitting of the inner plexiform layer. It is of note that there appears to be no good genotype-phenotype correlation. The severity of ERG abnormalities does not appear to correlate with clinical findings, age, or the type of mutation. Responses may even differ between affected males within the same family.[8]

Although the electroretinogram is a key diagnostic test for X-linked retinoschisis, Sieving et al.[68] have documented a normal electroretinogram scotopic b-wave in a male with molecularly confirmed X-linked retinoschisis. Caution is therefore advised in placing too much reliance on the electroretinogram to exclude the diagnosis.

RETINITIS PIGMENTOSA Most patients with advanced RP of many subtypes will have an electronegative ERG with greater relative loss of b-wave than a-wave (figure 72.3). The selective loss of the b-wave probably occurs from the secondary remodeling effects of the retinal degeneration on middle and inner retinal neurons and Müller cells. These stress-induced reorganizational responses to the degeneration and death of photoreceptors lead to neuronal cell death, neuronal and glial migration, elaboration of new neurites and synapses, rewiring of retinal circuits, glial hypertrophy, and the evolution of a fibrotic glial seal that isolates the remnant neural retina from the surviving RPE and choroid.[30,41] Other patients with early retinitis pigmentosa (RP) with otherwise typical clinical features have been found to have the unusual electroretinographic finding of a negative waveform to a bright flash in the dark-adapted state (figure 72.4). The ERG findings in this subset of RP patients indicate there is relatively early dysfunction not only at the level of the photoreceptor outer segment but also at or prox-

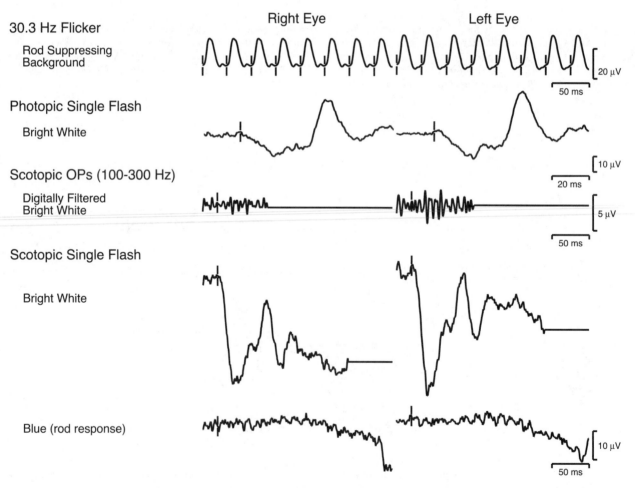

FIGURE 72.3 ISCEV standard ERG for the right and left eyes of a 35-year-old patient with autosomal-dominant RP, compared to a normal. The fundus appearance was typical for moderately advanced RP.

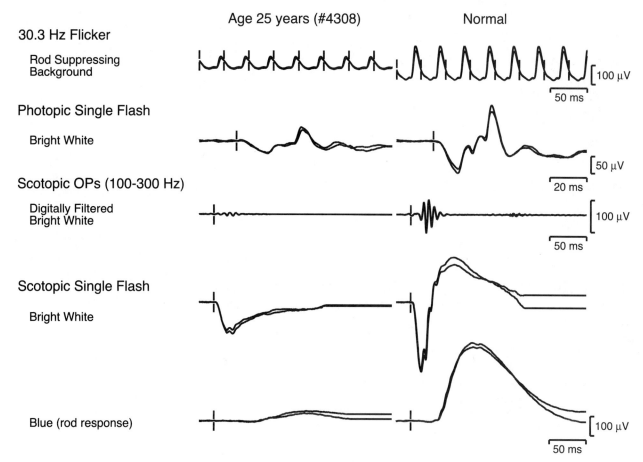

Age 25 years (#4308)   **Normal**

30.3 Hz Flicker

Rod Suppressing
Background

100 µV
50 ms

Photopic Single Flash

Bright White

50 µV
20 ms

Scotopic OPs (100-300 Hz)

Digitally Filtered
Bright White

100 µV
50 ms

Scotopic Single Flash

Bright White

Blue (rod response)

100 µV
50 ms

FIGURE 72.4 ISCEV standard ERG for a patient with autosomal-dominant RP, compared to a normal. The fundus showed a bull's-eye maculopathy with minimal pigment in the periphery.

imal to the photoreceptor terminal region.[16] Even patients with molecular defects limited to rods, for example, RP from the P23H mutation of rhodopsin, may show an electronegative ERG (figure 72.5). The possibility of autoimmune retinopathy should be considered in patients with RP and electronegative ERG (see chapter 58).

CONE, CONE-ROD AND MACULAR DYSTROPHIES WITH ELECTRONEGATIVE ERGS   A progressive cone dystrophy has been described in which negative scotopic and photopic full-field ERGs were recorded. The authors comment that this is most unusual and raise the possibility that the retinal and electrophysiological defects may be inherited separately.[34] More likely, the defective gene product is required for maintenance of health and function of photoreceptor (cone) inner segments and/or middle retinal neurons (bipolar cells). Electronegative ERGs have also been noted in three families with dominantly inherited cone-rod dystrophies.[20,24,72]

Miyake et al.[48] studied four patients with a bull's-eye maculopathy and otherwise normal fundus. Acuity and color

vision losses were progressive, though visual fields were unaffected. A dark-adapted single-flash ERG with an intense white light stimulus was electronegative. Cone responses were relatively well preserved. The 30-Hz flicker ERG and EOG were normal.

FUNDUS ALBIPUNCTATUS   Fundus albipunctatus is a rare autosomal-recessive condition characterized by numerous yellow-white punctate lesions at the level of the retinal pigment epithelium.[42,49] Although originally considered a stationary disorder, Miyake et al. have reported that patients of all ages may develop atrophic macular lesions.[49] Scotopic and photopic ERG responses are subnormal following conventional dark adaptation but reach normal or near-normal amplitudes following extended dark adaptation.[14,42,47] However, what is not addressed in any of these studies is the negative waveform of the scotopic maximal responses with conventional dark adaptation.[49]

MÜLLER CELL SHEEN RETINAL DYSTROPHY   Kellner and colleagues have described a negative ERG in a family with

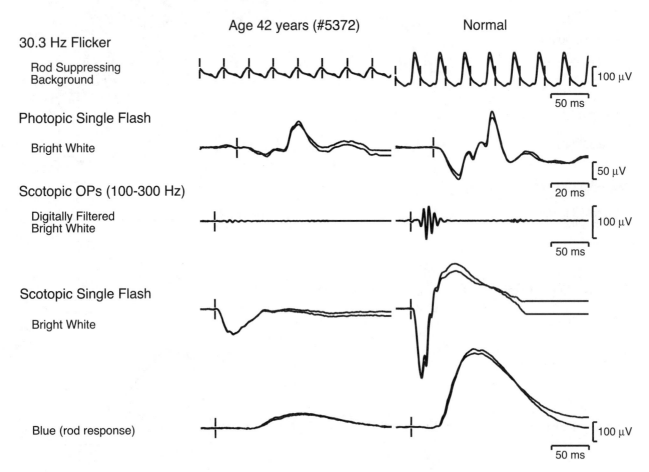

Age 42 years (#5372)   Normal

30.3 Hz Flicker

   Rod Suppressing
   Background   100 µV

                                                                  50 ms

Photopic Single Flash

   Bright White   50 µV

                                                                  20 ms

Scotopic OPs (100-300 Hz)

   Digitally Filtered
   Bright White   100 µV

                                                                  50 ms

Scotopic Single Flash

   Bright White

   Blue (rod response)   100 µV

                                                                  50 ms

FIGURE 72.5 ISCEV standard ERG for a patient with autosomal-dominant RP from the P23H mutation of rhodopsin, compared to a normal. An early regional pigmentary retinopathy was evident on fundus examination. The visual fields showed a ring scotoma in each eye.

Müller cell sheen dystrophy. Light-adapted responses showed an unusually delayed b-wave, broad and delayed ON and OFF responses, and a missing flicker response, suggesting Müller cell dysfunction.[35]

FAMILIAL OPTIC ATROPHY Dominant optic atrophy has been reported with an electronegative ERG, presumably representing a newly appreciated genetic disorder.[77] Such electrophysiological abnormalities are not seen with other familial optic atrophies.

AUTOSOMAL-DOMINANT INHERITANCE OF A NEGATIVE ERG PHENOTYPE Electrophysiologic studies were performed in an infant who presented with moderate myopia, nystagmus, visual developmental delay, and an electronegative ERG.[18] These findings prompted investigation of other family members who showed similar electrophysiological abnormalities, apparently inherited as a dominant trait. Rod thresholds were normal, as were acuities and visual fields. The infant's nystagmus resolved by age 5 years, at which point the fundi remained normal and there was no evidence

of systemic disease. The authors speculated that a mutation within the gene encoding metabotropic glutamate receptor subtype 6 might be causative but found no sequence changes.

BIETTI CRYSTALLINE DYSTROPHY Jurklies et al.[31] have reported a single case of an individual with Bietti crystalline dystrophy, whom they followed over a 30-year course. Serial ERG recordings progressed from low normal amplitudes to extinction. However, during his third decade, electronegative scotopic ERG waveforms were noted.

AUTOSOMAL-DOMINANT NEOVASCULAR INFLAMMATORY VITREORETINOPATHY Autosomal-dominant neovascular inflammatory vitreoretinopathy is a rare genetic eye disorder first described in 1990 and linked in 1992 in a large family to the long arm of chromosome 11 (11q13).[5,70] Affected patients may be asymptomatic in early adulthood but eventually acquire vitreous cells and selective loss of the b-wave of the scotopic ERG. They eventually develop cystoid macular edema, cataracts, and glaucoma as well as peripheral arteriolar closure, peripheral neovascularization, and peripheral retinal pigmentary retinopathy. Retinal detachments can ensue, and these patients react to surgery with a marked inflammatory response.

Neurodegenerative disorders

NEURONAL CEROID LIPOFUSCINOSES   The neuronal ceroid lipofuscinoses (NCL, Batten's disease) are neurodegenerative disorders with psychomotor deterioration, seizures, visual failure, and premature death, all associated with abnormal storage of lipoproteins within lysosomes (see chapter 80). The most common forms of NCL are an infantile form (INCL, *CLN1*), a late infantile form (LINCL, *CLN2*) and a juvenile-onset form (JNCL, *CLN3*). The ERG is abnormal early in all three of these forms, and may take on an electronegative configuration, and eventually is totally ablated. Patients with JNCL invariably showed severe to profound ERG abnormalities when first tested, usually with no discernible rod-mediated activity and marked loss of a-wave

amplitudes with even greater loss of b-wave amplitudes, creating electronegative configuration waveforms (figure 72.6). Differences in the ERG responses were thus found that provide further clues to the earliest site of pathology within the retina.[74]

MUCOLIPIDOSIS IV   The finding of electronegative ERGs in two cases of mucolipidosis IV suggests that the primary retinal disturbance in mucolipidosis IV may occur at or proximal to the photoreceptor terminals.[59] For children with corneal cloudiness and developmental delays, the finding of an electronegative ERG (figure 72.7) should trigger the consideration of this disorder.

INFANTILE REFSUM'S DISEASE   Infantile Refsum's disease (IRD) represents a disorder of peroxisomal biogenesis and is distinct from the classical later-onset or classic form of Refsum's disease (reviewed in Weleber[79]). The biochemical abnormalities in IRD are more extensive and reflect the expected multiple biochemical defects and deficiencies

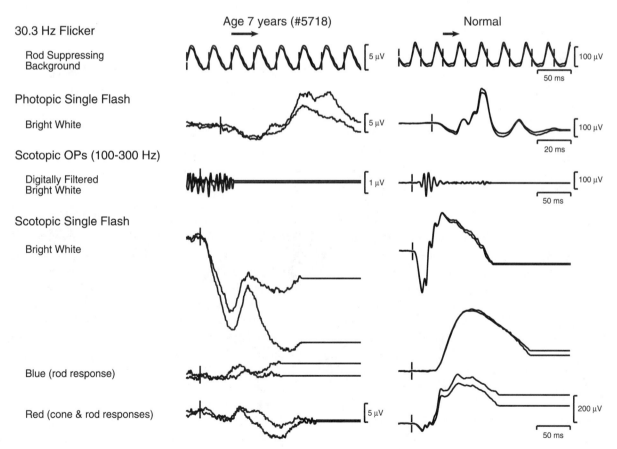

FIGURE 72.6   ISCEV standard ERG for a 7-year-old patient with juvenile-onset neuronal ceroid lipofuscinosis, compared to an age-similar normal. Tracings from the right and left eyes are superimposed. Note the differences in the vertical scale. The patient was heterozygous for the 1.02-kb deletion of *CLN3*.

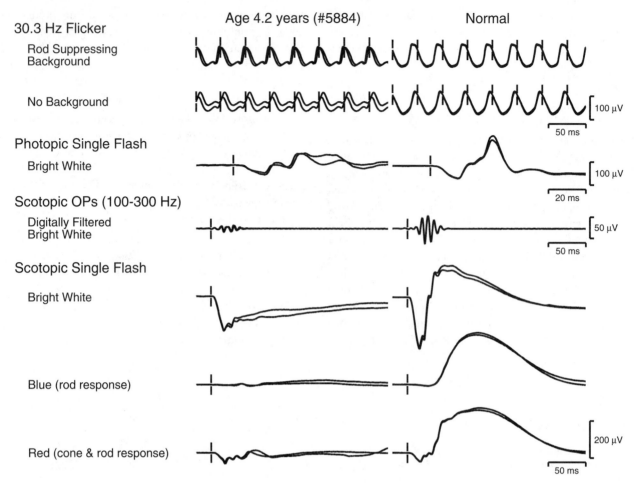

FIGURE 72.7 ISCEV standard ERG for a 4-year-old patient with type IV mucolipidosis, compared to an age-similar normal. Tracings from the right and left eyes are superimposed.

resulting from the near total absence of functional peroxisomes. Abnormal laboratory findings in IRD include elevated plasma levels of very long chain fatty acids, phytanic acid, and pipecolic acid. Patients are deficient in docosahexaenoic acid, precursors of plasmalogens, and the biliary dihydroxycholestanoic and trihydroxycholestanoic acids. Features include early-onset mental retardation, facial dysmorphism, RP, sensorineural hearing loss, hepatomegaly, osteoporosis, failure-to-thrive, and hypocholesteremia. The ERG is severely abnormal early in the course of the disease and shows an electronegative configuration (figure 72.8). The reason why an electronegative ERG is observed in some patients remains to be elucidated but may involve a function of peroxisomes that is critical for maintenance and survival of middle retinal neuronal as well as photoreceptors.[75,79]

DUCHENNE/BECKER MUSCULAR DYSTROPHIES Duchenne muscular dystrophy (DMD) and Becker muscular dystrophy (BMD) patients have mutations in the dystrophin gene that result in progressive muscle degeneration. The ERG often will be electronegative for these patients as well as patients with the contiguous gene deletion involving dystrophin known as Oregon eye disease, even in the absence of defective dark adaptation.[27,55,56,69,78] At least four isoforms of dystrophin have been shown to be present in the outer plexiform layer of the human retina.[55] Although most patients have no ocular symptoms, a reduced b-wave amplitude is typically seen in the dark-adapted ERG in individuals with mutations that result in the loss of function of these isoforms.[57] Unfortunately, it appears that although ERG findings in DMD and BMD patients may correlate with molecular analysis, such testing is not discriminatory in DMD and BMD carriers.[73]

Acquired diseases of the eye

RETINOVASCULAR DISORDERS An electronegative ERG can be seen in situations in which the retinal capillary circula-

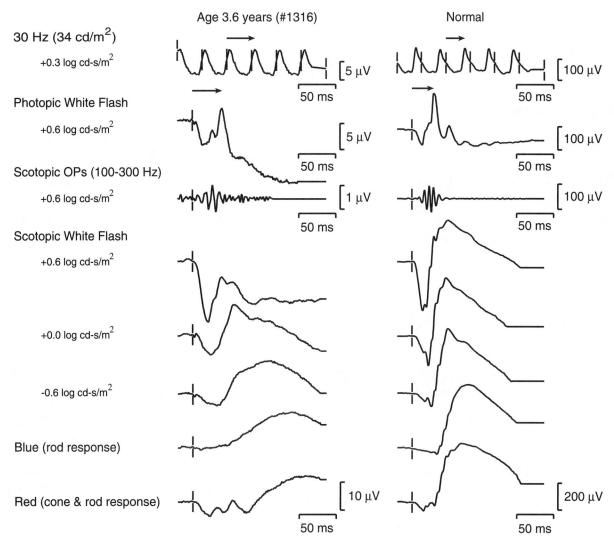

30 Hz (34 cd/m²)
+0.3 log cd-s/m²

Photopic White Flash
+0.6 log cd-s/m²

Scotopic OPs (100-300 Hz)
+0.6 log cd-s/m²

Scotopic White Flash
+0.6 log cd-s/m²

+0.0 log cd-s/m²

-0.6 log cd-s/m²

Blue (rod response)

Red (cone & rod response)

Age 3.6 years (#1316)　　　Normal

FIGURE 72.8 ISCEV standard ERG for a 3-year-old patient with infantile Refsum disease, compared to an age-similar normal. Tracings from the right and left eyes are superimposed.

tion is extensively disrupted, such as occurs in central retinal artery occlusion[32] or hemorrhagic (or ischemic) central retinal vein occlusion (CRVO) (figure 72.9).[32,64] Central retinal vein occlusion can be associated with good capillary perfusion, termed *nonischemic CRVO*, and poorly perfused eyes, termed *ischemic CRVO*. Ischemic CRVO conveys a great risk of iris neovascularization (with subsequent neovascular glaucoma). Panretinal photocoagulation can prevent or ameliorate neovascular glaucoma, but questions persist as to when to offer this treatment. Various techniques (fluorescein angiography, quantitative measures of the afferent pupillary defect, and the ERG) have been evaluated to assess the extent of capillary nonperfusion in eyes with CRVO in an attempt to predict which patients with CRVO are at great-

est risk for iris neovascularization (for a review, see Bresnick[9]). In a retropective study of 45 patients with CRVO, Sabates, Hirose, and McMeel[64] found that six patients with hemorrhagic (ischemic) disease, who had an ERG that was initially electronegative, with on average a b/a ratio of 0.84, developed neovascular glaucoma; conversely, the 27 venous stasis retinopathy (nonischemic) CRVO patients (with an average b/a ration of 1.67) did not develop neovascular glaucoma. Five of the 12 patients with undetermined retinopathy had electronegative ERGs, and two of these developed neovascular glaucoma; three had normal or near-normal ERGs, none of whom developed glaucoma. Overall, no patient with a b/a ratio greater than 1.0 developed neovascular glaucoma. Several investigators have studied the ERG in

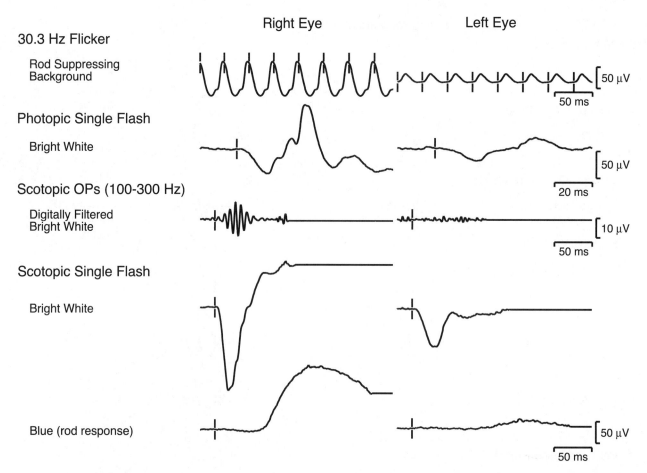

30.3 Hz Flicker

Rod Suppressing Background

Right Eye   Left Eye

50 µV

50 ms

Photopic Single Flash

Bright White

50 µV

20 ms

Scotopic OPs (100–300 Hz)

Digitally Filtered Bright White

10 µV

50 ms

Scotopic Single Flash

Bright White

Blue (rod response)

50 µV

50 ms

FIGURE 72.9   ISCEV standard ERG for the right and left eyes of an 84-year-old male with an ischemic central retinal vein occlusion of the left eye. The b/a ratios were 1.4 OD and 0.9 OS. Rod and cone b-wave implicit times for the left eye were prolonged for single flash and 30 Hz flicker responses. The left eye developed neovascular glaucoma.

CRVO to determine which components are most sensitive and specific for development of iris neovascularization and hence which patients would need consideration for early panretinal photocoagulation.[10–12,28,29,33,37,44,45,82] Debate persists with regard to which protocol is most helpful in the clinical setting; however, the finding of an electronegative ERG in an eye with CRVO is accepted as being highly predictive of iris neovascularization.

MELANOMA-ASSOCIATED RETINOPATHY   Melanoma-associated retinopathy (MAR) is a paraneoplastic retinopathy that commonly presents after the diagnosis of melanoma has been made, often at the stage of metastases. Symptoms include shimmering, photopsias, night blindness, and mild peripheral visual field loss. The fundus may appear normal.[7,15] Histologically, there is evidence of ganglion cell transsynaptic atrophy, a marked decrease in bipolar neurons in the inner nuclear layer, and relative preservation of the photoreceptors themselves.[22] It appears that there is an antibody cross-reactivity between an antigen on melanoma cells and a pro-

tein or lipid on ON bipolar cells.[38] It has recently been suggested that the antigen may be transducin.[58] Such a pattern of retinal degeneration explains intuitively the preferential amplitude reduction in the b-wave of the scotopic full-field ERG that results in the electronegative waveform, characteristic of patients with MAR.

Rarely, individuals present with symptoms, signs, and electrophysiologic abnormalities consistent with a diagnosis of MAR but with no evidence of malignancy. In these instances, similar autoimmune phenomena are hypothesized.[17,51]

BIRDSHOT CHORIORETINOPATHY   Birdshot chorioretinopathy (BSCR) is a bilateral posterior uveitis characterized by the development of cream-colored depigmented chorioretinal lesions that, untreated, result in progressive visual loss from optic atrophy and chronic cystoid macula edema.[53] Electrophysiology typically may show an initially electronegative ERG (figure 72.10) and may be associated with a diminished a-wave; however, both components of the ERG can eventually become extinguished.[39,60]

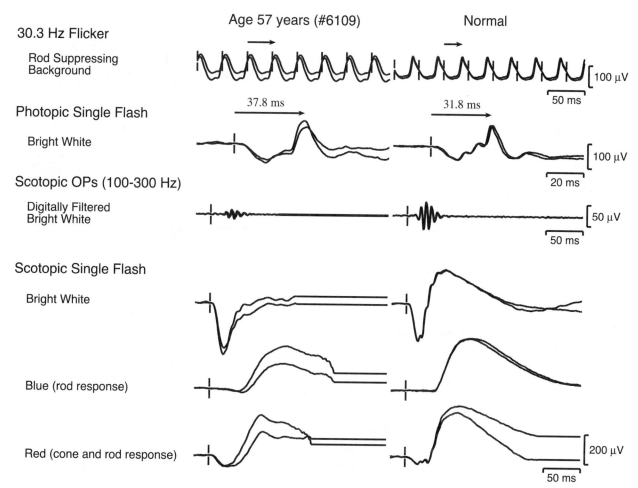

FIGURE 72.10   ISCEV standard ERG for a 5-year-old female with birdshot choroidopathy, compared to an age-similar normal. Tracings from the right and left eyes are superimposed. The disease responded slowly to immunosuppression therapy with modest ERG improvement.

TOXIC RETINOPATHIES   The clinician should be aware that several pharmacological agents can be associated with the generation of negative ERGs and that, in some cases, prompt cessation of treatment may prevent further damage. These include quinine toxicity (figure 72.11),[2] vincristine,[62] methanol,[46] and MS222 (fish anesthetic).[6] A negative ERG has also been documented in ocular siderosis resulting from intraocular ferric foreign bodies.[65]

Concluding comments: The electronegative ERG in clinical practice

Electrophysiological testing is often performed to rule out or add weight to a suspected clinical diagnosis. In instances in which the clinical diagnosis is suspected, the appearance of a negative ERG is useful in providing confirmation. An example is X-linked juvenile retinoschisis. The diagnosis of XLRS may be difficult in instances in which the foveal abnormalities are subtle or late in the disease, when non-specific macular atrophy may supervene. In these instances, an ERG will prove incisive.

However, clinicians are not infrequently confronted with a patient with unexplained subnormal acuity or symptoms, and the ERG is unexpectedly found to be electronegative, providing valuable information in narrowing the possible diagnoses. In some cases, the finding of an electronegative ERG in the face of normal or nonspecific clinical findings warrants prompt further evaluation of the patient for such conditions as melanoma or pharmacological toxicity.

ACKNOWLEDGMENTS   Supported by the Foundation Fighting Blindness, Research to Prevent Blindness, and the Frost Charitable Trust.

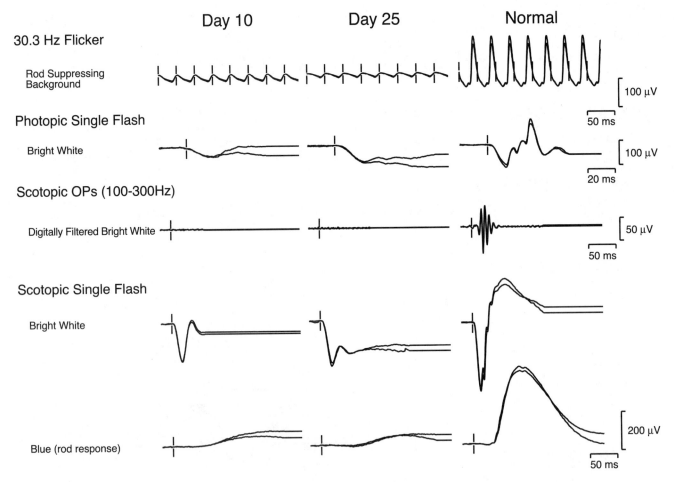

FIGURE 72.11 ISCEV standard ERG for a 15-year-old patient with severe quinine toxicity at day 10 and day 25, compared to an age-similar normal. Tracings from the right and left eyes are superimposed. The visual acuity returned to near normal, but the patient had marked residual field constriction.

REFERENCES

1. Alitalo T, Kruse TA, Forsius H, Eriksson AW, de la Chapelle A: Localization of the Åland island eye disease locus to the pericentromeric region of the X chromosome by linkage analysis. *Am J Hum Genet* 1991; 48:31–38.

2. Bacon P, Spalton D, Smith S: Blindness from quinine toxicity. *Br J Ophthalmol* 1988; 72:219–224.

3. Bech-Hansen NT, Naylor MJ, Maybaum TA, Pearce WG, Koop B, Fishman GA, Mets M, Musarella MA, Boycott KM: Loss-of-function mutations in a calcium-channel alpha1-subunit gene in Xp11.23 cause incomplete X-linked congenital stationary night blindness. *Nat Genet* 1998; 19:264–267.

4. Bech-Hansen NT, Naylor MJ, Maybaum TA, Sparkes RL, Koop B, Birch DG, Bergen AA, Prinsen CF, Polomeno RC, Gal A, Drack AV, Musarella MA, Jacobson SG, Young RS, Weleber RG: Mutations in *NYX*, encoding the leucine-rich proteoglycan nyctalopin, cause X-linked complete congenital stationary night blindness. *Nat Genet* 2000; 26:319–323. [Erratum 2001; 27:125.]

5. Bennett SR, Folk JC, Kimura AE, Russell SR, Stone EM, Raphtis EM: Autosomal dominant neovascular inflammatory vitreoretinopathy. *Ophthalmology* 1990; 97:1125–1135; discussion 35–36.

6. Bernstein PS, Digre KB, Creel DJ: Retinal toxicity associated with occupational exposure to the fish anesthetic MS-222. *Am J Ophthalmol* 1997; 124:843–844.

7. Berson E, Lessell S: Paraneoplastic night blindness with malignant melanoma. *Am J Ophthalmol* 1988; 106:307–311.

8. Bradshaw K, George N, Moore A, Trump D: Mutations of the XLRS1 gene cause abnormalities of photoreceptor as well as inner retinal responses of the ERG. *Doc Ophthalmol* 1999; 98:153–173.

9. Bresnick GH: Following up patients with central retinal vein occlusion. *Arch Ophthalmol* 1988; 106:324–326.

10. Breton ME, Montzka DP, Brucker AJ, Quinn GE: Electroretinogram interpretation in central retinal vein occlusion. *Ophthalmology* 1991; 98:1837–1844.

11. Breton ME, Quinn GE, Keene SS, Dahmen JC, Brucker AJ: Electroretinogram parameters at presentation as predictors of rubeosis in central retinal vein occlusion patients. *Ophthalmology* 1989; 96:1343–1352.

12. Breton ME, Schueller AW, Montzka DP: Electroretinogram b-wave implicit time and b/a wave ratio as a function of intensity in central retinal vein occlusion. *Ophthalmology* 1991; 98:1845–1853.

13. Carlson S, Vesti E, Raitta C, Donner M, Eriksson AW, Forsius H: Clinical and electroretinographic comparison between

Åland island eye disease and a newly found related disease with X-chromosomal inheritance. *Acta Ophthalmol (Copenh)* 1991; 69:703–710.

14. Carr RE, Margolis S, Siegel IM: Fluorescein angiography and vitamin A and oxalate levels in fundus albipunctatus. *Am J Ophthalmol* 1976; 82:549–558.

15. Chan J: Paraneoplastic retinopathies and optic neuropathies. *Surv Ophthalmol* 2003; 48:12–38.

16. Cideciyan AV, Jacobson SG: Negative electroretinograms in retinitis pigmentosa. *Invest Ophthalmol Vis Sci* 1993; 34:3253–3263.

17. Fishman GA, Alexander KR, Milam AH, Derlacki DJ: Acquired unilateral night blindness associated with a negative electroretinogram waveform. *Ophthalmology* 1996; 103:96–104.

18. Fitzgerald KM, Hashimoto T, Hug TE, Cibis GW, Harris DJ: Autosomal dominant inheritance of a negative electroretinogram phenotype in three generations. *Am J Ophthalmol* 2001; 131:495–502.

19. Forsius H, Eriksson A: Tapeto-retinal degenerations with varying clinical features in Åland islanders. *J Med Genet* 1970; 7:200–212.

20. Fujii N, Shiono T, Wada Y, Nakazawa M, Tamai M, Yamada N: Autosomal dominant cone-rod dystrophy with negative electroretinogram. *Br J Ophthalmol* 1995; 79:916–921.

21. George N, Yates J, Moore A: Clinical features in affected males with X-linked retinoschisis. *Arch Ophthalmol* 1996; 114:274–280.

22. Gittinger J, Smith T: Cutaneous melanoma-associated paraneoplastic retinopathy: Histopathologic observations. *Am J Ophthalmol* 1999; 127:612–614.

23. Glass IA, Good P, Coleman MP, Fullwood P, Giles MG, Lindsay S, Nemeth AH, Davies KE, Willshaw KE, Fielder HA, Kilpatrick M, Farndon PA: Genetic mapping of a cone and rod dysfunction (Åland Island eye disease) to the proximal short arm of the human X chromosome. *J Med Genet* 1993; 30:1044–1051.

24. Gregory-Evans K, Kelsell RE, Gregory-Evans CY, Downes SM, Fitzke FW, Holder GE, Simunovic M, Mollon JD, Taylor R, Hunt DM, Bird AC, Moore AT: Autosomal dominant cone-rod retinal dystrophy (CORD6) from heterozygous mutation of *GUCY2D*, which encodes retinal guanylate cyclase. *Ophthalmology* 2000; 107:55–61.

25. Hirose T, Wolf E, Hara A: Electrophysiological and psychophysiological studies in congenital retinoschisis of X-linked recessive inheritance. *Doc Ophthalmol Proc Series* 1977; 13:173–184.

26. Hood DC, Birch DG: Beta wave of the scotopic (rod) electroretinogram as a measure of the activity of human on-bipolar cells. *J Opt Soc Am A* 1996; 13:623–633.

27. Jensen H, Warburg M, Sjö O, Schwartz M: Duchenne muscular dystrophy: Negative electroretinograms and normal dark adaptation. Reappraisal of assignment of X linked incomplete congenital stationary night blindness. *J Med Genet* 1995; 32:348–351.

28. Johnson MA, Marcus S, Elman MJ, McPhee TJ: Neovascularization in central retinal vein occlusion: Electroretinographic findings. *Arch Ophthalmol* 1988; 106:348–352.

29. Johnson MA, McPhee TJ: Electroretinographic findings in iris neovascularization due to acute central retinal vein occlusion. *Arch Ophthalmol* 1993; 111:806–814.

30. Jones BW, Watt CB, Frederick JM, Baehr W, Chen CK, Levine EM, Milam AH, Lavail MM, Marc RE: Retinal remodeling triggered by photoreceptor degenerations. *J Comp Neurol* 2003; 464:1–16.

31. Jurklies B, Jurklies C, Schmidt U, Wessing A: Bietti's crystalline dystrophy of the retina and cornea. *Retina* 1999; 19:168–171.

32. Karpe G, Uchermann A: The clinical electroretinogram: IV. The electroretinogram in circulatory disturbances of the retina. *Acta Ophthalmol (Copenh)* 1955; 33:493–516.

33. Kaye SB, Harding SP: Early electroretinography in unilateral central retinal vein occlusion as a predictor of rubeosis iridis. *Arch Ophthalmol* 1988; 106:353–356.

34. Kellner U, Foerster MH: Cone dystrophies with a negative photopic electroretinogram. *Br J Ophthalmol* 1993; 77:404–409.

35. Kellner U, Kraus H, Heimann H, Helbig H, Bornfeld N, Foerster MH: Electrophysiological evaluation of visual loss in Müller cell sheen dystrophy. *Br J Ophthalmol* 1998; 82:650–654.

36. Koh AH, Hogg CR, Holder GE: The incidence of negative ERG in clinical practice. *Doc Ophthalmol* 2001; 102:19–30.

37. Larsson J, Andréasson S, Bauer B: Cone b-wave implicit time as an early predictor of rubeosis in central retinal vein occlusion. *Am J Ophthalmol* 1998; 125:247–249.

38. Lei B, Bush R, Milam A, Sieving P: Human melanoma-associated retinopathy (MAR) antibodies alter the retinal ON-response of the monkey ERG in vivo. *Invest Ophthalmol Vis Sci* 2000; 41:262–266.

39. Levinson R, Gonzales C: Birdshot retinochoroidopathy: Immunopathogenesis, evaluation and treatment. *Ophthalmol Clin North Am* 2002; 15:343–350.

40. Li S, Mizota A, Adachi-Usami E: Alterations of the electroretinogram by intravitreal kainic acid in the rat. *Jpn J Ophthalmol* 1999; 43:495–501.

41. Marc RE, Jones BW, Watt CB, Strettoi E: Neural remodeling in retinal degeneration. *Prog Retin Eye Res* 2003; 22:607–655.

42. Marmor MF: Fundus albipunctatus: A clinical study of the fundus lesions, the physiologic deficit, and the vitamin A metabolism. *Doc Ophthalmol* 1977; 43:277–302.

43. Marshman W, Lee J, Jones B, Schalit G, Holder G: Duane's retraction syndrome and juvenile Batten's disease: A new association? *Aust N Z J Ophthalmol* 1998; 26:251–254.

44. Matsui Y, Katsumi O, McMeel JW, Hirose T: Prognostic value of initial electroretinogram in central retinal vein obstruction. *Graefes Arch Clin Exp Ophthalmol* 1994; 232:75–81.

45. Matsui Y, Katsumi O, Mehta MC, Hirose T: Correlation of electroretinographic and fluorescein angiographic findings in unilateral central retinal vein obstruction. *Graefes Arch Clin Exp Ophthalmol* 1994; 232:449–457.

46. McKellar M, Hidajat RR, Elder M: Acute ocular methanol toxicity: Clinical and electrophysiological features. *Aust N Z J Ophthalmol* 1997; 25:225–230.

47. Miyake Y, Asano T, Sakai T, Watanabe I: [ERG and EOG in retinitis punctata albescens.] *Nippon Ganka Gakkai Zasshi* 1972; 76:247–256.

48. Miyake Y, Shiroyama N, Horiguchi M, Saito A, Yagasaki K: Bull's-eye maculopathy and negative electroretinogram. *Retina* 1989; 9:210–215.

49. Miyake Y, Shiroyama N, Sugita S, Horiguchi M, Yagasaki K: Fundus albipunctatus associated with cone dystrophy. *Br J Ophthalmol* 1992; 76:375–379.

50. Miyake Y, Yagasaki K, Horiguchi M, Kawase Y, Kanda T: Congenital stationary night blindness with negative electroretinogram: A new classification. *Arch Ophthalmol* 1986; 104:1013–1020.

51. Mizener JB, Kimura AE, Adamus G, Thirkill CE, Goeken JA, Kardon RH: Autoimmune retinopathy in the absence of cancer. *Am J Ophthalmol* 1997; 123:607–618.

52. Mooy C, Born LVD, Baarsma S, Paridaens D, Kraaijenbrink T, Bergen A, Weber B: Hereditary X-linked juvenile retinoschisis: A review of the role of Müller cells. *Arch Ophthalmol* 2002; 120:979–984.

53. Oh K, Christmas N, Folk J: Birdshot retinochoroiditis: Long term follow-up of a chronically progressive disease. *Am J Ophthalmol* 2002; 133:622–629.

54. Peachey NS, Fishman GA, Derlacki DJ, Brigell MG: Psychophysical and electroretinographic findings in X-linked juvenile retinoschisis. *Arch Ophthalmol* 1987; 105:513–516.

55. Pillers DM, Bulman DE, Weleber RG, Sigesmund DA, Musarella MA, Powell BR, Murphey WH, Westall C, Panton C, Becker LE, et al: Dystrophin expression in the human retina is required for normal function as defined by electroretinography. *Nat Genet* 1993; 4:82–86.

56. Pillers DM, Seltzer WK, Powell BR, Ray PN, Tremblay F, La Roche GR, Lewis RA, McCabe ER, Eriksson AW, Weleber RG: Negative-configuration electroretinogram in Oregon eye disease: Consistent phenotype in Xp21 deletion syndrome. *Arch Ophthalmol* 1993; 111:1558–1563.

57. Pillers DM, Weleber RG, Green DG, Rash SM, Dally GY, Howard PL, Powers MR, Hood DC, Chapman VM, Ray PN, Woodward WR: Effects of dystrophin isoforms on signal transduction through neural retina: Genotype-phenotype analysis of Duchenne Muscular Dystrophy mouse mutants. *Mol Genet Metab* 1999; 66:100–110.

58. Potter MJ, Adamus G, Szabo SM, Lee R, Mohaseb K, Behn D: Autoantibodies to transducin in a patient with melanoma-associated retinopathy. *Am J Ophthalmol* 2002; 134:128–130.

59. Pradhan SM, Atchaneeyasakul LO, Appukuttan B, Mixon RN, McFarland TJ, Billingslea AM, Wilson DJ, Stout JT, Weleber RG: Electronegative electroretinogram in mucolipidosis IV. *Arch Ophthalmol* 2002; 120:45–50.

60. Priem H, Rouck AD, De Laey JJ, Bird A: Electrophysiologic studies in birdshot chorioretinopathy. *Am J Ophthalmol* 1988; 106:430–436.

61. Pusch CM, Zeitz C, Brandau O, Pesch K, Achatz H, Feil S, Scharfe C, Maurer J, Jacobi FK, Pinckers A, Andreasson S, Hardcastle A, Wissinger B, Berger W, Meindl A: The complete form of X-linked congenital stationary night blindness is caused by mutations in a gene encoding a leucine-rich repeat protein. *Nat Genet* 2000; 26:324–327.

62. Ripps H, Carr R, Siegel I, Greenstein V: Functional abnormalities in vincristine induced night blindness. *Invest Ophthalmol Vis Sci* 1984; 25:787–794.

63. Ruether K, Grosse J, Matthiessen E, Hoffmann K, Hartmann C: Abnormalities of the photoreceptor-bipolar cell synapse in a substrain of C57BL/10 mice. *Invest Ophthalmol Vis Sci* 2000; 41:4039–4047.

64. Sabates R, Hirose T, McMeel JW: Electroretinography in the prognosis and classification of central retinal vein occlusion. *Arch Ophthalmol* 1983; 101:232–235.

65. Schechner R, Miller B, Merksamer E, Perlman I: A long term follow up of ocular siderosis: Quantitative assessment of the electroretinogram. *Doc Ophthalmol* 1991; 76:231–240.

66. Schwartz M, Rosenberg T: Åland eye disease: Linkage data. *Genomics* 1991; 10:327–332.

67. Shiells RA, Falk G: Contribution of rod, on-bipolar, and horizontal cell light responses to the ERG of dogfish retina. *Vis Neurosci* 1999; 16:503–511.

68. Sieving PA, Bingham EL, Kemp J, Richards J, Hiriyanna K: Juvenile X-linked retinoschisis from XLRS1 Arg213Trp muta-

tion with preservation of the electroretinogram scotopic b-wave. *Am J Ophthalmol* 1999; 128:179–184.

69. Sigesmund DA, Weleber RG, Pillers D-AM, Westall CA, Panton CM, Powell BR, Héon E, Murphey WH, Musarella MA, Ray PN: Characterization of the ocular phenotype of Duchenne and Becker muscular dystrophy. *Ophthalmology* 1994; 101:856–865.

70. Stone EM, Kimura AE, Folk JC, Bennett SR, Nichols BE, Streb LM, Sheffield VC: Genetic linkage of autosomal dominant neovascular inflammatory vitreoretinopathy to chromosome 11q13. *Hum Mol Genet* 1992; 1:685–689.

71. Strom TM, Nyakatura G, Apfelstedt-Sylla E, Hellebrand H, Lorenz B, Weber BH, Wutz K, Gutwillinger N, Ruther K, Drescher B, Sauer C, Zrenner E, Meitinger T, Rosenthal A, Meindl A: An L-type calcium-channel gene mutated in incomplete X-linked congenital stationary night blindness. *Nat Genet* 1998; 19:260–263.

72. Swain PK, Chen S, Wang Q-L, Affatigato LM, Coats CL, Brady KD, Fishman GA, Jacobson SG, Swaroop A, Stone E, Sieving PA, Zack DJ: Mutations in the cone-rod homeobox gene are associated with the cone-rod dystrophy photoreceptor degeneration. *Neuron* 1997; 19:1329–1336.

73. Ulgenalp A, Oner FH, Soylev MF, Bora E, Afrashi F, Kose S, Ercal D: Electroretinographic findings in Duchenne/Becker muscular dystrophy and correlation with genotype. *Ophthalmic Genet* 2002; 23:157–165.

74. Weleber RG: The dystrophic retina in multisystem disorders: The electroretinogram in neuronal ceroid lipofuscinoses. *Eye* 1998; 12(3b):580–590.

75. Weleber RG: Peroxisomal disorders. In Traboulsi EI (ed): *Genetic Diseases of the Eye*. Oxford, UK: Oxford University Press, 1998, pp 663–696.

76. Weleber RG: Infantile and childhood retinal blindness: A molecular perspective (The Franceschetti Lecture). *Ophthalmic Genet* 2002; 23:71–97.

77. Weleber RG, Miyake Y: Familial optic atrophy with negative electroretinogram. *Arch Ophthalmol* 1992; 110:640–645.

78. Weleber RG, Pillers DM, Powell BR, Hanna CE, Magenis RE, Buist NRM: Åland island eye disease (Forsius-Eriksson syndrome) associated with contiguous deletion syndrome at Xp21. *Arch Ophthalmol* 1989; 107:1170–1179.

79. Weleber RG, Tongue AT, Kennaway NG, Budden SS, Buist NRM: Ophthalmic manifestations of infantile phytanic acid storage disease. *Arch Ophthalmol* 1984; 102:1317–1321.

80. Weleber RG, Tongue AC: Congenital stationary night blindness presenting as Leber's congenital amaurosis. *Arch Ophthalmol* 1987; 105:360–365.

81. Williamson TH, Keating D, Bradnam M: Electroretinography of central retinal vein occlusion under scotopic and photopic conditions: What to measure? *Acta Ophthalmol Scand* 1997; 75:48–53.

82. Wu WW, Molday RS: Defective discoidin domain structure, subunit assembly, and endoplasmic reticulum processing of retinoschisin are primary mechanisms responsible for X-linked retinoschisis. *J Biol Chem* 2003; 278:28139–28146.

83. Wurziger K, Lichtenberger T, Hanitzsch R: On-bipolar cells and depolarising third-order neurons as the origin of the ERG-b-wave in the RCS rat. *Vision Res* 2001; 41:1091–1101.

84. Wutz K, Sauer C, Zrenner E, Lorenz B, Alitalo T, Broghammer M, Hergersberg M, de La Chapelle A, Weber BH, Wissinger B, Meindl A, Pusch CM: Thirty distinct *CACNA1F* mutations in 33 families with incomplete type of XLCSNB and *Cacna1f* expression profiling in mouse retina. *Eur J Hum Genet* 2002; 10:449–456.

73 Juvenile X-Linked Retinoschisis

PAUL A. SIEVING, IAN M. MACDONALD, AND NAHEED W. KHAN

JUVENILE X-LINKED retinoschisis (XLRS, OMIM 31270) is a vitreoretinal dystrophy that manifests early in life (as early as 3 months of age)[22] and has no associated nonocular findings. Intraretinal cysts form in the macula, and splitting of the retinal layers occurs in peripheral retina (figures 73.1 and 73.2). The macular changes frequently are in the form of a spoke-wheel pattern of perifoveal cysts and may result in a visual acuity of 20/60 or less. Patients tend to be hyperopic.[11] Substantial peripheral visual field loss can occur. The term *retinoschisis* was introduced by Wilczek in 1935.[28]

The condition is limited nearly exclusively to males. Female carriers essentially never show macular or retinal pathology or suffer visual symptoms, but in rare cases, carriers may have macular or peripheral retinal changes, presumably on the basis of Lyonization of the trait.[9]

XLRS is one of the more common causes of juvenile macular degeneration in males, with a prevalence of 1:5,000 to 1:25,000. Affected males typically are identified by early grade-school age owing to reduced visual acuity. Males initially complain of reduced visual acuity, not poor night vision or loss of peripheral vision. In many cases, the reduced visual acuity stabilizes by the teenage years in affected males and then remains constant into middle age. Macular atrophy may begin in late middle age and progress toward legal blindness (20/200) in affected males. Vitreous hemorrhage and full-thickness retinal detachment occurs occasionally, and successful surgical repair is infrequent.

While the fundus appearance of XLRS may be diagnostic in affected males, the presentation can be confusing in some cases, requiring additional testing with electroretinography. This will be most helpful in the males who have progressed beyond the typical spoke-wheel pattern and present with a bilateral maculopathy, with or without areas of peripheral schisis. A fluorescein angiogram may also be helpful in differentiating XLRS from autosomal-recessive Stargardt macular dystrophy, which exhibits a silent or dark choroid. Younger patients typically show a normal angiogram, although older patients with XLRS may exhibit changes in the retinal pigment epithelium, including relative window defects in the macula (figure 73.3). Occasionally, patients exhibit a change in color immediately or shortly after light onset with dark adaptation (Mizuo phenomenon).[5] This phenomenon disappears with vitrectomy and removal of the posterior vitreous face.[15]

Differential diagnosis

A careful review of the family history will assist in establishing a diagnosis in which an index case presents with a bilateral maculopathy and an electronegative ERG. Cone-rod dystrophy and Stargardt macular dystrophy have a macular phenotype but do not show either an X-linked pattern of inheritance or selective b-wave reduction of the ERG that occurs with XLRS.

Goldmann-Favre syndrome is an autosomal-recessive vitreoretinal disorder in which macular cysts and peripheral lattice degeneration are seen. Patients complain of nyctalopia, unlike in XLRS, and have a markedly reduced ERG.[6] Wagner disease is an autosomal-dominant disorder that maps to 5q13–14[3] and is characterized by myopia, vitreous syneresis, and frequent retinal detachment. The macula may show pigmentary changes. While the ERG may be abnormal in patients with Wagner disease, selective b-wave reduction is not seen.

Gene identification

XLRS was mapped to Xp22.1–22.3 by linkage analysis of many pedigrees.[1,4,17,18,24,26,27] The XLRS gene was cloned in 1997 and was designated RS1.[22] RS1 gene structure consists of six exons coding for 224 amino acid residues. The C-terminal discoidin domain mediates cell-cell adhesion. The RS1 protein is heavily expressed in inner segments of both rod and cone photoreceptors and is also seen in cells of the inner nuclear layer.[7]

Penetrance of mutations is virtually 100%. There is significant intrafamilial variability in the phenotype. Clinically useful genotype-phenotype correlations have not been found. Mutations result in loss of function. Exons 1–3 tend to have nonsense mutations, whereas exons 4–6 (encoding the discoidin domain) have missense mutations, which draws attention to its functional importance.[20]

Classical ERG studies

The electroretinogram (ERG) is the single most useful test for confirming a diagnosis of XLRS. Significant abnormality of dark-adapted thresholds is uncommon. The Arden ratio of the electro-oculogram is usually normal in affected

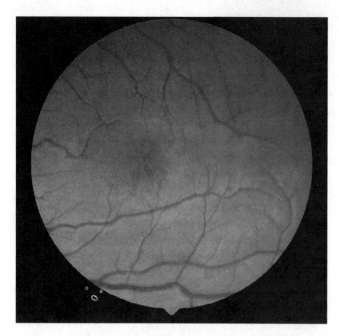

FIGURE 73.1 Fundus photograph of XLRS-affected male with juvenile retinoschisis showing spoke-wheel pattern of foveal cysts covering an area of approximately one disk diameter. (See also color plate 47.)

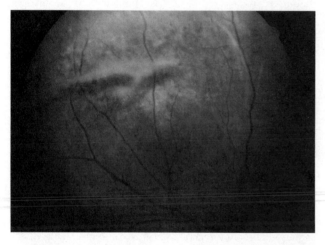

FIGURE 73.2 Fundus photograph of XLRS-affected male with peripheral schisis cavity, which occurs in 50% of affected males. (See also color plate 48.)

individuals.[12,19] The ERG frequently shows an electronegative configuration, in which a-wave amplitude remains substantially normal but the b-wave is reduced (figure 73.4A). Since the b-wave historically was thought to arise from Müller cell depolarization following release of potassium by activity of depolarizing bipolar cells,[10] the presumption was that Müller cells might harbor the primary defect in XLRS. Other diseases that can cause an electronegative ERG configuration include congenital stationary night blindness,[2] which has a normal fundus, whereas XLRS has an abnor-

mal fundus and is not associated with symptomatic night blindness. Other ERG abnormalities in XLRS include the scotopic threshold response (STR).[16] The STR originates in the proximal retina owing to potassium release by amacrine cells and a subsequent depolarization of the Müller cells from this excess potassium. One study suggested that the STR was a sensitive test for identifying XLRS.[16] Despite this apparent sensitivity, however, female carriers exhibited no STR abnormality. Female carriers have normal a- and b-waves. Consequently, female carriers can be identified only by pedigree analysis (daughter of an affected father or woman having an XLRS-affected son).

Although an electronegative ERG is the most frequent presentation in XLRS, exceptions have been reported. In one study of an XLRS family with an Arg213Trp mutation, one affected male retained a normal scotopic b-wave response (figure 73.4B).[23] This indicates that caution is advised in placing complete reliance on the ERG for differential diagnosis of this condition. In this case, genotyping was particularly helpful to confirm the diagnosis of XLRS.

Analysis of photoreceptor and inner retinal responses in XLRS

In a study of 15 males with retinoschisis who had been genotyped for RS1 mutations,[8,20] the ERG was evaluated to determine whether RS1 protein expression in photoreceptors affected their function.[13] When the phototransduction model was applied to dark-adapted a-wave responses elicited by high-intensity flashes, no significant differences were found in XLRS subjects for the parameters R_{max} and $\log S$ compared with normal subjects. Seven of these affected males had normal rod values of R_{max} and $\log S$. This indicated that the photoreceptors were not inherently affected, even though these cells express the RS1 protein. Dark-adapted b-wave responses were considerably reduced under rod-isolating conditions, implicating defective signaling by the depolarizing bipolar cells of the rod pathway.[21]

Normal cone phototransduction in XLRS was demonstrated by normal scaling of the photopic cone a-wave compared with the leading edge of the normals' a-wave (figures 73.5 and 73.6).[13] However, the XLRS a-wave amplitudes were significantly lower than normals by a relatively consistent amount across all intensities, suggesting that second-order hyperpolarizing neurons (hyperpolarizing bipolar cells and horizontal cells) were not contributing to the response. This effect is also found in the monkey a-wave after applying APB + PDA, which isolates the photoreceptor activity.

Additional studies were then performed to investigate possible ON- and OFF-pathway sites of dysfunction by recording photopic ON-OFF responses to 150-ms long-duration

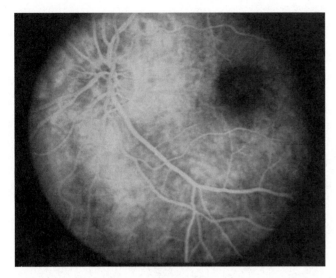

FIGURE 73.3 Intravenous fluoroscein angiogram of XLRS-affected male with abnormal RPE and showing a typical central fluoroscein staining due to RPE thinning.

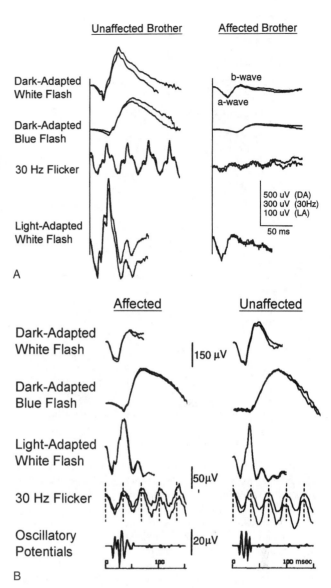

FIGURE 73.4 Electronegative full-field ERG in XLRS. A, Twelve-year-old XLRS-affected male shows typical ERG, with selective b-wave reduction but a-wave preservation in dark-adapted recordings, compared with unaffected brother. Photopic b-wave and flicker are also reduced. (Figure modified from Pawar et al: *Hum Hered* 1996; 46:329–335.) Used by permission from S. Karger AG, Basel.) B, Atypical ERG in XLRS male with an ARG213Trp mutation in the RS1 gene shows preservation of b-wave for dark-adapted and light-adapted conditions, compared with unaffected male relative. All parameters were recorded according to International Society for Clinical Electrophysiology of Vision standards. (Figure modified from Sieving PA, Bingham EL, Kemp J, et al: *Am J Ophthalmol* 1999; 128:179–184. Used by permission from Elsevier Science, UK).

stimuli. This demonstrated reduced b-wave amplitude but normal d-wave amplitude, which caused the ratio of the b/d amplitudes to be less than 1, which is invariably abnormal for this particular stimulus condition.[25] However, we also found a similar reduction of the b/d ratio in a number of other retinal degenerations; consequently, this appears to be a nonspecific finding in retinal degenerations and is nonspecific for localizing the defect in retinal signaling to either the ON or the OFF pathway.

Photopic flicker ERG responses were elicited at 32 Hz, and the fundamental component showed reduced amplitude and delayed phase, consistent with abnormal signaling by both the ON and OFF pathway components.[14] This may be useful in the clinical assessment of XLRS.

The aggregate of these results indicated that, although the expression of RS1 protein is heavily concentrated in the inner segments of both rods and cones, it does not inherently affect the photoreceptor function of either cell type. Immunohistochemical studies localizing the RS1 protein show involvement of retinal cells in the inner nuclear layer, but precise subcellular localization has not yet been performed to learn whether both depolarizing and hyperpolarizing bipolar cells are involved. However, from these ERG studies, it currently is reasonable to propose that retinal signaling by ERG generators associated with both the ON and OFF pathways is defective.

ACKNOWLEDGMENTS   The authors thank Dr. Deborah Carper, Ms. Terry Green, and Ms. Maria Macotto for technical and editorial assistance.

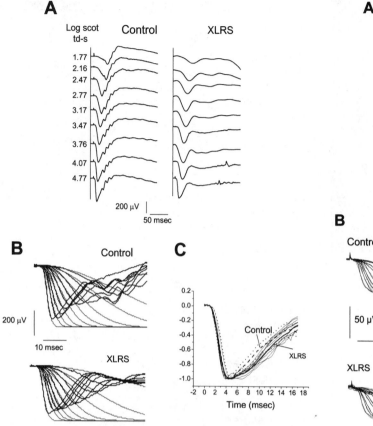

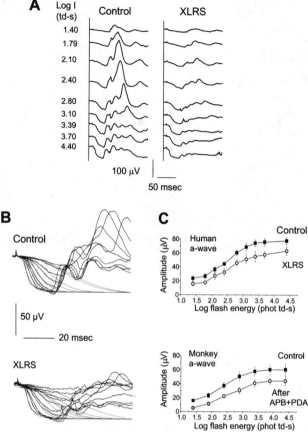

FIGURE 73.5 Rod-driven a-wave analysis in XLRS. A, Dark-adapted ERG responses from a representative XLRS-affected male show preservation of the a-wave but suppression or loss of the b-wave. B, Phototransduction modeling of rod a-wave responses (after subtraction of cone-driven components) elicited by high-intensity flashes gave normal R_{max} and log S parameters for XLRS. C, Normalized rod a-wave XLRS responses (averaged from nine affected males, heavy solid curve) at the brightest flash intensity (4.77 log scot td s) overlapped that of 12 control subjects (heavy dashed curve). The data indicated no functional impairment of rod photoreceptor activity compared with normals. (Modified from Khan NW, Jamison JA, Kemp JA, Sieving PA: *Vision Res* 2001; 41:3931–3942. Used by permission from Elsevier Science, UK.)

FIGURE 73.6 Photopic ERG analysis in XLRS. A, Photopic cone-driven ERG shows relative loss of b-wave versus a-wave. B, Phototransduction modeling of cone a-wave responses. C, Human XLRS a-wave responses are subnormal by a constant amount across the intensities elicited, consistent with the absence of a contribution from hyperpolarizing bipolar and/or horizontal cells, implicating impaired signaling of the retinal OFF pathway. This effect is mirrored in the monkey a-wave (average of four animals) on blocking synaptic output from cones, using APB + PDA. (Modified from Khan NW, Jamison JA, Kemp JA, Sieving PA: *Vision Res* 2001; 41:3931–3942. Used by permission from Elsevier Science, UK.)

REFERENCES

1. Alitalo T, Kurse TA, de la Chapelle A: Refined localization of the gene causing X-linked juvenile retinoschisis. *Genomics* 1991; 9:505–510.

2. Bornschein H, Schubert G: Das photopische flimmer-elektroretinogramm des menschen. *Zeit Biol* 1953; 106:229–238.

3. Brown DM, Graemiger RA, Hergersberg M, Schinzel A, Messmer EP, Niemeyer G, Schneeberger SA, Streb LM, Taylor CM, Kimura AE, Weingeist TA, Sheffield VC, Stone EM: Genetic linkage of Wagner disease and erosive vitreoretinopathy to chromosome 5q13–14. *Arch Ophthal* 1995; 113:671–675.

4. Browne D, Barker D, Litt M: Dinucleotide repeat polymorphisms at the DXS365, DXS443 and DXS451 loci. *Hum Mol Gen* 1992; 1:213.

5. de Jong PT, Zrenner E, van Meel GJ, Keunen JE, van Norren D: Mizuo phenomenon in X-linked retinoschisis: Pathogenesis of the Mizuo phenomenon. *Arch Ophthalmol* 1991; 109:1104–1108.

6. Fishman GA, Jampol LM, Goldberg MF: Diagnostic features of the Favre-Goldmann syndrome. *Br J Ophthalmol* 1976; 60:345–353.

7. Grayson C, Reid SN, Ellis JA, Rutherford A, Sowden JC, Yates JR, Farber DB, Trump D: Retinoschisin, the X-linked retinoschisis protein, is a secreted photoreceptor protein, and is expressed and released by Weri-Rb1 cells. *Hum Mol Genet* 2000; 9:1873–1879.

8. Hiriyanna KT, Bingham EL, Yashar BM, Ayyagari R, Fishman G, Small KW, Weinberg DV, Weleber RG, Lewis RA, Andreasson S, Richards JE, Sieving PA: Novel mutations in XLRS1 causing retinoschisis, including first evidence of putative leader sequence change. *Hum Mutat* 1999; 14:423–427.

9. Kaplan J, Pelet A, Hentati H, Jeanpierre M, Briard ML, Journel H, Munnich A, Dufier JL: Contribution to carrier detection and genetic counselling in X-linked retinoschisis. *J Med Genet* 1991; 28:383–388.

10. Karwoski CJ, Proenza LM: Relationship between Muller cell responses, a local transretinal potential, and potassium flux. *J Neurophysiol* 1977; 40:244–259.

11. Kato K, Miyake Y, Kachi S, Suzuki T, Terasaki H, Kawase Y, Kanda T: Axial length and refractive error in X-linked retinoschisis. *Am J Ophthalmol* 2001; 131:812–814.

12. Kellner U, Brummer S, Foerster MH, Wessing A: X-linked congenital retinoschisis. *Graefes Arch Clin Exp Ophthalmol* 1990; 228:432–437.

13. Khan NW, Jamison JA, Kemp JA, Sieving PA: Analysis of photoreceptor function and inner retinal activity in juvenile X-linked retinoschisis. *Vision Res* 2001; 41:3931–3942.

14. Kondo M, Sieving PA: Primate photopic sine-wave flicker ERG: Vector modeling analysis of component origins using glutamate analogs. *Invest Ophthalmol Vis Sci* 2001; 42:305–312.

15. Miyake Y, Terasaki H: Golden tapetal-like fundus reflex and posterior hyaloid in a patient with x-linked juvenile retinoschisis. *Retina* 1999; 19:84–86.

16. Murayama K, Kuo C, Sieving PA: Abnormal threshold ERG response in X-linked juvenile retinoschisis: Evidence for a proximal retinal origin of the human STR. *Clin Vis Sci* 1991; 6:317–322.

17. Oudet C, Weber C, Kaplan J, Segues B, Croquette MF, Roman EO, Hanauer A: Characterisation of a highly polymorphic microsatellite at the *DXS207* locus: Confirmation of very close linkage to the retinoschisis disease gene. *J Med Genet* 1993; 30:300–303.

18. Pawar H, Bingham EL, Hiriyanna K, Segal M, Richards JE, Sieving PA: X-linked juvenile retinoschisis: Localization between (DXS1195, DXS418) and AFM291 wf5 on a single YAC. *Hum Hered* 1996; 46:329–335.

19. Peachey NS, Fishman GA, Derlacki DJ, Brigell MG: Psychophysical and electroretinographic findings in X-linked juvenile retinoschisis. *Arch Ophthalmol* 1987; 105:513–516.

20. Retinoschisis Consortium: Functional implications of the spectrum of mutations found in 234 cases with X-linked juvenile retinoschisis (XLRS). *Hum Mol Genet* 1998; 7:1185–1192.

21. Robson JG, Frishman LJ: Response linearity and kinetics of the cat retina: The bipolar cell component of the dark-adapted electroretinogram. *Vis Neurosci* 1995; 12:837–850.

22. Sauer CG, Gehrig A, Warneke-Wittstock R, Marquardt A, Ewing CC, Gibson A, Lorenz B, Jurklies B, Weber BH: Positional cloning of the gene associated with X-linked juvenile retinoschisis. *Nat Genet* 1997; 17:164–170.

23. Sieving PA, Bingham EL, Kemp J, Richards J, Hiriyanna K: Juvenile X-linked retinoschisis from XLRS1 Arg213Trp mutation with preservation of the electroretinogram scotopic b-wave. *Am J Ophthalmol* 1999; 128:179–184.

24. Sieving PA, Bingham EL, Roth MS, Young MR, Boehnke M, Kuo CY, Ginsburg D: Linkage relationship of X-linked juvenile retinoschisis with Xp22.1–p22.3 probes. *Am J Hum Genet* 1990; 47:616–621.

25. Sieving PA: AOS Thesis: Photopic ON- and OFF-pathway abnormalities in retinal dystrophies. *Trans Am Ophthalmol Soc* 1993; 91:701–773.

26. Weber BH, Janocha S, Vogt G, Sander S, Ewing CC, Roesch M, Gibson A: X-linked juvenile retinoschisis (RS) maps between DXS987 and DXS443. *Cytogenet Cell Genet* 1995; 69:35–37.

27. Wieacker P, Wienker TF, Dallapiccola B, Bender K, Davies KE, Ropers HH: Linkage relationships between retinoschisis, Xg and a cloned DNA sequence from the distal short arm of the X chromosome. *Hum Genet* 1983; 64:143–145.

28. Wilczek M: Ein der netzhautspaltung (retinoschisis) mit einer offnung. *Zeit Augenhlkd* 1935; 85:108–116.

74 Congenital Stationary Night Blindness

YOZO MIYAKE

THE PATHOPHYSIOLOGY of several kinds of congenital stationary night blindness (CSNB) has been clarified in the last years, following the analysis of the visual function and molecular genetics. This chapter reviews recent knowledge of four kinds of CSNB: complete CSNB, incomplete CSNB, fundus albipunctatus, and Oguchi's disease. All these types of CSNB show the negative waveform in the dark-adapted single bright-flash (mixed rod-cone) electroretinogram (ERG) after 20–30 minutes of dark adaptation (see below). The identification of the mutant genes causing forms of CSNB in combination with the electrophysiological analysis refines the classification of these diseases and enhances our understanding of the underlying pathophysiology.

Complete CSNB (CSNB 1) and incomplete CSNB (CSNB 2)

The Schubert-Bornschein type of CSNB[35] has normal fundi and the mixed rod-cone ERG recorded with a single bright flash shows negative configuration (normal a-wave with smaller b-wave). The associated hereditary pattern can be either X-linked or autosomal-recessive. In 1986, we reported that the X-linked Schubert-Bornschein type CSNB can be divided into two different subtypes: complete CSNB, which has also been termed CSNB 1, and incomplete CSNB, which has also been termed CSNB.[24] The distinction between the complete and incomplete types was based on the rod function, evaluated by routine dark adaptometry and rod-mediated ERG; the complete type lacks rod function, while the incomplete type shows residual rod function. Other significant differences between two types include cone ERG,[24] long-flash photopic ERG,[23] changes of 30-Hz flicker ERG under the light adaptation,[16] oscillatory potentials,[10,24] scotopic threshold response (STR),[19] S-cone ERG,[18] refractive error,[24] and color vision.[42] These differences lead us to confirm that these two types are different clinical entities. Our clinical hypothesis was validated by molecular genetics. In 1998, the α-1-subunit of L-type voltage-gated calcium channel gene (*CACNA1F*) was identified as the mutated gene in X-linked incomplete CSNB,[1,40] and in 2000, NYX gene mutation was identified to cause X-linked complete CSNB.[2,33]

INITIAL COMPLAINTS OF PATIENTS   Table 74.1 shows the initial complaints of our 49 complete CSNB patients and 41 incomplete CSNB patients.[15] Many patients visited our clinic with the initial complaint of low visual acuity. It should be noted that only one of the 41 incomplete CSNB patients complained of night blindness, which causes us to overlook this disease because we then tend not to perform the ERG testing.

VISUAL ACUITY   The distribution of corrected visual acuity is shown in figure 74.1. In both types, the visual acuity ranged from 0.1 to 1.0, with a mean of 0.4–0.5. There was no statistical difference in visual acuity between two types.[15,24]

REFRACTIVE ERROR   Figure 74.2 shows the distribution of refractive error in patients in the two groups. Many patients with complete CSNB have high or moderate myopic refractive error, while those with incomplete CSNB have mild myopic or hyperopic refractive error. The mean refractive errors are −8.7 and −2.5 diopters in complete CSNB and incomplete CSNB, respectively. The difference in refractive error between the two groups is statistically significant ($P < 0.001$)[15,24] and helps to distinguish the two types of CSNB.

SUBJECTIVE DARK ADAPTATION CURVE   Figure 74.3 shows the representative subjective dark adaptation curves in patients with complete CSNB, incomplete CSNB, fundus albipunctatus, and Oguchi's disease. Compared with a normal curve, the rod adaptation is absent, and the cone adaptation shows an elevated threshold in complete CSNB. In incomplete CSNB, rod adaptation is present, although the final threshold is elevated by approximately 1.0–1.5 log units.[24]

FULL-FIELD ROD AND CONE ERG   Representative examples of standard full-field ERGs are shown in figure 74.4. The mixed rod-cone ERG in a single bright-flash stimulus reveals negative configuration with normal a-wave in both types, but the incomplete CSNB has on the rising b-wave much more prominent oscillatory potentials.[24] The rod ERG is absent in complete CSNB but is subnormally present in incomplete CSNB.[24] The normal a-wave and subnormal or absent rod

TABLE 74.1
Initial complaints of the patients

	Complete CSNB	Incomplete CSNB
Low visual acuity	30	29
Night blindness	15	1
Strabismus	13	5
Nystagmus	10	8
Familial survey	2	5
Others	4	1

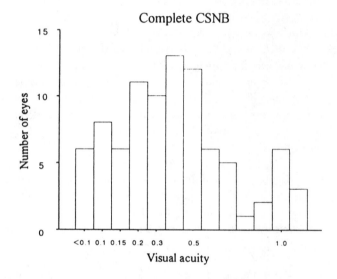

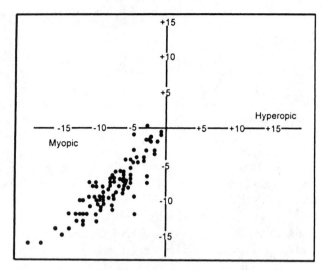

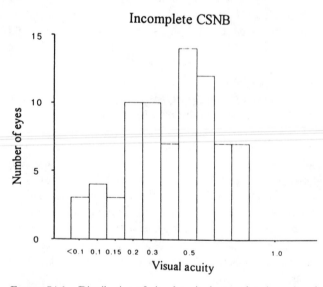

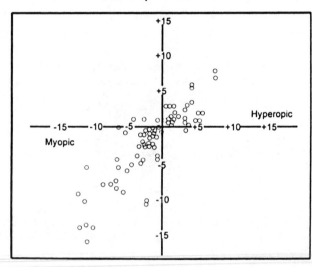

FIGURE 74.2   Distribution of refractive error in complete (upper) and incomplete (lower) CSNB patients. Minus and plus signs indicate myopic and hyperopic refraction, respectively. Vertical and horizontal axes correspond to axes in skiascopy.

FIGURE 74.1   Distribution of visual acuity in complete (upper) and incomplete (lower) CSNB patients. Vertical and horizontal axes indicate number of eyes and visual acuity, respectively.

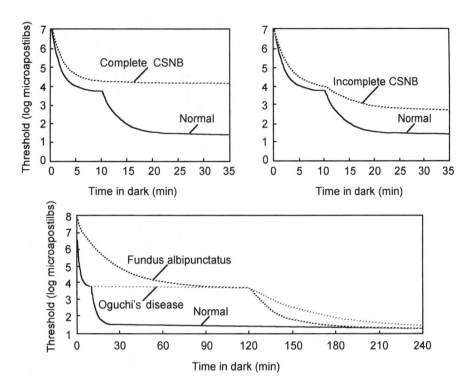

FIGURE 74.3 Subjective dark adaptation curve in a normal subject, complete CSNB, incomplete CSNB, fundus albipunctatus and Oguchi's disease. Each vertical and horizontal axes indicate threshold (log) and dark adaptation time, respectively.

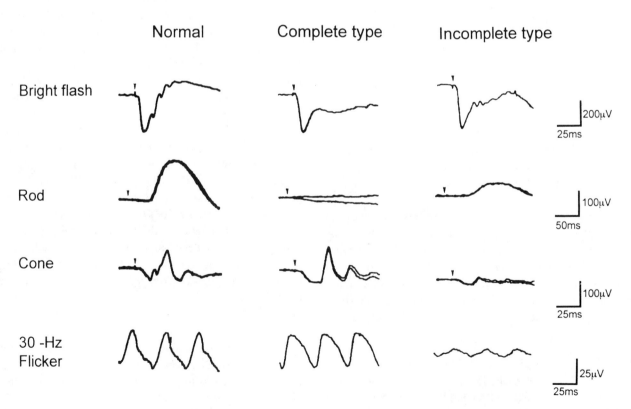

FIGURE 74.4 The standard full-field ERG in a normal subject and a patient with complete and incomplete CSNB. Arrowheads indicate stimulus onset.

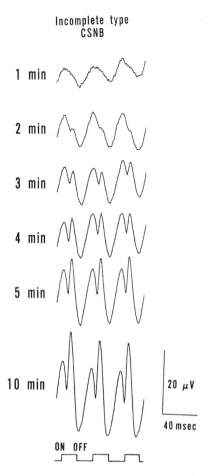

Incomplete type
CSNB

1 min

2 min

3 min

4 min

5 min

10 min

20 μV

40 msec

ON   OFF

FIGURE 74.5   Exaggerated enhancement of amplitude and change of wave shape of 30-Hz flicker ERG during light adaptation in incomplete CSNB.

the peak time shortened as the stimuli intensity increased. At the intensity of −5.8 log units, the b-wave becomes clearly visible for the first time. At the intense stimuli (lower panel), the b-wave had saturated at −1.4 log units, and the a-wave (−1.7 log units) and oscillatory potentials (−0.8 log units) started to appear. In complete CSNB, neither STR nor b-wave was recorded when the stimulus intensity was low (upper panel). At the moderate stimulus intensity of −4.4 log units (lower panel), both a- and b-waves began to appear, the former presenting normal and increasing amplitude. However, the b-wave saturated quickly, resulting in a negative configuration when the stimulus intensity was relatively strong. Oscillatory potentials were undetectable. In incomplete CSNB, the STR started to appear at −7.6 log units, showing a slightly higher threshold than that of a normal subject; however, the peak time was approximately 80 ms longer than normal. The b-wave began to appear at −5.8 log units as in the normal subject, with normal amplitude and peak time. At greater intensities, the b-wave amplitude became lower than normal, saturating at −3.4 log units, whereas the a-wave amplitude continued to increase progressively, resulting in a negative configuration. The oscillatory potentials were clearly visible.

LONG-FLASH PHOTOPIC ERG   The photopic ERG to square wave light simulation (long-flash) have shown that the cone ON response, which is generated by depolarizing bipolar cells,[36] is severely disturbed in complete CSNB, showing the hyperpolarizing pattern[23] (figure 74.7). This waveform is similar to the monkey's ERG when the neurotransmitter blocking agent APB[38] was applied to the retina.[36] The OFF response, on the other hand, which is generated by hyperpolarizing bipolar cells,[36] is intact in complete CSNB, leading us to hypothesize that complete CSNB has a complete defect of ON function in both rod and cone visual pathways.[18,36] The incomplete CSNB showed the reduction of ON and OFF responses, and our analysis of large series of patients suggested that incomplete CSNB has an incomplete defect on both ON and OFF responses,[23] but the OFF responses are perhaps more severely disturbed.[18]

Significant differences exist between S- and ML-cones ERG. S-cones connect only with the ON bipolar cells, whereas ML-cones connect with both ON and OFF bipolar cells.[41] The full-field S-cone ERG was absent in complete CSNB,[14,18] while it was recordable in incomplete CSNB.[18]

EOG   The electro-oculogram (EOG) is normal in both types of CSNB.[24] This is a very important finding to differentiate the CSNB with progressive disorder, such as retinitis pigmentosa, which shows abnormal or flattened EOG. The EOG may not be as helpful in differentiating cone-rod dystrophy from incomplete CSNB.

ERG suggest that both types of CSNB have a defect not in the rod itself but in the second-order neuron or the synapsis to the second-order neuron in the rod visual pathway. The defect is almost complete in complete CSNB and incomplete in incomplete CSNB.

The cone and 30-Hz flicker ERG appears nearly normal in complete CSNB except for the finding of flattening appearance of the bottom of cone ERG a-wave but are severely deteriorated in incomplete CSNB.[24] Although the amplitude of 30-Hz flicker ERG recorded after 30 minutes of dark adaptation is very small in incomplete CSNB, it increases exaggeratedly after 10 minutes of light adaptation[16] (figure 74.5).

ERG INTENSITY SERIES   Figure 74.6 shows ERG intensity series, elicited by relatively dim (upper) and intense (lower) stimuli, of a normal subject, a complete CSNB patient, and an incomplete CSNB patient.[19] In the normal subject, the cornea-negative STR[37] was recorded at −8.2 log units, and

Dim Stimulus Range

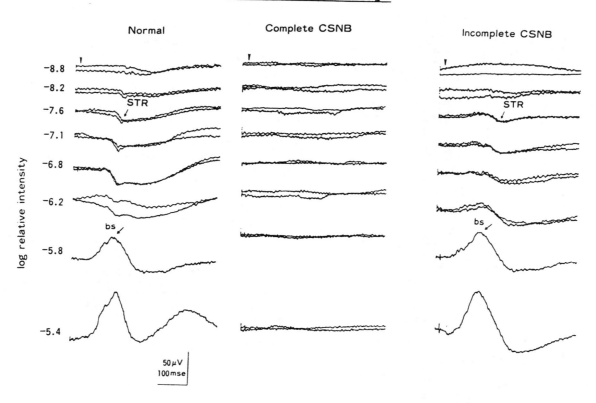

Relatively Intense Stimulus Range

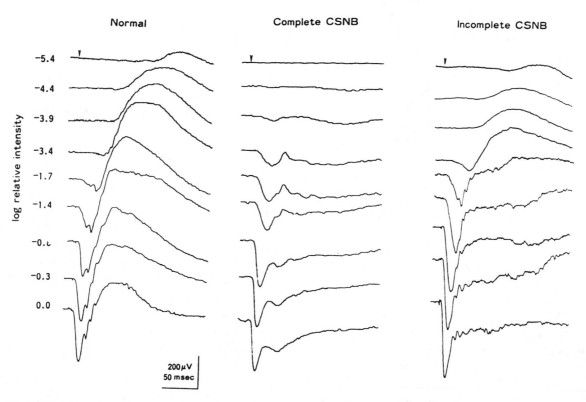

FIGURE 74.6 ERG intensity series with relatively dim stimuli (upper) and relatively intense stimuli (lower) in a normal subject and a patient with complete and incomplete CSNB. STR: scotopic threshold response, bs: scotopic b-wave.

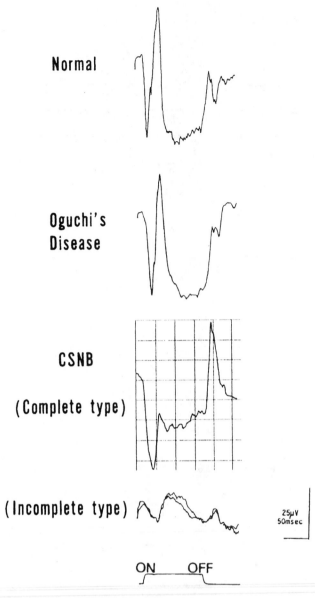

Normal

Oguchi's
Disease

CSNB

(Complete type)

(Incomplete type)

25μV
50msec

ON   OFF

FIGURE 74.7   Long-flash photopic ERG in a normal subject, a patient with Oguchi's disease, complete and incomplete CSNB.

COLOR VISION   The color vision in both complete and incomplete type patients is essentially normal.[24] It appears curious that in spite of nonrecordable S-cone ERG, psychophysical color vision is essentially normal in complete CSNB. We found that S-cone function in complete CSNB is preserved only in the fovea and becomes abnormal toward the peripheral retina.[42] This accounts for the normal color vision that tests mainly foveal function and the nonrecordable S-cone ERGs that arise mainly from peripheral retina.

MOLECULAR GENETICS   Linkage studies of X-linked complete CSNB localized the gene for complete CSNB to the short arm of the X chromosome.[26] In 2000, the gene, which is called *NYX*, was cloned from the Xp11 region by Bech-Hansen et al.[2] and Meindl et al.[33] The *NYX* gene, which encodes the glycosylphosphatidyl (GTP)-anchored extracellular protein nyctalopin. Nyctalopin is a new and unique member of the small leucine-rich proteoglycan family, which may be the gene product that guides and promotes the formation and function of the ON pathway within the retina. This mutation was also found in our six original Japanese patients with X-linked complete CSNB.[15] The mouse mutant of a natural occurring model of X-linked complete CSNB, the no b-wave (nob), was recently found by Pardue et al.[32] The ERG abnormalities are similar to those of complete CSNB patients.

In 1998, the gene for the X-linked incomplete CSNB was identified by Bech-Hansen et al.[1] and Strom et al.[40] It codes for the pore-forming subunit of an L-type voltage-gated calcium channel (*CACNA1F*) that is found in the retina. The mutation of *CACNA1F* was also found in all 15 patients examined in our original study of Japanese patients with incomplete CSNB[15,29] (figure 74.8). The loss of the functional channel impairs the calcium flux into photoreceptors (rods and cones) that is needed for sustaining the tonic neurotransmitter release from presynaptic terminals. The knock-out mice without a functional beta subunit of the channel were found to have marked loss of the ribbon synapses of photoreceptor inner segments.[34]

POSSIBLE PATHOGENESIS   Above-mentioned pathophysiological studies using clinical patients, animal models, and molecular genetics suggested that X-linked complete CSNB has an almost complete defect of the ON bipolar cells or its synapsis in both rod and cone visual pathways, leaving the OFF pathway intact. On the other hand, the X-linked incomplete CSNB has an incomplete defect of the ON and OFF bipolar cells or their synapsis in the rod and cone visual pathways.

Fundus albipunctatus

The fundus albipunctatus is a type of CSNB with autosomal-recessive inheritance. This type of CSNB was first differentiated from retinitis punctata albescens, one of the varieties of progressive tapetoretinal degeneration, by Lauber[12] in 1910. The fundi of typical patients have a characteristic appearance with a large number of discrete, round or elliptical, yellowish-white lesions at the level of the retinal pigment epithelium. These lesions may change in appearance during long-term follow-up, and some may fade.[13] The subjective dark adaptation (see figure 74.3)[39] and the dark adaptation time to obtain the maximum ERG response[11] is quite delayed. We found that the fundus albipunctatus can

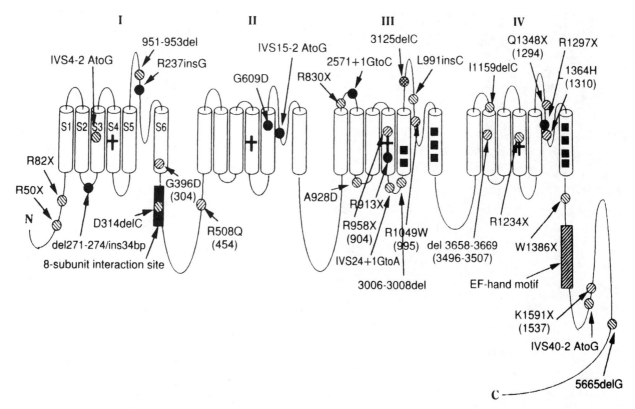

FIGURE 74.8 Putative topology of the human retina-specific calcium channel L-type. All mutations found in our study and in other reports. Solid circles: mutations found in our study; circles with left oblique lines: mutations found by Strom et al.[40]; circles with right oblique lines: mutations found by Bach-Hansen et al.[1]

be associated with cone dystrophy in many patients.[20] In this chapter, the typical fundus albipunctatus and the fundus albipunctatus associated with cone dystrophy are described separately.

TYPICAL FUNDUS ALBIPUNCTATUS The representative fundus picture is shown in figure 74.9 (top). As is shown in the subjective dark adaptation in figure 74.3, the ERG and EOG are also distinctive because an unusually long dark adaptation is needed to obtain the maximum normal scotopic ERG responses (figure 74.10) and normal EOG light rise.[5,22] The cone-mediated ERG as well as subjective cone visual functions such as visual acuity, color vision, and visual field is essentially normal. Patients with typical fundus albipunctatus complain of night blindness from early childhood, and the clinical course has been considered to be stationary.

FUNDUS ALBIPUNCTATUS ASSOCIATED WITH CONE DYSTROPHY We found that fundus albipunctatus can be associated with cone dystrophy.[20] Such patients often show bull's-eye maculopathy (figure 74.9, bottom) with progressive decrease of visual acuity and color vision deficiency. Although the

maximum responses are obtained after prolonged dark adaptation, as seen in typical fundus albipunctatus, the maximum amplitude is smaller than normal in some patients, indicating that rod function after a long period of dark adaptation does not recover to a normal level. The cone-mediated ERGs were very abnormal or essentially absent (see figure 74.10).

MOLECULAR GENETICS It has been unclear whether the fundus albipunctatus associated with cone dystrophy represents an advanced stage of fundus albipunctatus, a distinct disease entity, or a chance combination of two different diseases. In 1999, the 11-*cis*-retinol dehydrogenase gene, RDH5, was identified as the mutated gene in patients with typical fundus albipunctatus.[44] We analyzed many patients with fundus albipunctatus with or without cone dystrophy. We found either homozygous or compound heterozygous mutations in the *RDH5* gene in all of the patients.[28] Because some mutations were detected in both groups and because a progressive decline of visual functions was observed in some of the older patients, we concluded that mutations of the *RDH5* gene can lead to progressive cone dystrophy as well as congenital night blindness. This result indicates that

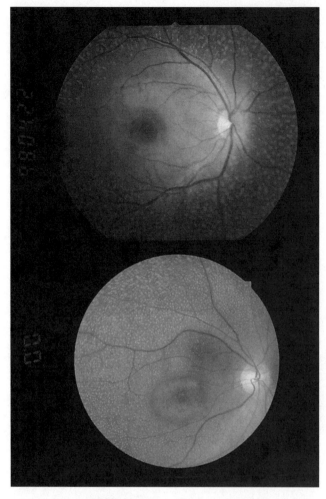

FIGURE 74.9 Fundus photograph in fundus albipunctatus (upper) and fundus albipunctatus associated with cone dystrophy (lower). (See also color plate 49.)

white discoloration of the fundus (figure 74.11). In 1913, Mizuo found that this fundus coloration disappeared after a long period of dark adaptation (Mizuo's phenomenon)[25] (see figure 74.11).

Although the rod function is absent both subjectively and electroretinographically after 30 minutes of dark adaptation, it may reappear after 2–3 hours of dark adaptation[3,27] (see figures 74.3 and 74.10). It has been reported that mutations in either the arrestin gene[9] or the rhodopsin kinase gene[45] cause a recessive form of Oguchi's disease.

FULL-FIELD ERG Figure 74.10 shows the full-field ERGs in an Oguchi's disease patient with the mutation in the arrestin gene. When recorded after 30 minutes of dark adaptation, the rod ERG is absent, and cone-mediated (cone, 30-Hz flicker) ERGs are essentially normal. The mixed rod-cone ERG shows a negative configuration with relatively preserved oscillatory potentials, and the a-wave amplitude is reduced in comparison with a normal control. After 3 hours of dark adaptation, however, the mixed rod-cone ERG shows increases in the a-wave and b-wave. Including our seven patients, the ERGs of 26 patients with Oguchi's disease recorded after 15–30 minutes of dark adaptation were reported in past Japanese literature. All of those ERGs have reduced a-waves, nearly absent b-waves, and relatively preserved oscillatory potentials.[17] The pathogenesis of the cone visual system in Oguchi's disease is different from those of complete CSNB and incomplete CSNB. Unlike in complete and incomplete CSNB, the long-flash photopic ERG shows a normal amplitude and waveform, indicating that the ON and OFF systems in cone visual pathway are functioning normally[17,23] (see figure 74.7).

EOG Including our six patients, 16 of 21 Japanese patients have had an extremely low Arden ratio (<1.4) in the EOG (normal > 1.8).[17] It should also be noted that even in patients with a normal to subnormal Arden ratio, the a-wave amplitude was significantly smaller than normal.

OTHER OCULAR FINDINGS The visual acuity and color vision are normal. Reviewing all Japanese patients with Oguchi's disease reported so far, I got the impression that the refractive error in Oguchi's disease is minor, if any, and I found neither patients with high myopia nor patients with high hyperopia.

MOLECULAR GENETICS Rhodopsin kinase and arrestin, of which genes have been proved to be mutated in Oguchi's disease, act in sequence to deactivate rhodopsin to stop the phototransduction cascade. Most patients reported in the literature with mutations in the arrestin gene are Japanese.

the fundus albipunctatus is not always stationary but is progressive in about one third of the patients, associating with diffuse cone dysfunction in old age.

POSSIBLE PATHOGENESIS The delayed dark adaptation in subjective threshold ERG and EOG in fundus albipunctatus either with or without cone dystrophy is understandable in view of the mutations leading to a deficiency of 11-*cis*-RDH. Accordingly, the production of 11-*cis*-retinal in the retinal pigment epithelium is compromised, and the deficient supply of chromophore to the photoreceptors delays the rate at which they can recover after bleaching.[6]

Oguchi's disease

Oguchi's disease, first described by Oguchi[31] in 1907, is an unusual form of CSNB characterized by a peculiar gray-

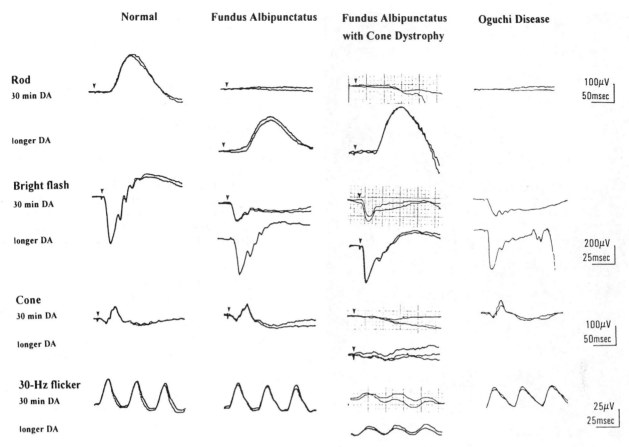

FIGURE 74.10   Full-field ERG in a normal subject, a patient with fundus albipunctatus, a patient with fundus albipunctatus associated with cone dystrophy, and a patient with Oguchi's disease. The standard ERG was recorded after 30 minutes of dark adaptation, but some ERGs were recorded with longer dark adaptation of 2–3 hours.

Although the patients with mutations of rhodopsin kinase gene showed no signs of photoreceptor degeneration in literature, some patients with mutations of arrestin were reported to be associated with photoreceptor degeneration similar to retinitis pigmentosa.[30] The animal model is not essentially the same as the findings in Oguchi's disease patients. Elimination of the function of arrestin in fruit flies uniformly causes photoreceptor degeneration, which is dependent on exposure of light.[8] Transgenic mice that were homozygous for an arrestin mutation showed prolonged photoresponses.[43]

POSSIBLE PATHOGENESIS   In 1965, Carr and Gouras[3] reported detailed ERG findings in four Caucasian patients with Oguchi's disease. Their patients' ERGs, when recorded with a relatively intense stimulus after 10 minutes of dark adaptation, showed a negative form with normal a-waves and small b-waves, similar to those in complete CSNB. In a later study, Carr and Ripps[4] restudied one of these patients and found, in addition to the normal a-wave, a normal EOG and normal concentrations and kinetics of visual pigments.

The authors concluded that a defect in the postreceptor signals is the cause of night blindness. In 1997, two of their patients were examined by Yamamoto et al.[45] in terms of the molecular genetics and the mutations of rhodopsin kinase were detected. It appears slightly difficult to explain the normal a-wave and normal EOG in relation to the mutations of rhodopsin kinase.

In Japanese patients, however, the a-wave amplitude of mixed rod-cone ERG was significantly lower than normal when recorded after 20–30 minutes of dark adaptation.[17] Our analysis of three patients with Oguchi's disease indicated that the rod a-wave is absent.[17] Also, many Japanese patients showed abnormal EOG.[17] Since most Japanese patients with Oguchi's disease have mutations of arrestin, these differences may be caused by different gene mutations.

The mechanism of the Mizuo phenomenon is also unknown. Some authors speculate that it is the result of elevated extracellular potassium levels generated in the retina in response to an excessive stimulation of rod photoreceptors.

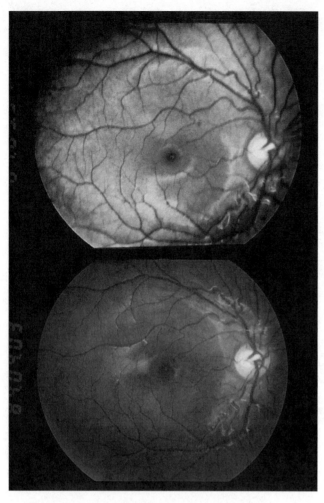

FIGURE 74.11 Fundus photographs of Oguchi's disease in light adaptation (upper) and after a long period of dark adaptation (lower). (See also color plate 50.)

REFERENCES

1. Bech-Hansen NT, Naylor MJ, Maybaum TA, Pearce WG, Koop B, Fishman GA, et al: Loss-of-function mutation in a calcium-channel alphal-subunit gene in Xp11.3 cause incomplete X-linked congenital stationary night blindness. *Nat Genet* 1998; 19:264–267.
2. Bech-Hansen NT, Naylor MJ, Maybaum TA, Sparkes RL, Koop B, Birch DG, et al: Mutations in NYX, encoding the leucine-rich proteoglycan nyctalopin, cause X-linked complete congenital stationary night blindness. *Nat Genet* 2000; 26:319–323.
3. Carr RE, Gouras P: Oguchi's disease. *Arch Ophthalmol* 1965; 73:646–656.
4. Carr RE, Ripps H: Rhodopsin kinetics and rod adaptation in Oguchi's disease. *Invest Ophthalmol* 1967; 6:426–436.
5. Carr RE, Ripps H, Siegel IM: Visual pigment kinetics and adaptation in fundus albipunctatus. *Doc Ophthalmol* 1974; 4:193–204.
6. Cideciyan AV, Haeseleer F, Fariss RN, Aleman TS, Jang GF, Verlinde CL, Marmor MF, Jacobson SG, Palczewski K: Rod and cone visual cycle consequences of a null mutation in the 11-cis-retinol dehydrogenase gene in man. *Vis Neurosci* 2000; 17:667–678.
7. de Jong PTVM, Zrenner E, van Meel GJ, Keunen JE, van Norren D: Mizuo phenomenon in X-linked retinoschisis. *Arch Ophthalmol* 1991; 109:1104–1108.
8. Dolph PJ, Ranganathan R, Colley NJ, et al: Arrestin function in inactivation of G protein-coupled receptor rhodopsin in vivo. *Science* 1993; 260:1910–1916.
9. Fuchs S, Nakazawa M, Maw M, Tamai M, Oguchi Y, Gal A: A homozygous 1-base pair deletion in the arrestin gene is a frequent cause of Oguchi's disease in Japanese. *Nat Genet* 1995; 10:360–362.
10. Heckenlively JR, Martin DA, Rosebaum AL: Loss of oscillatory potentials, optic atrophy, and dysplasia in congenital stationary night blindness. *Amer J Ophthalmol* 1983; 96:526–534.
11. Krill AE, Fork MR: Retinitis punctata albescens: A functional evaluation of an unusual case. *Am J Ophthalmol* 1962; 53:450–455.
12. Lauber H: Die sogenannte Retinitis punctata albescens. *Klin Monatsbl Augenheilkd* 1910; 48:133–148.
13. Marmor MF: Long-term follow-up of the physiological abnormalities and fundus changes in fundus albipunctatus. *Ophthalmology* 1990; 97:380–384.
14. McKay CJ, Saeki M, Gouras P, Roy M: Congenital and acquired nyctalopia eliminate the S-cone ERG without disturbing color vision. *Invest Ophthalmol Vis Sci* Suppl 1995; 36:8925.
15. Miyake Y: Establishment of the concept of new clinical entities: Complete and incomplete form of congenital stationary night blindness. *J Jpn Ophthalmol Soc* 2002; 106:737–756.
16. Miyake Y, Horiguchi M, Ota I, Shiroyama N: Characteristic ERG flicker anomaly in incomplete congenital stationary night blindness. *Invest Ophthalmol Vis Sci* 1987; 28:1816–1823.
17. Miyake Y, Horiguchi M, Suzuki S, Kondo M, Tanikawa A: Electrophysiological findings in patients with Oguchi's disease. *Jpn J Ophthalmol* 1996; 40:511–519.
18. Miyake Y, Horiguchi M, Suzuki S, Kondo M, Tanikawa A: Complete and incomplete type congenital stationary night blindness as a model of "OFF-retina" and "ON-retina." In LaVail MM, Hollyfield JG, Anderson RE (eds): *Degenerative Retinal Diseases*. New York, Plenum, 1997, pp 31–41.
19. Miyake Y, Horiguchi M, Terasaki H, Kondo M: Scotopic threshold response in complete and incomplete types of congenital stationary night blindness. *Invest Ophthalmol Vis Sci* 1994; 35:3770–3775.
20. Miyake Y, Shiroyama N, Sugita S, Horiguchi M, Yagasaki K: Fundus albipunctatus associated with cone dystrophy. *Br J Ophthalmol* 1992; 76:375–379.
21. Miyake Y, Terasaki H: Golden tapetal-like fundus reflex and posterior hyaloid in a patient with X-linked juvenile retinoschisis. *Retina* 1999; 19:84–86.
22. Miyake Y, Watanabe I, Asano T, Sakai T: Further studies on EOG in retinitis punctata albescens: Effects of change of dark adaptation time on EOG. *Folia Ophthalmol Jpn* 1974; 25:518–527.
23. Miyake Y, Yagasaki K, Horiguchi M, Kawase T: On- and Off-responses in photopic electroretinogram in complete and incomplete types of congenital stationary night blindness. *Jpn J Ophthalmol* 1987; 31:81–87.
24. Miyake Y, Yagasaki K, Horiguchi M, Kawase Y, Kanda T: Congenital stationary night blindness with negative electroretinogram: A new classification. *Arch Ophthalmol* 1986; 104:1013–1020.

25. Mizuo G: On a new discovery in the dark adaptation on Oguchi's disease. *Acta Soc Ophthalmol Jpn* 1913; 17:1148.

26. Musarella MA, Weleber RG, Murphey WH, Young RS, Anson-Cartwright L, Mets M, et al: Assignment of the gene for complete X-linked congenital stationary night blindness (CSNB 1) to Xp 11.3. *Genomics* 1989; 5:727–737.

27. Nakamura B: Ueber ein neues Phanomen der Farbenveranderung des menschlichen Augenhintergrundes in Zusammenhang mit der fortschreitenden Dunkeladaptaton. *Klin Monatsbl Augenheilkd* 1920; 65:883.

28. Nakamura M, Hotta Y, Tanikawa A, Terasaki H, Miyake Y: A high association with cone dystrophy in fundus albipunctatus caused by mutations of the RDH5 gene. *Invest Ophthalmol Vis Sci* 2000; 41:3925–3932.

29. Nakamura M, Ito S, Terasaki H, Miyake Y: Novel CACNA1F mutations in Japanese patients with incomplete congenital stationary night blindness. *Invest Ophthalmol Vis Sci* 2001; 42:1610–1616.

30. Nakazawa M, Wada Y, Tamai M: Arrestin gene mutations in autosomal recessive retinitis pigmentosa. *Arch Ophthalmol* 1998; 116:498–501.

31. Oguchi C: Ueber einen Fall von eigenartiger Hemeralopie. *Acta Soc Ophthalmol Jpn* 1907; 11:123.

32. Pardue MT, McCall MA, La Vail MM, Gregg RG, Peachey NS: A naturally occurring mouse model of X-linked congenital stationary night blindness. *Invest Ophthalmol Vis Sci* 1998; 39:2443–2449.

33. Pasch CM, Zeitz C, Brandau O, Pesch K, Achatz H, Feil S, et al: The complete form of X-linked congenital stationary night blindness is caused by mutations in a gene encoding a leucine-rich repeat protein. *Nat Genet* 2000; 26:324–327.

34. Read DS, Ball SL, Pardue MT, Morgans CW, Peachey NS, McCall MA, Gregg RG: Photoreceptor L-type voltage-dependent Ca^{2+} channels are required for formation and or maintenance of ribbon synapses in the OPL. *Invest Ophthalmol Vis Sci* 2001; 42:S365 (Abstract #1972).

35. Schubert G, Bornschein H: Beitrag zur Analyse des menshlichen Electroretinograms. *Ophthalmologica* 1952; 123:396–412.

36. Sieving PA: Photopic on- and off-pathway abnormalities in retinal dystrophies. *Trans Amer Ophthalmol Soc* 1993; 91:701–773.

37. Sieving PA, Frishman LJ, Steinberg RH: Scotopic threshold response of proximal retina in cat. *J Neurophysiol* 1986; 56:1049–1061.

38. Slaughter MM, Miller RF: 2-amino-4-phosphonobutyric acid: A new pharmacological tool for retina research. *Science* 1981; 211:181–185.

39. Smith BF, Ripps H, Goodman G: Retinitis punctata albescens, a functional and diagnostic evaluation. *Arch Ophthalmol* 1959; 61:93–101.

40. Strom TM, Nyakatura G, Apfelstedt-Sylla E, Hellebrand H, Lorenz B, Weber BH, et al: An L-type calcium channel gene mutated in incomplete X-linked congenital stationary night blindness. *Nat Genet* 1998; 19:260–263.

41. Swanson WH, Birch DG, Anderson JL: S-cone function in patients with retinitis pigmentosa. *Invest Ophthalmol Vis Sci* 1993; 33:3045–3055.

42. Terasaki H, Miyake Y, Nomura R, Horiguchi M, Suzuki S, Kondo M: Blue-on-yellow perimetry in the complete type of congenital stationary night blindness. *Invest Ophthalmol Vis Sci* 1999; 40:2716–2764.

43. Xi J, Donald RL, Makino CL, Simon MI, Baylor DA, Chen J: Prolonged photoresponses in transgenic mouse rods lacking arrestin. *Nature* 1997; 389:505–509.

44. Yamamoto H, Simon A, Eriksson U, Harris E, Berson EL, Dryja TP: Mutations in the gene encoding 11-cis retinol dehydrogenase cause delayed dark adaptation and fundus albipunctatus. *Nat Genet* 1999; 22:188–191.

45. Yamamoto S, Sippel KC, Berson EL, Dryja TP: Defects in the rhodopsin kinase gene in patients with Oguchi's form of stationary night blindness. *Nat Genet* 1997; 14:175–178.

75 Quinine Retinopathy

GRAHAM E. HOLDER

QUININE, ORIGINALLY made from the bark of the cinchona tree, is an alkaloid with a long history of medicinal use and has been available in synthetic form since the 1940s. It is perhaps best known for the treatment of malaria (e.g., Mandel et al.[8]) but is also prescribed for night cramps,[9] with a dosage of 200–300 mg. In the past, it was used as an abortifacient.[4] Acute quinine toxicity, or cinchonism, may be characterized by blindness, tinnitus, nausea, vomiting, cardiac dysrrhythmias, coma, and even death. Symptoms of cinchonism are likely with doses above 4 g, and as little as 8 g may be fatal.[10] There is marked interindividual variation in susceptibility to quinine that may give rise to so-called idiosyncratic toxic reactions.[2,5,11] Serum quinine levels are a poor prognostic indicator.[2] In addition, this author has experience of one patient (unpublished data) who had been taking therapeutic doses of quinine for night cramps but who was a covert alcoholic and developed a typical retinopathy presumed consequent upon impaired liver function.

Acute visual disturbances occur in approximately 40% of patients, but less than a third of those suffer permanent visual impairment.[2] There is usually severe visual loss with gradual recovery over the subsequent days or weeks. These improvements in visual function, often dramatic, may incorrectly be ascribed to the effects of treatment. However, even though visual symptoms are common, patients usually present to physicians with a history of attempted suicide by quinine overdose, often in association with alcohol and/or other medication. This may delay referral to ophthalmologists and thence to electrophysiologists. Ocular quinine toxicity in humans has therefore been difficult to study in the acute phase.

In early presentation, fluorescein angiography shows attenuated retinal arteries with a return of normal choroidal fluorescence as the initial masking from acute retinal edema subsides. Histological examination may reveal collapse of retinal architecture, early gliosis, and vascular narrowing.[3,6] The pathological process in the chronic phase is due to either delayed or secondary ischemia, although clinically, the onset of vascular attenuation often heralds the return of central visual function. The acute effects are less well characterized; one group has suggested the possibility of retinal toxicity, being unable to find histological evidence of acute ischemic changes in an experimental model.[3]

There does not appear to have been an electrophysiological study of quinine retinopathy since the introduction of the International Society for Clinical Electrophysiology of Vision (ISCEV) standard to electroretinography. However, early studies report an electronegative response to a single bright white flash under dark adaptation, similar to the maximal mixed rod-cone response in the current ISCEV standard. There is preservation of the photoreceptor derived a-wave but marked reduction in the postreceptoral b-wave.[1,5,12] This appearance is superficially similar to that which occurs in association with ischemic damage to the inner nuclear layer consequent on central retinal artery occlusion. Typical findings appear in figure 75.1. In addition to the electronegative electroretinogram (ERG), note the marked delay and amplitude reduction in the 30-Hz flicker ERG. A further feature of note is the highly distinctive appearance when long-duration stimulation is used to assess ON and OFF pathway function. There is a profoundly electronegative ON response with virtually no b-wave, and an extended plateau to the OFF response d-wave, giving an overall waveform reminiscent of a sawtooth. This highly unusual waveform has been present in all cases of quinine retinopathy examined by the author in which ON and OFF response recording has been performed, but has not been recognized in other disorders and may be specific to quinine toxicity.

In the acute phase, there is marked generalized retinal abnormality involving all ERG waveforms but not accompanied by the electronegative waveform, which only becomes apparent some weeks later (unpublished data). It is postulated that the initial disturbance reflects the known effects of quinine on cell membranes (e.g., Malchow et al.[7]). The acute effects, in which there may be reduction of vision down to no light perception, can then be ascribed to generalized retinal dysfunction involving all retinal cell types, including the retinal ganglion cells. The visual evoked potential (VEP) at this stage may be undetectable. As the acute effects resolve, visual acuity may recover, and the a-wave of the ERG may show recovery. The characteristic negative ERG waveform is then a feature. The VEP may show recovery, presumably reflecting recovery of ganglion cell function, but tends not to be of normal latency. The VEP delay can be assumed to be secondary to continuing macular dysfunction, as the pattern ERG at this stage may be

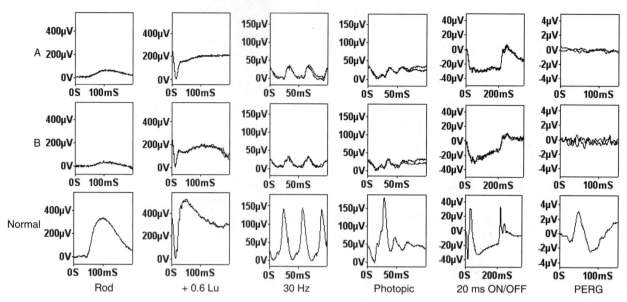

FIGURE 75.1 ERGs and PERGs in two patients with quinine retinopathy following overdose. Data are shown from the right eye. Patient A is a 72-year-old female who took an overdose of quinine as an abortifacient some 40 years prior to investigation. Visual acuity was 6/18. Patient B is a 55-year-old male with an 11-month history and visual acuity of 6/6. Both patients show very similar ERG findings. The rod-specific ERG is subnormal; there is an electronegative bright-flash ERG; cone flicker and single-flash ERGs are delayed and markedly subnormal; and ON-OFF response recording shows almost complete ON b-wave loss with an elevated and extended plateau to the d-wave. PERGs are undetectable despite the normal visual acuity in patient B.

undetectable despite normal visual acuity (see figure 75.1). It is uncertain whether the negative ERG reflects inner retinal damage consequent upon vascular spasm and vessel attenuation or whether the vessel narrowing reflects loss of demand from inner retinal structures.

To conclude, the presence of a profoundly electronegative ERG in a patient with marked field constriction, pale disks, and attenuated retinal vasculature raises the question of quinine toxicity. Directed questioning of the patient may be necessary to reveal the relevant history, usually of an overdose. The nature of the ON and OFF response abnormality seems characteristic.

REFERENCES

1. Bacon P, Spalton DJ, Smith SE: Blindness from quinine toxicity. *Br J Ophthalmol* 1988; 72:219–224.
2. Boland ME, Brennand Roper SM, Henry JA: Complications of quinine poisoning. *Lancet* 1985; 1:384–385.
3. Buchanan TAS, Lyness RW, Collins AD, Gardiner TA, Archer DB: An experimental study of quinine blindness. *Eye* 1987; 1:522–524.
4. Dannenberg A, Dorman SF, Johnson J: Use of quinine for self induced abortion. *South Med J* 1983; 76:846–849.
5. Gangitano JL, Keltner JL: Abnormalities of the pupil and VEP in quinine amblyopia. *Am J Ophthalmol* 1980; 89:425–430.
6. Gass JDM: *Stereoscopic Atlas of Macular Diseases: Diagnosis and Treatment*, vol. 2, ed 3. St. Louis, CV Mosby, 1987.
7. Malchow RP, Qian H, Ripps H: A novel action of quinine and quinidine on the membrane conductance of neurons from the vertebrate retina. *J Gen Physiol* 1994; 104:1039–1055.
8. Mandell GL, Douglas RG, Bennet JE (eds): *Anti-infective Therapy*. New York, Wiley, 1985.
9. Man-Son-Hing M, Wells G: Meta-analysis of efficacy of quinine for treatment of nocturnal leg cramps in elderly people. *Br Med J* 1995; 310:13–17.
10. Polson CJ, Tattersal RN: *Clinical Toxicology*. London, English Universities Press, 1959.
11. Wanwimolruk S, Chalcroft S, Coville PF, Campbell AJ: Pharmacokinetics of quinine in young and elderly subjects. *Trans R Soc Trop Med Hyg* 1991; 85:714–717.
12. Zahn JR, Brinton GF, Norton E: Ocular quinine toxicity followed by electroretinogram, electro-oculogram and pattern evoked potential. *Am J Optometry Physiol Optics* 1981; 58:492–498.

XIV OPTIC NERVE AND CENTRAL NERVOUS SYSTEM DYSFUNCTION

76 Leber's Hereditary Optic Neuropathy

YOSHIHISA OGUCHI

LEBER'S HEREDITARY optic neuropathy (LHON) is a disease of optic atrophy first reported by Theodor Leber in 1871.[9] This disease has an acute or subacute onset in both eyes, and it typically appears in young men in their teens and twenties. It causes a severe optic atrophy with severe visual loss within one year. The disease was considered to be hereditary because their patients showed a similar family history, in which male patients did not seem to transit the disease to their offspring, while children of female carriers always inherit the disease. Its hereditary type was unknown until in 1936. Imai and Moriwaki reported that it was a cytoplasmic inheritance.[6] Nikoskelainen and his group proposed that mitochondrial DNA inheritance explained the hereditary patterns seen in LHON families.[17,18]

In 1988, Wallace et al. reported a new mutation of 11778 base pairs of mtDNA of patients with LHON.[22] Since then, more than 20 primary or secondary mtDNA mutations have been associated with LHON. The 3460, 11778, and 14484 mtDNA mutations are considered to be the most important in the pathogenesis of this disease and are classified as primary mutations.[1,4,5,8] Among the three mutations, the 11778 mutation is most frequently seen in patients with LHON. But the frequencies of the primary LHON mutations reportedly differ among ethnic groups.[15,23]

The characteristics of fundus are blurred disk margins, tortuous retinal vessels, irregular telangiectatic dilation of capillaries in peripapillary and prepapillary networks in the acute stage. In spite of such microangiopathy, fluorescein angiography shows no leakage around the optic nervehead. As the disease progresses, the microangiopathy disappears, and optic atrophy develops after at least two months. In the visual field, a relative centrocecal scotoma is detected in the acute stage, and then a large central scotoma is observed. In LHON, spontaneous recovery has been well known, but it does not occur often. Johns et al. have reported that patients with the 14484 mutation show a higher incidence of visual recovery than did patients with the 11778 or 3460 mutations and that visual loss may depend more on epigenetic factors in patients with the 14484 mutation than in patients with the other primary mutations.[7] At the present time, no effective treatment is known for LHON.

In 1992, the authors reported the results of treatment with idebenone, a quinol compound that may contribute to stimulation of the formation of ATP, in a 10-year-old Japanese boy with LHON and homoplasmic 11778 mutation.[10] The authors studied the effectiveness of idebenon combined with vitamin B2, vitamin C, and isopropyl unoprostone (Rescula) for recovery of the circulation of the optic nervehead for patients in the acute stage.[13] In patients with visual acuity of 0.3 or more, there was no statistical difference between treated and untreated groups. But the recovery interval up to 0.3 was significantly shorter in the treated group than in the untreated group.

Electrophysiological study for LHON

Pathogenesis of LHON has been considered to be damage of the optic nerve. Smith et al.,[21] and Nikoskeleinen et al. described the typical signs and appearance of fluorescein angiography.[16] From their study, they assumed LHON to be caused by damage of retinal nerve fiber layer and proposed that this disease should be called Leber's hereditary optic neuroretinopathy. In electrophysiological examination, electro-oculograms (EOGs), electroretinograms (ERGs), and visual evoked potentials (VEPs) are used in daily eye clinic. EOGs and ERGs have been reported to be normal in patients with LHON. In flash ERG, Riordan-Eva et al. reported the electrophysiological results of 34 patients with LHON; in three patients, the b-wave of the ERG was low in amplitude.[19] They also showed the results of pattern ERGs for seven LHON patients. Pattern ERGs were normal in two patients, showed a low response in three patients, and in two others had normal P50 components but absent N95 components. Shibata et al. reported an ERG and VEP study for a 49-year-old male patient with LHON.[20] The recordings of the VEPs and ERGs, four weeks after onset, showed attenuation of the pattern VEPs and P50 component and absence of N95 component in pattern ERGs bilaterally. However, the flash VEPs and flash ERGs were normal. Six months after the onset, the pattern ERGs and flash VEPs showed severe attenuation; however, the a- and b-waves in flash ERGs were normal. Mondelli et al. reported a VEP study in 11 patients at the atrophic stage of LHON.[14] Two patients showed no response bilaterally. Three patients showed no response of one eye and delayed latency and decreased amplitude of the other eye. In six patients, both latency and amplitude were abnormal. Dorfman et al. studied the pattern VEP in two brothers with early LHON.[3] One month after onset, the latency of VEP was normal. Then the response developed prolonged latency and reduced amplitude, with the waveform developing a bifid positivity in a W configuration. The pattern size that was used in this study was a check of 1° 50′ of arc.

Carroll and Mastaglia also found that pattern VEPs in patients with LHON were less delayed in P100 latency but showed a greater reduction in amplitude and were disorganized.[2] The pattern size used was a check of 12′ of arc. The authors reported the electrophysiological results of a 28-year-old male patient with LHON in the relatively acute stage.[12] The single-flash ERG was normal in each eye. The pattern ERG showed normal latency of P50 in each eye, and the amplitude from the right eye decreased to 3.6 μV and that from the left eye to 2.5 μV. The flash VEP responses, though less delayed, were markedly reduced in amplitude in the relatively acute stage. The authors reported VEPs in a patient with the 11778 mutation who developed LHON at the age of 23 years.[11] VEPs were recorded in the right eye at the presymptomatic and symptomatic stages. Pattern VEPs were not recorded in the left eye that had developed LHON 4 months earlier. In the presymptomatic stage (figure 76.1A) when the visual acuity of right eye was 1.0, N80 latency was the upper limit of normal, P100 was slightly delayed, and the amplitudes were in the normal range at three check sizes but not at the check size of 5′. Three days after the onset of LHON (figure 76.1B), the patient's visual

acuity was still 1.0. The amplitude was markedly reduced, but N80 and P100 were unchanged. Two weeks after onset (figure 76.1C), his visual acuity had decreased to 0.6. The amplitude showed a significant reduction, and N80 and P100 were further delayed. Pattern VEPs were not recordable one month after onset. During onset of LHON, there was a marked reduction in amplitude, followed by a delay in latency.

Figure 76.2 shows the waveforms of flash VEPs in the same patient as shown in figure 76.1. Flash VEPs were recorded at four different intensities of stimulus using red and ND filters. The visual stimulus was a xenon flash light of 0.3 joule (J) and 2.0 J. The four stimulus intensities were 0.3×10^{-2} J (−2.0 log unit), 0.3×10^{-1} J (−1.0 log unit), 0.3 J (0 log unit), and 2.0 J (0.8 log unit). The intensity-latency curve and the intensity-amplitude curve served as critical variables. Three days and two weeks after onset, flash VEPs were slightly attenuated in the stimulus of low intensity compared in the presymptomatic stage. But N80 latency and P100 were not delayed, although pattern VEPs deteriorated rapidly. These results of VEPs by pattern and flash light stimuli suggested that in early LHON, the dissociation of damage to spatial and luminance channels existed.

To investigate the dissociation of damage between spatial luminance channels in early stage of LHON, patients with LHON were examined by use of pattern VEP and flash VEP, and the findings were compared with those in patients with optic neuritis (ON), including MS. Twenty-eight Japanese patients were investigated; 12 (18 eyes) with LHON and 16 (18 eyes) with ON, including eight patients of MS. Thirty normal volunteers (30 eyes) served as controls. In pattern VEP, the check size–amplitude curve and the check size–latency curve are shown in figure 76.3. Pattern VEPs

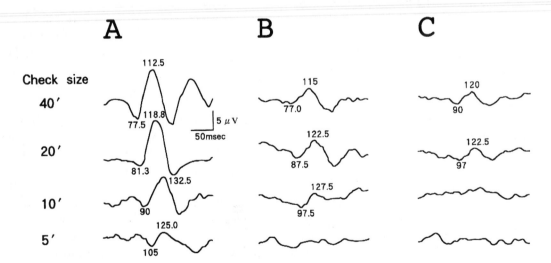

FIGURE 76.1　Waveforms of pattern VEPs from the right eye in a 23-year-old-patient with LHON. A, In the presymptomatic stage, visual acuity was 25/20. B, Three days after onset, visual acuity was 20/20. C, Two weeks after onset, visual acuity was 20/30. Numerals represent latency times of N80 and P100. (From Mashima Y, Imamura Y, Oguchi Y.[11] Used by permission.)

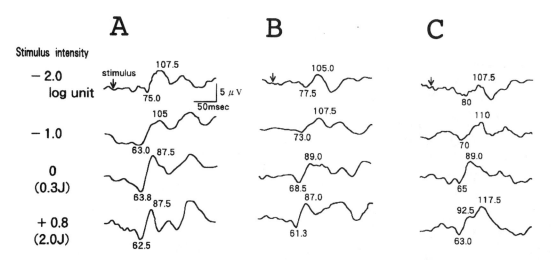

Stimulus intensity

A **B** **C**

FIGURE 76.2 Waveforms of flash VEPs from the right eye in the same patient as shown in figure 76.1. A, Presymptomatic stage. B, Three days after onset. C, Two weeks after onset. Numerals represent latency times of N80 and P100. Stimulus delay was 20 ms after a trigger signal (vertical arrows). (From Mashima, Imamura Y, Oguchi Y.[11] Used by permission.)

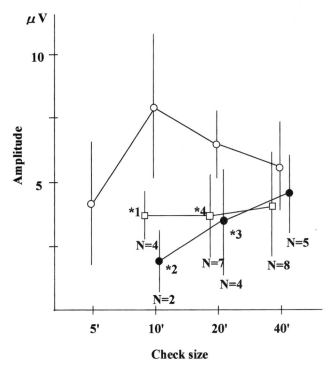

FIGURE 76.3 Check size–amplitude curve in pattern VEPs. Open circles and bars represent the mean plus or minus standard deviation (S.D.) in normal subjects (30 eyes). Solid circles and bars represent the mean ± S.D. in patients with LHON, and open squares represent the mean ± S.D. in patients with optic neuritis (ON). N shows the number of eyes. Mean amplitude was significantly reduced in both LHON and ON patients compared with normal subjects in check sizes 10′ and 20′. There was no difference in amplitude between LHON and ON. (From Mashima Y, Imamura Y, Oguchi Y.[11] Used by permission.)

were recordable in 5 of the 12 patients with LHON and in 8 of the 16 patients with ON.

In normal subjects, the check size–amplitude curve represented a maximum response produced by check sizes of 10′ to 20′, which suggested a band-pass function. In patients with LHON and ON, however, the curve was linear. In LHON, as well as in ON, the mean amplitude was significantly reduced in comparison with normal subjects; except for a larger check size of 40′ (see figure 76.3), there was no difference in amplitude between patients with LHON and ON ($p > .05$). The N80 latency in LHON as well as in ON was significantly delayed in comparison with normal subjects (figure 76.4). Moreover, the delay in the ON exceeded that in LHON. In flash VEP, the intensity-amplitude curve and the intensity-latency curve are shown in figures 76.5 and 76.6. Flash VEP were recordable in all patients with LHON and in all 16 patients with ON. Mean amplitude was significantly reduced in both patients with LHON and ON compared with normal subjects (see figure 76.5). There was no difference in amplitude between patients with LHON and ON ($p > .05$). Mean latency time was not delayed in LHON in comparison with normal subjects, but in ON the mean latency time was markedly delayed in comparison with normal subjects as well as with LHON patients (see figure 76.6).

From these results, it may be suggested that most of the nerve fibers in the luminance channels were less affected by LHON than nerve fibers in the spatial frequency channels. In an acute stage of LHON, luminance-related fibers may be less affected than the spatial frequency–related fibers are, whereas in patients with ON, all these types of fibers are damaged by inflammation or demyelination of the optic nerve.

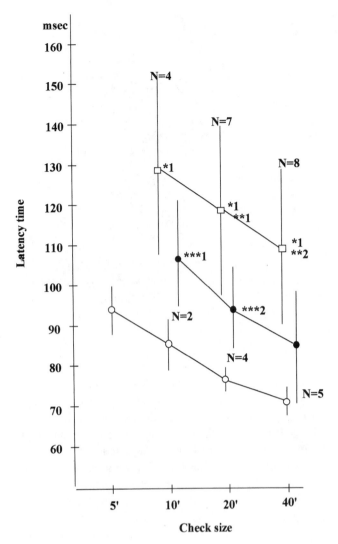

FIGURE 76.4 Check size–latency curve in pattern VEPs. In patients with LHON, mean latency was delayed in comparison with normal subjects in two check sizes: 10′ and 20′. In patients with ON, mean latency was delayed in comparison with normal subjects in check sizes 10′, 20′, and 40′ and patients with LHON in check sizes 20′ and 40′. (From Mashima Y, Imamura Y, Oguchi Y.[11] Used by permission.)

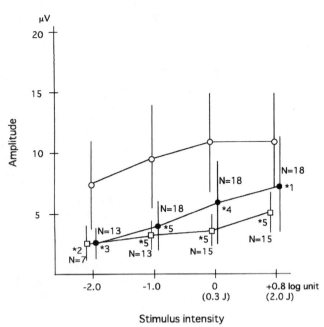

FIGURE 76.5 Intensity-amplitude curve in flash VEPs. Open circles and bars represent the mean ± S.D. in normal subjects (30 eyes). Solid circles and bars represent the mean ± S.D. in patients with LHON, and open squares represent the mean ± S.D. in patients with ON. Mean amplitude was significantly reduced in both LHON and ON patients compared with normal subjects. There was no difference in amplitude between LHON and ON patients. (From Mashima Y, Imamura Y, Oguchi Y.[11] Used by permission.)

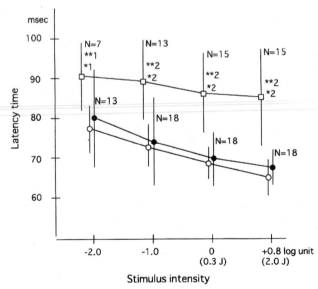

FIGURE 76.6 Intensity-latency curve in flash VEPs. In patients with LHON, mean latency time was not delayed in comparison with normal subjects. In patients with ON, mean latency time was markedly delayed in comparison with normal subjects as well as with LHON patients. (From Mashima Y, Imamura Y, Oguchi Y.[11] Used by permission.)

REFERENCES

1. Brown MD, Wallace DC: Spectrum of mitochondrial DNA mutations in Leber's hereditary optic neuropathy. *Clin Neurosci* 1994; 2:138–145.

2. Carroll WM, Mastaglia FL: Leber's optic neuropathy: A clinical and visual evoked potential study of affected and asymptomatic members of a six generation family. *Brain* 1979; 102:559–580.

3. Dorfman LJ, Nikoskeleinen E, Rosenthal AR, Sogg RL: Visual evoked potentials in Leber's hereditary optic neuropathy. *Ann Neurol* 1977; 1:565–568.

4. Houponen K, Vikki J, Aula P, Nikoskeleinen EK, Savontaus ML: A new mtDNA mutation associated with Leber hereditary optic neuroretinopathy. *Am J Hum Genet* 1991; 48:1147–1153.

5. Howell N, Bindoff LA, McCullough DA, Kubacka I, Poulton J, Mackey D, et al: Leber hereditary optic neuropathy: Identification of the same mitochondrial ND1 mutation in six pedigrees. *Am J Hum Genet* 1991; 49:939–950.

6. Imai Y, Moriwaki D: A possible case of cytoplasmic inheritance in man: A critique of Leber's disease. *J Genet* 1936; 33:163–167.

7. Johns DR, Heher KL, Miller NR, Smith KH: Leber's hereditary optic neuropathy: Clinical manifestations of the 14484 mutation. *Arch Ophthalmol* 1993; 111:495–498.

8. Johns DR, Neufeld MJ, Park RD: An ND-6 mitochondrial DNA mutation associated with Leber's hereditary optic neuropathy. *Biochem Biophys Res Commun* 1992; 187:1551–1557.

9. Leber T: Uber hereditare und congenital-angelegte Sehnervenleiden. *Graefes Arch Ophthalmol* 1871; 17:249–291.

10. Mashima Y, Hiida Y, Oguchi Y: Remission of Leber's optic neuropathy with idebenone. *Lancet* 1992; 340:368–369.

11. Mashima Y, Imamura Y, Oguchi Y: Dissociation of damage to spatial and luminance channels in early Leber's hereditary optic neuropathy manifested by the visual evoked potential. *Eye* 1997; 11:707–712.

12. Mashima Y, Kigasawa K, Oguchi Y, Fujino T: Leber's optic neuropathy—Electrophysiological studies. *Folia Ophthalmol Jpn* 1987; 38:1046–1053.

13. Mashima Y, Kigasawa K, Wakakura M, Oguchi Y: Do idebenone and vitamin therapy shorten the time to achieve visual recovery in Leber hereditary optic neuropathy? *J Neuro-ophthalmol* 2000; 20:166–170.

14. Mondelli M, Rossi A, Scarpini C, Dotti MT, Federico A: BAEP changes in Leber's hereditary optic atrophy: Further confirmation of multisystem involvement. *Acta Neurol Scand* 1990; 81:349–353.

15. Newman NJ: Leber's optic neuropathy: New genetic consideration. *Arch Neurol* 1993; 50:540–548.

16. Nikoskeleinen E, Hoyt WF, Nummelin K: Ophthalmoscopic findings in Leber's hereditary optic neuropathy: I. Fundus findings in asymptomatic family members. *Arch Ophthalmol* 1982; 100:1597–1620.

17. Nikoskelainen E, Parjarvi E, Lang H, Kalimo H: Leber's hereditary optic neuropathy: A mitochondrial disease? Proceedings of the 25th Scandiavian Congress. *Neurology* 1984; 69 (suppl 98):172–173.

18. Nikoskelainen E, Savontaus M-J, Wanne OP, Katila MJ, Nummelin KU: Leber's hereditary optic neuroretinopathy a maternally inherited disease: A genealogic study in four pediages. *Arch Ophthalmol* 1987; 105:665–671.

19. Riordan-Eva P, Sanders MD, Govan GG, Sweeney MG, Da Costa J, Harding AE: The clinical features of Leber's hereditary optic neuropathy defined by the presence of a pathogenic mitochondrial DNA mutation. *Brain* 1995; 118:319–337.

20. Shibata K, Shibagaki Y, Nagai C, Iwata M: Visual evoked potentials and electroretinograms in early stage of Leber's hereditary optic neuropathy. *J Neurol* 1999; 246:847–849.

21. Smith LJ, Hoyt WF, Sausac JO: Ocular fundus in acute Leber optic neuropathy. *Arch Ophthalmol* 1973; 90:349–354.

22. Wallace DC, Singh G, Lott MT, Hodge JA, Schurr G, Lezza MS, Elsas LJ II, Nikoskelainen EK: Mitochondrial DNA mutation associated with Leber's hereditary optic neuropathy. *Science* 1988; 242:1427–1430.

23. Yamada K, Oguchi Y, Hotta Y, Nakamura M, Isashiki Y, Mashima Y: Multicenter study on the frequency of three primary mutations of mitochondrial DNA in Japanese pedigees with Leber's hereditary optic neuropathy: Comparison with American and British counterparts. *J Neuro-ophthalmol* 1999; 22:187–193.

77 The Pattern Electroretinogram in Glaucoma and Ocular Hypertension

GARY L. TRICK

PRIMARY OPEN-ANGLE glaucoma (POAG) is a chronic visual disorder characterized by elevated intraocular pressure (IOP) in the presence of an anatomically open anterior chamber angle, excavation and/or pallor of the optic disc along with the nerve fiber layer defects, and visual field loss. Visual loss in chronic glaucoma results from the destruction of the retinal ganglion cell axons that form the optic nerve. The optic nerve damage in POAG occurs over a protracted period of time (often months or years) and appears to be due to an increase in IOP to an intolerable level. Individuals with elevated IOP who do not exhibit optic disk, nerve fiber layer, or visual field defects (i.e., ocular hypertensives) are considered glaucoma suspects because they are at risk of developing the disease. However, the relationship between elevated IOP and the development of glaucoma remains unclear since many ocular hypertensives may not develop the disease while other individuals with apparently normal IOP develop the optic disk, nerve fiber layer, and visual field abnormalities that are characteristic of glaucoma (i.e., low-tension glaucoma). This suggests that there is considerable interindividual variability in the IOP level necessary to produce optic nerve damage.

The mechanism by which elevated IOP induces optic nerve damage is not known. The two primary hypotheses suggest that elevated IOP either interferes with blood flow at the optic nerve head (the vascular theory) or produces mechanical compression of the retinal ganglion cell axons in the region of the lamina cribrosa (mechanical theory). In either case, there is a slowly progressive loss of retinal ganglion cell axons that eventually results in the development of a characteristic visual field defect (figure 77.1), upon which the diagnosis of glaucoma is often made. However, the manifestation of a visual field defect may represent a relatively late stage in the progression of the disease, a time when retinal ganglion cell loss is virtually irreversible. Recent estimates suggest that 40% to 50% of the optic nerve axons can be lost prior to the development of a visual field defect that is detectable with manual perimetry.[31] As a result there has been considerable interest in developing more sensitive and more reliable methods for studying the pathogenesis and pathophysiology of retinal ganglion cell damage in glaucoma. The pattern electroretinogram (PERG) is one method that is being used in these studies.

The original suggestion by Maffei and Fiorentini[24] that the PERG could be used to monitor the bioelectrical response of the retinal ganglion cells provided the impetus for a large number of studies on patients with glaucoma. In a general sense these investigations can be characterized as either (1) testing the hypothesis that the PERG has a ganglion cell origin by studying individuals with a disease that is known to directly affect these cells or (2) evaluating the possible clinical value of the PERG for detecting glaucoma. Taken together, these diverse studies have provided considerable insight concerning both the basic properties of the human PERG and the pathophysiology of retinal ganglion cell dysfunction in glaucoma.

Earlier electrophysiological studies of the pathogenesis and pathophysiology of visual dysfunction in glaucoma were hampered by the lack of an appropriate technique for directly evaluating the functional integrity of the neural elements in the proximal retina and, in particular, the retinal ganglion cells. Studies of the flash electroretinogram (ERG) in patients with glaucoma clearly illustrated that the more distal neural elements in the retina were unaffected,[14,21] at least until relatively late in the disease process.[3,12] The results of visual evoked potential (VEP) studies in glaucoma patients, on the other hand, indicated that the latency of the bioelectrical responses generated in the primary visual cortex was often increased.[17,37] Therefore, the flash ERG and VEP results implied that there was a significant deficit within the primary visual pathway of glaucoma patients that was not the result of dysfunction in the neural elements of the distal retina. However, the mechanism whereby a loss in retinal ganglion cell axons would produce an increase in VEP latency remains unclear. Furthermore, the relationship between the VEP latency increase and the nature and extent

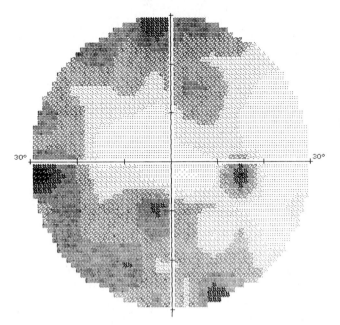

30°   30°

FIGURE 77.1 The diagnosis of chronic open-angle glaucoma is often based upon evidence of a visual field defect similar to the visual field loss apparent in this 65-year-old white male. This result was obtained by automated perimetry (Humphrey 30–2).

of the early damage to the optic nerve in glaucoma has not been established, perhaps because the VEP is an indirect reflection of retinal ganglion cell function that is dominated by the bioelectrical response of neural elements within the central 5 to 10 degrees of the visual field.[36] Thus the availability of an electrophysiological technique to monitor a bioelectrical response that includes a component (or components) that originates in the proximal retina and possibly reflects the functional integrity of the retinal ganglion cells that themselves filled an obvious void.

There now have been numerous studies of the PERG in glaucoma patients, and the clear consensus of these studies is that PERG abnormalities frequently are evident in individuals with well-diagnosed POAG (table 77.1). Both PERG amplitude reductions and latency increases (or phase shifts) have been reported in various studies (figure 77.2), but because the latency increase is relatively small (about 5 to 8 ms) although statistically significant, the more robust amplitude reductions have drawn the most interest. The results of these investigations indicate that in glaucoma patients PERG amplitude reductions occur in the presence of normal flash and flicker ERGs. Some evidence also indicates that the PERG amplitude reductions become more profound when other signs of glaucoma (i.e., cupping and field loss) indicate an increase in the severity of the disease.[19,45]

Important confirmation of the conclusions drawn from studies of patients with glaucoma has come from studies of experimental glaucoma that is induced in primates by argon laser application to the trabecular meshwork.[11,26,27] In this glaucoma model the aqueous outflow facility is decreased, IOP is increased, and there are consequent changes in cupping of the optic nervehead and loss of optic nerve axons that are quite similar to the changes that occur in the human condition.[27,30] Results from the primate model indicate that PERG amplitude reductions (1) precede the development of significant changes in the optic nervehead, (2) are related to the degree of cupping and nerve fiber loss, and (3) are not diminished when IOP is reduced pharmacologically.[11,26,27]

Estimates of the magnitude of the PERG amplitude reductions observed in glaucoma patients vary from 10% to 80% (or more), partially depending upon the spatial and temporal characteristics of the stimulus. Our studies[40] of the spatial and temporal tuning of the PERG abnormality in glaucoma patients indicate that the magnitude of the deficit is greatest when high–temporal frequency stimuli are used to elicit steady-state PERGs (figure 77.3). Based upon these results and the histological observation that the larger retinal ganglion cell fibers appear to be most susceptible to glaucomatous damage early in the course of the disease,[32] Trick

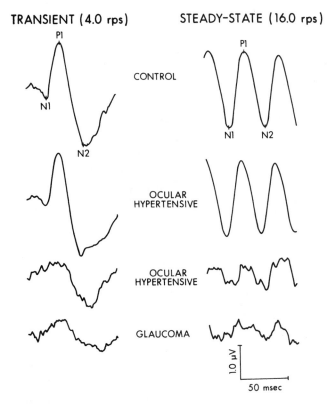

FIGURE 77.2 Representative PERGs for low–temporal frequency (transient) and high–temporal frequency (steady-state) conditions are illustrated for an age-matched visual normal (control), two patients with diagnosed ocular hypertension and normal visual fields, and a patient with diagnosed POAG. Note that one ocular hypertensive produced good responses for both test conditions while in the other ocular hypertensive both responses were poor.

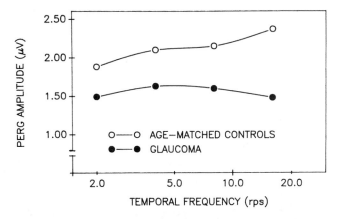

FIGURE 77.3 PERG amplitude is plotted as a function of temporal frequency. The data points have been replotted from Trick[40] and represent values for 32 patients with chronic open-angle glaucoma and 32 age-matched controls average across check size.

further suggested that this represented a selective loss of the type A retinal ganglion cells that underlie the magnicellular stream of the primary visual pathway.[22] Similarly, in the primate model of glaucoma the largest PERG deficits are

observed with high–temporal and low–spatial frequency stimuli, once again supporting the concept of a selective deficit in the magnicellular system.[26,27] Possible variations in the extent of this selective damage associated with progression of the disease is a topic that requires further investigation.

More recently it has been suggested[15] that the transient PERG includes two semi-independent processes that are evident as the N1-P1 and the P1-N2 components of the waveform (see figure 77.2). In diseases where damage is localized in the proximal retina and/or optic nerve only the P1-N2 component of the transient PERG is reduced. In diseases that affect the distal retina the N1-P1 component of the transient PERG is reduced (due to the direct influence of the disease on the retinal generators of this component), and the P1-N2 component is also reduced (since the input to the neural elements in the proximal retina/optic nerve is distorted by the effect on the distal retina). Based upon this observation the large-magnitude reduction Trick noted in the steady-state PERG also could be interpreted as resulting from the merging of the N1-P1 and N2-P2 components due to the high temporal frequency. In one study it was observed that the P1-N2 component of the transient PERG was more reduced than the N1-P1 component in glaucoma patients.[48] Certainly, this relationship between the waveform components of both the transient and the steady-state PERG should be more completely evaluated.

Studies of the PERG in patients with ocular hypertension (see table 77.1) suggest that this retinal potential may provide a sensitive measure of retinal ganglion cell dysfunction that could be used to detect visual loss in ocular hypertensives prior to the development of glaucomatous visual field loss. PERG amplitude reductions are apparent in some, although not all ocular hypertensives (see figure 77.2). In different studies, however, the percentage of ocular hypertensives with abnormal PERGs has varied considerably. Porciatti et al.[29] reported significant PERG amplitude reductions in 11 of 12 (91.6%) ocular hypertensives who had normal visual fields, while Wanger and Persson[46] observed significant amplitude reduction in four of seven (57.1%) patients with unilateral ocular hypertension. Ambrosio et al.[4] detected PERG amplitude reductions in 75% of the ocular hypertensives tested in their study but failed to indicate whether all of these were significant statistically. On the other hand, Trick et al.[41] found significant PERG amplitude reductions in only 15 of 130 (11.5%) ocular hypertensives.

The high percentage of ocular hypertensives with PERG abnormalities that has been observed in some studies suggests that this retinal potential may be sensitive to early changes in visual processing that are associated with elevated IOP. However, this high figure also raises questions about the utility of the technique for predicting which patients will develop glaucoma. Epidemiological evidence suggests that 0.5% to 2.0% of patients with mild to moderately elevated IOP (21 to 35 mm Hg) will develop visual loss each year.[20] Long-term follow-up of ocular hypertensives suggests similar values.[18,23] Thus the high percentages observed in some studies could also suggest that this technique has inadequate specificity (i.e., poorly discriminates the patients with impending glaucomatous visual field loss from other ocular hypertensives). The high percentage of abnormal responses observed in some studies may be partially the result of the small size of the samples tested and a loose definition of a significant deficit. In addition, it is likely that the sample selection criteria influenced the percentage of patients observed to have abnormal responses. Trick[39] demonstrated that over 50% of ocular hypertensives who are considered to be at high risk of developing POAG (based upon a weighted combination of the following risk factors: age, IOP, family history of glaucoma, and cup-to-disk ratio) exhibit significant PERG amplitude reductions while less than 10% of low-risk ocular hypertensives exhibit these deficits. The larger group of ocular hypertensives later tested by Trick et al.[41] were unselected for these risk factors and may have been composed of a large percentage of individuals who were at lower risk than the patients included in other investigations (e.g., Weinstein et al.[48]). Therefore, a prospective study will be necessary to eventually determine whether PERG amplitude reductions reliably precede the development of a glaucomatous visual field defect in these patients.

The exact relationship between IOP elevations and PERG amplitude reductions has not been determined. There is evidence that large, acute elevations in IOP (as might occur in angle-closure glaucoma or glaucoma secondary to ocular trauma) do produce reductions in PERG amplitude. However, in these cases the PERG amplitude reductions may not reflect only retinal ganglion cell dysfunction since the functional integrity of neural elements in the distal retina, the elements that provide input to the ganglion cells, is also disrupted by acute IOP elevations. It is uncertain whether smaller, chronic changes in IOP produce PERG alterations that are similar to the changes that occur as a result of acute IOP elevation. Among ocular hypertensives the correlation between IOP and PERG amplitude is weak (figure 77.4), while the association of other factors (such as age and blood pressure) with PERG amplitude may be as strong or stronger. This may simply reflect the variability in pressure tolerance of retinal ganglion cells between individuals, in which case evidence of intraindividual effects of elevated pressure may become obvious when prospective studies are completed. However, in an interesting study designed to separate the influence of IOP and retinal vascular perfusion on the PERG, Siliprandi et al.[35] demonstrated that perfusion pressure rather than IOP plays the major role influencing the PERG. Perhaps, therefore, the

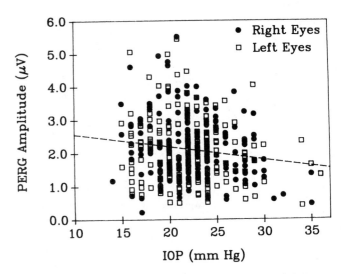

FIGURE 77.4   Among ocular hypertensives there is a weak, but statistically significant correlation between PERG amplitude and IOP ($r = -0.16$). The dashed line represents the best-fit linear regression (least squares) based upon the data for 153 patients.

PERG amplitude reductions associated with chronic glaucoma and ocular hypertension are more directly the result of retinal vascular changes and only indirectly result from elevated IOP.

Visual dysfunction in glaucoma and ocular hypertension has also been revealed in a variety of psychophysical studies. Color vision,[1,42] contrast sensitivity,[6] and temporal resolution[43] deficits have all been observed in some ocular hypertensives as well as in glaucoma patients. The collective results of these studies suggest that the visual dysfunction associated with the development of glaucomatous damage is not constrained to the retinal areas where the characteristic visual field defects are observed; the damage often involves other retinal areas including the macula. Only color vision deficits have been demonstrated to precede visual field loss in prospective studies of patients developing glaucoma,[10] but many glaucoma patients do not exhibit abnormal color vision,[2,9] and the percentage of ocular hypertensive patients with color vision deficits exceeds the proportion expected to develop glaucoma.[42] The relationship between these visual deficits and the visual dysfunction underlying the PERG abnormalities of glaucoma patients and ocular hypertensives has been explored incompletely. There is some evidence that the association between the color vision and the PERG deficits in ocular hypertensives is weak, a finding that could imply that different physiological mechanisms are involved in each deficit.

In a recent study Drance et al.[9] examined the sensitivity and specificity of a variety of psychophysical, electrophysiological, and fundus imaging techniques in glaucoma patients, glaucoma suspects, and controls. The results indicated that both sensitivity and specificity were higher for the

PERG than for either color vision or contrast sensitivity. Several measures derived from optic disk imaging techniques, however, had higher sensitivity and specificity than did the PERG.

In conclusion, the PERG is a tool that has promise for investigating the pathophysiology of retinal ganglion cell dysfunction in glaucoma. Although it is doubtful that PERG will ever replace perimetry as the method of choice for detecting visual loss in glaucoma patients, it is clear that the technique can be a complement to the visual field in confirming a diagnosis of glaucoma. In addition, PERG studies should be considered in cases where it is difficult to obtain a reliable visual field. Nevertheless, it is important to remember that the precise sensitivity and specificity of the technique for detecting glaucomatous damage remains to be established. The clinical value of PERG for detecting retinal ganglion cell dysfunction in the ocular hypertensives who will develop glaucoma also remains an open question. However, prospective studies of the utility of the PERG in ocular hypertension are underway, so perhaps this issue will be resolved in the not too distant future.

REFERENCES

1. Adams AJ, Heron G, Husted R: Clinical measures of central visual function in glaucoma and ocular hypertension. *Arch Ophthalmol* 1987; 105:782.
2. Adams AJ, Rodic R, Husted R, Stamper R: Spectral sensitivity and color discrimination changes in glaucoma and glaucoma-suspect patients. *Invest Ophthalmol Vis Sci* 1982; 23:516.
3. Alvis DL: Electroretinographic changes in controlled chronic open-angle glaucoma. *Am J Ophthalmol* 1966; 62:121–131.
4. Ambrosio G, Arienzo G, Aurilia P, et al: Pattern electroretinograms in ocular hypertension. *Doc Ophthalmol* 1988; 69:161–165.
5. Arden GB, Vaegan, Hogg CR: Clinical and experimental evidence that the pattern electroretinogram (PERG) is generated in more proximal retinal layers than the focal electroretinogram (FERG). *Ann NY Acad Sci* 1982; 388:580–601.
6. Atkin A, Wolkstein M, Bodis-Wollner I, et al: Interocular comparison of contrast sensitivities in glaucoma patients and suspects. *Br J Ophthalmol* 1980; 64:858.
7. Bach M, Hiss P, Rover J: Check-size specific changes of pattern electroretinogram in patients with early open-angle glaucoma. *Doc Ophthalmol* 1987; 69:315–322.
8. Bobak P, Bodis-Wollner I, Harnois C, et al: Pattern electroretinograms and visual evoked potentials in glaucoma and multiple sclerosis. *Am J Ophthalmol* 1983; 96:72.
9. Drance SM, Airaksinen PJ, Price M, et al: The use of psychophysical, structural and electro-diagnostic parameters to identify glaucomatous damage. *Graefes Arch Clin Exp Ophthalmol* 1987; 225:365.
10. Drance SM, Lakowski R, Schulzer M, Douglas GR: Acquired color vision changes in glaucoma: Use of 100-hue test and Pickford anomaloscope as predictors of glaucomatous field change. *Arch Ophthalmol* 1981; 99:829.
11. Drum B, Johnson MA, Quigley HA, et al: Pattern ERG and optic nerve histology in monkeys with unilateral laser induced glaucoma. *Invest Ophthalmol Vis Sci* 1986; 27 (suppl):40.
12. Fazio D, Heckenlively JR, Martin DA, Christensen RE: The electroretinogram in advanced glaucoma. *Doc Ophthalmol* 1986; 63:45–54.
13. Fiorentini A, Maffei L, Pirchio M, et al: The ERG in response to alternating gratings in patients with diseases of the peripheral visual pathway. *Invest Ophthalmol Vis Sci* 1981; 21:490.
14. Henkes H: Electroretinography. *Am J Ophthalmol* 1957; 43:67.
15. Holder GE: Significance of abnormal pattern electroretinography in anterior visual pathway dysfunction. *Br J Ophthalmol* 1987; 71:166.
16. Howe JW, Mitchell KW: Simultaneous recording of pattern electroretinogram and visual evoked cortical potential in a group of patients with chronic glaucoma. *Doc Ophthalmol Proc Ser* 1984; 40:101–107.
17. Huber C: Pattern evoked cortical potentials and automated perimetry in chronic glaucoma. *Doc Ophthalmol Proc Ser* 1981; 27:87–94.
18. Jensen JE: Glaucoma screening: A 16-year follow-up of ocular normotensives. *Acta Ophthalmol* 1984; 62:203.
19. Korth M, Horn F, Storck B, Jonas J: Pattern electroretinograms in normal and glaucomatous eyes. *Invest Ophthalmol Vis Sci* 1987; 28 (suppl):129.
20. Leske MC: The epidemiology of open-angle glaucoma: A review. *Am J Epidemiol* 1983; 118:166.
21. Leydhecker G: The electroretinogram in glaucomatous eyes. *Br J Ophthalmol* 1950; 34:550–554.
22. Livingstone MS, Hubel DH: Segregation of form, color, movement and depth: Anatomy, physiology and perception. *Science* 1988; 240:740–749.
23. Lundberg L, Wettrell K, Linear E: Ocular hypertension: A prospective twenty-year follow-up study. *Acta Ophthalmol* 1987; 65:705.
24. Maffei L, Fiorentini A: Electroretinographic responses to alternating gratings before and after section of the optic nerve. *Science* 1981; 211:953–955.
25. Markoff JI, Breton ME, Shakin E, Franz J: Pattern reversal electroretinogram in glaucoma, glaucoma suspects and normals. *Invest Ophthalmol Vis Sci* 1983; 24 (suppl):102.
26. Marx MS, Podos SM, Bodis-Wollner I, et al: Flash and pattern electroretinograms in normal and laser-induced glaucomatous primate eyes. *Invest Ophthalmol Vis Sci* 1986; 27:378–386.
27. Marx MS, Podos SM, Bodis-Wollner I, et al: Signs of early damage in glaucomatous monkey eyes: Low spatial frequency losses in the pattern ERG and VEP. *Exp Eye Res* 1988; 46:173–184.
28. Papst N, Bopp M, Schnaudigel OE: Pattern electroretinogram and visually evoked cortical potentials in glaucoma. *Graefes Arch Clin Exp Ophthalmol* 1984; 222:29.
29. Porciatti V, Falsini B, Brunori S, et al: Pattern electroretinogram as a function of spatial frequency in ocular hypertension and early glaucoma. *Doc Ophthalmol* 1987; 65:349–355.
30. Quigley HA, Hohman RM: Laser energy levels for trabecular meshwork damage in the primate eye. *Invest Ophthalmol Vis Sci* 1983; 24:1305–1307.
31. Quigley HA, Hohman RM, Addicks EM, et al: Morphologic changes in the lamina cribrosa correlated with neural loss in open-angel glaucoma. *Am J Ophthalmol* 1983; 95:673–691.
32. Quigley HA, Sanchez RM, Dunkelberger GR, et al: Chronic glaucoma selectively damages large optic nerve fibers. *Invest Ophthalmol Vis Sci* 1987; 28:913–920.
33. Ringens PJ, Viifvinkel-Bruinenga S, van Lith GHM: The pattern elicited electroretinogram I. A tool in the early detection of glaucoma? *Ophthalmologica* 1986; 192:171–175.

34. Seiple W, Price MJ, Kupersmith M, Carr RE: The pattern electroretinogram in optic nerve disease. *Ophthalmology* 1983; 90:1127.

35. Siliprandi R, Bucci MG, Canella R, Cormignoto G: Flash and pattern electroretinograms during and after acute intra-ocular pressure elevation in cats. *Invest Ophthalmol Vis Sci* 1988; 29:558–565.

36. Sokol S: Visually evoked potentials: Theory, technique and clinical application. *Surv Ophthalmol* 1976; 21:18.

37. Towle VL, Moskowitz A, Sokol S, Schwartz B: The visual evoked potential in glaucoma and ocular hypertension: Effects of check size, field size, and stimulation rate. *Invest Ophthalmol Vis Sci* 1983; 24:175.

38. Trick GL: Anomalous PRRP spatial-temporal frequency tuning characteristics in glaucoma. *Invest Ophthalmol Vis Sci* 1983; 24 (suppl):102.

39. Trick GL: PRRP abnormalities in glaucoma and ocular hypertension. *Invest Ophthalmol Vis Sci* 1986; 27:749.

40. Trick GL: Retinal potentials in patients with primary open-angle glaucoma: Physiological evidence for temporal frequency tuning defects. *Invest Ophthalmol Vis Sci* 1985; 26:1750–1758.

41. Trick GL, Bickler-Bluth M, Cooper DG, et al: Pattern reversal electroretinogram (PRERG) abnormalities in ocular hypertension: Correlation with glaucoma risk factors. *Curr Eye Res* 1988; 7:201–206.

42. Trick GL, Nesher RN, Cooper D, et al: Dissociation of visual deficits in ocular hypertension. *Invest Ophthalmol Vis Sci* 1988; 29:1486–1491.

43. Tyler CW: Specific deficits of flicker sensitivity in glaucoma and ocular hypertension. *Invest Ophthalmol Vis Sci* 1981; 20:204.

44. van Lith GHM, Ringens P, de Heer LJ: Pattern electroretinogram and glaucoma. *Dev Ophthalmol* 1984; 9:133–139.

45. Wanger P, Persson HE: Pattern-reversal electroretinograms from normotensive, hypertensive and glaucomatous eyes. *Ophthalmologica* 1987; 195:205–208.

46. Wanger P, Persson HE: Pattern reversal electroretinograms in ocular hypertension. *Doc Ophthalmol* 1985; 61:27–31.

47. Wanger P, Persson HE: Pattern reversal electroretinograms in unilateral glaucoma. *Invest Ophthalmol Vis Sci* 1983; 24: 749.

48. Weinstein GW, Arden GB, Hitchings RA, et al: The pattern electroretinogram (PERG) in ocular hypertension and glaucoma. *Arch Ophthalmol* 1988; 106:923–928.

78 Chiasmal and Retrochiasmal Lesions

GRAHAM E. HOLDER

Chiasmal lesions

The principal cause of chiasmal dysfunction is pituitary tumor, the anatomical relationship between the optic chiasm and the pituitary gland making the chiasm susceptible to compression by lesions expanding from the pituitary fossa. The classic triad of neuro-ophthalmic signs in pituitary tumors of reduced visual acuity, visual field defects, and optic atrophy arises from suprasellar tumor extension with resulting compression of the chiasm. Other types of tumor, aneurysm, inflammation, demyelination, and trauma can also affect chiasmal function. A bitemporal hemianopia is the classic visual field defect due to a disturbance of the decussating fibers from the nasal retinae but occurs in less than 50% of patients with pituitary tumors and visual loss.[42,78] Other types of visual field defect can result, including central scotoma. Approximately 13% of patients present with unilateral visual loss.[25]

The investigation of choice in patients with suspected chiasmal compression is neuroradiology, either magnetic resonance imaging (MRI) or high-resolution computed tomography (CT) scanning. There are probably two roles for electrophysiological testing. The first is in the initial assessment and diagnosis of patients with visual symptoms; the delayed or misdiagnosis of chiasmal dysfunction can result in severe irreversible visual loss, and it is therefore of critical importance that the correct diagnosis be reached promptly. Reports of misdiagnoses in the literature include (atypical) retrobulbar neuritis, glaucoma, cataract, hysteria, macular degeneration, refractive error, choroidal sclerosis, and vascular lesions.[31,41,59,65] The second role for electrophysiology is in the follow-up and management of patients with radiologically confirmed lesions that might or might not show suprasellar extension and signs of visual pathway dysfunction and encompasses postoperative monitoring.

The likely involvement of the crossing fibers enables the use of hemifield stimulation in the visual evoked potential (VEP) assessment of chiasmal function, but adequate consideration of registration parameters is critical to VEP interpretation. A hemifield VEP abnormality may be the most sensitive electrophysiological index of early chiasmal involvement, but some patients with reduced visual acuity have difficulty in maintaining accurate fixation, and it might not be possible to perform hemifield stimulation adequately in all patients. Full-field stimulation also gives accurate localization of chiasmal lesions but is slightly less sensitive.[15,28] Multichannel recording is indicated; assessment of chiasmal function should not be attempted with a single midline channel.

An understanding of the results of hemifield pattern stimulation in normal individuals is important to accurate interpretation of the electrophysiological abnormalities in chiasmal dysfunction. Use of a large hemifield stimulus, for example, greater than a 12-degree radius, gives "paradoxical" lateralization of the normal P100 component of the pattern-reversal VEP ipsilateral to the stimulated hemifield.[6] There is a contralateral N105/P135 complex. However, as the size of the stimulus field is progressively reduced, the P100 firstly becomes bilateral in distribution and then contralateral with a small hemifield stimulus (e.g., 2.5-degree radius[36]). Similar changes occur in patients with hemifield defects[39] (see below). In general, when Fz is used as a reference, a small-field, small-check stimulus will show anatomical lateralization, whereas a large-check, large-field stimulus will show paradoxical lateralization. Bipolar recordings using ipsilateral hemisphere reference electrodes do not show paradoxical lateralization with any stimulus parameters, and the contribution to paradoxical lateralization of the signal recorded via the Fz "reference" is thus apparent.

Following the initial report by Muller[52] that the flash VEP (FVEP) could be of abnormal latency in chiasmal dysfunction, other workers noted that the maximum FVEP abnormality was localized contralateral to the visual field defect.[27,43,48,73] The first reports using contrast stimuli appeared in 1976. Van Lith's group[76] used both full-field and hemifield steady-state (8 Hz) stimulation in six patients with bitemporal hemianopia due to tumor, and found both phase and amplitude abnormalities contralateral to the stimulated eye.

The first detailed report of transient pattern VEP (PVEP) was that of Halliday's group.[34] Using a 16-degree radius, 50-minute check stimulus, they found markedly asymmetrical

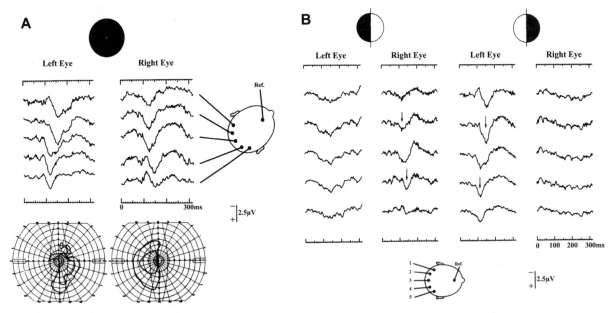

FIGURE 78.1   Crossed VEP asymmetry in a 48-year-old male with bitemporal hemianopia from a suprasellar mass (16-degree radius, 50-minute checks). A, With full-field stimulation, the normal P100 component is recorded over the right hemisphere when the left eye is stimulated and over the left hemisphere when the right eye is stimulated, that is, contralateral to the impaired temporal visual field and showing the phenomenon of paradoxical lateralization.

B, The use of hemifield recording demonstrates that the full-field responses reflect preservation of the responses to the preserved nasal fields. (From Halliday AM, Barrett G, Blumhardt LD, et al: The macular and paramacular subcomponents of the pattern evoked response. In Lehman D, Calloway E (eds): *Human Evoked Potentials: Applications and Problems.* New York, Plenum, 1975, pp 135–151. Used by permission.)

scalp distribution in ten patients with chiasmal dysfunction. In particular, they described the "crossed" asymmetry typical of chiasmal lesions in which the findings from one eye are more abnormal over one hemisphere but the distribution of abnormality changes such that findings from the fellow eye are more abnormal over the other hemisphere. Unexpectedly, the maximum abnormality was localized ipsilateral to the visual field defect, that is, the "paradoxical" lateralization referred to above (figure 78.1). PVEP abnormalities were present from some eyes with normal (kinetic) visual fields. The findings were contrasted to those in demyelination, in which preservation of waveform, a generally greater latency delay, and symmetry across the scalp were much more frequent. The use of hemifield stimulation was further elaborated in another publication by the same group.[8]

Holder[38] confirmed this "crossed" asymmetry in ten patients, but when full-field stimulation (11-degree full-field, 26-minute checks, bipolar recording) was used, the maximal PVEP abnormality was always contralateral to the stimulated eye (figure 78.2). Although apparently contradictory, these findings are in fact consistent with those of Halliday's group, the alternate abnormality lateralization reflecting the use of a smaller stimulating field/check size (see above). The abnormality lateralization was enhanced with a 4-degree radius, 13-minute check stimulus. It was confirmed that the

asymmetrical scalp distribution was atypical for demyelination and that abnormal VEPs could occur in eyes with full visual fields. Equally, normal PVEPs could occur in eyes with field defects. Latency delays were a frequent occurrence.

Those findings were extended in a study of 34 patients with histologically confirmed nonfunctioning chromophobe adenomas.[41] The PVEP results were compared with clinical, radiological, and surgical findings. There were four eyes with normal PVEPs; one had a full visual field, one had a paracentral scotoma, and two had superior temporal quadrant defects. It is of interest that FVEPs in the latter two eyes were abnormal. Full fields but abnormal PVEPs occurred in two eyes. The PVEPs often indicated marked functional asymmetry when the neuroradiology (CT scan) suggested symmetrical midline suprasellar extension. The PVEPs were usually more sensitive than the conventional clinical tests of visual acuity and visual fields.

A number of other studies reported PVEP findings in chiasmal dysfunction, mostly (those using multichannel recording techniques) confirming the "crossed" PVEP asymmetry to be pathognomonic of chiasmal dysfunction but describing clinical and electrophysiological findings in varying degrees of detail.[13–16,28,32,33,51,55,58,68,71] Gott and colleagues examined 83 patients with tomographically demonstrated pituitary tumors.[32] Most were intrasellar and had normal fields and PVEPs. Suprasellar extension was radiologically

Pattern VEP

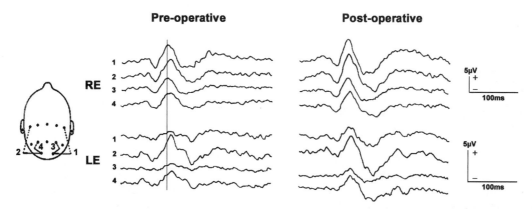

Pre-operative   **Post-operative**

FIGURE 78.2 Crossed VEP asymmetry in a 48-year-old male with a nonfunctioning chromophobe adenoma showing crossed asymmetry of the VEPs. Use of a small field (11 degrees), small check stimulus (26 minutes), gives "anatomical" rather than "paradoxical" distribution of abnormality. The preoperative findings from the right eye show increased latency in the left hemisphere traces, in keeping with dysfunction of the decussating fibers from the right eye to the left hemisphere. Preoperative stimulation of the left eye shows an overall longer latency compared to the right eye, in keeping with a degree of optic nerve dysfunction; the right hemisphere traces are more abnormal than the left, in keeping with the chiasmal compression. Note the improvement after surgery such that the right eye findings no longer show any abnormality and the left eye findings now show no delay and less interhemispheric asymmetry.

demonstrated in 12 cases; all had abnormal PVEPs, but visual fields were normal in eight patients. The abnormality was usually an increased P100 latency, but asymmetrical scalp amplitude distribution was also observed (22-degree full field, abnormality ipsilateral to the field defect).

The ability of the PVEP to influence management was noted by Stark and Lenton,[68] who cite one case with a radiologically confirmed pituitary tumor but unreliable clinical testing in which an abnormal PVEP prompted surgical intervention. Haimovic and Pedley[33] found a delayed P100 (19 × 13.5-degree hemifield, 31-minute checks, abnormality ipsilateral to the field defect) in one of 15 patients with hemifield stimulation but in four patients when full-field stimulation was used. This illustrates the difficulty in component identification with large-field stimuli, which can lead to spurious "delays." Blumhardt[7] forcefully argued this point. Others concluded that the VEP was not a suitable means of detecting subtle field defects following a study of eight patients[51] with 5-degree hemifield, 50-minute checks: two patients who were normal, four with ipsilateral abnormality, and two with no lateralization. This failure to reveal abnormalities may relate to the choice of stimulus parameters and emphasizes the importance of this factor. The two patients with normal PVEPs were presumably postoperative because the visual field defects had "resolved." There was, however, subjective desaturation to red. Flanagan and Harding[28] carefully examined the effects of various stimulus parameters in nine patients with pituitary tumors; hemifield stimulation with a large-check, large-field stimulus was more sensitive than full-field stimulation in the early detec-

tion of chiasmal dysfunction. This observation was later confirmed.[13,15]

Optimal use of medical therapy, such as bromocriptine, for pituitary lesions is aided by a sensitive, objective assessment of chiasmal function. Wass et al.[74] first described PVEP improvement during bromocriptine therapy in patients with large pituitary tumors but did not supply full details. Pullan and colleagues examined hemifield PVEPs in five nonfunctioning and five functioning tumors (prolactinomata) before and after bromocriptine treatment.[60] Suprasellar extension on CT scan was a criterion for patient selection. All patients with radiological evidence of tumor shrinkage showed PVEP improvement, as did one patient without evident radiological change. The author's laboratory has also monitored patients with intrasellar lesions (unpublished data). Changes in the VEP may be the first indicator of functional involvement of the chiasm, preceding field loss, and thus precipitate a change from medical to surgical management. Serial postoperative VEP recording can also monitor the functional state of the optic nerves and chiasm in a patient following tumor excision (figure 78.3) and may help detect tumor recurrence prior to deterioration in visual fields or acuity. Similarly, some patients decline surgery when offered, and additional objective evidence of increasing visual pathway dysfunction may help them to reconsider.

VEP recording has also been used to monitor chiasmal function during surgery.[2,17,20,26,54,61,77] There is no consensus in relation to the contribution of intraoperative recording to surgical outcome. There are inevitable limitations of the technique owing to the need for diffuse flash stimulation.

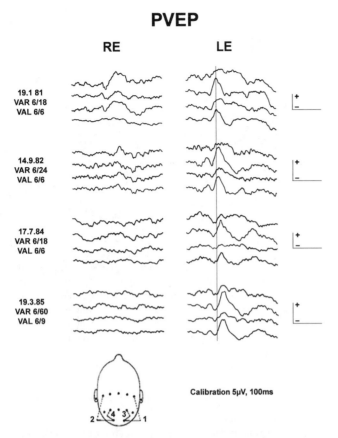

PVEP

RE   **LE**

19.1 81
VAR 6/18
VAL 6/6

14.9.82
VAR 6/24
VAL 6/6

17.7.84
VAR 6/18
VAL 6/6

19.3.85
VAR 6/60
VAL 6/9

Calibration 5µV, 100ms

2   1

FIGURE 78.3   Serial VEPs in a patient with recurrence of a non-functioning chromophobe adenoma (11-degree full-field stimulus; 26-minute checks). The patient was aware of the recurrence but declined further surgical intervention. Initial findings from the right eye show a P100 component that is markedly delayed and is better seen in the ipsilateral hemisphere traces than the right in keeping with the lateralization expected with a small-field, small-check stimulus. The PVEP had become undetectable by March 1984 but without change in visual acuity. Right eye visual acuity dropped to 6/60 approximately one year later. The initial findings from the left eye show a well-formed PVEP in the ipsilateral hemisphere traces but marked abnormality in the right hemisphere traces in keeping with dysfunction of the decussating chiasmal fibers. The latency of the P10 component in the ipsilateral hemisphere traces increases by ~20 ms over a 4-year period with no deterioration in visual acuity. Note the continuing interhemispheric asymmetry. Visual fields were abnormal throughout but showed no significant deterioration. Neuroradiological investigation (CT scan) showed tumor expansion during the period of follow-up.

Chiasmal hypoplasia or aplasia can also be detected by using VEP techniques.[4,70]

The PERG has been suggested to be a useful prognostic indicator for visual outcome in the preoperative assessment of optic nerve compression in pituitary tumor.[45,63] That has been confirmed in the author's laboratories.[57] An abnormal PERG correlates with a lack of postoperative recovery, presumably by demonstrating significant retrograde degeneration to the retinal ganglion cells.

The VEP is also of major importance in the demonstration of abnormal chiasmal routing in patients suspected of albinism.[23] That issue is addressed elsewhere in this volume (see chapter 25).

Retrochiasmal lesions

UNILATERAL DYSFUNCTION   The typical VEP appearance in unilateral retrochiasmal dysfunction is an "uncrossed" asymmetry in which there is an abnormal scalp distribution that is similar for each eye. The comments in the previous section regarding the influence of registration parameters on PVEP abnormality lateralization and component identification are equally applicable to retrochiasmal dysfunction and are of paramount importance to accurate interpretation of the findings. Although there are many reports of VEP changes, the development of improved neuroradiological techniques such as high-resolution CT scanning and MRI has greatly reduced any role that electrodiagnostic evaluation may have played in the diagnosis and management of these patients.

The PVEP is more sensitive than the FVEP in most conditions but needs a cooperative patient who is able and willing to fixate and concentrate. If this is not possible, the FVEP may give useful information. Equally, the two techniques can provide complementary information about the intracranial visual pathways (figure 78.4). A brief review of FVEP reports is therefore presented. There is consensus in the FVEP studies that any abnormality detected is lateralized to the side of the lesion (contralateral to the field defect) in unilateral hemisphere dysfunction, most differences relating to the incidence of abnormality in relation to the visual field defect. In summarizing the results of a number of studies with unilateral lesions, it seems that some 70–75% of patients with homonymous hemianopic defects have abnormal FVEPs, an abnormality being more likely to occur with complete homonymous hemianopia than with a quadrantanopia.[30,43–45,56,72,73] Some patients have FVEP abnormalities with lesions that do not produce a field defect.[22,44,56] Abnormalities have also been reported to occur ipsilateral to the lesion with flashed pattern stimulation.[64]

The first report of contrast stimulation is that of Regan and Heron.[62] By using a technique involving Fourier analysis, they found that the response to sine wave–modulated light was reduced, but that to pattern stimulation was normal, in a patient with a macular-sparing homonymous hemianopia. Wildberger et al.[76] studied steady-state VEPs, both full-field and hemifield, in six patients with homonymous hemianopia and found abnormalities contralateral to the field defect but no difference between those with and without macular involvement.

Halliday's group described the typical "uncrossed" asymmetry in homonymous hemianopia.[8] When using full-field stimulation (50-minute checks, 16-degree radius), they found

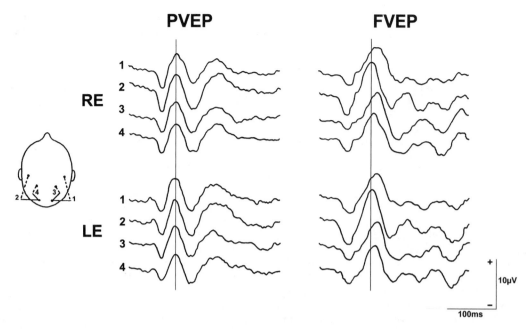

FIGURE 78.4 Pattern (PVEP) and flash (FVEP) evoked potentials in a patient with a macular-sparing left homonymous hemianopia. PVEPs show no significant abnormality, but flash VEPs from both right and left eyes show an "uncrossed" asymmetry such that both eyes show relative latency delay in the traces from the affected right hemisphere. Note that the flash VEP is not subject to the phenomenon of paradoxical lateralization.

a markedly asymmetrical scalp distribution, the normal P100 component being recorded only over the damaged hemisphere, in keeping with the "paradoxical lateralization" originally described by the same group.[6] Hemifield stimulation confirmed that the responses obtained with the full-field stimulus were due to preservation of the normal responses from the residual hemifield. Holder[39] confirmed the "uncrossed" asymmetry in homonymous hemianopia but found the abnormality ipsilateral to the lesion when using small full-field stimulation (26- or 13-minute checks, 5.5- or 4-degree radius) (figure 78.5). Although the cause of some controversy at the time, the apparently contradictory findings reflect the different registration parameters[35,36] (see the previous section), in particular the size of the stimulating field and the avoidance of Fz as a "reference" electrode position. The lateralization of Halliday's group was also demonstrated in a patient following unilateral occipital lobectomy for glioma by using similar techniques.[39] Note that with an Fz "reference," the abnormality lateralization is dependent on stimulus parameters, changing from paradoxical to anatomical with progressive reduction in stimulus field and check size (see figure 78.5).

Subsequent reports confirmed the "uncrossed" asymmetry in retrochiasmal dysfunction.[9,10,16,19,21,33,37,40,49–51,55,69] The main conclusions are that hemifield stimulation is more sensitive than full-field stimulation,[19,33,49,55] that ear reference recording is unsatisfactory,[37] and that, in general, the more severe the hemianopic defect, the more likely the PVEP to

be abnormal. Normal PVEPs will often be found in quadrantic field defects.[9,19,33,40] A dense, macular-splitting hemianopia can be expected to give an abnormal PVEP. The percentage of abnormal PVEPs in the presence of known field defects is in the region of 80–90%. Latency delay may be found, even with hemifield stimulation, in up to 25% of cases[49] but does not approach the magnitude of that regularly seen in anterior visual pathway dysfunction. The problems of accurate component identification in the assessment of "delays" are again noted.

A particularly interesting report examined both P100 and the late P3 component in four patients with homonymous hemianopia, including one with clinical evidence of blindsight.[66] The P3 was well formed to target stimuli in the preserved field for all four patients, but it was additionally present for target stimuli in the hemianopic field of the patient with "blindsight." In contrast, the P100 component could only be recorded with stimulation of the preserved field in this patient. The authors suggested that cognitive processing could occur in the absence of subjective perception, presumably via a mechanism independent of the geniculostriate pathway.

BILATERAL DYSFUNCTION AND CORTICAL BLINDNESS Bilateral occipital lobe disease will result in bilateral homonymous hemianopic defects of variable severity; in its most severe form, there is complete cortical blindness. However, this may be denied by the patient (Anton's syndrome). There

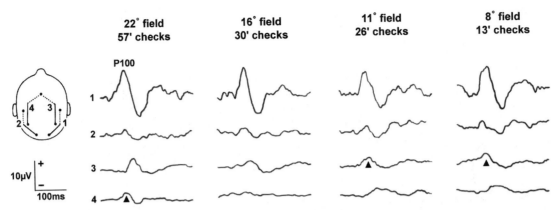

| 22° field 57' checks | 16° field 30' checks | 11° field 26' checks | 8° field 13' checks |

FIGURE 78.5 Pattern VEPs in a patient following left occipital lobectomy for glioma show the effects of variations in stimulus and recording parameters. The right occipital lobe is thus the main cortical origin of the potentials recorded. Channels 1 and 2 use occipital electrodes at O1 and O2 referred to an ipsilateral sylvian reference electrode. Channels 3 and 4 use the "Queen Square" montage (QS) with electrodes 5 cm anterior and lateral to the inion referred to Fz. Using a large stimulus field and check size, the QS montage shows "paradoxical" lateralization of the normal P100 component (arrowhead) such that it is recorded over the lobectomized left hemisphere. On reduction in field and check size, there is a shorter latency response over the right hemisphere but no clearly identifiable component in the left hemisphere trace. Further reduction in field size results in the emergence of a normal P100 component in the right hemisphere trace and the appearance of a later positivity in the left hemisphere traces similar to that previously present in the right hemisphere traces with a large stimulus field. The exact stimulus parameters at which the transition from paradoxical to anatomical lateralization occurs can show marked interindividual variation. Note that the lateralization of the abnormality is constant using the sylvian reference montage, consistently showing the abnormality over the damaged hemisphere.

are few reports of PVEPs in patients with bilateral occipital infarction. Streletz et al.[69] describe the PVEPs in two cases as being of grossly abnormal waveform. Halliday's group cite two cases, one with low-amplitude PVEPs of normal latency.[9] Three personal cases[39] all showed amplitude reductions, with latency changes seen in two of the three patients. Subsequent experience suggests that reduced amplitude responses are usually seen but that waveform abnormalities or mild latency changes can also occur depending on the degree of visual field preservation.

A later report describes PVEP findings in nine cases, some with bilateral occipital infarction.[3] No response was seen in five cases, an increased latency in two, and normal findings in two. The findings correlated poorly with outcome. FVEPs were studied in ten patients, some with bilateral occipital infarction; these also showed poor correlation with outcome. There are even fewer reports of PVEPs in complete cortical blindness. Bodis-Wollner's group[11] report the case of a 6-year-old boy with normal PVEPs to high-contrast gratings and preservation of area 17 but destruction of areas 18 and 19 (partial in one hemisphere, complete in the other). Another single case is described with normal PVEPs yet bilateral destruction of area 17, with preservation of areas 18 (partial) and 19.[18] They postulated that the PVEPs were mediated by extrageniculocalcarine pathways. A further patient had complete cortical blindness but normal latency PVEPs.[3] Bodis-Wollner and Mylin[12] studied the VEPs in two patients during recovery from cortical blindness with both monocular (gratings) and binocular (random dot correlo-grams) simulation. The recovery of binocular vision occurred later than that of monocular vision. One further case is reported in which 1-degree 20-minute checks "sometimes" gave a response over one hemisphere 2–4 months following cortical blindness, but the exact nature of the stimulus is not defined and may be flashed pattern.[56]

Many more cases have been investigated using flash stimulation. Preserved FVEPs in cortical blindness have been described by some authors in adults,[1,3,47,67] one group concluding that the FVEP was of prognostic value in basilar artery occlusion.[1] Others examined childhood cortical blindness.[5,24,29,52] In one series of 30 children, only one child with cortical blindness had extinguished FVEPs; some had abnormal FVEPs but appeared to have normal vision.[29] The VEP was not thought a good method for diagnosing cortical blindness in children.

A recent study examined a group of children, some developmentally normal (DN; $N = 14$) and some developmentally delayed (DD; $N = 16$), who were "visually unresponsive."[75] The DN infants had normal visual function, with a small subset having normal VEPs and were considered to have visual inattention (VI). Sixteen infants had abnormal VEPs and abnormal neuroimaging studies (CT, MRI, or both) or microcephaly and thus were diagnosed as having cortical visual impairment. Visual acuity in these infants ranged from normal to no visual orienting to the low-vision Teller Acuity Cards. The inability to "fix and follow" in three further infants was attributed to oculomotor apraxia, and adjunctive oculomotor testing was recommended.

Electrophysiological examination is therefore of limited value in the clinical management of patients with retrochiasmal dysfunction, particularly with ever-improving neuroradiological techniques. However, the functional assessment provided by careful serial VEP recording can be valuable in the objective monitoring of disease progression or resolution and may add significantly to the clinician's understanding of the underlying pathophysiological processes. Also, valuable information can be obtained by using electrophysiology as a research tool in the investigation of higher visual function.

REFERENCES

1. Abraham FA, Melamed E, Lavy S: Prognostic value of visual evoked potentials in occipital blindness following basilar artery occlusion. *Appl Neurophysiol* 1975; 38:126–135.
2. Albright AL, Sclabassi RJ: Cavitron ultrasonic aspirator and visual evoked potential monitoring for chiasmal glioma in children. *J Neurosurg* 1985; 63:138–140.
3. Aldrich MS, Alessi AG, Beck RW, et al: Cortical blindness: Etiology, diagnosis and prognosis. *Ann Neurol* 1987; 21:149–158.
4. Apkarian P, Bour L, Barth PG: A unique achiasmatic anomaly detected in non-albinos with misrouted retinal-fugal projections. *Eur J Neurosci* 1994; 6:501–507.
5. Barnet AB, Manson Jl, Wilner E: Acute cerebral blindness in childhood. *Neurology* 1970; 20:1147–1156.
6. Barrett G, Blumhardt LD, Halliday AM, et al: A paradox in the lateralisation of the visual evoked response. *Nature* 1976; 261:253–255.
7. Blumhardt LD: Visual field defects and pathological alterations in topography: Factors complicating the estimation of visual evoked response "delay" in multiple sclerosis. In Cracco RQ, Bodis-Wollner I (eds): *Evoked Potentials.* New York, Alan R Liss, 1986, pp 354–365.
8. Blumhardt LD, Barrett G, Halliday AM: The asymmetrical visual evoked potential to pattern reversal in one half field and its significance for the analysis of visual field defects. *Br J Ophthalmol* 1977; 61:454–461.
9. Blumhardt LD, Barrett G, Kriss A, et al: The pattern evoked potential in lesions of the posterior visual pathways. *Ann N Y Acad Sci* 1982; 388:264–289.
10. Blumhardt LD, Halliday AM: Cortical abnormalities and the visual evoked response. *Doc Ophthalmol Proc Ser* 1981; 27:347–365.
11. Bodis-Wollner I, Atkin A, Raab E, et al: Visual association cortex and vision in man: Pattern-evoked occipital potentials in a blind boy. *Science* 1977; 198:629–631.
12. Bodis-Wollner I, Mylin L: Plasticity of monocular and binocular vision following cerebral blindness: Evoked potential evidence. *Electroencephalogr Clin Neurophysiol* 1987; 68:70–74.
13. Brecelj J: A VEP study of the visual pathway function in compressive lesions of the optic chiasm: Full-field versus half-field stimulation. *Electroencephalogr Clin Neurophysiol* 1992; 84:209–218.
14. Brecelj J: Electrodiagnostics of chiasmal compressive lesions. *Int J Psychophysiol* 1994; 16:263–272.
15. Brecelj J, Denislic M, Skrbec M: Visual evoked potential abnormalities in chiasmal lesions. *Doc Ophthalmol* 1989; 73:139–148.
16. Camacho LM, Wenzel W, Aschoff JC: The pattern reversal visual evoked potential in the clinical study of lesions of the optic chiasm and visual pathway. In Courjon J, Mauguiere F, Revol M (eds): *Clinical Applications of Evoked Potentials in Neurology.* New York, Raven Press, 1982, pp 49–59.
17. Cedzich C, Scramm J, Mengedohr CF, Fahlbusch R: Factors that limit the use of flash visual evoked potentials for surgical monitoring. *Electroencephalogr Clin Neurophysiol* 1988; 71:142–145.
18. Celesia GG, Archer CR, Kuroiwa Y, et al: Visual function of the extrageniculo-calcarine system in man: Relationship to cortical blindness. *Arch Neurol* 1980; 37:704–706.
19. Celesia GG, Meredith JT, Pluff K: Perimetry, visual evoked potentials and visual evoked spectrum array in homonymous hemianopia. *Electroencephalogr Clin Neurophysiol* 1983; 56:16–30.
20. Chacko AG, Babu KS, Chandy MJ: Value of visual evoked potential monitoring during trans-sphenoidal pituitary surgery. *Br J Neurosurg* 1996; 10:275–278.
21. Chain F, Lesevre N, Pinel JF, et al: Spatio-temporal study of visual evoked potentials in patients with homonymous hemianopia. In Courjon J, Mauguiere F, Revol M (eds): *Clinical Applications of Evoked Potentials in Neurology.* New York, Raven Press, 1982, pp 61–70.
22. Crighel E, Poilici L: Photic evoked responses in patients with thalamic and brain stem lesions. *Confin Neurol (Basel)* 1968; 30:301–312.
23. Dorey SE, Neveu MM, Burton L, Sloper JJ, Holder GE: The clinical features of albinism and their correlation with visual evoked potentials. *Br J Ophthalmol* 2003; 87:767–772.
24. Duchowny MS, Weiss IP, Majlessi H, et al: Visual evoked responses in childhood cortical blindness after trauma and meningitis: A longitudinal study of six cases. *Neurology* 1974; 24:933–940.
25. Fahlbusch R, Marguth F: Optic nerve compression by pituitary adenomas. In Sarnii M, Jannetta PJ (eds): *The Cranial Nerves: Anatomy, Pathology, Pathophysiology, Diagnosis, Treatment.* Berlin, Springer-Verlag, 1981, pp 140–147.
26. Feinsod M, Selhorst JB, Hoyt WF, Wilson CB: Monitoring optic nerve function during craniotomy. *J Neurosurg* 1976; 44:29–31.
27. Fisher NF, Jampolsky A, Scott AB, et al: Traumatic bitemporal hemianopsia: III. Nasal versus temporal retinal function. *Am J Ophthalmol* 1968; 65:578–581.
28. Flanagan JG, Harding GFA: Multi-channel visual evoked potentials in early compressive lesions of the optic chiasm. *Doc Ophthalmol* 1987; 69:271–282.
29. Frank Y, Torres F: Visual evoked potentials in the evaluation of "cortical blindness" in children. *Ann Neurol* 1979; 6:126–129.
30. Galkina NS, Gnezditskii VV, Aleksandrova AA, et al: Investigation of evoked potentials to photic stimulation in man after deafferentation of the visual cortex. *Biull Eksp Biol Med* 1975; 79:23–26.
31. Garfield J, Neil-Dwyer G: Delay in diagnosis of optic nerve and chiasmal compression presenting with unilateral failing vision. *Br Med J* 1975; 1:22–25.
32. Gott PS, Weiss MH, Apuzzo M, et al: Checkerboard visual evoked response in evaluation and management of pituitary tumours. *Neurosurgery* 1979; 5:553–558.
33. Haimovic IC, Pedley TA: Hemi-field pattern reversal visual evoked potentials: II. Lesions of the chiasm and posterior visual pathways. *Electroencephalogr Clin Neurophysiol* 1982; 54:121–131.
34. Halliday AM, Halliday E, Kriss A, et al: The pattern evoked potential in compression of the anterior visual pathways. *Brain* 1976; 99:357–374.

35. Halliday AM, Holder GE, Harding GFA: Abnormalities of the pattern visual evoked potential in patients with homonymous visual field defects (discussion). In Barber C (ed): *Evoked Potentials*. Lancaster, UK, MTP Press, 1980, pp 292–298.

36. Harding GFA, Smith GF, Smith PA: The effect of various stimulus parameters on the lateralization of the VEP. In Barber C (ed): *Evoked Potentials*. Lancaster, UK, MTP Press, 1980, pp 213–218.

37. Hoeppner TJ, Bergen D, Morrell F: Hemispheric asymmetry of visual evoked potentials in patients with well-defined occipital lesions. *Electroencephalogr Clin Neurophysiol* 1984; 57:310–319.

38. Holder GE: The effects of chiasmal compression on the pattern visual evoked potential. *Electroencephalogr Clin Neurophysiol* 1978; 45:278–280.

39. Holder GE: Abnormalities of the pattern visual evoked potential in patients with homonymous visual field defects. In Barber C (ed): *Evoked Potentials*. Lancaster, UK, MTP Press, 1980, pp 285–291.

40. Holder GE: Pattern visual evoked potentials in patients with posteriorly situated space-occupying lesions. *Doc Ophthalmol* 1985; 59:121–128.

41. Holder GE, Bullock PR: Visual evoked potentials in the assessment of patients with non-functioning chromophobe adenomas. *J Neurol Neurosurg Psychiatry* 1989; 52:31–37.

42. Hollenhorst RW, Younge BR: Ocular manifestations produced by adenomas of the pituitary gland: Analysis of 1000 cases. In Kohler PO, Ross GT (eds): *Diagnosis and Treatment of Pituitary Tumours*. New York, Elsevier Science, 1973, pp 53–64.

43. Jacobsen JH, Hirose T, Suziki TA: Simultaneous ERG and VER in lesions of the optic pathway. *Invest Ophthalmol* 1968; 7:279–292.

44. Jonkman EJ: The Average Cortical Response to Photic Stimulation (thesis). University of Amsterdam, 1967.

45. Kaufmann D, Wray SH, Lorance R, Woods M: An analysis of the pathophysiology and the development of treatment strategies for compressive optic nerve lesions using pattern electroretinograms and visual evoked potential. *Neurol* 1986; 36:232.

46. Kooi KA, Guvener M, Bagchi BK: Visual evoked responses in lesions of the higher optic pathways. *Neurology* 1965; 15:841–854.

47. Kooi KA, Sharbrough FW: Electrophysiological findings in cortical blindness. *Electroencephalogr Clin Neurophysiol* 1966; 20:260–263.

48. Kooi KA, Yamada T, Marshall RE: Field studies of monocularly evoked cerebral potentials in bitemporal hemianopsia. *Neurology* 1973; 23:1217–1225.

49. Kuroiwa Y, Celesia GG: Visual evoked potentials with hemifield pattern stimulation: Their use in the diagnosis of retrochiasmatic lesions. *Arch Neurol* 1981; 38:86–90.

50. Maccolini E, Andreoli A, Valde G, et al: Hemi-field pattern-reversal evoked potentials (VEPs) in retrochiasmal lesions with homonymous visual field defect. *Ital J Neurol Sci* 1986; 7:437–442.

51. Maitland CG, Aminoff MJ, Kennard C, et al: Evoked potentials in the evaluation of visual field defects due to chiasmal or retrochiasmal lesions. *Neurology* 1982; 32:986–991.

52. Makino A, Soga T, Obayashi M, et al: Cortical blindness caused by acute general cerebral swelling. *Surg Neurol* 1988; 29:393–400.

53. Muller W: Untersuchungen uber das Verhalten der Corticalzeit bei bitemporaler Hemianopsie. *Graefes Arch Ophthalmol* 1962; 165:214–218.

54. Newer M: *Evoked Potentials in the Operating Room*. New York: Raven Press, 1982.

55. Onofrj M, Bodis-Wollner I, Mylin L: Visual evoked potential diagnosis of field defects in patients with chiasmatic and retrochiasmatic lesions. *J Neurol Neurosurg Psychiatry* 1982; 45:294–302.

56. Oosterhuis HJGH, Ponsen L, Jonkman EJ, et al: The average visual evoked response in patients with cerebrovascular disease. *Electroencephalogr Clin Neurophysiol* 1969; 27:23–34.

57. Parmar DN, Sofat A, Bowman R, Bartlett JR, Holder GE: Prognostic value of the pattern electroretinogram in chiasmal compression. *Br J Ophthalmol* 2000; 84:1024–1026.

58. Pietrangeli A, Jandolo B, Occhipinti E, Carapella CM, Morace E: The VEP in evaluation of pituitary tumors. *Electromyogr Clin Neurophysiol* 1991; 31:163–165.

59. Pruett RC, Wepsic JG: Delayed diagnosis of chiasmal compression. *Am J Ophthalmol* 1973; 76:229–236.

60. Pullan PT, Carroll WM, Chakera TMH, et al: Management of extra-sellar pituitary tumours with bromocriptine: Comparison of prolactin secreting and non-functioning tumours using half-field visual evoked potentials and computerised tomography. *Aust N Z J Med* 1985; 15:203–208.

61. Raudzens PA: Intraoperative monitoring of evoked potentials. *Ann N Y Acad Sci* 1982; 388:308–325.

62. Regan D, Heron JR: Clinical investigation of lesions of the visual pathway: A new objective technique. *J Neurol Neurosurg Psychiatry* 1969; 32:479–483.

63. Ruther K, Ehlich P, Philipp A, Eckstein A, Zrenner E: Prognostic value of the pattern electroretinogram in cases of tumors affecting the optic pathway. *Graefes Arch Clin Exp Ophthalmol* 1998; 236:259–263.

64. Samson-Dollfus D, Parain D, Weber J, et al: The visually evoked potential in retrochiasmatic lesions of the optic pathways: An attempt to interpret the responses obtained by flash pattern stimulation and the results of the calculation of the correlation coefficient between visual evoked potentials. In Courjon J, Mauguiere F, Revol M (eds): *Clinical Applications of Evoked Potentials in Neurology*. New York, Raven Press, 1982, pp 71–80.

65. Segal AJ, Fishman RS: Delayed diagnosis of pituitary tumours. *Am J Ophthalmol* 1975; 79:77–81.

66. Shefrin SL, Goodin DS, Aminoff MJ: Visual evoked potentials in the investigation of "blindsight." *Neurology* 1988; 38:104–109.

67. Spehlmann R, Gross RA, Ho SU: Visual evoked potentials and post mortem findings in a case of cortical blindness. *Ann Neurol* 1977; 2:531–534.

68. Stark DJ, Lenton L: Electrophysiological assessment of compressive lesions of anterior visual pathways. *Aust J Ophthalmol* 1981; 9:135–141.

69. Streletz LJ, Bae SH, Roeshman RM, et al: Visual evoked potentials in occipital lobe lesions. *Arch Neurol* 1981:38:80–85.

70. Thompson DA, Kriss A, Chong K, Harris C, Russell-Eggitt I, Shawkat F, Neville BGR, Aclimandos W, Taylor DSI: Visual-evoked potential evidence of chiasmal hypoplasia. *Ophthalmology* 1999; 106:2354–2361.

71. Van Lith GHM, Vijfvinkel-Bruinenga S, Graniewski-Wijnands H: Pattern evoked cortical potentials and compressive lesions along the visual pathways. *Doc Ophthalmol* 1982; 52:347–353.

72. Vaughan HG, Katzman R: Evoked response in visual disorders. *Ann N Y Acad Sci* 1964; 112:305–319.

73. Vaughan HG, Katzman R, Taylor J: Alterations of visual evoked response in the presence of homonymous visual

defects. *Electroencephalogr Clin Neurophysiol* 1963; 15:737–746.

74. Wass JAH, Thorner MO, Charletworth M, et al: Bromocriptine in management of large pituitary tumours. *Br Med J* 1982; 284:1908–1911.

75. Weiss AH, Kelly JP, Phillips JO: The infant who is visually unresponsive on a cortical basis. *Ophthalmology* 2001; 108:2076–2087.

76. Wildberger HGH, Van Lith GHM, Wijngaarde R, et al: Visually evoked cortical potentials in the evaluation of homonymous and bitemporal visual field defects. *Br J Ophthalmol* 1976; 60:273–278.

77. Wilson WB, Kirsch WM, Neville H, Stears J, Feinsod M, Lehman RA: Monitoring of function during parasellar surgery. *Surg Neurol* 1976; 5:323–329.

78. Wray SH: Neuro-ophthalmologic manifestations of pituitary and parasellar lesions. *Clin Neurosurg* 1977; 24:86–117.

79 Optic Nerve and Central Nervous Dysfunctions: Parkinson's Disease and Multiple Sclerosis

IVAN BODIS-WOLLNER AND ANDREA ANTAL

CLINICAL ELECTROPHYSIOLOGICAL measurements have a long history in the assessment of visual disorders caused by ocular pathology. Starting from the seminal studies of Halliday and his group of visual electrophysiological studies in multiple sclerosis (MS),[90] other neurological disorders were investigated, using techniques of electroretinogram (ERG) and visual evoked potentials (VEPs) (figure 79.1). Surprisingly, visual studies not only in MS but also in Parkinson's disease (PD) have allowed new insights into the pathophysiology of these neurological diseases and have revealed hitherto unknown aspects of visual system organization.

PD is generally known as a movement disorder, neuropharmacologically as a dopaminergic deficiency syndrome affecting the basal ganglia, and anatomically as loss of dopaminergic neurons of these structures. However, in the last two decades, anatomical, biochemical, neurophysiological, and clinical studies have demonstrated involvement of the central nervous system (CNS) beyond the basal ganglia. One of the affected areas is the visual system from the lowest level, from the retina up to the frontoparietal cognitive centers of the brain.

Because PD is predominantly a disease of the elderly, it is not surprising that many patients have visual complaints, such as tired eyes, blurred vision, and difficulty in reading. They may represent various etiologies and clinicians do not relate these nonspecific complaints to a disease known to be a "movement disorder." Visual abnormalities specific to PD are usually hidden and not likely to be uncovered during a routine neurological examination or by ordinary high-contrast visual acuity (VA) testing. Contrast sensitivity (CS), a measure that can be affected independently from VA, provides a sensitive test for vision impairment in neurodegenerative diseases.[26,28] Nonspecific visual complaints may, however, be related to impaired CS. Intact CS is very important for most visual functions,[139] for example, for the normal perception and discrimination of depth.[160] It is determined by the inverse of the minimal contrast necessary to distinguish objects of patterns presented at a given spatial frequency (SF). CS is abnormal in PD.[24,30,39,58,60,105,157] However, reduced CS in PD goes undocumented in the majority of patients, as many vision care specialists are not aware of testing for a potentially profound CS deficit in a patient with near normal VA. In CNS lesions, a VA score no worse than 20/40 may go along with a 20-fold reduction in CS to size of targets of considerable practical significance for everyday vision.[26,28] The spatial and temporal selectivity of visual losses detected with CS in PD is consistent with the results of electrophysiological tests (electroretinogram [ERG] and visual evoked potentials [VEP]). Additionally, it has been shown that idiopathic PD patients, subjects with drug-induced parkinsonism,[109] and animals with experimentally induced parkinsonism[81,82,84,110] exhibit similar visual impairments. The specificity of the common visual loss is likely to be due to dopaminergic deficiency. In all of these conditions, the visual impairment has been established with psychophysical and electrophysiological measures and supported by the results of neuropharmacological and histochemical studies.

MS commonly involves the visual pathways, as was noted as early as 1890 by Uhthoff.[167] A spectrum of visual complaints exists, ranging from the manifestations of acute temporary demyelination of the optic nerve, resulting in sudden visual loss, to subtle clinical disturbance, which could be discovered only with neurophysiological or psychophysical testing. One of the breakthroughs in establishing the clinical value of VEP occurred when Halliday et al.[90] first described that in carefully examined MS patients who have never suffered optic neuritis, commonly over 90% of subjects had abnormal, delayed VEPs. The original results, with slightly different percentages, were proven many times (see, for example, Logi et al.[114]). It is an established interpretation of visual deficits in MS that many patients may have suffered an asymptomatic involvement of the visual pathway.[71,115] An understanding of this type of subclinical disease has been much aided by the availability of magnetic resonance imaging (MRI). Nearly all of the studies provide

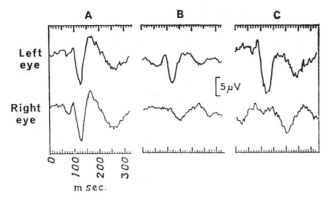

FIGURE 79.1 Pattern visual evoked potentials, recorded from a midline occipital electrode from the left and right eyes of a healthy subject (A) and two patients who were recovering from acute attacks of optic neuritis in the right eye with onset four weeks (B) and three weeks (C) previously. (From Halliday AM, McDonald WI, Mushin J: Visual evoked response in diagnosis of multiple sclerosis. *Br Med J* 1973; 4:661–664; with permission of *Lancet*.)

evidence of more or less continuous disease activity,[111,125,200] suggesting that even acute MS lesions do not give rise to symptoms or clinical signs. Recent data suggest that the damage caused by progressive subclinical lesions have a larger impact on the visual pathways than the damage caused by acute optic neuritis itself.[115] Besides simple visual loss, MS patients are known to have heterogeneous neurocognitive disturbances, such as dysfunction of attention, visuospatial perception, memory, and executive mechanisms.[141,153]

In this chapter, electrophysiological studies of visual impairment in PD and MS are supplemented by psychophysical and imaging data when appropriate. We shall focus our discussion on the known physiology of neuronal receptive fields in the retina and cortex and on the relationship between the physiology of the visual pathways and the known or putative pathogenesis of PD and of MS. For each disease, we first discuss retinal, optic nerve, and primary visual cortical causes of visual impairment. Second, we discuss visual electrophysiological measurements that address cognitive aspects of visual processing, most likely involving extrastriate and nonoccipital cortices. We emphasize the clinical importance of new or newer versions of electrophysiological techniques that have emerged in the last decades as the result of physiological and pathophysiological studies of the visual system.

Electrophysiology and visual psychophysics of visual deficits caused by retinal and primary visual pathway involvement

PARKINSON'S DISEASE The deficiency of the neurotransmitter dopamine (DA) involves several CNS areas that subserve vision. In the retina, DA is localized within amacrine and interplexiform cells.[74] Dopaminergic neurons subserve a modulatory role in the retina and mediate center-surround interaction for establishing the receptive field structure of ganglion cells.[33] Autopsy studies have shown decreased retinal DA concentration in PD[93] but not in patients who received levodopa therapy shortly before their death. In the monkey retina, dopaminergic deficiency is achieved by systemic administration of 1-methyl-4-phenyl-1,2,3,6-tetrahydropyridine (MPTP), which causes a PD-like picture in nonhuman mammals.[110] Furthermore, systemic MPTP and intraocular 6-hydroxydopamine, a known selective toxin of dopaminergic neurons, cause comparable retinal effects,[82] as shown by neurohistochemistry and in vivo pattern ERG (PERG) recordings.

Spatial and temporal frequency contingent visual loss in PD: The importance of stimulus selection in clinical electrophysiology Following the original report of Bodis-Wollner and Yahr[36] demonstrating delayed VEP in PD patients, there has been considerable controversy concerning visual changes in PD. However, in the ensuing decades, many electrophysiological and psychophysical studies have provided evidence for the validity of visual impairment in PD (for a review, see Bodis-Wollner[24]). To demonstrate visual dysfunction, it is important to use visual stimuli that are optimal for foveal ganglion cells with strong center-surround organization, as dopamine appears to act as an essential neurotransmitter for receptive field organization.[34] PERG records the activity of retinal ganglion cells (optic nerve cell body)[116] and hence indirectly reflects the preganglionic retinal circuitry, which is essential for the center-surround organization of the mammalian retinal ganglion cells.[34] Both PERG[11] and VEP[45] vary as a function of spatial and temporal parameters of the stimulation. Therefore, the visual electrophysiological abnormalities in PD remained controversial until studies critically evaluated electrophysiological responses to these parameters of stimulation.[22,132,144,183] It became apparent that specific visual stimulus constraints are necessary for demonstrating dopaminergic deficits. These studies revealed that the VEP and PERG abnormality in PD is most evident for foveal stimuli of medium and high SFs—above 2 cycles per degree (cpd)—where normal observers are most sensitive for the visual stimuli,[22] as shown by CS testing. Using stimuli of sinusoidal gratings of 50% contrast that were counterphase modulated at 7.5 Hz with a SF ranging from 0.5 to 6.9 cpd, Tagliati et al.[181] have shown that aging and PD lead to different types of losses in the retina. In aged normal subjects, the PERG reflects a loss, compared to younger observers, at all the studied SFs, while PD patients showed a specific loss peaking at 5 cpd. Consequently, all PD patients had an attenuated PERG "tuning ratio," calculated as the PERG amplitude of ratio of medium (5 cpd) to low (1 cpd) SF amplitudes

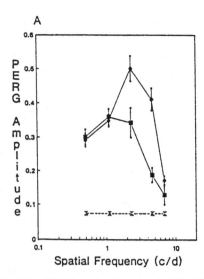

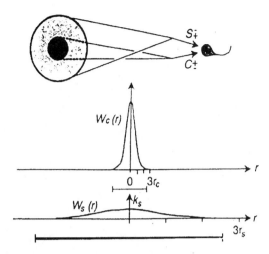

FIGURE 79.2 The PERG tuning function in PD: PERG spatial transfer function obtained in patients (squares) and age-matched subjects (diamonds). The functions are parallel at lower SF and very close at the higher SF tested (6.9 cpd). (From Tagliati M, Bodis-Wollner I, Yahr MD: The pattern electroretinogram in Parkinson's disease reveals lack of retinal spatial tuning. *Electroencephalogr Clin Neurophysiol* 1996; 100:1–11; with permission.)

FIGURE 79.3 The receptive field model representing signal summation over a retinal ganglion cell receptive field, as described by Enroth-Cugell and Robson.[70] Upper diagram illustrates the concentric center and surround region. Signal from the center (C) and surround (S) have an antagonistic effect on the ganglion cell, expressed by the opposite sign of the C and S signals, either an on-center (+C) or an off-center (–C). Lower diagram shows the Gaussian profiles, assumed to describe the sensitivity of the center surround. (Adapted from Enroth-Cugell C, Robson JG: The contrast sensitivity of retinal ganglion cells of the cat. *J Physiol (Lond)* 1966; 187:517–552; with permission.)

(figure 79.2). The tuning ratio of the PERG covaried with the severity (Hoehn and Yahr scale) of PD. Because lack of tuning of the spatial CS in PD shows some similarity to the CS in normal subjects at reduced (scotopic) light levels, it has been suggested that DA is involved in the process of dark adaptation and the parkinsonian retina behaves as though inappropriately dark-adapted.[201] However, PD patients do not show high SF losses when properly refracted, while the scotopic CS is not only low-pass, but also narrowed in spatial bandwidth. This is not the case in PD owing to the fact that DA deficiency has a specific and predictable effect on center-surround interaction of the receptive field and is responsible for the band-pass shape of spatial tuning in the retina at photopic levels. Indeed, light onset can increase the metabolism, or it can increase the DA release in the retina.[51,65] Constant light exposure decreases the D2 receptor sites, which is associated with the decrease of sensitivity of presynaptic melatonin receptors.[63] It is likely that enhanced DA release will augment the cell's luminance contrast response by weakening the strength of the surround on the final retinal ganglion cell output, which is the difference of center and surround responses (as discussed below).

The role of DA in spatial processing in the retina The data above imply that the function of DA is rather complex. Indeed, animal and human physiological and pathophysiological studies have revealed a specific role of DA in neural signal processing.[24,146,173] Pharmacological studies using D1 and D2 antagonists or a D1 agonist suggested that D1 and D2 recep-

tors synergistically optimize the spatial properties of retinal ganglion cells (for reviews, see Bodis-Wollner and Tagliati,[33] Bodis-Wollner and Tzelepi[34]). The response of most retinal ganglion cells are based on center-surround antagonism of the receptive field, which was quantitatively described by the difference of two Gaussian functions[70] (figure 79.3). Pharmacological studies have shown that D1 deficiency weakens the surround response and enhances low spatial frequencies, while D2 antagonists reduce the center response and suppress peak SF responses. The net result of D1 and D2 activation is therefore an enhanced center response to stimuli that have dimensions of the center diameter of the largest foveal ganglion cells (figure 79.4). On the basis of the results of human pharmaco-ERG studies, it has been also suggested that presynaptic D2 "autoreceptors" are involved in the surround D1 dopaminergic pathway.[34] This interpretation is based on the fact that a high dose of L-sulpiride (a D2 receptor blocker) allows greater DA effect on D1 receptors and enhances surround signals and therefore attenuates low SF responses.[180] The results of experimental manipulations of DA on visual processing converge to an understanding of changed CS functions in dopaminergic deficiency, as has been described in PD.

In PD, foveal spatial vision is affected, as shown by impaired CS and electrophysiological measures to patterns with a SF above 2 cpd.[30,175,181] On the basis of studies in PD and in the monkey model of PD, which show that the

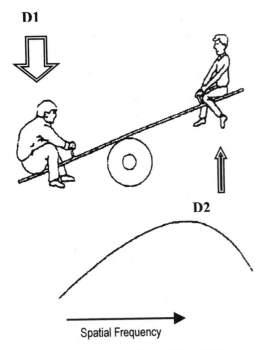

D1

D2

Spatial Frequency

FIGURE 79.4 The antagonistic effect of D1 and D2 receptor activation acting on different arms of the seesaw. As a consequence, the doubly opposite effects produce an overall synergistic action. The space underneath the curve represents the overall spatial frequency transfer function of the retina: Low-frequency decline occurs where D1 receptors are active. The peak of the curve is created by the seesaw pointing to the right. (Adapted from Bodis-Wollner I, Tzelepi A: Push-pull model of dopamine's action in the retina. In Hung GK, Ciuffreda KC (eds): Models of the visual system. Kluwer Academic Publishers, 2002, pp 191–214; with permission.)

normal primate CS curve changes into a low pass function, the physiological spatial CS curve cannot represent a single type of ganglion cell in the primate retina. Nearly 40 years ago, Enroth-Cugell and Robson[70] established the properties of cat retinal ganglion cells, describing their output as reflecting the linear interaction of center and surround organization for X cells and as a nonlinear process for Y cells. It was later shown by Hochstein and Shapley[97] that Y cells have the same basic linear properties as X cells with the addition of nonlinearities originating from receptive field subunits. Another difference, originally pointed out by Enroth-Cugell and Robson,[70] was a difference in the ratio of center versus surround receptive field diameter. It was also shown that center and surround mechanisms are cocentered; that is, the same very central photoreceptors contribute to both center and surround. Many later physiological studies, also in primates, have shown additional anatomical and functional differences in the properties of these two major classes of foveal ganglion cells. However, it remained uncontested that the retinal contribution to the normal foveal CS function relies on two types of retinal ganglion cells. For

understanding the role of DA in retinal processing, Bodis-Wollner and Tzelepi[34] reached back to the classical description of the retinal ganglion cell output as reflecting the linear interaction of two mechanisms, the center and surround, each of the two represented by a Gaussian profile of different size and height but cocentered and having different size ratios for the two classes of foveal ganglion cell (figure 79.5).

The results of vision studies in dopaminergic deficiency syndromes suggest that the two major foveal retinal ganglion cell classes are different concerning the predominant role of DA in their respective receptive field organization. This difference emanates from the role of D1 and D2 receptors, which have differential roles in the surround and center organization. On the basis of the role of dopaminergic mechanisms, it has been suggested that one class of ganglion cells has a dominant surround mechanism and strong D1 receptor–coupled dopaminergic mechanisms, mediating the response to low spatial frequencies. The receptive field of the second class of foveal neurons is dominated by the center organization, which is aided by strong D2 receptor activation by DA, which can amplify the response of the center through photoreceptor coupling. This type of neuron mediates the response to middle and high SF stimuli. D1 DA receptors themselves are at the front end of the retina, mediating horizontal cell coupling strength, important for the surround mechanism. Center photoreceptors themselves of course contribute to both. The signals of the receptors that feed into the center and into the surround organization remain most likely separate until they converge on their ganglion cells. Accordingly, Dacey et al.[56] described two types of bipolar cells, which exhibit two types of center-surround organization. Smaller bipolars have stronger centers, while larger ones have stronger surrounds. It is possible that each type of ganglion cells receives input from similar bipolar input but is under the influence of neuropharmacologically different presynaptic organization.

Parallel pathways and vision in PD It should be emphasized that the pathophysiological evidence of separating foveal retinal ganglion cells into two classes, based on their dominant DA receptor and receptive field organization, is consistent with the notion of parallel pathways originating in the retina. However, there is no evidence that dopaminergic deficiency selectively affects one of these pathways. Rather, the opposite is true: Dopaminergic deficiency causes reduced activity of both classes of DA receptors. The reduction in the activity of both types of receptors, reducing the strength of the center and the subtractive surround, results in the low-pass retinal spatial transfer function in dopaminergic deficiency.

The effect of L-dopa on vision in PD CS loss does respond (at least acutely) to levodopa therapy in PD.[40,99] Acute visual

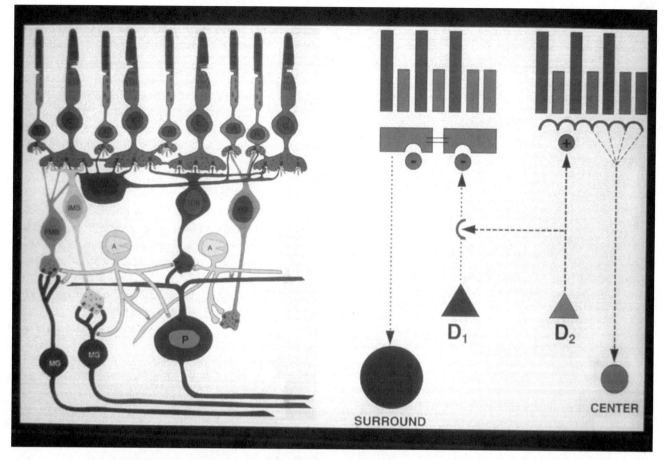

FIGURE 79.5 Simplified schema of the D1–D2 interaction of the retina. The D1 DA pathway enhances the surround signal, while the D2 pathway enhances the center signal. Experimental results suggest that these two DA pathways are not independent of each other: D2 is involved in the D1 pathway participating in a negative feedback loop, providing a greater D1 effect when D2 receptors are blocked. (Adapted from Bodis-Wollner I, Tzelepi A: Push-pull model of dopamine's action in the retina. In Hung GK, Ciuffreda KC (eds): Models of the visual system. Kluwer Academic Publishers, 2002, pp 191–214; with permission.) (See also color plate 51.)

changes are especially striking in chronically treated patients who develop ON-OFF motor phenomena, having dyskinetic-akinetic motor fluctuations on a daily basis, according to the DA replaced or depleted state. In the OFF state, visual abnormalities are prominent, while they are less evident in the ON state.[32] In ON-OFF patients, CS changes in tandem with motor fluctuations,[30] revealing a normally tuned CS function in the ON state and a low-pass shape in the OFF state, suggesting that SF tuning is under dopaminergic modulation. A marked effect of levodopa therapy has been demonstrated on the PERG tuning ratio between patients treated and not treated with L-dopa.[181] PD patients receiving L-dopa had higher PERG amplitude and improved SF tuning compared to untreated patients, although they have rarely achieved normal values (figure 79.6). These results suggest that L-Dopa therapy has a lasting effect on retinal processing.

Generally, both VEP and PERG impairments are sensitive to levodopa therapy,[142,143] although there is an apparent difference: Levodopa therapy improves PERG abnormalities to a higher degree than it does VEP deficits. One possible interpretation is that VEP changes in PD represent secondary, nondopaminergic and therefore more chronic alterations in visual processing. An essential proof of visual system involvement in PD and the relationship of visual and motor changes was recently provided by a longitudinal study of visual dysfunction in PD patients: CS is impaired in parallel with the worsening of motor score.[60] These results therefore suggest that the visual system shares with the motor system progressive degeneration of dopaminergic neurons and/or progressive failure of the effect of L-dopa therapy.

Visual losses in PD that may not be direct consequences of dopaminergic deficiency The foregoing discussion makes a case for the conclusion that visual dysfunction is an integral part of PD: The deficit fluctuates with motor symptoms in ON-OFF patients and worsens with the progression of motor symptoms. While the role of DA deficiency is strongly implied by

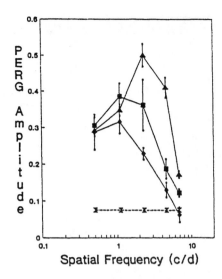

FIGURE 79.6 Effects of L-dopa therapy on PERG amplitude. PERG amplitude obtained in age-matched subjects (triangles) and PD patients receiving (squares) and not receiving (diamonds) L-dopa are plotted as a function of SF. PD patients receiving L-dopa show higher values and better tuning compared to untreated patients, although they rarely achieve normal values. The dashed line represents the mean noise level during recordings. Error bars indicate standard error. (From Tagliati M, Bodis-Wollner I, Yahr MD: The pattern electroretinogram in Parkinson's disease reveals lack of retinal spatial tuning. *Electroencephalogr Clin Neurophysiol* 1996; 100:1–11; with permission.)

all these studies, DA deficiency may not be exclusively responsible for visual changes in PD.

It has been noted that in dopaminergic deficiency, the spatial CS abnormality is even more profound when the grating is temporally modulated at 4–8 Hz,[32,157] suggesting that a dopaminergic deficiency state also affects temporal processing.[119] However, little is known of the relationship of the two types of retinal DA receptors to dynamic processing in the retina.

Compared to the clinically standardized pattern reversal stimulation, pattern onset/offset VEP is rarely used in patient studies, although it has been extensively studied physiologically.[172,188,193] Onset versus offset VEP amplitude differs in healthy normals: The onset VEP amplitude is factors larger than the offset response. This is not so in PD, and the onset/offset amplitude ratio provides a simple measure to quantify one specific aspect of impaired vision.[12] When horizontal sinusoidal gratings with 1 and 4 cpd were used, the evoked P1 offset amplitude was significantly larger in PD patients than in controls, particularly for 1 cpd, while onset P1 values and offset P1 latency did not show significant differences between patients and controls. It is known that onset versus offset retinal responses may be separated by using selective glutamate receptor blockers.[166] The relevance of dopaminergic deficiency or other neurotransmitter alteration, such as the involvement of selective glutamate recep-

tor subtypes in the retina and beyond in generating the "supernormal" offset VEP in PD, has not yet been established. Although the findings appear robust and intriguing, no other studies have yet addressed the ramifications of these challenging results in PD.

There is a potential pathophysiological role of serotonin in the retina. Tremor is one of the cardinal symptoms of PD, but its treatment with dopaminergic agents is less than satisfactory. Recently, Doder et al.[62] have shown that serotonergic dysfunction in PD, more precisely 5-HT1A receptor binding in the nucleus raphe, correlates with tremor severity. The original studies by Mangel and Brunken[118] have revealed retinal dopaminergic amacrine cells with high affinity to 5-HTT. While it is not inconceivable that some visual dysfunction related to retinal serotonergic dysfunction, there have been no studies concerning this area.

Color vision deficits in PD Color vision abnormalities have frequently been reported in PD patients,[18,41,42,60,94,95,129,147,152] most prominently in the blue-yellow axis (tritan). These short-wavelength sensitive cones are relatively scarce in number in the retina and therefore are more separated than middle- and long-wavelength cones. Also, their behavior differs in many aspects from that of the other cones, providing input to the red-green pathway. Thus, the preservation of their receptive fields is mainly dependent on the interactions among dopaminergic interplexiform and amacrine cells, which are dysfunctional in PD.[94,95] It is also possible that there is a loss of inhibitory inputs from dysfunctional dopaminergic interplexiform cells through D1 receptors to GABA-ergic horizontal cells. The diminished action of DA on D2 receptors also can diminish coupling and hence the overall sensitivity of cones. However, color test results should be handled very carefully because commercially available tests are often unlikely to be helpful in identifying the color deficiency in PD.[18] For example, it was observed that general performance on some of these color tests is age related.[18] Therefore, it is very important to use an age-matched control group for these experiments.

The abnormality of color vision (on both the blue-yellow and red-green axes) can be reversed by dopaminergic drugs.[42] Impairment of color (red-green) VEP was more responsive to levodopa therapy than VEP evoked by luminance contrast stimuli.[14] Although color vision abnormalities were not correlated with dopaminergic nigral degenerations as measured by single photon emission computer tomography (SPECT),[128] the severity of parkinsonian symptoms and scores on the United Parkinson's Disease Rating Scale (UPDRS), a generally accepted clinical measuring tool of motor impairment in PD, showed significant correlation with the error score of certain color vision tests.[128]

It has been thought that color vision impairment may be partially determined by motor deficiency in PD[155] because when the response does not require a motor action, then color vision impairments are not significant. However, the noted ERG and color VEP abnormalities are not consistent with this explanation.[18,41,42,94,95,152] Furthermore, Diederich et al.[59] found worse color discrimination in PD patients with visual hallucinations compared with patients without hallucinations. Further studies are necessary to clarify the relationship of color vision and motor abnormalities in PD.

Are there visual cortical deficits in PD? The evidence is that PERG changes in PD are linked to retinal dopaminergic deficiency. However, the retina may not be the only site of visual pathology in PD. The lateral geniculate nucleus[2] and the visual cortex have dopaminergic innervation.[154] Asymmetrically lateralized primary visual cortex glucose hypometabolism has been demonstrated in PD. The most severe abnormalities are contralateral to the most severe motoric dysfunction.[37] It is therefore possible that occipital hypometabolism indirectly reflects basal ganglia dysfunction rather than being a consequence of disordered retinal input. Another possibility is that occipital hypometabolism reflects intrinsic cortical pathology.

Consistent with the notion of intrinsic cortical pathology is that CS losses in PD depend on pattern orientation. Orientation selectivity of visual neurons is first established in the primary visual cortex of primates and most mammals.[19,202] The deficit in PD is more severe for horizontal patterns than for vertical patterns.[38,157] This finding does not fit into the concept of retinal dopaminergic deficiency as the cause. One possible explanation may be visual cortical pathology in PD. The presence of intraocular differences in CS and VEP in PD is consistent with either retinal pathology[58] or pathology affecting monocular columns in V1. However, it is difficult to explain the orientation-dependent CS abnormality in PD on the basis of retinal mechanisms. On the other hand, contrast adaptation, which has a cortical origin, is spared in PD.[184] Studying the effect of dopaminergic therapy on orientation selective losses in PD may be valuable.

MULTIPLE SCLEROSIS

The PERG in MS The PERG depends on the normal functioning of the intraretinal cell body of the optic nerve;[116] therefore, one may expect an abnormal PERG in patients with optic nerve pathology. However, the intraretinal optic nerve fibers are myelinated in only 10% of humans; therefore, one would expect the PERG to be abnormal if there is primary axonal or preganglionic retinal pathology. From the known pathology of MS, the initial effect on the optic nerve is not at the cell body but at the myelinated optic nerve. Therefore, in MS or in any other demyelinating disease, PERG changes may perhaps occur only some months after acute optic neuritis as a secondary consequence of demyeli-

nation and retrograde degeneration of the retinal ganglion cells and axons. Indeed, it is a fact that normal PERG can be recorded during the acute stage of optic neuritis, and PERG abnormalities occur only after recovery from the symptoms of optic neuritis.[163] In MS patients who were previously affected by optic neuritis, a correlation exists between PERG changes and the degree of optic nerve fiber loss (representing intraretinal axonal death). This result is consistent with the notion that a PERG abnormality in MS is secondary to demyelination.[140]

While several studies reported normal PERG amplitude and latency in the majority of MS patients with or without signs of optic neuritis,[102,168] other investigators have shown decreased PERG amplitude in MS patients.[71] PERG spatial tuning in MS was studied with sinusoidal grating stimuli with 8-Hz temporal modulation over a range (0.6–4.8 cpd) of spatial frequencies.[71] MS patients with a previous history of optic neuritis or without optic neuritis showed general amplitude decreases that were worse at medium and high SFs. Thus, both groups had a low-pass shaped SF response curve; however, the PERG phase was delayed only in the optic neuritis group independently from the SF used. This is particularly important since several studies[48,49,69] attempted to show that one of the two major classes of retinal ganglion cells, each sensitive to a slightly different range of spatial frequencies, are selectively vulnerable in MS.

All in all, PERG studies in MS are contradictory.[71,102,140,168] It appears that the PERG has not proven itself in providing essential clinical information concerning the optic nerve in MS.

Stimulus specificity and diagnosis of MS: Pattern orientation–dependent abnormalities and electrophysiological diagnosis In MS, as in PD or in any other disease with select involvement of certain types of neurones, appropriate pattern stimuli need to be selected for the best diagnostic yield. Pattern presentation (reversal versus on/off), stimulus details, such as element size or SF composition, orientation, and luminance do influence VEP diagnosis: Different stimuli may stimulate different and differentially vulnerable neuronal channels. Surprisingly, despite this physiological constraint, different stimulation parameters provide somewhat similar diagnostic yields of the VEP, suggesting that MS does not preferentially attack one or another stimulus-specific visual pathway. Employing more than one stimulus condition results in increased diagnostic yield.[20,21,48,50] This increase in diagnostic yield can be understood as a simple result of increasing the probability of "hitting" different stimulus specific pathways that are unselective as far as the pathology of MS is concerned. These results are probably due to the fact that MS affects the nervous system haphazardly in a patchy manner.

Increasing the diagnostic yield by exploring the response to more than one type of stimulus was first shown by Camisa

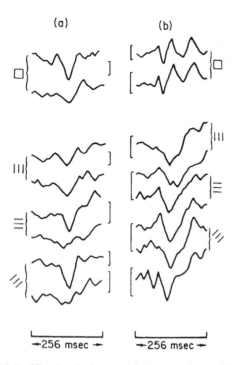

←256 msec→   ←256 msec→

FIGURE 79.7 Visual evoked potentials in two patients with definite (A) and possible (B) MS. A, The latencies are normal for check stimulus and for oblique gratings. With the vertical grating there is a considerable delay in the left eye. B, The patient has normal and symmetrical latencies for all stimuli except vertical gratings, for which there is a 24- to 30-ms interocular difference. (From Camisa J, Mylin LH, Bodis-Wollner I: The effect of stimulus orientation on the visual evoked potential in multiple sclerosis. *Ann Neurol* 1981; 10:532–539; with permission.)

et al.,[41] who used pattern orientation as a variable (figure 79.7). Celesia et al.[48] have obtained steady-state VEPs to sinusoidal gratings of several SFs and determined that applying more than one SFs can increase the diagnostic yield by 17%. Using checkerboard stimuli, different studies have found abnormal VEP latencies in 30–95% of patients with suspected MS, depending on the degree of clinical signs and symptoms.[149] The main drawback in using conventional checkerboard VEP stimulation methods is that the results are less specific.[31] Both false negatives and false positives are more likely with checkerboard pattern stimulation. Checkerboard pattern evoked responses are predictably more degraded by pure optical factors (undercorrection);[20] hence, a poor checkerboard pattern evoked VEP might not be due to MS. Alternatively a false negative result may occur because the checkerboard pattern contains energy at many different spatial frequencies and orientations; hence, the response may be dominated by the responses of a healthy neuronal channel.[27] In addition to spatial and temporal stimulus factors, pattern presentation (reversal versus on/off) and response component selection all influence the diagnosis. Ghilardi et al.[83] have demonstrated that even the different

components of pattern VEP (N70 and P100) can be independently affected in patients with MS. Indirectly, this evidence suggests that the VEP latency is determined by intrinsic cortical processing and not only by optic nerve conduction.

VEP delay and cortical pathology in MS   Consistent with earlier suggestions[21,44,131] that VEP abnormalities in ON and MS have a postretinal origin, there is no correlation between VEP abnormalities and optic nerve fiber layer thickness in MS.[140] The original theory, that VEP abnormalities in MS may represent intracortical pathology, emanated from findings concerning orientation selective visual losses.[44,159] Orientation-specific effects in MS were originally demonstrated with psychophysical determination of CS as a function of grating orientation. These impairments were commonly observed at medium spatial frequencies.[114,159,190] Camisa, Mylin and Bodis-Wollner[44] reported that while the specific orientation (e.g., vertical versus horizontal) of a grating stimulus did not appreciably influence VEP latency of control observers, over half of MS patients exhibited orientation-dependent delays of the VEP. This original finding was supported by several subsequent studies.[43,54,103,104,114,190]

Kupersmith and his colleagues estimated CS functions on the basis of VEP amplitude in MS patients.[103,104] Four different orientations (0, 45, 90, and 135 degrees) and three spatial frequencies (low, medium, and high) were used. The study shows that more orientation-specific rather than SF-specific VEP abnormalities exist in MS. Moreover, orientation and SF abnormalities do not covary (they might be independently abnormal and different in MS patients). Logi et al.[114] measured VEP and CS, comparing vertical and horizontal gratings using 1 and 4 cpd. They found that the use of vertical grating in clinical routine is more reliable for both VEP and CS measurements independently from the SF. However, Celesia et al.[48] determined that using more SFs is equally important and can significantly increase the diagnostic yield in MS.

In summary, optic nerve pathology is not sufficient to explain orientation-dependent VEP latency changes in MS. Several electrophysiological studies have demonstrated that directional-selective circuitry exits in rat and rabbit mammalian retina (for the most recent, see Fried et al.[76]) and suggested that amacrine cells have a key role in the modulation of this circuit. However, pathology of amacrine cells of the retina in MS has never been demonstrated, and there is no evidence of directionally selective retinal circuits in the primate retina. In the cat,[185] retinal ganglion cell receptive fields are not perfectly round; rather, they have an ovoid shape along the principal meridians. However, their aspect ratio is less than 1.3, while the human VEP latency orientational asymmetry can be well over 30%. Bodis-Wollner et al.[29] suggested that orientation-dependent selective impair-

874   OPTIC NERVE AND CENTRAL NERVOUS SYSTEM DYSFUNCTION

ment may occur if myelinated intracortical axonal branches, which "zip" together monocular orientation columns of neighboring visual field, suffer from patchy demyelinating processes. Thus, at present, the best explanation for orientation-dependent VEP losses in MS is demyelination of intracortical branching axons, connecting monocular orientation columns representing contiguous chunks of the visual field (figure 79.8).

The relationship of VEP and psychophysical measures of visual sensitivity in MS How close is the relationship between delayed VEP and visual acuity (VA)? An attack of optic neuritis starts with a sudden visual loss and decrease to a very low VA level (1/10), such as light perception. At this acute stage, the VEP is found to be nonrecordable.[1] Delayed VEP is generally found in patients with VA remaining higher than 2/10. Delayed VEP recovers to normal with time in accordance with the recovery of VA; however, the recovery of subjective vision that time is still not perfect.[9] Sanders et al.[163] have reported that impairment in VEP amplitude is more related to decreased VA than VEP delay. However, a recent study has reported significantly decreased VEP amplitudes in MS patients with normal VA.[61] In addition, a slight latency increase of VEP was also observed.

How close is the relationship between delayed VEP latency and reduced contrast sensitivity (CS)? CS and VEP are independently affected in MS[29] (see figure 79.8). For one, CS is obtained at low contrast (threshold contrast), while the VEP is elicited with high-contrast patterns. It was suggested that CS is more sensitive than VEP because abnormal CS with normal VEP or less impaired VEP compared to the significantly reduced CS were observed.[108,114] Additionally, CS measurements show a higher rate of abnormalities in MS and optic neuritis fellow eyes compared even to visual field testing,[10,123,134,158,170] suggesting the diagnostic advantage of low-contrast patterns. Second, CS measurements test all "points" in the central 4–8 degrees of the retina, but deficits may lie outside the central 8 degrees.[26,28,29,158,170]

Advantages of visual field (VF) and CS testing were combined in a new test, called contrast perimetry (CP), to detect visual impairment in MS.[3] With this method, as opposed to customary VF testing with punctuate stimuli, all "points" in the paracentral retina are tested with grating patterns covering several degrees of the visual field. In this study, the stimuli ranged in diameter from 1 to 8 degrees and were Gaussian apertured vertical sinusoidal gratings of 1 cpd, randomly presented in four paracentral VF quadrants. The independent variable was stimulus (grating patch) size, the independent variable being contrast. The largest CS decrease was found not with small but with large-sized stimuli (figure 79.9). This is different from CP changes in glaucomatous optic neuropathy (GOND). In GOND, the deficit is best seen with small stimuli.[25] The explanation of this specific result in MS may

be that the mechanism of cortical interneuronal connections necessary for spatial summation suffers and is responsible for some visual deficits in MS, as was suggested by Bodis-Wollner et al.[29] to explain orientation-dependent VEP changes in MS. Myelinated lateral cortical interconnections establish binding between neurons covering the same area of the VF but belonging in different functional groups. In the parafoveal area, optimal binding may occur over an area representing 2 to 4 degrees of visual space. Additionally, previous studies have established that myelinated axons of the visual cortex make like-with-like connections of monocular, orientation-selective columns.[121,189] Pattern VEP studies use extended visual stimuli as stimuli. When demyelinization affects intracortical like-with-like connections, then monocular deficits would be predicted to stimuli, which are oriented and extended patterns, as was shown by several VEP and CS studies.[44,83,103,104,158]

Parallel pathways and MS There is little cellular-pathological evidence the affinity of MS to select visual pathways. However, there have been many attempts to evaluate whether MS functionally affects selective visual pathways.

Several studies[57,73,120,126,145,150,156,195,196,203] have examined the demyelination process of so-called parvocellular pathway and ventral stream projections and magnocellular pathway and dorsal stream connections, respectively. These parallel routes are segregated from both morphological and functional points of view. Magnocellular channels are responsible mainly for the analysis of motion and spatial location, whereas parvocellular channels are related to the processing of pattern and color. Physiological data from animals and humans demonstrated that certain experimental parameters allow a relatively predominant stimulation of the parallel pathways.[112,169] It was inferred by some[145,156,208] that magnocellular functions are more affected in MS and optic neuritis; others found that chromatic (parvocellular) function is more sensitive to MS.[126,150,196] A third group of studies reported that luminance and chromatic responses are unselectively affected in MS.[57,73,120,195]

In a detailed study, steady-state (2–24 Hz) and transient chromatic and achromatic PERGs and VEPs were recorded by using high-contrast (90%) stimuli at low (0.3 cpd) SF.[150] Chromatic CS was also measured at 5 Hz as a function of color ratio. Both transient and steady-state chromatic and achromatic VEPs and PERGs were delayed and decreased; however, chromatic PERGs displayed abnormalities to a higher degree. Chromatic VEP delays were remarkable also in the fellow, clinically normal eyes. CSs were reduced in the optic neuritis eyes for both luminance and chromatic gratings. On the basis of the results, it was suggested that the parvocellular stream probably is more impaired in optic neuropathy than the magnocellular stream. The observations of a recent MRI study support this hypothesis.[46] Patients with

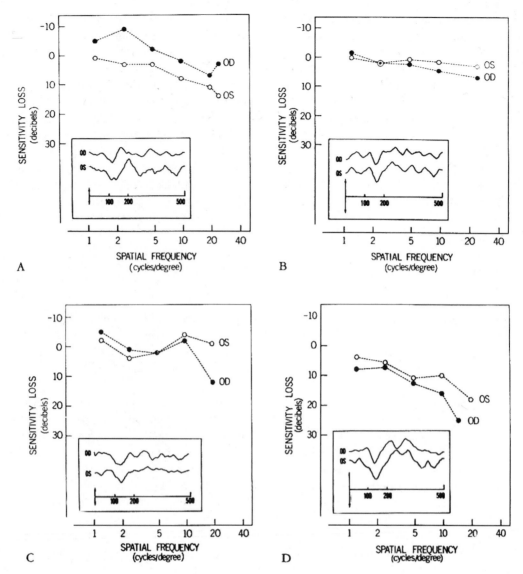

FIGURE 79.8 Contrast detection threshold measurements were taken for several gratings of different spatial frequencies. The patient's contrast threshold was compared to the normal subject's and charted as a visuogram. A, Normal VEP latency (122 ms) and normal visuogram OD, prolonged VEP latency (146 ms) and borderline visuogram OS, in a patient with probable MS. VAs were 20/20 OD and 20/25 OS. B, Normal visuogram in a 54-year-old woman with the spinal form of MS. VA was 20/20 OU. The VEPs had increased latencies (158 and 162 ms) in both eyes. C, Visuogram of a patient with definite MS who had cerebellar symptoms and blurred vision in each eye separately and occurring episodically. The visuogram shows a high SF loss in the right eye only. VA was 20/20 OU. The evoked potential latency, on the other hand, is more prolonged in the left eye (144 ms as opposed to 134 ms in the right eye). (D) Bilaterally increased latency (140 ms OD, 150 ms OS) in a patient with probable MS. VA was 20/20 OU. The visuogram is abnormal in OD and borderline in OS. (From Bodis-Wollner I, Hendley CD, Mylin LH, Thornton J: Visual evoked potentials and the visuogram in multiple sclerosis. *Ann Neurol* 1979; 5:40–47; with permission.)

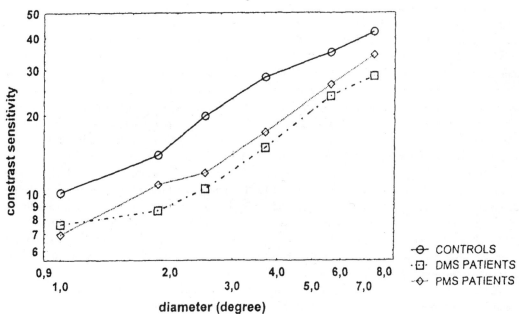

Contrast Perimetry Results

FIGURE 79.9 Mean CSs as a function of the diameter (size) of the Gaussian limited patch of a grating pattern (so-called *GABOR*) in 26 normal observers, 23 definite MS patients, and eight probable MS patients. The increase of CS as a function of the *size* of a sinusoidal grating of a fixed spatial frequency (1 cpd) was explored in four quadrants of the VF field. The central 16 degrees of the VF were tested, and Gabor patches were localized to a point 4 degrees along the diagonal from fixation without crossing the midline. Note that the CS decrease in patients was most pronounced at intermediate sizes of 2.5 and 3.7 degrees in both patient groups. The greatest number of eyes with abnormal CS was also found at these diameters. (From Antal A, Aita JF, Bodis-Wollner I: The paracentral visual field in multiple sclerosis: evidence for a deficit in interneuronal spatial summation? *Vision Res* 2001; 41:1735–1742; with permission.)

secondary progressive MS were studied by using isoluminant red and green sinusoidal gratings of the same SFs combined out of phase for the stimulation of the parvocellular system and in phase for the stimulation of the magnocellular system. CS loss was highly correlated with lesion area seen on proton density MRI sequences of the postchiasmal pathway. Additionally, the parvocellular pathway was more affected than the magnocellular pathway.

Sartucci et al.[164] compared the relative involvement of chromatic visual subsystems (parvocellular and koniocellular), recording VEPs to onset and offset of equiluminant sinusoidal gratings. According to VEP data, the red-green and yellow-blue axes appear to be equally involved.

A recent longitudinal study (for nine years) employed the visual testing technique, called high-pass resolution perimetry (HPRP). The study found that asymptomatic visual losses could be discovered already at the onset of relapsing-remitting MS, and these losses progress only slowly during the course of MS.[115] HPRP primarily tests high SF contrast sensitivity. Therefore, resolution perimetry losses in MS were attributed to the impairment of neurons selective for high spatial frequencies. High SF resolution is synonymous with good visual acuity. Therefore, if MS selectively affected high SF sensitive neurons, patients who have resolution perime-

try losses should have lowered VA, correlating with the magnitude of the high SF loss. However, many MS patients have normal VA. There is little physiopathological evidence that demyelination affects the select class of parvocellular neurons. An explanation for high SF loss is not reconcilable with nonselective demyelination of the optic nerve, however, and it is unlikely to be caused by demyelination of the cortical like-with-like connections for the following reasons. Spatial summation area is inversely related to SF; that is, for normal detection of different SF gratings, the number of cycles is constant.[80] A larger area is therefore needed for the detection of low SF gratings, and one would predict that pathology affecting intracortical connections would first affect the detectability of low, and not of high, SF gratings. To explain high SF losses in resolution perimetry by the process of demyelination, one would have to assume that the area necessary for the detection of gratings is actually larger for high rather than for low spatial frequencies. This is contrary to the psychophysical results, although no direct data exist on the spatial extent of intralaminar connections for different classes of SF selective neurons of the visual cortex.

The CP results,[3] along with VEP results obtained with oriented pattern stimuli, suggest that the optic nerve demyelination affecting only one type of optic nerve fibers could not be the sole source of visual defects in MS. MS pathology probably also causes scattered lesions of the network relying on myelinated lateral connections of the visual cortex, which may be detected with CP.

One possible resolution of the conflicting results and suggestions concerning MS selectivity for parallel pathways could come forth if visual studies critically selected patients on the basis of the duration and course of their disease. The summarized data provide some suggestion that MS imparts different vulnerability and damage to one of the two systems, depending on the chronicity of the disease. By using a spectrum of neuropsychological tests to quantify visuo-perceptual dysfunctions in MS, it has been suggested that magnocellular pathway impairment occurs earlier in the course of MS,[194] while apparently, a more profound parvocellular pathway deficit may exist in advanced MS; a short time course of MS may led to an opposite conclusion regarding the selective involvement of parallel pathways of vision. Taken together, these data do not suggest an easy pathophysiological explanation concerning selective neuronal involvement in the visual pathways in MS.

Higher visuocognitive abnormalities: Electrophysiology and psychophysics

PARKINSON'S DISEASE   Many aspects of consciously controlled information processing, such as planning, problem solving, decision making, and response selection are associated with the functions of frontostriatal circuits.[78,85,86,135–137] A dopaminergic dysregulation of this subcorticocortical system in PD leads to apparent higher-level cognitive dysfunctions.[53,78,122,136–138]   Recent electrophysiological, neurophysiological, and functional imaging studies have attempted to link impaired and selective aspects of cognitive processing and related neuronal mechanism to the pathological anatomy and pathophysiology of PD. There is a considerable number of studies that have used visual stimuli to evaluate higher-order visuocognitive dysfunction in PD. Some of these studies controlled for the possibly contributing effect of lower-order (primary) visual dysfunction to cognitive defects. The most commonly used electrophysiological method to evaluate cognitive defects utilizes the power of event-related potentials (ERPs).

ERPs are thought to index the timing of stages of information processing such as stimulus evaluation, response selection, and context updating.[107] ERPs are recorded in response to an external stimulus or event to which the subject is consciously paying attention. They are often elicited in the so-called oddball paradigm, in which subjects distinguish one rarely presented stimulus (target) from other stimuli (nontargets).[176] The most extensively studied ERP component is the P300, appearing 300–400 ms after the onset of the target stimulus. P300 amplitude is maximal at the midline electrodes (Cz and Pz) and is inversely related to the probability of the eliciting event.

Many visual ERP studies yielded a delayed P300 latency only in demented PD patients,[87,174,175,179,187,198] although several studies reported a prolonged P300 latency in nondemented patients.[8,161,177] This suggests that the slowness of visual information processing may be independent of or precede global dementia. However, it is uncertain why P300 latency is affected in some but not in all studies of nondemented PD patients. First, differences in visual paradigms should be taken into account. Wang et al.[197] have observed that different interstimulus intervals (ISI) could differentiate PD patients from controls: Cognitive processes reflected by P300 latency to rare target stimuli were influenced by longer ISI in PD patients but not in control subjects. Second, P300 latency during the oddball paradigm in PD was also influenced by age at test, age at onset, and duration of illness.[8,161,197]

Is a delayed visual P300 the passive consequence of primary visual delay? It is known that in the primary visual evoked potential (VEP), the P100 component, is delayed in PD.[36] However, while P100 is delayed to patterns of spatial frequencies above 2.3 cpd in nondemented PD patients, the most evident P300 delay occurs to lower spatial frequencies.[8] The possibility that a prolonged visual P300 latency is only a passive consequence of the P100 delay was ruled out by concurrently obtaining P100 and P300 measures in a visual ERP paradigm in PD.[8,161] A prolongation of the normalized P300 latency (P300 − P100 latency difference, called *central processing time*) differentiated younger PD patients from controls.[8] These data suggest that younger PD patients could be differentiated from other types of PD by using a concurrent VEP and visual P300 recording. These data were confirmed in non-Caucasian PD patients, who again conspicuously were the younger and not older patients.[161] There is also neuropharmacological evidence that the visual P300 in PD is affected directly in PD. Amantidine shortened the latency of the visual P300 with little or no effect on the primary VEP component.[13]

Apparently, functional changes in visual cognition are reflected in separate electrophysiological mechanisms: Not only P100 and P300 are independently affected in PD; the analysis of earlier cognitive ERP components, such as N200, showed that its abnormality is uncorrelated with a change in P300.[8] The visual N200 that follows P100 and precedes P300 is probably a visual form of the auditory mismatch negativity.[182] This component is more negative for the infrequent deviant stimuli and is distributed over the extrastriate visual areas and the posterior-temporal cortex. N200 latency was delayed in nondemented PD patients, even when P300 was not prolonged using a simple visual paradigm.[8] In a semantic discrimination task, the same result was found.[177] These data further suggest that visual deficits and processes indexed by various components of the visual ERP may reflect parallel processing.

The clinical neuropharmacology of P300 delays in PD In interpreting P300 delays in PD, the type of medication the patient is receiving should also be considered. Studies in MPTP-treated monkeys suggest that levodopa therapy alone does not affect the visual P300,[84] although D2 receptor blockade could influence it.[5] In patients, levodopa treatment has been found to shorten the latency of P300.[171,174] However, some investigators have described a prolonged P300 latency in medicated patients.[91,151] Accordingly, it has even been suggested that cognitive slowing in PD is related to abnormalities of nondopaminergic systems.[148] A recent study is consistent but does not prove this hypothesis: P300 latency decreased in PD patients treated with amantidine, a low-affinity, uncompetitive NMDA receptor antagonist, even if they were on chronic levodopa therapy.[13] However, amantidine's effect might not be confined to glutamate receptors. It is thought that amantidine also acts as a dopaminomimetic substance, whether directly or indirectly, such as disinhibiting DA pathways. It is known that D1 receptor is involved in visual working memory in the prefrontal area (for a review, see Goldman-Rakic[85]). In the classical oddball paradigm, which is commonly used to elicit the P300 component, a target stimulus has to be stored in the working memory to be compared with subsequently presented stimuli for decision making. In addition, the prefrontal cortex was identified as one of the generators of P300.[89] However, a recent study has found that the lateral occipital cortex also plays an important role in visual working memory,[17] but there is no information about the neuropharmacological background of these processes.

Cholinergic agents are thought to enhance cognition and improve memory functions in healthy subjects and in several neurodegenerative disorders (for a recent review, see Freo et al.[75]). Therefore, it is not surprising that PD patients treated with anticholinergic drugs usually show poorer performance on different short- and long-term memory tests and have impaired cognitive shifting in card-sorting tests.[64,113] It was determined by several studies (for a review, see Frodl-Bauch et al.[77]) that cholinergic substrates influence P300. However, there are no published studies of modifying the P300 in PD with anticholinergics.

Although numerous studies have analyzed P300 latency, only a few have examined P300 amplitude in PD. P300 amplitude increases when more attention is allocated, as in the case of unexpected or complex tasks. However, it is conceivable that raw P300 amplitude is misleading, since a nonspecific, age-related low voltage EEG recording could cause low P300 amplitude.[8] Measuring the P300/P100 amplitude ratio could give a more reliable measure of the nature of amplitude alterations. Indeed, it was found that by this measure, the individually normalized P300 amplitude provides a robust separation of younger nondemented PD patients from older patients and from age-matched control subjects[8,161] (figure 79.10). It was observed that P300 amplitude changes parallel with the difficulty level the task, accordingly to the load on working memory;[79] therefore, the detailed analysis of P300 amplitude gives also information about the impaired functioning of prefrontal areas.

Electrophysiological differential diagnosis of PD and related disorders Most event-related potential (ERP) studies have used an active condition to evoke the P300 component (silent count or button press to the visual or auditory target stimuli). However, there is another positive wave, called *P3a* or *passive P300*, that is elicited by unexpected neutral stimuli under conditions of passive attention. This component is thought to reflect automatic cognitive processing. While P3a amplitude did not distinguish between demented PD patients and age-matched controls, it separated the group of demented PD patients from Alzheimer's disease patients.[179] This result suggests that an abnormality of the passive P300 may depend on the specific underlying neuropathology of dementia.

Differentiating between multiple system atrophy (MSA) with striatonigral degeneration and idiopathic PD is often difficult, since autonomic failures or signs of pyramidal and cerebellar dysfunction may develop only late in the course of the disease. However, vision is usually less affected in MSA compared with PD, since the DA deficiency in the latter is generally recognized to be more pronounced. According to this evidence, visual tests may have significant values in the differential diagnosis of MSA and PD.

Although cognitive dysfunction was not considered a main feature of MSA, mild cognitive deficits are not uncommon. A recent study[100] has found that the early negative components (N1 and N2) of the visual ERP were normal in the MSA group; however, the P3a component was frequently undetectable in the MSA group. Significant difference in P3b latency and P3b amplitude was found only in the MSA group, showing dominantly cerebellar features, not parkinsonian symptoms. In the MSA group, P3b latency significantly correlated with the size on MRI of the pons and the cerebellum.

In the future, a better differentiation of idiopathic PD and overlapping dementing illnesses such as diffuse Lewy body disease may be possible by using selective cognitive paradigms for visual electrophysiological studies.

Electrophysiological evidence of visual categorization impairment in PD The vast majority of human mental activities are based on categorical processes. In everyday life, we classify the components of our environment into discrete categories as a cornerstone of adaptive and purposeful behavior.[92] Electrophysiological evidence suggests that in the temporal

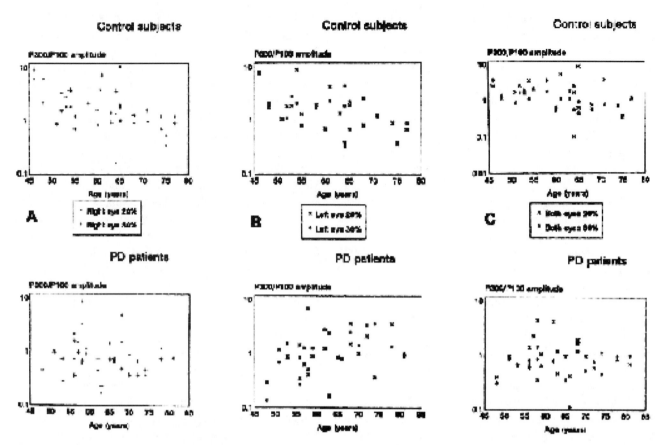

FIGURE 79.10 The P300/P100 (cognitive against primary ERP) amplitude ratio in normal subjects and in PD patients. A, Right eye. B, Left eye. C, Both eyes. To avoid confounding factors of absolute amplitude differences due to generally low-voltage recordings or poor primary visual responses, P300 amplitudes normalized to P100 amplitudes were evaluated. Individually normalized P300/P100 ratios provided significant distinction of younger PD patients from age-matched controls. (From Antal A, Pfeiffer R, Bodis-Wollner I: Simultaneously evoked primary and cognitive visual evoked potentials distinguish younger and older patients with Parkinson's disease. *J Neural Transm* 1996; 103:1053–1067; with permission.)

domain, categorization processes can be divided into early and late phases. Basic visual feature encoding and initial stages of perceptual categorization take place in the first 200 ms poststimulus, whereas conceptual and semantic properties are represented in later stages of information processing.[96,165] There is growing evidence that the motor symptoms first observed in PD are also accompanied by progressive neuropsychological deficits, including impairment of semantic memory and categorization processes. Thorpe and his associates found that nonanimal scenes elicited more negative responses than did images with animals even at 150 ms following stimulus onset (N1).[186,192] In spite of relatively preserved basic-level visual functions, this difference was not observable in the PD group.[6,7] Previous studies suggested that the striatofrontal system not only is necessary for higher-level cognitive functions, including planning, attentional set-shifting, and problem solving,[137] but also seems to be responsible for learning new categories and for generalization to novel exemplars of well-learned categories. The electrophysiological results above suggest that dopaminergic

deficiency in the striatal and prefrontal areas may lead to the impairment of natural scene classification even when the mechanisms of visual analysis (occipito-temporal regions) are relatively spared. In this view, posterior visual areas do not distinguish between natural categories; a cooperation of the striatofrontal system is necessary for such functions.

Wang and his coworkers also measured the amplitude difference of N1 component using a delayed matching S1–S2 task.[199] In this paradigm, first a simple geometric design is presented (S1), followed by another stimulus (S2), which can be the same or different as S1. ERP recorded only for S2 stimuli. Similarly to the above-mentioned studies, Wang et al.[199] found a smaller amplitude difference in the patient group compared to normal subjects.

The N400 component of ERPs has been extensively investigated as an indicator of semantic relatedness: Pictures and words appearing in an incongruent semantic context elicit more negative N400.[106] However, only a few studies investigated N400 in PD.[124,178] Despite the methodological differences, reduced N400 amplitudes have been reported.

Electrophysiological evidence of impaired corticocortical interactions in PD The "binding" hypothesis of visual perception assumes that it is not feasible to provide specialized brain areas for each of the multitude of different tasks. Rather, different areas have to be "bound" together within very short time intervals to solve perceptual tasks.[68] The binding mechanism is reflected in high-frequency, so-called gamma rhythms, representing neuronal synchrony. Gamma rhythms were originally revealed by intracerebral recordings and more recently in humans by advanced methods of analysis of the surface-recorded electroencephalogram (EEG).

Since the EEG represents nonstationary potentials, its frequency content changes as a function of time. Consequently, fast Fourier transform (FFT), which misses information about time, is not the ideal way to analyze short time bursts of electrophysiological rhythms. Techniques that are able to track frequency changes over time are necessary to analyze nonstationary potentials. The evaluation of visuocognitive dysfunction in PD was therefore extended, using wavelet analysis[117] of the oscillatory brain activities, which occur at around 20–40 Hz and are known as *gamma-band activity*.[35] This rhythm exists spontaneously and/or can be evoked, induced, or emitted in different structures of the CNS in response to olfactory, auditory, somatosensory, and visual stimuli or in connection with attentional/perceptual-cognitive processes. In normal observers, gamma range activity is enhanced during the N70 of the VEP and suppressed during the P300 time period.[72,127,191] This cortical suppression is thought to reflect competitive hippocampal gamma activation associated with P300 target processing.[191] In this case, hippocampal gamma activation may be due to short-term memory updating. Alternatively, according to the threshold regulation model by Elbert and Rockstroh,[66] the P300 component of the ERP could represent an inhibition of the cortical pyramidal neurons responsible for gamma oscillation. In PD patients, the lack of "cognitive" gamma suppression may reflect visuocognitive processing deficits during the performance of the task. Gamma is known to be prevalent, for instance, in bistable conditions, such as ambiguous figures,[101] which promote switching percepts. At this point, no such studies have been published on PD patients.

Levodopa therapy increases corticocortical coherence in PD patients.[47] Using simple visual tracking, a task-related coherence increased after levodopa therapy, while without levodopa, coherence was reduced. It appears that ascending dopaminergic projections from the mesencephalon may modulate the pattern and extent of corticocortical coupling in visuomotor tasks.

MULTIPLE SCLEROSIS

Electrophysiological correlates of visuocognitive deficits Visuocognitive deficits in MS are rarely selective. Complex impairments in attention, memory, and cognitive skills are frequently noted, however, and they tend to vary from patient to patient (for a review, see Comi et al.[52]). In the early phases of the disease, the mental disturbances are usually absent or subtle, but they tend to progress with the disease, with phases of stability, which can last months or years. However, some patients can present severe cognitive dysfunctions at the beginning of the disease, and some have normal mental abilities even in the more advanced phases. Little is known about the natural history or characteristics of progression of these cognitive dysfunctions. Similar patterns in impairments of visuocognitive processes have been described in patients with lesions involving the white matter of the frontal lobes and also in patients with basal ganglia disorders.[55] Recently, attempts have been made to identify the connections between lesion locations and visuocognitive deficits; however, the results have been contradictory owing to several factors: MS lesions are very heterogeneous and may have different functional consequences, such as that a neuropsychological test rarely addresses only the function of one area but draws on interconnections with other areas as well.

It has been suggested that auditory ERPs are more sensitive markers of cognitive dysfunctions in MS;[88,141] however, several visual ERP studies found latency increase of late ERP components,[67,130,133,141] amplitude reduction of the N2–P3 components,[130] abnormal topography of P300,[133] or even the absence of ERPs.[133] Delayed ERPs are more common in patients with secondary progressive MS compared to other subgroups.[67]

There are too few studies that evaluate whether the ERP is predictive for the development of cognitive dysfunction during the course of the disease. A 31-year-old patient with ON only on the left eye was observed for five months.[15] Auditory and visual ERPs were within normal limits 8 days after the onset of symptoms, at which time MRI showed several lesions of cerebral white matter. Twenty-eight days later, the number of MRI lesions had increased, and the auditory ERPs showed amplitude reductions; however, the visual ERPs remained well defined, with an N2-P3 amplitude increase parietally. Reaction times and performance were unchanged. Two week, later there were new lesions on MRI; however, some of the previous ones had disappeared or become smaller. While the auditory ERPs returned toward normal, there was no significant change in visual ERPs. Two weeks later, the patient developed optic neuropathy in the previously unaffected eye, and the MRI showed new cerebral lesions. Yet, the auditory ERPs were similar to the first (normal) recording; however, all of the visual ERP components showed significant delay. (Visual acuity was poor at that time, so it is possible that the delayed visual ERP delay was related to poor central vision.)

Correlation with imaging results There have been a number of studies designed to determine the connection between ERP abnormalities and MRI lesion volumes.[98,130,162] A high correlation was found between the MRI score and the incidence of abnormality on the ERP tests.[130] MRI total lesion volume correlated with reduced N2 amplitude, which had mainly frontal distribution in this visual task.[162] This study suggests that the total lesion volume probably is a more important factor in neurocognitive changes than the lesion location.

Conclusions

Neurophysiological, electrophysiological, and anatomical studies of the past decade provided new information of visual and visuocognitive changes in PD and MS. Until fairly recently, PD was traditionally characterized as a motor disorder resulting from a deficiency of the nigrostriatal dopaminergic system. Only in the last decades has its systematic classification been extended to incorporate visuospatial, visual perceptual, visuomotor, and visuocognitive impairments next to other sensory and vegetative dysfunctions. Abnormalities of electrophysiological and psychophysical tests, such as VEP, PERG, and CS, have provided evidence that the visual system is directly affected by dopaminergic deficiency. Animal models of PD have established a link between the visual abnormalities observed in PD and dopaminergic deficiency. In PD patients and in the monkey model of the disease, visual deficits improve acutely by L-dopa therapy. As PD progresses, L-dopa therapy seems to be less effective, and the clinical progression of the disease is paralleled by chronic progressive visual impairment, despite continued therapy. Although it is known that a dopaminergic dysregulation of the corticosubcortical system in PD patients may lead to higher-level visuocognitive dysfunctions,[4] it is likely that underlying cognitive changes are codetermined by noradrenergic and cholinergic deficits and the appearance of cortical Lewy bodies.[137]

While one form of MS is characterized by intermittent appearance of clinical symptoms, compelling new evidence suggests continuous disease activity. Thus, despite the presence of new symptoms, it appears that many MS lesions are subclinical.[111,125,200] While subclinical pathological changes are probably present earlier than clinical signs in MS, they can be detected with selective, sensitive visual tests, such as with contrast perimetry (CP), which combines the advantages of conventional contrast sensitivity and perimetry testing. It has in fact been shown that GOND, directly affecting the retinal ganglion cells, and demyelinating optic neuropathy, as in MS, have different CP signatures. The evidence is that GOND affects a type of ganglion cell with a broad spatial tuning profile, while MS affects overall (large scale) spatial summation. This result, suggesting the impairment of myelinated interconnections of neurons responding to adjacent visual spaces, is consistent with suggestions derived from VEP studies. It was shown that the VEP delay in MS is pattern orientation dependent. VEP provides a near-selective and sensitive test for MS if it is elicited with at least two principal orientations of the visual stimulus grating patterns of medium (around 5 cpd) SF. This result is inconsistent with precortical pathology and suggests the involvement of the myelinated like-with-like horizontal interconnecting system of monocular columns of the visual cortex. These interconnections are likely candidates to supply ocular and orientation specific "zipping" of neuronal receptive fields to provide a unitary percept of the VF.

The relevance of primary (retinal) visual pathology to higher-level visuocognitive deficits in MS is not yet evident. There are so far few studies that have explored visuocognitive changes in reference to the notion that cortical interconnections are affected in this disease. Elucidating their relationship would be of pathophysiological and clinical interest. In both PD and MS, the role of other than dopaminergic processes involved in distributed parallel processing provides an area for future research, using modern techniques of clinical electrophysiology, such as wavelet transform of the EEG, transcranial magnetic stimulation, and event-related functional MRI.

In summary, in PD a specific retinopathy affecting center/surround interactions contributes to visual dysfunction. In MS the visual dysfunction is not entirely due to the demyelination of the optic nerve; rather, intracortical processing is also affected.

REFERENCES

1. Adachi-Usami E: Facially distributed pattern-evoked potentials in multiple sclerosis. *Doc Ophthalmol* 1987; 65:259–269.
2. Albrecht D, Quaschling U, Zippel U, Davidowa H: Effects of dopamine on neurons of the lateral geniculate nucleus: An iontophoretic study. *Synapse* 1996; 23:70–78.
3. Antal A, Aita JF, Bodis-Wollner I: The paracentral visual field in multiple sclerosis: Evidence for a deficit in interneuronal spatial summation? *Vision Res* 2001; 41:1735–1742.
4. Antal A, Bandini F, Keri S, Bodis-Wollner I: Visuo-cognitive dysfunctions in Parkinson's disease. *Clin Neurosci* 1998; 5:147–152.
5. Antal A, Keri S, Bodis-Wollner I: Dopamine D2 receptor blockade alters the primary and cognitive components of visual evoked potentials in the monkey, Macaca fascicularis. *Neurosci Lett* 1997; 232:179–181.
6. Antal A, Keri S, Dibo G, Benedek G, Janka Z, Vecsei L, Bodis-Wollner I: Electrophysiological correlates of visual categorization: Evidence for cognitive dysfunctions in early Parkinson's disease. *Brain Res Cogn Brain Res* 2000; 13:153–158.
7. Antal A, Keri S, Kincses T, Kalman J, Dibo G, Benedek G, Janka Z, Vecsei L: Corticostriatal circuitry mediates fast-track visual categorization. *Brain Res Cogn Brain Res* 2000; 13:53–59.
8. Antal A, Pfeiffer R, Bodis-Wollner I: Simultaneously evoked primary and cognitive visual evoked potentials distinguish younger and older patients with Parkinson's disease. *J Neural Transm* 1996; 103:1053–1067.

9. Asselman P, Chadwick DW, Marsden DC: Visual evoked responses in the diagnosis and management of patients suspected of multiple sclerosis. *Brain* 1975; 98:261–282.

10. Augustinus B, Van den Bergh L, Zeyen T: VISTECH contrast sensitivity and pattern-VEP in multiple sclerosis patients. *Bull Soc Belge Ophtalmol* 1990; 236:89–96.

11. Baker CL Jr, Hess RF: Linear and nonlinear components of human electroretinogram. *J Neurophysiol* 1984; 51:952–967.

12. Bandini F, Pierantozzi M, Bodis-Wollner I: Parkinson's disease changes the balance of onset and offset visual responses: An evoked potential study. *Clin Neurophysiol* 2001; 112:976–983.

13. Bandini F, Pierantozzi M, Bodis-Wollner I: The visuo-cognitive and motor effect of amantidine in non-Caucasian patients with Parkinson's disease: A clinical and electrophysiological study. *J Neural Transm* 2002; 109:41–51.

14. Barbato L, Rinalduzzi S, Laurenti M, Ruggieri S, Accornero N: Color VEPs in Parkinson's disease. *Electroencephalogr Clin Neurophysiol* 1994; 92:169–172.

15. Barrett G, Feinstein A, Jones S, Turano G, Youl B: Event-related potentials in the assessment of cognitive function in multiple sclerosis. *Electroencephalogr Clin Neurophysiol Suppl* 1999; 50:469–479.

16. Basar-Eroglu C, Basar E: A compound P300-40 Hz response of the cat hippocampus. *Int J Neurosci* 1991; 60:227–237.

17. Berman RA, Colby CL: Spatial working memory in human extrastriate cortex. *Physiol Behav* 2002; 77:621–627.

18. Birch J, Kolle RU, Kunkel M, Paulus W, Upadhyay P: Acquired colour deficiency in patients with Parkinson's disease. *Vision Res* 1998; 38:3421–3426.

19. Blakemore C, Campbell FW: On the existence of neurons in the human visual system selectively sensitive to the orientation and size of retinal images. *J Physiol* 1969; 203:237–260.

20. Bobak P, Bodis-Wollner I, Guillory S: The effect of blur and contrast on VEP latency: Comparison between check and sinusoidal and grating patterns. *Electroencephalogr Clin Neurophysiol* 1987; 68:247–255.

21. Bobak P, Bodis-Wollner I, Harnois C, Maffei L, Mylin L, Podos SM, Thornton J: Pattern electroretinograms and visual-evoked potentials in glaucoma and multiple sclerosis. *Am J Ophthalmol* 1983; 96:72–83.

22. Bodis-Wollner I: Pattern evoked potential changes in Parkinson's disease are stimulus-dependent. *Neurology* 1985; 35:1675–1676.

23. Bodis-Wollner I: Visual contrast sensitivity. *Neurology* 1988; 38:336–337.

24. Bodis-Wollner I: The visual system in Parkinson's disease. *Res Publ Assoc Res Nerv Ment Dis* 1990; 67:297–316.

25. Bodis-Wollner I, Brannan JR: Hidden visual loss in optic neuropathy is revealed using Gabor patch contrast perimetry. *Clin Neurosci* 1997; 4:284–291.

26. Bodis-Wollner I, Diamond S: The measurement of spatial contrast sensitivity in cases of blurred vision associated with cerebral lesions. *Brain* 1976; 99:695–710.

27. Bodis-Wollner I, Ghilardi MF, Mylin MH: The importance of stimulus selection in VEP practice: The clinical relevance of visual physiology. In Cracco RQ, Bodis-Wollner I (eds): *Frontiers of Clinical Neuroscience, Vol 3: Evoked Potentials.* New York, Alan R. Liss, 1986, pp 15–27.

28. Bodis-Wollner I, Hendley CD, Kulikowski JJ: Electrophysiological and psychophysical responses to modulation of contrast of a grating pattern. *Perception* 1972; 1:341–349.

29. Bodis-Wollner I, Hendley CD, Mylin LH, Thornton J: Visual evoked potentials and the visuogram in multiple sclerosis. *Ann Neurol* 1979; 5:40–47.

30. Bodis-Wollner I, Marx MS, Mitra S, Bobak P, Mylin L, Yahr M: Visual dysfunction in Parkinson's disease: Loss in spatiotemporal contrast sensitivity. *Brain* 1987; 110(6):1675–1698.

31. Bodis-Wollner I, Onofrj M: System diseases and visual evoked potential diagnosis in neurology: Changes due to synaptic malfunction. *Ann N Y Acad Sci* 1982; 388:327–348.

32. Bodis-Wollner I, Piccolino M: *Dopaminergic Mechanisms in Vision.* New York, A. R. Liss, 1988.

33. Bodis-Wollner I, Tagliati M: The visual system in Parkinson's disease. *Adv Neurol* 1993; 60:390–394.

34. Bodis-Wollner I, Tzelepi A: Push-pull model of dopamine's action in the retina. In Hung GK, Ciuffreda KC (eds): *Models of the Visual System.* Amsterdam, Kluwer, 2002, pp 191–214.

35. Bodis-Wollner I, Tzelepi A, Sagliocco L, Bandini F, Mari Z, Pierantozzi MA, Bezerianos A, Ogliastro EC, Kim J, Ko Chr, Gulzar J: Visual processing deficit in Parkinson's disease. In Koga Y, Nagata K, Hirata K (eds): *Brain Topography Today.* Amsterdam, Elsevier, 1998, pp 606–611.

36. Bodis-Wollner I, Yahr MD: Measurements of visual evoked potentials in Parkinson's disease. *Brain* 1978; 101:661–671.

37. Bohnen NI, Minoshima S, Giordani B, Frey KA, Kuhl DE: Motor correlates of occipital glucose hypometabolism in Parkinson's disease without dementia. *Neurology* 1999; 52:541–546.

38. Bulens C, Meerwaldt JD, Van der Wildt GJ: Effect of stimulus orientation on contrast sensitivity in Parkinson's disease. *Neurology* 1988; 38:76–81.

39. Bulens C, Meerwaldt JD, van der Wildt GJ, Keemink CJ: Contrast sensitivity in Parkinson's disease. *Neurology* 1986; 36:1121–1125.

40. Bulens C, Meerwaldt JD, van der Wildt GJ, Keemink CJ: Visual contrast sensitivity in drug-induced Parkinsonism. *J Neurol Neurosurg Psychiatry* 1989; 52:341–345.

41. Büttner T, Kuhn W, Müller T, Patzold T, Heidbrink K, Przuntek H: Distorted color discrimination in "de novo" parkinsonian patients. *Neurology* 1995; 45:386–387.

42. Büttner T, Kuhn W, Patzold T, Przuntek H: L-dopa improves colour vision in Parkinson's disease. *J Neural Transm Park Dis Dement Sect* 1994; 7:13–19.

43. Camisa J, Bodis-Wollner I: Stimulus parameters and visual evoked potential diagnosis. *Ann N Y Acad Sci* 1982; 388:645–647.

44. Camisa J, Mylin LH, Bodis-Wollner I: The effect of stimulus orientation on the visual evoked potential in multiple sclerosis. *Ann Neurol* 1981; 10:532–539.

45. Campbell FW, Maffei L: Electrophysiological evidence for the existence of orientation and size detectors in the human visual system. *J Physiol* 1970; 207:635–652.

46. Caruana PA, Davies MB, Weatherby SJ, Williams R, Haq N, Foster DH, Hawkins CP: Correlation of MRI lesions with visual psychophysical deficit in secondary progressive multiple sclerosis. *Brain* 2000; 123(7):1471–1480.

47. Cassidy M, Brown P: Task-related EEG-EEG coherence depends on dopaminergic activity in Parkinson's disease. *Neuroreport* 2001; 12:703–707.

48. Celesia GG, Brigell M, Gunnink R, Dang H: Spatial frequency evoked visuograms in multiple sclerosis. *Neurology* 1992; 42:1067–1070.

49. Celesia GG, Kaufman D, Cone SB: Simultaneous recording of pattern electroretinography and visual evoked potentials in multiple sclerosis: A method to separate demyelination from axonal damage to the optic nerve. *Arch Neurol* 1986; 43:1247–1252.

50. Chiapa KH: Evoked potentials in multiple sclerosis and optic neuritis. In Luders H (ed): *Advanced Evoked Potentials*. Boston, Kluwer, 1989, pp 161–180.

51. Cohen J, Hadjiconstantinou M, Neff NH: Activation of dopamine-containing amacrine cells of retina: Light-induced increase of acidic dopamine metabolites. *Brain Res* 1983; 260:125–127.

52. Comi G, Leocani L, Locatelli T, Medaglini S, Martinelli V: Electrophysiological investigations in multiple sclerosis dementia. *Electroencephalogr Clin Neurophysiol Suppl* 1999; 50:480–485.

53. Cools R, Stefanova E, Barker RA, Robbins TW, Owen AM: Dopaminergic modulation of high-level cognition in Parkinson's disease: The role of the prefrontal cortex revealed by PET. *Brain* 2002; 125:584–594.

54. Coupland SG, Kirkham TH: Orientation-specific visual evoked potential deficits in multiple sclerosis. *Can J Neurol Sci* 1982; 9:331–337.

55. Cummings JL, Benson DF: Subcortical dementia: Review of an emerging concept. *Arch Neurol* 1984; 41:874–879.

56. Dacey D, Packer OS, Diller L, Brainard D, Peterson B, Lee B: Center-surround receptive field structure of cone bipolar cells in primate retina. *Vision Res* 2000; 40:1801–1811.

57. Dain SJ, Rammohan KW, Benes SC, King-Smith PE: Chromatic, spatial, and temporal losses of sensitivity in multiple sclerosis. *Invest Ophthalmol Vis Sci* 1990; 31:548–558.

58. Delalande I, Hache JC, Forzy G, Bughin M, Benhadjali J, Destee A: Do visual-evoked potentials and spatiotemporal contrast sensitivity help to distinguish idiopathic Parkinson's disease and multiple system atrophy? *Mov Disord* 1998; 13:446–452.

59. Diederich NJ, Goetz CG, Raman R, Pappert EJ, Leurgans S, Piery V: Poor visual discrimination and visual hallucinations in Parkinson's disease. *Clin Neuropharmacol* 1998; 21:289–295.

60. Diederich NJ, Raman R, Leurgans S, Goetz CG: Progressive worsening of spatial and chromatic processing deficits in Parkinson disease. *Arch Neurol* 2002; 59:1249–1252.

61. Diem R, Tschirne A, Bahr M: Decreased amplitudes in multiple sclerosis patients with normal visual acuity: A VEP study. *J Clin Neurosci* 2003; 10:67–70.

62. Doder M, Rabiner EA, Turjanski N, Lees AJ, Brooks DJ: Tremor in Parkinson's disease and serotonergic dysfunction: An (11) C-WAY 100635 PET study. *Neurology* 2003; 60:601–605.

63. Dubocovich ML: Melatonin is a potent modulator of dopamine release in the retina. *Nature* 1983; 306:782–784.

64. Dubois B, Pilon B, Lhermitte F, Agid Y: Cholinergic deficiency and frontal dysfunction in Parkinson's disease. *Ann Neurol* 1990; 28:117–121.

65. Ehinger B: Connexions between retinal neurons with identified neurotransmitters. *Vision Res* 1983; 23:1281–1291.

66. Elbert T, Rockstroh B: Threshold regulation: Key to understanding of the combined dynamics of EEG activity and event related potentials. *J Psychophysiol* 1987; 4:317–333.

67. Ellger T, Bethke F, Frese A, Luettmann RJ, Buchheister A, Ringelstein EB, Evers S: Event-related potentials in different subtypes of multiple sclerosis: A cross-sectional study. *J Neurol Sci* 2002; 205:35–40.

68. Engel AK, Konig P, Kreiter AK, Schillen TB, Singer W: Temporal coding in the visual cortex: New vistas on integration in the nervous system. *Trends Neurosci* 1992; 15:218–226.

69. Enoch JM, Fitzgerald CR, Campos EC, Temme LA: Different functional changes recorded in open angle glaucoma and anterior ischemic optic neuropathy. *Doc Ophthalmol* 1980; 50:169–184.

70. Enroth-Cugell C, Robson JG: The contrast sensitivity of retinal ganglion cells of the cat. *J. Physiol (Lond)* 1966; 187:517–552.

71. Falsini B, Porrello G, Porciatti V, Fadda A, Salgarello T, Piccardi M: The spatial tuning of steady state pattern electroretinogram in multiple sclerosis. *Eur J Neurol* 1999; 6:151–162.

72. Fell J, Hinrichs H, Roschke J: Time course of human 40 Hz EEG activity accompanying P3 responses in an auditory oddball paradigm. *Neurosci Lett* 1997; 235:121–124.

73. Foster DH, Snelgar RS, Heron JR: Nonselective losses in foveal chromatic and luminance sensitivity in multiple sclerosis. *Invest Ophthalmol Vis Sci* 1985; 26:1431–1441.

74. Frederick JM, Rayborn ME, Laties AM, Lam DM, Hollyfield JG: Dopaminergic neurons in the human retina. *J Comp Neurol* 1982; 210:65–79.

75. Freo U, Pizzolato G, Dam M, Ori C, Battistin L: A short review of cognitive and functional neuroimaging studies of cholinergic drugs: Implications for therapeutic potentials. *J Neural Transm* 2002; 109:857–870.

76. Fried SI, Munch TA, Werblin FS: Mechanisms and circuitry underlying directional selectivity in the retina. *Nature* 2002; 420:411–414.

77. Frodl-Bauch T, Bottlender R, Hegerl U: Neurochemical substrates and neuroanatomical generators of the event-related P300. *Neuropsychobiology* 1999; 40:86–94.

78. Gabrieli JD: Memory systems analyses of mnemonic disorders in aging and age-related diseases. *Proc Natl Acad Sci U S A* 1996; 93:13534–13540.

79. Garcia-Larrea L, Cezanne-Bert G: P3, positive slow wave and working memory load: A study on the functional correlates of slow wave activity. *Electroencephalogr Clin Neurophysiol* 1998; 108:260–273.

80. Georgeson MA, Sullivan GD: Contrast constancy: Deblurring in human vision by spatial frequency channels. *J Physiol* 1975; 252:627–656.

81. Ghilardi MF, Chung E, Bodis-Wollner I, Dvorzniak M, Glover A, Onofrj M: Systemic 1-methyl,4-phenyl,1-2-3-6-tetrahydropyridine (MPTP) administration decreases retinal dopamine content in primates. *Life Sci* 1988; 43:255–262.

82. Ghilardi MF, Marx MS, Bodis-Wollner I, Camras CB, Glover AA: The effect of intraocular 6-hydroxydopamine on retinal processing of primates. *Ann Neurol* 1989; 25:357–364.

83. Ghilardi MF, Sartucci F, Brannan JR, Onofrj MC, Bodis-Wollner I, Mylin L, Stroch R: N70 and P100 can be independently affected in multiple sclerosis. *Electroencephalogr Clin Neurophysiol* 1991; 80:1–7.

84. Glover A, Ghilardi MF, Bodis-Wollner I, Onofrj M: Alterations in event-related potentials (ERPs) of MPTP-treated monkeys. *Electroencephalogr Clin Neurophysiol* 1988; 71:461–468.

85. Goldman-Rakic PS: The cortical dopamine system: Role in memory and cognition. *Adv Pharmacol* 1998; 42:707–711.

86. Goldman-Rakic PS, Lidow MS, Smiley JF, Williams MS: The anatomy of dopamine in monkey and human prefrontal cortex. *J Neural Transm Suppl* 1992; 36:163–177.

87. Goodin DS, Aminoff MJ: Electrophysiological differences between demented and nondemented patients with Parkinson's disease. *Ann Neurol* 1987; 21:90–94.

88. Goodin DS, Squires KC, Starr A: Long latency event-related components of the auditory evoked potential in dementia. *Brain* 1978; 101:635–648.

89. Halgren E, Marinkovic K, Chauvel P: Generators of the late cognitive potentials in auditory and visual oddball tasks. *Electroencephalogr Clin Neurophysiol* 1998; 106:156–164.

90. Halliday AM, McDonald WI, Mushin J: Visual evoked response in diagnosis of multiple sclerosis. *Br Med J* 1973; 4:661–664.

91. Hansch EC, Syndulko K, Cohen SN, Goldberg ZI, Potvin AR, Tourtellotte W: Cognition in Parkinson disease: An event-related potential perspective. *Ann Neurol* 1982; 11:599–607.

92. Harnad S: *Categorical Perception: The Groundwork of Cognition.* New York, Cambridge University Press, 1987.

93. Harnois C, Di Paolo T: Decreased dopamine in the retinas of patients with Parkinson's disease. *Invest Ophthalmol Vis Sci* 1990; 31:2473–2475.

94. Haug BA, Kolle RU, Trenkwalder C, Oertel WH, Paulus W: Predominant affection of the blue cone pathway in Parkinson's disease. *Brain* 1995; 118(3):771–778.

95. Haug BA, Trenkwalder C, Arden GB, Oertel WH, Paulus W: Visual thresholds to low-contrast pattern displacement, color contrast, and luminance contrast stimuli in Parkinson's disease. *Mov Disord* 1994; 9:563–570.

96. Hillyard SA, Teder-Salejarvi WA, Münte TF: Temporal dynamics of early perceptual processing. *Curr Opin Neurobiol* 1998; 8:202–210.

97. Hochstein S, Shapley RM: Linear and nonlinear spatial subunits in Y cat retinal ganglion cells. *J Physiol* 1976; 262:265–284.

98. Honig LS, Ramsay RE, Sheremata WA: Event-related potential P300 in multiple sclerosis: Relation to magnetic resonance imaging and cognitive impairment. *Arch Neurol* 1992; 49:44–50.

99. Hutton JT, Morris JL, Elias JW: Levodopa improves spatial contrast sensitivity in Parkinson's disease. *Arch Neurol* 1993; 50:721–724.

100. Kamitani T, Kuroiwa Y, Wang L, Li M, Suzuki Y, Takahashi T, Ikegami T, Matsubara S: Visual event-related potential changes in two subtypes of multiple system atrophy, MSA-C and MSA-P. *J Neurol* 2002; 249:975–982.

101. Keil A, Müller MM, Ray WJ, Gruber T, Elbert T: Human gamma band activity and perception of a gestalt. *J Neurosci* 1999; 19:7152–7161.

102. Kirkham TH, Coupland SG: The pattern electroretinogram in optic nerve demyelination. *Can J Neurol Sci* 1983; 10: 256–260.

103. Kupersmith MJ, Nelson JI, Seiple WH, Carr RE: Electrophysiological confirmation of orientation-specific contrast losses in multiple sclerosis. *Ann N Y Acad Sci* 1984; 436:487–491.

104. Kupersmith MJ, Seiple WH, Nelson JI, Carr RE: Contrast sensitivity loss in multiple sclerosis: Selectivity by eye, orientation, and spatial frequency measured with the evoked potential. *Invest Ophthalmol Vis Sci* 1984; 25:632–639.

105. Kupersmith MJ, Shakin E, Siegel IM, Lieberman A: Visual system abnormalities in patients with Parkinson's disease. *Arch Neurol* 1982; 39:284–286.

106. Kutas M, Hillyard SA: Brain potentials during reading reflect word expectancy and semantic association. *Nature* 1984; 307:161–163.

107. Kutas M, McCarthy G, Donchin E: Augmenting mental chronometry: The P300 as a measure of stimulus evaluation time. *Science* 1977; 197:792–795.

108. Langheinrich T, Tebartz van Elst L, Lagreze WA, Bach M, Lucking CH, Greenlee MW: Visual contrast response functions in Parkinson's disease: Evidence from electroretinograms, visually evoked potentials and psychophysics. *Clin Neurophysiol* 2000; 111:66–74.

109. Langston JW, Ballard P, Tetrud JW, Irwin I: Chronic Parkinsonism in humans due to a product of meperidine-analog synthesis. *Science* 1983; 219:979–980.

110. Langston JW, Langston EB, Irwin I: MPTP-induced parkinsonism in human and non-human primates: Clinical and experimental aspects. *Acta Neurol Scand Suppl* 1984; 100:49–54.

111. Lee KH, Hashimoto SA, Hooge JP, Kastrukoff LF, Oger JJ, Li DK, Paty DW: Magnetic resonance imaging of the head in the diagnosis of multiple sclerosis: A prospective 2-year follow-up with comparison of clinical evaluation, evoked potentials, oligoclonal banding, and CT. *Neurology* 1991; 41:657–660.

112. Lennie P: Parallel visual pathways: A review. *Vision Res* 1980; 20:561–594.

113. Levin BE, Tomer R, Rey GJ: Cognitive impairments in Parkinson's disease. *Neurol Clin* 1992; 10:471–485.

114. Logi F, Pellegrinetti A, Bonfiglio L, Baglini O, Siciliano G, Ludice A, Sartucci F: Effects of grating spatial orientation on visual evoked potentials and contrast sensitivity in multiple sclerosis. *Acta Neurol Scand* 2001; 103:97–104.

115. Lycke J, Tollesson PO, Frisen L: Asymptomatic visual loss in multiple sclerosis. *J Neurol* 2001; 248:1079–1086.

116. Maffei L, Fiorentini A, Bisti S, Hollander H: Pattern ERG in the monkey after section of the optic nerve. *Exp Brain Res* 1985; 59:423–425.

117. Mallat S: A theory for multiresolution signal decomposition: The wavelet representation. *IEEE Trans Patt Anal Mach Intel* 1989; 7:674–693.

118. Mangel SC, Brunken WJ: The effects of serotonin drugs on horizontal and ganglion cells in the rabbit retina. *Vis Neurosci* 1992; 8:213–218.

119. Marx M, Bodis-Wollner I, Bobak P, Harnois C, Mylin L, Yahr M: Temporal frequency-dependent VEP changes in Parkinson's disease. *Vision Res* 1986; 26:185–193.

120. Mason RJ, Snelgar RS, Foster DH, Heron JR, Jones RE: Abnormalities of chromatic and luminance critical flicker frequency in multiple sclerosis. *Invest Ophthalmol Vis Sci* 1982; 23:246–252.

121. Matsubara J, Cynader M, Swindale NV, Stryker MP: Intrinsic projections within visual cortex: Evidence for orientation-specific local connections. *Proc Natl Acad Sci U S A* 1985; 82:935–939.

122. Mattay VS, Tessitore A, Callicott JH, Bertolino A, Goldberg TE, Chase TN, Hyde TM, Weinberger DR: Dopaminergic modulation of cortical function in patients with Parkinson's disease. *Ann Neurol* 2002; 51:156–164.

123. Medjbeur S, Tulunay-Keesey U: Suprathreshold responses of the visual system in normals and in demyelinating diseases. *Invest Ophthalmol Vis Sci* 1986; 27:1368–1378.

124. Miyata Y, Tachibana H, Sugita M: [Memory function in aging and Parkinson's disease: An event-related potential study.] *Nippon Ronen Igakkai Zasshi* 1998; 35:464–471.

125. Morrissey SP, Miller DH, Kendall BE, Kingsley DP, Kelly MA, Francis DA, MacManus DG, McDonald WI: The significance of brain magnetic resonance imaging abnormalities at presentation with clinically isolated syndromes suggestive of multiple sclerosis: A 5-year follow-up study. *Brain* 1993; 116(1):135–146.

126. Mullen KT, Plant GT: Colour and luminance vision in human optic neuritis. *Brain* 1986; 109(1):1–13.

127. Müller M, Rockstroh B, Berg P, Wagner M, Elbert T, Makeig S: SSR-modulation during slow cortical potentials. In Pantev C, et al (eds): *Oscillatory Event-Related Brain Dynamics*. New York, Plenum, 1994, pp 325–343.

128. Müller T, Kuhn W, Büttner T, Eising E, Coenen H, Haas M, Przuntek H: Colour vision abnormalities do not correlate with dopaminergic nigrostriatal degeneration in Parkinson's disease. *J Neurol* 1998; 245:659–664.

129. Müller T, Woitalla D, Peters S, Kohla K, Przuntek H: Progress of visual dysfunction in Parkinson's disease. *Acta Neurol Scand* 2002; 105:256–260.

130. Newton MR, Barrett G, Callanan MM, Towell AD: Cognitive event-related potentials in multiple sclerosis. *Brain* 1989; 112(6):1637–1660.

131. Onofrj M, Bazzano S, Malatesta G, Gambi D: Pathophysiology of delayed evoked potentials in multiple sclerosis. *Funct Neurol* 1990; 5:301–319.

132. Onofrj M, Ghilardi MF, Basciani M, Gambi D: Visual evoked potentials in parkinsonism and dopamine blockade reveal a stimulus-dependent dopamine function in humans. *J Neurol Neurosurg Psychiatry* 1986; 49:1150–1159.

133. Onofrj M, Gambi D, Del Re ML, Fulgente T, Bazzano S, Colamartino P, Malatesta G: Mapping of event-related potentials to auditory and visual odd-ball paradigms in patients affected by different forms of dementia. *Eur Neurol* 1991; 31:259–269.

134. Optic Neuritis Study Group: The clinical profile of optic neuritis: Experience of the Optic Neuritis Treatment Trial. *Arch Ophthalmol* 1991; 109:1673–1678.

135. Owen AM, Downes JJ, Sahakian BJ, Polkey CE, Robbins TW: Planning and spatial working memory following frontal lobe lesions in man. *Neuropsychologia* 1990; 28:1021–1034.

136. Owen AM, Doyon J, Dagher A, Sadikot A, Evans AC: Abnormal basal ganglia outflow in Parkinson's disease identified with PET: Implications for higher cortical functions. *Brain* 1998; 121(5):949–965.

137. Owen AM, Iddon JL, Hodges JR, Summers BA, Robbins TW: Spatial and non-spatial working memory at different stages of Parkinson's disease. *Neuropsychologia* 1997; 35:519–532.

138. Owen AM, James M, Leigh PN, Summers BA, Marsden CD, Quinn NP, Lange KW, Robbins TW: Fronto-striatal cognitive deficits at different stages of Parkinson's disease. *Brain* 1992; 115(6):1727–1751.

139. Owsley C, Sloane ME: Contrast sensitivity, acuity, and the perception of "real-world" targets. *Br J Ophthalmol* 1987; 71:791–796.

140. Parisi V, Manni G, Spadaro M, Colacino G, Restuccia R, Marchi S, Bucci MG, Pierelli F: Correlation between morphological and functional retinal impairment in multiple sclerosis patients. *Invest Ophthalmol Vis Sci* 1999; 40:2520–2527.

141. Pelosi L, Geesken JM, Holly M, Hayward M, Blumhardt LD: Working memory impairment in early multiple sclerosis: Evidence from an event-related potential study of patients with clinically isolated myelopathy. *Brain* 1997; 120(11):2039–2058.

142. Peppe A, Stanzione P, Pierantozzi M, Semprini R, Bassi A, Santilli AM, Formisano R, Piccolino M, Bernardi G: Does pattern electroretinogram spatial tuning alteration in Parkinson's disease depend on motor disturbances or retinal dopaminergic loss? *Electroencephalogr Clin Neurophysiol* 1998; 106:374–382.

143. Peppe A, Stanzione P, Pierelli F, De Angelis D, Pierantozzi M, Bernardi G: Visual alterations in de novo Parkinson's disease: Pattern electroretinogram latencies are more delayed and more reversible by levodopa than are visual evoked potentials. *Neurology* 1995; 45:1144–1148.

144. Peppe A, Stanzione P, Pierelli F, Stefano E, Rizzo PA, Tagliati M, Morocutti C: Low contrast stimuli enhance PERG sensitivity to the visual dysfunction in Parkinson's disease. *Electroencephalogr Clin Neurophysiol* 1992; 82:453–457.

145. Phillips ML, Foster DH, Honan WP, Edgar GK, Heron JR: Optic neuritis. Differential losses of luminance and chromatic function near a scotoma. *Brain* 1994; 117(4):767–773.

146. Piccolino M, Witkovsky P, Trimarchi C: Dopaminergic mechanisms underlying the reduction of electrical coupling between horizontal cells of the turtle retina induced by d-amphetamine, bicuculline, and veratridine. *J Neurosci* 1987; 7:2273–2284.

147. Pieri V, Diederich NJ, Raman R, Goetz CG: Decreased color discrimination and contrast sensitivity in Parkinson's disease. *J Neurol Sci* 2000; 172:7–11.

148. Pillon B, Dubois B, Cusimano G, Bonnet AM, Lhermitte F, Agid Y: Does cognitive impairment in Parkinson's disease result from non-dopaminergic lesions? *J Neurol Neurosurg Psychiatry* 1989; 52:201–206.

149. Polich J, Romine JS, Sipe JC, Aung M, Dalessio DJ: P300 in multiple sclerosis: A preliminary report. *Int J Psychophysiol* 1992; 12:155–163.

150. Porciatti V, Sartucci F: Retinal and cortical evoked responses to chromatic contrast stimuli: Specific losses in both eyes of patients with multiple sclerosis and unilateral optic neuritis. *Brain* 1996; 119(3):723–740.

151. Prasher D, Findley L: Dopaminergic induced changes in cognitive and motor processing in Parkinson's disease: An electrophysiological investigation. *J Neurol Neurosurg Psychiatry* 1991; 54:603–609.

152. Price MJ, Feldman RG, Adelberg D, Kayne H: Abnormalities in color vision and contrast sensitivity in Parkinson's disease. *Neurology* 1992; 42:887–890.

153. Rao SM: Neuropsychology of multiple sclerosis: A critical review. *J Clin Exp Neuropsychol* 1986; 8:503–542.

154. Reader TA, Quesney LF: Dopamine in the visual cortex of the cat. *Experientia* 1986; 42:1242–1244.

155. Regan BC, Freudenthaler N, Kolle R, Mollon JD, Paulus W: Colour discrimination thresholds in Parkinson's disease: Results obtained with a rapid computer-controlled colour vision test. *Vision Res* 1998; 38:3427–3431.

156. Regan D, Kothe AC, Sharpe JA: Recognition of motion-defined shapes in patients with multiple sclerosis and optic neuritis. *Brain* 1991; 114(3):1129–1155.

157. Regan D, Maxner C: Orientation-selective visual loss in patients with Parkinson's disease. *Brain* 1987; 110(2):415–432.

158. Regan D, Silver R, Murray TJ: Visual acuity and contrast sensitivity in multiple sclerosis—hidden visual loss: An auxiliary diagnostic test. *Brain* 1977; 100:563–579.

159. Regan D, Whitlock JA, Murray TJ, Beverley KI: Orientation-specific losses of contrast sensitivity in multiple sclerosis. *Invest Ophthalmol Vis Sci* 1980; 19:324–328.

160. Rohaly AM, Wilson HR: The effects of contrast on perceived depth and depth discrimination. *Vision Res* 1999; 39:9–18.

161. Sagliocco L, Bandini F, Pierantozzi M, Mari Z, Tzelepi A, Ko C, Gulzar J, Bodis-Wollner I: Electrophysiological evidence for visuocognitive dysfunction in younger non Caucasian patients with Parkinson's disease. *J Neural Transm* 1997; 104:427–439.

162. Sailer M, Heinze HJ, Tendolkar I, Decker U, Kreye O, von Rolbicki U, Munte TF: Influence of cerebral lesion volume and lesion distribution on event-related brain potentials in multiple sclerosis. *J Neurol* 2001; 248:1049–1055.

163. Sanders EA, Reulen JP, Van der Velde EA, Hogenhuis LA: The diagnosis of multiple sclerosis: Contribution of non-clinical tests. *J Neurol Sci* 1986; 72:273–285.

164. Sartucci F, Murri L, Orsini C, Porciatti V: Equiluminant red-green and blue-yellow VEPs in multiple sclerosis. *J Clin Neurophysiol* 2001; 18:583–591.

165. Schendan HE, Ganis G, Kutas M: Neurophysiological evidence for visual perceptual categorization of words and faces within 150 ms. *Psychophysiology* 1998; 35:240–251.

166. Schiller PH: The ON and OFF channels of the visual system. *Trends Neurosci* 1992; 15:86–92.

167. Selhorst JB, Saul RF: Uhthoff and his symptom. *J Neuroophthalmol* 1995; 15:70–78.

168. Serra G, Carreras M, Tugnoli V, Manca M, Cristofori MC: Pattern electroretinogram in multiple sclerosis. *J Neurol Neurosurg Psychiatry* 1984; 47:879–883.

169. Shapley R: Parallel pathways in the mammalian visual system. *Ann N Y Acad Sci* 1982; 388:11–20.

170. Sjostrand J, Abrahamsson M: Suprathreshold vision in acute optic neuritis. *J Neurol Neurosurg Psychiatry* 1982; 45:227–234.

171. Sohn YH, Kim GW, Huh K, Kim JS: Dopaminergic influences on the P300 abnormality in Parkinson's disease. *J Neurol Sci* 1998; 158:83–87.

172. Spekreijse H, Van der Tweel LH, Zuidema T: Contrast evoked responses in man. *Vision Res* 1973; 13:1577–1601.

173. Stanzione P, Bodis-Wollner I, Pierantozzi M, Semprini R, Tagliati M, Peppe A, Bernardi G: A mixed D1 and D2 antagonist does not replay pattern electroretinogram alterations observed with a selective D2 antagonist in normal humans: Relationship with Parkinson's disease pattern electroretinogram alterations. *Clin Neurophysiol* 1999; 110:82–85.

174. Stanzione P, Fattapposta F, Giunti P, D'Alessio C, Tagliati M, Affricano C, Amabile G: P300 variations in parkinsonian patients before and during dopaminergic monotherapy: A suggested dopamine component in P300. *Electroencephalogr Clin Neurophysiol* 1991; 80:446–453.

175. Stanzione P, Fattapposta F, Tagliati M, D'Alessio C, Marciani MG, Foti A, Amabile G: Dopaminergic pharmacological manipulations in normal humans confirm the specificity of the visual (PERG-VEP) and cognitive (P300) electrophysiological alterations in Parkinson's disease. *Electroencephalogr Clin Neurophysiol Suppl* 1990; 41:216–220.

176. Sutton S, Braren M, Zubin J, John ER: Evoked potentials correlate of stimulus uncertainty. *Science* 1965; 150:1187–1188.

177. Tachibana H, Aragane K, Miyata Y, Sugita M: Electrophysiological analysis of cognitive slowing in Parkinson's disease. *J Neurol Sci* 1997; 149:47–56.

178. Tachibana H, Miyata Y, Takeda M, Sugita M, Okita T: Event-related potentials reveal memory deficits in Parkinson's disease. *Brain Res Cogn Brain Res* 1999; 8:165–172.

179. Tachibana H, Toda L, Sugita M: Actively and passively evoked P3 latency of event-related potentials in Parkinson's disease. *J Neurol Sci* 1992; 111:134–142.

180. Tagliati M, Bodis-Wollner I, Kovanecz I, Stanzione P: Spatial frequency tuning of the monkey pattern ERG depends on D2 receptor-linked action of dopamine. *Vision Res* 1994; 34:2051–2057.

181. Tagliati M, Bodis-Wollner I, Yahr MD: The pattern electroretinogram in Parkinson's disease reveals lack of retinal spatial tuning. *Electroencephalogr Clin Neurophysiol* 1996; 100:1–11.

182. Tales A, Newton P, Troscianko T, Butler S: Mismatch negativity in the visual modality. *Neuroreport* 1999; 10:3363–3367.

183. Tartaglione A, Pizio N, Bino G, Spadavecchia L, Favale E: VEP changes in Parkinson's disease are stimulus dependent. *J Neurol Neurosurg Psychiatry* 1984; 47:305–307.

184. Tebartz van Elst L, Greenlee MW, Foley JM, Lucking CH: Contrast detection, discrimination and adaptation in patients with Parkinson's disease and multiple system atrophy. *Brain* 1997; 120(12):2219–2228.

185. Thibos LN, Levick WR: Spatial frequency characteristics of brisk and sluggish ganglion cells of the cat's retina. *Exp Brain Res* 1983; 51:16–22.

186. Thorpe S, Fize D, Marlot C: Speed of processing in the human visual system. *Nature* 1996; 381:520–522.

187. Toda K, Tachibana H, Sugita M, Konishi K: P300 and reaction time in Parkinson's disease. *J Geriatr Psychiatry Neurol* 1993; 6:131–136.

188. Török B, Meyer M, Wildberger H: The influence of pattern size on amplitude, latency and wave form of retinal and cortical potentials elicited by checkerboard pattern reversal and stimulus onset-offset. *Electroencephalogr Clin Neurophysiol* 1992; 84:13–19.

189. Ts'o DY, Gilbert CD: The organization of chromatic and spatial interactions in the primate striate cortex. *J Neurosci* 1988; 8:1712–1727.

190. Tulunay-Keesey U, Brooks BR, Kukuljan R, Ver Hoeve JN: Effect of orientation on spatiotemporal contrast sensitivity in multiple sclerosis. *Vision Res* 1994; 34:123–136.

191. Tzelepi A, Bezerianos T, Bodis-Wollner I: Functional properties of sub-bands of oscillatory brain waves to pattern visual stimulation in man. *Clin Neurophysiol* 2000; 111:259–269.

192. VanRullen R, Thorpe SJ: The time course of visual processing: From early perception to decision-making. *J Cogn Neurosci* 2001; 13:454–461.

193. Vassilev A, Manahilov V, Mitov D: Spatial frequency and the pattern onset-offset response. *Vision Res* 1983; 23:1417–1422.

194. Vleugels L, Lafosse C, van Nunen A, Charlier M, Ketelaer P, Vandenbussche E: Visuoperceptual impairment in MS patients: Nature and possible neural origins. *Mult Scler* 2001; 7:389–401.

195. Vleugels L, van Nunen A, Lafosse C, Ketelaer P, Vandenbussche E: Temporal and spatial resolution in foveal vision of multiple sclerosis patients. *Vision Res* 1998; 38:2987–2997.

196. Wall M: Loss of P retinal ganglion cell function in resolved optic neuritis. *Neurology* 1990; 40:649–653.

197. Wang L, Kuroiwa Y, Kamitani T: Visual event-related potential changes at two different tasks in nondemented Parkinson's disease. *J Neurol Sci* 1999; 164:139–147.

198. Wang L, Kuroiwa Y, Li M, Kamitani T, Wang J, Takahashi T, Suzuki Y, Ikegami T, Matsubara S: The correlation between P300 alterations and regional cerebral blood flow in

non-demented Parkinson's disease. *Neurosci Lett* 2000; 282:133–136.

199. Wang L, Kuroiwa Y, Li M, Wang J, Kamitani T: Do P1 and N1 evoked by the ERP task reflect primary visual processing in Parkinson's disease? *Doc Ophthalmol* 2001; 102:83–93.

200. Willoughby EW, Grochowski E, Li DK, Oger J, Kastrukoff LF, Paty DW: Serial magnetic resonance scanning in multiple sclerosis: A second prospective study in relapsing patients. *Ann Neurol* 1989; 25:43–49.

201. Wink B, Harris J: A model of the Parkinsonian visual system: Support for the dark adaptation hypothesis. *Vision Res* 2000; 40:1937–1946.

202. Zeki S: The distribution of wavelength and orientation selective cells in different areas of monkey visual cortex. *Proc R Soc Lond B Biol Sci* 1983; 217:449–470.

203. Zisman F, King-Smith PE, Bhargava SK: Spectral sensitivities of acquired color defects analyzed in terms of color opponent theory. *Mod Probl Ophthalmol* 1978; 19:254–257.

80 Diseases of Fatty Acid Storage and Metabolism: Neuronal Ceroid Lipofuscinoses and the Long-Chain 3-Hydroxyacyl-CoA Dehydrogenase Deficiency

DAVID G. BIRCH AND RICHARD G. WELEBER

RETINAL DEGENERATION is an early consequence of the lysosomal storage diseases that are collectively referred to as the neuronal ceroid lipofuscinoses (NCLs) and the fatty acid oxidation disorder long-chain 3-hydroxyacyl CoA dehydrogenase (LCHAD) deficiency. This review summarizes recent developments that have been made in diagnosing and understanding the molecular bases of these disorders. The first symptoms of many of the NCLs often relate to visual loss from retinal degeneration. The resulting decrease in vision is typically evident at an early age, and the ophthalmologist may be the first specialist to examine the patient. Since the fundus of a young patient may be normal or not diagnostic of specific disease, the eventual diagnosis of the NCL often must come from additional testing. Since the retina is a readily accessible portion of the central nervous system, tests of retinal function have potential value not only for diagnosis, but also for future treatment trials in NCLs and LCHAD deficiency as rational interventions become available. This review will summarize ERG findings in young children with these metabolic disorders. Because the degeneration is often severe, even at an early age, specialized techniques developed for patients with retinitis pigmentosa are also necessary for analyzing the very small (submicrovolt) electroretinograms (ERGs).[1,2]

The neuronal ceroid lipofuscinoses (NCLs) are a group of progressive neurodegenerative disorders characterized by the accumulation of complex storage material within lysosomes. As a class, the NCLs are the most common neurodegenerative disorders affecting children. In a recent survey of the causes of intellectual and neurological deterioration in childhood, the NCLs represented the largest category with 16% of cases. All storage diseases combined accounted for 63% of cases. The worldwide incidence is 1:12,500 live births.[14] The disease is characterized by severe psychomotor deterioration that progresses to a vegetative state, seizures, visual failure from retinal degeneration, and premature death.[5,8,18] Four classical forms exist—three childhood-onset forms, which are all autosomal-recessive, and one adult-onset form, which may be autosomal-recessive or -dominant:

1. An infantile-onset form (INCL, *CLN1*), also called Haltia-Santavuori disease, Hagberg-Santavuori disease, or simply the Finnish form. This usually manifests at 8–24 months of age with severe psychomotor retardation, blindness, and microcephaly.
2. A late infantile-onset form (LINCL, *CLN2*), also called Jansky-Bielschowsky disease. This condition manifests at 2–4 years of age with ataxia, loss of speech, regression of developmental milestones, seizures, and later gradual loss of vision.
3. A juvenile-onset form (JNCL, *CLN3*), also called Batten-Mayou syndrome, Spielmeyer-Vogt disease, or Spielmeyer-Sjögren syndrome, which manifests at 4–8 years of age with visual acuity loss that progresses to loss of virtually all useful vision over a year or two. Seizures, cognitive decline, and motor disturbances follow.
4. The adult-onset disorder (ANCL, *CLN4*), also called Kufs' disease, usually manifests as a motor disturbance usually without visual symptoms or findings. Although Kufs' disease is believed to be an autosomal-recessive trait, autosomal-dominant inheritance has been described.

In addition, as many as 15 atypical forms have been described, some of which may be allelic to certain of the classical forms. One of the variant forms (vLINCL, *CLN5*) occurs essentially only in the Finnish population and shows linkage to a site (13q22) distinct from the three classic forms of childhood NCL.[16] In Europe, the term *Batten's disease* is often used collectively for all forms of NCL.

All forms of NCL show accumulation of storage material that is autofluorescent, sudanophilic, and PAS-positive within lysosomes in neurons and other cells. Because of its osmophilic nature and appearance on light microscopy, the storage material resembles ceroid and lipofuscin but actually is a complex mixture of lipoproteins and other hydrophobic peptides. The lipoprotein deposits within cells on electron microscopy take on characteristic patterns that are used for diagnosis and classification. Granular inclusions are seen in INCL, Kufs' disease, and some atypical forms of JNCL. Curvilinear inclusions predominate in classic LINCL. Variant forms of LINCL often show a mixture of curvilinear and fingerprint profiles. Fingerprint inclusions are seen in JNCL (with occasional to rare curvilinear inclusions). Historically, the diagnosis of this group of disorders has been established by looking for inclusion bodies in cells from brain biopsy or full-thickness rectal biopsy. More recently, skin or bulbar conjunctival biopsies have supplanted these more invasive surgical procedures. Buffy coat leukocytes can be used but may include a wider range of inclusions that may represent other storage disorders, such as the mucopolysaccharidoses. Muscle biopsy appears to be the only tissue suitable for diagnosis for ANCL or Kuf's disease.

The defective gene *CLN1* for INCL encodes the enzyme palmitoyl-protein thioesterase-1 (PPT-1), an enzyme that removes long-chain fatty acids, mostly palmitate residues, from S-acylated proteins. As such, this enzyme is necessary for the reversible palmitoylation-depalmitoylation cycles used by signal transport proteins. Patients with INCL accumulate fatty acid esters of cysteine in their cells.[7,18] The most common mutation is R122W, which accounts for 98% of disease chromosomes in Finland but is rare in other parts of the world. In the United States, R151X is the most common CLN1 mutation, accounting for about 40% of mutant alleles. The gene *CLN2* for LINCL encodes a pepstatin-insensitive lysosomal peptidase (TPP-1), which cleaves tripeptides from the N-terminus of small proteins before their degradation by other lysosomal proteases.[6] The gene for the Finnish variant form of LINCL (*CLN5*) has been found to be a transmembrane protein that shows no homology to previous proteins and is distinct from the proteins defective in the other forms of NCL. The gene *CLN3* for JNCL has been cloned and mutations have been defined, although the function of the gene is not known. The most frequent mutation for JNCL is a 1.02-kb deletion that is present in 90% of abnormal alleles in Finland and in 81–85% of abnormal alleles worldwide.[18]

Vision loss in the three classic childhood forms (INCL, LINCL, and JNCL) typically involves central vision initially and eventually results in profound visual loss, often with complete blindness, within a few years after the onset of symptoms. The ERG becomes abnormal early in all forms of the disease and within a few years is usually totally abolished to standard single-flash recording techniques. Functional testing of patients with retinal degeneration involves both psychophysical and electrophysiological measures. Among psychophysical measures, visual acuity and visual fields quantify the degree of visual impairment from the disease and are important for determining the necessity of, and eligibility for, a variety of low-vision services. Determinations of legal blindness (20/200 or worse, or field diameter less than 20 degrees, in the better eye) also rely on these two measures. While acuity is typically measured with Snellen eye charts in the clinic, treatment trials for retinal disease often employ standardized measures of acuity based on the Bailey-Lovie eye charts.[4] These charts have a number of advantages for clinical trials, such as a constant number of letters on each line and a logarithmic progression between lines. Similarly, while Goldmann perimetry has historically been used to quantify field loss, clinical trials are increasingly utilizing the additional quantification available with automated static perimetry. Among the earliest complaints in patients with retinal degeneration is night blindness. Devices such as the Goldmann-Weekers dark adaptometer (Haag Streit AG, Berne, Switzerland) have traditionally been used to measure the full time course of dark adaptation, but such measures are time consuming and laborious for both the patient and the examiner. An alternative is to measure the final dark-adapted threshold. Typically, this can be accomplished in less than 5 minutes after patching one eye of the patient for 45 minutes. Smaller and less expensive alternatives to the Goldmann-Weekers dark adaptometer, such as the SST-1 (LKC Technologies, Gaithersburg, MD), are now available for this purpose.[13]

The primary electrophysiological test for patients with retinal degeneration is the full-field ERG. The core of the full-field ERG protocol is a set of responses adhering to the International Society for the Clinical Electrophysiology of Vision (ISCEV) standards established in 1989.[12] The standard specifies stimulus conditions and recording parameters to ensure that responses are comparable among test centers. Standardization has been a key development in ensuring that reports can be readily transferred and interpreted at centers around the country (or world) when a patient moves. It is also crucial for planning and implementing multicenter trials as rational therapeutic intervention becomes available.

The ISCEV standard specifies four responses of particular relevance to hereditary retinal degeneration (figure 80.1). The rod response is recorded following 45 minutes of dark adaptation, utilizing a flash (either blue or dim white) that is below the threshold for eliciting a cone ERG. Rods are affected at an early age in many forms of RP and allied retinal degenerations, so it is not unusual for the response to be non-

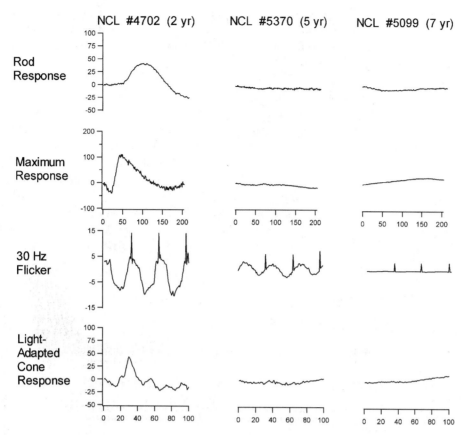

Rod Response

Maximum Response

30 Hz Flicker

Light-Adapted Cone Response

FIGURE 80.1 Computer-averaged ERGs to ISCEV standard protocol in patients with NCL. Top row, Rod responses to blue flash of −0.1 log scot td s. Second row, Maximal response to standard achromatic flash (2.0 log phot td s). Third row, 30-Hz flicker response to standard achromatic flash. Spikes are superimposed markers for stimulus onset. Bottom row, Light-adapted (1.5 log cd/m² background) cone response to standard achromatic flash.

detectable even in a young patient. To obtain a response that can be followed over time, the standard specifies a maximal response to a specified achromatic flash. The maximal response is a mix of rod-mediated and cone-mediated components; in a normal subject, approximately 70% of the amplitude is generated by rods. Two stimulus conditions are used to isolate the cones. An achromatic stimulus flickering at 30 Hz exceeds the flicker fusion frequency of rods; that is, only cones can respond. Similarly, an achromatic background of 34 cd/m² (lower right panel) saturates the rods; cones alone mediate stable responses following 10 minutes of light adaptation. These four responses should be incorporated into any protocol designed to assess patients with hereditary retinal degeneration. When the patient is dark adapted ahead of time, either by patching the eye or by sitting in total darkness, the core protocol takes less than 20 minutes, allowing ample time for additional, more specialized testing.

The rate of progression of the retinal degeneration in patients with NCL is extremely rapid in comparison to typical forms of RP. As shown in figure 80.1, ERG responses may be significantly reduced in amplitude in patients as young as 2 years of age (#4702). This young girl was subsequently found to have an active epileptic focus and diagnosed with juvenile NCL at age 4. The ERGs shown in the second column were obtained from a 5-year-old boy (#5370) with JNCL. Rod responses at this age are barely detectable, and the cone response to 31-Hz flicker is reduced by 80%. The patient tested at age 7 (#5099) had a nondetectable rod response and a cone response that was less than 1.0 μV in amplitude.

Specialized recording techniques, including the selective filtering of responses to periodic stimuli through narrowband amplification, can resolve ERG signals in the submicrovolt range.[1] The need is particularly acute within the population of patients with RP and NCL. The requirements of following these patients and conducting clinical studies in RP and NCL have led to unique approaches to recording small signals. These techniques have evolved in conjunction with the availability of powerful but inexpensive computers to acquire and process the signals. Selective filtering of responses to periodic stimuli through narrowband amplification shares many advantages with Fourier analysis but is generally more commercially available. A key property of any system for acquiring submicrovolt signals is that the analysis be conducted on-line so that the quality of the recording can be evaluated before the patient leaves. Another is the utilization of an artifact-reject window. Narrowband filtering removes the high-frequency components of blinks and the low-frequency components of movement. With this prefiltering, the artifact-reject window can be narrowed to two to three times the stimulus amplitude, further eliminating those components of noise at the stimulus frequency. With the techniques used here, signals greater than $0.05\,\mu V$ can be reliably distinguished from noise.[2]

The ERGs in patients with INCL, LINCL, and JNCL (figures 80.2, 80.3, and 80.4) have been found to be abnormal early in the course of all three disease types.[17] For a patient with INCL (figure 80.2), rod responses were severely subnormal; the ISCEV standard rod and bright-flash ERG showed a normal a-wave and a profoundly subnormal b-wave, indi-

cating that the earliest manifestations of this disease appear not to directly affect phototransduction. The electronegative ERG was interpreted as evidence for an effect on neurotransmission from proximal photoreceptors to ON bipolar cells. This appeared to occur at one of three possible sites: a disturbance of proximal photoreceptor function that interfered with presynaptic neurotransmission, a disturbance of the post-synaptic plate region, or some other effect on the bipolar cells, with subsequent reduction of the generation of the b-wave.

The ERGs of young patients with LINCL (figure 80.3) had mildy abnormal rod amplitudes, mildly prolonged rod implicit times, and severely subnormal, prolonged cone responses.[17] Patients with more advanced stages of LINCL also had a greater loss of b-wave than a-wave, again consistent with loss of signal transmission from photoreceptor

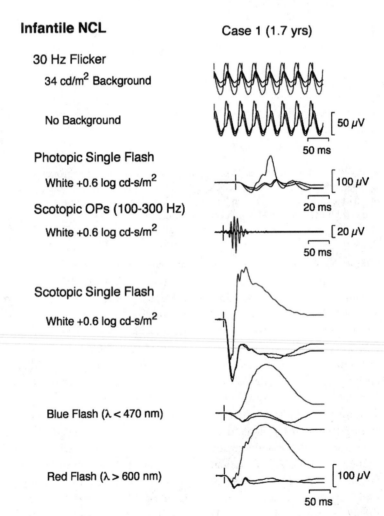

Infantile NCL

Case 1 (1.7 yrs)

30 Hz Flicker

34 cd/m² Background

No Background

[50 μV

50 ms

Photopic Single Flash

White +0.6 log cd-s/m²

[100 μV

20 ms

Scotopic OPs (100-300 Hz)

White +0.6 log cd-s/m²

[20 μV

50 ms

Scotopic Single Flash

White +0.6 log cd-s/m²

Blue Flash (λ < 470 nm)

Red Flash (λ > 600 nm)

[100 μV

50 ms

FIGURE 80.2 Computer-averaged ERGs, using intravenous propofol sedation, to a modified ISCEV protocol in a patient with infantile NCL from the Arg151 stop mutation of the *CLN1* gene that encodes PPT1. The tracings from the right and left eyes are shown in black; the red tracings show the average of both eyes from a normal subject age 1.6 years. The scotopic blue and red flash stimuli were matched in normal control subjects to produce equal

rod amplitudes. Note the sizable rod a-wave and profoundly subnormal rod b-wave for the blue flash, the electronegative configuration of the scotopic ERG to the bright white flash, and the subnormal, prolonged photopic cone response. (Reproduced with permission from Weleber RG: The dystrophic retina in multisystem disorders: The electroretinogram in neuronal ceroid lipofuscinosis. *Eye* 1998; 12:580–590.) (See also color plate 52.)

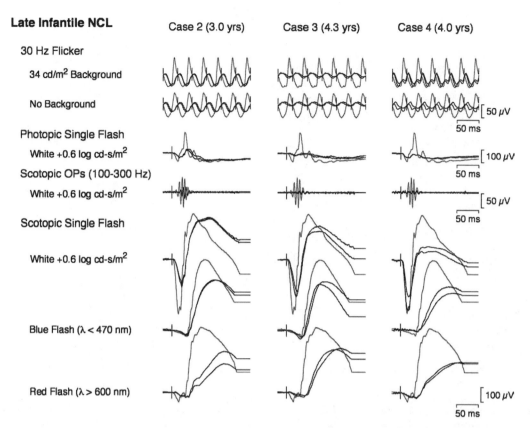

Late Infantile NCL

Case 2 (3.0 yrs)   Case 3 (4.3 yrs)   Case 4 (4.0 yrs)

30 Hz Flicker

34 cd/m² Background

No Background

Photopic Single Flash
White +0.6 log cd-s/m²

Scotopic OPs (100-300 Hz)
White +0.6 log cd-s/m²

Scotopic Single Flash

White +0.6 log cd-s/m²

Blue Flash (λ < 470 nm)

Red Flash (λ > 600 nm)

50 μV / 50 ms
100 μV / 50 ms
50 μV / 50 ms
100 μV / 50 ms

FIGURE 80.3 Computer-averaged ERGs to modified ISCEV protocol in three patients with late infantile NCL. The tracings from the right and left eyes are shown in black; the red tracings show the average of both eyes from an age-similar normal subject. Note the sizable but delayed rod responses, the prolongation of the scotopic oscillatory potentials, and the subnormal, prolonged cone responses. (Reproduced with permission from Weleber RG: The dystrophic retina in multisystem disorders: The electroretinogram in neuronal ceroid lipofuscinosis. *Eye* 1998; 12:580–590.) (See also color plate 53.)

inner segments to bipolar cells. Unlike the ERG in either INCL or in JNCL, the rod responses in early LINCL were only mildly subnormal and prolonged but with much more preserved amplitude, even though cone responses were severely subnormal and delayed.

Patients with JNCL invariably showed severe ERG abnormalities when first tested (figure 80.4), with essentially no rod-mediated activity and marked loss of a-wave amplitudes.[17] They showed even greater loss of b-wave amplitudes, creating electronegative configuration waveforms. Greater loss of b-wave than a-wave amplitude for patients with JNCL would be consistent with the inner retinal localization of the gene product for *CLN3*.[16]

Patients with inherited long-chain fatty acid oxidation disorders, such as long-chain 3-hydroxyacyl-CoA dehydrogenase (LCHAD) deficiency, are deprived of an essential source of energy during fasting or metabolic stress when carbohydrate stores become depleted. The patients are typically treated with a modified diet consisting of medium-chain triglycerides or simply through restriction of dietary fat (low-fat/high-carbohydrate diet). These treatments dramatically reduce the progressive deterioration of cardiac, muscular,

hepatic, and neurologic function associated with this disorder. Without treatment, patients with LCHAD deficiency have severe disease that usually results in death during the first two years of life. Now that patients are living longer with dietary interventions, it has become apparent that retinal degeneration often is associated with LCHAD.

The LCHAD activity resides in the mitochondrial trifunctional protein (MTP). Enzyme activities of subunits of this protein are responsible for distinct steps within the β-oxidation cycle. Genes for both subunits of MTP have been localized to the p23 region of chromosome 2.[10,19] The MTP deficiency can result from a mutation in either subunit, whereas LCHAD deficiency has only been reported with mutations in the α-subunit.[3,9,11]

The fundus appears to be normal in LCHAD deficiency at birth. Between the ages of 4 months and 5 years, some patients develop a granular appearance to the retinal pigment epithelium. This can occur with or without pigment clumping within the retina (figure 80.5).[15] The patients subsequently show vessel attenuation and retinal atrophy (figure 80.6). ERGs in this subset of patients are characteristic of severe retinal degeneration (figure 80.7). Other patients with

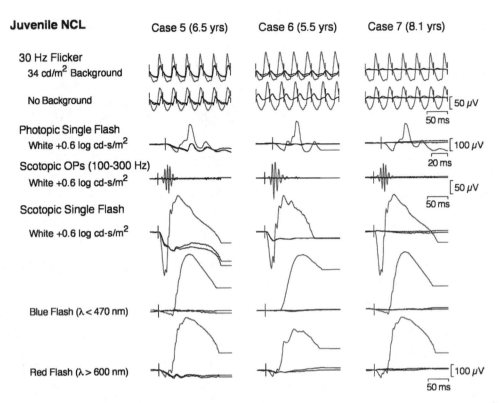

Juvenile NCL Case 5 (6.5 yrs) Case 6 (5.5 yrs) Case 7 (8.1 yrs)

30 Hz Flicker
34 cd/m² Background

No Background

Photopic Single Flash
White +0.6 log cd-s/m²

Scotopic OPs (100–300 Hz)
White +0.6 log cd-s/m²

Scotopic Single Flash
White +0.6 log cd-s/m²

Blue Flash (λ < 470 nm)

Red Flash (λ > 600 nm)

FIGURE 80.4 Computer-averaged ERGs to a modified ISCEV protocol in three patients with juvenile NCL from mutation of the *CLN3* gene. The tracings from the right and left eyes are shown in black; the red tracings show the average of both eyes from an age-similar normal subject. All responses were elicited using the same Ganzfeld stimulator, but because a different computer system was used for recording the responses for Case 6, a different normal is shown. Note the profoundly subnormal rod responses, the electronegative configuration of the scotopic ERG to the bright white flash for Cases 5 and 6, and the subnormal photopic responses, which were greater for the b-wave than the a-wave for Case 5. (Reproduced with permission from Weleber RG: The dystrophic retina in multisystem disorders: The electroretinogram in neuronal ceroid lipofuscinosis. *Eye* 1998; 12:580–590.) (See also color plate 54.)

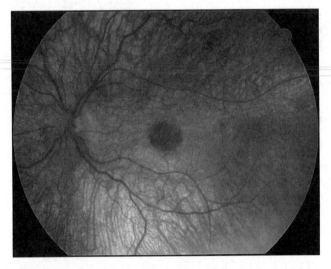

FIGURE 80.5 Fundus appearance in 4-year-old patient with LCHAD deficiency and early retinal degeneration. Note the characteristic dark brown spot in the fovea, the early thinning and atrophy of the retinal pigment epithelium (RPE), and the early pigment dispersion with fine clumping. The ERG was still normal at this stage. (See also color plate 55.)

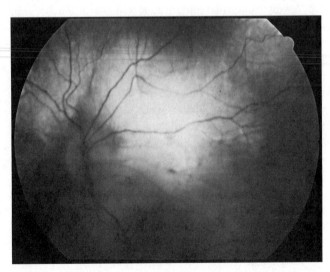

FIGURE 80.6 Fundus appearance in a patient with later stage LCHAD deficiency and retinal degeneration. Note the more extensive atrophy of the RPE and choroid in the posterior pole. (See also color plate 56.)

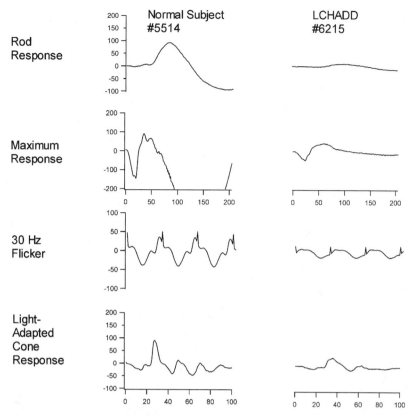

FIGURE 80.7 Computer-averaged ERGs to ISCEV standard protocol in a normal subject (first column) and a patient with LCHAD deficiency (second column). Rod responses are severely reduced in amplitude, while cone responses have delay characteristic of progressive retinal degeneration.

LCHAD deficiency do not seem to develop retinal degeneration and may retain entirely normal ERGs. Whether the presence or absence of retinal degeneration is related to the particular genetic mutation is currently under investigation.

Conclusion

Retinal degeneration is an early manifestation of the NCLs and is often seen in LCHAD deficiency. The techniques that have been developed for assessing and following the progression of retinal degeneration in RP should also be of considerable value in managing patients with these storage and metabolic disorders. Single-center treatment trials for these rare hereditary diseases are enormously difficult to conduct. However, the international acceptance of a standardized full-field ERG protocol should lead to an increase in multi-center clinical trials aimed at slowing the progression of retinal degeneration in both NCLs and LCHAD deficiency. The past decade has also seen dramatic advances in our understanding of the molecular biological bases of NCLs and LCHAD deficiency. With the identification of disease-causing gene mutations comes the promise of gene therapy, which is the ultimate route to a cure. In the meantime, medical therapy with nutritional and environmental modifying factors has the potential for slowing the rate of disease progression in metabolic diseases that include hereditary retinal degeneration.

ACKNOWLEDGMENTS Supported by EY05235, the Foundation Fighting Blindness, and Research to Prevent Blindness.

REFERENCES

1. Andreasson SO, Sandberg MA, Berson EL: Narrow-band filtering for monitoring low-amplitude cone electroretinograms in retinitis pigmentosa. *Am J Ophthalmol* 1988; 105(5):500–503.
2. Birch DG, Sandberg MA: Acquisition of submicrovolt full-field cone ERGs; artifacts and reproducibility. *Doc Ophthalmol* 1997; 92:269–280.
3. Brackett JC, et al: Two a subunit donor splice site mutations cause human trifunctional protein deficiency. *J Clin Invest* 1995; 95:2076–2082.
4. Ferris FL, et al: New visual acuity charts for clinical research. *Am J Ophthalmol* 1982; 94(1):91–96.
5. Gardiner RM: Clinical features and molecular genetic basis of the neuronal ceroid lipofuscinoses. *Adv Neurol* 2002; 89:211–215.
6. Gupta P, Hofmann SL: Neuronal ceroid lipofuscinoses/Batten disease: The lysosomal proteinoses. *Mol Psychiatry* 2002; 7:434–436.

7. Hofmann SL, et al: Positional candidate gene cloning of CLN1. *Adv Genet* 2001; 45:69–92.

8. Hofmann SL, et al: Neuronal ceroid lipofuscinoses caused by defects in soluble lysosomal enzymes (CLN1 and CLN2). *Curr Mol Med* 2002; 2:423–437.

9. Ijlst L, et al: Long-chain 3-hydroxyacyl-CoA dehydrogenase deficiency: High frequency of the G1528C mutation with no apparent correlation with the clinical phenotype. *J Inherit Metab Dis* 1995; 18:241–244.

10. Ijlst L, et al: Common missense mutation G1528C in long-chain 3-hydroxyacyl-CoA dehydrogenase deficiency: Characterization and expression of the mutant protein, mutation analysis on genomic DNA and chromosomal localization of the mitochondrial trifunctional protein alpha sub-unit gene. *J Clin Invest* 1996; 98:1028–1033.

11. Jackson S, et al: Combined enzyme defect of mitochondrial fatty acid oxidation. *J Clin Invest* 1992; 90:1219–1225.

12. Marmor MF, et al: Standard for clinical electroretinography. *Arch Ophthalmol* 1989; 107:816–819.

13. Peters AY, Locke KG, Birch DG: Comparison of the Goldmann-Weekers Dark Adaptometer and LKC Technologies Scotopic Sensitivity Tester. *Doc Ophthalmol* 2000; 101:1–10.

14. Rider JA, Rider DL: Thirty years of Batten disease research: Present status and future goals. *Mol Genet Metab* 1999; 66:231–233.

15. Tyni T, et al: Ophthalmologic findings in long-chain 3-hydroxyacyl-CoA dehydrogenase deficiency caused by the G1528C mutation. *Ophthalmology* 1998; 105:810–824.

16. Vesa J, Peltonen L: Mutated genes in juvenile and variant late infantile neuronal ceroid lipofuscinoses encode lysosomal proteins. *Curr Mol Med* 2002; 2:439–444.

17. Weleber RG: The dystrophic retina in multisystem disorders: The electroretinogram in neuronal ceroid lipofuscinosis. *Eye* 1998; 12:580–590.

18. Wisniewski KE, Zhong NA, Philippart M: Pheno/genotypic correlations of neuronal ceroid lipofuscinoses. *Neurology* 2001; 57:576–581.

19. Yang BZ, et al: The genes for the a and b subunits of the mitochondrial trifunctional protein are both located in the same region of human chromosome 2p23. *Genomics* 1996; 37:141–143.

XV ANIMAL TESTING

81 Evaluating Retinal Function in the Mouse Retina with the Electroretinogram

STEVEN NUSINOWITZ AND JOHN R. HECKENLIVELY

The electroretinogram

As described in previous chapters, the electroretinogram (ERG) recorded from the corneal surface of the eye represents the massed response of the retina to light stimulation. The ERG is easily recorded from the mouse eye with minor modifications of the general methodologies that have been employed for humans for many years. The basic methodology for recording the ERG in the mouse has been described in detail elsewhere.[34] The solid curve shown in figure 81.1 is an example of an ERG recording from a normal C57BL/6J mouse in response to a bright flash of light. The major components of the response are the a-wave, which is the first negative corneal potential, and the b-wave, which is the first positive corneal potential. ERGs to bright flashes presented in the dark also contain a high-frequency oscillatory component on the ascending limb of the b-wave, collectively called the oscillatory potentials (OPs). An example record of dark-adapted OPs obtained from a normal C57BL/6J mouse are shown in the lower left panel of figure 81.2. After the onset of steady illumination, the relatively fast a- and b-waves are followed by a slower positive-going c-wave (not shown in figure 81.1). Other components of the ERG not shown in figure 81.1 will be described below.

The cellular origins of ERG components

Under dark-adapted conditions, the leading edge of the a-wave is generally associated with rod photoreceptor activity.[13,14,39] The b-wave is associated with the combined activity of depolarizing bipolar cells and bipolar cell–dependent K^+ currents affecting Muller cells.[18,30,32,42,51,58] The cellular origin of the OPs is not completely understood, although they are likely generated by amacrine cells and other inner retinal cells interacting with bipolar and ganglion cells.[19,25,35,54,55] The c-wave of the ERG is a corneal positive potential recorded across the retinal pigment epithelium (RPE) and results from an increase in the RPE's transepithelial potential.[16] Because of the technical difficulties in recording the c-wave, it has not found general use in the mouse, although a recent studies have demonstrated its potential usefulness as an analytic tool (see, e.g., Wu et al.[56]).

Contributions from amacrine and ganglion cells have also been identified in the scotopic threshold response (STR), which is a negative-going potential in the dark-adapted ERG that is present at threshold and with dim illumination.[49] The STR has been recorded from human, primate, cat, and rat retinas, but so far, there are no publications demonstrating such recordings from the mouse (for rats, see Bush, Hawks, and Sieving,[5] and Sugawara, Sieving, and Bush[53]).

Rod- and cone-mediated ERGs

The mouse retina is dominated by rod photoreceptors with a peak sensitivity at 510 nm, corresponding to the spectral absorption characteristics of rhodopsin. Estimates of cone percentages in the mouse retina range from 1% to 10%, with most studies suggesting that approximately 3% of photoreceptors are cones.[7,29,47] Morphologically, the cones of the mouse are indistinguishable from those of higher mammals.[7] Molecular biological, histological, and flicker electroretinographic results have established that mice have two cone photopigments: one peaking near 350 nm (UV-cone pigment) and a second near 510 nm (midwave [M]-cone pigment).[23,24,53] ERG techniques for isolating the action spectra and absolute sensitivities of the UV-cone and M-cone driven signals have been described.[27] The properties of the cone driven light-adapted murine ERG have also been described,[9,37] as have regional variations in cone function.[6]

ERG responses obtained to dim flashes of light after a period of dark adaptation are generally presumed to derive from rod photoreceptors. Care must be exercised to ensure sufficient time to completely dark-adapt rods, as some recent studies suggest differences in the time necessary to achieve a fully dark-adapted state. Overnight dark adaptation is usually sufficient for most standard inbred strains. ERG responses obtained after a period of light adaptation are generally presumed to be driven by cone photoreceptors.

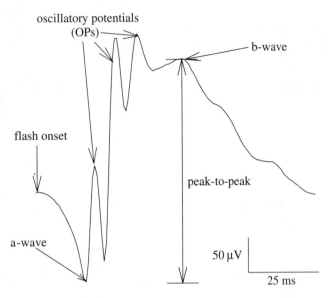

oscillatory potentials
(OPs)

b-wave

flash onset

peak-to-peak

a-wave

50 µV

25 ms

FIGURE 81.1 Representative ERG response to a bright flash obtained from a normal adult C57BL6 mouse. (See text for details.)

When the light stimulus does not emit a significant amount of ultraviolet (UV) light, then the response to a light flash on a rod-saturating background is mediated primarily by the middle-wavelength-sensitive cone (M-cone). Light sources with broad emission spectra are required to isolate the UV-sensitive cone. As with humans, the period of light adaptation suppresses the contribution from rods, thereby yielding a cone-dominated signal. Further, presenting stimuli at a temporal frequency above the critical fusion frequency (CFF) for rods is an additional method that is sometimes used to isolate a cone response. In a recent study in our own laboratory, the rod CFF was found to be 6–7 Hz (Nusinowitz, unpublished data).

A note of caution should be added to the above discussion. Responses under a variety of conditions that theoretically suppress the contribution from rods do not always derive from cone photoreceptors. ERG studies in a mouse model of Leber's congenital amaurosis (LCA) caused by mutations in the gene encoding RPE65, a protein vital for regeneration of the visual pigment rhodopsin in the retinal pigment epithelium, produce a severe retinal phenotype in which residual function is usually attributed to cones in the light-adapted state. However, in an elegant study, the rod system was shown to be the source of vision in the RPE65-deficient mouse, not cones, even under conditions that would normally completely suppress rods.[45]

Representative rod- and cone-mediated ERGs from a normal C57BL/6J mouse are shown in the upper left and right panels of figure 81.2. Each trace shows the response to a different light intensity, which is varied in 0.3 log unit steps. The b-wave of the rod-mediated response increases in amplitude, and implicit times (time from flash onset to peak of b-wave) are shortened with increasing intensity (compare

the heavy solid curves). The b-wave amplitude versus intensity (I-R) series for the rod-mediated responses is summarized in the inset. Note that the b-wave amplitude saturates at the highest intensities. The I-R series can be fitted with a Naka-Rushton function to obtain the maximum saturated b-wave amplitude, V_{max}; the semisaturation intensity, k; a measure of sensitivity; and the ERG threshold intensity. In contrast, cone-mediated responses collected under the conditions employed in our laboratory increase in amplitude but have relatively constant timing (compare the heavy solid curve in the upper right panel of figure 81.2). The I-R series for the cone responses are shown in the inset. At flash intensities beyond those used to generate the data shown, cone amplitudes also saturate, thereby allowing fits with the Naka-Rushton equation as for rod-mediated function.

Basic ERG recording technique

In laboratories where mouse ERGs are currently recorded, different recording techniques (e.g., electrodes), methods of stimulating the eye (e.g., Ganzfeld versus Maxwellian view), and experimental protocols are employed (see, e.g., Green et al.,[15] Marti et al.,[28] Peachey et al.,[38] Ruether et al.,[44] Shaaban et al.,[46] and Smith and Hamasaki[50]). In principle, the techniques for recording the ERG from the mouse are virtually identical to those used in human studies. The major components of a typical ERG system are (1) a light source for stimulating the retina, (2) electrodes for recording the signal generated by the retina in response to light, (3) a signal amplification system, and (4) a data acquisition system to accumulate, condition, and display data. Most commercial systems have integrated all of these elements into a single unit. A comparison of physiological recording systems that can be used for mouse ERGs are described in chapter 19. In addition, a comprehensive description of ERG recording methodologies can be found in Nusinowitz et al.[34]

Factors affecting the ERG

There are many variables that affect the ERG, and standard and consistent techniques are imperative to reduce the sometimes wide variability seen in mouse ERG recordings. Improper technique strongly affects the ERG and greatly reduces the reliability and reproducibility of data. Increased variability within ERG responses decreases the test's ability to detect differences between strains and within strains over time, particularly when these changes are subtle. Variables that can affect the ERG include the improper use of anesthetics, variations in body temperature, insufficient dilation, inadequate light or dark adaptation, and prolonged testing, all of which can lead to a decrease in response amplitude. Location of the electrode on the eye can alter the amplitude of a signal by up to 30–40%, and a decrease in mouse body

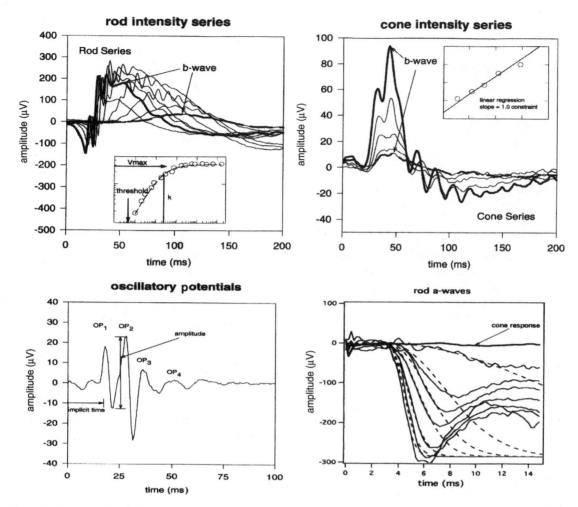

FIGURE 81.2   Rod (upper left panel) and cone (upper right panel) ERGs obtained from a normal C57BL6/J mouse. Each trace displays the response to increasing light intensities. Upper left inset, Peak-to-peak amplitude versus retinal illuminance fitted with a Naka-Rushton function to obtain the maximum saturated b-wave amplitude, V_{max}, the semisaturation intensity, k, and the rod ERG threshold. Right inset, Cone b-wave amplitude versus intensity series fitted with a linear regression to derive the cone ERG threshold intensity. Lower left, A single ERG recording filtered to illustrate the major oscillatory potentials. Lower right, Representative a-wave ERG recordings to a range of flash intensities for a normal mouse. The smooth dotted curves are the fit of a rod model (see text for details) from which estimates for Rm_{P3}, the maximum saturated photoreceptor response, and S, a sensitivity parameter, were derived. (See text for details.)

temperature by just a few degrees is associated with a virtually nondetectable ERG. Repeated flashing, commonly used in signal averaging, reduces rod-mediated (but not cone-mediated) ERG response amplitudes by about 20% at high flash intensities unless flash presentation rate is slowed to allow sufficient recovery of rod function. The consequences on the ERG of inappropriate control of extraneous variables are described in Nusinowitz et al.[34] and Ridder et al.[41]

Specialized ERG recording techniques

By setting specific stimulus conditions, the ERG can be used to index the functional status of a wide range of cell types and can provide information to better understand the site and mechanisms of disease action (see figure 81.4 later in the chapter).

Long-duration stimuli have been reported suitable for dissecting the contribution of ON and OFF bipolar cells to the photopic ERG.[48] For example, while the photopic b-wave is largely generated by cones and the depolarizing ON bipolar cells, the activity of the hyperpolarizing OFF bipolar cells can limit the size and shape of the b-wave. These different components can be evaluated separately with long-duration flashes that produce distinct waveform components at flash onset and offset. While standard ERG recordings are in response to brief flashes less than 10 ms in duration, the separation of ON and OFF components requires longer flashes that are typically 100–200 ms in duration. Clinical application of the long-duration stimulus to such disease entities as congenital stationary night blindness[31] and paraneoplastic night blindness[1] have been reported in humans.

a-Wave analyses: Studies of activation and inactivation steps of phototransduction

Photoreceptor structure and function can be studied by analyzing the leading edge of the ERG (called the a-wave) obtained to bright flashes.[3,4,8,20,21] Prior research suggests that current quantitative rod models have the potential to discriminate structural from functional abnormalities as the underlying mechanism of disease action in retinal disease (see, e.g., Birch et al.[2] and Hood and Birch[22]). These techniques have been used extensively in the mouse.[10–12,26,33,36,38,40,43,57] However, this type of a-wave analysis requires stimulus intensities that are substantially higher than are available with conventional photic stimulators. Intensities that clearly saturate the a-wave of the ERG are required. High-output xenon arc lamps and photographic flash heads can be adapted for this purpose and can provide intensities 2.0–4.0 log units higher than a standard flash.

An example of recordings to high-intensity flashes is shown in figure 81.2 (lower right panel) for a normal mouse. Dark-adapted ERGs were recorded to blue light flashes up to 3.1 log scot td s in 0.3 log unit steps. The first 30 ms of each of the responses is shown in the figure. Note that the amplitude of the a-wave is fairly stable at the highest intensities and that the time to the peak of the a-wave is shortened. The leading edge of the rod a-waves was fitted with a model of the activation phase of phototransduction.[22] The fit of the model to the raw data is indicated by the dotted lines. Generated by the model are three parameters: S, Rm_{P3}, and t_d. S is a sensitivity parameter that scales flash energy. In general, any factor that decreases quantal catch or affects the gain at one or more of the steps involved in phototransduction will result in a reduction in the estimate of S. Rm_{P3} is propor-

tional to the magnitude of the circulating current in the rod outer-segment membrane at the time of flash presentation.[4,8,20,21] A number of factors can affect this circulating current, including the ionic driving force within the cell (perhaps determined by the number of mitochondria), the electrical resistance and/or leakage of the photoreceptor layer, immaturities in membrane proteins that mediate the permeability of the outer limiting membrane, and/or the density of light-sensitive channels distributed along the rod outer segment (ROS). The parameter t_d is a brief delay before response onset.

The kinetics of recovery to bright flashes can be studied using a two-flash technique. Recovery cannot be measured directly in the ERG because of the intrusion of postreceptor components. However, recovery can be inferred from the amplitude of the a-wave response to a second saturating test flash. An example of rod a-wave responses to a test flash at varying interstimulus intervals (ISIs) following a bright conditioning flash is shown in figure 81.3 (left panel). The test flash response in isolation is shown as the tracing labeled baseline. The other tracings show the a-wave response to the same test flash but with different ISIs ranging from 50 to 250 ms. Note that the a-wave amplitude increases as the ISI is elongated, consistent with rod functional recovery. Repetition of this two-flash paradigm with variations of the interval (ISIs) between the first and subsequent saturating flash allows determination of the recovery time course for a given conditioning flash intensity and T_c, the critical delay before the onset of recovery. Examples of normalized a-wave amplitudes to a test flash at varying ISIs are shown in figure 81.3 (right panel) for a dim and a bright conditioning flash (first flash). Note the faster recovery to baseline for the dim conditioning flash. We have previously reported that

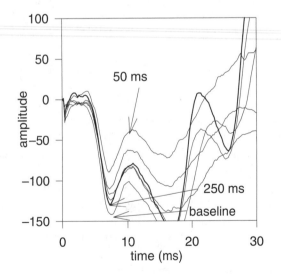
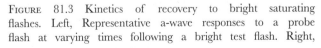
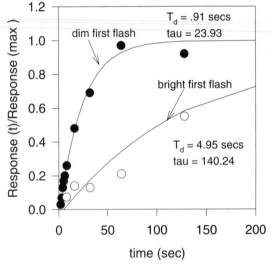

FIGURE 81.3 Kinetics of recovery to bright saturating flashes. Left, Representative a-wave responses to a probe flash at varying times following a bright test flash. Right, Normalized a-wave amplitudes to a probe flash at varying ISIs for a dim and a bright test flash. (See text for details.)

patients with retinitis pigmentosa and a *Pro23His* rhodopsin mutation not only had a decrease in the gain of activation but also had significantly slower recovery times to bright saturating flashes.[2] More recently, we have used this technique to demonstrate a slowed photoreceptor recovery following an intense bleach in albino mice with a MET450 variant in RPE65.[34] A modification of this technique can be used to obtain the full time course of the rod response in vivo to test flashes of subsaturating intensity.[17]

Interstrain differences in ERG parameters for normal inbred mouse strains

Standard inbred mouse strains provide a stable genetic background for the study of specific genes and their role in retinal degeneration. However, little has been published about retinal function across (normal) inbred strains without known retinopathy *when tested with a standardized protocol and at the same age.* In our laboratory, we characterized retinal function in normal inbred mouse strains using the ERG to provide normative data for a broad range of physiological parameters. These data are intended to provide a standard against which transgenic and knock-out mice on similar backgrounds can be evaluated.

GENERAL TESTING PROTOCOL We recorded intensity-response series to evaluate both rod- and cone-mediated function (examples are shown in the upper panels of figure 81.2). Rod-mediated ERGs were recorded to brief flashes of short-wavelength (W47A; 8_{max} = 470 nm) light presented to the dark-adapted eye. Cone-mediated responses were obtained with white flashes on a rod-saturating background. The Naka-Rushton parameters, V_{max}, the saturated b-wave amplitude, k, retinal sensitivity, and rod ERG threshold were derived from the intensity-response series. Oscillatory potentials (OP) were recorded in the dark-adapted eye using bright flashes of white light. Amplitude and timing were determined for each of the first four major OPs, as shown in figure 81.2. Flash intensity was extended to record rod-mediated photoresponses in the mouse as shown in the lower left panel of figure 81.2. Rod photoresponse parameters were derived from the fit of a rod model to the leading edge of the a-wave. From these photoresponses, we derived Rm_{P3}, the maximum saturated photoreceptor amplitude, and S, photoreceptor sensitivity, as previously described.[33] Finally, cone-mediated maximum amplitude and ERG threshold were also determined.

STANDARD STRAINS ERGs were recorded from 11 normal inbred mouse strains (mean age 13 ± 3 weeks). The strains investigated were C57BL/6J, NZB/BlNJ, A/J, C57BL/6J[c2J], BALB/cJ, NZW/LacJ, AKR, CBA/CaJ, DBA/2J, DBA/1j, and LP/J. All mice were obtained from the Jackson Laboratory.

ROD-MEDIATED RESPONSES The results for the Naka-Rushton analysis of the b-wave intensity-response series are shown in figures 81.4 and 81.5. Across all strains, V_{max}, the saturated b-wave amplitude, ranged from 194 mV ($\pm$ 77) to 374 ($\pm$ 99) mV. The albino strains on average produced the highest-amplitude signals, with marginally significant differences across strains (V_{max} for albino strains = 314 ± 90 mV, $P = 0.061$). The two black strains on average produced amplitudes that were lower than those of the albino strains but that were not significantly different from those of either the albino or agouti strains (V_{max} for black strains = 280 ± 63 mV, $P = 0.395$). However, the agouti, or mixed coat, strains produced saturated amplitudes with wide variation across the strains (V_{max} for brown/agouti strains = 278 [$\pm$ 99] mV, $P = 0.0002$). Multiple comparisons suggested that the largest difference among the agouti strains occurred for the CBA and LP/J strains ($P < 0.01$).

The retinal sensitivity parameter, k, derived from the Naka-Rushton fit, also varied across strains, ranging from 0.0015 ± 0.008 to 0.032 ± 0.033 scotopic tds (lower panel of figure 81.4). Again, the albino strains produced the lowest values of k (highest sensitivity), with significant variation across strains (k for albino strains = 0.0062 ± 0.008), $P < 0.0001$), the agouti strains producing the lowest sensitivity (k for brown/agouti strains = 0.0195 ± 0.009, $P = 0.32$) and the black strains producing intermediate sensitivity (k for black strains = 0.0166 ± 0.008, $P = 0.10$). In general, the parameters V_{max} and k were loosely correlated, with the higher saturated amplitudes also producing higher sensitivity values. Finally, ERG threshold intensity and k were highly correlated, as shown in figure 81.5.

OSCILLATORY POTENTIALS An analysis of the oscillatory potentials is shown in figure 81.6. The upper panel shows the summed amplitudes (OP_{sum}) of the four dominant components of the ERG waveform. The lower panel shows the individual amplitudes for each of the four components. OP_{sum} amplitudes were significantly different across the three coat colors. OP_{sum} amplitude was 56.5 ± 35.0, 35.5 ± 13.0, and $79.8 + 28.0$ mV for the black, albino, and brown/agouti strains, respectively ($P < 0.0001$). Surprisingly, the albino strains produced the lowest OP amplitudes despite generating the highest V_{max} amplitudes. Statistically significant differences within the black and agouti strains were present, but no such differences were observed across the albino strains. Finally, the timing of OP peak components was not significantly different across all strains ($P > 0.05$).

a-WAVE PARAMETERS As previously described,[33] the leading edge of the rod ERG was fitted with a rod model to derive parameters of photoreceptor structure and function. The parameters, Rm_{P3}, the photoreceptor saturated amplitude, and S, photoreceptor sensitivity, were calculated. The results are shown in figure 81.7. An analysis of a-wave revealed that

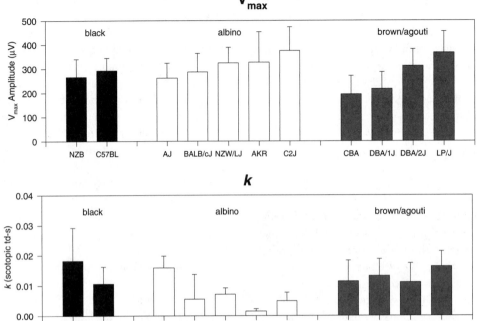

FIGURE 81.4 Naka-Rushton parameters derived from rod-mediated intensity versus b-wave amplitude response series. Upper panel, Mean (± 1 standard error) saturated b-wave amplitudes across strains. Lower panel, Mean (± 1 standard error) retinal sensitivity across strains.

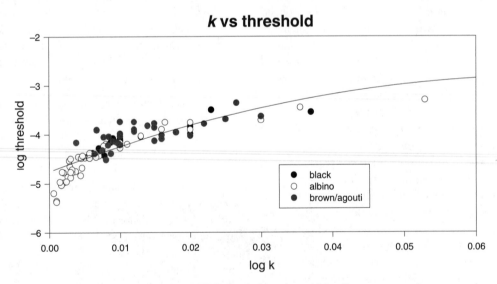

FIGURE 81.5 Correlation between rod ERG threshold and sensitivity (k) across normal mouse strains.

Oscillatory Potentials (OPs)

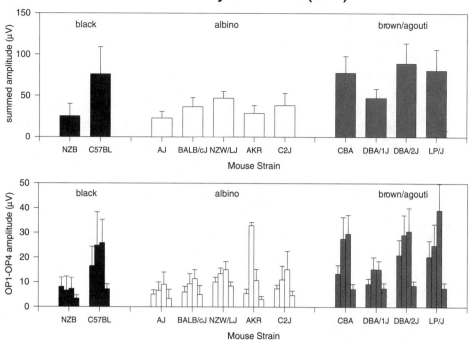

FIGURE 81.6   Upper panel, Summed oscillatory potentials (± 1 standard error) across strains. Lower panel, Mean amplitude (± 1 standard error) of each of the first four major oscillatory potentials.

a-wave parameters

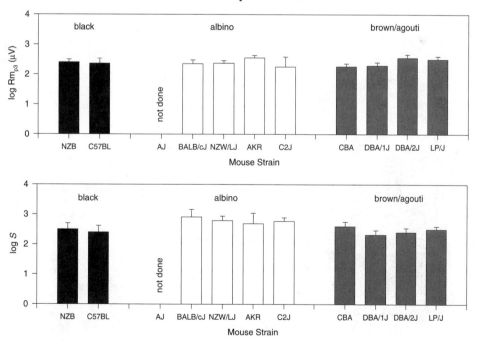

FIGURE 81.7   Rod photoreceptor structure and function. Upper panel, Saturated a-wave amplitude (± 1 standard error) across strains. Lower panel, Mean (± 1 standard error) values of photoreceptor sensitivity, S, across strains.

Rm_{P3} was not statistically different across or within strains (mean Rm_{P3} = 266.4 ± 89.0 mV, P = 0.342). In contrast, S, the photoresponse sensitivity, differed across the three coat colors. Log S was found to be 2.43 (± 0.21), 2.84 (± 0.18), and 2.45 (± 0.16) for the black, albino, and brown/agouti strains, respectively (P < 0.0001). In addition, significant differences were found among strains for the albino and agouti strains but not among the black strains (P > 0.10).

CONE-MEDIATED RESPONSES   A summary of cone-mediated responses is given in figure 81.8. Cone maximal amplitude across all strains ranged from 32.9 (± 21.0) mV to 116.5 (± 32.0) mV. Statistically different responses were not found across the black strains (77.8 ± 32 mV, P = 0.014). However, substantial differences in cone amplitude were found for the albino strains (69.6 ± 34 mV, P < 0.0001) and for the brown/agouti strains (95.4 ± 29 mV, P < 0.0001). As shown in figure 81.9, cone maximum amplitude and ERG threshold intensity were highly correlated (r = −0.93, P < 0.0001). Finally, implicit time of the major b-wave peak was not significantly different across strains (44.0 ± 5.4 ms).

ROD- VERSUS CONE-MEDIATED COMPARISONS   A comparison of maximal rod- and cone-mediated amplitudes is shown in figure 81.10. In general, rod- and cone-mediated amplitudes were correlated across all strains (r = 0.60, P < 0.0001). Within individual strains, correlations ranged from +0.43 to +0.93. However, for AJ and LP/j mice, rod function and cone function were uncorrelated. This means that for these strains, cone function could not be predicted from the responses that were rod-mediated. In addition, for strains with weak correlations, a high rod amplitude did not necessarily predict a high cone amplitude. For example, in figure 81.10, the albino strain with the highest rod amplitude (V_{max}) had only intermediate cone amplitudes.

General conclusions

The electrophysiological and analytical techniques based on the ERG can be powerful tools to better understand the sites and mechanisms of disease action in mouse models of ocular disease. The ERG is a commonly used technique to assess panretinal function and can be dissected to quantify and evaluate the functional integrity of different retinal layers. The ERG has been used extensively to describe the retinal phenotype in mouse models of human retinal disease and has been used to evaluate the efficacy of a broad spectrum of genetic and pharmaceutical interventions. At the present time, however, there are no internationally accepted standards for recording ERGs in mice.

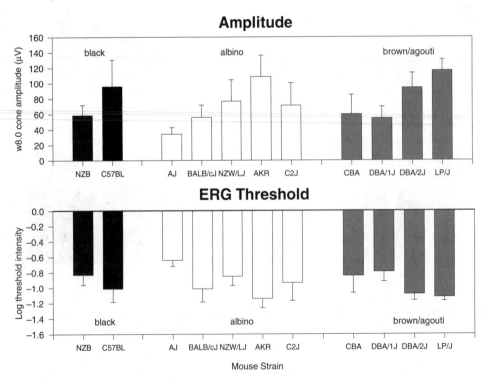

FIGURE 81.8   Upper panel, Mean (± 1 standard error) cone-mediated b-wave maximal amplitudes across strains. Lower panel, Mean (± 1 standard error) cone ERG threshold intensity across strains.

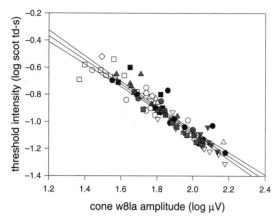

FIGURE 81.9 Correlation between cone ERG threshold and the maximal cone b-wave amplitude across strains.

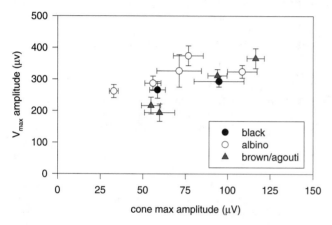

FIGURE 81.10 Rod- versus cone-mediated function. Each data point represents the mean response with error bars for each strain. (See text for discussion.)

While there are abundant published ERG data on mutant mice, little has been published that documents retinal function across normal inbred strains without known retinopathy. In addition, little is known about how retinal function in the normal mouse alters during the aging process. Within the context of our understanding of the cellular origins of different components of the ERG, such studies could provide insights into which cells in the retina are most susceptible to aging and disease.

As a first step, we have characterized retinal function with the ERG across a range of normal inbred strains that are commonly used in vision science. While there were many subtle differences between strains that could be dismissed as normal variability, some differences were substantial and statistically significant, suggesting differences in cellular function. Some of the differences can be relatively easily

explained. For example, the albino strains were generally more sensitive to light than the pigmented and agouti strains. These differences in sensitivity are largely due to differences in ocular melanin, which absorbs light, thereby reducing the amount of light reaching the photoreceptors. The underlying mechanisms responsible for other differences in ERG parameters are not yet understood. Ongoing work in our own laboratory is focused on determining the reliability and replicability of these differences, how ERG parameters are altered during aging, and the underlying cellular variations that could cause such differences.

REFERENCES

1. Alexander K, Fishman GA, Peachy NS, Marchese AL, Tso MO: "On" response defect in paraneoplastic night blindness with cutaneous malignant melanoma. *Invest Ophthalmol Vis Sci* 1992; 33:477.
2. Birch DG, Hood DC, Nusinowitz S, Pepperberg DR: Abnormal activation and inactivation mechanisms of rod transduction of patients with autosomal dominant retinitis and the PRO-23-HIS mutation. *Invest Ophthalmol Vis Sci* 1996; 36:1603.
3. Breton ME, Montzka D: Empiric limits of rod photocurrent component underlying a-wave response in the electroretinogram. *Doc Ophthalmol* 1992; 79:337.
4. Breton ME, Schueller AW, Lamb TD, Pugh EN Jr: Analysis of ERG a-wave amplification and kinetics in terms of the G-protein cascade of phototransduction. *Invest Ophthalmol Vis Sci* 1994; 35:295.
5. Bush RA, Hawks KW, Sieving PA: Preservation of inner retinal responses in the aged Royal College of Surgeons rat: Evidence against glutamate excitotoxicity in photoreceptor degeneration. *Invest Ophthalmol Vis Sci* 1995; 36:2054.
6. Calderone JB, Jacobs GH: Regional variations in the relative sensitivity to UV light in the mouse retina. *Vis Neurosci* 1995; 12:463.
7. Carter-Dawson L, LaVail MM: Rods and cones in the mouse retina: I. Structural analysis using light and electron microscopy. *J Comp Neurol* 1979; 188:245.
8. Cideciyan AV, Jacobson SG: Negative electroretinograms in retinitis pigmentosa. *Invest Ophthalmol Vis Sci* 1993; 34:3253.
9. Ekesten B, Gouras P, Moschos M: Cone properties of the light-adapted murine ERG. *Doc Ophthalmol* 1998; 97:23.
10. Goto Y, Peachey NS, Ripps H, Naash MI: Functional abnormalities in transgenic mice expressing a mutant rhodopsin gene. *Invest Ophthalmol Vis Sci* 1995; 36:62.
11. Goto Y, Peachey NS, Ziroli NE, Seiple WH, Gryczan C, Pepperberg DR, Naash MI: Rod phototransduction in transgenic mice expressing a mutant opsin gene. *J Opt Soc Am A Opt Image Sci* 1996; 13:577.
12. Goto Y, Peachey NS, Ziroli NE, Seiple WH, Gryczan C, Pepperberg DR, Naash MI: Rod phototransduction in transgenic mice expressing a mutant opsin gene. *J Opt Soc Am A Opt Image Sci* 1996; 13:577.
13. Granit R: Two types of retinae and their electrical responses to intermittent stimuli in dark and light adaptation. *J Physiol* 1935; 85:421.
14. Granit R: *Receptors and Sensory Perception.* New Haven, CT, Yale University Press, 1955.

15. Green DG, Kapousta-Bruneau NV, Hitchcock PF, Keller SA: Electrophysiology and density of retinal neurons in mice with a mutation that includes the Pax2 locus, *Invest Ophthalmol Vis Sci* 1997; 38:919.

16. Griff ER: Electroretinographic components arising in the distal retina. In Heckenlively JR, Arden GB (eds): *Principles and Practice of Clinical Electrophysiology of Vision*. St. Louis, Mosby, 1991, pp 91–98.

17. Hetling JR, Pepperberg DR: Sensitivity and kinetics of mouse rod flash responses determined in vivo from paired-flash electroretinograms. *J Physiol* 1999; 516:593.

18. Heynen H, Van Norren D: Origin of the electroretinogram in the intact macaque eye: I. *Vision Res* 1985; 25:697.

19. Heynen H, Wachtmeister L, Van Norren D: Origin of the oscillatory potentials in the primate retina. *Vision Res* 1985; 25:1365.

20. Hood DC, Birch DG: The a-wave of the human electroretinogram and rod receptor function. *Invest Ophthalmol Vis Sci* 1990; 31:2070.

21. Hood DC, Birch DG: A quantitative measure of the electrical activity of human rod photoreceptors using electroretinography. *Vis Neurosci* 1990; 5:379.

22. Hood DC, Birch DG: Rod phototransduction in retinitis pigmentosa: Estimation and interpretation of parameters derived from the rod a-wave. *Invest Ophthalmol Vis Sci* 1994; 35: 2948.

23. Jacobs GH: Ultraviolet vision in vertebrates. *Am Zool* 1992; 32:544.

24. Jacobs GH, Neitz J, Deegan JF III: Retinal receptors in rodents maximally sensitive to ultraviolet light. *Nature* 1991; 353:655.

25. Karwoski C, Kawasaki K: Oscillatory potentials. In Heckenlively JH, Arden GB (eds): *Handbook of Clinical Electrophysiology of Vision Testing*. St Louis, Mosby Year Book, 1991, pp 125–128.

26. Kedzierski W, Lloyd M, Birch D, Bok D, Travis G: Generation and analysis of transgenic mice expressing P216L-substituted Rds/Peripherin in rod photoreceptors. *Invest Ophthalmol Vis Sci* 1997; 38:498.

27. Lyubarsky AL, Falsini B, Pennesi ME, Valentini P, Pugh EN Jr: UV- and midwave-sensitive cone-driven retinal responses of the mouse: A possible phenotype for coexpression of cone photopigments. *J Neurosci* 1999; 19:442.

28. Marti A, Hafezi F, Lansel N, Hegi ME, Wenzel A, Grimm C, Niemeyer G, Remae CE: Light-induced cell death of retinal photoreceptors in the absence of p53. *Inv Ophthal Vis Sci* 1998; 39:846.

29. Menner E: Untersuchunger uber die Retina mit besonderer Berucksichtigung der ausseren Kornerschichte. *Z vergl Physiol* 1928; 8:761.

30. Miller RF, Dowling JE: Intracellular responses of Muller (glial) cells of the mudpuppy retina: Their relation to the b-wave of the electroretinogram. *J Neurophysiol* 1970; 33:323.

31. Miyake Y, Yagasaki K, Horiguchi M, Kawase Y: On- and off-responses in photopic electroretinogram in complete and incomplete types of congenital stationary night blindness. *Jpn J Ophthalmol* 1987; 31:81.

32. Newman EA, Odette LL: Model of electroretinogram b-wave generation: A test of the K+ hypothesis. *J Neurophysiol* 1984; 51:164.

33. Nusinowitz S, Nguyen L, Farber D, Danciger M: Electroretinographic evidence for reduced phototransduction gain and slowed photoreceptor recovery in albino mice with a MET450 variant in RPE65. *Exp Eye Res* 2003; 77(5):627–638.

34. Nusinowitz S, Ridder W, Heckenlively JR: Electrodiagnostic techniques for visual function testing in mice. In Smith R, John SWM, Nishina PM, Sundberg JP (eds): *Systematic Evaluation of the Mouse Eye: Anatomy, Pathology, and Biomethods*. New York, CRC Press, 2002, pp 320–344.

35. Ogden TE: The oscillatory waves of the primate electroretinogram. *Vision Res* 1973; 13:1059.

36. Pardue MT, McCall MA, LaVail MM, Gregg RG, Peachey NS: A naturally occurring mouse model of X-linked congenital stationary night blindness. *Invest Ophthal Vis Sci* 1998; 39:2443.

37. Peachey NS, Goto Y, al-Ubaidi MR, Naash MI: Properties of the mouse cone-mediated electroretinogram during light adaptation. *Neurosci Lett* 1993; 162:9.

38. Peachey NS, Roveri L, Messing A, McCall MA: Functional consequences of oncogene-induced horizontal cell degeneration in the retinas of transgenic mice. *Vis Neurosci* 1997; 14:627.

39. Penn RD, Hagins WA: Signal transmission along retinal rods and the origin of the electroretinographic a-wave. *Nature* 1969; 223:201.

40. Ren JC, LaVail MM, Peachey NS: Retinal degeneration in the nervous mutant mouse: III. Electrophysiological studies of the visual pathway. *Exp Eye Res* 2000; 70:467.

41. Ridder W, Azimi A, Heckenlively JH, Nusinowitz S: Cataractogenesis in anesthetized mice. *Curr Eye Res* 2002; 75(3):365–370.

42. Robson JG, Frishman LJ: Response linearity and kinetics of the cat retina: The bipolar cell component of the dark-adapted electroretinogram. *Vis Neurosci* 1995; 12:837.

43. Rohrer B, Korenbrot JI, LaVail MM, Reichardt LF, Xu B: Role of neurotrophin receptor TrkB in the maturation of rod photoreceptors and establishment of synaptic transmission to the inner retina. *J Neurosci* 1999; 19:8919.

44. Ruether K, van de Pol D, Jaissle G, Berger W, Tornow RP, Zrenner E, Retinoschisis-like alterations in the mouse eye caused by gene targeting of the Norrie disease gene. *Invest Ophthal Vis Sci* 1997; 38:710.

45. Seeliger MW, Grimm C, Stahlberg F, Friedburg C, Jaissle G, Zrenner E, Guo H, Reme CE, Humphries P, Hofmann F, Biel M, Fariss RN, Redmond TM, Wenzel A: New views on RPE65 deficiency: The rod system is the source of vision in a mouse model of Leber congenital amaurosis. *Nat Genet* 2001; 29(1):70–74.

46. Shaaban SA, Crognale ME, Calderone JB, Huang J, Jacobs G, Deeb SS: Transgenic mice expressing a functional human photopigment. *Invest Ophthalmol Vis Sci* 1998; 39:1036.

47. Sidman RL, Histochemical studies on photoreceptor cells. *Ann N Y Acad Sci* 1958; 74:182.

48. Sieving P: Photopic "ON" and "OFF" pathway abnormalities in retinal dystrophies. *Trans Am Ophthalmol Soc* 1993; 91: 701.

49. Sieving PA, Frishman LJ, Steinberg RH: Scotopic threshold response of proximal retina in cat. *J Neurophysiol* 1986; 56:1049.

50. Smith SB, Hamasaki DI: Electroretinographic study of the C57BL/6-mivit/mivit mouse model of retinal degeneration. *Invest Ophthalmol Vis Sci* 1994; 35:3119.

51. Stockton RA, Slaughter MM: B-wave of the electroretinogram: Reflection of ON bipolar cell activity. *J Gen Physiol* 1989; 93:101.

52. Sugawara T, Sieving PA, Bush RA: Quantitative relationship of the scotopic and photopic ERG to photoreceptor cell loss in light damaged rats. *Exp Eye Res* 2000; 70:693.

53. Sun H, Macke JP, Nathans J: Mechanisms of spectral tuning in the mouse green cone pigment. *Proc Natl Acad Sci U S A* 1997; 94:8860.

54. Wachtmeister L: Oscillatory potentials in the retina: What do they reveal. *Prog Retin Eye Res* 1998; 17:485.

55. Wachtmeister L, Dowling JE: The oscillatory potentials of the mudpuppy retina. *Invest Ophthalmol Vis Sci* 1978; 17:1176.

56. Wu J, Peachey NS, Marmorstein AD: Light-evoked responses of the mouse retinal pigment epithelium. *J Neurophysiol* 2004; 91(3):1134–1142.

57. Yang RB, Robinson SW, Xiong WH, Yau KW, Birch DG, Garbers DL: Disruption of a retinal guanylyl cyclase gene leads to cone-specific dystrophy and paradoxical rod behavior, *J Neurosci* 1999; 19:5889.

58. Xu XJ, Karwoski CJ: Current source density analysis of retinal field potentials: 2. Pharmacological analysis of the b-wave and m-wave. *J Neurophysiol* 1994; 72:96.

82 Electroretinograms of Dog and Chicken

SIMON PETERSEN-JONES, NALINEE TUNTIVANICH, FABIANO MONTIANI-FERREIRA, AND NAHEED W. KHAN

LARGER ANIMAL COLONIES with retinal dystrophy are increasing in importance as models of human conditions, particularly for the testing of therapeutic strategies. Spontaneously occurring retinal dystrophies are recognized in both dogs and chickens. Hereditary disease that leads to vision loss in the dog is also important because this species plays a valuable role in human life, not only as a working and service animal, tasks for which vision is required, but also as a companion animal. In addition to its use as a laboratory model for the study of retinal disease, the chicken is widely used for the study of ametropias.

This chapter will elucidate some practical aspects of canine and chicken ERGs, give examples, and show some of the changes that can be seen in inherited retinal diseases.

The canine electroretinogram

The dog is becoming more widely recognized as an important model for human retinal dystrophies. There are a number of different spontaneously occurring hereditary retinal degenerations in the dog, and this coupled with the fact that the dog eye is very similar in size to the human eye makes the canine retinal dystrophies important for the study of retinal dysfunction and the therapeutic approaches to save vision.

Electroretinography is commonly performed on dogs by veterinary ophthalmologists to investigate retinal disease in working and companion dogs and by researchers utilizing the dog as a model for human disease. The increased utilization of the dog as a model of human disease demands that the normal canine electroretinogram (ERG) is fully characterized so that this technique can be most effectively utilized.

There are some important differences between the dog and human retina. For example, the dog does not appear to have an area with predominance of cones and does not have a fovea. The dog retina does have a region called the visual streak (or area centralis) in which there is greater ganglion cell density,[58] and it is this region that is used for most detailed vision. As with humans, there are many more rods in the canine retina than cones, but the exact rod-to-cone ratio has not been reported. There are some reports describing how the distribution of cones varies across the retina

although the results vary between the publications (see the review by Miller and Murphy[42]). The dog has dichromatic color vision having two types of cone: one with peak spectral absorbance at 429–435 nm and the other at 555 nm.[31,53] Peak spectral absorption of the canine rod photopigment rhodopsin is 508 nm.[31]

The following section gives examples of ERGs in the normal dog and in dogs with hereditary retinal disease.

METHODS OF RECORDING CANINE ERGS   Techniques used to record the canine ERG are described in chapter 83. The ERGs shown in the current chapter were recorded from anesthetized dogs (typically sedated with acepromazine, induced with thiopentone, and anesthesia maintained with halothane or isoflurane delivered in oxygen). Although anesthetic agents can alter the ERG responses,[36,84] anesthesia is required to immobilize the dog. Ganzfeld flash ERGs were recorded with an LKC UTAS E-3000 electrophysiology unit (LKC Technologies, Gaithersburg, MD). Although 20 minutes of dark adaptation is recommended by the standards established by the European College of Veterinary Ophthalmologists (ECVO) ERG committee,[51] we find that dark-adapting the eye for at least 45–60 minutes results in greater amplitudes in the scotopic ERG. We have also shown that if a dog is examined by indirect ophthalmoscopy or fundus photographs are taken immediately prior to the ERG session, the period of dark adaptation time must be increased to at least 60 minutes to achieve ERG amplitudes comparable to those that can be recorded after 20 minutes of dark adaptation[76] (if examination with bright lights had not been performed.) Typically, the pupil is maximally dilated by topical application of tropicamide or a combination of tropicamide and phenylephrine. The pupil diameter is monitored before and after the procedure because some drugs used for premedication or anesthesia can result in pupillary constriction and some individual dogs develop miosis after anesthesia, despite repeated application of mydriatics.

The selection of recording lens can influence the amplitudes and also, to some extent, the shape of the ERG recorded from dogs. In a study comparing three different electrodes, we found that significantly higher amplitudes were recorded using either a DTL fiber electrode or an ERG-Jet lens electrode compared to the amplitudes recorded by using a bipolar Burian-Allen lens.[40] This finding differs from the results obtained in human patients, in which the Burian-Allen lens tended to result in greater amplitudes compared to the other electrodes.[21] Additionally, we demonstrated that in using monopolar electrodes, choosing a consistent position of the reference electrode is very important. When we compared amplitudes obtained by using the ERG-Jet lens electrode and a skin reference electrode positioned 1, 3, or 5 cm caudal to the lateral canthus of the eye we found that between the three reference electrode positions, the further caudally the electrode, the greater the amplitude.[40] A study of canine perfused eyes found that the greatest ERG could be recorded in that system with a corneal contact electrode when the reference electrode was placed on the posterior sclera adjacent to the optic nerve.[17] The lack of a complete bony wall to the lateral orbit in the dog may mean that there is less electrical resistance between a skin electrode positioned more posteriorly and the current generated in the retina than there would be in a human with a complete bony orbit, given that bone offers greater electrical resistance than soft tissues. These studies demonstrate the importance of standardization of equipment and technique if ERGs are to be comparable.

In addition to the effect of recording technique on ERG amplitudes, the breed and age of dog are important. Dogs represent one of the most phenotypically diverse species (compare a chihuahua with a Great Dane, for example), so it is perhaps not surprising that normal ERG amplitudes can differ considerably between breeds of dog. Amplitudes also tend to decrease with age. For any study using a particular breed of dog, it is important that an appropriate breed- and age-matched control is available, particularly in trying to detect the early stages of retinal disease.

MATURATION OF THE CANINE ERG   The retina of the dog is not fully developed at birth. Retinal maturation occurs over the first couple of months of age (figure 82.1). When the eyes of puppies open at between 10 and 14 days of age, the ERG is just a low-amplitude negative waveform in response to brighter flashes of light. By 4 weeks of age, the ERG waveform is adultlike with an a-wave, a b-wave, and oscillatory potentials. Maximal amplitudes are achieved by about 7 weeks of age and appear to decrease slightly after that age as the animal matures; a- and b-wave response thresholds are at their lowest intensity by a similar age (7 weeks).

COMPONENTS OF THE CANINE ERG   In addition to the a- and b-waves and oscillatory potentials (figure 82.1), other components of the canine ERG have been described. The scotopic threshold response (STR) can be recorded under specific recording conditions with good dark adaptation[85,86] but can be reduced by the use of some anesthetic agents.[84]

The early receptor potential described in other species has not been reported in the dog, probably because of the technical difficulties in recording this response.[48] Similarly, there are no reports of investigation of the canine M-wave. Averaging several flashes of red light has been reported to allow the separation of a cone-derived x-wave from the b-wave.[50] A photopic i-wave can be seen in the dog,[66] although we have found that the selection of recording electrode is important in being able to record this response. See figure 82.5C later in the chapter for an example of a canine i-wave. Consideration of the d-wave is included in the section about canine long-flash responses.

ANALYSIS OF THE CANINE ERG   Canine ERGs can be analyzed similarly to those of other species. a- and b-wave amplitudes and implicit times can be measured. Scotopic and photopic intensity-response curves can be plotted, and a- and b-wave thresholds can be calculated. To allow for consistent comparison, a criterion threshold value can be selected. The Naka-Rusthon formula can be applied to fit the b-wave intensity-response curve and used to derive a value for maximal rod photoreceptor response (Vb_{max}), and a value for retinal sensitivity (k) may be calculated (k = the intensity that gives a response of $1/2\ Vb_{max}$).

LONG-FLASH ERG IN THE DOG   Figure 82.2 shows a typical example of a canine long-flash ERG. The stimulus for photopic ON-OFF recordings (long-flash ERGs) were as described by Sieving.[73] A stimulus of $200\,cd/m^2$ (typically, a 150- to 200-ms flash duration was chosen) was presented on a background light of $34\,cd/m^2$. The ON response has typical a- and b-waves. Following the b-wave is a plateau that varies between slightly rising (as in figure 82.4 later in the chapter) and slightly decreasing. At the onset of the OFF response, there is often a small positive deflection that is then followed by a large negative deflection similar in amplitude to the b-wave. At the trough of the negative deflection, there is a small positive deflection followed by a large positive waveform that returns to baseline. The OFF response of the dog is thus similar to that of the rat.[49] This represents a response from what Granit[25] classified as an excitatory (E-type) retina rather than an inhibitory (I-type) retina as in the human and the chicken (see below). It is not clear whether the small positive wave seen at the onset of the OFF response represents the equivalent of the d-wave recorded in other species, such as primates, or whether the large negative response is the equivalent of the d-wave.

EXAMPLES OF ERG CHANGES IN CANINE RETINAL DYSTROPHIES   Canine retinal dystrophies include models for retinitis pigmentosa and for Leber congenital amaurosis. The retinitis pigmentosa models in dogs are known as the progressive retinal atrophies and occur in several different

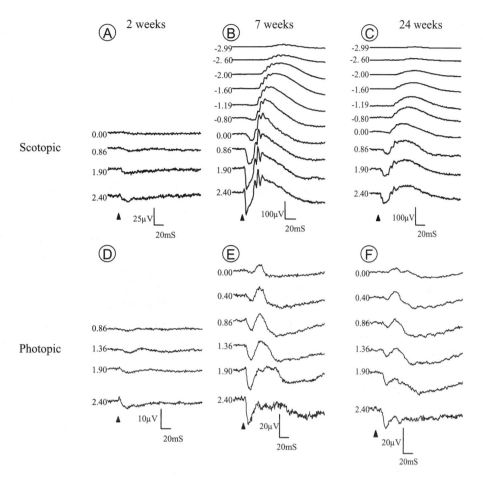

FIGURE 82.1 Maturation of the canine ERG. The tracings are from the same dog. Panels A, B, and C show scotopic intensity series responses, while panels D, E, and F are photopic intensity series responses. Panels A and D are at 2 weeks of age, panels B and E at 7 weeks of age, and panels C and F at 24 weeks of age. Arrowheads indicate the onset of flash.

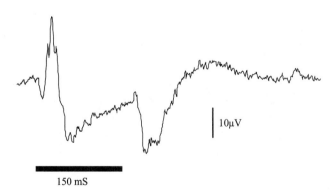

FIGURE 82.2 Long-flash ERG from a dog. This shows the photopic long-flash ERG from a normal adult dog. This is the result of a 150-ms flash of 200 cd/m^2 superimposed on a background light of 34 cd/m^2. The ON response is characterized by an a- and a b-wave. There is a plateau region while the light remains on. The OFF response is characterized by a small positive deflection followed by a large negative response, similar in amplitude to the b-wave. At the trough of the negative OFF response, there is often a small positive deflection, which is followed by a larger positive waveform that passes the baseline before returning to baseline.

breeds of dog. The progressive retinal atrophies show genetic heterogeneity. The gene mutations underlying some of the forms have been identified. Phenotypically, the progressive retinal atrophies can be divided into early- and late-onset forms.

Progressive retinal atrophies Some of the early-onset forms are given the phenotypic description *rod-cone dysplasias* because photoreceptor development becomes halted during development, and this is followed by a rapid loss of rod photoreceptors with a much slower loss of cones. The first form was described in the Irish setter breed and is known as rod-cone degeneration type 1 (*rcd1*),[9,14] the second form was described in the collie (*rcd2*),[81] and the third form was described in the Cardigan Welsh corgi (*rcd3*).[32] *Rcd1* is caused by a point mutation resulting in a premature stop codon in the gene encoding the rod cyclic GMP phosphodiesterase beta subunit (*PDE6B*).[16,74] The gene mutation underlying *rcd2* has not been identified, and that underlying *rcd3* is a 1-bp deletion in the gene encoding the rod cyclic

GMP phosphodiesterase alpha subunit (*PDE6A*) leading to a premature stop codon.[60] The mutations in *PDE6A* and *PDE6B* are most likely functional *null* mutations. The rod cyclic GMP phosphodiesterase enzyme requires the presence of both alpha and beta excitatory subunits for normal activity. When one subunit is missing or is nonfunctional, phosphodiesterase activity is much reduced,[62] so the substrate cyclic GMP accumulates. In similar animal models, such as the *rd1* mouse, it has been shown that the accumulation of cyclic GMP and the resulting opening of an increased proportion of cyclic GMP-gated channels in the cell membrane trigger apoptosis in the rod photoreceptor.[34] Cones, although genetically normal, are affected by the loss of surrounding rods and are halted in their development and then degenerate slowly.[9,14,15] Figure 82.3 shows representative scotopic and photopic ERG intensity series from an *rcd3*-affected dog. The *rcd3* dogs lack rod-mediated responses at all ages. This very-early-onset abnormality suggests, as would be expected given the lack of functional rod cyclic GMP phosphodiesterase alpha subunit, that normal rod phototransduction does not develop in the affected dogs. The developmental abnormalities of cones are reflected functionally in a significant reduction of the photopic a-wave amplitude as early as 3 weeks of age (figure 82.3F). The photopic b-wave of the affected dogs is not significantly different from that of breed-matched normal controls until later in the disease process.[61] Although cone function is abnormal

from a very early age, the loss of cones is relatively slow (unpublished histological findings), and sufficient vision in good lighting conditions to allow negotiation of obstacle courses is maintained for two to four years. It is of note that only a small photopic b-wave remains in these animals, and histological examination of the retina of affected dogs in this age range that still have some residual vision reveals that they have only isolated areas with residual cone photoreceptor cells apparently with just stunted inner segments.

Of the later-onset forms of progressive retinal atrophy in dogs, one form called *progressive rod-cone degeneration* (*prcd*) is known to be present in several different breeds.[3–5] *Prcd* maps to canine chromosome 9,[2,24,41,72] although the actual gene defect underlying it had not been published at the time of writing. In *prcd*, the photoreceptors mature normally, but then there is a progressive rod-led loss of photoreceptors.[6] The loss of photoreceptors is reflected in a progressive reduction in ERG amplitudes. Figure 82.4 shows an example of a dog presented for early diagnosis of *prcd*. The rod responses are affected first,[8,67] but changes are not seen until after normal maturation and probably reflect a loss of total number of photoreceptors rather than a generalized abnormality in photoreceptor function. The shape of the dark-adapted waveforms are essentially normal; however, the response threshold is elevated, and the a- and b-wave amplitudes are both reduced to a similar extent (compare figure 82.4B with figure 82.4A). The photopic responses are still

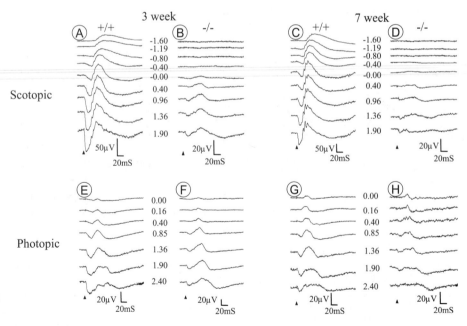

FIGURE 82.3 ERGs from an *rcd3* dog. Representative scotopic (A–D) and photopic (E–H) inensity series responses from a normal control dog (A, C, E, and G) compared to a PDE6A mutant/*rcd3* dog (B, D, F, and H) at 3 weeks (A, B and E, F) and 7 weeks (C, D and G, H) of age. Arrowheads indicate the onset of flash.

well preserved at this stage (compare figure 82.4D with figure 82.4C).

Dog model of Leber congenital amaurosis Leber congenital amaurosis (LCA) is an early-onset severe retinal dystrophy with vision loss in childhood.[59] Similarly to retinitis pigmentosa, it shows genetic heterogeneity.[28] LCA type II results from mutations in *RPE65*,[19,26,46,75] a gene encoding a 65-kDa protein expressed in retinal pigment epithelium (RPE) that plays a role in the visual cycle.[64] A spontaneously occurring dog model of LCA type II in the briard breed has been investigated.[52,82,83] The original colony that was characterized and in which the mutation in *RPE65* was identified was established in Sweden; hence, the name *Swedish briard dog* came into use, although "Swedish briard" is not a separate breed from the briard. The mutation identified in the briard dog is a 4-bp deletion leading to a premature stop codon.[78] The affected dogs have a lack of dim light vision and a variable degree of daytime vision loss. Studies in mice

have shown that the lack of *RPE65* protein activity means that 11-*cis*-retinal is not recycled from the RPE to the photoreceptors.[64] There is therefore a lack of formation of visual pigment and a resultant failure in normal rod phototransduction.[64] In affected dogs, there is only a slow degeneration of photoreceptors, and as the animals get older, there is a progressive accumulation of retinyl esters in the RPE.[82,83] The lack of phototransduction is reflected in the ERG of affected dogs,[54] as can be seen in the representative ERGs in figure 82.5. Comparison of dark-adapted with light-adapted ERG waveforms in the *RPE65* dog reveal that the intensity-matched responses are very similar in amplitude, suggesting that the majority of the response recorded in the *RPE65* mutant dog at this age is cone-mediated; similar findings are reported in children with *RPE65* mutations[37] and *RPE65* knock-out mice.[64] An ERG study using *RPE65* knock-out mice suggested that the mutant mice have a pronounced loss of UV cone function with preservation of M cone function.[20] Similar studies have not been reported in dogs. However a study utilizing double knockout mice that had a lack or functional *RPE65* with either a lack of functional

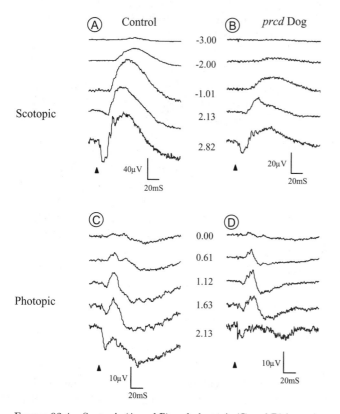

FIGURE 82.4 Scotopic (A and B) and photopic (C and D) intensity series responses from a *prcd* dog (B and D) compared to a normal control (A and C). The dog being tested had been observed to have some subtle bilateral fundoscopic changes that were not considered to be diagnostic for PRA and was referred for ERG testing. The ERGs clearly showed a marked decrease in ERG amplitudes compared to the normal control dog, showing that the test dog had a generalized retinal dysfunction. Arrowheads indicate the onset of flash.

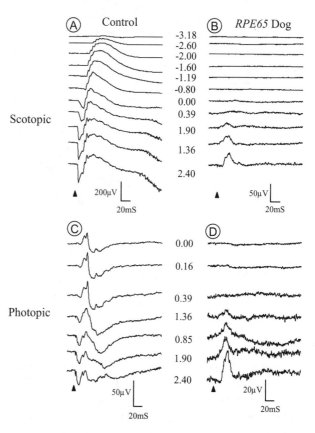

FIGURE 82.5 Scotopic (A and B) and photopic (C and D) intensity series responses from an *RPE65* mutant dog (B and D) compared with a normal control (A and C). Arrowheads indicate the onset of flash.

rods or a lack of functional cones showed that the major ERG response was due to a response from desensitized rods,[68] although it was subsequently shown that a small cone derived response was also recordable.[65]

OTHER CANINE MODELS This article has given only some selected examples of ERGs of dog retinal dystrophy models. There are other canine retinal dystrophy models in which the gene mutation has been described, such as X-linked PRA (due to mutations in RP GTPase regulator; *RPGR* mutations),[87] dominantly inherited PRA (due to a mutation in the rod opsin gene),[33] and achromatopsia in the cone dysplasia dog (due to a mutation in cyclic nucleotide-gated channel beta-subunit gene; *CNGB3*).[10,68,69] There are also other canine models that have been phenotypically characterized but for which the causal gene mutation has not been identified, such as the rod dysplasia (*rd*) Norwegian elkhound,[7] the early retinal degeneration (*erd*) Norwegian elkhound,[1] and the photoreceptor dysplasia (*pd*) miniature schnauzer.[57] Many other naturally occurring canine retinal dystrophies remain to be characterized. The publishing of the canine genome[35] and the development of tools for disease mapping mean that it is becoming progressively easier to identify the gene mutations underlying the myriad of genetic diseases that occur in pure-bred dogs. This will provide the opportunity to establish further colonies of experimental dogs for study and investigation of potential therapies for homologues of human disease.

SUMMARY This article has emphasized the canine ERG in hereditary retinal disease. ERG studies in dogs are performed for other reasons, such as the investigation of ocular disease in veterinary medicine and in toxicology studies. Although the ERG of the dog has been well described in several studies, there is a need for further characterization, particularly in view of the emergence of the dog as an important model species of human diseases.

Electroretinography in the chicken

There are a few spontaneously occurring retinal dystrophies in chickens, although thus far, the gene mutation underlying only one of these diseases has been identified.

The chicken retina has a number of differences from the human retina. The retina is avascular, receiving its nutrition from the vitreous and via the choroid. Birds have a highly vascular structure called the pecten that protrudes from the surface of the optic nerve head into the vitreous. There are several theories as to the purpose of the pecten, one of which is that it is involved in supplying nutrition to the inner retina via the vitreous. The chicken has a relatively cone-rich retina compared to humans and canines. Most of the cones

contain colored oil droplets within the photoreceptor inner segments. These droplets act as spectral filters for the light that reaches the outer segments. The cones are divided into single cones and double cones. Double cones consist of a principal cone (similar in structure to a normal single cone), which contains an oil droplet, and an accessory cone, which curves around the inner segment of the principal cone and, according to some authors, only rarely contains a miniscule oil droplet,[11] whereas others report that it has one or more oil droplets.[79] On the basis of morphological appearance, three separate forms of double cone have been described.[80] Four cone visual pigments are recognized: ultraviolet, short-wavelength, middle-wavelength, and long-wavelength. A different type of oil droplet is matched with each of the four visual pigments.[11] The visual pigment in both members of the double cone is the same as that found in the long-wavelength-sensitive single cone. The reported proportion of each of the photoreceptor types in the chicken retina differs between studies. For example, Bowmaker and Knowles[12] reported that double cones account for 50–60% of photoreceptors, whereas Morris[47] reported that in the central retina, the ratios were 14% rods, 32% double cones, and 54% single cones and peripherally, 33% rods, 30% double cones, and 37% single cones.

METHODS OF RECORDING THE CHICKEN ERG The chicken ERGs shown in this chapter were recorded from anesthetized chickens (typically with isoflurane delivered in oxygen). The flash ERGs were recorded by using an LKC Utas 3000 electrophysiology unit (LKC) with a Ganzfeld unit. A bipolar Burian-Allen lens (Hansen Ophthalmic Development Laboratories, Coralville, Iowa) was used with the ground electrode placed in the hind leg. Conjunctival stay sutures were used to stabilize the globe and keep the recording lens in position. Hypromellose (0.25–0.5%) was used as a coupling solution for the lens. Birds have striated muscle in their iris; therefore, the pupil does not dilate with the topical parasympatholytic or sympathomimetic drugs used in mammals. Topical neuromuscular blocking drugs were used to induce mydriasis; for example, topical 1% vecuronium bromide given 20 minutes prior to the procedure.

NORMAL CHICKEN ERG The chick retina is well developed at hatch. The ERG can be recorded from the chick embryo by the eighteenth day of incubation.[55] After hatch, the ERG continues to mature over the first week or so.[56] We have found that over the first 2–3 weeks post hatch, the a- and b-wave thresholds decrease. Figures 82.6A and 82.6C show representative scotopic and photopic ERG tracings, respectively, from a normal 7-day-old chick. The cone dominance of the chicken retina means that there is a significant cone component to the dark-adapted ERG, particularly

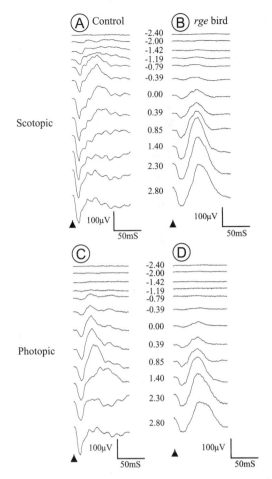

FIGURE 82.6   Representative scotopic (A and B) and photopic (C and D) intensity series responses from normal (A and C) and *rge* (B and D) 7-day-old chicks. There is a major cone component to the dark-adapted ERG in response to brighter flashes of light. The *rge* chicks have elevated response thresholds, a lack of oscillatory potentials, and enhanced b-waves to brighter flashes of light. The photopic and scotopic ERGs are very similar, indicating that rod function is more severely affected than cone function at this stage of the disease. Arrowheads indicate the onset of flash.

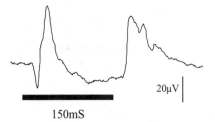

FIGURE 82.7   Long-flash ERG of a chicken. A photopic ON-OFF response to a 150-ms flash (200 cd/m^2) superimposed on a white background light of 34 cd/m^2. The ON response consists of an a- and a b-wave followed by a plateau. The OFF response consists of a positive d-wave typical of the response from an I-type retina.

those in response to brighter flashes. The light-adapted responses are of proportionally greater amplitude than would be recorded from a species with a rod-dominated retina (e.g., Mears et al.[39]).

LONG-FLASH ERG   The stimulus for the photopic ON-OFF recording (long-flash ERGs) was as described by Sieving.[73] A long-flash stimulus of 200 cd/m^2 (typically of 150-ms duration) was presented on a background light of 34 cd/m^2.

Utilization of a long-flash protocol to investigate ON and OFF responses shows that the chicken has a positive OFF response (d-wave) (figure 82.7) similar to that of humans and primates (an I-type response) but unlike rats and dogs.

CHICKEN ERGS IN DISEASE   The ERG changes that characterize some of the different forms of hereditary retinal degeneration have been reported in the chicken. These include retinal degeneration (*rd*), retinal dysplasia and degeneration (*rdd*), delayed amelanotic (*dam*), and retinopathy, globe enlarged (*rge*).

The *rd* phenotype is caused by a *null* mutation in the photoreceptor guanylate cyclase (*GUCY2D*) gene and is therefore a model of Leber congenital amaurosis type 1 in humans.[69] The *rd* birds have a severe phenotype with nonrecordable ERGs under light- or dark-adapted conditions from the time of hatch.[77]

The *rdd* chicken phenotype is sex-linked and characterized by a progressive degeneration of the retina, culminating in blindness. By 3 weeks of age, homozygotes have a flat ERG, indicative of their severe loss of visual function.[63] Linkage analysis mapped the *rdd* locus to a small region of the chicken Z chromosome with homologies to human chromosomes 5q and 9p.[13]

The *dam* chicken is characterized by a postnatal, spontaneous cutaneous amelanosis and a high incidence of blindness.[22] The main ERG change observed in this phenotype is a generalized decrease in a- and b-wave amplitudes.[23]

Retinopathy, globe enlarged chick (*rge*) is autosomal-recessive[18] and is due to a mutant locus on chicken chromosome one.[30] *Rge* chicks have unusual ERG changes.[44] The homozygous affected chicks have reduced vision, particularly in dim light, from hatch and lose functional vision at about one month after hatch.[44] The retina slowly degenerates but has some early ultrastructural abnormalities of photoreceptor synaptic terminals.[43] The ERGs are abnormal in shape from hatch, slowly deteriorate, and yet maintain relatively large amplitudes for some months after functional vision loss.[45] Examples of the affected birds' scotopic and photopic ERGs are shown in figures 82.6B and 82.6D, respectively. a- and b-wave thresholds are elevated for both the dark- and light-adapted ERGs (figure 82.8). The shape of the b-wave is abnormal, partly owing to the lack of oscillatory potentials. Interestingly, in response to very bright flashes of light, both the scotopic and photopic b-wave amplitudes of *rge* birds are supernormal for the first 6 or 7 weeks of age (see figure 82.8). Supernormal ERG amplitudes are reported in certain retinal dystrophies, including enhanced S-cone syndrome.[29,38] In this condition, there is a lack of rods and a marked increase in numbers of S-cones.[27] However, histological studies showed that *rge* chicks do not have marked alterations in photoreceptor ratios.[43] Drug dissections of the ERG of *rge* chicks revealed that intravitreous APB (2-amino-4-phosphonobutyric acid) does not block this abnormal b-wave. In the normal control chick, APB almost completely eliminates the b-wave (figure 82.9). This finding suggests that the "b-wave" of *rge* chicks may be generated

differently from the normal chicken b-wave or from different cellular components. The true basis for the ERG changes in this interesting dystrophy remains to be elucidated.

SUMMARY   The chicken ERG reflects the fact that this species has a cone-dominated retina. Spontaneously occurring retinal dystrophies have been described in this species. The only one of these to be characterized at the molecular level, the *rd* mutation, provides a model for Leber congenital amaurosis type 1. Other chicken retinal dystrophies have been characterized to varying degrees at the phenotypic level, and the chromosomal locations of the underlying genetic mutation of some forms have been mapped. The presence of naturally occurring retinal dystrophies in chickens, coupled with the large size of the eye, the cone-dominated retina, and the ease of access and manipulation of the embryo, makes this an attractive model system for studying retinal gene function in higher vertebrates.

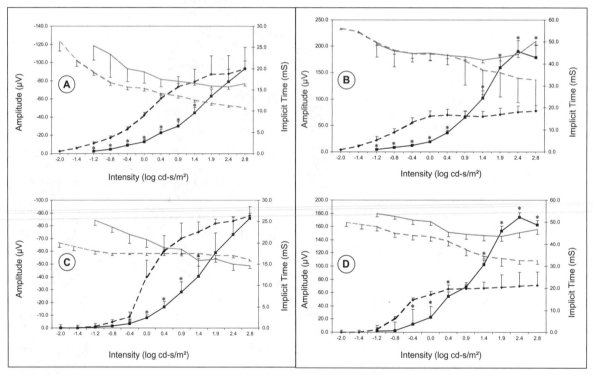

FIGURE 82.8   Scotopic and photopic a- and b-wave intensity-response and implicit time plots form normal and *rge* chicks at 7 days of age. Mean scotopic (A) and photopic (C) a-wave amplitude and implicit times and mean scotopic (B) and photopic (D) b-wave amplitude and implicit times. In each graph, the black solid curve represents the mean intensity-response curve of the *rge* birds, and the black dashed curve represents that of the control birds. The gray solid curve represents the intensity-implicit time curve of the *rge* birds, and the gray dashed curves represent the a-wave implicit time curve from normal birds. Note the increased a- and b-wave threshold of the *rge* birds compared to control birds. The scotopic and photopic b-wave amplitudes are supernormal in response to the brighter light intensities (above $1.4 \log cd\,s/m^2$). Seven control and seven *rge* birds' standard error bars are shown. (* = a significant difference at $P < 0.05$.)

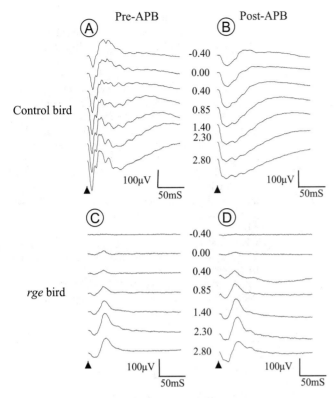

FIGURE 82.9 The effect of intravitreal APB on a normal (A and B) and a *rge* (C and D) chick flash ERG. Panels A and C are preinjection intensity-response series in dark-adapted birds. Panels B and D are post injection. Note that in the normal bird APB (which blocks on-bipolar cells) eliminates the b-wave. In the *rge* chick, APB has very little effect on the abnormal b-wave. Arrowheads indicate the onset of flash.

REFERENCES

1. Acland GM, Aguirre GD: Retinal degenerations in the dog: IV. Early retinal degeneration (erd) in the Norwegian elkhound. *Exp Eye Res* 1987; 44:491–521.
2. Acland GM, Ray K, Mellersh CS, Gu W, Langston AA, Rine J, et al: Linkage analysis and comparative mapping of canine progressive rod-cone degeneration (prcd) establishes potential locus homology with retinitis pigmentosa (RP17) in humans. *Proc Natl Acad Sci U S A* 1998; 95:3048–3053.
3. Aguirre GD, Acland GM: Progressive retinal atrophy in the English cocker spaniel. *Trans Am Coll Vet Ophthalmol* 1983; 14:104.
4. Aguirre GD, Acland GM: Variation in retinal degeneration phenotype inherited at the prcd locus. *Exp Eye Res* 1988; 46:663–687.
5. Aguirre GD, Acland GM: Progressive retinal atrophy in the Labrador retriever is a progressive rod-cone degeneration (PRCD). *Trans Am Coll Vet Ophthalmol* 1989; 20:150.
6. Aguirre GD, O'Brien P: Morphological and biochemical studies of canine progressive rod-cone degeneration. *Invest Ophthalmol Vis Sci* 1986; 27:635–655.
7. Aguirre GD, Rubin LF: An electrophysiologic approach for the early diagnosis of progressive retinal atrophy in the Norwegian elkhound. *J Am Anim Hosp Assoc* 1971; 7:136.
8. Aguirre GD, Rubin LF: Progressive retinal atrophy in the miniature poodle: An electrophysiologic study. *J Am Vet Med Assoc* 1972; 160:191–201.
9. Aguirre GD, Rubin LF: Rod-cone dysplasia (progressive retinal atrophy) in Irish setters. *J Am Vet Med Assoc* 1975; 166:157–164.
10. Aguirre GD, Rubin LF: The electroretinogram in dogs with inherited cone degeneration. *Investigative Ophthalmol Vis Sci* 1975; 14:840–847.
11. Bowmaker JK, Heath LA, Wilkie SE, Hunt DM: Visual pigments and oil droplets from six classes of photoreceptor in the retinas of birds. *Vision Res* 1997; 37:2183–2194.
12. Bowmaker JK, Knowles A: The visual pigments and oil droplets of the chicken retina. *Vision Res* 1977; 17:755–764.
13. Burt DW, Morrice DR, Lester DH, Robertson GW, Mohamed MD, Simmons I, et al: Analysis of the rdd locus in chicken: A model for human retinitis pigmentosa. *Mol Vis* 2003; 9:164–170.
14. Buyukmihci N, Aguirre GD, Marshall J: Retinal degenerations in the dog: II. Development of the retina in rod-cone dysplasia. *Exp Eye Res* 1980; 30:575–591.
15. Chader GJ, Liu YP, Fletcher RT, Aguirre G, Santos-Anderson R, Tso M: Cyclic-GMP phosphodiesterase and calmodulin in early-onset inherited retinal degenerations. *Curr Topics Membranes Transport* 1981; 15:133–156.
16. Clements PJM, Gregory CY, Petersen-Jones SM, Sargan DR, Bhattacharya SS: Confirmation of the rod cGMP phosphodiesterase β-subunit (PDEβ) nonsense mutation in affected rcd-1 Irish setters in the UK and development of a diagnostic test. *Curr Eye Res* 1993; 12:861–866.
17. Cringle SJ, Alder VA, Brown MJ, Yu DY: Effect of scleral recording location on ERG amplitude. *Curr Eye Res* 1986; 5:959–965.
18. Curtis R, Baker JR, Curtis PE, Johnston AR: An inherited retinopathy in commercial breeding chickens. *Avian Pathol* 1988; 17:87–89.
19. Dharmaraj SR, Silva ER, Pina AL, Li YY, Yang JM, Carter CR, et al: Mutational analysis and clinical correlation in Leber congenital amaurosis. *Ophthalmic Genet* 2000; 21:135–150.
20. Ekesten B, Gouras P, Salchow DJ: Ultraviolet and middle wavelength sensitive cone responses in the electroretinogram (ERG) of normal and Rpe65 −/− mice. *Vision Res* 2001; 41:2425–2433.
21. Esakowitz L, Kriss A, Shawkat F: A comparison of flash electroretinograms recorded from Burian Allen, JET, C-glide, gold foil, DTL and skin electrodes. *Eye* 1993; 7(1):169–171.
22. Fite KV, Bengston L, Doran P: Retinal pigment epithelial correlates of avian retinal degeneration: Electron microscopic analysis. *J Comp Neurol* 1985; 231:310–322.
23. Fulton AB, Fite KV, Bengston L: Retinal degeneration in the delayed amelanotic (DAM) chicken: An electroretinographic study. *Curr Eye Res* 1982; 2:757–763.
24. Goldstein O, Nelson J, Kijas J, Sidjanin D, Acland G, Aguirre G: A linkage disequilibrium map of the progressive rod cone degeneration interval [ARVO abstract]. *Invest Ophthalmol Vis Sci* 2004; 45:4756.
25. Granit R: Two types of retinas and their electrical responses to intermittent stimuli in light and dark adaptation. *J Physiol (Lond)* 1935; 85:421–428.
26. Gu SM, Thompson DA, Srikumari CR, Lorenz B, Finckh U, Nicoletti A, et al: Mutations in RPE65 cause autosomal recessive childhood-onset severe retinal dystrophy. *Nat Genet* 1997; 17:194–197.

27. Haider NB, Naggert JK, Nishina PM: Excess cone cell proliferation due to lack of a functional NR2E3 causes retinal dysplasia and degeneration in rd7/rd7 mice. *Hum Mol Genet* 2001; 10:1619–1626.

28. Hanein S, Perrault I, Gerber S, Tanguy G, Barbet F, Ducroq D, et al: Leber congenital amaurosis: Comprehensive survey of the genetic heterogeneity, refinement of the clinical definition, and genotype-phenotype correlations as a strategy for molecular diagnosis. *Hum Mut* 2004; 23:306–317.

29. Hood DC, Cideciyan AV, Roman AJ, Jacobson SG: Enhanced S cone syndrome: Evidence for an abnormally large number of S cones. *Vision Res* 1995; 35:1473–1481.

30. Inglehearn CF, Morrice DR, Lester DH, Robertson GW, Mohamed MD, Simmons I, et al: Genetic, ophthalmic, morphometric and histopathological analysis of the retinopathy globe enlarged (rge) chicken. *Mol Vis* 2003; 9:295–300.

31. Jacobs GH, Deegan JF, Crognale MA, Fenwick JA: Photopigments of dogs and foxes and their implications for canid vision. *Vis Neurosci* 1993; 10:173–180.

32. Keep JM: Clinical aspects of progressive retinal atrophy in the Cardigan Welsh corgi. *Aust Vet J* 1972; 48:197–199.

33. Kijas JW, Cideciyan AV, Aleman TS, Pianta MJ, Pearce-Kelling SE, Miller BJ, et al: Naturally occurring rhodopsin mutation in the dog causes retinal dysfunction and degeneration mimicking human dominant retinitis pigmentosa. *Proc Natl Acad Sci U S A* 2002; 99:6328–6333.

34. Kim DH, Kim JA, Choi JS, Joo CK: Activation of caspase-3 during degeneration of the outer nuclear layer in the rd mouse retina. *Ophthalmic Res* 2002; 34:150–157.

35. Kirkness EF, Bafna V, Halpern AL, Levy S, Remington K, Rusch DB, et al: The dog genome: Survey sequencing and comparative analysis. *Science* 2003; 301:1898–1903.

36. Kommonen B: The DC-recorded dog electroretinogram in ketamine-medetomidine anaesthesia. *Acta Vet Scand* 1988; 29:35–41.

37. Lorenz B, Gyurus P, Preising M, Bremser D, Gu S, Andrassi M, et al: Early-onset severe rod-cone dystrophy in young children with RPE65 mutations. *Invest Ophthalmol Vis Sci* 2000; 41:2735–2742.

38. Marmor MF, Tan F, Sutter EE, Bearse MA Jr: Topography of cone electrophysiology in the enhanced S cone syndrome. *Invest Ophthalmol Vis Sci* 1999; 40:1866–1873.

39. Mears AJ, Kondo M, Swain PK, Takada Y, Bush RA, Saunders TL, et al: Nrl is required for rod photoreceptor development. *Nat Gen* 2001; 29:447–452.

40. Mentzer AL, Eifler D, Montiani-Ferreira F, Tuntivanich N, Forcier JQ, Petersen-Jones SM: Influence of recording electrode type and reference electrode position on the canine electroretinogram. *Doc Ophthalmol* 2006; in press.

41. Miller BJ, Sidjanin DJ, Kijas J, McElwee J, Acland GM, Aguirre G: Physical and transcription mapping of the canine prcd region syntenic to human chromosome 17q24–25[ARVO abstract]. *Invest Ophthalmol Vis Sci* 2002; 43:3672.

42. Miller PE, Murphy CJ: Vision in dogs. *J Am Vet Med Assoc* 1995; 207:1623–1634.

43. Montiani-Ferreira F, Fischer A, Cernuda-Cernuda R, DeGrip WJ, Sherry D, Cho SS, et al: Detailed histopathologic characterization of the retinopathy, globe enlarged (rge) chick phenotype. *Mol Vis* 2005; 11:11–27.

44. Montiani-Ferreira F, Li T, Kiupel M, Howland H, Hocking P, Curtis R, et al: Clinical features of the retinopathy, globe enlarged (rge) chick phenotype. *Vision Res* 2003; 43:2009–2018.

45. Montiani-Ferreira F, Petersen-Jones SM: Characterization of electroretinographic abnormalities in the retinopathy, globe enlarged (RGE) chick [ARVO abstract]. *Invest Ophthalmol Visual Sci* 2003; 44:4534.

46. Morimura H, Fishman GA, Grover SA, Fulton AB, Berson EL, Dryja TP: Mutations in the RPE65 gene in patients with autosomal recessive retinitis pigmentosa or Leber congenital amaurosis. *Proc Natl Acad Sci U S A* 1998; 95:3088–3093.

47. Morris VB: Symmetry in a receptor mosaic demonstrated in the chick from the frequencies, spacing and arrangement of the types of retinal receptor. *J Comp Neurol* 1970; 140:359–398.

48. Muller W, Topke H: The early receptor potential (ERP). *Doc Ophthalmol* 1987; 66:35–74.

49. Naarendorp F, Williams GE: The d-wave of the rod electroretinogram of rat originates in the cone pathway. *Vis Neurosci* 1999; 16:91–105.

50. Narfström K, Ekesten B: Electroretinographic evaluation of papillons with and without hereditary retinal degeneration. *Am J Vet Res* 1998; 59:221–226.

51. Narfström K, Ekesten B, Rosolen SG, Spiess BM, Pecicot CL, Ofri R: Guidelines for clinical electroretinography in the dog. *Doc Ophthalmol* 2002; 105:83–92.

52. Narfström K, Wrigstad A, Nilsson SEG: The briard dog: A new animal model of congenital stationary night blindness. *Br J Ophthalmol* 1989; 73:750–756.

53. Neitz J, Geist T, Jacobs GH: Color-vision in the dog. *Vis Neurosci* 1989; 3:119–125.

54. Nilsson SE, Wrigstad A, Narfström K: Changes in the DC electroretinogram in briard dogs with hereditary congenital night blindness and partial day blindness. *Exp Eye Res* 1992; 54:291–296.

55. Ookawa T: On the ontogenetic study of the chick ERG. *Nippon Seirigaku Zasshi* 1971; 33:317–318.

56. Ookawa T: The onset and development of the chick electroretinogram: The A- and B-waves. *Poult Sci* 1971; 50:601–608.

57. Parshall CJ, Wyman M, Nitroy S, Acland G, Aguirre G: Photoreceptor dysplasia: An inherited progressive retinal atrophy of miniature schnauzer dogs. *Prog Vet Comp Ophthalmol* 1991; 1:187–203.

58. Peichl L: Topography of ganglion cells in the dog and wolf retina. *J Comp Neurol* 1992; 324:603–620.

59. Perrault I, Rozet JM, Gerber S, Ghazi I, Leowski C, Ducroq D, et al: Leber congenital amaurosis. *Mol Genet Metab* 1999; 68:200–208.

60. Petersen-Jones SM, Entz DD, Sargan DR: cGMP phosphodiesterase-α mutation causes progressive retinal atrophy in the Cardigan Welsh corgi dog. *Invest Ophthalmol Vis Sci* 1999; 40:1637–1644.

61. Petersen-Jones SM, Grosjean N, Ramsey DT, Tuntivanich N: Preliminary characterization of the clinical and electroretinographic features of a PDE6A mutation in the dog [ARVO abstract]. *Invest Ophthalmol Vis Sci Suppl* 2000; 41:1063.

62. Piriev NI, Yamashita C, Samuel G, Farber DB: Rod photoreceptor cGMP-phosphodiesterase: Analysis of alpha and beta subunits expressed in human kidney cells. *Proc Natl Acad Sci U S A* 1993; 90:9340–9344.

63. Randall CJ, Wilson MA, Pollock BJ, Clayton RM, Ross AS, Bard JB, et al: Partial retinal dysplasia and subsequent degeneration in a mutant strain of domestic fowl (rdd). *Exp Eye Res* 1983; 37:337–347.

64. Redmond TM, Yu S, Lee E, Bok D, Hamasaki D, Chen N, et al: Rpe65 is necessary for production of 11-cis-vitamin A in the retinal visual cycle. *Nat Genet* 1998; 20:344–351.

65. Rohrer B, Lohr HR, Humphries P, Redmond TM, Seeliger MW, Crouch RK: Cone opsin mislocalization in Rpe65-/- mice: A defect that can be corrected by 11-cis retinal. *Invest Ophthalmol Vis Sci* 2005; 46:3876–3882.

66. Rosolen SG, Rigaudiere F, Legargasson JF, Chalier C, Rufiange M, Racine J, et al: Comparing the photopic ERG i-wave in different species. *Vet Ophthalmol* 2004; 7:189–192.

67. Sandberg MA, Pawlyk BS, Berson EL: Full-field electroretinograms in miniature poodles with progressive rod-cone degeneration. *Invest Ophthalmol Vis Sci* 1986; 27:1179–1184.

68. Seeliger MW, Grimm C, Stahlberg F, Friedburg C, Jaissle G, Zrenner E, Guo H, Reme CE, Humphries P, Hofmann F, Biel M, Fariss RN, Redmond TM, Wenzel A: New views on RPE65 deficiency: the rod system is the source of vision in a mouse model of Leber congenital amaurosis. *Nat Genet* 2001; 29:70–74.

69. Semple-Rowland SL, Lee NR, Van Hooser JP, Palczewski K, Baehr W: A null mutation in the photoreceptor guanylate cyclase gene causes the retinal degeneration chicken phenotype. *Proc Natl Acad Sci U S A* 1998; 95:1271–1276.

70. Sidjanin DJ, Lowe JK, McElwee JL, Milne BS, Phippen TM, Sargan DR, et al: Canine CNGB3 mutations establish cone degeneration as orthologous to the human achromatopsia locus ACHM3. *Hum Molec Genet* 2002; 11:1823–1833.

71. Sidjanin DJ, Lowe J, Mellersh C, Ostrander EA, Milne B, Sargan D, et al: Identification of a mutation responsible for hereditary cone degeneration in dog. *Invest Ophthalmol Vis Sci* 2002; 43:3671.

72. Sidjanin DJ, Miller B, Kijas J, Pillardy J, Malek J, Pai G, et al: Radiation hybrid map, physical map and low-pass genomic sequence of the canine prcd region on CFA9, and comparative mapping with the syntenic region on human chromosome 17. *Invest Ophthalmol Vis Sci* 2003; 44:1502.

73. Sieving PA: Photopic ON- and OFF-pathway abnormalities in retinal dystrophies. *Trans Am Ophthalmol Soc* 1993; 91:701–773.

74. Suber ML, Pittler SJ, Quin N, Wright GC, Holcombe N, Lee RH, et al: Irish setter dogs affected with rod-cone dysplasia contain a nonsense mutation in the rod cGMP phosphodiesterase beta-subunit gene. *Proc Natl Acad Sci U S A* 1993; 90:3968–3972.

75. Thompson DA, Gyurus P, Fleischer LL, Bingham EL, McHenry CL, Apfelstedt-Sylla E, et al: Genetics and phenotypes of RPE65 mutations in inherited retinal degeneration. *Invest Ophthalmol Vis Sci* 2000; 41:4293–4299.

76. Tuntivanich N, Mentzer AL, Eifler D, Montiani-Ferreira F, Forcier JQ, Johnson C, et al: Assessment of the dark-adaptation time required for recovery of electroretinographic responses in dogs after fundus photography and indirect ophthalmoscopy. *Am J Vet Res* 2005; 66:1798–1804.

77. Ulshafer RJ, Allen C, Dawson WW, Wolf ED: Hereditary retinal degeneration in the Rhode Island Red chicken: I. Histology and ERG. *Exp Eye Res* 1984; 39:125–135.

78. Veske A, Nilsson SE, Narfström K, Gal A: Retinal dystrophy of Swedish briard/briard-beagle dogs is due to a 4-bp deletion in RPE65. *Genomics* 1999: 57:57–61.

79. Wai SM, Yew DT: A cytological study on the development of the different types of visual cells in the chicken (Gallus domesticus). *Cell Mol Neurobiol* 2002; 22:57–85.

80. Wai SM, Kung LS, Yew DT: Novel identification of the different types of cones in the retina of the chicken. *Cell Mol Neurobiol* 2002; 22:177–184.

81. Wolf ED, Vainisi SJ, Santos-Anderson RM: Rod cone dysplasia in the collie. *J Am Vet Med Assoc* 1978; 173:1331–1333.

82. Wrigstad A, Nilsson SE, Narfström K: Ultrastructural changes of the retina and the retinal pigment epithelium in briard dogs with hereditary congenital night blindness and partial day blindness. *Exp Eye Res* 1992; 55:805–818.

83. Wrigstad A, Narfström K, Nilsson SE: Slowly progressive changes of the retina and retinal pigment epithelium in briard dogs with hereditary retinal dystrophy: A morphological study. *Doc Ophthalmol* 1994; 87:337–354.

84. Yanase J, Ogawa H: Effects of halothane and sevoflurane on the electroretinogram of dogs. *Am J Vet Res* 1997; 58:904–909.

85. Yanase J, Ogawa H, Ohtsuka H: Rod and cone components in the dog electroretinogram during and after dark adaptation. *J Vet Med Sci* 1995; 57:877–881.

86. Yanase J, Ogawa H, Ohtsuka H: Scotopic threshold response of the electroretinogram of dogs. *Am J Vet Res* 1996; 57:361–366.

87. Zhang Q, Acland GM, Wu WX, Johnson JL, Pearce-Kelling S, Tulloch B, et al: Different RPGR exon ORF15 mutations in canids provide insights into photoreceptor cell degeneration. *Hum Mol Genet* 2002; 11:993–1003.

83 Electroretinographic Testing in Larger Animals

KRISTINA NARFSTRÖM

MANY ELECTROPHYSIOLOGICAL studies have been performed in animals as a means to describe basic physiological response mechanisms of the retina to light stimulation. The recordings have served to expand our knowledge, not only of the normal anatomy and physiology of the retinal cells and their interactions, but also of pathological and disease processes of the eye. For the latter purpose, there have been a number of animal retinal diseases to study. In addition, there are now genetically modified animals, that is, knock-out animals, that are used to examine the role of single genes and amino acids or as direct models of human retinal diseases.

Electroretinogram (ERG) testing in animals larger than rats and mice has been performed for research purposes in guinea pigs,[11] pigeons,[25] ground squirrels,[26] chickens,[21,74] rabbits,[73,75,79] cats,[38,56,67,76,77] dogs,[4,28,32,58,69,84] sheep,[29] and monkeys,[20,24,68,78] as well as other species. It appears that animals larger than these, such as pigs, cows, and horses, are seldom used for pure research, owing to impracticalities, such as the higher housing costs and the increased risks for both investigators and animals in conjunction with the testing procedures.

Virtually all kinds of objective ERG studies that are routinely done in humans can be performed in larger animals. One major difference is the need for anesthetics in these animals,[1,52,71] which can have a direct effect on the configuration of the ERG recordings. Depending on the choice of anesthetics, the effects range from minimal, when using only hypnotics, to more severe when using barbiturates or volatile anesthetics such as halothane.[33,41]

Another difference in larger animals (mammals), except primates, is that they are dichromats. Two types of cones are prevalent, varying in numbers and topographic location in the retina.[64] Rods dominate most retinas of larger animals, although cones dominate for lizards, birds, and squirrels. These variations in photoreceptor types and distribution between species cause the resultant normal ERG curves to vary markedly between species. Another anatomic variable is the "extra" refractile cell layer located in the inner part of the choroid of many domestic species. It is called *tapetum lucidum* (dogs and cats) or *tapetum cellulosum* (horse and cattle) and is found in the superior half of the fundus. This layer increases the effect of incident light on the photoreceptors

and results in increased retinal illuminance.[60] It also increases stray light, effects that significantly affect ERG recordings.[66]

Today, the application for electroretinography in larger animals has broadened, due to the objective nature of the test. This is true especially in the field of veterinary ophthalmology, in which electrophysiological studies in domesticated animals such as dogs, cats, and horses are more or less routinely performed. Although more sophisticated studies such as pattern,[58] focal, multifocal,[66] bright-flash, double-flash, and ON and OFF[17] and d.c. ERGs[31,33] are used only in a few specialized centers across the world in larger animals, most veterinary ophthalmology specialty clinics today have equipment to record flash ERGs.[57]

Flash ERGs are most commonly used in dogs in veterinary medicine. For example, ERGs are used as a routine screening procedure for quick evaluation of retinal function, prior to cataract surgery, and in the evaluation of acute blinding diseases or trauma.[2,52] There is an increasing need for flash ERGs to be performed more frequently in horses as well.[30] Complete cataracts, especially in foals, is a frequent indication for equine ERGs. Also in trauma cases, ERGs are indicated and in conjunction with intraocular inflammatory disease entities such as uveitis, the most common cause of blindness in the horse.

ERGs are also used for the screening of hereditary eye disease, mainly in dogs, sometimes in cats, and less frequently in Appaloosa horses. In the pedigree dog population, there is a high incidence of generalized, hereditary photoreceptor disorders, collectively termed *progressive retinal atrophy* (PRA) (table 83.1). Among photoreceptor disorders that have been more specifically studied and documented in dogs are rod-cone dysplasias,[12,37,82] rod dysplasia,[5] early rod degeneration,[2] photoreceptor dysplasia,[59] progressive rod-cone degeneration,[7,45] cone degeneration,[4] and congenital retinal dystrophy.[55]

Some of these photoreceptor disorders are congenital and cause early-onset severe visual impairment or blindness.[55] Others do not cause blindness until the animal is several years old and are often not diagnosed until late in the disease process.[1,4,13,54] Early diagnosis of these bilateral, generalized hereditary retinal diseases is advocated. It is recommended that such studies be used prior to breeding, thus reducing the

Species	Breed	Disease Name	Onset of Fundus Abnormalities	ERG Diagnostically Informative
Canine	Irish setter	Rod-cone dysplasia type 1	3–4 months	6 weeks
	Collie	Rod-cone dysplasia type 2	3–4 months	6 weeks
	Norwegian elkhound	Rod dysplasia	5 months	6 weeks
	Norwegian elkhound	Early rod degeneration	6 months	6 weeks
	Miniature schnauzer	Photoreceptor dysplasia	2–5 years	6 weeks
	Belgian shepherd	Unclassified	11 weeks	4 weeks
	Portuguese waterdog	Progressive rod-cone degeneration	3–6 years	1.5 years
	Miniature and toy poodle	Progressive rod-cone degeneration	3–5 years	9–10 months
	English cocker spaniel	Progressive rod-cone degeneration	4–8 years	18–24 months
	American cocker spaniel	Progressive rod-cone degeneration	3–5 years	9 months
	Labrador retriever	Progressive rod-cone degeneration	4–6 years	12–15 months
	Tibetan terrier	Progressive retinal atrophy	12–18 months	10 months
	Miniature longhaired dachshund	Progressive retinal atrophy	5–7 months	4 months
	Alaskan malamute	Cone degeneration	NR	6 weeks
	Akita-inu	Progressive retinal atrophy	5–18 months	10 months
	Irish wolfhound	Progressive retinal atrophy	2–3 years	NR
	English setter	Progressive retinal atrophy	<7 years	NR
	Tibetan spaniel	Progressive retinal atrophy	3–4 years	NR
	Papillon	Progressive retinal atrophy	2–6 years	18 months
	Siberian husky	X-linked progressive retinal atrophy	6–12 months	18 months
	Samoyed	X-linked progressive retinal atrophy	2–4 years	16–24 months
	Briard	Congenital retinal dystrophy (*RPE65* mutation)	4–6 years	5 weeks
	Cardigan Welsh corgi	Progressive retinal atrophy	NR	NR
Feline	Abyssinian	Rod-cone dysplasia	4–5 weeks	5 weeks
	Abyssinian	Rod-cone degeneration	1–2 years	8–12 months
Equine	Appaloosa	Congenital stationary night blindness	NR	1 month

NR = Not recorded.

For further reading, see references 13, 14, 45, 47, 50, and 81.

frequency of affected animals with genetic defects prevalent in the population.[1,50]

Owing to an increasing awareness among clinicians and pedigree dog and cat owners and breeders, it is likely that diagnostic ERGs will be performed more frequently in the future. In this regard, there has been debate regarding the use and misuse of ERGs in dogs,[6] and ways have been proposed to resolve this problem: the establishment of referral centers with specific competency in ERG procedures where more comprehensive procedures are routinely performed, enabling researchers and clinicians a more focused approach to diagnostics of retinal disease processes in companion animals.[46]

Specific procedures needed in working with larger animals

ERGs in awake, restrained, or even freely moving animals have also been described.[36,62,72] Although the recording of ERG should not be a painful procedure by itself, it requires patient cooperation. This cooperation is not attainable in conscious animals and therefore, to obtain reliable results, heavy sedation or general anesthesia is advocated. This not only prevents movement artifacts, such as blinks, but also reduces stress. Further, it allows for positioning of the eye in relation to the light source and recording electrodes without causing discomfort or pain.

A number of anesthetics have been used for electrophysiological studies in larger animals and specific effects shown on various electrophysiological parameters. It is not the aim of this chapter to give detailed recommendations regarding specific anesthetic procedures for various species or breeds. The choice of anesthetic regime depends on many factors, such as the user's experience with a specific anesthetic, the training of involved personnel, equipment availability, the species of animal being studied, and the electrophysiological effects to be investigated. See table 83.2 for a list of anesthetic protocols used in documented studies in larger animals.

Assessment of vision is performed prior to sedation or the induction of anesthesia. This is not always an easy procedure, given the lack of verbal communication and the animal's ability to compensate for reduced visual capacity by increased use of tactile and auditory sensations. The behavior in walking a maze and the cotton ball test in both dark and lighted environments are integral parts of the visual examination procedure.[49] A general examination of the

TABLE 83.2

Anesthetics used and described in the literature for some larger animal species in conjunction with ERG studies

Species	Ref. No.	Anesthetics	Dosage and Route of Application
Canine	63	Short-acting barbiturate	IV (NR)
		+ succinyl chloride	10–20 mg/kg IV**
	23	Thiamylal sodium	17.5 mg/kg IV
		+ succinylcholine chloride	10–20 mg IV**
	65	Acepromazine maleate	1 mg/kg IM
		+ numorphan	0.4 mg/kg IV*
	33, 35	Ketamine hydrochloride	1.04–1.32 mg/kg IM
		& xylazine	8.6–10.5 mg/kg
	31	Glycopyrrolate bromide	0.01 mg/kg IV
		+ medetomidine hydrochloride	15 μg/kg IM
		+ ketamine hydrochloride	1.5 mg/kg (after 20 minutes) IV
		+ vecuronium bromide	0.2 mg/kg IV**
	43	Pentobarbital sodium	26 mg/kg IV
		+ halothane	Inhalation*
	7	Short-acting thiobarbiturate	IV (NR)
		+ halothane	Inhalation*
	82, 44	Acepromazine maleate	1 mg/kg IV
		+ halothane	Inhalation*
	70	Acepromazine maleate	0.22 mg/kg IV
		+ isoflurane	Inhalation*
	71	Acepromazine maleate	0.1 mg/kg IM
		+ thiamylal sodium	10 mg/kg IV
		+ halthane	Inhalation*
	69	Oxymorphone	0.02 mg/kg IM
		+ isoflurane	Inhalation*
	32	Glycopyrrolate bromide	0.01 mg/kg IV
		+ thiamylal sodium	15 mg/kg IV
		+ pancuronium bromide	0.1 mg/kg/45 min**
	59	Thiamylal sodium	15 mg/kg IV (NR)
		+ halothane	Inhalation*
	58	Glycopyrrolate bromide	0.01 mg/kg IV
		+ thiamylal sodium	15 mg/kg IV
		+ pancuronium bromide	0.1 mg/kg IV
		+ 25% oxygen & 75% nitrous oxide	Inhalation**
	28	Isoflurane	Inhalation*
		& nitrous oxide	
	16	Glycopyrrolate bromide	0.01 mg/kg IV
		+ thiamylal sodium	15 mg/kg IV
		+ pancuronium bromide	0.1 mg/kg IV**
	83, 84	Ketamine	5 mg/kg IV
		+ vecuronium bromide	40 μg/kg IV
		+ 25% oxygen & 75% nitrous oxide	Inhalation**
	34	Glycopyrrolate bromide	0.01 mg/kg IV
		+ thiopental sodium	15–20 mg/kg IV
		+ pancuronium bromide	0.1–0.2 mg/kg/h
		+ 70% nitrous oxide & 30% oxygen	Inhalation**
	1, 39	Halothane or isoflurane	Inhalation*
	9	Sodium thiopental	15 mg/kg IV
		+ halothane	Inhalation*
	61	Ketamine hydrochloride	5 mg/kg
		+ medetomidine hydrochloride	0.04 ml/kg IM
	14, 19	Propofol	6 mg/kg IV
		+ isoflurane or halothane	Inhalation*

TABLE 83.2 (continued)

Species	Ref. No.	Anesthetics	Dosage and Route of Application
Feline	15, 37	Alphaxalone	IV (to effect)
		& alphadolone acetate	
		+ halothane	Inhalation*
	41, 77	Urethane	1.0–1.3 g/kg, Infusion: 1.92 g/h
		+ halothane + nitrous	Inhalation
		oxide/carbon gas mixture	For long term (up to 3 days):
		+ heparin, atropine,	50 IU, 2.5 mg, 4.7 g, & 240 mg/kg;
		anhydrous D-glucose &	4 ml/h of 100 ml solution for infusion†
		urethane mixture	
	8, 68	Ketamine hydrochloride	10–25 mg/kg IM
		& xylazine	1–2.5 mg/kg IM
	17, 48	Thiopental sodium	8 mg/kg IV
		+ isoflurane or halothane	Inhalation*
	76	Ketamine hydrochloride	10–20 mg/kg IM
		+ xylazine	0.33 mg/kg IM
		+ ketamine hydrochloride	Infusion: 10 mg/kg,
		& glucose & sodium chloride	10 g, 0.45 g & 0.56 g in 250 ml of solution
		& potassium chloride	
	10	Medetomidine hydrochloride	0.1 ml/kg IM
		+ ketamine hydrochloride	5 mg/kg IM
		(50 mg/ml)	
Equine	30	Detomidine hydrochloride	0.015 mg/kg IV
Rabbit	44	Ketamine hydrochloride	30 mg/kg IV
		+ urethane	1.4 g/kg IP
	73	Pentobarbital (60 mg/ml)	1.25–1.75 IV
		+ pentobarbital in Ringer's	Infusion: 20–30 ml/h
		solution (2 mg/ml)	
Guinea pig	11	Xylazine	5 mg/kg
		& ketamine hydrochloride	35 mg/kg IM
Ground squirrel	26	Xylazine	7 mg/kg
		& ketamine hydrochloride	70 mg/kg IM
Rat	18	Fluanisonum (10 mg/ml)	0.3 ml/kg
		& fentanyl (0.1315 mg/ml)	of mixture IP
	27	Sodium pentobarbital	5 mg/100 g IP
Pigeon	25	Chloral hydrate	410 mg/kg IM
Chicken	74	Ethyl carbamate	1.5 g/kg IP
Pig	80	Halothane	Inhalation*

Note: Glycopyrrolate and atropine are both anticholinergic drugs used primarily to prevent salivary secretions and to inhibit the bradycardic effect of vagal stimulation often seen in conjunction with general anesthesia in dogs and cats. The dose of atropine is not indicated in the table but is routinely used at 0.02–0.04 mg/kg IV, IM, or SQ in the dog and cat. For further information and instructions, see Muir WW, Hubbell JAE, Skarda R (eds): *Handbook of Veterinary Anesthesia*, ed 2. St. Louis, Mosby-Year Book, 1995.

+= Given after induction or after a specific time.

&= Given in combination.

*= Intubation needed.

**= Intubation and artificial respiration needed.

†= For terminal procedures.

NR= Not recorded.

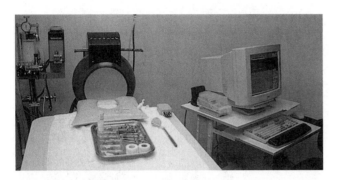

FIGURE 83.1 Computerized Ganzfeld ERG system for use in larger animals. Suitable adjunct utilities are demonstrated on the table: a deflatable cushion that aids in apposition of the head, a tray for electrodes, instruments used for stay suturing, and ophthalmic medications (methyl cellulose, phenylephrine hydrochloride, and atropine).

animal and more specific eye exams are thereafter performed. The latter includes menace testing, testing of dazzle and pupillary light reflexes, ophthalmoscopy, and slit-lamp biomicroscopy. The ERG requires dilatation, and ophthalmoscopy and biomicroscopy are best done in the dilated eye. These initial examinations can be performed prior to premedication, after premedication, or after the induction of general anesthesia. In dogs and cats, these examinations are easily performed with the animal sitting on a table in a calm, dark environment. Induction of general anesthesia or deep sedation is then performed, the pupils are dilated if this was not done previously, and the animal is moved to the ERG facility (figure 83.1).

For larger animals such as horses, it is recommended to provide sedation before any specific eye exams are performed. Due to higher risks in relation to general anesthesia in this species, it is recommended that ERGs be performed in the heavily sedated standing horse.[30] After light sedation and eye exams, deeper sedation is provided and possibly regional anesthesia (topical anesthesia and auriculopalpebral nerve block for eyelid akinesia) in order for the corneal electrodes to be inserted.

It is important to be aware of species variation as to type of anesthetics that are suitable to use as well as dosages (see table 83.2). Species may differ in their reactions to anesthetic agents, which also results in variations in the ERG responses obtained. Interpretation of the recorded ERG response must therefore always be done with the type of animal species studied and type of anesthesia used. ERG signals of animals also vary with age, as in human patients, with higher amplitudes in younger animals compared to those of older individuals and smaller amplitudes in animals of advanced age. Further, as was previously pointed out, there are species and breed variations as to the general configuration of the ERG responses mainly due to anatomic and physiological variations between species. It is not possible to directly compare

ERG recordings from a miniature poodle to those of a Labrador retriever, even when the same anesthetic protocol is used in both breeds of dog. Similarly, ERG recordings from dogs are different from those of cats, even when the same type of anesthetic is used. Cats have higher amplitudes and shorter implicit times in their a- and b-wave responses compared to similar recordings in dogs. Species variations are clearly seen when rodent ERGs are compared to recordings in some larger animals. Rats, for instance, have marked oscillatory potentials (OPs), while the OPs are prevalent but not as marked in cats under similar recording conditions, that is, similar state of retinal adaptation, color of light stimuli, intensity of light stimuli, and type of anesthesia.

Individual testing protocols, therefore, need to be established for each animal species studied by ERG. Normal baseline values should be obtained for each laboratory where ERG studies are performed in each species, each breed, and at least three age groups (juvenile, adult, and elderly).

Indications for flash a.c. (alternating current) ERGs may vary from simple preoperative recordings to evaluate gross retinal function in dogs with complete cataracts to extensive studies of newly discovered retinal disease processes. ERGs are often needed in conjunction with toxicological screening of the effects of various drugs and compounds and, as was previously described, in the early diagnosis of hereditary retinal disease. For these indications, except the first type, precise and standardized procedures are needed, a minimum being the evaluation of rod and cone function and the process of dark adaptation.[1,4,22,47] More extended testing procedures are often also used, such as the study of scotopic threshold responses, OPs, and retinal sensitivity. These more extended studies should, however, be performed as adjunct tests to a standardized testing procedure.

Guidelines for larger animals

Guidelines for larger animals have so far been published only for dogs. The International Society for Veterinary Ophthalmology initiated this work and, together with the European College of Veterinary Ophthalmology, established a working committee for this endeavor. The procedures for ERGs in dogs were approved at the First European Conference of Veterinary Visual Electrophysiology in Vienna in 2000, and the guidelines were published in *Documenta Ophthalmologica* in 2002.[52] These guidelines take the varying needs, previously described, for ERGs into account by providing two sets of recommendations for use in dogs: one short protocol, which is intended for rapid evaluation of gross retinal function in animals that are about to undergo cataract surgery or, for instance, to evaluate retinal versus central blindness, and a more elaborate protocol that is intended as part of a diagnostic process in the evaluation of retinal function. The second, more elaborate protocol is a longer procedure in

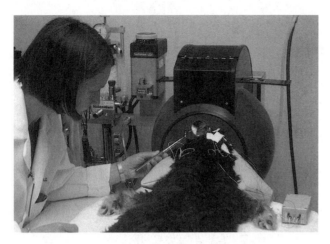

FIGURE 83.2 Preparation for simultaneous bilateral ERGs. The dog is lying on its chest with the electrodes connected. Three conjunctival stay sutures have been placed at the limbus and fastened to the skin with surgical tape. The apposition of the contact lens electrodes and the position of the eyes are checked by using a large dentists' mirror.

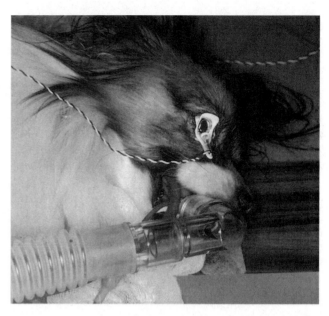

FIGURE 83.3 The dog is under general anesthesia and intubated. A bipolar Burian Allen corneal contact lens is in place and cushioned on the cornea with methylcellulose.

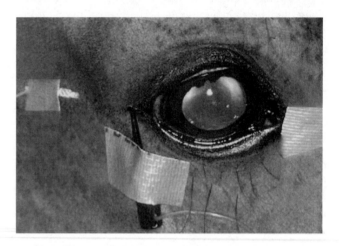

FIGURE 83.4 A DTL microfiber electrode is used in the standing horse. Note the thin microfiber stretched in the tearfilm along the lower eyelid margin. (Source: Komaromy AM, et al: *Vet Ophthalmol* 2003; 6:27–33. Used by permission.)

which rod function and cone function are tested separately. This diagnostic ERG test protocol can be used for studies of newly discovered photoreceptor disorders, in toxicological studies, and in the early diagnosis and testing for generalized inherited photoreceptor disorders (see table 83.1). It is the author's opinion that the same set of guidelines that have been described and published for dogs can be used in cats owing to physiological and anatomical similarities of retinal function and structure between the two species. The second, longer type of ERG protocol has many similarities to the human protocol published as the standard for clinical ERG (latest version published in 2004).[40]

The guidelines include the use of short white-flash ERGs, no more than 5 ms long, utilizing full-field light stimulation. Commercial or custom-made Ganzfeld stimulators are used that aim at obtaining a uniform distribution of the stimulating light across the retina in order to be able to measure the contributions of the entire rod and cone populations (figure 83.2). Pupils are maximally dilated during the recording session using mydriatics; 1% atropine (Isopto-Atropin) will produce dilation lasting over days, depending on animal species and frequency of instillation. If shorter dilation is required, 1% tropicamide hydrochloride (Mydriacyl) and 10% phenylephrine hydrochloride (Neosynephrine) work well and last only 3–5 hours. The use of white light is recommended. Neutral-density filters are used to attenuate the light. The choice of unilateral or simultaneous bilateral ERG recordings will depend on the species, the capacity of the equipment, and the indication for performing the ERG.

Contact lens electrodes are recommended. The most frequently used ones are gold-ring electrodes (ERG Jet Lens,

Universo Plastique, La Chaus-de-Fonds, Switzerland) and Burian Allen bipolar lens electrodes built specifically for the species and age (Hansen Ophthalmic Development Laboratory, Iowa), especially in dogs and cats (figure 83.3). Several laboratories design their own monopolar or bipolar lens electrodes. DTL microfiber electrodes (Retina Technologies, Scranton, PA) are useful because they do not need to be fitted onto the eye (figure 83.4). If the electrode is stretched across the cornea, the responses are large but sensitive to the position of the fiber on the cornea, which will change if the animal blinks. When the electrode is placed in the palpebral sac, DTL electrode recordings are stable, but amplitudes are lower. For reference and ground electrodes, platinum subdermal needle electrodes are often used (Grass Instrumental Division, Astro-Med., Inc., West Warwick, RI).

The use of conjunctival stay sutures at the limbus to stabilize the globe, or other adequate means, is recommended during the ERG procedure. Both eyelids must be open during the examination, and the corneas must be protected by using a nonirritating protective and wetting solution, such as 0.5% methyl cellulose.

Proper oxygenation and ventilation must be maintained throughout the examination, and orotracheal intubation is used when the animals are under general anesthesia. Body temperature must be controlled and kept stable at 38–39°C. As was previously pointed out, pupils must be fully dilated throughout the examination, and evaluation of pupil size must be conducted at the beginning and at the end of the testing procedure.

For both the short and longer protocols, the dogs (and cats) are prepared and anesthetized in ambient light. The recommended short protocol is as follows:

1. Test retinal function in ambient light using a white standard flash (SF = 2–3 cd s/m^2).
2. Turn off the light and test retinal function within the first minute of dark adaptation using white SF.
3. Test retinal function again after 5 minutes of dark adaptation using white SF.

Using this short protocol in a normal animal provides the examiner with a low-amplitude photopic ERG recording and low- and higher-amplitude scotopic recordings. This protocol does not allow for separation of rod function and cone function but gives an answer to the question of whether there is retinal function or not. Every lab will have to evaluate its ERG responses obtained from animal patients in comparison with those obtained under similar conditions in a group of previously tested normal animals of the same species and age group.

For a more elaborate diagnostic ERG protocol, rod function and cone function are tested separately. It is important to note that prior to the ERG examination, the animal should not have undergone fundus photography or fluorescein angiography or have been out in bright sunlight. Although the currently recommended protocol for dogs starts with evaluation of the dark-adapted responses, the choice of whether to begin with scotopic or photopic conditions is up to the user, as long as the adaptation times are met. The longer protocol is as follows:

1. Dark-adapt the animal for 20 minutes while evaluating rod function and the dynamic process of dark adaptation every 4 minutes (at 1, 4, 8, 12, 16, and 20 minutes of

dark adaptation) using a low level of white light (0.02–0.03 cd s/m^2).
2. Test the mixed rod and cone responses to a single high-intensity flash of white light (using 2–3 cd s/m^2).
3. Light-adapt the animal for 10 minutes, using white background light in a Ganzfeld dome or similar equipment, with an intensity of 30–40 cd/m^2 at the level of the stimulated eye. Thereafter, test cone function using white SF stimulus.
4. Perform the cone flicker test using 30 Hz of white light stimuli or higher-intensity frequencies.

The OPs can be extracted from the high-intensity white light stimulus response, with filtering of the signals, using a low filter setting at 70–100 Hz. This can be done as a separate recording or, it the software is available, mathematically during analysis.

Testing sessions using the second, more elaborate testing protocol result in a set of ERGs (figure 83.5) that are evaluated as to a- and b-wave amplitude and timing characteristics. Further, the process of dark adaptation is studied. These parameters are compared to the responses of normal animals of the same species, breed, and age group. To compare results of recordings from normal and tested animals, similar anesthetic procedures must have been used in the patient and in all animals of the test group.

A scheme for rapid evaluation of obtained results has been proposed involving a flowchart for the various procedures.[47,51] The amplitude and implicit time parameters for the studied animal are plotted on a chart, in which the median level for each testing parameter for normal dogs is given and the first and ninety-ninth or fifth and ninety-fifth percentiles are indicated as limits of normality.

Reports of ERGs should include a display of the animal's own ERG traces alongside the traces of a normal, age-matched animal of the same breed and anesthetized by using the same anesthetic protocol.

Correlation of ERG test results with clinical findings

It is important to realize that electrophysiological testing is a complementary way of obtaining a diagnosis in relation to a possible retinal functional problem and that ERGs cannot be interpreted in isolation. The results from a thorough history of the patient and knowledge of the specific hereditary diseases prevalent in the breed are important factors to take into account. Also, the results from visual behavior testing and the general and more specific ocular examinations performed are needed in order to obtain a correct diagnosis.

In dogs and cats with known hereditary disease entities, the majority of animals that are tested by using ERGs have a normal fundus appearance, are relatively young, and are

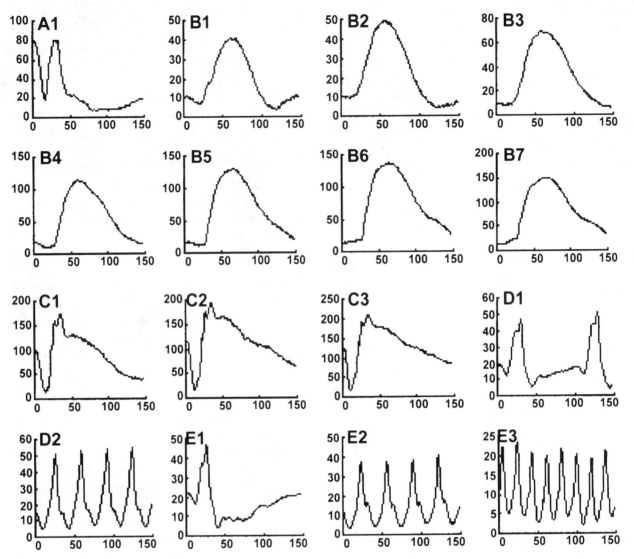

FIGURE 83.5   Results from an actual ERG recording session using the recommended protocol in a normal 2-year-old Labrador retriever dog but extending the recording session. A1, Photopic single flash recording after preparation of the dog. B1–B7, Scotopic ERGs recorded at 1, 4, 8, 12, 16, 20, and 24 minutes using $-2.0 \log \text{cd s/m}^2$ of white light, respectively. Note the increase in b-wave amplitudes during the recording session. C1–C3, Scotopic ERGs using 0, 0.3, and $0.6 \log \text{cd s/m}^2$, respectively. D1–D3, Scotopic 10- and 30-Hz flicker recordings, respectively. E1–E3, Photopic recordings at 5, 30, and 50 Hz, respectively, after 10 minutes of light adaptation (background light: 37cd/m^2) using white light stimuli at $0 \log \text{cd s/m}^2$.

often in their first years of breeding. For these, diagnostic ERGs, specifically evaluating rod and cone function, are of utmost importance. The papillon dog breed is an example of a breed that is affected by a hereditary rod-cone degeneration of late onset and slow progression. Fundus appearance and behavioral testing can be normal up to 2–6 years of age, but electrophysiologically, rod function is abnormal at the age of 0.8–1.5 years. In the papillon retinal disease, it appears that cone function is normal for several years, until late in the disease process, allowing the dog normal visual behavior in daylight conditions and thus hiding clinical symptoms of this progressively blinding disease. Moreover, fundus appearance is difficult to evaluate in many papillon dogs, owing to great variations in the normal fundus appearance of this breed, varying from generalized darkly pigmented fundus to a subalbinotic fundus. Both types of fundi have no or only very small numbers of tapetal cells, making the ophthalmoscopic evaluation difficult. This is an example in which ERG testing is essential in order to obtain an accurate and comparably early diagnosis.[51]

In the briard dog retinal dystrophy, with the *RPE65* null mutation, the situation is different. Affected dogs are night blind from birth and are severely visually impaired also in daylight. A quivering nystagmus is usually observed in affected dogs after the age of 6–7 weeks. Fundus appearance is normal until early middle age (3–4 years), when there is a

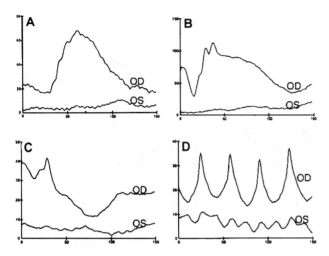

FIGURE 83.6 Actual, bilateral ERGs in an *RPE65* null mutation dog treated in the right eye (OD) by subretinal gene transfer 6 weeks previously.[53] The left eye (OS) was not treated. Panels A and B are low- and high-intensity scotopic responses, respectively, and panels C and D are photopic responses (5 and 30 Hz, respectively).

generalized vascular attenuation and sometimes fundus color changes and spotting. Scotopic ERGs are nonrecordable, and photopic responses are severely reduced or nonrecordable. A tentative diagnosis can, in most cases, be made by using clinical observations, such as behavioral studies and ophthalmic exams. The diagnosis is then verified by using ERG testing in 5- to 7-week-old puppies.[55]

Hereditary photoreceptor diseases in companion animals are most often bilateral and progressive. Thus, unilateral focal or generalized retinopathies are in general due to inflammatory or circulatory causes, and not hereditary. Various nondiagnostic ERG changes may be observed in the affected eye. In cases in which ERG results are borderline as to limits of normality, it is wise to recommend a follow-up ERG in most animals, within 6–12 months, owing to the progressive nature of most of these disorders.

Simultaneous bilateral ERG recordings are valuable to perform in conjunction with screening for hereditary eye disease,[61] since the diseases are mostly bilateral but can be asymmetric. Bilateral recordings are also valuable in conjunction with unilateral treatment studies[53] (figure 83.6).

ACKNOWLEDGMENTS   I would like to thank the following for valuable discussions, comments, and advice on this chapter: Doctors Vaegan, Bertel Kommonen, Ron Ofri, and John Dodam. I am grateful for the secretarial assistance provided by Debbie Becker.

REFERENCES

1. Acland G: Diagnosis and differentiation of retinal diseases in small animals by electroretinography. *Semin Vet Med Surg (Small Animal)* 1988; 3:15–27.

2. Acland GM, Aguirre GD: Retinal degeneration in the dog: IV. Early retinal degeneration (ERD) in Norwegian elkhounds. *Exp Eye Res* 1987; 44:491–521.

3. Aguirre GD: Electroretinography in veterinary ophthalmology. *J Am Anim Hosp Assoc* 1973; 9:234–237.

4. Aguirre GD: *Rod and cone contributions to the canine electroretinogram.* PhD thesis. University of Pennsylvania, Philadelphia, 1975.

5. Aguirre G: Retinal degeneration in the dog: I. Rod dysplasia. *Exp Eye Res* 1978; 26:233–253.

6. Aguirre G: Electroretinography: Are we misusing an excellent diagnostic tool? *Vet Comp Ophthalmol* 1995; 5:2–3.

7. Aguirre GD, Acland GM: Variation in retinal degeneration phenotype inherited at the prcd locus. *Exp Eye Res* 1988; 46:663–687.

8. Baro JA, Lehmkuhle S, Dratz KE: Electroretinograms and visual evoked potentials in long-term monocularly deprived cats. *Invest Ophthalmol Vis Sci* 1990; 31:1405–1409.

9. Beltran WA, Chahory S, Gnirs K, Escriou C, Blot S, Clerc B: The electroretinographic phenotype of dogs with golden retriever muscular dystrophy. *Vet Ophthalmol* 2001; 4:277–282.

10. Bragadottir R, Narfström K: Lens sparing pars plana vitrectomy and retinal transplantation in cats. *Vet Ophthalmol* 2003; 6:135–139.

11. Bui BV, Armitage JA, Vingrys AJ: Extraction and modeling of oscillatory potentials. *Doc Ophthalmol* 2002; 104:17–36.

12. Buyukmihci N, Aguirre G, Marshall J: Retinal degeneration in the dog: II. Development of the retina in rod-cone dysplasia. *Exp Eye Res* 1980; 30:575–591.

13. Clements PJM, Sargan DR, Gould DJ, Petersen-Jones SM: Recent advances in understanding the spectrum of canine generalized progressive retinal atrophy. *J Small Anim Pract* 1996; 37:155–162.

14. Curtis R, Barnett KC: Progressive retinal atrophy in miniature longhaired dachshund dogs. *Br Vet J* 1993; 149:71–85.

15. Curtis R, Barnett KC, Leon A: An early-onset retinal dystrophy with dominant inheritance in the Abyssinian cat: Clinical and pathological findings. *Invest Ophthalmol Vis Sci* 1987; 28:131–139.

16. Dawson WW, Kommonen B: The late positive retinal potential in dogs. *Exp Eye Res* 1995; 60:173–179.

17. Ekesten B, Narfström K: Cone positive off-response in normal and dystrophic cats. *Doc Ophthalmol* 1999; 97:9–21.

18. El Azazi M, Wachtmeister L: The postnatal development of the oscillatory potentials of the electroretinogram: I. Basic characteristics. *Acta Ophthalmol* 1990; 68:401–409.

19. Ford MM, Bragadottir R, Rakoczy EP, Narfström K: Gene transfer in the RPE65 null mutation dog: Relationship between construct volume, visual behavior and electroretinographic (ERG) results. *Doc Ophthalmol* 2003; 107:79–86.

20. Fortune B, Cull G, Wang L, Buskirk MV, Cioffi GA: Factors affecting the use of multifocal electroretinography to monitor function in a primate model of glaucoma. *Doc Ophthalmol* 2002; 105:151–178.

21. Gallemore RP, Steinberg RH: Light-evoked modulation of basolateral membrane Cl⁻ conductance in chick retinal pigment epithelium: The light peak and fast oscillation. *J Neurophysiol* 1993; 70:1669–1680.

22. Gouras P: Electroretinography: Some basic principles. *Invest Ophthalmol* 1970; 9:557–569.

23. Gum GG, Gelatt KN, Samuelson DA: Maturation of the retina of the canine neonate as determined by electroretinography and histology. *Am J Vet Res* 1983; 45:1166–1171.

24. Hare WA, Ton H: Effects of APB, PDA, and TTX on ERG responses recorded using both multifocal and conventional methods in monkey. *Doc Ophthalmol* 2002; 195:189–222.

25. Hodos W, Ghim MH, Potocki A, Fields JN, Storm T: Contrast sensitivity in pigeons: A comparison of behavioral and pattern ERG methods. *Doc Ophthalmol* 2002; 104:107–118.

26. Jacobs GH, Calderone JB, Sakai T, Lewis GP, Fisher SK: An animal model for studying cone function in retinal detachment. *Doc Ophthalmol* 2002; 104:119–132.

27. Jiang CJ, Hansen RM, Reynaud X, Fulton AB: Background adaptation in a rat model of retinopathy of prematurity. *Doc Ophthalmol* 2002; 104:97–105.

28. Jones RD, Brenneke CJ, Hoss HE, Loney ML: An electroretinogram protocol for toxicological screening in the canine model. *Toxicol Lett* 1994; 70:223–234.

29. Knave B, Persson HE, Nilsson SEG: The effect of barbiturate on the retinal functions: II. Effect on the c-wave of the electroretinogram and the standing potential of the sheep eye. *Acta Physiol Scand* 1974; 91:180–186.

30. Komaromy AM, Andrew SE, Sapp HL Jr, Brooks DE, Dawson WW: Flash electroretinography in standing horses using the DTL™ microfiber electrode. *Vet Ophthalmol* 2003; 6:27–33.

31. Kommonen B: The DC-recorded dog electroretinogram in ketamine-medetomidine anesthesia. *Acta Vet Scand* 1988; 29:35–41.

32. Kommonen B, Dawson WW, Parmer R: Pigment epithelial function in canine retina. *Am J Vet Res* 1991; 52:1341–1344.

33. Kommonen B, Karhunen U, Raitta C: Effects of thiopentone, halothane-nitrous oxide anesthesia compared to ketamine-xylazine anesthesia on the DC-recorded dog electroretinogram. *Acta Vet Scand* 1988; 29:23–33.

34. Kommonen BK, Kylma T, Karhunen U, Dawson WW, Penn JS: Impaired retinal function in young Labrador retriever dogs heterozygous for late onset rod-cone degeneration. *Vision Res* 1997; 37:365–370.

35. Kommonen B, Raitta C: Electroretinography in Labrador retrievers given ketamine-xylazine anesthesia. *Am J Vet Res* 1987; 48:1325–1331.

36. Kotani T, Kurosawa T, Numata Y, Izumisawa Y, Satoh H, Brooks DE: The normal electroretinogram in cattle and its clinical application in calves with visual defects. *Prog Vet Comp Ophthalmol* 1993; 3:37–44.

37. Leon A, Hussain AA, Curtis R: Autosomal dominant rod-cone dysplasia in the Rdy cat: II. Electrophysiological findings. *Exp Eye Res* 1991; 53:489–502.

38. Linsenmeyer RA, Steinberg RH: Delayed basal hyperpolarization of cat retinal pigment epithelium and its relation to the fast oscillation of the DC electroretinogram. *J Gen Physiol* 1984; 83:213–232.

39. Majji AB, Humayun MS, Weiland JD, Suzuki A, D'Anna SA, de Juan E: Long-term histological and electrophysiological results in an inactive epiretinal electrode array implantation in dogs. *Invest Ophthalmol Vis Sci* 1999; 40:2073–2081.

40. Marmor MF, Holder GE, Seeliger MW, Yamamoto S: Standard for clinical electroretinography (2004 update). *Doc Ophthalmol* 2004; 108:107–114.

41. Millar TJ, Vaegan, Arora A: Urethane as a sole general anaesthetic in cats used for electroretinogram studies. *Neurosci Lett* 1989; 103:108–112.

42. Millichamp NJ, Arden GB: Transretinal mass receptor potentials recorded from the canine retina in vitro. *Am J Vet Res* 1989; 50:1710–1714.

43. Millichamp NJ, Curtis R, Barnett KC: Progressive retinal atrophy in Tibetan terriers. *J Am Vet Med Assoc* 1988; 192:769–776.

44. Mori T, Pepperberg DR, Marmor MF: Dark adaptation in locally detached retina. *Invest Ophthalmol Vis Sci* 1990; 31:1259–1263.

45. Narfström K: Progressive retinal atrophy in the Abyssinian cat: Clinical characteristics. *Invest Ophthalmol Vis Sci* 1985; 26:193–200.

46. Narfström K: Electroretinography in veterinary medicine: Easy or accurate? *Vet Ophthalmol* 2002; 5:249–251.

47. Narfström K, Andersson B-E, Andreasson S, Gouras P: Clinical electroretinography in the dog using Ganzfeld stimulation: A practical method of examining rod and cone function. *Doc Ophthalmol* 1995; 90:279–290.

48. Narfström K, Arden G, Nilsson SEG: Retinal sensitivity in hereditary retinal degeneration in Abyssinian cats: Electrophysiological similarities to man and cat. *Br J Ophthalmol* 1989; 73:516–521.

49. Narfström K, Bjerkas E, Ekesten B: Visual impairment. In Peiffer RL, Peterson-Jones S (eds): *Small Animal Ophthalmology: A Problem Oriented Approach*, ed 3. London, Saunders, 2001, pp 103–176.

50. Narfström K, Ekesten B: Diseases of the canine ocular fundus. In Gelatt KN (ed): *Veterinary Ophthalmology*, ed 3. Philadelphia, Lippincott, Williams & Wilkins, 1991, pp 887–910.

51. Narfström K, Ekesten B: Electroretinographic evaluation of papillon dogs with and without hereditary retinal degeneration. *Am J Vet Res* 1998; 59:221–226.

52. Narfström K, Ekesten B, Rosolen S, Spiess BM, Percicot CL, Ofri R: Guidelines for clinical electroretinography in the dog. *Doc Ophthalmol* 2002; 105:83–92.

53. Narfström K, Katz M, Bragadottir R, Seeliger M, Boulanger A, Redmond TM, Lai C-M, Rakoczy EP: Functional and structural recovery of the retina after gene therapy in the RPE65 null mutation dog. *Invest Ophthalmol Vis Sci* 2003; 44:1663–1672.

54. Narfström K, Wrigstad A: Clinical, electrophysiological and morphological changes in a case of hereditary retinal degeneration in the papillon dog. *Vet Ophthalmol* 1999; 2:67–74.

55. Narfström K, Wrigstad A, Ekesten B, Nilsson SE: Hereditary retinal dystrophy in the briard dog: Clinical and hereditary characteristics. *Prog Vet Comp Ophthalmol* 1994; 4:85–92.

56. Nelson R, Kolb H, Famiglietti EV Jr, Gouras P: Neural responses in the rod and cone systems of the cat retina: Intracellular records and procion stains. *Invest Ophthalmol* 1976; 15:946–953.

57. Ofri R: Clinical electrophysiology in veterinary ophthalmology: The past, present and future. *Doc Ophthalmol* 2002; 104:5–16.

58. Ofri R, Dawson WW, Gelatt KN: Visual resolution in normal and glaucomatous dogs determined by pattern electroretinogram. *Prog Vet Comp Ophthalmol* 1993; 3:111–116.

59. Parshall CJ, Wyman M, Nitroy S, Acland G, Aguirre G: Photoreceptor dysplasia: An inherited progressive retinal atrophy of miniature Schnauzer dogs. *Prog Vet Comp Ophthalmol* 1991; 1:187–203.

60. Rodiek RW: *The Vertebrate Retina*. San Francisco, WH Freeman, 1973, p 259.

61. Rosolen SG, Rigaudiere F, Lachapelle P: A practical method to obtain reproducible binocular electroretinograms in dogs. *Doc Ophthalmol* 2002; 105:93–103.

62. Rosolen SG, Rigaudiere F, Saint-Macary G, Lachapelle P: Recording of photopic electroretinogram from conscious adult Yucutan micropigs. *Doc Ophthalmol* 1990; 98:197–205.

63. Rubin LF: Clinical electroretinography in dogs. *J Am Vet Med Assoc* 1967; 151:1456–1469.

64. Samuelson DA: Ophthalmic anatomy. In Gelatt KN (ed): *Veterinary Ophthalmology*, ed 3. Philadelphia, Lippincott, Williams & Wilkins, 1991, pp 117–134.

65. Sandberg MA, Pawlyk BS, Berson EL: Full-field electroretinograms in miniature poodles with progressive rod-cone degeneration. *Invest Ophthalmol Vis Sci* 1986; 27:1179–1184.

66. Seeliger MW, Narfström K: Functional assessment of the regional distribution of disease in a cat model of hereditary retinal degeneration. *Invest Ophthalmol Vis Sci* 2000; 41:1998–2005.

67. Sieving A, Frishman LJ, Steinberg RH: Scotopic threshold response (STR) of the proximal retina in the cat. *J Neurophys* 1986; 56:1048–1061.

68. Sieving P, Wakabayashi K: Comparison of rod threshold ERG from monkey, cat and human. *Clin Vision Sci* 1991; 6:171–179.

69. Sims MH, Brooks DE: Changes in oscillary potentials in the canine electroretinogram during dark adaptation. *Am J Vet Res* 1990; 51:1580–1586.

70. Sims MH, Laratta LJ, Bubb WJ, Morgan RV: Waveform analysis and reproducibility of visual-evoked potentials in dogs. *Am J Vet Res* 1989; 50:1823–1828.

71. Spiess B: *Elektroretinographie beim Beagle: Methodik und normalwerte.* Inaugural-dissertation, University of Zurich, Schwitzerland, 1990, p 34.

72. Strain GM, Claxton MS, Olcott BM, Turnquist SE: Visual-evoked potentials and electroretinograms in ruminant with thiamine-responsive polioencephalomalacia or suspected listerioris. *Am J Vet Res* 1990; 51:1513–1517.

73. Textorius O, Gottvall E: The c-wave of the direct-current-recorded electroretinogram and the standing potential of the albino rabbit in response to repeated series of light stimuli of different intensities. *Doc Ophthalmol* 1992; 80:91–103.

74. Ulshafer RJ, Allen C, Dawson WW, Wolf ED: Hereditary retinal degeneration in the Rhode Island red chicken: I. Histology and ERG. *Exp Eye Res* 1984; 39:125–135.

75. Vaegan: Electroretinograms and pattern electroretinograms of pigmented and albino rabbits. *Clin Vision Sci* 1992; 7:305–311.

76. Vaegan, Anderton PJ, Millar TJ: Multifocal, pattern and full field electroretinograms in cats with unilateral optic nerve section. *Doc Ophthalmol* 2000; 100:207–229.

77. Vaegan, Graham SL, Goldberg I, Millar TJ: Selective reduction of oscillatory potentials and pattern electroretinograms after retinal ganglion cell damage by disease in human or by kainic acid toxicity in cats. *Doc Ophthalmol* 1991; 77:237–253.

78. Viswanathan S, Frishman LJ, Robson JG: Inner-retinal contributions to the photopic sinusoidal flicker electroretinogram of macaques. *Doc Ophthalmol* 2002; 105:223–242.

79. White MP, Hock PA: Effects of continuous darkness on ERG correlates of disc shedding in rabbit retina. *Exp Eye Res* 1992; 54:173–180.

80. Witzel DA, Smith EL, Beerwinkle KR, Johnson JH: Arsanilic acid-induced blindness in swine: Electroretinographic and visually evoked responses. *Am J Vet Res* 1976; 37:521–524.

81. Witzel DA, Smith EL, Wilson RD, Aguirre GD: Congenital stationary night blindness: An animal model. *Invest Ophthalmol Vis Sci* 1978; 17:788–795.

82. Wolf ED, Vainisi SJ, Santos-Anderson R: Rod-cone dysplasia in the collie. *J Am Vet Med Assoc* 1978; 173:1331–1333.

83. Yanase J, Ogawa H, Ohtsuka H: Rod and cone components in the dog electroretinogram during and after dark adaptation. *J Vet Med Sci* 1995; 57:877–881.

84. Yanase J, Ogawa H, Ohtsuka H: Scotopic threshold response of the electroretinogram of dogs. *Am J Vet Res* 1996; 57:361–366.

84 Visual Evoked Potentials in Animals

WILLIAM RIDDER

THE VISUAL EVOKED potential (VEP) is used to assess visual performance in a wide variety of animals. A recent literature search found that in the last 25 years, VEPs were recorded from mice,[35,44,61,67,85,89,97,121] rats,[9,33,36,68,72,87,94,137] guinea pigs,[118,119] turtles,[79] fish,[12] birds,[88] rabbits,[81,82] cats,[84,86,215] dogs,[4,113,132] swine,[134] sheep,[16,111] cows,[112,120] monkeys,[10,133,138] baboons,[107] and great apes.[11] A small subset of the references is listed for each species. The specific species chosen for investigation was based on the experimental question asked and the availability of the species. For example, rats are a readily accessible lab animal with a short growth cycle and were used extensively to study the effects of drugs on the visual system. Because of this, the most common species employed in VEP studies was the rat. Monkeys, the second most common species investigated with VEPs, was studied because of its close anatomical relationship to humans. Thus, the VEP has been investigated in many different species for many different reasons.

Because of the extensive literature on VEPs in animals, this chapter will focus on only two species: mice and monkeys. The monkey literature will be reviewed because it reveals important information concerning the recording of VEPs in humans. The origin of the individual VEP components under various stimulus conditions has been investigated in monkeys. The mouse has recently become the model for many different retinal diseases. The reasons for this are many. For example, the mouse has a short life span, so the course of a disease can be followed in a relatively short time. Furthermore, mice can be bred with different retinal diseases, and treatments for these retinal diseases can be perfected in these mice models. The visual evoked potential has the potential to be employed to follow the course and treatment of diseases that affect the visual system. Thus, these two species appear to be the most pertinent to the understanding of the visual system of the human.

The visual evoked potential

The visual evoked potential is a gross electrical potential recorded from the visual cortex in response to a visual stimulus. That is, a visual stimulus results in the excitation of many cells in the cortex, and the summed activity of these cells is recorded as the VEP on the scalp. In all species, two anatomical constraints determine the location in the visual field from which a VEP can be recorded: the location of the visual cortex with respect to the surface of the skull and the number of cortical cells devoted to a given region of the visual field.

Owing to the cortical magnification factor (M) and the anatomy of the visual cortex, the majority of the VEP response is from the central visual field in mice, monkeys, and humans. The M determines the number of cells in the visual cortex devoted to analyzing a specific area of the visual field. The M is the linear extent of cortex in millimeters corresponding to one degree of visual angle. In animals with retinas that have a concentrated area of cones (e.g., monkeys and humans), the M is the greatest where the cone concentration is the highest and decreases with eccentricity. In humans, M at the fovea is 5.6 mm per degree (mm/deg), and at 10 degrees from the fovea, the M is 1.5 mm/deg.[99] Other estimates of M for the human fovea range up to 15.1 mm/deg.[17,24,99] Estimates of M in monkeys range from 13 to 30 mm/deg at the fovea.[18,20,122] In mice, the cortical magnification factor is about 0.016 mm of cortex per degree of visual field.[21, 89] Wagor et al.[130] demonstrated that the M in the mouse is the highest near the vertical midline and decreases by a factor of 2 at 30 degrees from the midline (i.e., from 0.027 to 0.013 mm/deg). They suggested that this results from a higher concentration of ganglion cells devoted to the visual field near the midline. This could result in more cortical space being devoted to the central visual field.

The cortical anatomy can also play a role in the VEP response. In humans, the peripheral visual field is found at deeper locations in the calcarine fissure. The central visual field projects to the most posterior aspect of the striate cortex. This is the area closest to the scalp, and so electrodes placed over this area would be more effective at recording activity from the central visual field. In mice and monkeys, the striate cortex (area 17 or V1) is relatively flat and exposed on the surface of the brain.[18,21,122, 130] This allows for VEP recordings in mice and monkeys from a large extent of the visual field. Thus, in mice and monkeys, the VEP depends more on M than on the cortical anatomy. Since the VEP depends on the number of cells in the visual cortex responding and M is the greatest near the vertical midline for mice and the fovea in monkeys, the VEP is principally a function of the central visual field in the mouse and monkey.

Visual pathway anatomy

To understand the visual evoked potential, a brief review of the anatomy and physiology of the mouse and monkey visual pathway is necessary. A more complete summary can be found in texts devoted to anatomy and physiology.[40,65,110] The following paragraphs will summarize information that is known about the retina, lateral geniculate nucleus, and striate visual cortex that are important in the origin of the visual evoked potential.

RETINA   The photoreceptors of the retina are stimulated by light that passes through the cornea, the lens, the vitreous, and several layers of the retina (figure 84.1). The primary function of the photoreceptors is phototransduction, the conversion of the energy of light into a neuroelectrical

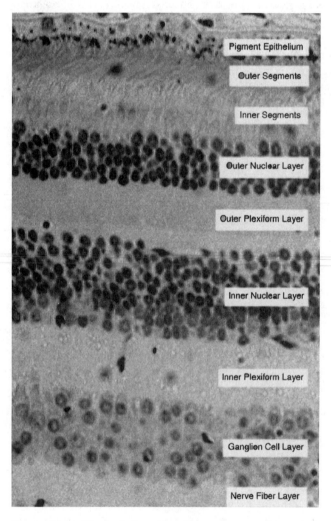

FIGURE 84.1   Histological section of a macaque monkey retina. (Courtesy of MLJ Crawford.)

response. The photoreceptors alter their membrane potential (i.e., hyperpolarize) in response to light stimulation. There are roughly 120 million photoreceptors scattered across the primate retina, each responsive to stimulation of a discrete area of the visual field. There are four types of photoreceptors (i.e., rods and S-, M-, and L-cones) in the primate retina (i.e., old world primates and humans), which respond optimally to different wavelengths of light. The cones have their highest concentration in the fovea of the retina. The cone concentration decreases with distance from the fovea but never reaches zero. Rods are not found in the center of the fovea but are most concentrated about 20 degrees from the fovea. Owing to the anatomy of the fovea, this area is specialized for processing high spatial frequency and color information.

The mouse retina is rod dominated with few cones identified. Estimates of cone percentages in the mouse retina range from 1% to 10%, with newer techniques suggesting approximately 3% of the photoreceptors are cones.[14,69,106] Morphologically, the cones of the mouse are indistinguishable from those of higher mammals.[14] The mouse retina does not have an area centralis (i.e., an area of concentrated cones) or a visual streak. Carter-Dawson and LaVail,[14] after examining the posterior pole, equator, and periphery, concluded that the cone concentration was about 3% in all areas. A study employing both electroretinograms and psychophysical testing suggested that there are two different cone types in the mouse.[48] One cone has a peak spectral sensitivity at 510 nm, and the other is in the ultraviolet region of the spectrum at about 370 nm. Using the same ERG methodology as with the mouse, Jacobs et al.[48] also identified these two cone types in gerbils, rats, and gophers.

The information from the photoreceptors is then processed though the retina, and finally, retinal ganglion cells are stimulated. This processing of visual information in the retina results in electrical changes in the tissue that can be recorded as a mass potential called the electroretinogram. Under certain recording conditions, the electroretinogram can be observed in the visual evoked potential waveform.

There are approximately 1.2 million retinal ganglion cells that give rise to the primate optic nerve. Thus, there is a convergence of information from the photoreceptors to the retinal ganglion cells. Each retinal ganglion cell processes a specific set of visual properties (e.g., spatial, temporal, color, and luminance information) and relays that information to higher visual centers. The primate has two broad classes of retinal ganglion cells: M (Pα) and P (Pβ) ganglion cells. The cells in each class process similar types of visual information. In general, M cells carry information specific for low-spatial-frequency, high-temporal-frequency, low-contrast luminance objects, and P cells carry information specific for high-spatial-frequency, low-temporal-frequency, high-contrast color objects. About 80% of retinal ganglion cells are P cells. P cells are concentrated in the fovea, where there is little convergence of information.[131] That is, one cone may project to a single retinal ganglion cell in the fovea, whereas in the periphery, many cones may project to a single ganglion cell. The percentage of M cells increases with retinal eccentricity. The P cells project to the parvocellular layers of the LGN, and the M cells project to the magnocellular layers of the LGN.

Each mouse retina has from 48,000 to 65,000 ganglion cells.[23,37] Similar to primates, it has been suggested that mice have different classes of ganglion cells based on their cell body size.[23] The receptive fields of the retinal ganglion cells of the mouse have the classic center-surround arrangement found in other mammals. The size of the mouse ganglion cell receptive field is more than a log unit larger than that of the primate. This would suggest that the visual acuity of the mouse is more than 1 log unit less than that of primates.

LATERAL GENICULATE NUCLEUS The lateral geniculate nucleus (LGN) of the primate is a small nucleus, containing roughly 1.3 million neurons, located in the lateral and posterior aspect of the thalamus. Thus, there is roughly a 1:1 correspondence of retinal ganglion cells to LGN cells. The LGN of old-world primates and humans has six layers. The layers are numbered 1 to 6 starting ventrally (figure 84.2). Layers 1 and 2 are the magnocellular layers (M), and layers 3–6 are the parvocellular layers (P). Each layer lies in register with those above and below it. Between these layers and ventral to the LGN are a small number of cells referred to as intercalated or I neurons.[139] The receptive field properties of LGN cells are primarily determined by their inputs, that is, the retinal ganglion cells. Thus, the magnocellular layers

process visual information concerned with low spatial frequencies, high temporal frequencies, low contrast, and luminance. The parvocellular layers process visual information concerned with high spatial frequencies, low temporal frequencies, high contrast, and color. The parvocellular layers developed later evolutionarily than the magnocellular layers.

In general, retinal ganglion cells located in the nasal retina project to the contralateral LGN, and those found in the temporal retina project to the ipsilateral LGN. The ipsilateral fibers terminate in layers 2, 3, and 5, while the contralateral fibers terminate in layers 1, 4, and 6. Thus, approximately 50% of the retinal ganglion cells decussate at the optic chiasm to innervate the contralateral LGN. This results in the monocular VEPs having similar amplitudes at the cortex.

Ganglion cells from the macula project to the most posterior aspect of the LGN. The anterior LGN receives input from ganglion cells located in the peripheral retina. The ganglion cells in the superior retina project to the medial LGN, and those in the inferior retina project to the temporal LGN. Thus, the LGN has a retinotopic arrangement that results in neighboring cells in the LGN processing information from contiguous areas of the visual field.

In the mouse, Drager and Olsen[23] and Balkema and Drager[7] identified 2.6% of the total ganglion cell axons that projected to the ipsilateral lateral geniculate nucleus of the thalamus. Thus, over 97% of the axons decussate at the optic chiasm in the mouse. However, those ganglion cells with receptive fields located in binocular regions of the visual field (i.e., the central 30–40 degrees) had a somewhat higher percentage (approximately 9%) of axons that remained ipsilateral. The ipsilaterally projecting axons

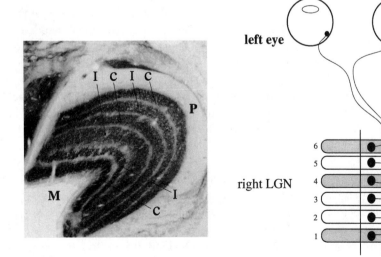

FIGURE 84.2 Left, Vertical section of a macaque monkey LGN. Right, Interconnections with the retinas. (See text for details.) (LGN section courtesy of MLJ Crawford.) (See also color plate 57.)

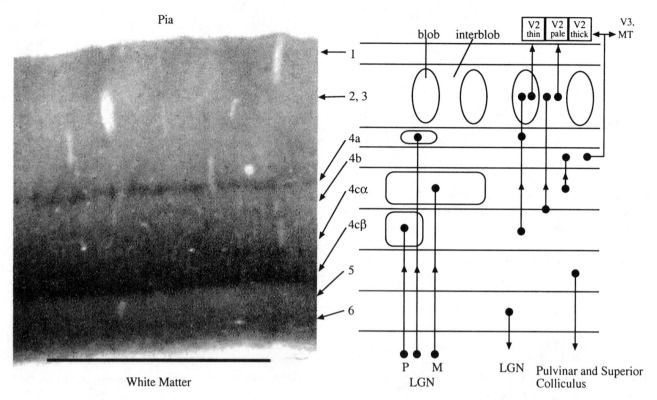

FIGURE 84.3 Left, Striate cortex of a macaque monkey. Right, Interconnections with the LGN and the extrastriate cortex. (Cortex section courtesy of MLJ Crawford.)

demonstrate a divergence of connections in the LGN and occupy 14–18% of its volume.[58] The divergence of the axons at the level of the LGN may be responsible for the amplitude of the VEP from the ipsilateral eye being as much as half that of the contralateral eye.[89] As in higher mammals, the projection onto the LGN follows a retinotopic arrangement.[31]

STRIATE CORTEX The primate striate cortex is about 2 mm thick and can be divided into six layers (figure 84.3). The striate cortex of macaques covers roughly 1300 mm² of total surface area[47] and has roughly 200,000 neurons per square millimeter of cortex.[83] There is a large amount of information divergence from the LGN to the estimated 260 million neurons in the cortex. This divergence has a significant impact on the VEP recording.

The different layers of the LGN (i.e., magnocellular and parvocellular) project to specific layers in the cortex.[13,62] The six layers of the cortex are numbered 1–6, starting at the pial surface and proceeding to the white matter. Some of these layers are further subdivided. The magnocellular layers of the LGN project to layer 4cα of the striate cortex, and the parvocellular layers project to layers 4cβ and 4a. LGN inputs to layer 4 alternate from the right and left eyes, producing ocular dominance columns. Cells above and below layer 4 typically receive input from both eyes.

A significant amount of information is available concerning the intricacies of the striate cortical pathways in primates. The following is a brief summary. The superficial layers receive input from layer 4 and relay this information to higher cortical areas. The deeper layers (5 and 6) project back to subcortical nuclei (e.g., LGN and pulvinar). Layer 4cα projects to layer 4b and then to areas V2 and V5 (MT). Layer 4cβ projects to superficial layers 2 and 3, which then project to area V2. Cells in layers 2 and 3 can be further grouped on the basis of their response to cytochrome oxidase staining.[135] Cells that stain for cytochrome oxidase have a high metabolic rate, and these cells are grouped together in clusters referred to as blobs. The projection from layer 4cβ terminates in blobs in layers 2 and 3. A third projection channel originates in the middle of layer 4 (i.e., contains both M and P pathway input) and projects to the interblob zones (i.e., areas between the blobs) of layers 2 and 3. The information is then relayed to area V2. Thus, several parallel channels of information flow through the striate cortex. These pathways carry different types of information and terminate in different extrastriate areas.

Cells in the striate cortex are arranged retinotopically as in the LGN. Thus, two cells located next to one another in the cortex process information from areas of the visual field located next to one another. Furthermore, there is a significant divergence of information from the macula to the cortex (i.e., cortical magnification or M). The divergence results in more cortical cells devoted to processing macular information than peripheral information. Approximately half of the striate cortex is devoted to processing information from the central 10 degrees of visual field.[122] Since most of the cortical cells are devoted to the macula, the VEP is principally a macular response.

In the human, the macula projects to the most posterior aspect of the calcarine fissure in the occipital lobe. The peripheral visual field projects to more anterior locations in the calcarine fissure. This results in the macular projection on the striate cortex being closest to the surface of the brain and producing the major component of the VEP. In the monkey, more of the striate cortex is exposed on the surface of the brain lateral to the midline. Thus, in the monkey, the macular projection also produces a major component of the VEP.

The mouse geniculocortical afferents project from the LGN to the primary visual cortex or area V1.[21,22,130] Area V1, like the LGN, has a retinotopic arrangement.[21,32,108,130] Single-cell microelectrode studies have indicated that as the midline is approached in area V1, the cells' receptive fields move temporally in the visual field. Additionally, the superior visual field is represented posteriorly in area V1. The lateral one third of area V1 receives binocular input from the central 30–40 degrees of the upper portion of each visual hemifield.

Several studies have delineated the extent of area V1 in the mouse.[21,23,32,108,126,130] Drager[26] showed a map of area V1 with relation to external landmarks of the skull. Area V1 is located at the most posterior edge of the cerebral cortex. It is about 2 mm wide and 1.5–2.0 mm in the anteroposterior direction. The medial edge of area V1 is about 2 mm from the sagittal suture. Surrounding area V1 is area V2. All published maps of area V1 agree with Drager.[32,108,126,130]

All of the physiological classes of striate cortical cells that have been identified in cats and monkeys (i.e., center-surround cells, simple cells, complex cells, and hypercomplex cells) have also been observed in the mouse.[21,45,46,63] The receptive field properties of these cells are similar in the different species.

Based on single-cell recordings, extrastriate areas have also been identified in the mouse cortex. Wagor et al.[130] identified two extrastriate areas (V2 and V3) having complete or near complete representations of the contralateral visual field. However, the cortical map that he displayed (Figure 8 in Wagor et al.[130]) indicates that areas V2 and V3 are considerably smaller than area V1. Thus, their contribution to the VEP is limited. Based on the mouse and monkey anatomy, a normal VEP requires a normal central visual pathway from the retina to the striate cortex.

Monkey visual evoked potential

The visual evoked potential has been used as a tool to study the visual system of normal and abnormal monkeys. Initially, the effects of different stimuli were determined on the VEP in monkeys.[51,74,127,129] Subsequently, the effects of different treatments on the monkey visual system were determined with the VEP. Animal models of amblyopia,[6,10,124,138] encephalitis,[80,96] glaucoma,[49,64] Parkinson's disease,[26] laser retinal damage,[92,93,100–103] and lead and PCP toxicity[60,66] have been investigated.

FLASH VEP Several different kinds of stimuli have been employed to produce the VEP. The stimulus chosen will depend on the question being asked. Stimuli can consist of flashes of light, checkerboard patterns, square wave gratings, or sine gratings. Examples of normal VEP responses from monkeys to several stimuli are shown in figures 84.4, 84.5, and 84.6. Electrode placement can have a significant impact on the waveform. For these data, the active electrode was placed 2 cm lateral to the midline and 1 cm anterior to the nuchal crest. The reference electrode was placed at the vertex, and the ground was placed on the midline of the forehead. The monkey (*Macaca fasicularis*) was anesthetized with ketamine (10 mg/kg IM) and paralyzed with Norcuron (30 μg/kg IV). Supplemental doses of Norcuron (10 μg/kg) were used as needed. The animal was artificially ventilated (Engler 1000), and the body temperature was maintained with a heating pad. The pupils were dilated with 2.5% phenylephrine and 1% tropicamide. Heart rate, blood pressure, and expired CO_2 were monitored.

Figure 84.4 shows the VEP response to a flash of light (i.e., the fVEP; $N = 100$). The stimulus was a 1-Hz flash of light (8

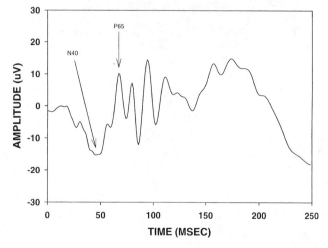

MONKEY FLASH VEP

FIGURE 84.4 Flash visual evoked potential (fVEP) from a monkey. (See text for details.) (Recordings were made in the lab of James Burke, Allergan, Inc.)

MONKEY PATTERN VEP

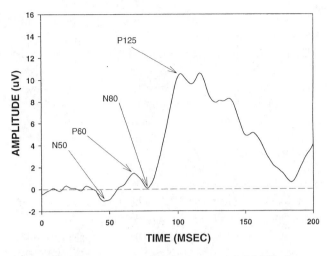

FIGURE 84.5 Pattern visual evoked potential (pVEP) from a monkey. (See text for details.) (Recordings were made in the lab of James Burke, Allergan, Inc.)

MONKEY SWEEP VEP

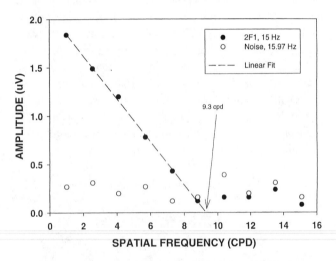

FIGURE 84.6 Sweep visual evoked potential (sVEP) from a monkey. (See text for details.) (Recordings were made in the lab of James Burke, Allergan, Inc.)

cd s/m²) produced in a Ganzfeld. The data were acquired with an Espion system (Diagnosys LLC, Littleton, MA). The VEP recorded in response to a flash of light can be a complicated waveform consisting of several negative- and positive-going waves.[15] These waves have been given many different names by different investigators.[38] For our purposes, the waveforms will be labeled P or N for positive- or negative-going waveforms, respectively. To conform to the monkey fVEP literature, following the P or N will be the approximate latency of the peak of the waveform (e.g., P100 for a positive waveform with a peak latency of about 100 ms).

Several different positive- and negative-going waveforms have been identified in the fVEP.[28,52,53] The largest are a negative-going wave at about 40 ms (N40), a positive-going wave at about 65 ms (P65), and a second negative-going wave at about 95 ms (N95) after the flash of light. For figure 84.4, the peaks are N44, P67, and N86. The amplitude from N44 to P67 is 25.2 µV. As flash intensity increases, the amplitude of the response increases and the latency decreases.[29] The stimulus wavelength also has a significant effect on the amplitude and latency of the response.

The origin of the fVEP response was assessed by combining VEP recordings, multiunit activity response profiles, and current source density analysis in the same animals.[28,52,53,104] The findings indicate that the early components of the fVEP (N40 and P65) originate in the striate cortex and later components are generated in the extrastriate cortex (e.g., possibly V4).[28] Peaks recorded before N40 may arise from LGN activity[104] or the optic radiations.[52,105] The N40 peak may originate from EPSP (excitatory postsynaptic potential) activity of stellate cells and depolarization of thalamic axons in layer 4c of the striate cortex.[105] The P65 component results from the hyperpolarization of the stellate cells in layer 4c. The human fVEP is composed of a negative-going wave at 70 ms (N70) and a positive-going wave at about 100 ms (P100) after the flash of light. Kraut et al.[52] have suggested that the monkey fVEP N40 and P65 peaks correlate with the human fVEP N70 and P100 peaks, respectively. Very early components of the fVEP in humans (less than 65 ms after the flash onset) may be from the electroretinogram.[5] Thus, the fVEP may be used to assess the function of specific layers of the striate cortex in monkeys and humans.

PATTERN VEP Figure 84.5 contains an example of a pattern VEP (pVEP). The stimulus was a checkerboard pattern (100% contrast) square wave modulated at 1 Hz. Each check subtended 0.5 degree of visual angle at a 1-m viewing distance. The graph is the average of 200 phase reversals. Electrode placement is the same as in the fVEP in figure 84.4. The pVEP to gratings usually consist of a positive-going wave at 60 ms (P60), a negative-going wave at about 80 ms (N80), and a second positive-going wave at about 125 ms (P125) after stimulus alternation.[105] Typically, pattern stimuli consist of checkerboard patterns or gratings (sine or square wave). The size, contrast, and temporal modulation of the pattern will affect the amplitude and latency of the response.[18,26,30,51,64,73,74,127] The location of the recording electrode over the striate cortex may also influence the waveform that is recorded.[18] The closer the electrode is placed to the foveal projection, the higher the amplitude of the response.[127] In figure 84.5, the peak waveform latencies are P33, N46, P68, N78, and P105. The amplitude from N78 to P105 is 10.4 µV.

The origin of the pVEP has also been investigated.[18,105,127] These investigations utilized pVEP recordings, multiunit activity response profiles, and current source density analysis. In addition to the peaks listed above for the pVEP, Schroeder et al.[105] have identified an earlier set of peaks (P40 and N50) in some animals. Their findings indicate that the N50 results from activation of stellate cells in layer 4c of the striate cortex. The P60 arises from the activation of supragranular (i.e., layers 2 and 3 of the striate cortex) neurons, possibly pyramidal cells. Later waves appear to arise from multiple generators that may include extrastriate regions. Schroeder et al.[105] suggest that the N50, P60, and N80 peaks of the monkey pVEP are equivalent to the N70, P100, and post-P100 negativity in the human pVEP.

The pVEP was used to assess conditions that may affect the spatial or temporal processing of the visual pathway.[26,49,64] Marx et al.[64] found that in monkeys with glaucoma, the pVEP was reduced in amplitude to low-spatial-frequency stimuli. Johnson et al.[49] found reductions in the pVEP amplitude in glaucoma monkeys, but there was not a spatial frequency effect. These differences might be the result of the different methodologies employed. Marx et al.[64] used a square wave grating, while Johnson et al.[49] used a checkerboard pattern. Additionally, the temporal and spatial frequencies presented were different. Spatial-frequency-dependent changes in the pVEP have also been observed in a Parkinsonian-induced syndrome in monkeys.[26]

Amblyopia is a common visual condition that was investigated with the pVEP.[123,133] These investigations indicated that strabismic amblyopic monkeys and humans have similar abnormalities of the visual pathway. Normal visual processes such as color vision[54,55] and texture segregation[57] were also investigated with the pVEP. Thus, the pVEP can be used to assess normal visual processes (i.e., spatial, temporal, contrast, and color mechanisms), as well as conditions that alter visual processing (e.g., glaucoma, amblyopia, and Parkinson's disease).

A modification of the pattern VEP is the sweep VEP (sVEP). The sVEP technique was developed to rapidly obtain visual acuity estimates in humans.[77,78,125] This technique utilizes sine wave or square wave gratings. Several different spatial frequencies, centered on the subject's visual acuity, are presented in rapid succession, and the individual responses are partitioned out on the basis of the stimulus spatial frequency. A plot of spatial frequency versus response amplitude is then obtained. Visual acuity can then be determined from this plot. This technique can be used to estimate visual acuity much more quickly than a pVEP technique. The sVEP can also be used to determine thresholds for other visual parameters (e.g., contrast and temporal frequency).

Figure 84.6 shows the sVEP results for one monkey (*Macaca fasicularis*). The electrode placement is the same as

in figures 84.4 and 84.5. The sVEP technique was described by Norcia et al.[76] The horizontal axis displays spatial frequency, and the vertical axis displays the amplitude of the response. The solid symbols display the Fourier amplitude at twice the fundamental frequency (15 Hz), and the open symbols display the noise (15.97 Hz). The phase lag of the response increased slightly as the spatial frequency was increased until the response fell to noise (not shown). At higher spatial frequencies, the change in phase was random. Norcia and Tyler[77] determined acuity by fitting a line to the high-spatial-frequency limb of the function and extrapolating this to 0 μV. The extrapolated acuity for this animal was 9.3 cpd, or about 20/65.

The sVEP was used in monkeys to measure visual acuity.[10,30,56,104,129,138] The monkey sVEP acuity is typically between 15 and 30 cpd.[30,129,138] Squirrel monkeys (*Saimiri sciureus*) have lower visual acuities than macaque monkeys (*Macaca mulatta*).[138] The visual acuity obtained with the sVEP is similar to that obtained with the steady-state VEP and by psychophysical methods.[3,19,30,41,50,70,71] Furthermore, the sVEP acuity is similar with or without propofol anesthesia.[3] The sVEP was also used to examine acuity in monkey models of amblyopia,[10,56,138] as well as to examine short-term fluctuations in acuity after laser exposure.[104]

The mouse visual evoked potential

FLASH VEP   The fVEP has been examined in mice to determine the effects of various drugs on the cortex,[1,2,42,121] examine the effects of albinism or aging on the visual pathway,[1,42,43] determine the absolute light sensitivity,[35] and examine ultradian rhythms.[67] Recent studies have examined the effect of various stimulus parameters on the flash VEP response.[61,114]

A typical fVEP response recorded from a light-adapted mouse is displayed in figure 84.7. The effect of a series of flash intensities is shown. The animal was anesthetized with a mixture of ketamine and xylazine (15 μg/g body weight and 7 μg/g body weight, respectively) injected intraperitoneally. The active electrode was a stainless steel bolt implanted 3 mm lateral to the lambda. The tip of the bolt rested on the dura. The reference electrode was a gold wire placed against the roof of the mouth, and the ground was a needle under the skin near the tail. The mouse was placed in a stereotaxic apparatus (Stoelting, Wood Dale, IL) that held the snout. The stereotaxic apparatus was placed in a Ganzfeld, and the stimulus was produced by a photostimulator set at a temporal frequency of 1 Hz. Each waveform is the average of 100 repetitions. In agreement with previous publications on fVEPs, the initial positive-going wave is referred to as P1, and the subsequent negative-gong wave is N1. The second large positive waveform is P2.[42,43,121] The

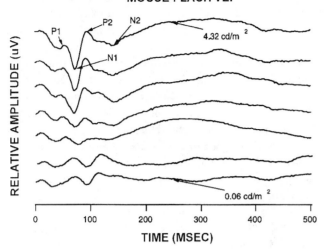

FIGURE 84.7   Flash visual evoked potential from a mouse. (See text for details.)

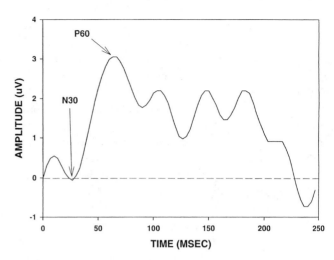

FIGURE 84.8   Pattern visual evoked potential from a mouse. (See text for details.)

latency of the P1, N1, and P2 peaks and the amplitude of the response are typically determined. In this example, the latencies of the P1, N1, and P2 waves for the top response are approximately 54, 75, and 96 ms, respectively. The amplitude from N1 to P2 is 82 μV. As the stimulus intensity decreases, the amplitude of the response decreases and the latency increases (i.e., similar to monkey results).

Early studies of the fVEP in mice examined the extent of the visual cortex[136] or the effects of anesthetics.[2,42] Later studies of the fVEP have examined the effect of stimulus parameters such as temporal frequency[1,114] and flash intensity.[35] These studies demonstrated that certain anesthetics (e.g., pentobarbitol, chlorprothixene, and haloperidol) could alter the latency of the VEP response. Increasing the temporal frequency of the stimulus resulted in an increase in the latency of the response and a decrease in the amplitude. The most recent studies have used the fVEP to examine the effects of specific genetic mutations in mice.[59,85,97]

In conclusion, early studies of the fVEP in mice have demonstrated the basic waveform. Recently, the fVEP has been used to assess physiological functions of the mouse visual pathway. Future studies are needed to assess the effects of various stimulus attributes (e.g., background and stimulus intensity, wavelength, and temporal frequency) so that a complete picture of the fVEP response can be obtained. Additionally, studies should be carried out to determine the optimal recording technique (e.g., electrode locations and anesthesia) for the mouse fVEP. The electrode configuration and the anesthetic employed have a significant effect on the shape and timing of the VEP waveform. These studies will be necessary before the fVEP can be used to routinely assess the mouse visual pathway and comparisons between labs can be made.

PATTERN VEP   The pVEP can be used to assess several aspects of the visual system. The field size, pattern size, contrast, retinal location, and rate of stimulus presentation all affect the response. Thus, with the pVEP, the visual acuity, contrast sensitivity, and motion sensitivity can be determined.[89–91,114] There is a good correlation between these parameters that are determined psychophysically and electrophysiologically.[27,95,109]

The waveform for the pVEP has a simpler morphology than the fVEP. A typical pVEP recorded from a mouse is displayed in figure 84.8. The electrode positions are the same as those for the fVEP in figure 84.7. The stimulus is a checkerboard pattern reversing (square wave) at a temporal frequency of 4 Hz. Each check subtended an angle of 6.2 degrees at the mouse eye. The pVEP consists of a negative-going wave at about 30 ms and a positive-going wave at about 60 ms. The amplitude from the first negative-going wave to the positive-going wave is 3.1 μV.

Several different pattern stimuli have been used to assess the mouse visual system.[89,90,114] Porciatti et al.[89] assessed the visual acuity, cortical magnification factor (M), ocularity, contrast threshold, temporal tuning function, motion sensitivity, and luminance effect with the pVEP. Their stimuli were horizontal sine wave gratings of different spatial frequencies that covered 81 × 86 degrees of the visual field. The mice were anesthetized with 20% urethane (Sigma, 8 ml/kg) and mounted in a stereotaxic apparatus. A craniotomy was made over the visual cortex, and the dura was left intact. The electrode (a resin-coated microelectrode) was placed approximately 3 mm lateral to the lambda (the intersection between the saggital and lambdoid sutures) overlying the binocular area of the striate visual cortex.[21]

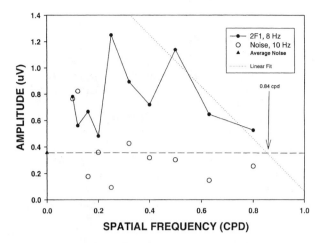

MOUSE SWEEP VEP

0.84 cpd

Legend:
- 2F1, 8 Hz (filled circles)
- Noise, 10 Hz (open circles)
- Average Noise (filled triangle)
- Linear Fit (dotted line)

Y-axis: AMPLITUDE (µV)

X-axis: SPATIAL FREQUENCY (CPD)

FIGURE 84.9   Sweep visual evoked potential from a mouse. (See text for details.)

The acuity obtained with the pVEP was similar to previous psychophysical measures of acuity in the mouse. Peak responses were obtained with stimuli of 0.06–0.1 c/deg. The acuity was determined by extrapolation of the high-spatial-frequency data to the x-axis or zero amplitude. Porciatti et al.[89] found an average acuity of 0.6 c/deg with the pVEP. Studies of optokinetic nystagmus have suggested that the acuity of mice is about 0.5 c/deg.[109] Forced choice, psychophysical techniques have also resulted in acuity estimates of 0.5–0.6 c/deg.[27,95] Thus, the acuity of mice is slightly more than 1 log unit less than that of primates.

Sweep VEP acuity estimates are similar to those obtained using psychophysical methods.[98] Figure 84.9 displays an sVEP response for a mouse. The electrode position and anesthesia are the same as previously described. Spatial frequency is plotted on the horizontal axis, and the response amplitude (the second harmonic of the discrete Fourier transform, 8 Hz) is plotted on the vertical axis (solid symbols). The open symbols represent the noise (10 Hz). The stimulus was a horizontally oriented sine wave grating. The stimulus contrast was 80%, and the temporal reversal rate (square wave) was 4 Hz. The screen luminance was 100 cd/m², and the screen subtended 100 degrees (H) by 82 degrees (V) at the mouse eye. Stimulus production and data collection were carried out with the Enfant (Neuroscientific Corp.) system.

The data in the figure display two peaks in the sVEP function: one peak at 0.24 cpd and a second peak at 0.50 cpd. This double-peaked function has been observed in human sVEP data.[34,77,116,117] In humans, it has been postulated that the double peak results from the interaction of two parallel channels (i.e., the proposed transient and sustained or M and P channels) of information flow reaching the cortex at different times. Thus, at intermediate spatial frequencies (0.3–0.4 cpd in this mouse), these two parallel channels may

interact destructively to produce a decrease in the response amplitude. Acuity can be determined by fitting a line to the high-spatial-frequency data and extrapolating this line to the noise. The horizontal dashed line depicts the average noise for the data set. By using this technique for this set of data (the dotted line in the figure), the acuity was estimated to be 0.84 cpd. This corresponds to an acuity of 20/714. This is similar to previous reports of acuity measured with the pVEP and using psychophysical techniques.

Contrast sensitivity has not been measured psychophysically in the mouse; however, pVEP data suggest that the peak contrast threshold is about 5%.[89] This is similar to the peak contrast threshold of the rat.[8] Temporal tuning functions for the mouse striate cortex determined from pVEPs suggest that there is a peak at 2–4 Hz.[89,114] On either side of this, the sensitivity is less. The temporal frequency cutoff is about 12 Hz. The peak of the temporal tuning function correlates with a stimulus velocity of about 67 deg/s. The temporal frequency cutoff correlates with a stimulus velocity of about 200 deg/s. These values agree well with the optimal stimulus velocities for the cortical cells in mice.[21] Drager[21] found that mouse cortical cells preferred stimulus velocities from 5 to 200 deg/s with some cells as high as 1000 deg/s. She speculated that this was the result of the anatomy of the mouse eye. The relationship between the mouse lens and the eye's axial length would result in a minimized image of the world on the retina. Thus, only rapidly moving objects would optimally stimulate retinal cells.

Porciatti et al.[89] also examined the effect of mean luminance on the amplitude of the pVEP. Over the range of 0.25 cd/m² to 25 cd/m², the VEP amplitude increased with the maximum amplitude obtained at the highest luminance. These luminance levels are in the mesopic and photopic ranges. Since the VEP amplitude is greatest at the highest luminance, the mouse VEP may be cone-driven.

By driving an electrode to various layers of the cortex and monitoring the pVEP, the source of the VEP can be determined. On either side of the source, the VEPs will have opposite polarities. Porciatti et al.,[89] using this technique in the mouse, determined that the source of the pVEP is in the supragranular layers of area V1. This agrees with work on the rat[25,87] and monkey.[105]

In conclusion, the pVEP has been used to assess several aspects of the mouse visual system. The pVEP results correspond to the psychophysical findings for the mouse and can be used to make these measurements more efficiently. Thus, the pVEP can be used to assess the visual pathway in mouse models of various visual system diseases.

General conclusions

International standards for VEP recordings in humans have recently been accepted.[39] Other standards for animals (e.g., electroretinograms in dogs) have also been proposed.[75] These standards were the result of many investigations into stimulus parameters and recording techniques and their effect on the specific electrophysiological test. The standards allow for predictable results based on a specific recording technique and stimulus. The groundwork for VEP recording in mice and monkeys has been done. It is clear that VEPs can be readily recorded from the central visual field of mice and monkeys. The fVEP can be employed to determine whether there are any lesions of the visual pathway from the retina to the striate cortex. Pattern VEPs can be employed to assess several aspects of the visual system (e.g., visual acuity, cortical magnification factor (M), ocularity, contrast threshold, temporal tuning function, motion sensitivity, and luminance effects). Multifocal VEPs, which have not been reported in mice or monkeys, may prove beneficial in assessing specific aspects of the visual field. Future studies are needed to extend this work so that the effect of various stimulus parameters on the VEP is clarified. These studies may allow for standards to be developed for mice and monkeys so that the visual effect of alterations in the visual system due to disease or experimental manipulation can be readily identified.

REFERENCES

1. Adachi-Usami E: Senescence of visual function as studied by visually evoked cortical potentials. *Jpn J Ophthalmol* 1990; 34:81–94.

2. Adachi-Usami E, Ikeda H, Satoh H: Haloperidol delays visually evoked cortical potentials but not electroretinograms in mice. *J Ocul Pharmacol Ther* 1990; 6(3):203–210.

3. Aiyer A, Wilson JR, Swenson B, Levi A, Boothe RG: Acuity assessment by behavioral and VEP methods: A comparison in monkeys [ARVO Abstract]. *Invest Ophthalmol Vis Sci* 1996; 37:S708.

4. Akabane A, Saito K, Suzuki Y, Shibuya M, Sugita K: Monitoring visual evoked potentials during retraction of the canine optic nerve: Protective effect of unroofing the optic canal. *J Neurosurg* 1995; 82(2):284–287.

5. Allison T, Matsumya Y, Goff GD, Goff WR: The scalp topography of human visual evoked potentials. *Electroencephalogr Clin Neurophysiol* 1977; 42:185–197.

6. Baitch LW, Ridder WH III, Harwerth RS, Smith EL III: Binocular beat VEPs: Losses of cortical binocularity in monkeys reared with abnormal visual experience. *Invest Ophthalmol Vis Sci* 1991; 32(12):3096–3103.

7. Balkema GW, Drager UC: Origins of uncrossed retinofugal projections in normal and hypopigmented mice. *Vis Neurosci* 1990; 4(6):595–604.

8. Birch D, Jacobs GH: Spatial contrast sensitivity in albino and pigmented rats. *Vision Res* 1979; 19:933–937.

9. Biro K, Palhalmi J, Toth AJ, Kukorelli T, Juhasz G: Bimoclomol improves early electrophysiological signs of retinopathy in diabetic rats. *Neuroreport* 1998; 9(9):2029–2033.

10. Boothe RG, Louden T, Aiyer A, Izquierdo A, Drews C, Lambert SR: Visual outcome after contact lens and intra-ocular lens correction of neonatal monocular aphakia in monkeys. *Invest Ophthalmol Vis Sci* 2000; 41(1):110–119.

11. Boysen ST, Berntson GG: Visual evoked potentials in the great apes. *Electroencephalogr Clin Neurophysiol* 1985; 62(2):150–153.

12. Bullock TH, Hofmann MH, New JG, Nahm FK: Dynamic properties of visual evoked potentials in the tectum of cartilaginous and bony fishes, with neuroethological implications. *J Exp Zool Suppl* 1990; 5:142–155.

13. Callaway EM: Local circuits in primary visual cortex of the macaque monkey. *Ann Rev Neurosci* 1998; 21:47–74.

14. Carter-Dawson LD, LaVail MM: Rods and cones in the mouse retina: I. Structural analysis using light and electron microscopy. *J Comp Neurol* 1979; 188(2):245–262.

15. Ciganek ML: The EEG response (evoked potential) to light stimulus in man. *Electroencephalogr Clin Neurophysiol* 1961; 13:165–172.

16. Coupland SG, Cochrane DD: Maturational topography of the visual evoked potential in fetal lambs. *Doc Ophthalmol* 1987; 66(4):337–346.

17. Cowey A, Rolls ET: Human cortical magnification factor and its relation to visual acuity. *Exp Brain Res* 1974; 21(5):447–454.

18. Dagnelie G, Spekreijse H, van Dijk B: Topography and homogeneity of monkey V1 studied through subdurally recorded pattern-evoked potentials. *Vis Neurosci* 1989; 3(6):509–525.

19. De Valois RL, Morgan H, Snodderly DM: Psychophysical studies of monkey vision: III. Spatial luminance contrast sensitivity tests of macaque and human observers. *Vision Res* 1974; 14(1):75–81.

20. Dow BM, Snyder AZ, Vautin RG, Bauer R: Magnification factor and receptive field size in foveal striate cortex of the monkey. *Exp Brain Res* 1981; 44(2):213–228.

21. Drager UC: Receptive fields of single cells and topography in mouse visual cortex. *J Comp Neurol* 1975; 160(3):269–290.

22. Drager UC: Observations on monocular deprivation in mice. *J Neurophysiol* 1978; 41(1):28–42.

23. Drager UC, Olsen JF: Origins of crossed and uncrossed retinal projections in pigmented and albino mice. *J Comp Neurol* 1980; 191(3):383–412.

24. Drasdo N: The neural representation of visual space. *Nature* 1977; 266(5602):554–556.

25. Fontanesi G, Siciliano R, Porciatti V, Bagnoli P: Somastatin depletion modifies the functional activity of the visual cortex in the rat. *Vis Neurosci* 1996; 3:327–334.

26. Ghilardi MF, Bodis-Wollner I, Onofrj MC, Marx MS, Glover AA: Spatial frequency-dependent abnormalities of the pattern electroretinogram and visual evoked potentials in a parkinsonian monkey model. *Brain* 1988; 111(1):131–149.

27. Gianfranceschi L, Fiorentini A, Maffei L: Behavioural visual acuity of wild type and bc12 transgenic mouse. *Vision Res* 1999; 39(3):569–574.

28. Givre SJ, Schroeder CE, Arezzo JC: Contribution of extrastriate area V4 to the surface-recorded flash VEP in the awake macaque. *Vision Res* 1994; 34(4):415–428.

29. Givre SJ, Arezzo JC, Schroeder CE: Effects of wavelength on the timing and laminar distribution of illuminance-evoked activity in macaque V1. *Vis Neurosci* 1995; 12(2):229–239.

30. Glickman RD, Rhodes JW, Coffey DJ: Noninvasive techniques for assessing the effect of environmental stressors on visual function. *Neurosci Biobehav Rev* 1991; 15(1):173–181.

31. Godement P, Salaun J, Imbert M: Prenatal and postnatal development of retinogeniculate and retinocollicular projections in the mouse. *J Comp Neurol* 1984; 230:552–575.

32. Gordon JA, Stryker MP: Experience-dependent plasticity of binocular responses in the primary visual cortex of the mouse. *J Neurosci* 1996; 16(10):3274–3286.

33. Goto Y, Furuta A, Tobimatsu S: Magnesium deficiency differentially affects the retina and visual cortex of intact rats. *J Nutr* 2001; 131(9):2378–2381.

34. Gottlob I, Wizov SS, Odom JV, Reinecke RD: Predicting optotype visual acuity by swept spatial visual-evoked potentials. *Clin Vision Sci* 1993; 8:417–423.

35. Green DG, Herreros de Tejada P, Glover MJ: Electrophysiological estimates of visual sensitivity in albino and pigmented mice. *Vis Neurosci* 1994; 11(5):919–925.

36. Guire ES, Lickey ME, Gordon B: Critical period for the monocular deprivation effect in rats: Assessment with sweep visually evoked potentials. *J Neurophysiol* 1999; 81(1):121–128.

37. Gyllensten L, Malmfors T, Norrlin-Grettve ML: Developmental and functional alterations in the fiber composition of the optic nerve in visually deprived mice. *J Comp Neurol* 1966; 128:413–418.

38. Harding GFA: History of visual evoked cortical testing. In Arden GB (ed): *Principles and Practice of Clinical Electrophysiology of Vision*. St. Louis, Mosby, 1991, pp 17–22.

39. Harding GFA, Odom JV, Spileers W, Spekreijse H: Standard for visual evoked potentials. *Vision Res* 1996; 36:3567–3572.

40. Hart WM: *Adler's Physiology of the Eye*. St. Louis, Mosby, 1992.

41. Harwerth RS, Smith EL III, Boltz RL, Crawford ML, von Noorden GK: Behavioral studies on the effect of abnormal early visual experience in monkeys: Spatial modulation sensitivity. *Vision Res* 1983; 23(12):1501–1510.

42. Henry KR, Rhoades RW: Relation of albinism and drugs to the visual evoked potential of the mouse. *J Comp Physiol Psychol* 1978; 92(2):271–279.

43. Henry KR, Rhoades RW, Haythorn MM: Effects of ambient lighting and the albino gene on the developing visual evoked potential of the mouse. *Physiol Psychol* 1977; 5:204–208.

44. Herreros de Tejada P, Munoz Tedo C, Costi C: Behavioral estimates of absolute visual threshold in mice. *Vision Res* 1997; 37(17):2427–2432.

45. Hubel DH, Wiesel TN: Receptive fields, binocular interaction and functional architecture in the cat's visual cortex. *J Physiol* 1962; 160:106–154.

46. Hubel DH, Wiesel TN: Receptive fields and functional architecture of monkey striate cortex. *J Physiol* 1968; 195(1):215–243.

47. Hubel DH, Wiesel TN: Ferrier lecture: Functional architecture of macaque monkey visual cortex. *Proc R Soc Lond B Biol Sci* 1977; 198(1130):1–59.

48. Jacobs GH, Neitz J, Deegan JF II: Retinal receptors in rodents maximally sensitive to ultraviolet light. *Nature* 1991; 353(6345):655–656.

49. Johnson MA, Drum BA, Quigley HA, Sanchez RM, Dunkelberger GR: Pattern-evoked potentials and optic nerve fiber loss in monocular laser-induced glaucoma. *Invest Ophthalmol Vis Sci* 1989; 30(5):897–907.

50. Kiorpes L, Kiper DC: Development of contrast sensitivity across the visual field in macaque monkeys (Macaca nemestrina). *Vision Res* 1996; 36(2):239–247.

51. Klemm WR, Goodson RA, Allen RG: Steady-state visual evoked responses in anesthetized monkeys. *Brain Res Bull* 1984; 13(2):287–291.

52. Kraut MA, Arezzo JC, Vaughan HG Jr: Intracortical generators of the flash VEP in monkeys. *Electroencephalogr Clin Neurophysiol* 1985; 62(4):300–312.

53. Kraut MA, Arezzo JC, Vaughan HG Jr: Inhibitory processes in the flash evoked potential of the monkey. *Electroencephalogr Clin Neurophysiol* 1990; 76(5):440–452.

54. Kulikowski JJ, Robson AG, Murray IJ: Scalp VEPs and intracortical responses to chromatic and achromatic stimuli in primates. *Doc Ophthalmol* 2002; 105:243–279.

55. Kulikowski JJ, Walsh V, McKeefry D, Butler SR, Carden D: The electrophysiological basis of colour processing in macaques with V4 lesions. *Behav Brain Res* 1994; 60(1):73–78.

56. Lambert SR, Aiyer A, Grossniklaus H: Infantile lensectomy and intraocular lens implantation with long-term follow-up in a monkey model. *J Pediatr Ophthalmol Strabismus* 1999; 36(5):271–278.

57. Lamme VA, Van Dijk BW, Spekreijse H: Texture segregation is processed by primary visual cortex in man and monkey: Evidence from VEP experiments. *Vision Res* 1992; 32(5): 797–807.

58. LaVail JH, Nixon RA, Sidman RL: Genetic control of retinal ganglion cell projections. *J Comp Neurol* 1978; 182(3):399–421.

59. Lehman DM, Harrison JM: Flash visual evoked potentials in the hypomyelinated mutant mouse shiverer. *Doc Ophthalmol* 2002; 104(1):83–95.

60. Lilienthal H, Lenaerts C, Winneke G, Hennekes R: Alteration of the visual evoked potential and the electroretinogram in lead-treated monkeys. *Neurotoxicol Teratol* 1988; 10(5):417–422.

61. Lopez L, Brusa A, Fadda A, Loizzo S, Martinangeli A, Sannita WG, et al: Modulation of flash stimulation intensity and frequency: Effects on visual evoked potentials and oscillatory potentials recorded in awake, freely moving mice. *Behav Brain Res* 2002; 131(1–2):105–114.

62. Lund JS: Anatomical organization of macaque monkey striate visual cortex. *Ann Rev Neurosci* 1988; 11:253–288.

63. Mangini NJ, Pearlman AL: Laminar distribution of receptive field properties in the primary visual cortex of the mouse. *J Comp Neurol* 1980; 193(1):203–222.

64. Marx MS, Podos SM, Bodis-Wollner I, Lee PY, Wang RF, Severin C: Signs of early damage in glaucomatous monkey eyes: Low spatial frequency losses in the pattern ERG and VEP. *Exp Eye Res* 1988; 46(2):173–184.

65. Mason C, Kandel ER: Central visual pathways. In Jessell TM (ed): *Principles of Neural Science*, ed 3. Norwalk, CT Appleton & Lange, 1991, pp 420–439.

66. Matsuzaki M, Dowling KC: Effects of phencyclidine (PCP) on the visual evoked potentials in the rhesus monkey. *Brain Res Bull* 1983; 10(1):33–38.

67. Mazzucchelli A, Conte S, D'Olimpio F, Ferlazzo F, Loizzo A, Palazzesi S, et al: Ultradian rhythms in the N1-P2 amplitude of the visual evoked potential in two inbred strains of mice: DBA/2J and C57BL/6. *Behav Brain Res* 1995; 67(1):81–84.

68. Meeren HK, Van Luijtelaar EL, Coenen AM: Cortical and thalamic visual evoked potentials during sleep-wake states and spike-wave discharges in the rat. *Electroencephalogr Clin Neurophysiol* 1998; 108(3):306–319.

69. Menner E: Untersuchunger uber die Retina mit besonderer Berucksichtigung der ausseren Kornerschichte. *Z Vergl Physiol* 1928; 8:761–826.

70. Merigan WH, Katz LM: Spatial resolution across the macaque retina. *Vision Res* 1990; 30(7):985–991.

71. Merigan WH, Pasternak T, Zehl D: Spatial and temporal vision of macaques after central retinal lesions. *Invest Ophthalmol Vis Sci* 1981; 21(1, Pt 1):17–26.

72. Mutti DO, Ver Hoeve JN, Zadnik K, Murphy CJ: The artifact of retinoscopy revisited: Comparison of refractive error measured by retinoscopy and visual evoked potential in the rat. *Optom Vis Sci* 1997; 74(7):483–484.

73. Nakayama K, Mackeben M, Sutter E: Narrow spatial and temporal frequency tuning in the alert monkey VEP. *Brain Res* 1980; 193(1):263–267.

74. Nakayama K, Mackeben M: Steady state visual evoked potentials in the alert primate. *Vision Res* 1982; 22(10): 1261–1271.

75. Narfström K, Ekesten B, Rosolen SG, Spiess BM, Percicot CL, Ofri R: Guidelines for clinical electroretinography in the dog. *Doc Ophthalmol* 2002; 105:83–92.

76. Norcia AM, Clarke M, Tyler CW: Digital filtering and robust regression techniques for estimating sensory thresholds from the evoked potential. *IEEE Eng Med Biol* 1985; 4:26–32.

77. Norcia AM, Tyler CW: Infant VEP acuity measurements: Analysis of individual differences and measurement error. *Electroencephalogr Clin Neurophysiol* 1985; 61(5):359–369.

78. Norcia AM, Tyler CW: Spatial frequency sweep VEP: Visual acuity during the first year of life. *Vision Res* 1985; 25(10):1399–1408.

79. Northmore DP, Granda AM: Refractive state, contrast sensitivity, and resolution in the freshwater turtle, Pseudemys scripta elegans, determined by tectal visual-evoked potentials. *Vis Neurosci* 1991; 7(6):619–625.

80. Ochikubo F, Nagata T, Yoshikawa Y, Matsubara Y, Kai C, Yamanouchi Y: Electroencephalogram and evoked potentials in the primate model of viral encephalitis. *Electroencephalogr Clin Neurophysiol* 1993; 88(5):397–407.

81. Oku H, Sugiyama T, Kojima S, Watanabe T, Ikeda T: Improving effects of topical administration of iganidipine, a new calcium channel blocker, on the impaired visual evoked potential after endothelin-1 injection into the vitreous body of rabbits. *Curr Eye Res* 2000; 20(2):101–108.

82. Okuno T, Oku H, Sugiyama T, Yang Y, Ikeda T: Evidence that nitric oxide is involved in autoregulation in optic nerve head of rabbits. *Invest Ophthalmol Vis Sci* 2002; 43(3):784–789.

83. O'Kusky J, Colonnier M: A laminar analysis of the number of neurons, glia, and synapses in the visual cortex (area 17) of adult macaque monkeys. *J Comp Neurol* 1982; 210: 278–290.

84. Padnick LB, Linsenmeier RA: Properties of the flash visual evoked potential recorded in the cat primary visual cortex. *Vision Res* 1999; 39(17):2833–2840.

85. Peachey NS, Roveri L, Messing A, McCall MA: Functional consequences of oncogene-induced horizontal cell degeneration in the retinas of transgenic mice. *Vis Neurosci* 1997; 14(4):627–632.

86. Perez-Cobo JC, Lopez de Armentia M, Sanchez-Suero S, Perez-Arroyo M: Visual evoked potentials in response to pattern reversal in the cat cortex. *Rev Esp Fisiol* 1994; 50(4):205–210.

87. Pizzorusso T, Fagiolini M, Porciatti V, Maffei L: Temporal aspects of contrast visual evoked potentials in the pigmented rat: Changes with dark rearing. *Vision Res* 1996; 37:389–395.

88. Porciatti V, Fontanesi G, Raffaelli A, Bagnoli P: Binocularity in the little owl, Athene noctua: II. Properties of visually evoked potentials from the Wulst in response to monocular and binocular stimulation with sine wave gratings. *Brain Behav Evol* 1990; 35(1):40–48.

89. Porciatti V, Pizzorusso T, Maffei L: The visual physiology of the wild type mouse determined with pattern VEPs. *Vision Res* 1999; 39(18):3071–3781.

90. Porciatti V, Pizzorusso T, Maffei L: Vision in mice with neuronal redundancy due to inhibition of developmental cell death. *Vis Neurosci* 1999; 16(4):721–726.

91. Porciatti V, Pizzorusso T, Maffei L: Electrophysiology of the postreceptoral visual pathway in mice. *Doc Ophthalmol* 2002; 104(1):69–82.

92. Previc FH, Allen RG, Blankenstein MF: Visual evoked potential correlates of laser flashblindness in rhesus monkeys: II. Doubled-neodymium laser flashes. *Am J Optom Physiol Opt* 1985; 62(9):626–632.

93. Previc FH, Blankenstein MF, Garcia PV, Allen RG: Visual evoked potential correlates of laser flashblindness in rhesus monkeys: I. Argon laser flashes. *Am J Optom Physiol Opt* 1985; 62(5):309–321.

94. Prospero-Garcia O, Huitron-Resendiz S, Casalman SC, Sanchez-Alavez M, Diaz-Ruiz O, Navarro L, et al: Feline immunodeficiency virus envelope protein (FIVgp120) causes electrophysiological alterations in rats. *Brain Res* 1999; 836(1–2):203–209.

95. Prusky GT, West PW, Douglas RM: Behavioral assessment of visual acuity in mice and rats. *Vision Res* 2000; 40(16):2201–2209.

96. Raymond LA, Wallace D, Raghavan R, Marcario JK, Johnson JK, Foresman LL, et al: Sensory evoked potentials in SIV-infected monkeys with rapidly and slowly progressing disease. *AIDS Res Hum Retroviruses* 2000; 16(12):1163–1173.

97. Ren JC, LaVail MM, Peachey NS: Retinal degeneration in the nervous mutant mouse: III. Electrophysiological studies of the visual pathway. *Exp Eye Res* 2000; 70(4):467–473.

98. Ridder WH III, Nusinowitz S: Sweep VEP (sVEP) acuity in mice [abstract]. Abstract 1802. *2002 Annual Meeting Abstract and Program Planner* [on CD-ROM]. Association for Research in Vision and Ophthalmology, 2002.

99. Rovamo J, Virsu V: An estimation and application of the human cortical magnification factor. *Exp Brain Res* 1979; 37:495–510.

100. Schmeisser ET: Flicker electroretinograms and visual evoked potentials in the evaluation of laser flash effects. *Am J Optom Physiol Opt* 1985; 62(1):35–39.

101. Schmeisser ET: Laser flash effects on laser speckle shift visual evoked potential. *Am J Optom Physiol Opt* 1985; 62(10): 709–714.

102. Schmeisser ET: Laser-induced chromatic adaptation. *Am J Optom Physiol Opt* 1988; 65(8):644–652.

103. Schmeisser ET: Acute laser lesion effects on acuity sweep VEPs. *Invest Ophthalmol Vis Sci* 1992; 33(13):3546–3554.

104. Schroeder CE, Tenke CE, Givre SJ: Subcortical contributions to the surface-recorded flash-VEP in the awake macaque. *Electroencephalogr Clin Neurophysiol* 1992; 84(3):219–231.

105. Schroeder CE, Tenke CE, Givre SJ, Arezzo JC, Vaughan HG Jr: Striate cortical contribution to the surface-recorded pattern-reversal VEP in the alert monkey. *Vision Res* 1991; 31(7–8):1143–1157.

106. Sidman RL: Histochemical studies on photoreceptor cells. *Ann N Y Acad Sci* 1958; 74:182–195.

107. Silva-Barrat C, Menini C: The influence of intermittent light stimulation on potentials evoked by single flashes in photo-

sensitive and non-photosensitive Papio papio. *Electroencephalogr Clin Neurophysiol* 1984; 57(5):448–461.

108. Simmons PA, Pearlman AL: Retinotopic organization of the striate cortex (area 17) in the reeler mutant mouse. *Brain Res* 1982; 256(1):124–126.

109. Sinex DG, Burdette LJ, Pearlman AL: A psychophysical investigation of spatial vision in the normal and reeler mutant mouse. *Vision Res* 1979; 19(8):853–857.

110. Smith RS, John SWM, Nishina PM: The posterior segment and orbit. In Smith RS (ed): *Systematic Evaluation of the Mouse Eye: Anatomy, Pathology, and Biomethods.* Boca Raton, FL, CRC Press, 2002, pp 25–44.

111. Strain GM, Claxton MS, Prescott-Mathews JS, LaPhand DJ: Electroretinogram and visual-evoked potential measurements in sheep. *Can J Vet Res* 1991; 55(1):1–4.

112. Strain GM, Graham MC, Claxton MS, Olcott BM: Postnatal development of brainstem auditory-evoked potentials, electroretinograms, and visual-evoked potentials in the calf. *J Vet Intern Med* 1989; 3(4):231–237.

113. Strain GM, Jackson RM, Tedford BL: Visual evoked potentials in the clinically normal dog. *J Vet Intern Med* 1990; 4(4):222–225.

114. Strain GM, Tedford BL: Flash and pattern reversal visual evoked potentials in C57BL/6J and B6CBAF1/J mice. *Brain Res Bull* 1993; 32(1):57–63.

115. Strain GM, Tedford BL, Littlefield-Chabaud MA, Trevino LT: Air- and bone-conduction brainstem auditory evoked potentials and flash visual evoked potentials in cats. *Am J Vet Res* 1998; 59(2):135–137.

116. Strasburger H, Murray IJ, Remky A: Sustained and transient mechanisms in the steady-state visual evoked potential: Onset presentation compared to pattern reversal. *Clin Vision Sci* 1993; 8:211–234.

117. Strasburger H, Scheidler W, Rentschler I: Amplitude and phase characteristics of the steady-state visual evoked potential. *Appl Optics* 1988; 27:1069–1088.

118. Suzuki M, Sitizyo K, Takeuchi T, Saito T: Visual evoked potential from scalp in guinea pigs. *J Vet Med Sci* 1991; 53(2):301–305.

119. Takeuchi T, Suzuki M, Sitizyo K, Isobe R, Saito T, Umemura T, et al: Visual evoked potentials in guinea pigs with brain lesion. *J Vet Med Sci* 1992; 54(5):813–820.

120. Takeuchi T, Suzuki M, Sitizyo K, Saito T: Postnatal development of visual evoked potentials in Japanese black calves. *Jpn J Physiol* 1993; 43(6):809–815.

121. Tebano MT, Luzi M, Palazzesi S, Pomponi M, Loizzo A: Effects of cholinergic drugs on neocortical EEG and flash-visual evoked potentials in the mouse. *Neuropsychobiology* 1999; 40(1):47–56.

122. Tootell RB, Switkes E, Silverman MS, Hamilton SL: Functional anatomy of macaque striate cortex: II. Retinotopic organization. *J Neurosci* 1988; 8(5):1531–1568.

123. Tychsen L, Boothe RG: Latent fixation nystagmus and nasotemporal asymmetries of motion visually evoked potentials in naturally strabismic primate. *J Pediatr Ophthalmol Strabismus* 1996; 33(3):148–152.

124. Tychsen L, Burkhalter A, Boothe RG: [Functional and structural abnormalities in the visual cortex in early childhood strabismus.] *Klin Monatsbl Augenheilkd* 1996; 208(1):18–22.

125. Tyler CW, Apkarian P, Levi DM, Nakayama K: Rapid assessment of visual function: An electronic sweep technique for the pattern visual evoked potential. *Invest Ophthalmol Vis Sci* 1979; 18(7):703–713.

126. Valverde F, Esteban ME: Peristriate cortex of mouse: Location and the effects of enucleation on the number of dendritic spines. *Brain Res* 1968; 9(1):145–148.

127. Van der Marel EH, Dagnelie G, Spekreijse H: Subdurally recorded pattern and luminance EPs in the alert rhesus monkey. *Electroencephalogr Clin Neurophysiol* 1984; 57(4):354–368.

128. Van Essen DC, Lewis JW, Drury HA, Hadjikhani N, Tootell RB, Bakircioglu M, et al: Mapping visual cortex in monkeys and humans using surface-based atlases. *Vision Res* 2001; 41(10–11):1359–1378.

129. Ver Hoeve JN, Danilov YP, Kim CB, Spear PD: VEP and PERG acuity in anesthetized young adult rhesus monkeys. *Vis Neurosci* 1999; 16(4):607–617.

130. Wagor E, Mangini NJ, Pearlman AL: Retinotopic organization of striate and extrastriate visual cortex in the mouse. *J Comp Neurol* 1980; 193(1):187–202.

131. Wassle H, Grunert U, Rohrenbeck J, Boycott BB: Cortical magnification factor and the ganglion cell density of the primate retina. *Nature* 1989; 341:643–646.

132. Watanabe M, Ozaki T, Mushiroi T, Ukai Y, Ueda F, Kimura K, et al: Behavioral and electroencephalographic studies of beagles with an Eck's fistula: Suitability as a model of hepatic encephalopathy. *Pharmacol Biochem Behav* 1997; 57(1–2):367–375.

133. Wilson JR, Noyd WW, Aiyer AD, Norcia AM, Mustari MJ, Boothe RG: Asymmetric responses in cortical visually evoked potentials to motion are not derived from eye movements. *Invest Ophthalmol Vis Sci* 1999; 40(10):2435–2439.

134. Witzel DA, Smith EL III, Beerwinkle KR, Johnson JH: Arsanilic acid-induced blindness in swine: Electroretinographic and visually evoked responses. *Am J Vet Res* 1976; 37:521–524.

135. Wong-Riley M: Changes in the visual system of monocularly sutured or enucleated cats demonstrable with cytochrome oxidase histochemistry. *Brain Res* 1979; 171(1):11–28.

136. Woolsey TA: Somatosensory, auditory and visual cortical areas of the mouse. *Johns Hopkins Med J* 1967; 121(2):91–112.

137. Yargicoglu P, Agar A, Edremitlioglu M, Kara C: The effects of cadmium and experimental diabetes on VEP spectral data and lipid peroxidation. *Int J Neurosci* 1998; 93(1–2):63–74.

138. Yildirim C, Tychsen L: Effect of infantile strabismus on visuomotor development in the squirrel monkey (Saimiri sciureus): Optokinetic nystagmus, motion VEP and spatial sweep VEP. *Strabismus* 1999; 7(4):211–219.

139. Yoshioka T, Levitt JB, Lund JS: Independence and merger of thalamocortical channels within macaque monkey primary visual cortex: Anatomy of interlaminar projections. *Vis Neurosci* 1994; 11(3):467–489.

INDEX

Page numbers followed by *f* or *t* indicate figures or tables, respectively.

E

Retinal pigment epithelium (RPE) (*continued*)
  transport by, 27, 37–42
    ion, 37–42, 41*f*
    lactic acid, 40, 41*f*, 42
  voltage difference across, 11, 123–126, 124*f*–125*f*. See also
      Electro-oculogram
Retinal vein occlusion
  branch, 681
  central, 675–681
    electroretinogram in, 675–681, 676*f*–680*f*, 816–818, 818*f*
      amplitudes in, 675–676, 676*f*–677*f*
      intensity-response analysis in, 677–678, 680*f*
      temporal factors in, 676–677, 678*f*–679*f*
    ischemic, 817, 818*f*
    multifocal ERG in, 677
    nonischemic, 817
    photoreceptor function in, 679–680, 680*f*
Retinitis pigmentosa, 781–792
  autoimmune retinopathy with, 691–697
  versus choroideremia, 777
  clinical features of, 781
  clinical-test result correlation in, 628–629, 628*t*
  Coats' reaction in, 427, 428*f*
  conditions associated with, 781
  electro-oculogram in, 624
  electroretinogram in, 506–507, 506*f*, 508*f*, 623, 784–791,
      812–813, 812*f*–813*f*
    amplitude-retinal illuminance functions in, 787–791,
        789*f*–790*f*
    a-wave analysis in, 506–507, 790*f*, 791
    c-wave in, 560*f*, 561
    extensions of protocol for, 787–791
    full-field, sensitivity of, 786–787, 787*f*
    paired-flash method in, 791, 791*f*
    protocol for, 784–786, 785*f*–787*f*
  flicker ERG in, 581, 582*f*–583*f*
  fluorescein angiogram of, 425, 426*f*, 427, 428*f*
  fundus appearance of, 781, 782*f*
  genetic analysis of, 781–784, 782*t*
  light adaptation in, 594–595, 595*t*
  mouse model of, 783
  multifocal electroretinogram in, 199, 202*f*, 334, 508*f*
  oscillatory potentials in, 576*f*, 577, 578*f*
  pattern ERG in, 506–507, 508*f*
  photoreceptor responses in, 496*f*–498*f*, 497, 506–507, 506*f*, 508*f*,
      783–784
  phototransduction cascade in, 783–784
  preserved para-arteriolar retinal pigment epithelial, 425, 426*f*
  prevalence of, 781
  psychophysical approaches in, 399
  suppressive rod-cone interaction in, 418–419
  visual cycle in, 784
  X-linked, 781
    alcohol electro-oculogram in, 134–135, 134*f*
    oscillatory potentials in, 576*f*, 577
Retinol, transport of, 27
Retinoschisis, juvenile (X-linked), 823–825
  a-wave analysis in, 824–825, 826*f*
  b-wave analysis in, 824–825, 825*f*–826*f*
  differential diagnosis of, 823
  electro-oculogram in, 823–824
  electroretinogram in, 810–812, 811*f*, 823–825, 825*f*–826*f*
  fluorescein angiogram of, 424, 425*f*, 823, 825*f*
  fundus appearance of, 823, 824*f*
  gene identification in, 823
  photoreceptor and inner retinal responses in, 824–825, 826*f*

scotopic threshold response in, 824
suppressive rod-cone interaction in, 419
Retinovascular disorders. *See also specific types*
  electroretinogram in, 816–818
Retrochiasmal dysfunction (lesions), 665, 860–863
  bilateral, 861–863
  cortical blindness in, 861–863
  unilateral, 860–861
  visual evoked potentials in, 231, 307, 515, 860–863, 861*f*–862*f*
Reverse correlation, 461–471
  in alert animal, 465–466, 466*f*–467*f*
  basics of, 462–463, 462*f*
  of color selectivity, 469–470, 469*f*
  of depth selectivity, 469–470
  early technical limitations of, 465
  of orientation selectivity, 469–470, 469*f*
  potential pitfalls in, 470–471
  of second-order kernels, 467*f*, 468
  of simple cell receptive fields, 463–465, 464*f*
  space-time maps in, 465, 466*f*
  suppression *versus* no response in, 470
Rhodopsin, 28–29, 47, 48*f*, 65
  activation of, 67–68, 68*f*
  cycle of, 69*f*
  and early receptor potential, 549–551
  inactivation of, 68–69, 69*f*
  in retinitis pigmentosa, 783–784
  vitamin A deficiency and, 803, 805*f*
Rhodopsin kinase, in Oguchi's disease, 836–837
Riddoch phenomenon, 111
"Rim" protein, 29
RLBP1 gene, and retinitis pigmentosa, 781
ROC (receiver operating characteristic) curve, 401, 434–435
Rod(s)
  activity of, clinical assessment of, 497–500
  biochemistry of, 29–30
  cell cytology of, 28–30
  cilia of, 65–66, 66*f*–67*f*
  currents of, and a-wave, 151–152, 151*f*–152*f*
  definition of, 47
  disc membranes of, 29
  in duplicity theory, 404–405
  embryological development of, 25–27
  functional organization of, 47–48
  health of, measuring with a-wave leading edge, 487–500
  image properties of, 49–50
  inner segments of, 24*f*, 25, 29, 65, 66*f*
  microfilaments of, 65, 67*f*
  microtubules of, 65, 67*f*
  morphology of, 28–30
  neurotransmitter release from, 79
  in nocturnal vision, 47
  outer segments of, 24*f*, 25, 28–29, 28*f*, 47, 48*f*, 65, 66*f*
  phototransduction in, 66–72
    paired-flash ERG analysis of, 519–530
  physiology of, 65–75
  protein migration/translocation in, 72–75, 74*f*
  recovery following bright illumination, 525–530, 527*f*–530*f*
  responses of. *See* Rod response
  spatial density of, 405
  suppressive interaction with cones, 417–420. *See also* Suppressive
      rod-cone interaction
  synaptic transmission in, 79–91
Rod-cone break, 406, 406*f*, 407, 407*f*
Rod-cone dysplasia, in dogs, 913–915, 914*f*–915*f*
Rod monochromatism, 795–796, 798*t*